NOTICE PURSUANT TO CHAPTER 12 (PAGE 172):

The Role of Preventive Multimodal Analgesia and Impact on Patient Outcome
(Scott S Reuben and Asokumar Buvanendran)

As this book was going to press, a number of papers involving nonopioid agents as part of multimodal analgesia have been withdrawn from the literature. Some of these papers are referenced in Chapter 12. Of the 155 references listed in the chapter, six have been retracted as of this date (March 24th 2009). These are the references numbered 38, 39, 67, 118, 146, and 154. Since it was impossible to remove these at such a late stage of production, the reader is cautioned to disregard these from the evidence presented in this chapter. Scientific literature continues to change over time but it is unfortunate that change in this instance comes as a result of retracted papers. At the time of this writing, approximately 20 papers have been retracted. It is not possible to determine if additional papers will be withdrawn. The reader is cautioned that these references may appear in other chapters of this book, as well as in the literature in general.

The principles upon which this chapter is written remain true; there are references by other authors supporting the concept discussed here. While it is important to be aware of the retracted articles, it is equally vital to appreciate that valid published studies demonstrating similar clinical outcome remain in the peer reviewed literature.

Asokumar Buvanendran
Oscar A. De Leon-Casasola
Brian Ginsberg
Raymond S. Sinatra
Eugene R Viscusi
March 24, 2009

5-14-10

To Joyce and Lyenka
I hope this textbook
will help with some of
the confusing aspects
of Acute Pain !

[signature]

5/14/10

To Joyce and Lyenka

What can I say, to be your
friend is a privilege, but to
be asked to sign this copy is an
honor. I hope that you enjoy it

[signature]

Acute Pain Management

This textbook is written as a comprehensive overview of acute pain management. It is designed to guide clinicians through the impressive array of different options available to them and to patients. Since the late 1990s, there has been a flurry of interest in the extent to which acute pain can become chronic pain and how we might reduce the incidence of such chronicity. This overview covers topics related to a wide range of treatments for pain management, including the anatomy of pain pathways, the pathophysiology of severe pain, pain assessment, therapeutic guidelines, analgesic options, organization of pain services, and the role of anesthesiologists, surgeons, pharmacists, and nurses in providing optimal care. It also discusses the use of patient-controlled analgesia and how this may or may not be effective and useful.

Dr. Raymond S. Sinatra currently serves as Professor of Anesthesiology at Yale University School of Medicine. He received his MD as well as a PhD in neuroscience at SUNY Downstate School of Medicine and completed his anesthesiology residency at the Brigham & Women's Hospital, Harvard Medical School. Dr. Sinatra joined the faculty at Yale in 1985 and organized one of the first anesthesiology-based pain management services in the United States. In addition to directing the service, he has served as principal investigator for dozens of clinical protocols evaluating novel analgesics and analgesic delivery systems. Dr. Sinatra has authored more than 130 scientific papers, review articles, and textbook chapters on pain management and obstetrical anaesthesiology and was senior editor of an earlier textbook titled *Acute Pain: Mechanisms and Management.* Dr. Sinatra annually presents papers and lectures at both national and international meetings and serves as a reviewer for several anaesthesiology and pain management journals.

Dr. Oscar A. de Leon-Casasola is Professor of Anesthesiology and Chief of Pain Medicine in the Department of Anesthesiology of the Roswell Park Cancer Institute. His research interests include advances in analgesic therapy, physiology and pharmacology of epidural opioids, perioperative surgical outcomes, thoracic and cardiac anesthesia, acute pain control, and chronic cancer pain. He is a member of the American Society of Regional Anesthesia, American Society of Anesthesiologists, New York State Society of Anesthesiologists, American Pain Society, and Eastern Pain Association. Dr. de Leon-Casasola has authored or coauthored 115 journal articles, abstracts, and book chapters. He serves as an associate editor for the *Latin American Journal of Pain*, the *Argentinian Journal of Anesthesiology*, the *Journal of the Spanish Society of Pain*, and the *Clinical Journal of Pain*. He also is editor-in-chief of *Techniques in Regional Anesthesia and Pain Management* and was listed as an exceptional practitioner by *Good Housekeeping* magazine in 2003.

Dr. Brian Ginsberg is Professor of Anesthesiology and Medical Director of the Division of Acute Pain Therapy in the Department of Anesthesiology of Duke University School of Medicine.

Dr. Eugene R. Viscusi is Director of Acute Pain Management and Regional Anesthesia in the Department of Anesthesiology at Thomas Jefferson University in Philadelphia, Pennsylvania, and Associate Professor of Anesthesiology. After receiving a medical degree from Jefferson Medical College, Dr. Viscusi completed a residency in anesthesiology at the University of Pennsylvania in Philadelphia. His research interests include the development of new pain management techniques, outcome studies with pain management, and the development of novel agents and delivery systems for pain management. He developed a novel "nurse-driven" model for delivering acute pain management with specially trained nurses that has served as a model for other institutions. Dr. Viscusi also has been a primary investigator for many emerging technologies in the perioperative arena.

Dr. Viscusi is a member of numerous professional associations, including the American Society of Anesthesiologists, the American Society of Regional Anesthesiology, and the International Anesthesia Research Society and serves on numerous society committees. Dr. Viscusi has lectured extensively both nationally and internationally, has authored more than 100 book chapters and abstracts, and has authored more than 50 peer-reviewed articles in journals including *Journal of the American Medical Association, Anesthesiology, Anesthesia & Analgesia,* and *Regional Anesthesia and Pain Medicine.* Dr. Viscusi currently serves on the editorial board of the *Clinical Journal of Pain* and regularly reviews for many journals. He also has appeared in articles in major media including, *Newsweek*, the *Wall Street Journal, USA Today,* and has appeared nationally on televised interviews.

Acute Pain Management

Edited by

Raymond S. Sinatra
Yale University

Oscar A. de Leon-Casasola
Roswell Park Cancer Institute

Brian Ginsberg
Duke University

Eugene R. Viscusi
Thomas Jefferson University

Foreword
Henry McQuay

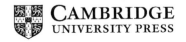
CAMBRIDGE
UNIVERSITY PRESS

CAMBRIDGE UNIVERSITY PRESS
Cambridge, New York, Melbourne, Madrid, Cape Town, Singapore, São Paulo, Delhi

Cambridge University Press
32 Avenue of the Americas, New York, NY 10013-2473, USA

www.cambridge.org
Information on this title: www.cambridge.org/9780521874915

First published 2009

Printed in the United States of America

A catalog record for this publication is available from the British Library

Library of Congress Cataloging in Publication data

Acute pain management / edited by Raymond Sinatra . . . [et al.].
p. ; cm.
Includes bibliographical references and index.
ISBN 978-0-521-87491-5 (hardback)
1. Pain – Treatment.   2. Analgesia.   I. Sinatra, Raymond S.   II. Title.
[DNLM: 1. Pain – therapy.   2. Acute Disease – therapy.
3. Analgesia – methods. WL 704 A1896 2009]
RB127.A323   2009
616′.0472–dc22   2008022660

ISBN   978-0-521-87491-5 hardback

Contents

Contributors

Chapter 1

Nalini Vadivelu, MD
    CA-3 Resident in Anesthesiology
    Department of Anesthesiology
    Yale University School of Medicine
    New Haven, CT

Christian J. Whitney, MD
    Associate Professor of Anesthesiology
    Department of Anesthesiology
    Yale University School of Medicine
    New Haven, CT

Raymond S. Sinatra, MD, PhD
    Professor of Anesthesiology
    Director of Acute Pain Management Service
    Department of Anesthesiology
    Yale University School of Medicine
    New Haven, CT

Chapter 2

M. Khurram Ghori, MD
    Assistant Professor of Anesthesiology
    Department of Anesthesiology
    Yale University School of Medicine
    New Haven, CT

Yu-Fan (Robert) Zhang, MD
    CA-3 Resident in Anesthesiology
    Department of Anesthesiology
    Yale University School of Medicine
    New Haven, CT

Raymond S. Sinatra, MD, PhD
    Professor of Anesthesiology
    Director of Acute Pain Management Service
    Department of Anesthesiology
    Yale University School of Medicine
    New Haven, CT

Chapter 3

Joshua Wellington, MD, MS
    Assistant Professor of Clinical Anesthesia and Physical
      Medicine and Rehabilitation
    Department of Anesthesia
    Indiana University Medical Center
    Indianapolis, IN

Yuan-Yi Chia, MD
    Associate Professor of Anesthesiology
    Kaohsiung Veterans General Hospital
    National Yang-Ming University, School of Medicine, and
      Institute of Health Care Management
    National Sun Yatsen University
    Kaohsiung, Taiwan

Chapter 4

Francis J. Keefe, PhD
    Pain Prevention and Treatment Research Program
    Duke University Medical Center
    Durham, NC

Chapter 5

Jon McCormack, MBChB, FRCA, MRCP
    Clinical and Surgical Sciences Anaesthesia
    Critical Care and Pain Medicine
    University of Edinburgh
    Royal Infirmary Little France
    Edinburgh, UK

Ian Power, MD
    Clinical and Surgical Sciences Anaesthesia
    Critical Care and Pain Medicine
    University of Edinburgh
    Royal Infirmary Little France
    Edinburgh, UK

Chapter 6

John Butterworth, MD
  Robert K. Stoelting Professor and Chairman
  Department of Anesthesia
  Indiana University School of Medicine
  Indianapolis, IN

Chapter 7

P. M. Lavand'homme, MD, PhD
  Department of Anesthesiology
  St Luc Hospital
  Université Catholique de Louvain
  Brussels, Belgium

M. F. De Kock, MD, PhD
  Department of Anesthesiology
  St Luc Hospital
  Université Catholique de Louvain
  Brussels, Belgium

Chapter 8

Bradley Urie, MD
  Fellow, Pain Management
  Department of Anesthesiology
  University at Buffalo, School of Medicine
  Buffalo, NY

Oscar A. de Leon-Casasola, MD
  Professor and Vice-Chair for Clinical Affairs
  Department of Anesthesiology
  University at Buffalo, School of Medicine
  Chief, Pain Medicine and Professor of Oncology
  Roswell Park Cancer Institute
  Buffalo, NY

Chapter 9

Frederick M. Perkins, MD
  Chief of Anesthesia
  Veterans Administration Medical Center
  White River Junction, VT

Chapter 10

Larry F. Chu, MD, MS (BCHM), MS (Epidemiology)
  Assistant Professor
  Department of Anesthesia
  Stanford University School of Medicine
  Palo Alto, CA

David Clark, MD, PhD
  Professor
  Department of Anesthesia and Pain
    Management
  Veterans Affairs Palo Alto Health Care System
  Palo Alto, CA

Martin S. Angst, MD
  Associate Professor
  Department of Anesthesia
  Stanford University School of Medicine
  Palo Alto, CA

Chapter 11

Cynthia M. Welchek, RPh, MS
  Clinical Pharmacist
  Department of Pharmacy Service
  Yale New Haven Hospital
  New Haven, CT

Lisa Mastrangelo, RN, BC, MS
  Nurse Coordinator
  Acute Pain Management Service
  Department of Anesthesiology
  Yale University School of Medicine
  New Haven, CT

Raymond S. Sinatra, MD, PhD
  Professor of Anesthesiology
  Director of Acute Pain Management Service
  Department of Anesthesiology
  Yale University School of Medicine
  New Haven, CT

Richard Martinez, MD
  CA-3 Resident in Anesthesiology
  Department of Anesthesiology
  Yale University School of Medicine
  New Haven, CT

Chapter 12

Scott S. Reuben, MD
  Director of Acute Pain Service
  Department of Anesthesiology
  Baystate Medical Center
  Springfield, MA
      and
  Professor of Anesthesiology and Pain Medicine
  Tufts University School of Medicine
  Boston, MA

Asokumar Buvanendran, MD
  Associate Professor of Anesthesiology
  Department of Anesthesiology
  Director of Orthopedic Anesthesia
  Rush University Medical Center
  Chicago, IL

Chapter 13

Raymond S. Sinatra, MD, PhD
  Professor of Anesthesiology
  Director of Acute Pain Management Service
  Department of Anesthesiology
  Yale University School of Medicine
  New Haven, CT

Chapter 14

Pamela E. Macintyre, BMedSc, MBBS, MHA, FANZCA,
FFPMANZCA
  Director of Acute Pain Service
  Consultant Anaesthetist
  Department of Anaesthesia, Pain Medicine and Hyperbaric
    Medicine
  Royal Adelaide Hospital and University of Adelaide
  Adelaide, Australia

Julia Coldrey, MBBS(Hons), FANZCA
 Consultant Anaesthetist
 Department of Anaesthesia, Pain Medicine and Hyperbaric
  Medicine
 Royal Adelaide Hospital and University of Adelaide
 Adelaide, Australia

Chapter 15

Daniel B. Maalouf, MD, MPH
 Instructor in Anesthesiology
 Department of Anesthesia
 Hospital for Special Surgery
 The Weill Medical College of Cornell University
 New York, NY

Spencer S. Liu, MD
 Clinical Professor of Anesthesiology, Director of Acute Pain
  Service
 Department of Anesthesia
 Hospital for Special Surgery
 The Weill Medical College of Cornell University
 New York, NY

Chapter 16

Susan Dabu-Bondoc, MD
 Assistant Professor of Anesthesiology
 Department of Anesthesiology
 Yale University School of Medicine
 New Haven, CT

Samantha A. Franco, MD
 CA-3 Resident in Anesthesiology
 Department of Anesthesiology
 Yale University School of Medicine
 New Haven, CT

Raymond S. Sinatra, MD, PhD
 Professor of Anesthesiology
 Director of Acute Pain Management Service
 Department of Anesthesiology
 Yale University School of Medicine
 New Haven, CT

Chapter 17

James Benonis, MD
 Assistant Professor of Anesthesiology
 Division of Orthopedic, Plastic and Regional
  Anesthesia
 Department of Anesthesiology
 Duke University Health System
 Durham, NC

Jennifer Fortney, MD
 Assistant Professor of Anesthesiology
 Division of Orthopedic, Plastic and Regional
  Anesthesia
 Department of Anesthesiology
 Duke University Health System
 Durham, NC

David Hardman, MD
 Assistant Professor of Anesthesiology
 Division of Orthopedic, Plastic and Regional
  Anesthesia
 Department of Anesthesiology
 Duke University Health System
 Durham, NC

Gavin Martin, MB, ChB, FRCA
 Associate Professor of Anesthesiology
 Division of Orthopedic, Plastic and Regional
  Anesthesia
 Department of Anesthesiology
 Duke University Health System
 Durham, NC

Chapter 18

Holly Evans, MD, FRCPC
 Assistant Professor
 Department of Anesthesiology
 University of Ottawa
 Ottawa, Ontario, Canada

Karen C. Nielsen, MD
 Assistant Professor
 Division of Ambulatory Anesthesiology
 Department of Anesthesiology
 Duke University Medical Center
 Durham, NC

Marcy S. Tucker, MD, PhD
 Assistant Professor
 Division of Ambulatory Anesthesiology
 Department of Anesthesiology
 Duke University Medical Center
 Durham, NC

Stephen M. Klein, MD
 Associate Professor
 Department of Anesthesiology
 Duke University Medical Center
 Durham, NC

Chapter 19

Benjamin Sherman, MD
 CA-3 Resident in Anesthesiology
 Department of Anesthesiology
 Acute Pain Management Section
 Yale University School of Medicine
 New Haven, CT

Ikay Enu, MD
 CA-3 Resident in Anesthesiology
 Department of Anesthesiology
 Acute Pain Management Section
 Yale University School of Medicine
 New Haven, CT

Raymond S. Sinatra, MD, PhD
    Professor of Anesthesiology
    Director of Acute Pain Management Service
    Department of Anesthesiology
    Yale University School of Medicine
    New Haven, CT

Chapter 20

James W. Heitz, MD
    Assistant Professor of Anesthesiology and Medicine
    Jefferson Medical College
    Thomas Jefferson University
    Philadelphia, PA

Eugene R. Viscusi, MD
    Jefferson Medical College
    Thomas Jefferson University
    Philadelphia, PA

Chapter 21

Jonathan S. Jahr, MD
    Professor of Clinical Anesthesiology
    David Geffen School of Medicine at UCLA
    Los Angeles, CA

Kofi N. Donkor, PharmD
    Staff Pharmacist
    Department of Pharmaceutical Services
    UCLA Medical Center
    Los Angeles, CA

Raymond S. Sinatra, MD, PhD
    Professor of Anesthesiology
    Director of Acute Pain Management Section
    Department of Anesthesiology
    Yale University School of Medicine
    New Haven, CT

Chapter 22

Manzo Suzuki, MD
    Instructor
    Department of Anesthesiology
    Second Hospital
    Nippon Medical School
    Kanagawa, Japan

Chapter 23

Johan Raeder, MD, PhD
    Professor in Anesthesiology
    Chairman of Ambulatory Anesthesia Medical Faculty
    University of Oslo
    Ullevaal University Hospital
    Oslo, Norway

Vegard Dahl, MD, PhD
    Head
    Department of Anaesthesia and Intensive Care
    Professor in Anesthesiology
    University of Oslo
    Asker and Baerum Hospital
    Rud, Norway

Chapter 24

Stefan Erceg, MD
    CA-3 Resident in Anesthesiology
    Department of Anesthesiology
    Pain Management Service
    Yale University School of Medicine
    New Haven, CT

Keun Sam Chung, MD
    Associate Professor of Anesthesiology
    Department of Anesthesiology
    Pain Management Service
    Yale University School of Medicine
    New Haven, CT

Chapter 25

Kok-Yuen Ho, MBBS, MMed, FIPP, DAAPM
    Department of Anaesthesia and Surgical Intensive
        Care
    Singapore General Hospital
    Singapore, Singapore

Tong J. Gan, MB, FRCA, FFARCSI
    Department of Anesthesiology
    Duke University Medical Center
    Durham, NC

Chapter 26

Dermot R. Fitzgibbon, MD
    Associate Professor of Anesthesiology
    Adjunct Associate Professor of Medicine
    University of Washington School of Medicine
    Seattle, WA

Chapter 27

Paul Willoughby, MD
    Associate Professor
    Department of Anesthesiology
    Stony Brook Health Sciences Center
    Stony Brook, NY

Chapter 28

Brian E. Harrington, MD
    Staff Anesthesiologist
    Billings Clinic
    Billings, MT

Joseph Marino, MD
    Attending Anesthesiologist
    Director of Acute Pain Management Service
    Huntington Hospital
    Huntington, NY

Chapter 29

Tariq M. Malik, MD
    Assistant Professor of Anesthesiology
    University of Chicago School of Medicine
    Department of Anesthesia and Critical Care
    Chicago, IL

Raymond S. Sinatra, MD, PhD
    Professor of Anesthesiology
    Director of Acute Pain Management Service
    Department of Anesthesiology
    Yale University School of Medicine
    New Haven, CT

Chapter 30

Giorgio Ivani, MD
    Professor
    Chairman, Department for the Ladies Staff
        Doctors
    Department of Pediatric Anesthesiology and
        Intensive Care
    Regina Margherita Children's Hospital
    Turin, Italy

Valeria Mossetti, MD
    Department of Pediatric Anesthesiology and
        Intensive Care
    Regina Margherita Children's Hospital
    Turin, Italy

Simona Italiano, MD
    Department of Pediatric Anesthesiology and
        Intensive Care
    Regina Margherita Children's Hospital
    Turin, Italy

Chapter 31

Thomas M. Halaszynski, DMD, MD, MBA
    Associate Professor of Anesthesiology
    Department of Anesthesiology
    Yale University School of Medicine
    New Haven, CT

Nousheh Saidi, MD
    Assistant Professor of Anesthesiology
    Department of Anesthesiology
    Yale University School of Medicine
    New Haven, CT

Javier Lopez, MD
    CA-3 Resident in Anesthesiology
    Department of Anesthesiology
    Yale University School of Medicine
    New Haven, CT

Chapter 32

Kate Miller, MD
    Chief Resident in Anesthesiology
    Department of Anesthesiology
    Yale University School of Medicine
    New Haven, CT

Ferne Braveman, MD
    Professor
    Department of Anesthesiology
    Yale University School of Medicine
    New Haven, CT

Chapter 33

Jaya L. Varadarajan, MD
    Attending Physician
    Children's Hospital of Wisconsin
    Assistant Professor of Anesthesiology
    Medical College of Wisconsin
    Milwaukee, WI

Steven J. Weisman, MD
    Jane B. Pettit Chair in Pain Management
    Children's Hospital of Wisconsin
    Professor of Anesthesiology and Pediatrics
    Medical College of Wisconsin
    Milwaukee, WI

Chapter 34

Sukanya Mitra, MD
    Reader
    Department of Anaesthesia and Intensive Care
    Government Medical College & Hospital
    Chandigarh, India

Raymond S. Sinatra, MD, PhD
    Professor of Anesthesiology
    Director of Acute Pain Management Service
    Department of Anesthesiology
    Yale University School of Medicine
    New Haven, CT

Chapter 35

Theodore J. Saclarides, MD
    Professor of Surgery
    Head of the Section of Colon and Rectal Surgery
    Department of General Surgery
    Rush University Medical Center
    Chicago, IL

Chapter 36

Knox H. Todd, MD, MPH
    Professor of Emergency Medicine
    Albert Einstein College of Medicine
    Director of the Pain and Emergency Medicine
        Institute
    Department of Emergency Medicine
    Beth Israel Medical Center
    New York, NY

James R. Miner, MD, FACEP
    Associate Professor of Emergency Medicine
    University of Minnesota Medical School
    Department of Emergency Medicine
    Hennepin County Medical Center
    Minneapolis, MN

Chapter 37

Chris Pasero, MS, RN-BC, FAAN
    Pain Management Educator and Clinical Consultant
    El Dorado Hills, CA

Nancy Eksterowicz, MSN, RN-BC, APN
Advanced Practice Nurse in Pain Services
University of Virginia Health System
Charlottesville, VA

Margo McCaffery, MS, RN-BC, FAAN
Consultant in the Care of Patients with Pain
Los Angeles, CA

Chapter 38

Leslie N. Schechter, PharmD
Advanced Practice Pharmacist
Thomas Jefferson University Hospital
Philadelphia, PA

Chapter 39

Amr E. Abouleish, MD, MBA
Professor
Department of Anesthesiology
University of Texas Medical Branch
Galveston, TX

Govindaraj Ranganathan, MD, FRCA
Assistant Professor
Department of Anesthesiology
University of Texas Medical Branch
Galveston, TX

Chapter 40

Tee Yong Tan, MBBS, M Med (Anesthesiology)
Department of Anaesthesia
Alexandra Hospital
Singapore, Singapore

Stephan A. Schug, MD, FANZCA, FFPMANZCA
Department of Anaesthesia and Pain Medicine
Royal Perth Hospital
Perth, Australia

Chapter 41

Marie N. Hanna, MD
Associate Professor
Department of Anesthesiology and Critical Care Medicine
The Johns Hopkins University
Baltimore, MD

Spencer S. Liu, MD
Clinical Professor
Department of Anesthesia
Hospital for Special Surgery
The Weill Medical College of Cornell University
New York, NY

Christopher L. Wu, MD
Associate Professor
Department of Anesthesiology and Critical Care Medicine
The Johns Hopkins University
Baltimore, MD

Chapter 42

Craig T. Hartrick, MD, DABPM, FIPP
Anesthesiology Research
William Beaumont Hospital
Royal Oak, MI

Garen Manvelian, MD
Independent Pharmaceutical and Biotechnology Industry Consultant
San Diego, CA

Chapter 43

Christine Miaskowski, RN, PhD, FAAN
Professor and Associate Dean for Academic Affairs
Department of Physiological Nursing
University of California
San Francisco, CA

Chapter 44

Brian Durkin, DO
Director of Acute Pain Service
Assistant Professor of Clinical Anesthesiology
Department of Anesthesiology
Stony Brook University Medical Center
Stony Brook, NY

Peter S. A. Glass, MB, ChB
Professor and Chairman
Department of Anesthesiology
Stony Brook University Medical Center
Stony Brook, NY

Acknowledgments

To my wife Linda and daughters Kristin, Lauren, and Elizabeth who have encouraged and supported me during my academic career.

    Raymond S. Sinatra

To my family for all the support throughout life.

    Oscar A. de Leon-Casasola

To my wife Brenda and my children Nicki, Terri and Aaron. Thanks for your support and help.

    Brian Ginsberg

To my children, Christina and Andrew, my wife, Beverly, and my parents who have supported me throughout my career.

    Eugene R. Viscusi

Foreword: Historical Perspective, Unmet Needs, and Incidence

Henry McQuay

It is a delight and an honor to be asked to write the foreword for this text on acute pain management. We have an impressive array of different options for acute pain management (Figure F.1), and not all of them were available in the late 1970s.

As a simple example of the improvement in knowledge, compare the analgesic efficacy work of Moertel and colleagues[1] with that available to us now (Figure F.2). We can use these league tables of relative efficacy to say with some authority how well on average the different analgesics compare. This leaves us, of course, with the real-world issues of, for example, how the individual patient will react, prior experience, and drug-drug interactions.

Yet, we have the continued embarrassment of surveys that show that a substantial number of patients still endure severe pain after their surgery or trauma. This "unmet need" is a mixture of our failure to implement effective analgesic strategies and the inadequacy of those strategies. Acute pain teams date back to the early 1980s, and their policies and education of both patients and caregivers have made a difference. There is little excuse now for the failure to provide adequate analgesia for straightforward cases, but we need to acknowledge that there are also difficult cases. Many of the patients whose care causes problems for the teams seem, locally for us at least, to be the patients with chronic pain problems who are already on substantial analgesic therapy (e.g., chronic gastrointestinal disease) or substance abusers. Things the teams can do well include the education and patient advocacy roles within the institution. Things they may struggle with include changing behavior and provision of seamless care across nights and weekends.

Since the late 1990s there has been a flurry of interest in the extent to which acute pain can become chronic pain and how we might reduce the incidence of such chronicity.

Perhaps the most important thing this foreword points out is the sheer scale of the problem. From the chronic pain perspective, it appears now that surgery may be the most common cause of nerve damage pain and should perhaps be something that patients are warned about as a possibility in the consenting process. Mechanistically, one can ask what happens to cause this surgical pain to become chronic. I have always been skeptical that there is some psychological factor, pejoratively some weakness, that causes some patients to have the problem and others not. As an example, take a patient who had an inguinal herniorrhaphy 3 years ago: the procedure was performed perfectly and result was perfect. This year he had the other side done, and the same procedure was performed by the same surgeon. The patient described very severe postoperative pain, qualitatively and quantitatively quite different from the first operation, and this severe pain persisted. Something happened to cause the pain, and one cannot invoke a psychological explanation because of the perfect result the first time. What can we do about this? We still have no strong evidence that analgesia delivered before the pain does anything radically different from the same analgesia given after the pain, let alone that it preempts the development of this type of chronicity. It may be that unexpected severe pain is a red flag, but that is not easy to spot given the huge variations in pain intensity experienced after a given procedure. But it might be something we could pursue. Teasing apart precisely what happens during surgery would be another approach.

The measurement of the analgesic efficacy of preemptive strategies is another of the outstanding methodological issues in acute pain management. Our current methods allow us to measure the relative change in pain intensity. If the patient has no pain initially, then the method is invalid. This is the conundrum in measurement of the analgesic efficacy of preemptive strategies, because we have no idea whether the patient would have had no pain without the intervention. We claim that the patient had no pain because of the intervention, but they may not have had any pain without it.

A second cause of methodological angst is the use of patient-controlled analgesia (PCA) as an outcome measure. Many of the current crop of studies – for instance, those studying prophylactic antiepileptic drugs – use PCA in this way and report reduced PCA opioid consumption compared with controls. Unfortunately, this difference in consumption is not reported at valid equivalence in pain scores in the two groups. The control groups

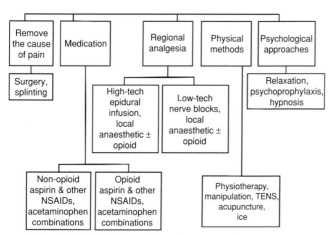

Figure F.1: The different options for acute pain management.

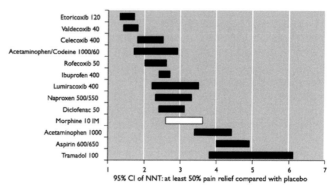

Figure F.2: Relative analgesic efficacy of analgesics in postoperative pain: number-needed-to-treat (NNT) for at least 50% pain relief over 6 hours compared with placebo in single-dose trials of acute pain.

commonly fail to use the PCA to lower their pain scores to the same level as is seen in the "active" group. Unless the pain scores are equivalent, it is very difficult to interpret the difference in PCA consumption. We need urgently to establish the validity of PCA as an outcome measure.

The editors and the authors of this book are to be congratulated on keeping academic and practical attention focused on acute pain, because there is room to both improve our current practice by learning from the best and try to answer some of the important outstanding issues.

Henry McQuay
Nuffield Professor of Clinical Anaesthetics
University of Oxford

REFERENCE

1. Moertel CG, Ahmann DL, Taylor WF, Schwartau N. Relief of pain by oral medications. *JAMA.* 1974;229:55–59.

Acute Pain Management

Pain Physiology and Pharmacology

1

Pain Pathways and Acute Pain Processing

Nalini Vadivelu, Christian J. Whitney, and
Raymond S. Sinatra

Understanding the anatomical pathways and neurochemical mediators involved in noxious transmission and pain perception is key to optimizing the management of acute and chronic pain. The International Association for the Study of Pain defines pain as "an unpleasant sensory and emotional experience associated with actual or potential tissue damage, or described in terms of such damage." Although acute pain and associated responses can be unpleasant and often debilitating, they serve important adaptive purposes. They identify and localize noxious stimuli, initiate withdrawal responses that limit tissue injury, inhibit mobility thereby enhancing wound healing, and initiate motivational and affective responses that modify future behavior. Nevertheless, intense and prolonged pain transmission,[1] as well as analgesic undermedication, can increase postsurgical/traumatic morbidity, delay recovery, and lead to development of chronic pain (see also Chapter 11, Transitions from acute to persistent pain). This chapter focuses on the anatomy and neurophysiology of pain transmission and pain processing. Particular emphasis is directed to mediators and receptors responsible for noxious facilitation, as well as to factors underlying the transition from acute to persistent pain.

CLASSIFICATION OF PAIN

Pain can be categorized according to several variables, including its duration (acute, convalescent, chronic), its pathophysiologic mechanisms (physiologic, nociceptive, neuropathic),[2] and its clinical context (eg, postsurgical, malignancy related, neuropathic, degenerative). Acute pain[3] follows traumatic tissue injuries, is generally limited in duration, and is associated with temporal reductions in intensity. Chronic pain[4] may be defined as discomfort persisting 3–6 months beyond the expected period of healing. In some chronic pain conditions, symptomatology, underlying disease states, and other factors may be of greater clinical importance than definitions based on duration of discomfort.[5] Clinical differentiation between acute and chronic pain is outlined in Table 1.1.

With regard to a more recent classification, pain states may be characterized as physiologic, inflammatory (nociceptive), or neuropathic. *Physiologic* pain defines rapidly perceived nontraumatic discomfort of very short duration. Physiologic pain alerts the individual to the presence of a potentially injurious environmental stimulus, such as a hot object, and initiates withdrawal reflexes that prevent or minimize tissue injury.

Nociceptive pain is defined as noxious perception resulting from cellular damage following surgical, traumatic, or disease-related injuries. Nociceptive pain has also been termed *inflammatory*[6] because peripheral inflammation and inflammatory mediators play major roles in its initiation and development. In general, the intensity of nociceptive pain is proportional to the magnitude of tissue damage and release of inflammatory mediators.

Somatic nociceptive pain is well localized and generally follows a dermatomal pattern. It is usually described as sharp, crushing, or tearing in character. Visceral nociceptive pain defines discomfort associated with peritoneal irritation as well as dilation of smooth muscle surrounding viscus or tubular passages.[7] It is generally poorly localized and nondermatomal and is described as cramping or colicky. Moderate to severe visceral pain is observed in patients presenting with bowel or ureteral obstructions, as well as peritonitis and appendicitis. Visceral pain radiating in a somatic dermatomal pattern is described as referred pain. Referred pain[8] may be explained by convergence of noxious input from visceral afferents activating second-order cells that are normally responsive to somatic sensation. Because of convergence, pain emanating from deep visceral structures may be perceived as well-delineated somatic discomfort at sites either adjacent to or distant from internal sites of irritation or injury.

The process of neural sensitization and the clinical term *hyperalgesia*[9] describe an exacerbation of acute nociceptive pain, as well as discomfort in response to sensations that normally would not be perceived as painful. These changes, termed *hyperpathia*[10] and *allodynia*,[11] although common following severe or extensive injuries, are most pronounced in patients developing persistent and neuropathic pain. Hyperalgesia can be

Table 1.1: Clinical Differentiations between Acute and Chronic Pain

Acute Pain	Chronic Pain
1. Usually obvious tissue damage	1. Multiple causes (malignancy, benign)
2. Distinct onset	2. Gradual or distinct onset.
3. Short, well characterized duration	3. Persists after 3–6 mo of healing
4. Resolves with healing	4. Can be a symptom or diagnosis.
5. Serves a protective function	5. Serves no adaptive purpose
6. Effective therapy is available	6. May be refractory to treatment

classified into primary and secondary forms (Table 1.2). Primary hyperalgesia[12] reflects sensitization of peripheral nociceptors and is characterized by exaggerated responses to thermal stimulation at or in regions immediately adjacent to the site of injury. Secondary hyperalgesia[13] involves sensitization within the spinal cord and central nervous system (CNS) and includes increased reactivity to mechanical stimulation and spread of the hyperalgesic area.[13] Enhanced pain sensitivity extends to uninjured regions several dermatomes above and below the initial site of injury. The stimulus response associated with primary and secondary hyperalgesia is outlined in Figure 1.1.

Neuropathic pain is defined by the International Association for the Study of Pain as "pain initiated or caused by a pathologic lesion or dysfunction" in peripheral nerves and CNS. Some authorities have suggested that any chronic pain state associated with structural remodeling or "plasticity" changes should be characterized as neuropathic.[1] Disease states associated with classic neuropathic sysmptoms include infection (eg, herpes zoster), metabolic derangements (eg, diabetic neuropathy), toxicity (eg, chemotherapy), and Wallerian degeneration secondary to trauma or nerve compression. Neuropathic pain is usually constant and described as burning, electrical, lancinating, and shooting. Differences between the pathophysiologic aspects of physiologic, nociceptive, and neuropathic pain are outlined in Table 1.3.

A common characteristic of neuropathic pain is the paradoxical coexistence of sensory deficits in the setting of increased noxious sensation.[14] By convention, symptoms related to peripheral lesions are termed *neuropathic*, whereas symptoms related to spinal cord injuries are termed *myelopathic*.[15] Causalgia or

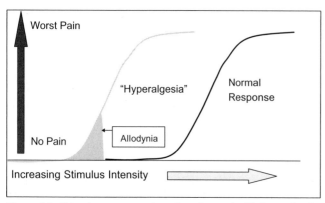

Figure 1.1: Stimulus response alteration observed with hyperalgesia.

Table 1.2: Characteristics of Hyperalgesia

Hyperalgesia

Defines a state of increased pain sensitivity and enhanced perception following acute injury that may persist chronically.

The hyperalgesic region may extend to dermatomes above and below the area of injury and is associated with ipsilateral (and occasionally contralateral) muscular spasm/immobility.

(Hyperalgesia is may be observed following incision, crush, amputation, and blunt trauma.)

Primary hyperalgesia

Increased pain sensitivity at the injury site

Related to peripheral release of intracellular or humoral noxious mediators

Secondary hyperalgesia

Increased pain sensitivity at adjacent, uninjured sites

Related to changes in excitability of spinal and supraspinal neurons

Abnormal sensations associated with hyperalgesia

Hyperpathia (increased or exaggerated pain intensity with minor stimulation)

Allodynia (nonnoxious sensory stimulation is perceived as painful)

Dysesthesia (unpleasant sensation at rest or movement)

Paresthesia [unpleasant often shock-like or electrical sensation precipitated by touch or pressure (CRPS-II causalgia)]

chronic regional pain syndrome II[16] describes pain following injury to sensory nerves, whereas discomfort associated with injury or abnormal activity of sympathetic fibers is termed *reflex sympathetic dystrophy* or *chronic regional pain syndrome I.*[17]

Finally, it is well recognized that certain acute traumatic and chronic pain conditions are associated with a mixture of nociceptive and neuropathic pain. Symptoms are proportional to the extent of neural versus nonneural tissue injuries. Clinical appreciation of the qualitative factors of the pain complaint helps guide the caregiver in differentiating between pain categories (Table 1.4).

PAIN PERCEPTION

A number of theories have been formulated to explain noxious perception.[18] One of the earliest ideas, termed the *specificity theory*, was proposed by Descartes.[19] The theory suggested that specific pain fibers carry specific coding that discriminates between different forms of noxious and nonnoxious sensation. The *intensity theory*, proposed by Sydenham,[20] suggested that the intensity of the peripheral stimulus determines which sensation is perceived. More recently, Melzack and Wall[21] proposed the *gate control theory* and suggested that sensory fibers of differing specificity stimulate second-order spinal neurons (dorsal horn transmission cell or wide dynamic range [WDR] neuron) that, depending on their degree of facilitation or inhibition, fire at varying intensity. Both large- and small-diameter afferents can activate "transmission" cells in dorsal horn; however, large sensory fibers also activate inhibitory substantia gelatinosa (SG) cells.[22] Indeed, it is the neurons and circuitry within the substantia gelatinosa that determine whether the "gate" is opened

Table 1.3: Pathophysiologic Representation of Pain

Category	Cause	Symptom	Examples
Physiologic	Brief exposure to a noxious stimulus	Rapid yet brief pain perception	Touching a pin or hot object
Nociceptive/inflammatory	Somatic or visceral tissue injury with mediators having an impact on intact nervous tissue	Moderate to severe pain, described as crushing or stabbing	Surgical pain, traumatic pain, sickle cell crisis
Neuropathic	Damage or dysfunction of peripheral nerves or CNS	Severe lancinating, burning or electrical shock like pain	Neuropathy, CRPS. Postherpetic Neuralgia
Mixed	Combined somatic and nervous tissue injury	Combinations of symptoms; soft tissue plus radicular pain	Low back pain, back surgery pain

Table 1.4: Qualitative Aspects of Pain Perception

1. Temporal: onset (when was it first noticed?) and duration (eg, acute, subacute, chronic)

2. Variability: constant, effort dependent (incident pain), waxing and waning, episodic "flare"

3. Intensity: average pain, worst pain, least pain, pain with activity of living

4. Topography: focal, dermatomal, diffuse, referred, superficial, deep

5. Character: sharp, aching, cramping, stabbing, burning, shooting

6. Exacerbating/Relieving: worse at rest, with movement or no difference; incident pain is worse with movement (stretching and tearing of injured tissue); intensity changes with touch, pressure, temperature

7. Quality of life: interfere with movement, coughing, ambulation, daily life tasks, work, etc.

or closed.[23] Substantia gelatinosa cells close the gate by directly suppressing transmission cells. In contrast, increased activity in small-diameter fibers decreases the suppressive effect of SG cells and opens the gate. Peripheral nerve injuries also open the gate by increasing small fiber activity and reducing large fiber inhibition.[24] Finally, descending inhibition from higher CNS centers and other inhibitory interneurons can also suppress transmission cells and close the gate. Some aspects of the gate control theory have fallen out of favor; nevertheless, pain processing in dorsal horn and, ultimately, pain perception are dependent on the degree of noxious stimulation, local and descending inhibition, and responses of second-order transmission cells. A schematic representation of the gate control system is presented in Figure 1.2.

Woolf and coworkers have proposed a new theory to explain pain processing.[27] They suggest that primary and secondary hyperalgesia as well as qualitative differences among physiologic, inflammatory, and neuropathic pain reflect sensitization of both peripheral nociceptors and spinal neurons (Figure 1.3). Noxious perception is the result of several distinct processes that begin in the periphery, extend up the neuraxis, and terminate at supraspinal regions responsible for interpretation and reaction. The process includes nociceptor activation, neural conduction, spinal transmission, noxious modulation, limbic and frontal-cortical perception, and spinal and supraspinal responses. The process of central sensitization, particularly within the SG, appears to be the key that unlocks the dorsal horn gate, thereby facilitating pain transmission. Identifying mediators that increase or diminish spinal sensitization and help close the gate will be important targets for treating pain in the near future.[23] The anatomic pathways mediating pain perception are outlined in Figure 1.4.

TRANSDUCTION

Transduction[27] defines responses of peripheral nociceptors to traumatic or potentially damaging chemical, thermal, or mechanical stimulation. Noxious stimuli are converted into a calcium ion– (Ca^{2+}) mediated electrical depolarization within the distal fingerlike nociceptor endings. Peripheral noxious mediators are either released from cells damaged during injury or as a result of humoral and neural responses to the injury. Cellular damage in skin, fascia, muscle, bone, and ligaments is associated with the release of intracellular hydrogen (H^+) and potassium (K^+) ions, as well as arachadonic acid (AA) from lysed cell membranes. Accumulations of AA stimulate and upregulate the cyclooxygenase 2 enzyme isoform (COX-2) that converts AA into biologically active metabolites, including prostaglandin E_2 (PGE_2), prostaglandin G_2 (PGG_2), and, later, prostaglandin H_2 (PGH_2). Prostaglandins[28] and intracellular H^+ and K^+ ions play key roles as primary activators of peripheral nociceptors. They also initiate inflammatory responses and peripheral sensitization that increase tissue swelling and pain at the site of injury.

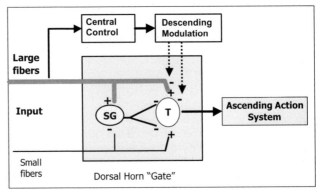

Figure 1.2: The gate control theory of pain processing. T = Second-order transmission cell; SG = substantia gelatinosa cell. (Modified from Melzack R and Wall PD, *Science.* 1965;150(699):971–979.).[21]

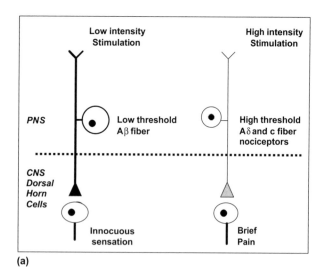
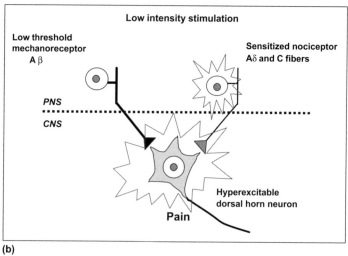

(a)   (b)

Figure 1.3: (a) The sensitization theory of pain perception suggests that brief high-intensity noxious stimulation in the absence of tissue injury activates the nociceptive endings of unmyelinated or thinly myelinated (high-threshold) fibers, resulting in physiologic pain perception of short duration. Other low-threshold sensory modalities (pressure, vibration, touch) are carried by larger-caliber (low-threshold) fibers. Large and small fibers make contact with second-order neurons in the dorsal horn. (b) Following tissue injuries and release of noxious mediators, peripheral nociceptors become sensitized and fire repeatedly. Peripheral sensitization occurs in the presence of inflammatory mediators, which in turn increases the sensitivity of high-threshold nociceptors as well as the peripheral terminals of other sensory neurons. This increase in nociceptor sensitivity, lowering of the pain threshold, and exaggerated response to painful and nonpainful stimuli is termed *primary hyperalgesia*. The ongoing barrage of noxious impulses sensitizes second-order transmission neurons in dorsal horn via a process termed *wind-up*. Central sensitization results in secondary hyperalgesia and spread of the hyperalgesic area to nearby uninjured tissues. Inhibitory interneurons and descending inhibitory fibers modulate and suppress spinal sensitization, whereas analgesic under medication and poorly controlled pain favors sensitization. In certain settings central sensitization may then lead to neurochemical/neuroanatomical changes (plasticity), prolonged neuronal discharge and sensitivity (long-term potentiation), and the development of chronic pain. (Modified from Woolf CJ, Salter MW. Neuronal plasticity: increasing the gain in pain. *Science*. 2000;288(5472):1765–1769.)[1]

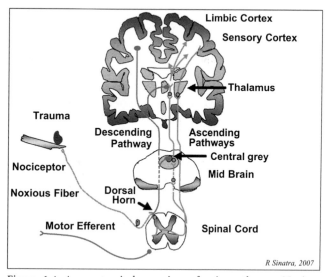

Figure 1.4: An anatomical overview of pain pathways. Noxious information is conveyed from peripheral nociceptors to the dorsal horn via unmeylinated and myelinated noxious fibers. Second-order spinal neurons send impulses rostrally via two distinct pathways, the neospinothalamic and paleospinothalamic tracts. These cells also activate motor and sympathetic efferents within the spinal cord. Ascending tracts make contacts in the brainstem and midbrain, central gray, and thalamus. Projections are then made with the frontal and limbic cortex. Descending fibers emanating from cortex, hypothalamus, and brainstem project to the spinal cord to modulate pain transmission.

In addition to PGEs, leukotrienes,[29] 5-hydroxytryptamine (5-HT),[30] bradykinin (BK),[31] and histamine[32] released following tissue injury are powerful primary and secondary noxious sensitizers. 5-hydroxytryptamine released after thermal injury sensitizes primary afferent neurons and produces mechanical allodynia and thermal hyperalgesia via peripheral 5-HT2a receptors.[33] Bradykinin's role in peripheral sensitization is mediated by G-protein-coupled receptors,[1] B1 and B2, that are expressed by the primary nociceptors. When activated by BK and kallidin, the receptor-G-protein complex strengthens inward Na^+ flux, whereas it weakens outward K^+ currents, thereby increasing nociceptor excitability. These locally released substances increase vascular permeability, initiate neurogenic edema, increase nociceptor irritability, and activate adjacent nociceptor endings. The resulting state of peripheral sensitization is termed *primary hyperalgesia*.

In addition to locally released and humoral noxious mediators, neural responses play an important role in maintaining both peripheral sensitization and primary hyperalgesia. Bradykinin, 5-HT, and other primary mediators stimulate orthodromic transmission in sensitized nerve endings and stimulate the release of peptides and neurokinins, including calcitonin gene-related protein (CGRP),[34] substance P (sP),[35] and cholocystokinin (CCK),[36] in and around the site of injury. Substance P, via a feedback loop mechanism, enhances peripheral sensitization by facilitating further release of bradykinin, histamine from mast cells, and 5-HT. Calcitonin gene-related protein is a 37-amino-acid peptide found in the peripheral and central terminals of more than 50% of C fibers and 35% of Aδ fibers.[37]

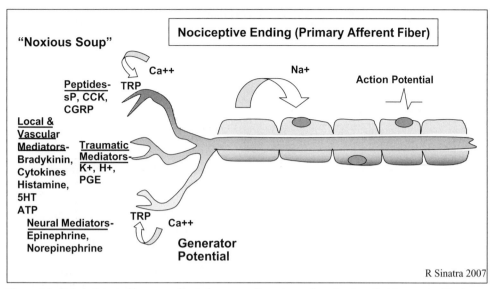

Figure 1.5: Pain is detected by unmyelinated nerve endings, termed *nociceptors*, that innervate skin, bone, muscle, and visceral tissues. Nociceptor activation initiates a depolarizing Ca^{2+} current or generator potential. Generator potentials depolarize the distal axonal segment and initiate an inward Na^+ current and self-propagating action potential. Following tissue injury, cellular mediators (potassium, hydrogen ions, and prostaglandin released from damaged cells, as well as bradykinin [BK] released from damaged vessels) activate the terminal endings (nociceptors) of sensory afferent fibers. Prostaglandin (PGE), synthesized by cyclooxygenase 2, is responsible for nociceptor sensitization and plays a key role in peripheral inflammation. Orthodromic transmission in sensitized afferents leads to the release of peptides (substance P (sP), cholycystokinin (CCK), and calcitonin gene-related peptide (CGRP) in and around the site of injury. Substance P is responsible for further release of BK and also stimulates release of histamine from mast cells and 5HT from platelets, which further increases vascular permeability (neurogenic edema) and nociceptor irritability. The release of these mediators and others, such as serotonin (5HT) and cytokines, creates a "noxious soup" that exacerbates the inflammatory response, recruits adjacent nociceptors, and results in primary hyperalgesia. Reflex sympathetic efferent responses may further sensitize nociceptors by releasing noradrenaline and, indirectly, by stimulating further release of BK and sP and leading to peripheral vasoconstriction and trophic changes.

Like sP, CGRP[38] is produced in the cell bodies of primary nociceptors located in the dorsal root ganglion. Following axonal transport to peripheral and central terminals, these substances initiate mechanical and thermal hyperalgesia. When released at peripheral endings, CGRP enhances PGE[39] and histamine-induced vasodilation and inflammatory extravasation. It also prolongs the effect of sP by inhibiting its peripheral metabolic breakdown.[40] Finally, reflex-sympathetic efferent responses also sensitize nociceptors by releasing norepinephrine, which produces peripheral vasoconstriction at the site of injury. Norepinephrine also stimulates release of BK and sP and leads to atrophic changes in bone and muscle.

Peripheral sensitization is also associated with release of nerve growth factor, which alters intracellular signaling pathways and initiated posttranslational regulatory changes, including phosphorylation of tyrosine kinase and G proteins. These alterations markedly increase the sensitivity and excitability of distal nociceptor terminals.[41] For example, nociceptors are activated at lower temperatures ($< 40^\circ C$) and in response to lower concentrations of PGE_2 and other primary mediators.

Acute tissue injury results in an increased synthesis and extravasation of humoral proinflammatory cytokines, such as interleukin- (IL) 1β and IL-6. These cytokines play an important role in exacerbating edematous and irritative components of inflammatory pain.[42] Studies have shown that elevated levels of IL-1β result in allodynia and the development of persistent pain,[42] whereas effective postoperative analgesia decreases proinflammatory cytokines levels.[43,44] According to Bessler et al,[42] genetic polymorphisms influence production of proinflammatory cytokines and may contribute to observed interindividual differences in postoperative pain intensity scores and variations in morphine consumption.

The inflammatory mediators and proinflammatory cytokines described above activate transducer molecules such as the transient receptor potential (TRP) ion channel.[1] At least 8 different TRP ion channels have been identified and respond differentially to thermal, traumatic, and chemical 14 evoked mediators within the microenvironment. The TRP-VI/capsaicin ion channel has been well described. This 4-unit receptor contains a central ion channel that permits inward Ca^{2+} and Na^+ currents following stimulation by H^+ ions, heat, and direct application of capsaicin,[45] the active chemical compound found in hot pepper. The inward flux of Ca^{2+} via TRP ion channels is responsible for the generator potential.[31] Generator potentials summate and depolarize the distal axonal segment and the resulting action potential is then conducted centrally to terminals in the dorsal horn. The "noxious soup" of local humoral and neural mediators released following acute tissue injury as well as the nociceptor response to peripheral injury are summarized in Figure 1.5.

Table 1.5: Classification of Primary Afferent Nerve Fibers

Characteristic	Aβ	Aδ	C fibers
Diameter size	Largest	Small	Very small
Degree of myelination	Myelinated	Thinly myelinated	Unmyelinated
Conduction velocity	Very Fast	Fast	Slow
	30–50 m/s	5–25 m/s	<2 m/s
Threshold level	Low	High	High
Activated by	Light touch movement and vibration	Brief noxious stimulation; also intense and prolonged noxious stimuli	Intense and prolonged noxious stimuli
Located in	Skin, joints	Skin and superficial tissues; deep somatic and visceral structures	Skin and superficial tissues; deep somatic and visceral structures

CONDUCTION

Conduction refers to the propagation of action potentials from peripheral nociceptive endings via myelinated and unmyelinated nerve fibers. Central terminals of these fibers make synaptic contact with second-order cells in the spinal cord. Nociceptive and nonnoxious nerve fibers are classified according to their degree of myelination, diameter, and conduction velocity (Table 1.5). The largest-diameter sensory fibers, termed Aβ fibers, are generally nonnoxious special sensory axons that innervate somatic structures of the skin and joints. Two classes of nociceptive fibers include the thin myelinated Aδ and unmyelinated C fibers that innervate skin and a wide variety of other tissues. The Aδ fibers transmit the "first pain," a rapid-onset (<1 s) well-localized, sharp or stinging sensation of short duration. This perception of "first pain" alerts the person to actual or potential injury, localizes the site of injury, and initiates reflex withdrawal responses. The unmyelinated C fibers, also termed *high threshold polymodal nociceptive fibers*, respond to mechanical, chemical, and thermal injuries. They are responsible for the perception of "second pain," which has a delayed latency (seconds to minutes) and is described as a diffuse burning, stabbing sensation that is often prolonged and may become progressively more uncomfortable.[46] Ion channels found in nociceptive axons as well as their terminal endings appear to have selective roles in noxious conduction. Axonal Na$^+$ ion channels have been classified as being either sensitive or resistant (TTX-r) to the puffer fish biotoxin tetrodotoxin. The TTX-r isoform is upregulated in sensitized nerve fibers. Currently available local anesthetics block both forms; however, development of specific TTX-r channel blockers may provide more selective therapy for neuropathic and chronic inflammatory pain. Axonal conduction in nociceptive fibers culminates in the release of excitatory amino acids (EAAs) and peptidergic transmitters from presynaptic terminal endings in the dorsal horn. Neuronal-type (N-type) calcium channels are concentrated in these terminal endings and open in response to action potential induced depolarization. Following depolarization, these 4-subunit voltage-gated channels allow a rapid influx of Ca^{2+} ions that facilitates release of EAAs. N-type calcium channels may be blocked by conotoxins such as ziconotide. Specific ion channels that facilitate or suppress pain transmission are presented in Table 1.6.

TRANSMISSION

Transmission refers to the transfer of noxious impulses from primary nociceptors to cells in the spinal cord dorsal horn. Aδ and C fibers are the axons of unipolar neurons that have distal projections known as nociceptive endings. Their proximal terminals enter the dorsal horn of the spinal cord, branch within Lissauer's tract, and synapse with second-order cells located predominantly in Rexed's laminae II (substantia gelatinosa) and V (nucleus proprius). The second-order dorsal horn neurons are of two main types. The first type, termed *nociceptive-specific neurons* (NS), are located in lamina I and respond exclusively to noxious impulses from C fibers. The second type, known as *WDR*, are primarily localized in lamina V and respond to both noxious and innocuous stimuli. Wide dynamic range neurons have variable response characteristics such that low-frequency C fiber stimulation results in nonpainful sensory transmission, whereas higher frequency stimulation leads to gradual increases in WDR neuronal discharge and transmission of painful impulses.[47] WDR neurons can also be suppressed by local inhibitory cells and descending synaptic contacts. The inhibitory actions of SG cells, as well as the ability of WDR neurons to function as "transmission cells" that differentially process noxious and innocuous stimuli, provide the physiologic foundation of the gate control theory. Synaptic connections made within the spinal cord are presented in Figure 1.6.

Excitatory amino acids such as glutamate (Glu) and aspartate are responsible for fast synaptic transmission and rapid neuronal depolarization. Excitatory amino acids activate ionotropic amino-3-hydroxyl-5-methyl-4-propionic acid (AMPA) and kainite (KAR) receptors that regulate Na$^+$ and K$^+$ ion influx and intraneuronal voltage. AMPA and KAR are relatively impermeable to Ca^{2+} and other cations.

Each AMPA receptor contains 4 subunits with integral glutamate binding sites that surround a central cation channel. Agonist binding at two or more sites activates the receptor, opening the channel and allowing passage of Na$^+$ ions into the cell.[48] This brief increase in Na$^+$ ion flux depolarizes second-order spinal neurons, allowing noxious signals to be rapidly transmitted to supraspinal sites of perception. Kainate receptors are also involved in postsynaptic excitation. The KAR cation channel regulates both Na$^+$ and K$^+$ flux; however, unlike AMPA,

Table 1.6: Receptors Associated with Noxious Transmission in the Dorsal Horn

Receptor	Type	Ligand	Voltage Gated	Action	Function	Onset
AMPA	Ionotropic	Glu	No	Excitatory	Na^+ flux	Rapid
NMDA	Ionotropic	Glu	Yes	Excitatory	Ca^2 flux	Delayed
KAR	Ionotropic	Glu	No	Excitatory	Na^+, K^+ flux	Rapid
NK-1	Metabotropic	sP	No	Excitatory	Activates 2nd messengers	Delayed
Glycine	Ionotropic	Gly	No	Inhibitory	Cl- Flux	Rapid
GABA	Iontropic	GABA	No	Inhibitory	Inhibits K^+ flux	Rapid
ENK	Metabotropic	ENK	No	Inhibitory	Inhibits K^+ flux and 2nd messengers	Rapid

Abbreviations: Glu = glutamate; sP = substance P; Gly = glycine; GABA = γ-aminobutyric acid; ENK = enkephalin.

these receptors appear to play a minor role in synaptic signaling following brief noxious stimulation. Once activated, KARs may improve synaptic efficacy by increasing the likelihood of second-order neuronal discharge in settings of ongoing stimulation.

In the setting of continued high-frequency noxious stimulation, activated AMPA and KAR receptors initiate voltage mediated priming of *N*-methyl-D-aspartic acid (NMDA) receptors.[49,50] The NMDA receptor is a 4-subunit (2 NR1 subunits and 1 NR2A and 1 NR2B subunit) membrane protein that regulates inflow of Na^+ and Ca^{2+} and cellular outflow of K^+ via an intrinsic ion channel. The extracellular portion of NR2 subunit contains a Glu binding site, whereas a glycine (Gly) binding site is located on the NR1 subunit. Each subunit has an extensive cytoplasmic portion that can be modified by protein kinases and an external allosteric portion that may be altered by zinc ions. NMDA receptors are both ligand dependent and voltage gated. Activation requires AMPA-induced membrane depolarization and a positive change in intracellular voltage, as well as binding of glutamate or aspartate to the receptor (Figure 1.7).

Activated AMPA receptors initiate slow excitatory postsynaptic potentials (EPSPs) lasting several hundred milliseconds.[51] These <5-Hz potentials accumulate and produce a summated depolarization that in turn dislodges a magnesium ion "plug" that normally blocks the NMDA ion channel. Following dislodgement of Mg^{2+}, a rapid influx of Ca^{2+} ions is initiated. Activated NMDA receptors (NMDARs) are further sensitized by direct effects of glutamate at the glutamate binding site.[52]

Accumulation of intracellular Ca^{2+} initiates a series of neurochemical and neurophysiologic changes that influence acute pain processing. Second-order spinal neurons become highly sensitized and fire rapidly and independently of further sensory stimulation. This process, termed *wind-up*, refers specifically to transcription-independent excitation of dorsal horn neurons. (Refer to section on transition from acute to chronic pain.)

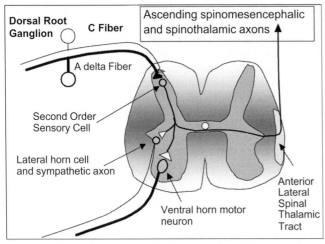

Figure 1.6: Synaptic contacts and pain transmission between primary afferent fibers and second-order cells in the dorsal horn. Projections from second-order cells contact efferent motor and sympathetic cell bodies in the spinal cord and also ascend to supraspinal sites.

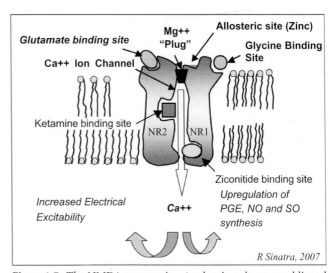

Figure 1.7: The NMDA receptor is a 4-subunit, voltage-gated ligand specific ion channel. The 4 subunits include 2 NR2 units, which contain glutamate binding sites, and 2 NR1 units, which contain glycine binding sites and an allosteric site that is sensitive to zinc ions. Glutamate is the primary agonist of NMDA, whereas glycine functions as a modulator. The central ion channel is normally blocked by a magnesium ion. Once dislodged, Ca^{2+} ions can pass through the channel and induce neuronal excitability.

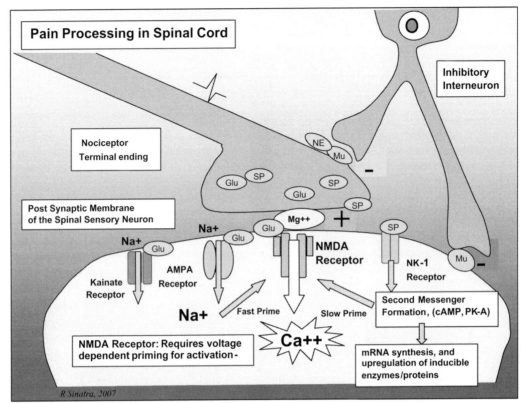

Figure 1.8: Targets of excitatory noxious mediators on second-order cells. Glutamate is the primary excitatory agonist for noxious transmission. Glutamate activates specific binding sites located on AMPA, kainate, and NMDA receptors. Ion channels on activated AMPA and kainate receptors allow Na^+ to enter and depolarize the cell. Changes in intracellular voltage rapidly prime the NMDA receptor and allows an Mg^{2+} plug to be dislodged. Following dislodgement, an inward flux of Ca^{2+} is initiated. Glutamate binding to NMDARs maintains the inward Ca^{2+} flux. Substance P binds and activates NK-1 receptors. This receptor upregulates second messengers, including cAMP and PKA, which slowly prime and maintain excitability of NMDARs. Activation of second messengers in turn upregulates inducible enzymes, initiates transcription of mRNA, and mediates synthesis of acute reaction proteins. These changes increase neuronal excitability and underlie subsequent plasticity.

Woolf and others have shown that NMDA activation, wind-up, and central sensitization are responsible for clinical hyperalgesia and can occur following nerve injury as well as trauma and inflammation,[1] Central sensitization is also observed in supraspinal regions of the CNS, including rostroventral medulla, amygdala, and anterior cingulate gyrus.[53]

Intracellular Ca^{2+} ions also activate inducible enzymes, including nitric oxide synthase (NOS) and COX-2. Peptides such as sP and CGRP are responsible for delayed and long-lasting depolarization of second-order dorsal horn neurons. Substance P binding at metabotrophic neurokinin 1 (NK-1) receptors synergistically activates NMDARs and appears necessary for the development of long-term potentiation (LTP).[54] Following activation of NK-1, second messengers cyclic adenosine monophosphate (cAMP) and phosphokinase A (PKA) are synthesized and mediate a number of cellular changes, including slow priming of NMDARs, second-messenger cascades, and genome activation. Synthesis of acute phase proteins together with increased intracellular and extracellular PGE and NO are responsible for transcription-dependent central sensitization and associated neural plasticity changes and responses that facilitate pain transmission. The process of NMDA activation and its consequences are presented in Figure 1.8.

MODULATION

The concept of modulation refers to pain-suppressive mechanisms within the spinal cord dorsal horn and at higher levels of the brainstem and midbrain. In the spinal cord, this intrinsic "breaking mechanism" inhibits pain transmission at the first synapse between the primary noxious afferent and second-order WDR and NS cells, thereby reducing spinothalamic relay of noxious impulses. Spinal modulation is mediated by the inhibitory actions of endogenous analgesic compounds released from spinal interneurons and terminal endings of inhibitory axons that descend from central gray locus ceruleus and other supraspinal sites. Endogenous analgesics, including enkephalin (ENK), norepinephrine (NE), and γ-aminobutyric acid (GABA), activate opioid, alpha adrenergic, and other receptors that either inhibit release of Glu from primary nociceptive afferents or diminish postsynaptic responses of second-order NS or WDR neurons (Figure 1.9). The balance between excitatory mediators and the inhibitory effects of endogenous analgesics adjusts K^+ ion flux and the firing frequency of dorssal horn cells.[55]

Endogenous opioids, including the ENKs and endorphins, modulate pain transmission by activating pre- and postsynaptic

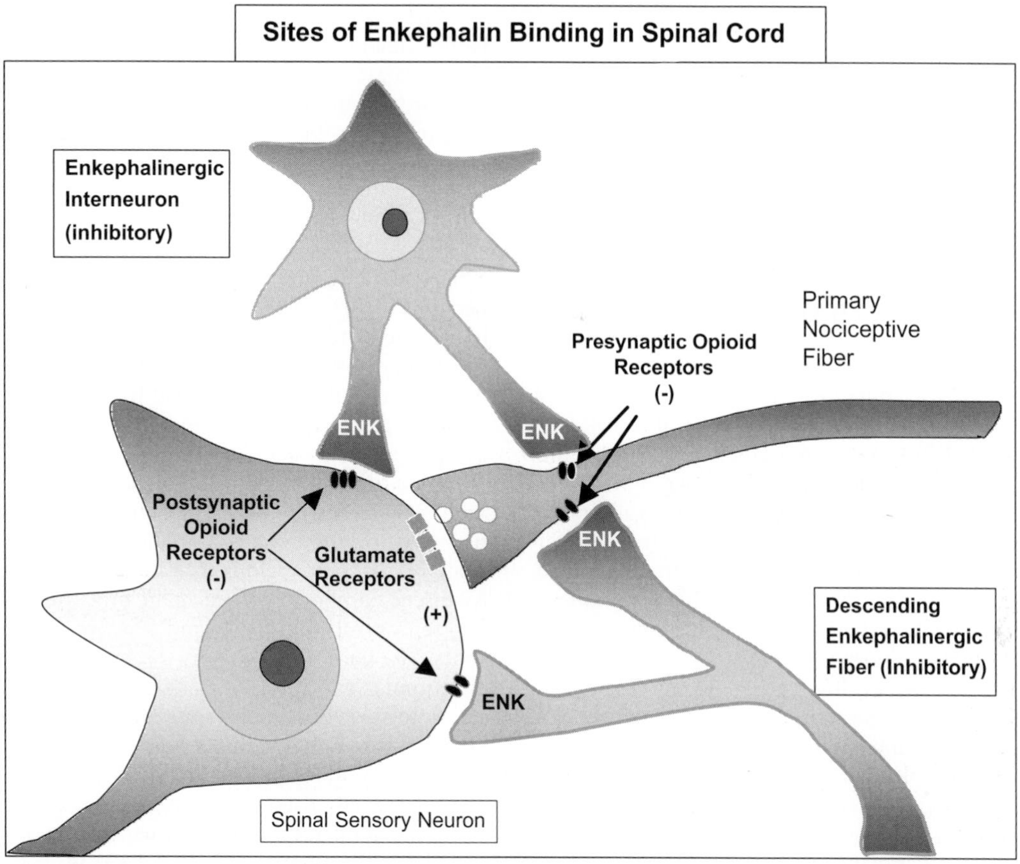

Sites of Enkephalin Binding in Spinal Cord

Enkephalinergic Interneuron (inhibitory)

Presynaptic Opioid Receptors (-)

Primary Nociceptive Fiber

ENK

ENK

Postsynaptic Opioid Receptors (-)

Glutamate Receptors

(+)

ENK

Descending Enkephalinergic Fiber (Inhibitory)

ENK

Spinal Sensory Neuron

Figure 1.9: Enkephalinergic modulation of noxious transmission. Both local interneurons and descending axons suppress synaptic transmission between the primary nociceptor and second-order sensory cells. Enkephalins activate both pre- and postsynaptic opioid receptors. Opioid receptors inhibit either release of noxious transmitters such as glutamate or second-order responses.

μ-, κ-, and δ-receptor subtypes. These subtypes belong to a large superfamily of transmembrane-spanning G-protein-coupled receptors.[56] μ-opioid receptors are primarily responsible for mediating spinal and supraspinal analgesia, euphoria, and respiratory depression. Kappa subtypes mediate spinal analgesia, as well as sedative/hypnotic effects of opioids. Delta receptors appear to potentiate mu-mediated analgesia, whereas activation of σ receptors may be responsible for dysphoria.[57] Opioid binding at μ receptors activates coupled G proteins (Gi/o), which in turn inhibit the neuronal cAMP pathway. Adenylate cyclase is suppressed, and production of cAMP PKA are markedly reduced. Reductions in cAMP and inhibition of potassium (K^+) influx decrease neuronal excitability (Figure 1.10). The structure of μ-opioid receptors (μ-opioid receptor peptide or MOP) is coded by the MOP gene, which is part of the opioid receptor μ 1 (*OPRM1*) gene. The *OPRM1* gene has 4 exons that determine the amino acid constituents and tertiary configuration of the external and internal portions of the MOP.[29] At least 10 single nucleotide polymorphisms (SNP) in the coding or open reading frames and more than 100 polymorphisms in the noncoding frames of the human *OPRM1* gene have been identified.[58] Polymorphic variations influence transcriptional regulation, expression, and functionality of the mu receptor.[59] With regard to expression, polymorphisms of *OPRM1* neither influence the conformation of the external binding site nor affect the binding affinity of opioid ligands. They do, however, alter

the internal segment and c-terminus of MOP and may influence secondary proteins, such as G proteins and adenylate cyclase, that modulate receptor efficacy.[60] In clinical settings, these polymorphisms may explain interindividual differences in opioid

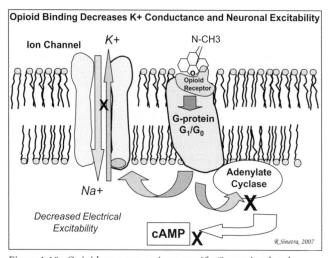

Figure 1.10: Opioid receptors activate specific G proteins that decrease neuronal excitability either by inhibiting K^+ ion conductance or decreasing intracellular cAMP.

sensitivity, incomplete cross tolerance, and improved efficacy associated with opioid rotation.

The modulatory effects of NE are mediated by activation of postsynaptic α-adrenergic receptors. The ability of α-adrenergic receptors to suppress noxious transmission in the spinal cord is nearly equivalent to that observed following binding and activation of opioid receptors binding and forms the basis of tricyclic antidepressant and neuraxial clonidine mediated analgesia.[61]

ASCENDING PAIN PATHWAYS

Axons from NS and WDR dorsal horn cells may either synapse with sympathetic anterolateral horn cells, anterior horn motor neurons, or project to the brainstem, midbrain, and thalamus (Figure 1.6). These cells also make important connections within the spinal cord. Synapses made with ventral horn motor neurons are responsible for reflexive musculoskeletal withdrawal responses observed with physiologic pain and important for minimizing tissue damage during traumatic injury. Increased excitability of motor neurons is also responsible for segmental ipsilateral and contralateral increases in skeletal muscle tone termed hyperreflexia or splinting. Telologically, muscle splinting and hyperreflexia have evolved to inhibit movement and encourage wound healing; however, these same responses can also impair pulmonary function and rehabilitation following surgical and traumatic injuries. In addition, severe muscle spasm and accumulation of lactic acid may further worsen some aspects of acute pain. Synapses with anterolateral cells are responsible for noxious segmental sympathetic responses, including vasoconstriction, vasodilation, and effects on gastrointestinal and cardiac function. These important "fight or flight" responses increase perfusion to heart, brain, and skeletal musculature, whereas reducing blood flow and hemorrhage at the site of injury. (Please see Chapter 2, *Pathophysiology of Acute Pain*).

Several ascending tracts are responsible for transmitting nociceptive impulses from the dorsal horn to supraspinal targets. These include the spinomesencephalic, spinoreticular, and spinothalamic tracts. However, the spinothalamic tract (STT) is considered the primary perception pathway. The STT is divided into two distinct projections; the lateral neospinothalamic tract (nSTT) and the more medial paleospinothalamic tract (pSTT). The nSTT projects directly to the neothalamus, whereas the pSTT is a slow multisynaptic pathway that projects to the reticular activating system and periaqueductal gray (PAG) and ascends to the medial thalamus.

CORTICAL PERCEPTION AND RESPONSES

Projections of the nSTT ascend directly and terminate within the ventroposterior lateral and ventroposterior medial (VPL, VPM) regions of the neothalamus. The laterally placed neothalamus is a highly somatotopically organized region. Axons from dorsal horn cell synapse with thalamic cells, which in turn transmit nociceptive impulses directly to the somatosensory cortex. This 3-neuron pathway is responsible for rapid perception, localization, and prompt withdrawal from the noxious stimulus. Thalamocortical connections made with other sites are discriminative in terms of intensity and account for sensory qualities, such as throbbing or burning.[62]

Distal projections of the pSTT contact neurons in medial thalamus. In contrast to the VPL connections made in the medial thalamus are not somatotopically organized. Medial thalamic cells in turn project to the various regions in the limbic system, including the amygdala, cingulate gyrus, and frontal cortex. Connections made within the limbic system are responsible for the suffering aspects of acute and persistent pain and the diffuse, unpleasant emotions that develop and persist long after an injury has occurred. Projections from the limbic cortex also activate motor cortex, hypothalamus, and pituitary gland. Connections to these areas mediate persistent supraspinal, hypothalamic, and pituitary effective responses that affect muscle tone, circulatory, respiratory, and endocrine function. Activation of μ-opioid receptors in the medial thalamus modulates thalamocortical pain transmission and reduces cognitive and affective components of pain.[63]

Brain functional MRI (fMRI) and positive emission tomography (PET) have helped clinicians better understand central sites of pain processing by revealing, in real time, discrete cortical and thalamic regions that are activated by noxious input. As discussed above, cortical pain processing may be divided into sensory-discriminative and affective-motivational components. The neocortical sensory discriminative domain localizes the stimulus and determines its intensity. This domain can be assessed using visual analog scales or numerical rating scales. The limbic affective-motivational domain determines the unpleasantness and other qualities of pain. Connections made with cells in frontal cortex and amygdala also underlie emotional and behavioral responses such as fear, anxiety, helplessness, and learned avoidance. Affective-motivational or unpleasantness domains can be assessed using multidimensional and qualitative pain scales such as the McGill pain questionnaire. (Please see Chapter 11, *Qualitative and Quantitative Measurement of Pain*.)

Cortical sensory, behavioral, cognitive, and motor responses to peripheral noxious stimuli can be studied by brain imaging. Brain imaging studies, including fMRI and PET scanning and brain spectroscopy, offer a bridge between basic research and understanding mechanisms underlying clinical pain states. These techniques have provided evidence that experimental pain is processed at interconnected cortical regions, with each having distributed functions. Functional imaging (PET scan and fMRI) techniques allow clinicians to visualize neuronal targets associated with pain modulation and perception in real time. Considering the multidimensional subjective experience of pain, functional imaging studies have revealed those CNS regions that are primarily involved in controlling the sensory discriminative, attentional cognitive aspects, behavioral/affective reactions, and motor responses to pain. Positron emission scan images can be used to visualize changes in regional cerebral blood flow (rCBF) induced by localizing and subjective aspects of noxious perception, whereas fMRI has higher spatial and temporal resolution and can measure both the change in rCBF as well as the change in neuronal activity in response to pain perception. Considering that the PET scan is the gold standard for rCBF measurement, regions identified or linked to pain perception have demonstrated fairly consistent noxious-induced alterations across several studies. In these trials, a standardized nociceptive stimulus consistently activated several well-connected regions in the CNS, including the contralateral insula, secondary somatosensory cortex (S2), and the anterior cingulate cortex (ACC)

Functional measures

A. Brain areas functionally related to pain processing.

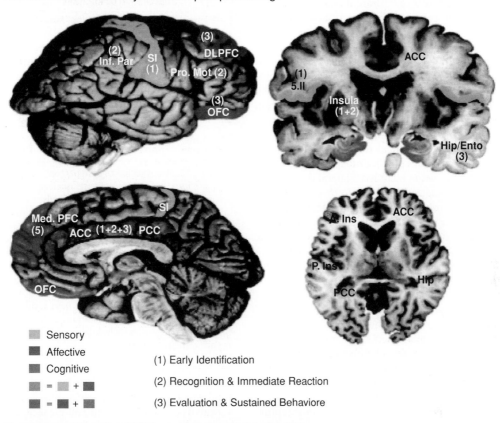

Sensory
Affective
Cognitive
■ = ■ + ■
■ = ■ + ■

(1) Early Identification

(2) Recognition & Immediate Reaction

(3) Evaluation & Sustained Behaviore

B. Example of functional MRI response to painful stimulation.

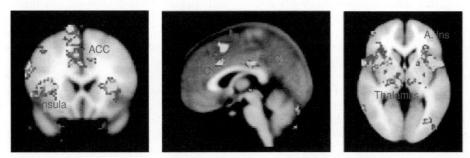

Figure 1.11: Cortical regions related to pain processing as determined by function magnetic resonance imaging (fMRI). The highlighted areas have been found to be particularly active ACC = anterior cingulate cortex, S1 = primary somatosensory cortex (Primarily involved in pain localization), S2 = secondary somatosensory cortex, OFC = orbitofrontal cortex, DLPFC = dorsolateral prefrontal cortex, Pre-Mot = premotor cortex, Med.PFC = medial prefrontal cortex, P.Ins = posterior insula, A.Ins = anterior insula, Hip = hippocampus, Ento = entorhinal cortex. From: Borsook, et al. *Molecular Pain* 2007; 3:25. See color plates.

Figure 1.11.[64] Primary somatosensory cortex (S1), is primarily responsible for acute noxious localization, whereas the insular cortex plays a role in pain anticipation. Thalamus, brain stem, cerebellum (CBLM), supplementary motor area (SMA), and the primary motor cortex are some of the other regions that become activated, although not as consistently as the insula, S1, and ACC.

In human studies of experimental electrical pain using fMRI,[65] regional blood flow in the anterior cingulate gyrus, parietoinsula cortex, and somatosensory cortex was markedly increased. Increased blood flow in the parietoinsular cortex cor-responded to the physical sensation of pain and its intensity (pain thresholds). Activity in the cingulate cortex, specifically the dorsal anterior cingulate gyrus, was related to the unpleasantness of pain and emotional affective responses to severe discomfort.[66] The posterior aspect of the anterior cingulate gyrus (PAACG) is located in the medial frontal cortex and processes pain thresholds and affective components of pain such as its unpleasantness.[67,68] Using fMRI to study experimental electrical pain, Davis and co-workers[69] noted that the PAACG responds to variations in pain intensity; however, significant activity was detected only after exposure to moderately intense or intense pain. Several other sites, including the amygdala and striatum, are activated at the same time the PAACG is activated.[70] Brain imaging techniques have also been employed to characterize cortical sites of pain modulation.

μ-opioid receptors are involved in regulating the experience of pain in specific thalamic and cortical regions. Zubieta and coworkers[71] utilized PET scanning with the selective μ-receptor agonist carfentanil to evaluate sites of opioid uptake. They also studied whether opioid suppression of masseter muscle pain reduced metabolic activation in specific regions of the brain. They found that carfentanil binding at μ receptors uniquely reduced metabolic activity in cortical regions responsible for sensory and affective dimensions of pain. Affective regions with diminished metabolic activation included bilateral dorsal anterior cingulate cortex and lateral prefrontal cortex as well as the contralateral insular cortex. Sensory regions demonstrating opioid-induced metabolic suppression included the ipsilateral thalamus and amygdala; however, opioid binding and metabolic alterations were not observed in the primary sensory cortex.

Metabolic changes have been studied with brain chemistry studies in pain states. Grachev et al[72] studied the brain chemistry changes in patients with chronic back pain in vivo single-voxel proton magnetic resonance spectroscopy (H-MRS). The concentration of several substances, including *N*-acetyl aspartate, creatine, choline, Glut, glutamine, GABA, inositol, glucose, and lactate, was studied. They found direct abnormal brain chemistry in chronic back pain as compared to volunteers that could be useful in the diagnosis and development of effective drugs for the treatment of pain

Understanding the variability of the μ-opioid-receptor-mediated antinociceptive responses and stress responses with functional neuroimaging may offer an important tool to help us understand why individuals respond differently to similar painful stimuli.

DESCENDING PATHWAYS

Descending modulatory neural pathways function to reduce pain perception and efferent responses by inhibiting pain transmission in the dorsal horn, PAG, brainstem (rostroventromedial medulla, RVM), and other regions of the CNS. The cerebral cortex, hypothalamus, thalamus, PAG, nucleus raphe magnus (NRM), and locus coeruleus (LC) all send descending axons that synapse with, and modulate pain transmission in, noxious cells located in the brainstem and spinal cord dorsal horn. Components of the descending system that play critical roles in modulating pain transmission include the previously mentioned endogenous opioid system, the descending noradrenergic system, and serotonergic neurons.

The PAG is an enkephalinergic brainstem nucleus responsible for both morphine- and stimulation-produced analgesia. Descending axons from the PAG project to nuclei in the reticular formation of the medulla, including NRM, and then descend to the dorsal horn, where they synapse with and inhibit WDR and NS neurons. Axon terminals from NRM project to the dorsal horn, where they release serotonin and NE. Stimulation of the RVM activates the serotonergic system descending to the spinal dorsal horn, resulting in analgesia. Although serotonin plays an important role in pain, the multiple subtypes of these receptors have confounded development of analgesics acting via these

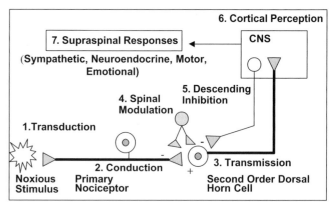

Figure 1.12: An overview of pain perception and response. (1) Peripheral noxious mediators activate nociceptor endings via a process termed *transduction*. (2) Noxious impulses are delivered to the spinal cord dorsal horn via the process of conduction in afferent fibers. (3) The process of transmission describes synaptic transfer of noxious impulses from primary afferents to second-order cells in the dorsal horn. (4) Modulation describes inhibitory and facilitory effects of spinal interneurons on noxious transmission. (5) Descending inhibition refers to descending brainstem, midbrain, and cortical inhibitor nerve endings that supress pain transmission. (6) Cortical perception includes neocortical sites of pain localization and limbic centers responsible for emotional and suffering components of pain. (7) Supraspinal responses include sympathetic, neuromuscular, and neuroendocrine responses to pain.

receptors.[73] Axons descending from LC modulate nociceptive transmission in dorsal horn primarily via release of NE and activation of postsynaptic α_2-adrenergic receptors. The role of NE in this pathway explains the analgesic effects of tricyclic antidepressants and clonidine. GABAergic and enkephalinergic interneurons in the dorsal horn also provide local suppression of pain transmission. Descending inhibition is enhanced during periods of inflammation because of an overall increased descending inhibitory flow and increased sensitivity of neurons to descending noradrenergic and opioid mediated inhibition.[74] Unlike the other senses, pain has important subjective and emotional components. Outflow of descending inhibitory impulses from the frontal cortex, cingulate gyrus, and hypothalamus are influenced by the patient's psychological and emotional state. Anxiety, psychological stressors, and depression can reduce descending inhibition, thereby lowering the threshold for central sensitization and increasing pain intensity scores.[75] Conversely psychological support, including imagery, biofeedback, and music therapy, can reduce pain intensity by either facilitating descending pathways or inhibiting cortical perception.[75] This may explain the beneficial role of cognitive therapies, which marshal descending inhibitory mechanisms to reduce long-term synaptic strength in acute and persistent pain states. The processes of pain transmission, perception, and associated responses are presented in Figure 1.12.

TRANSITIONS FROM ACUTE
TO PERSISTENT PAIN

The concept of neural plasticity, "that being the capacity of neurons to change their function, chemical profile, or structure," provides the basis for learning and memory and is also responsible for alterations in noxious perception.[1] Research performed since the mid-1990s has focused on nociception-induced pathophysiologic and plasticity changes that underlie peripheral and central sensitization. Peripheral sensitization is mediated in large part by locally released and humorally derived inflammatory mediators that increase nociceptor excitability either directly by activating ion channels or indirectly through second-messenger signaling. This facilitation of nociceptor discharge leads to spontaneous firing both in damaged and transected peripheral endings as well as second-order receiving cells in the dorsal horn.[41]

Activation of spinal and supraspinal NMDA receptors and increased intraneuronal Ca^{2+} ion influx are major requisites for the development of central sensitization and LTP.[76] Moreover, sensitization of CNS neurons underlies the transition from acute to persistent pain. Central sensitization can be divided into transcription-dependent and transcription-independent processes.[27] Transcription-independent sensitization reflects neurochemical and electrical alterations that follow acute traumatic and experimentally induced pain. It includes stimulus-dependent neuronal depolarization and stimulus-independent long-term potentiation.

Brief mild to moderately painful noxious impulses conveyed by high-threshold afferents are generally too weak to sustain action potentials in second-order NS or WDR neurons.[3] However, following an intense noxious conditioning stimulus, the synaptic efficacy and firing rate of dorsal horn cells are increased. This phenomenon, termed EPSP, has been related to upregulation of AMPA receptors.[77] Synaptic efficiency at contacts made with low-threshold nonnoxious Aβ fibers is also enhanced. The resulting increase in noxious perception, and development of tactile allodynia can outlast the conditioning stimulus for several hours.[78] A clinical example of this form of sensitization is observed following sunburn or paper cuts.

Wind-up and LTP represent a second form of transcription-independent central sensitization that is rapid in onset and reversible. In experimental settings, patients exposed to noxious heat or mechanical stimuli of constant intensity report increasing pain intensity with each repetitive stimulation.[79] In animal models, repetitive stimulation of high-threshold nociceptive fibers leads to progressive increases in action potential firing frequency ("wind up")[80] and stimulus-independent discharges in second-order dorsal horn neurons. Of importance were findings that the increased excitability of spinal cells far outlasted the stimulus duration and that local anesthetics applied to the site of nerve injury could not terminate the response. These observations suggested that wind-up and neuronal potentiation reflected altered receptor functionality and persistent excitatory ion flux rather than the effects of continued noxious stimulation.[24,81] Receptor-associated alterations mediating wind-up include upregulation and phosphorylation of AMPA receptors,[82] as well as subtle conformational changes in AMPA GluR2 subunits and cation channels that facilitate Na^+ flux. Several modulating proteins, including extracellular signal regulated kinase[83] and calmodulin-dependent protein kinase,[84] are responsible for activating tyrosine and threonine kinases that phosphorylate AMPA and NMDA and receptors.

Transcription-dependent sensitization describes delayed-onset, long-lasting, noxious facilitation that follows genomic activation, transcription of mRNA, and subsequent translational modifications. Activation of NMDA and metabotrophic NK-1 receptors and continued influx of Ca^{2+} leads to enhanced production of cAMP, protein kinases, and phosphokinases. Phosphokinases and other nuclear activators initiate transcrip-

tional processes over a period of several hours to several days. Following transcription of mRNA, inducible enzymes and reactive proteins are synthesized that mediate neuroanatomical and neuropathologic plasticity. It is now recognized that transcription-dependent sensitization is mediated by inflammation and inflammatory alterations in dorsal root ganglion and the dorsal horn, as well as potentially irreversible structural modifications within the CNS.[75] For example, cellular apoptosis, including glial and interneuronal cell death, diminish pain-suppressive mechanisms. In contrast, axonal sprouting and new afferent connections facilitate homosynaptic and heterosynaptic noxious transmission and potentiate discharge of second-order neurons in the dorsal horn.

Excitotoxicity defines the pathological alterations observed in nerve cells stimulated by overactivation of NMDA.[85] Important aspects of transcription-dependent central sensitization correlate with excitotoxic alterations within sensitized neurons, interneurons, and reactive microglial cells. Excitotoxicity is also mediated by Ca^{2+}-induced upregulation of COX-2, NOS, and superoxide desmutase (SOD) and enhanced synthesis of PGE, NO, and superoxides (SO). Elevated concentrations of intracellular Ca^{2+} also activate phospholipases, proteases, kinases, and other lytic enzymes that can damage cellular and nuclear membranes. Calcium also effects mitochondrial permeability, resulting in swelling loss of ATP production and subsequent neuronal apoptosis.[86] Glutamate in high concentrations functions as a direct excitotoxin. High concentrations of glutamate activate cAMP,[87] cAMP response element binding protein and brain-derived neurotrophic factor (BDNF), which alter genomic function and also initiate chromatolysis, or Nissil body disruption, and neuronal apoptosis.[88]

Engblom et al[89] were among the first to propose that some aspects of central sensitization observed following peripheral inflammation were dependant on increased production of PGE within the CNS. In animal models, intrathecal application of PGE_2 facilitated noxious excitation of dorsal horn cells and also caused profound hyperalgesia and allodynia.[39] Prostanoid synthesis[90] within the CNS is controlled by both neural and humoral signals. Within sensitized spinal neurons a specific transcription factor known as nuclear factor-κB (NFκB), upregulates COX-2 expression.[58] The major humoral inducer of central COX-2 is IL-1β. In this regard, inhibitors of IL-1β prevent upregulation of COX-2 in CNS and limit the development of central sensitization to peripheral inflammatory pain. Locally synthesized and humorally delivered PGE mediate a number of presynaptic and postsynaptic plasticity changes that facilitate noxious perception. Prostanoids increase release of Gly and activate a specific glycine receptor subtype GlyRα3.[91] Glycine binding at the NR2 subunit functions as a coagonist that facilitates opening of the NMDA ion channel.[92] Extracellular release of PGE also incites reactive changes in microglial cells. The inflammatory and destructive actions of reactive microglial cells resemble the activity of peripheral macrophages. Microglia synthesize and release additional PGE, NO, and SO and are responsible for removal of inhibitory synaptic contacts and dedifferentiation and death of inhibitory interneurons. Reactive microglia also induce sprouting of noxious terminal endings and facilitate new contacts with second-order cells. They also stimulate and guide nonnoxious afferents to make new synaptic contacts with sensitized spinal cells.[3,57,61] Plasticity changes associated with NMDA activation and central sensitization are presented in Figure 1.13.

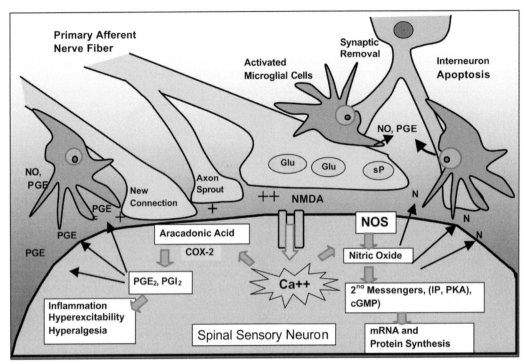

Figure 1.13: Mediators responsible for central sensitization and associated plasticity changes. Inflow of Ca^{2+} ions initiates upregulation of COX-2, NOS, and second messengers that initiate transcriptional and translational changes. Second-order neurons dedifferentiate and increase their excitability. Plasticity changes mediated by PGE and NO include axonal sprouting and new afferent connections. Extracellular release of PGE leads to inflammatory changes in the neuropil. These changes include activation of microglial cells synaptic retraction and interneuron apoptosis.

Inhibition of spinal cord PGE provides measurable antinociception. Samad et al found that in animals exposed to peripheral inflammatory lesions, intrathecal administration of a COX-2 inhibitor reduced spinal cord synthesis of PGE_2 and some aspects of central sensitization.[92–94] Koppert et al studied the effects of two intravenous COX-2 inhibitors, parecoxib and paracetamol, and provided evidence for their central antihyperalgesic effect.[95] Nitric oxide also plays an important role in central sensitization and secondary hyperalgesia. Preclinical studies have found that intrathecal application of NO initiates and maintains both neuropathic and inflammatory pain.[96] Nitric oxide is produced by three isoforms of the enzyme NOS. The isoforms that are constitutively present within endothelial NOS (eNOS) and neuronal NOS (nNOS) cells. Inducible NOS (iNOS) is generated by immunologic and inflammatory mechanisms and is found in macrophages, immunological cells, and microglia.[96] Ding and Weinberg[97] found that NK1 receptors in lamina I were the major target for NO. Following nerve injury, upregulation of iNOS and synthesis of NO in dorsal horn induces hyperalgesia and allodynia.[98] Furthermore, selective inhibition of iNOS produced antinociception.[96]

Superoxide has also been identified as a novel mediator of central sensitization. SOD is an intracellular antioxidant enzyme that controls the biological reactivity of SO.[99] In the inflammatory process, superoxide is produced at such a rapid rate that SOD is unable to remove it. Superoxide-mediated injury includes endothelial cell damage, increased microvascular permeability, release of cytokines, recruitment of reactive cells, and apoptosis.[100] Wang and coworkers[100] found that the synthetic compound (M40403) that mimics SOD prevents the development of inflammation and hyperalgesia after injection of noxious mediators. The results suggest SO is a vital component in the nociceptive-signaling cascade.[100] Furthermore, Muscoli et al[101] showed that SO may contribute to various forms of pain events that are driven by NMDA receptor activation.

NEUROPATHIC PAIN

Chronic neuropathic pain is not adaptive and appears to serve no purpose. Some have hypothesized that the anatomical and physiologic abnormalities associated with neuropathic pain as well as clinical symptoms may be related to misprogramed neural regenerative efforts of irritated or damaged neurons and reactive glial cells. Several mechanisms play roles in the development of neuropathic pain, including spontaneously generated action potentials, sympathetic stimulation, glial reaction, neuroimmune modulation, and disinhibition. The endogenous opioid modulatory system[102] also appears to be altered. The role of the immune system in the development of neuropathic pain has been proposed[103] because half of all cases are associated with clinical infection or inflammation of peripheral nerves. The major immune cells involved are neutrophils and macrophages; however, reactive microglial cells have also been implicated. The activation of the complement cascade causes disruption of the blood-nerve barrier, immune cell recruitment, and the formation of membrane attack complexes that causes nerve lesions.

Research on neuropathic pain has focused on the activation of microglia and the release of BDNF. Brain-derived neurotrophic factor[104] appears to switch off GABA-inhibitory mechanisms on second-order neurons in spinal lamina I. GABA and glycine hyperpolarize spinal neurons by increasing intracellular chloride and inhibiting pain transmission. BDNF is a crucial signaling molecule for microglia and neurons. It activates postsynaptic tyrosine kinase b (TrkB) receptors, resulting in chloride outflow, neuronal depolarization, and enhanced pain transmission. In animal models, intrathecally administered BDNF produced neuronal depolarization and allodynia,[105] whereas blocking the action of BDNF on the TrkB receptor reversed symptoms of neuropathic pain.[105,106]

Neuropathic pain states are also associated with impaired suppression of noxious transmission. In addition to reductions in endogenous opioid and nonopioid modulators, partial to complete resistance to opioid-mediated analgesia may be observed.[107] Injury to peripheral axons is associated with downregulation of μ-opiate receptors and activation of NMDA receptors that indirectly reduce opioid sensitivity.[108,109] In addition, CCK, a peptide with known antiopioid activity, is dramatically upregulated following nerve injury and may explain why opioids are less effective in the treatment of neuropathic pain.[110]

At the level of the spinal cord, dynorphin functions as a noxious facilitator and maintains experimental neuropathic pain.[99,111] Following peripheral nerve injuries, increased amounts of dynorphin are released by spinal modulatory cells and also by descending nerve fibers. The importance of prostanoids in peripheral inflammatory-induced central sensitization has been demonstrated[90]; however, their role in the elaboration of neuropathic pain remains unproven, and therapeutic benefits of nonsteroidal anti-inflammatory drugs or treatment with coxibs are limited.[112] In summary, persistent neurochemical and structural modifications that underlie transitions to chronic pain and the development of neuropathic pain are difficult, if not impossible, to reverse. In general, chronic and neuropathic pain are not maintained by the continued release of acute mediators and clinical symptoms are not easily controlled with opioid analgesics. Both forms of neuropathic pain result from transcription-dependent synthesis of neuronal sensitizers, including PGE and NO, as well as degradation of endogenous pain-suppressive mechanisms. As a result a new generation of analgesics, including ion channel blocking agents,[113] α_2 δ-membrane stabilizers,[114] selective serotonin reuptake inhibitors,[115] and COX-2 inhibitors[116] offer patients more effective pain relief, although complete elimination of noxious perception is unlikely to occur.

CONCLUSION

Advances in our understanding of noxious transmission and pain processing[117] have uncovered key mechanisms and molecular mediators responsible for specific syndromes, as well as improved treatment options for acute, persistent, and neuropathic pain. Mediators that trigger peripheral and central sensitization are responsible for opening the dorsal horn gate,[21,118] thereby facilitating pain transmission and subsequent perception. Peripheral TRPs and central NMDARs, as well as influx of intracellular Ca^{2+}, are among the key targets and transducing ions responsible for peripheral and central sensitization.

Because all chronic pain begins as an acute inflammatory or neuropathic event, aggressive multimodal acute pain management[119] is essential to minimize development of central sensitization, and the potentially irreversible neurochemical and neuropathologic changes that may follow. The development of diagnostic tools, including neuroimaging, allows direct visualization of pain processing that correlates with clinical changes in noxious perception. Future treatment options, including selective TRP, NMDAR, MAP-Kinase, and ion flux antagonists, and receptor polymorphism screening to optimize drug development, will enable physicians to develop rational analgesic treatment guidelines that will supercede the traditional trial-and-error approaches currently employed.[108]

REFERENCES

1. Woolf CJ, Salter MW. Neuronal Plasticity: Increasing the Gain in Pain. *Science*. 2000;288:1765–1769.
2. Cherny NI, Thaler HT, Friedlander-Klar H, et al. Opioid responsiveness of cancer pain syndromes caused by neuropathic or nociceptive mechanisms: a combined analysis of controlled, single-dose studies. *Neurology*. 1994;44(5):857–861.
3. Woolf CJ, King AE. Subthreshold components of the cutaneous mechanoreceptive fields of dorsal horn neurons in the rat lumbar spinal cord. *J Neurophysiol*. 1989;62(4):907–916.
4. Andersson GB. Epidemiological features of chronic low-back pain. *Lancet*. 1999;354(9178):581–585.
5. Smith BH, Elliott AM, Chambers WA, Smith WC, Hannaford PC, Penny K. The impact of chronic pain in the community. *Fam Pract*. 2001;18(3):292–299.
6. Mannion RJ, Costigan M, Decosterd I, et al. Neurotrophins: peripherally and centrally acting modulators of tactile stimulus-induced inflammatory pain hypersensitivity. *Proc Natl Acad Sci USA*. 1999;96(16):9385–9390.
7. Keay KA, Clement CI, Owler B, Depaulis A, Bandler R. Convergence of deep somatic and visceral nociceptive information onto a discrete ventrolateral midbrain periaqueductal gray region. *Neuroscience*. 1994;61(4):727–732.
8. Donelson R, Silva G, Murphy K. Centralization phenomenon: its usefulness in evaluating and treating referred pain. *Spine*. 1990;15(3):211–213.
9. Treede RD, Meyer RA, Raja SN, Campbell JN. Peripheral and central mechanisms of cutaneous hyperalgesia. *Prog Neurobiol*. 1992;38(4):397–421.
10. Lourie H, King RB. Sensory and neurohistological correlates of cutaneous hyperpathia. *Arch Neurol*. 1966;14(3):313–320.
11. Chaplan SR, Malmberg AB, Yaksh TL. Efficacy of spinal NMDA receptor antagonism in formalin hyperalgesia and nerve injury evoked allodynia in the rat. *J Pharmacol Exp Ther*. 1997;280(2):829–938.
12. Chen J, Luo C, Li H, Chen H. Primary hyperalgesia to mechanical and heat stimuli following subcutaneous bee venom injection into the plantar surface of hindpaw in the conscious rat: a comparative study with the formalin test. *Pain*. 1999;83(1):67–76.
13. Ziegler EA, Magerl W, Meyer RA, Treede RD. Secondary hyperalgesia to punctate mechanical stimuli: central sensitization to A-fibre nociceptor input. *Brain*. 1999;122 (Pt 12)(Pt 12):2245–2257.
14. Woolf CJ, Mannion RJ. Neuropathic pain: aetiology, symptoms, mechanisms, and management. *Lancet*. 1999;353(9168):1959–1964.

15. Wong TM, Leung HB, Wong WC. Correlation between magnetic resonance imaging and radiographic measurement of cervical spine in cervical myelopathic patients. *J Orthopaed Surg (Hong Kong)*. 2004;12(2):239–242.

16. Rommel O, Malin JP, Zenz M, Janig W. Quantitative sensory testing, neurophysiological and psychological examination in patients with complex regional pain syndrome and hemisensory deficits. *Pain*. 2001;93(3):279–293.

17. Sandroni P, Low PA, Ferrer T, Opfer-Gehrking TL, Willner CL, Wilson PR. Complex regional pain syndrome I (CRPS I): prospective study and laboratory evaluation. *Clin J Pain*. 1998;14(4):282–289.

18. McGrath PA. Psychological aspects of pain perception. *Arch Oral Biol*. 1994;39 Suppl:55S–62S.

19. Duncan G. Mind-body dualism and the biopsychosocial model of pain: what did Descartes really say? *J Med Philos*. 2000;25(4):485–513.

20. Sabatowski R, Schafer D, Kasper SM, Brunsch H, Radbruch L. Pain treatment: a historical overview. *Curr Pharmaceutl Des*. 2004;10(7):701–716.

21. Melzack R, Wall PD. Pain mechanisms: a new theory. New York, NY: Science. 1965;150(699):971–979.

22. Ataka T, Kumamoto E, Shimoji K, Yoshimura M. Baclofen inhibits more effectively C-afferent than Adelta-afferent glutamatergic transmission in substantia gelatinosa neurons of adult rat spinal cord slices. *Pain*. 2000;86(3):273–282.

23. Basbaum AI. A new way to lose your nerve: science of aging knowledge environment: SAGE KE. 2004 Apr 14;2004(15):pe15.

24. Mendell LM, Wall PD. Responses of single dorsal cord cells to peripheral cutaneous unmyelinated fibres. *Nature*. 1965;206:97–99.

25. Kehlet H. Surgical stress: the role of pain and analgesia. *Br J Anaesth*. 1989;63(2):189–195.

26. Vane JR, Botting RM. New insights into the mode of action of anti-inflammatory drugs. *Inflamm Res*. 1995;44(1):1–10.

27. Ji RR, Woolf CJ. Neuronal plasticity and signal transduction in nociceptive neurons: implications for the initiation and maintenance of pathological pain. *Neurobiol. Dis*. 2001;8(1):1–10.

28. Ito S, Okuda-Ashitaka E, Minami T. Central and peripheral roles of prostaglandins in pain and their interactions with novel neuropeptides nociceptin and nocistatin. *Neurosci Res*. 2001;41(4):299–332.

29. Funk CD. Prostaglandins and leukotrienes: advances in eicosanoid biology. *Science*. 2001;294(5548):1871–1875.

30. Millan MJ. Serotonin and pain: evidence that activation of 5-HT1A receptors does not elicit antinociception against noxious thermal, mechanical and chemical stimuli in mice. *Pain*. 1994;58(1):45–61.

31. Wang H, Kohno T, Amaya F, et al. Bradykinin produces pain hypersensitivity by potentiating spinal cord glutamatergic synaptic transmission. *J Neurosci*. 2005;25(35):7986–7992.

32. Mobarakeh JI, Sakurada S, et al. Role of histamine H(1) receptor in pain perception: a study of the receptor gene knockout mice. *Eur J Pharmacol*. 2000;391(1–2):81–89.

33. Sasaki M, Obata H, Kawahara K, Saito S, Goto F. Peripheral 5-HT2A receptor antagonism attenuates primary thermal hyperalgesia and secondary mechanical allodynia after thermal injury in rats. *Pain*. 2006;122(1–2):130–136.

34. Bennett AD, Chastain KM, Hulsebosch CE. Alleviation of mechanical and thermal allodynia by CGRP(8–37) in a rodent model of chronic central pain. *Pain*. 2000;86(1–2):163–175.

35. Liu H, Mantyh PW, Basbaum AI. NMDA-receptor regulation of substance P release from primary afferent nociceptors. *Nature*. 1997;386(6626):721–724.

36. Noble F, Derrien M, Roques BP. Modulation of opioid antinociception by CCK at the supraspinal level: evidence of regulatory mechanisms between CCK and enkephalin systems in the control of pain. *Br J Pharmacol*. 1993;109(4):1064–1070.

37. McCarthy PW, Lawson SN. Cell type and conduction velocity of rat primary sensory neurons with calcitonin gene-related peptide-like immunoreactivity. *Neuroscience*. 1990;34(3):623–632.

38. Evans BN, Rosenblatt MI, Mnayer LO, Oliver KR, Dickerson IM. CGRP-RCP, a novel protein required for signal transduction at calcitonin gene-related peptide and adrenomedullin receptors. *J Biol Chem*. 2000;275(40):31438–31443.

39. Ahmadi S, Lippross S, Neuhuber WL, Zeilhofer HU. PGE(2) selectively blocks inhibitory glycinergic neurotransmission onto rat superficial dorsal horn neurons. *Nat Neurosci*. 2002;5(1):34–40.

40. Tzabazis AZ, Pirc G, Votta-Velis E, Wilson SP, Laurito CE, Yeomans DC. Antihyperalgesic effect of a recombinant herpes virus encoding antisense for calcitonin gene-related peptide. *Anesthesiology*. 2007;106(6):1196–1203.

41. Julius D, Basbaum AI. Molecular mechanisms of nociception. *Nature*. 2001 13;413(6852):203–210.

42. Bessler H, Shavit Y, Mayburd E, Smirnov G, Beilin B. Postoperative pain, morphine consumption, and genetic polymorphism of IL-1beta and IL-1 receptor antagonist. *Neurosci Lett*. 2006;404(1–2):154–158.

43. Beilin B, Bessler H, Mayburd E, et al. Effects of preemptive analgesia on pain and cytokine production in the postoperative period. *Anesthesiology*. 2003;98(1):151–155.

44. Beilin B, Shavit Y, Trabekin E, et al. The effects of postoperative pain management on immune response to surgery. *Anesth Analges*. 2003;97(3):822–827.

45. Winter J, Bevan S, Campbell EA. Capsaicin and pain mechanisms. *Br J Anaesth*. 1995;75(2):157–168.

46. Djouhri L, Koutsikou S, Fang X, McMullan S, Lawson SN. Spontaneous pain, both neuropathic and inflammatory, is related to frequency of spontaneous firing in intact C-fiber nociceptors. *J Neurosci*. 2006;26(4):1281–1292.

47. Hogan QH, Abram SE. Neural blockade for diagnosis and prognosis: a review. *Anesthesiology*. 1997;86(1):216–241.

48. Malinow R, Malenka RC. AMPA receptor trafficking and synaptic plasticity. *Ann Rev Neurosci*. 2002;25:103–126.

49. Woolf CJ. An overview of the mechanisms of hyperalgesia. *Pulm Pharmacol*. 1995;8(4–5):161–167.

50. Mannion RJ, Woolf CJ. Pain mechanisms and management: a central perspective. *Clin J Pain*. 2000;16(3 Suppl):S144–S156.

51. Sivilotti LG, Thompson SW, Woolf CJ. Rate of rise of the cumulative depolarization evoked by repetitive stimulation of small-caliber afferents is a predictor of action potential windup in rat spinal neurons in vitro. *J Neurophysiol*. 1993;69(5):1621–1631.

52. Patel J, Zinkand WC, Thompson C, Keith R, Salama A. Role of glycine in the *N*-methyl-D-aspartate-mediated neuronal cytotoxicity. *J Neurochem*. 1990;54(3):849–854.

53. Porreca F, Ossipov MH, Gebhart GF. Chronic pain and medullary descending facilitation. *Trends Neurosci*. 2002;25(6):319–325.

54. Ikeda H, Heinke B, Ruscheweyh R, Sandkuhler J. Synaptic plasticity in spinal lamina I projection neurons that mediate hyperalgesia. *Science*. 200321;299(5610):1237–1240.

55. Derjean D, Bertrand S, Le Masson G, Landry M, Morisset V, Nagy F. Dynamic balance of metabotropic inputs causes dorsal horn neurons to switch functional states. *Nat Neurosci*. 2003;6(3):274–281.

56. Waldhoer M, Bartlett SE, Whistler JL. Opioid receptors. *Ann Rev Biochem*. 2004;73:953–990.

57. Raynor K, Kong H, Chen Y, et al. Pharmacological characterization of the cloned kappa-, delta-, and mu-opioid receptors. *Mol Pharmacol.* 1994;45(2):330–334.

58. Margas W, Zubkoff I, Schuler HG, Janicki PK, Ruiz-Velasco V. Modulation of Ca2+ channels by heterologously expressed wild-type and mutant human micro-opioid receptors (hMORs) containing the A118G single-nucleotide polymorphism. *J Neurophysiol.* 2007;97(2):1058–1067.

59. Stamer UM, Bayerer B, Stuber F. Genetics and variability in opioid response. *Eur J Pain.* 2005;9(2):101–104.

60. Pasternak GW. Multiple opiate receptors: deja vu all over again. *Neuropharmacology.* 2004;47(Suppl 1):312–323.

61. Sonohata M, Furue H, Katafuchi T, et al. Actions of noradrenaline on substantia gelatinosa neurones in the rat spinal cord revealed by in vivo patch recording. *J Physiol.* 2004;555(2):515–526.

62. LaMotte RH, Thalhammer JG, Robinson CJ. Peripheral neural correlates of magnitude of cutaneous pain and hyperalgesia: a comparison of neural events in monkey with sensory judgments in human. *J Neurophysiol.* 1983;50(1):1–26.

63. Bushnell MC, Duncan GH. Sensory and affective aspects of pain perception: is medial thalamus restricted to emotional issues? *Exp Brain Res.* 1989;78(2):415–418.

64. Peyron R, Laurent B, Garcia-Larrea L. Functional imaging of brain responses to pain: a review and meta-analysis. *Clin Neurophysiol.* 2000;30(5):263–288.

65. Coghill RC, Sang CN, Berman KF, Bennett GJ, Iadarola MJ. Global cerebral blood flow decreases during pain. *J Cerebral Blood Flow Metab.* 1998;18(2):141–147.

66. Rainville P, Duncan GH, Price DD, Carrier B, Bushnell MC. Pain affect encoded in human anterior cingulate but not somatosensory cortex. *Science.* 1997;277(5328):968–971.

67. Craig AD, Reiman EM, Evans A, Bushnell MC. Functional imaging of an illusion of pain. *Nature.* 1996;384(6606):258–260.

68. Talbot JD, Marrett S, Evans AC, Meyer E, Bushnell MC, Duncan GH. Multiple representations of pain in human cerebral cortex. *Science.* 1991;251(4999):1355–1358.

69. Davis KD, Taylor SJ, Crawley AP, Wood ML, Mikulis DJ. Functional MRI of pain- and attention-related activations in the human cingulate cortex. *J Neurophysiol.* 1997;77(6):3370–3380.

70. Craig AD. Pain mechanisms: labeled lines versus convergence in central processing. *Ann Rev Neurosci.* 2003;26:1–30.

71. Zubieta JK, Smith YR, Bueller JA, et al. Regional mu opioid receptor regulation of sensory and affective dimensions of pain. *Science.* 2001;293(5528):311–315.

72. Grachev ID, Fredrickson BE, Apkarian AV. Abnormal brain chemistry in chronic back pain: an in vivo proton magnetic resonance spectroscopy study. *Pain.* 2000;89(1):7–18.

73. Besson JM. The neurobiology of pain. *Lancet.* 1999;353(9164):1610–1615.

74. Vanegas H, Schaible HG. Descending control of persistent pain: inhibitory or facilitatory? *Brain Res.* 2004;46(3):295–309.

75. Rygh LJ, Svendsen F, Fiska A, Haugan F, Hole K, Tjolsen A. Long-term potentiation in spinal nociceptive systems: how acute pain may become chronic. *Psychoneuroendocrinology.* 2005;30(10):959–964.

76. Zeilhofer HU. Synaptic modulation in pain pathways. *Rev Physiol Biochem Pharmacol.* 2005;154:73–100.

77. Yu XM, Askalan R, Keil GJ, 2nd, Salter MW. NMDA channel regulation by channel-associated protein tyrosine kinase Src. *Science.* 1997;275(5300):674–678.

78. Woolf CJ, Wall PD. Relative effectiveness of C primary afferent fibers of different origins in evoking a prolonged facilitation of the flexor reflex in the rat. *J Neurosci.* 1986;6(5):1433–1442.

79. Staud R, Cannon RC, Mauderli AP, Robinson ME, Price DD, Vierck CJ, Jr. Temporal summation of pain from mechanical stimulation of muscle tissue in normal controls and subjects with fibromyalgia syndrome. *Pain.* 2003;102(1–2):87–95.

80. Herrero JF, Laird JM, Lopez-Garcia JA. Wind-up of spinal cord neurones and pain sensation: much ado about something? *Prog Neurobiol.* 2000;61(2):169–203.

81. Woolf CJ. Evidence for a central component of post-injury pain hypersensitivity. *Nature.* 1983;306(5944):686–688.

82. Tan SE, Wenthold RJ, Soderling TR. Phosphorylation of AMPA-type glutamate receptors by calcium/calmodulin-dependent protein kinase II and protein kinase C in cultured hippocampal neurons. *J Neurosci.* 1994;14(3 Pt 1):1123–1129.

83. Ji RR, Baba H, Brenner GJ, Woolf CJ. Nociceptive-specific activation of ERK in spinal neurons contributes to pain hypersensitivity. *Nat Neurosci.* 1999;2(12):1114–1119.

84. Fang L, Wu J, Lin Q, Willis WD. Calcium-calmodulin-dependent protein kinase II contributes to spinal cord central sensitization. *J Neurosci.* 2002;22(10):4196–4204.

85. Rothman SM, Olney JW. Excitotoxicity and the NMDA receptor—still lethal after eight years. *Trends Neurosci.* 1995;18(2):57–58.

86. Lipton SA, Nicotera P. Calcium, free radicals and excitotoxins in neuronal apoptosis. *Cell Calcium.* 1998;23(2–3):165–171.

87. Dolan S, Nolan AM. Biphasic modulation of nociceptive processing by the cyclic AMP-protein kinase A signalling pathway in sheep spinal cord. *Neurosci Lett.* 2001;309(3):157–160.

88. Hardingham GE, Fukunaga Y, Bading H. Extrasynaptic NMDARs oppose synaptic NMDARs by triggering CREB shut-off and cell death pathways. *Nat Neurosci.* 2002;5(5):405–414.

89. Engblom D, Ek M, Saha S, Ericsson-Dahlstrand A, Jakobsson PJ, Blomqvist A. Prostaglandins as inflammatory messengers across the blood-brain barrier. *J Mol Med.* 2002;80(1):5–15.

90. Samad TA, Sapirstein A, Woolf CJ. Prostanoids and pain: unraveling mechanisms and revealing therapeutic targets. *Trends Mol Med.* 2002;8(8):390–396.

91. Harvey RJ, Depner UB, Wassle H, et al. GlyR alpha3: an essential target for spinal PGE2-mediated inflammatory pain sensitization. *Science.* 2004;304(5672):884–887.

92. Zeilhofer HU, Brune K. Analgesic strategies beyond the inhibition of cyclooxygenases. *Trends Pharmacol Sci.* 2006;27(9):467–474.

93. Broom DC, Samad TA, Kohno T, Tegeder I, Geisslinger G, Woolf CJ. Cyclooxygenase 2 expression in the spared nerve injury model of neuropathic pain. *Neuroscience.* 2004;124(4):891–900.

94. Samad TA, Moore KA, Sapirstein A, et al. Interleukin-1beta-mediated induction of Cox-2 in the CNS contributes to inflammatory pain hypersensitivity. *Nature.* 2001;410(6827):471–475.

95. Koppert W, Wehrfritz A, Korber N, et al. The cyclooxygenase isozyme inhibitors parecoxib and paracetamol reduce central hyperalgesia in humans. *Pain.* 2004;108(1–2):148–153.

96. LaBuda CJ, Koblish M, Tuthill P, Dolle RE, Little PJ. Antinociceptive activity of the selective iNOS inhibitor AR-C102222 in rodent models of inflammatory, neuropathic and post-operative pain. *Eur J Pain.* 2006;10(6):505–512.

97. Ding JD, Weinberg RJ. Localization of soluble guanylyl cyclase in the superficial dorsal horn. *Journal Comp Neurol.* 2006;495(6):668–678.

98. Ikeda H, Kusudo K, Murase K. Nitric oxide-dependent long-term potentiation revealed by real-time imaging of nitric oxide production and neuronal excitation in the dorsal horn of rat spinal cord slices. *Eur J Neurosci.* 2006;23(7):1939–1943.

99. Wang Z, Gardell LR, Ossipov MH, et al. Pronociceptive actions of dynorphin maintain chronic neuropathic pain. *J Neurosci.* 2001;21(5):1779–1786.

100. Wang ZQ, Porreca F, Cuzzocrea S, et al. A newly identified role for superoxide in inflammatory pain. *J Pharmacol Exp Ther.* 2004;309(3):869–878.

101. Muscoli C, Mollace V, Wheatley J, et al. Superoxide-mediated nitration of spinal manganese superoxide dismutase: a novel pathway in *N*-methyl-D-aspartate-mediated hyperalgesia. *Pain.* 2004;111(1–2):96–103.

102. Urban MO, Gebhart GF. Central mechanisms in pain. *Med Clin North Am.* 1999;83(3):585–596.

103. Marchand F, Perretti M, McMahon SB. Role of the immune system in chronic pain. *Nature.* 2005;6(7):521–532.

104. McLean Bolton M, Pittman AJ, Lo DC. Brain-derived neurotrophic factor differentially regulates excitatory and inhibitory synaptic transmission in hippocampal cultures. *J Neurosci.* 2000;20(9):3221–3232.

105. Coull JA, Beggs S, Boudreau D, et al. BDNF from microglia causes the shift in neuronal anion gradient underlying neuropathic pain. *Nature.* 2005;438(7070):1017–1021.

106. Torsney C, MacDermott AB. Neuroscience: a painful factor. *Nature.* 2005;438(7070):923–925.

107. Scholz J, Broom DC, Youn DH, et al. Blocking caspase activity prevents transsynaptic neuronal apoptosis and the loss of inhibition in lamina II of the dorsal horn after peripheral nerve injury. *J Neuroscience.* 2005;25(32):7317–7323.

108. Woolf CJ, American College of P, American Physiological S. Pain: moving from symptom control toward mechanism-specific pharmacologic management. *Ann Int Med.* 2004;140(6):441–451.

109. Takasu K, Honda M, Ono H, Tanabe M. Spinal alpha(2)-adrenergic and muscarinic receptors and the NO release cascade mediate supraspinally produced effectiveness of gabapentin at decreasing mechanical hypersensitivity in mice after partial nerve injury. *Br J Pharmacol.* 2006;148(2):233–244.

110. Vadivelu N, Sinatra R. Recent advances in elucidating pain mechanisms. *Curr Opin Anaesthesiol.* 2005;18(5):540–547.

111. Vera-Portocarrero LP, Xie JY, Kowal J, Ossipov MH, King T, Porreca F. Descending facilitation from the rostral ventromedial medulla maintains visceral pain in rats with experimental pancreatitis. *Gastroenterology.* 2006;130(7):2155–2164.

112. Hosl K, Reinold H, Harvey RJ, Muller U, Narumiya S, Zeilhofer HU. Spinal prostaglandin E receptors of the EP2 subtype and the glycine receptor alpha3 subunit, which mediate central inflammatory hyperalgesia, do not contribute to pain after peripheral nerve injury or formalin injection. *Pain.* 2006;126(1–3):46–53.

113. Eglen RM, Hunter JC, Dray A. Ions in the fire: recent ion-channel research and approaches to pain therapy. *Trends Pharmacol Sci.* 1999;20(8):337–342.

114. Francis DA, Christopher AT, Beasley BD. Conservative treatment of peripheral neuropathy and neuropathic pain. *Clin Podiatr Med Surg.* 2006;23(3):509–530.

115. Jung AC, Staiger T, Sullivan M. The efficacy of selective serotonin reuptake inhibitors for the management of chronic pain. *J Gen Intern Med.* 1997;12(6):384–389.

116. Buvanendran A, Kroin JS, Tuman KJ, et al. Effects of perioperative administration of a selective cyclooxygenase 2 inhibitor on pain management and recovery of function after knee replacement: a randomized controlled trial. *JAMA.* 2003;290(18):2411–2418.

117. Ploner M, Schmitz F, Freund HJ, Schnitzler A. Parallel activation of primary and secondary somatosensory cortices in human pain processing. *J Neurophysiol.* 1999;81(6):3100–3104.

118. Torsney C, MacDermott AB. Disinhibition opens the gate to pathological pain signaling in superficial neurokinin 1 receptor-expressing neurons in rat spinal cord. *J Neurosci.* 20068;26(6):1833–1843.

119. Fassoulaki A, Triga A, Melemeni A, Sarantopoulos C. Multimodal analgesia with gabapentin and local anesthetics prevents acute and chronic pain after breast surgery for cancer. *Anesth Analg.* 2005;101(5):1427–1432.

2

Pathophysiology of Acute Pain

M. Khurram Ghori, Yu-Fan (Robert) Zhang, and
Raymond S. Sinatra

In addition to the ethical and humanitarian reasons for minimizing pain and suffering is the recognition that both physiologic and pathophysiologic responses to poorly controlled pain may have deleterious effects on postsurgical outcomes. Consequences may be particularly serious in elderly and critically ill populations. In these individuals, pathophysiologic responses to large incisions, extensive dissection, or visceral manipulation negatively affect cardiovascular and pulmonary, and incite maladaptive behaviors (Table 2.1).[1–4]

Commonly observed pathophysiologic changes include, but are not limited to, the following: (1) Neurohumoral alterations termed *peripheral sensitization* occurring at the site and in regions immediately adjacent to injury, (2) alterations in synaptic function and nociceptive processing occurring within spinal cord and limbic cortex, (3) sympathoadrenal activation resulting in an elevation of heart rate and blood pressure and a diminution in regional blood flow, and (4) neuroendocrine responses mediating hyperglycemia and a negative nitrogen balance.

HYPERALGESIA

Acute surgical or traumatic injury is followed by a series of neurohumoral reactions originally described by Lewis[5] and termed the inflammatory *triple response*. The classical response is characterized by increased blood flow (*flare*), tissue edema (*wheal*), and sensitization of peripheral nociceptors (*hyperalgesia*). Hyperalgesia defines an altered state of sensibility in which the intensity of discomfort associated with repetitive noxious stimulation is markedly increased.[6–8] Allodynia refers to a condition in which ordinarily nonnoxious stimulation such as pressure and light touch is perceived as being exquisitely painful. Hyperalgesia accompanies most inflammatory processes, abrasions, incisions, and burn injuries. Two forms of hyperalgesia, primary and secondary, have been defined and are described in Chapter 1 (*Pain Pathways and Acute Pain Processing*).

Primary hyperalgesia reflects enhanced noxious sensitivity, which becomes evident within minutes of the injury and is characterized by increased responsiveness to light touch, heat, and mechanical stimuli.[6–8] The development of primary hyperalgesia correlates with a diminution in pain threshold and enhanced sensitivity of C and Aδ mechanoheat nociceptors.

At the site of injury, peripheral nociceptor endings are stimulated by release of intracelluar H^+ and K^+ ions and synthesis of prostaglandins. Nociceptors are further sensitized by locally released mediators such as bradykinin, serotonin, and histamine.[8,9,10–12] Humoral factors and proinflammatory cytokines, including interleukin-1 Beta (IL-1B) and IL-6, increase peripheral edema and allodynia.[4,10–12] Genetic polymorphisms that influence production of these proinflammatory cytokines may be responsible for interindividual differences in postoperative pain intensity scores and development of persistent pain.[6,11,49] Several antidromically delivered sensitizers, including substance P and norepinephrine, are released from activated sensory and sympathetic nerve endings and further enhance pain sensitivity.[4,10,12] Mediators responsible for nociceptor activation and inflammation are depicted in Figure 2.1.

Secondary hyperalgesia refers to delayed alterations in noxious sensitivity observed in nontraumatized regions surrounding the injury site.[13–15] It is now recognized that secondary hyperalgesia is mediated by neuronal sensitization and adaptive facilitatory changes in the spinal cord, brainstem, and limbic cortex. Central facilitation is initiated by the action of neuropeptides and excitatory amino acids (EAA), such as aspartate and glutamate on *N*-methyl-D-aspartate (NMDA) and α-amino-3-hydroxy-5-methyl-4-isoxazole propionic acid (AMPA) receptors.[14–17] Activation of NMDA receptors (NMDARs) increase the responsiveness of dorsal horn wide dynamic range (WDR) neurons to noxious input.[16,17] The initial phase, termed *wind-up*, is characterized by an immediate increase in WDR firing rate and associated behavioral responses lasting about 5 minutes.[14,16,17] This is followed 15 to 20 minutes later by a second phase, termed *long-term potentiation*, in which WDR neurons exhibit enhanced sensitivity for prolonged periods.[14–17] This second phase of excitability outlasts the initial barrage of sensory input, does not require further noxious stimulation to be maintained, and is not antagonized by inhalational anesthetics or moderate doses of parenteral opioids.[16–18,19] Secondary

Table 2.1: The Acute Injury Response: Potential Benefits after Traumatic Injury versus Disadvantages in Controlled Postsurgical Settings

Beneficial Effects after Traumatic Injury	*Adverse Effects in Patients Recovering from Surgery*
1. Maintenance of intravascular volume and mean arterial pressure	1. Hypertension, hypervolemia, increased risk of hemorrhage, stroke
2. Maintenance of cardiac output and cerebral perfusion	2. Tachycardia, arrhythmias, myocardial ischemia, congestive heart failure
3. Enhanced hemostasis	3. Hypercoagulable state, increased risk of arterial and deep venous thrombosis, substrate mobilization, enhanced energy production.
4. Immobilization, minimizing further tissue injury	4. Hyperglycemia, negative nitrogen balance
5. Learned avoidance	5. Reduction in respiratory volume and flow rates, hypoxia, pneumonia
	6. Anxiety, fear, demoralization, prolonged convalescence

hyperalgesia provides the neurochemical basis for splinting and other adaptive behaviors. These include elaboration of ipsilateral and contralateral flexion reflexes and alterations in regional sympathetic tone.[1,2,4,14,17,18] Pain is perceived at dermatomes above and below the site of injury and is worsened by ambulation or movement. The impact of primary and secondary analgesia on acute pain intensity and the development of persistent pain is depicted in Figure 2.2.

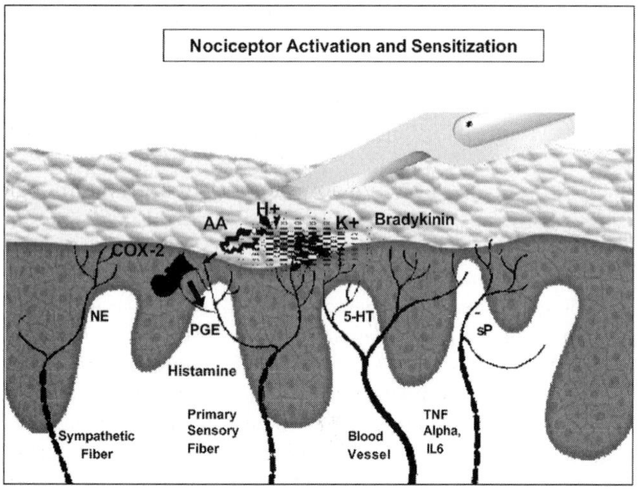

SYMPATHOADRENAL RESPONSES

The stress response to surgical or accidental trauma has been described as a general adaptation syndrome focused on tissue repair and improved survival. The sympathoadrenal response to traumatic injury evolves in three stages. The initial alarm stage or "fight-flight reaction" allows rapid withdrawal from the traumatic event and is followed by a "resistance stage," which maintains blood flow to critical organs, and later by an "exhaustion stage," which limits mobility and improves tissue repair.[1–4,20,21] Following extensive tissue injury, nociceptive impulses stimulate sympathetic cells in the hypothalamus and preganglionic neurons in the anterior lateral horn. Once stimulated, catecholamines released by these cells initiate cardiac inotropic and

Figure 2.1: Peripheral responses to acute injury. (1) Following tissue injury, potassium (K^+), hydrogen ions (H^+), and arachidonic acid (AA) released from damaged cells and bradykinin (BK) released from damaged vessels activate the terminal endings of sensory afferent fibers (nociceptors). Cyclooxygenase 2 (COX-2) is upregulated and is responsible for the conversion of AA into prostaglandin (PGE). Prostaglandin has been implicated in nociceptor sensitization and further increases in vascular permeability and primary hyperalgesia. (2) Orthodromic transmission in sensitized afferents leads to the release of substance P (sP) in and around the site of injury. Substance P is responsible for further release of BK. (3) Substance P also stimulates histamine release from mast cells and serotonin (5-HT) from platelets. These substances plus humoral factors TNF-α and IL-6β form a "noxious soup," which activates additional nociceptors and further exacerbates the inflammatory response. (4) Reflexes mediated by sympathetic efferents sensitize nociceptors directly via secretion of norepinephrine (NE), indirectly via further release of BK and PGE, and mediate peripheral vasoconstriction. (Modified from Sinatra RS, Bigham M: The anatomy and pathophysiology of acute pain. In: Grass JA, ed. *Problems in Anesthesiology*. Philadelphia, PA: Lippincott-Raven, 1997:10:8–22.[2])

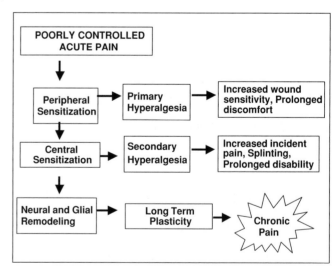

Figure 2.2: Following tissue injury, primary and secondary hyperalgesia increases the intensity of acute pain and may lead to the development of persistent pain.

chronotropic responses, increase peripheral vascular resistance, and redistribute blood flow away from peripheral tissues and viscera to the heart and brain.[1,2,20,21] These initially advantageous effects can become deleterious in time, particularly in at-risk or debilitated patients where myocardial activity and work of breathing may exceed the oxygen and metabolic supplies.[4,21–23]

Surgical trauma is promptly followed by increases in plasma concentrations of epinephrine and norepinephrine.[20,21] The magnitude and duration of catecholamine release is directly related to patient related factors such as the type of surgery, inherent sympathetic response, patient age, and genetic (inflammatory) polymorphisms. In general, highest elevations in plasma catecholamines are observed following extensive procedures and in younger individuals.[20,21] The earliest aspects of the catecholamine response reflect pronounced, but transient, increases in adrenal medullary secretion, whereas latter aspects reflect continued release of norepinephrine from sympathetic nerve endings.[21,22] Pathophysiological changes associated with increased sympathetic tone and altered regional perfusion include the following: (1) an increased incidence of postsurgical hypertension that ranges from 5% following minor, uncomplicated procedures to approximately 50% in patients recovering from more extensive vascular surgery.[21] (2) Increased peripheral vascular resistance is associated with increases in contractility and myocardial oxygen consumption as the organism attempts to maintain or augment cardiac output.[1,2,21]

Increases in oxygen consumption may precipitate myocardial ischemia in patients with coronary artery disease. Enhanced sympathetic tone may be especially deleterious in patients recovering from peripheral vascular surgery, because elevations in arterial pressure may risk rupture of vascular anastomoses, whereas intense vasospasm may compromise distal graft patency.[1,2,21,22]

(3) As perfusion is directed to high-priority organs, microcirculatory blood flow in injured tissues, adjacent musculature, and in the viscera may be significantly diminished.[3,21–23] Reductions in circulation have been associated with impaired wound healing, enhanced sensitization of nociceptors, increased muscle spasm, visceral/somatic ischemia, and acidosis.[21]

(4) Renal hypoperfusion results in activation of the renin-angiotensin-aldosterone axis. Angiotensin is a potent vasoconstrictor that, although capable of increasing renal perfusion, may further accentuate catecholamine-induced changes in regional blood flow and hypoperfusion of lower priority organs (injury site, skin, viscera, etc.).[1–3,21,22]

(5) Catecholamines, angiotensin, and other factors associated with surgical stress may increase platelet activation and accelerate coagulation.[22,23] Increased platelet-fibrinogen activation may be especially deleterious in patients with atherosclerotic vascular disease, because increased plasma viscosity, platelet aggregation, and platelet release of vasoconstrictive factors may significantly reduce blood flow in critically stenosed vessels.[21–23]

NEUROENDOCRINE RESPONSES

Following tissue injury, neurogenic stimuli affecting the hypothalamus, secretory target organs, or both, incite alterations in neuroendocrine response.[20–23] These well-described changes, termed the *stress response to injury*, are characterized by an increased secretion of catabolic hormones, including cortisol, glucagon, growth hormone, and catecholamines, and an inhibi-

tion of anabolic mediators, such as insulin and testosterone.[20–25] These mediators increase substrate mobilization, resulting in hyperglycemia and a negative nitrogen balance.[1,2,20–24] Associated metabolic changes, including gluconeogenesis, glycogenolysis, proteolysis, and breakdown of lipid stores, provide the injured organism with short-term benefits of enhanced energy production and availability; however, when amplified or prolonged, catabolic aspects of the stress response may adversely affect postsurgical outcome in the following ways: (1) excessive protein loss may lead to muscle wasting, fatigue, and prolonged convalescence and (2) impaired immunocompetence secondary to diminished immunoglobulin synthesis and impaired phagocytosis may decrease resistance to infection.[21,25–29]

Hume and Egdahl[30] were among the first to propose that nociceptive impulses (traveling up the spinal cord via the midbrain reticular formation) and conscious stimuli from the cerebral cortex were both capable of activating hypothalamic centers and initiating the neuroendocrine stress response. Activated cells in the preoptic region secrete pro-opiomelanocortin, which in turn facilitates release of adrenocorticotropic hormone (ACTH), β-endorphin, and other anterior pituitary hormones.[22,24,26,27] Sustained secretion of ACTH underlies the adrenocortical response to injury, which then heightens and continuously releases corticosteroids and mineral corticoids. In addition, trauma related release of IL-6 and IL-1β can also increase ACTH and cortisol secretion.[22,25,26,30] The relationship between plasma IL-6 and cortisol levels is linear in postsurgical patients.[25,26]

Significant hyperglycemia and a rise in plasma cortisol are commonly observed in the postsurgical period. Bromage and colleagues[31] noted in patients recovering from extensive abdominal procedures or thoracotomy that increases in blood sugar and cortisol reached a peak of 65% above control values and were maintained for more than 24 hours following surgery. Although the stress response in patients recovering from 1-day surgical procedures has not been evaluated, the same alterations may be expected to occur, but be less pronounced.

The negative nitrogen balance observed after surgical trauma has been related to the effects of starvation, release of catecholamines, and an altered insulin/glucagon ratio.[24–31,32,33] Prolonged negative nitrogen balance and sustained secretion of glucocorticoids are associated with impaired wound healing and immunocompetence.[25,27,32,33] Increased protein breakdown and diminutions in protein synthesis may inhibit cell division, production of collagen, and acute phase/leukocytic responses. Such inhibition results in stress-induced lymphopenia, granulocytosis, decreased natural killer and T-cell activity, and impaired synthesis/release of macrophage-derived peptides and immunoglobulins.[24,25,29] In animal models, and initial clinical trials, invasive surgery and poorly controlled pain are associated with profound immunosuppression and increased risk of tumor metastasis.[34,35] In surgical settings, immunologic suppression may have minimal consequences in subjects with normal immune function; however, diminished cellular and humoral immunity may predispose debilitated individuals and those with preexisting immune disorders to postoperative infections.[29,34]

Levels of β-endorphin increase 3-fold following surgical incision and remain elevated well into the postoperative period.[24,25,27,28] β-Endorphin mediates a number of systemic effects, including immunosuppression, complement release, decreased peripheral vascular resistance, and initiation of shock.[23,25,27,28] Finally, plasma levels of the posterior pituitary

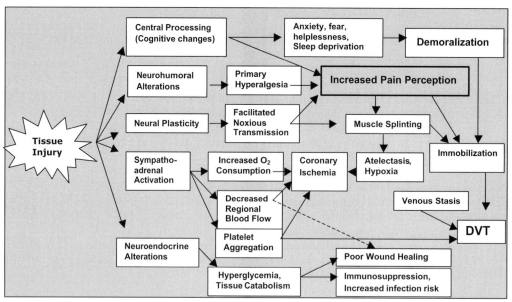

Figure 2.3: An outline of pathophysiological responses associated with surgical trauma and their effect on key target organs.

derived octapeptide, arginine vasopressin (AVP), rise dramatically and remain elevated for up to 5 days following extensive surgical trauma.[4,23,24,32] Increased secretion of AVP is responsible for postsurgical fluid retention, plasma hyposmolarity, and oliguria.[23] Figure 2.3 provides an overview of pathophysiologic responses to acute traumatic injuries.

EFFECTS ON KEY TARGET ORGANS

Pathophysiologic consequences related to poorly controlled pain include reduced functional capacity, increased sleep disturbance, and delayed wound healing; these consequences result in social burdens, such as decreased quality of life and increased cost of care.[22,36,37] Of even greater importance is the fact that in high-risk patients significant cardiovascular and pulmonary dysfunction may significantly increase postoperative morbidity and mortality risks

Heart

Despite considerable improvements in anesthetic technique and maintenance of intraoperative hemodynamic stability, cardiac dysfunction secondary to myocardial infarction, cardiac failure and arrhythmia continue to account for a significant percentage of postoperative deaths.[4,21,24,38,39] In high-risk populations, perioperative ischemia is most likely to occur following surgery, most commonly between postoperative days 1–3.[39] Although a variety of factors may contribute to the development of postoperative myocardial ischemia, including hypothermia, anemia, anxiety, and tracheal intubation/suctioning, responses to poorly controlled pain play a prominent role.[4,21,39,41,42] Catecholamine-induced tachycardia, enhanced myocardial contractility, increased afterload, and hypervolemia, secondary to enhanced release of AVP and aldosterone, are well-characterized factors responsible for increased oxygen demand. Increased oxygen demand, together with hypervolemia, may precipitate ischemia and acute cardiac failure, especially in patients

with poorly compensated coronary artery and/or valvular heart disease.[21,23,39,41]

Despite increased myocardial oxygen requirements, oxygen supply may be diminished because of alterations in pulmonary function (refer to the following section). Pulmonary alterations include atelectasis secondary to pain-induced hypoventilation and pulmonary edema resulting from stress-induced hypervolemia.[1,2,21,24] A second cause of reduced oxygen supply includes coronary artery occlusion. Coronary artery blockage may result from (1) high circulatory levels of catecholamines and increased coronary sympathetic tone, (2) stress-induced increases in plasma viscosity and platelet-induced thrombosis, and (3) coronary vasospasm secondary to platelet aggregation and release of serotonin.[4,21,24,40,42]

Lungs

Thoracic and upper abdominal injuries are associated with a high incidence of morbidity and mortality.[21,22,24] The causes of acute thoracic injury include blunt trauma, for example, deceleration injuries and penetrating etiologies, such as surgical scalpels, retractors, and other foreign bodies. Thoracic surgery and trauma are associated with a spectrum of injuries, including pneumothorax, hemothorax, myocardial, and pulmonary contusions and rib, scapular, and clavicular fractures.[21,22,43–45]

Thoracic and upper abdominal injuries and associated pain evoke significant pathophysiologic responses, which can adversely influence hospital course. In general, symptomatology is influenced by the extent of the injury and the physical status of the patient.[43,44] Depending on the mechanism of injury, patients may present with life-threatening alterations in pulmonary or cardiovascular mechanics and are troubled by severe skeletal, visceral, or neuralgic-type pain. Pain following division of the upper abdominal and thoracic musculature is effort dependent, reflecting rib, pleuritic, and diaphragmatic injury.[43–45] In contrast to resting pain, the intensity of effort dependent on dynamic pain markedly increases with inspiration and cough. The pain stimulus is also hyperalgesic in that severe discomfort and reflexive muscle splinting may be noted at many dermatomes above and below the site of injury. Chest wall and upper abdominal hyperalgesia are responsible for several pathophysiological alterations, including musculoskeletal and diaphragmatic dysfunction and impaired gas exchange.[21,43,44]

Pulmonary function is dramatically altered by surgically induced pain. Beecher[47] was first to describe the classical pulmonary response to upper abdominal surgery, which included an increased respiratory rate and decreased tidal volume (TV), vital capacity (VC), forced expiratory volume (FEV_1), and functional residual capacity (FRC). These pathophysiologic alterations reflect acute restrictive pulmonary dysfunction and, as such, may be associated with clinically significant hypoxia and hypocarbia.[21,43,44,47] Atelectasis, pneumonia, and arterial hypoxemia are common postoperative complications whose incidence approaches 70% in patients recovering from upper abdominal surgery.[47,48] Such complications have been related to the above-mentioned reductions in VC and a reduced ability to cough and clear secretions.[43–45]

Vital capacity is the first pulmonary parameter to change in the postoperative period. Significant reductions in VC are evident within the first 3 hours, and declines to 40%–60% of preoperative values have been reported. Following upper abdominal surgery, reductions in RV, FRC, and FEV_1 are greatest at 24 hours; thereafter, values gradually return to near normal levels by postoperative day 7.[48] In a classic study, Ali and coworkers[48] noted that postsurgical VC was most depressed from day 0 through day 7 following upper abdominal surgery, less depressed after lower abdominal surgery, and least affected in patients recovering from superficial procedures, including inguinal herniorrhaphy. Other factors that influence the magnitude of VC reduction include open vs laparoscopic procedures, duration of anesthesia, diaphragmatic injury, and patient history of chronic obstructive pulmonary disease.[43–45]

Reduction in FRC represents the most detrimental alteration in postsurgical lung volume.[43–46] As FRC declines, resting lung volume approaches closing volume. With further reduction, airway closure occurs resulting in atelectasis, ventilation/perfusion mismatch, and hypoxemia. In patients recovering from open cholecystectomy, a delay of 16 hours was noted until maximum reduction in FRC.[46] In these individuals, reductions in FRC were associated with progressive arterial hypoxemia, whereas a gradual improvement toward normal FRC was followed by a decrease in physiological shunt.

Following thoracotomy, alterations in chest wall motion reduce lung compliance and require an increased work of breathing if effectual respiration is to be achieved.[43–46] Splinting secondary to poorly controlled pain exaggerates this process by further decreasing respiratory effort. Perfusion is maintained in unventilated portions of the lung resulting in a shunt and ventilation/perfusion mismatch. Inhibition of diaphragmatic function represents an additional factor responsible for respiratory dysfunction and morbidity. Noxious impulses from the diaphragm, chest wall, and upper abdominal viscera result in reflex inhibition of phrenic nerve motor drive, which further compromises pulmonary function by increasing atelectasis, airway closure, alveolar ventilation (V) and pulmonary perfusion (Q) mismatch, and hypoxemia. If pneumonia or acute respiratory distress syndrome occurs, the risk of prolonged hospitalization and mortality increases.[43,44] Surgical induced alterations in VC, peak flow rate and alveolar–arterial (A-a) gradient are depicted in Figure 2.4.

Vascular System

As blood flow is directed to high-priority organs, perfusion in injured tissues, adjacent musculature, and in the viscera may be diminished. Reductions in circulation have been associated with impaired wound healing, increased muscle spasm, and visceral-somatic ischemia and acidosis.[21,22,44] Inadequately controlled pain can predispose patients to postsurgical deep venous thromboses (DVT) and pulmonary embolism. As previously discussed, catecholamines and angiotensin released in response to surgical stress may result in platelet-fibrinogen activation and the development of a hypercoagulable state.[21,42] Severe pain is commonly associated with an impaired ability to ambulate and decreased venous flow.[1,2,21,24] Surgical manipulation in and around the pelvis may damage venous conduits that return blood from the lower extremity. These factors make up Virchow's triad of hypercoagulability, venous stasis, and endothelial injury that underlie the development of DVT.[1,2]

In addition to concerns of local tissue swelling and venous stasis, is the worry that thromboembolism may lead to a more serious complication, pulmonary embolism. As thrombotic fragments travel to the heart and lungs, occlusions within pulmonary arteries result in varying degrees of ventilation perfusion mismatch and hypoxia. Because the initial thrombus incites vigorous local release of vasoactive and inflammatory cytokines, symptoms associated with pulmonary embolism generally worsen within a short period of time. If not recognized and promptly treated, this complication is associated with a 20%–30% mortality.

Finally it is well recognized that high plasma levels of norepinephrine levels lead to vascular constriction and platelet adhesion, which are factors that diminish peripheral limb perfusion and require reoperation for graft occlusion following vascular surgery.[1,2,21]

Injury Site

As discussed under *Heart*, humoral and neurochemical alterations in and around the site of injury play important roles in the development of persistent postsurgical pain and, in some cases, chronic pain. Continued sensitization of peripheral nociceptors and second-order spinal cells is responsible for prolonged hyperalgesia as well as qualitative differences among physiological, nociceptive, and neuropathic pain. Elevated levels of IL-1β and other cytokines exacerbate edematous and irritative components of inflammatory pain.[49] Cytokines, including IL-1β, IL-6, and tumor necrosis factor (TNF-α), also play a role in initiating allodynia and development of persistent pain.[50] These cytokines, initially released from neutrophils, macrophages, and other mediators, such as nerve growth factor (NGF) and nitric oxide (NO) that are also released at later stages from activated Schwann cells, further incite inflammatory neural injury and worsen neuropathic pain.[51–54] Lymphocytes, including T and NK cells, infiltrate into and further irritate injured nerves; they also play a role in the development of persistent neuropathic symptoms.

Chronic pain following surgical trauma is often related to poorly controlled acute pain, neuropathic pain secondary to neuromas, or myofascial pain syndromes created by procedural trauma.[53–56,65] Heightened reflex activity in sympathetic efferent fibers is responsible for vasoconstriction and nociceptor sensitization. Continued alteration in regional blood flow and

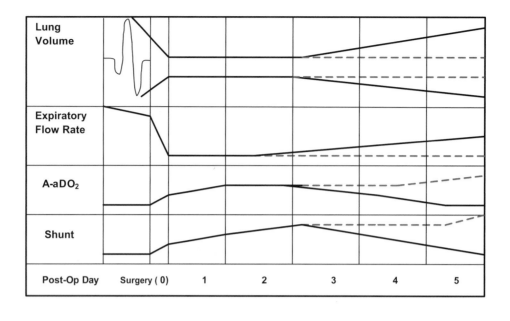

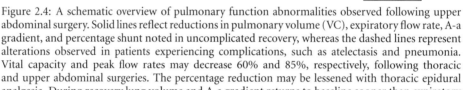

Figure 2.4: A schematic overview of pulmonary function abnormalities observed following upper abdominal surgery. Solid lines reflect reductions in pulmonary volume (VC), expiratory flow rate, A-a gradient, and percentage shunt noted in uncomplicated recovery, whereas the dashed lines represent alterations observed in patients experiencing complications, such as atelectasis and pneumonia. Vital capacity and peak flow rates may decrease 60% and 85%, respectively, following thoracic and upper abdominal surgeries. The percentage reduction may be lessened with thoracic epidural analgesia. During recovery lung volume and A-a gradient returns to baseline sooner than expiratory flow. Adapted from data reported in references: Brown DL, Carpenter RL. Perioperative analgesia: a review of risks and benefits. *J Cardiothorac Anesth.* 1990;4:368–383. Beecher HK: The measured effect of laparotomy on the respiration. *J Clin Invest.* 1933;12:639–650. Ali J, Weisel RD, Layug AB. Consequences of postoperative alterations in respiratory mechanics. *Am J Surg.* 1974;128:376–382.

development of nociceptive reflex arcs eventually result in sympathetic dystrophy or sympathetically maintained pain.[21,53–56]

Central Nervous System

Nociceptive input affects all levels of the central nervous system and results in neurochemical and neuroanatomical alterations. One of the more disturbing findings associated with analgesic undermedication and severe acute pain is the development of central sensitization. Central sensitization is not only responsible for secondary hyperalgesia, described under *Sympathoadrenal Responses*, but also sets in motion plasticity changes and prolonged enhancement in noxious sensitivity that may be difficult to reverse.[55–58] Many of these changes are mediated by activation of NMDARs and increased Ca^{2+} influx.[16,59] Subsequent neurochemical alterations include upregulation of COX-2 and NO synthetase and increased synthesis of prostaglandin (PGE) and NO within sensitized neurons and glial cells.[51,56,57] Synthesis of these and other inflammatory mediators induce neuroanatomical changes that, for reasons that remain unclear, appear designed to facilitate noxious transmission and pain processing.[54,55–57] These changes include pathophysiologic activation of microglia and neuronal apoptosis. Cells that are most vulnerable to atrophy and death include modulatory enkephalinergic and adrenergic interneurons that normally function to suppress noxious transmission.[56] Other neuroanatomical changes include nociceptor axonal sprouting and new connections with

dorsal horn cells and redirection of nonnoxious afferent fibers to sensitized second-order cells. These forms of plasticity are responsible for many of the allodynic and hyperpathic aspects of persistent somatic and neuropathic pain and also limit the effectiveness of pharmacological management.[53,56,57] Figure 2.5

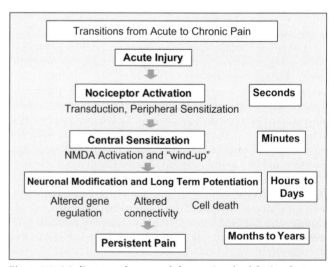

Figure 2.5: Mediators and temporal changes involved during the transition from acute to chronic pain. (Adapted from Woolf and Salter, *Science.* 2000;288:1765.)

Table 2.2: Incidences of Chronic Postoperative Pain and Disability[a,b]

Procedure	Estimated Incidence of Chronic Pain (%)	Estimated Incidence of Chronic Severe (Disabling) Pain[b] (%)	Number of Surgeries in the United States[a]
Amputation	30–50	5–10	159 000
Coronary artery bypass surgery	30–50	5–10	598 000
Thoracotomy	30–40	10	Unknown
Breast surgery (lumpectomy or mastectomy	20–30	5–10	479 000
Cesarean section	10	4	220 000
Inguinal hernia repair	10	2–4	609 000

[a] National Center for Health Statistics, United States of America, 1996.
[b] >5 of 10 pain scores.
Source: Kehlet H, et al. *Lancet.* 2006;367:1618–1625.[53]

provides a temporal outline describing the transition from acute to chronic pain. Other figures describing the neurochemical alterations and spinal plasticity changes responsible for this transition are presented in Chapter 1.

When one considers it, all chronic pain begins as acute pain. Kehlet and coworkers[53,60] found that a high percentage of patients recovering from commonly performed procedures were troubled by persistent somatic and neuropathic pain a year following surgery (Table 2.2). The highest incidence of persistent pain was noted in procedures where nerve injury is commonly observed, including thoracotomy, mastectomy, and inguinal hernia repair. Pluijms and coworkers[61] noted that patients most likely to develop persistent pain following thoracotomy were those who suffered the highest acute pain intensity during the first postoperative week. Sixty-seven percent of patients who developed chronic pain reported moderate to severe VAS pain scores, whereas 40% reported mild to moderate pain. Patients likely to develop chronic pain also reported a greater total amount of time spent having pain ($P = .02$).

Other risk factors linked to the development of persistent pain include patients with ongoing or preceding pain at the site of surgery, trauma occurring in younger individuals, and patients presenting with either psychosocial abnormalities or specific genetic susceptibilities (Figure 2.6).[53,62,63] These factors appear to have strong causality, because only a fraction of patients experiencing severe pain following traumatic neural injuries progress to a chronic pain state.[16,53] Effective pain management and close patient observation during recovery and rehabilitation may be the key to reducing long-term pain disability.[64] Those individuals experiencing extraordinary discomfort following routine procedures should be followed closely and may require a chronic pain consultation and treatment with antineuropathic agents (see also Chapter 9, *Transitions from Acute to Chronic Pain*).

Responses mediated via higher cortical centers and the limbic system can either modulate the intensity of noxious perception or exacerbate emotional distress, pain complaint, and patient anxiety.[21,27,41,66] Intense anxiety, fear, and loss of control that accompany traumatic injuries may have a profound effect on the hypothalamic-pituitary axis, further altering neuroendocrine response. Poorly controlled pain promotes sleep deprivation, reduced morale, and learned helplessness by affecting the limbic and cingulate cortices.

Patients suffering acute pain are commonly troubled by sleep disturbances that increase lethargy and negatively affect morale, mood, and motivation to participate in rehabilitation. Many patients require anxiolytics and sedatives to experience limited intervals of sleep and generally awake experiencing increased pain. In a study of 102 patients recovering from orthopedic surgery, increasingly severe postoperative pain resulted in greater interference with sleep.[66] Sleep quality and duration was most affected when pain scores were greater than 5 on a scale from 0 to 10. In settings of severe acute pain, sleep deprivation and behavioral alterations may diminish patient morale and their willingness to utilize incentive spirometry or participate in ambulation and physical therapy. In the setting of persistent pain, limbic cortical responses negatively affect quality of life and also mediate anxiety, depression, and other chronic pain behaviors.

ATTENUATION OF PAIN-INDUCED PATHOPHYSIOLOGY

Innovations in technology, such as neuraxial analgesia and continuous infusion of local anesthetics, have revolutionized postoperative pain management. Evidence-based practice suggests that epidural anesthesia, specially thoracic epidural anesthesia, improves postop myocardial infarction, deep venous thrombosis, pulmonary embolism, transfusion requirements, pneumonia, respiratory depression, and morbidity following major operative procedures.[67–73]

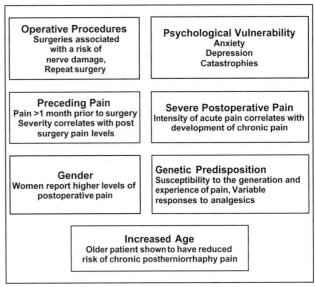

Figure 2.6: Risk factors for the development of persistent pain following routine surgery. Based on studies performed by Hanley MA, et al. *Disabil Rehabil.* 2004;26:882–893; Katz J, et al. *Pain.* 2005;119:16–25; Perkins FM, Kehlet H. *Anesthesiology.* 2000;93:1123–1133; Reuben SS, Buvanendran A. *J Bone Joint Surg Am.* 2007;89:1343–1358.

Vascular Surgery

Epidural infusions of local anesthetic combined with general anesthesia provide a significant cardioprotective effect for patients undergoing abdominal aortic aneurysm repair. Improvements in outcome are related to maintenance of hemodynamic stability and reduced arrhythmias following release of the aortic cross clamp.[71] Postsurgical hypertension found in up to 50% patients has been related to sympathetic nervous system hyperactivity and not adrenal epinephrine or pituitary secretion of arginine vasopressin is responsible for the development of hypertension following aortic and lower extremity vascular surgery.[40,70-72] The beneficial effect of epidural analgesia on sympathetic hypertensive response is mediated by blockade of noxious input as well as the sympatholytic effect of dilute local anesthetics.[71-73] Epidural morphine has no local anesthetic properties but may suppress sympathetic responses by providing effective pain control. Sympathetic hyperactivity and efferent outflow are more reliably blocked when local anesthetic is added to an epidural morphine infusion.[40,73] α_2 stimulation also inhibits sympathetic responses and release of catecholamine. Clonidine is an α_2 agonist that indirectly inhibits synaptic α-adrenergic receptors by decreasing central catecholamine ouflow. In a recent study, clonidine appeared to have a direct effect in modifying the sympathoadrenal response to surgical pain.[74]

Catecholamines released in response to surgical stress and poorly controlled pain incite vasospastic, vasoconstrictive, and thrombotic occlusive complications.[71,6,74] Vasospasm as a result of high plasma concentrations of epinephrine and locally released norepinephrine may compromise distal graft potency in patients recovering from vascular surgery and increase risk of deep venous thromboses in other forms of lower extremity procedures.[40,67,68,70] Compared with general anesthesia, epidural anesthesia followed by continuous epidural analgesia maintains fibrinolysis, reduces the risk of arterial thrombosis, and is associated with a lower incidence of reoperation for inadequate tissue perfusion.[74-76] Although local anesthetics directly inhibit platelet aggregation and have antithrombotic effects it remains unclear whether local anesthetics absorbed from peripheral or epidural sites of administration have clinically significant effects at the site of vascular surgery.[76,77]

Cardiac Surgery

Thoracic epidural analgesia allows specific blockade of nociceptive reflex arcs and may reduce or eliminate stress-induced alterations of organ dysfunction.[67] Untoward sympathetic effects on atherosclerotic vessels are suppressed and blood flow to at risk areas of myocardium is improved.[78] Understanding the pathophysiology of pain and providing optimal management has become important in cardiac surgery. The use of thoracic epidural anesthesia following coronary artery bypass graft surgery, although controversial from a safety point of view, has been shown to improve hemodynamic stability, reduces the release of troponin and the incidence of supraventricular arrhythmia and allows earlier extubation.[79,80] Epidural analgesia with local anesthetics plus opioids, but not opioids alone, blocks noxious impulses to and from the sympathetic ganglia and attenuates activation of the sympathoadrenal axis.[78-81] Such suppression helps to explain why a recent analysis of thoracic epidural analgesia continued for more than 24 hours was found to reduce mortality and postoperative myocardial infarction.[84]

Thoracic and Upper Abdominal Surgery

Clinically significant hypoxia and hypocarbia are commonly observed in patients recovering from chest wall trauma, thoracotomy, and upper abdominal surgery. Dynamic pain and associated restrictions in VC are difficult to control with either parenteral opioids or intravenous patient-controlled analgesia (IV PCA).[82] Cough-provoked dynamic pain is a more sensitive outcome measure for post upper abdominal and thoracotomy analgesia.[21,82,83] Several studies employing thoracic epidural infusions of opioid plus local anesthetic have documented improvement in pulmonary volume, flows, and cough-provoked dynamic pain as well as reductions in stress-induced hormonal, metabolic, and physiologic responses.[81-83] Improvements in pulmonary function observed with thoracic epidural anesthesia are related to several factors, including reduction in opioid exposure, superior relief of dynamic pain, and prevention of secondary hyperalgesia.[1,21]

Risk of Thromboembolism

Continuous infusions of epidural local anesthetics and continuous lower extremity neural blockade may be advantageous in patients at high risk for venous thromboembolism, particularly when DVT prophylaxis is inappropriate because of patient or surgical concerns.[75,76] A recent meta-analysis of all randomized studies,[84] including 141 trials in a total of 9559 patients, concluded that central neuraxial blockade reduces the risk of deep venous thrombosis by 44%, pulmonary embolism by 55%, transfusion requirements by 50%, pneumonia by 39%, respiratory depression by 59%, and myocardial infarction by 30%. Overall mortality was reduced by 30%. These positive findings were obtained predominantly after major orthopedic procedures, whereas no significant effects were found in other procedures (urological, abdominal, and thoracic).

Cytokine Response

Systemic opioids and IV PCA provide useful pain relief; however, they offer minimal to no suppressive effect on sympathetic and humoral responses to traumatic injury.[85] In contrast, continuous epidural or regional anesthesia/analgesia suppress sympathoadrenal responses and provide modest suppression of humoral-mediated responses and neuroendocrine reactivity.[53,67] Clonidine and other α_2-adrenergic receptor agonists offer an alternative pharmacologic approach that provides clinically effective pain relief while suppressing the sympathoadrenal responses to injury and intubation.[74,86]

Humoral mediators, including cytokines and IL-1β, and peripheral sensitizers, such as PGE, exacerbate peripheral inflammatory responses and inflammatory mediated pain. Interleukin 1β, IL-6, C-reactive protein, and TNF-α are increased in patients undergoing extensive and prolonged surgeries.[50,53,54] In a recent study, patients receiving epidural clonidine reported lower pain scores while coughing, required less intravenous morphine, and benefited from a more rapid return of bowel function throughout the 72-hour postoperative period.[86] Levels of the proinflammatory cytokines interleukin 1 receptor antagonist (IL-1ra), IL-6, and IL-8 were significantly reduced in the clonidine group at 12 and 24 hours after surgery. In a similarly designed study, patients treated with epidural PCA with opioids plus local anesthetics also experienced significant reductions in postsurgical cytokine response.[87]

Proinflammatory cytokines and PGE also have analgesic effects in the central nervous system.[11,88] In addition to their

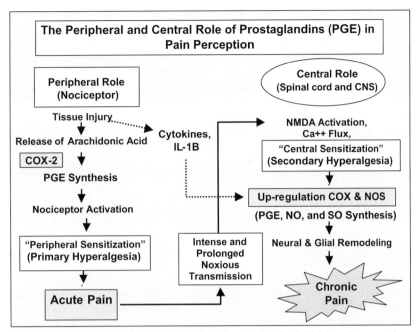

Figure 2.7: The peripheral and central roles of prostaglandin (PGE) in pain perception, hyperalgesia, and the development of chronic pain. In addition to their peripheral role in noxious stimulation and inflammation, PGEs incite central sensitization and plasticity changes by a variety of mechanisms, including (1) indirect effects following vascular delivery from the site of trauma to the CNS, (2) indirect effects mediated by cytokine-induced upregulation of COX-2 and PGE synthesis in the vascular endothelium, and (3) direct effects of COX-2 upregulation in microglial and sensitized neurons.

peripheral sites of activity, circulating cytokines are known to bind IL-1 receptors on the inner surface of cerebral endothelial cells.[88] Once activated these cells upregulate COX-2 and release PGE into brain tissue, resulting in irritation and heightened pain sensitivity.[89] Multimodal analgesics, including nonsteroidal anti-inflammatory drugs (NSAIDs) and COX-2 inhibitors, provide useful augmentation of epidural and regional analgesia and specifically reduce PGE synthesis as well as peripheral and central inflammatory responses. Peripheral and central effects of PGE in the development of primary and secondary hyperalgesia are presented in Figure 2.7.

Tissue Breakdown and Infection Risk

Parenteral and oral nutrition may compensate for catabolic hormonal stress responses and improve convalescence after major surgery.[90] Kehlet and Dahl[24] demonstrated that immediate postoperative administration of β-blockers, amino acids, insulin, and glucose improved nitrogen balance following major abdominal surgery. Further improvements in nitrogen balance may be gained by utilizing continuous epidural blockade.[31,91]

Impaired host defense mechanisms and immunosuppression caused by surgical trauma and hormonal stress responses may be reduced with epidural analgesia.[92] Postoperative epidural analgesia preserved lymphocyte reactivity to a significantly greater extent than IV opioids.[21,41,92] This improvement in immune status may improve postoperative resistance to infectious disease.

Sleep Disturbances and Return to Functionality

Epidural and continuous regional analgesia are associated with improved sleep quality and a more rapid return to functionality. Quality-of-life benefits provided by epidural opioid analgesia were evaluated in 100 patients recovering from major surgery.[93] Patients receiving epidural analgesia versus those receiving sham control plus parenteral opioids as required benefited from fewer sleep disturbances, a shorter hospital stay, and more rapid return to work (22 vs 30 days; $P < .05$). In a second study by Ilfeld et al,[94] postoperative pain management and sleep quality were assessed in patients receiving IV and oral opioids supplemented with either regional analgesia or saline control. Patients experiencing effective pain control benefited with significantly improved sleep pattern ($P < .05$). Pain relief was inferior and sleep disturbances 10-fold higher in the saline control group.

Epidural analgesia has also been shown to improve functionality following colon surgery.[95] While in the hospital, patients treated with epidural opioids plus local anesthetics experienced significant reductions in effort-related pain intensity scores than others using IV PCA morphine. These improvements continued following hospital discharge, as patients in the epidural group benefited from greater reductions in 6-minute walk test distance at 3 and 6 weeks postsurgery ($P < .01$). Capdevila and coworkers[96] found similar evidence that regional blockade and epidural analgesia were superior to IV PCA in reducing effort-dependent pain and improving knee flexion 24 and 48 hours following total knee replacement surgery. Of importance was the finding that these initial improvements continued 2 weeks and 3 months following hospital discharge.

Persistent Pain

In an effort to limit development of persistent pain, surgical and analgesic techniques that reduce the risk of neural and somatic injuries as well as the severity of acute pain and associated stress response have been advocated.[40,53,58,97] As discussed previously surgical and individual specific factors may increase patient susceptibility to developing chronic pain. Modification of surgical technique may reduce the development and severity of symptoms.[36,53,57,61] In patients at higher risk for developing persistent pain, the use of minimally invasive thoracoscopic, arthroscopic, and laproscopic procedures should be considered to minimize tissue injury, surgical stress, and risk of nerve damage. When performing mastectomy with axillary node dissection, care should be made to avoid damaging the intercostobrachial nerve that can result in upper arm neuropathy.[97] Anesthetic and analgesic management should employ a preemptive and multimodal approach that has been demonstrated to reduce pain intensity and opioid dose requirement[90,98–100] (see also Chapters 22 to 24, *Perioperative Ketamine for Better Postoperative Pain Outcome, Clinical Application of Glucocorticoids, Antineuropathics and Other Analgesic Adjuvants for Acute Pain Management* (Anticonvulsants and α_2 Agonists), and *Nonpharmacological Approaches for Acute Pain Management*), which describe several multimodal approaches for acute pain management). Preemptive and multimodal administration of coxibs, NSAIDs, anticonvulsant analgesics, and ketamine,[100] as well as presurgical initiation of neural blockade, not only reduce acute pain intensity but also may diminish wound hypersensitivity and residual pain intensity many months following surgery.[36,100–102]

CONCLUSION

Pathophysiologic responses and adaptive changes to extensive tissue injuries function to maintain hemodynamics, minimize tissue injury, and promote healing. However, the very same neural and hormonal catecholamine responses that promote recovery in healthy young adults worsen pain intensity, promote cardiovascular instability and pulmonary dysfunction and increase infection risk in American Society of Anesthesia highrisk patients. Anesthesiologists have traditionally been the physician specialists most familiar with pain physiology and pathophysiology and play the key role in initiating highly effective neuraxial, regional, and multimodal analgesia. Findings from randomized controlled trials and meta-analyses suggest that continuous epidural analgesia and regional analgesia can significantly reduce pain intensity scores, sympathoadrenal responses, and pulmonary complications. Although these techniques are more expensive, time-consuming, technically difficult to initiate and require continuous follow-up, their application in high-risk patients has been shown to reduce postsurgical morbidity, mortality, and time to hospital discharge.

REFERENCES

1. Cross SA. Pathophysiology of pain. *Mayo Clin. Proc.* 1994;69:375–383.
2. Sinatra RS, Bigham M. The anatomy and pathophysiology of acute pain. In: Grass JA, ed. *Problems in Anesthesiology.* Vol. 10. Philadelphia, PA: Lippincott-Raven; 1997:8–22.
3. Sinatra RS. The pathophysiology of acute pain. In: Sinatra RS, Hord A, Ginsberg B, Preble L, eds. *Acute Pain: Mechanisms and Management.* St. Louis, MO:Mosby; 1992.
4. Desborough JP. The stress response to trauma and surgery. *Br J Anaesth.* 2000;85:109–117.
5. Lewis T. Experiments relating to cutaneous hyperalgesia and its spread through somatic nerves. *Clin Sci.* 1936;2:373–416.
6. Julius D, Basbaum AI. Molecular mechanisms of nociception. *Nature.* 2001;413;203–210.
7. LaMotte RH, Thalhammer JG, Robinson CJ. Peripheral neural correlates of magnitude of cutaneous pain and hyperalgesia. *J Neurophysiol.* 1983;50:1–26.
8. Raja SN, Meyer RA, Campbell JN. Peripheral mechanisms of somatic pain. *Anesthesiology.* 1988;68:571–590.
9. Campbell, JN, Raja, SN, Cohen, RH, et al. Peripheral neural mechanisms of nociception. In: Wall PD, Melzack R, eds. *Textbook of Pain.* New York, NY: Churchill Livingston; 1989:22–45.
10. Coderre JJ, Melzack P. Cutaneous hyperalgesia contributions of the peripheral and central nervous system to the increase in pain sensitivity after injury. *Brain Res.* 1987;404:95–106.
11. Sinatra RS. Role of cox-2 inhibitors in the evolution of acute pain management. *J Pain Symptom Manage.* 2002;24:S18–S27.
12. Besson J-M, Chaouch A. Peripheral and spinal mechanisms of nociception. *Physiol. Rev.* 1987;67:67–186.
13. Bonica JJ. Anatomic and physiologic basis of nociception and pain. In: Bonica, JJ, eds. *The Management of Pain.* 2nd ed. Philadelphia, PA: Lea & Febiger; 1990:28–94.
14. Woolf CJ, Central sensitization: uncovering the relation between pain and plasticity. *Anesthesiology.* 2007;106:864–867.
15. Thompson SW, Woolf CJ. Primary afferent-evoked prolonged potentials in the spinal cord and their central summation: role of the NMDA receptor. In Bond MR, Charlton JE, Woolf CJ, eds. *Proceedings of the 6th World Congress on Pain.* Amsterdam: Elsevier: 1991.
16. Woolf CJ, Thompson SW. The induction and maintenance of central sensitization is dependent upon N-methyl-D-aspartic acid receptor activation. *Pain.* 1991;44:293–299.
17. Coderre TJ, Katz J, Vaccarino AL, Melzack R. Contribution of central neuroplasticity on pathological pain: review of clinical and experimental evidence. *Pain.* 1993;52:259–285.
18. Fields, HL, Basbaum AI. Endogenous pain control mechanisms. In: Wall PD, Melzack R, eds. Textbook of Pain. New York, NY: Churchill Livingston; 1989:206–217.
19. Abram SE, Olson EE. Systemic opioids do not supress spinal sensitization after subcutaneous formalin in rats. *Anesthesiology.* 1994;80:1114–1119.
20. Selye H. A syndrome produced by diverse nocuous agents. *J Neuropsych Clin Neurosci.* 1998;10:230–231.
21. Cousins MJ. Acute pain and the injury response: immediate and prolonged effects. *Reg Anesth.* 1989;16:162–176.
22. Kehlet H. Surgical stress: the role of pain and analgesia. *Br J Anaesth.* 1989;63:189–195.
23. Breslow MJ. Neuroendocrine responses to surgery. In Breslow MJ, Miller CF, Rogers MC, eds. *Perioperative Management.* St. Louis, MO: Mosby; 1990.
24. Kehlet H. Modification of responses to surgery by neural blockade: clinical implications. In: Cousins MJ, Bridenbaugh PO, eds. *Neural Blockade in Clinical Anesthesia and Management of Pain.* Philadelphia, PA: Lippincott; 1987.
25. Van der Poll T, Barbaza AE, Coyle SM. Hypercortisolemia increases plasma IL-10 during endotoxemia. *J Clin Endocrinol Metab.* 1996;81:3604–3606.
26. Lyons A, Kelly JL, Rodick ML, et al. Major injury induces increased production of interleukin-10 by cell of the immune system with a negative effect on infection resistance. *Ann Surg.* 1997:226;450–460.
27. Dubois M. Surgical stress in humans is accompanied by an increase in plasma beta-endorphin immunoreactivity. *Life Sci.* 1981;29:1249–1254.
28. Levy EM, McIntosh J, Black PH. Elevation of circulating endorphin levels with concomitant depression of immune parameters after traumatic injury. *J Trauma.* 1986;26:246–250.

Functional measures

A. Brain areas functionally related to pain processing.

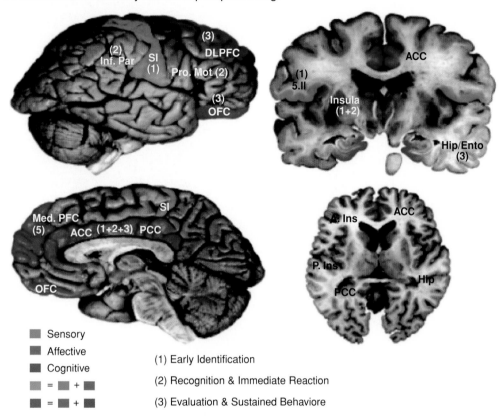

Sensory

Affective

Cognitive

■ = ■ + ■

■ = ■ + ■

(1) Early Identification

(2) Recognition & Immediate Reaction

(3) Evaluation & Sustained Behaviore

B. Example of functional MRI response to painful stimulation.

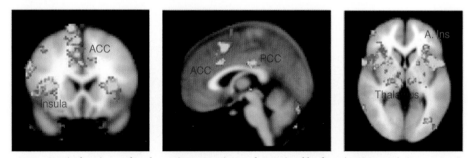

Figure 1.11: Cortical regions related to pain processing as determined by function Magnetic Resonance Imaging (fMRI). The highlighted areas have been found to be particularly active: (ACC) Anterior cingulate cortex, (S1) Primary somatosensory cortex (Primarily involved in pain localization), (S2) Secondary somatosensory cortex, (OFC) orbitofrontal cortex, (DLPFC) Dorsolateral prefrontal cortex, (Pre-Mot) Premotor cortex, (Med.PFC) Medial Prefrontal cortex, (P.Ins) Posterior insula, (A.Ins) Anterior insula, (Hip) Hippocampus, (Ento) Entorhinal cortex From: David Borsook, Eric A Moulton, Karl F Schmidt, Lino R Becerra Molecular Pain 2007, 3:25.

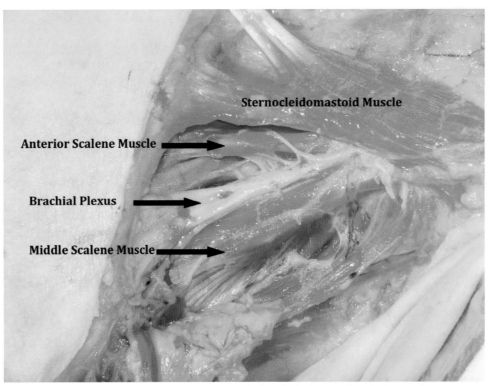

Figure 17.1: Anatomical dissection demonstrating the brachial plexus within the interscalene groove.

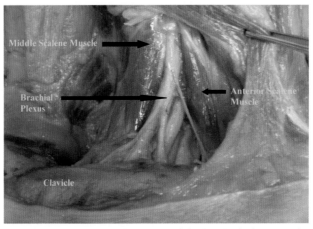

Figure 17.6: Anatomical dissection of the brachial plexus in the supraclavicular region.

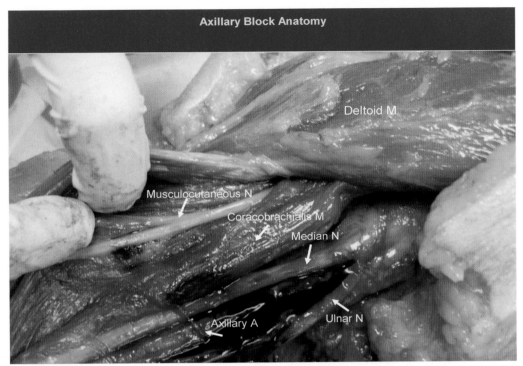

Figure 17.13: Axillary block anatomy.

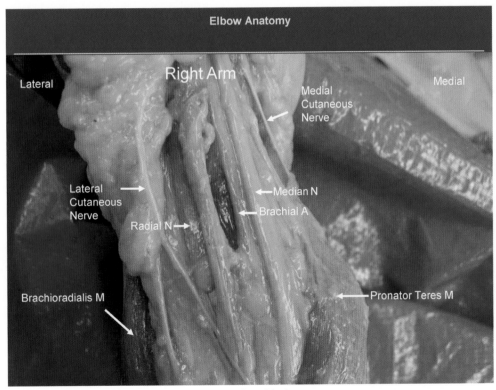

Figure 17.21: Elbow block anatomy.

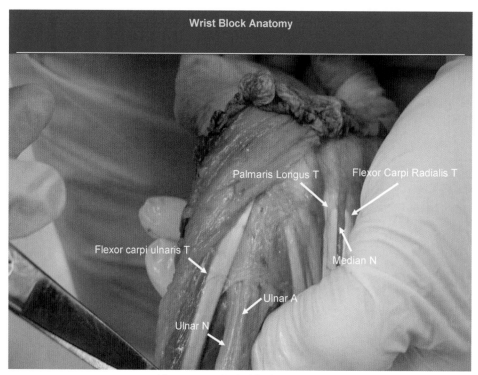

Figure 17.26: Wrist block anatomy.

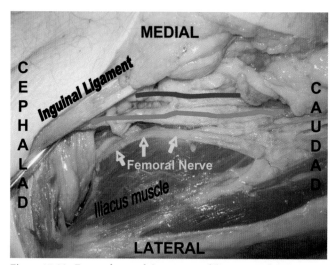

Figure 17.33: Femoral nerve lying on top of iliacus muscle as it passes under the inguinal ligament. Key: blue line = femoral vein; red line = femoral artery.

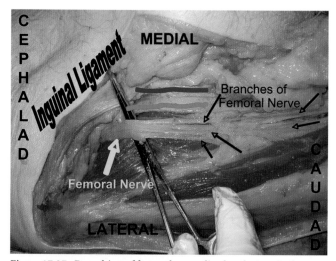

Figure 17.37: Branching of femoral nerve distal to the inguinal crease. Key: blue line = femoral vein; red line = femoral artery.

29. Redmond HP, Watson RW, Houghton K, et al. Immune function in patients undergoing open versus laproscopic surgery. *Arch Surg.* 1994;129:1240–1246.

30. Hume DM, Egdahl RH. The importance of the brain in the endocrine response to injury. *Ann Surg.* 1959;150:697–706.

31. Bromage PR, Shibata HR, Willoughby HW. Influence of prolonged epidural blockade and blood sugar and cortisol responses. *Surg Gynecol Obstet.* 1971;132:1051–1055.

32. Hagen C, Brandt MR, Kehlet H. Prolactin, LH, FSH, GH, and cortisol response to surgery and the effect of epidural analgesia. *Acta Endocrinol.* 1980;94:151–154.

33. Chernow B. Hormonal responses to a graded surgical stress. *Arch Intern Med.* 1987;147:1273–1278.

34. Allendorf JD, Bessler M, Kaylow ML, et al. Increased tumor establishment after laparotomy vs laparoscopy in a murine model. *Arch Surg.* 1995;130:649–653.

35. Georges C, Lo T, Alkofer B, et al. The effects of surgical trauma on colorectal liver metastasis. *Surg Endoscopy.* 2007;21:1817–1819.

36. Pavlin J, Chen C, Penaloza DA, Buckley P. A survey of pain and other symptoms that affect the recovery process after discharge from an ambulatory surgery unit. *J Clin Anesth.* 2004;16:200–206.

37. Wu C, Naqibuddin M, Rowlingson AJ, et al. The effect of pain on health related quality of life. *Anesth Analg.* 2003;97:1078–1085.

38. Tarhan S, Moffitt EA, Taylor WF, et al. Myocardial infarction after general anesthesia. *JAMA.* 1972;220:1451–1456.

39. Badner NH, Knoll RL, Brown JE, et al. Myocardial infarction after non cardiac surgery. *Anesthesiology.* 1998;88:572–578.

40. Breslow MJ, Jordan DA, Christopherson R, et al. Epidural morphine decreases postoperative hypertension by attenuating sympathetic nervous system hyperactivity. *JAMA.* 1989;261: 3577–3581.

41. Freeman LJ, Nixon PG, Sallabank P, et al. Psychological stress and silent myocardial ischemia. *Am Heart J.* 1987;114:477–482.

42. Willerson JT, Golino P, Eidt J, et al. Specific platelet mediators and unstable coronary artery lesions. *Circulation.* 1989;80:198–205.

43. Moulton AL, Greenburg AG. The pulmonary system. In: O'Leary JP ed. *The Physiologic Basis of Surgery.* Philadelphia, PA: William & Wilkins; 1993;512–514.

44. Sinatra RS, Ennevor S. Pain management following thoracic and upper abdominal trauma. In: Rosenberg AD, ed. *International Trauma Anesthesia and Critical Care Society.* Baltimore, MD: 1999.

45. Brown DL, Carpenter RL. Perioperative analgesia: a review of risks and benefits. *J Cardiothorac Anesth.* 1990;4:368–383.

46. Duggan J, Drummond GB. Activity of lower intercostal muscle function after upper abdominal surgery. *Anesth Analg.* 1987;66:852–855.

47. Beecher HK. The measured effect of laparotomy on the respiration. *J Clin Invest.* 1933;12:639–650.

48. Ali J, Weisel RD, Layug AB. Consequences of postoperative alterations in respiratory mechanics. *Am J Surg.* 1974;128:376–382.

49. Bessler H, Shavit Y, Mayburd E, et al. Post operative pain, morphine consumption and genetic polymorphism of IL 1B and IL receptor antagonists. *Neuroscience Lett.* 2006;404(1–2):154–158.

50. Flatters SJ, Fox AJ, Dickenson AH. Nerve injury alters the effects of interleukin-6 on nociceptive transmission in peripheral afferents. *Eur J Pharmacol.* 2004;484:183–191.

51. Meller ST, Gebhart GF. Nitric oxide (NO) and nociceptive processing in the spinal cord. *Pain.* 1993;52:127–136.

52. Thacker MA, Clark AK, Marchand F, McMahon SB. Pathophysiology of peripheral neuropathic pain: immune cells and molecules. *Anesth Analg.* 2007;105;838–847.

53. Kehlet H, Jensen TS, Woolf CJ. Persistent postsurgical pain: risk factors and prevention. Lancet 2006;367:1618–1625.

54. Sorkin LS, Xiao WH, Wagner R, Myers RR. Tumor necrois factor alpha induces ectopic activity in nociceptive primary afferent fibers. *Neuroscience.* 1997;81:255–263.

55. Kelly DJ, Ahmad M, Brull SJ. Pre-emptive analgesia II: recent advances and current trends.*Can J Anesth.* 2001:48(11):1091–1101.

56. Woolf CJ, Shortland P, Coggeshall RE. Peripheral nerve injury triggers central sprouting of myelinated afferents. *Nature.* 1992;355:75–78.

57. Jensen TS, Krebs B, Nielsen J, et al. Immediate and long-term phantom limb pain in amputees: incidence and clinical characteristics. *Pain.* 1988;21:267–278.

58. Woolf CJ, Chong MS. Preemptive analgesia-treating postoperative pain by preventing the establishment of central sensitization. *Anesth Analg.* 1993;77:362–379.

59. Mannion RJ, Woolf CJ. Pain mechanisms and management: a central perspective. *Clin J Pain.* 2000;16(suppl):144–156.

60. Perkins FM, Kehlet H. Chronic pain as an outcome of surgery: a review of predictive factors. *Anesthesiology.* 2000;93:1123–1133.

61. Pluijms WA, Steegers M, Verhagen A Scheffer GJ. Chronic postthoracotomy pain: a retrospective study. *Acta Anaesthesiol Scand.* 2006;50:804–808.

62. Diatchenko I, Slade GD, Nackley AG, et al. Genetic basis for individual variations in pain perception and the development of chronic pain conditions. *Hum Mol Genet.* 2005;14:135–143.

63. Mogil JS, Yu L, Basbaum AI. Pain Genes? Natural variation and transgenic mutants. *Ann Rev Neurosci.* 2000;23:777–811.

64. Reuben SS. Chronic pain after surgery: what can we do to prevent it. *Curr Pain Headache Rep.* 2007;11(1):5–13.

65. Katz J, Jackson M, Kavanaugh BP, Sandler AN. Acute pain after thoracic surgery predicts long term post thoracotomy pain. *Clin J Pain.* 1996;12:50–55.

66. Dihle A, Helseth S, Paul SM, Miaskowski C. The exploration of the establishment of cutpoints to categorize the severity of acute postoperative pain. *Clin J Pain.* 2006;22:617–624.

67. Kehlet H. Acute pain control and accelerated postoperative surgical recovery. *Surg Clin North Am.* 1999;79(2):431–443.

68. Beattie WS, Buckley DN, Forrest JB. Epidural morphine reduces the risk of postoperative myocardial ischemia in patients with cardiac risk factors. *Can J Anaesth.* 1993;40:523–541.

69. Liu S, Carpenter RL, Mackey DC, Thirlby RC, et al. Effects of perioperative analgesic technique on rate of recovery after colon surgery. *Anesthesiology.* 1995;83:757–765.

70. Tuman KJ, McCarthy RJ, March RJ, et al. Effects of epidural anesthesia and analgesia on coagulation and outcome after major vascular surgery. *Anesth Analg.* 1991;73:696–704.

71. Her C, Kizelshteyn G, Walker V. Combined epidural and general anesthesia for abdominal aortic surgery. *J Cardiothoracic Vasc Anesth.*1990;4(5):552–557.

72. Christopherson R, Beattie C, Meinert CL, et al. Perioperative morbidity in patients randomized to epidural or general anesthesia for lower extremity vascular surgery. *Anesthesiology.* 1993;79(3):422–434.

73. Akerman B, Arwenstrom E, Post C. Local anesthetic potentiates spinal morphine antinociception. *Anesth Analg.* 1988;67:943–947.

74. Dorman T, Clarkson K, Rosenfeld BA, et al. Effects of clonidine on prolonged postoperative sympathetic response. *Crit Care Med.* 1997;25(7):1147–1152.

75. Modig J, Borg T, Bagge L, Saldeen T. Role of extradural and general anesthesia in fibrinolysis and coagulation after total hip replacement. *Br J Anaesth.* 1983;55:625–631.

76. Rosenfeld BA, Beattie C, Christopherson R, et al. The effects of different anesthetic regimens on fibrinolysis and the development of postoperative arterial throbosis. *Anesthesiology.* 1993;79(3):435–443.

77. Lo B, Honemann CW, Kohrs R, et al. Local anesthetic actions on thrombxane-induced platelet aggregation. 2001;93(5):1240–1245.

78. Blomberg S, Emanuelsson H, Kvist H, et al. Effects of thoracic epidural anesthesia on coronary arteries and arterioles in patients with coronary artery disease. *Anesthesiology.* 1990;73:840–847.

79. Scott NB, Tufrey DJ, Ray DA, et al. A prospective randomized study of the potential benefits of thoracic epidural anesthesia and analgesia in patients undergoing coronary artery bypass grafting. *Anesth Analg.* 2001;93(3):528–535.

80. Royse C, Royse A, Soeding P, et al. Prospective randomized trial of high thoracic epidural analgesia for coronary artery bypass surgery. *Ann Thoracic Surg.* 2003;75(1):93–100.

81. Liu SS, Block B, Wu C. Effects of perioperative central neuraxial analgesia on outcome after coronary artery bypass surgery. *Anesthesiology.* 2004;101:153–161.

82. Bauer C, Hentz JG, Ducrocqx, et al. Lung function after lobectomy: a randomized, double blind trial comparing thoracic epidural ropivacaine/sufentanil and intravenous morphine for patient-controlled analgesia. *Anesth Analg.* 2007;105(1):238–244.

83. Jayr C, Thomas H, Rey A, et al. Postoperative pulmonary complications: epidural analgesia vs parenteral opioids. *Anesthesiology.* 1993;78:666–676.

84. Rodgers A, Walker N, Schung S, et al. Reduction of postoperative mortality and morbidity with epidural or spinal anesthesia. *BMJ* 2000;16;321(7275):1493.

85. Moller IW, Dinesen K, Sondergard S, et al. Effect of patient controlled analgesia on plasma catecholamine, cortisol and glucose concentrations after cholecystectomy. *Br J Anaesth.* 1988;61:160–164.

86. Wu CT, Jao SW, Borel CO, et al. The effect of epidural clonidine on prioperative cytokine response, postoperative pain and bowel function in patinets undergoing colorectal surgery. *Anesth Analg.* 2004;99(2):502–509.

87. Beilin B, Shavit Y, Trabekin, et al. The effects of postoperative pain management on immune response to surgery. *Anesth Analg.* 2003;97(3):822–827.

88. Samad TA, Moore KA, Saperstein A, et al. Interleukin 1-Beta mediated induction of Cox-2 in the CNS contributes to inflammatory pain hypersensitivity. *Nature.* 2001;410:471–475.

89. Ek M, Engblom D, Saha S, et al. Inflammatory response: pathway across the blood-brain barrier. *Nature.* 2001;410;425–427.

90. Kehlet H, Dahl JB: The value of "multimodal" or "balanced analgesia" in postoperative pain treatment. *Anesth Analg.* 1993;77:1048–1056.

91. Brandt MR, Fernandes A, Mondhorst R, et al: Epidural analgesia improves postoperative nitrogen balance. *Br Med J.* 1978;1:1106–1108.

92. Kawasaki T, Ogata M, Kawaski C, et al. Effects of epidural analgesia on stress induced immunosupression following abdominal surgery. *Br J Anaesth.* 2007;98:196–203.

93. Mastronardi L, Pappagallo M, Puzzilli F, Tatta C. Efficacy of the morphine-Adcon-L compound in the management of pain after lumbar microdiscectomy. *Neurosurgery.* 2002;50:518–524.

94. Ilfeld B, Morey T, Enneking FK. Continuous infraclavicular brachial plexus block for postoperative pain control at home. *Anesthesiology.* 2002;97:959–965.

95. Carli F, Mayo N, Klubien K, et al. Epidural analgesia enhances functional exercise capacity and health quality of life after colonic surgery. *Anesthesiology.* 2002;97:540–549.

96. Capdevila X, Bethelet Y, Biboulet P, et al. Effects of perioperative analgesic technique on the surgical outcome and duration of rehabilitation after major knee surgery. *Anesthesiology.* 1999;91:8–15.

97. Benedetti F, Vighetti S, Ricco C, et al. Neurophysiological assessment of nerve impairment in muscle sparing thoracotomy. *J Thorac Cardiovasc Surg.* 1998;115:841–847.

98. Sinatra RS, Boice J, Jahr J, Cavanaugh J, Reicin J. Multiple doses of rofecoxib in patients recovering from gynecological surgery: effects on pain intensity, morphine consumption, and bowel function. *Regional Anesth Pain Med.* 2006;31:134–142.

99. Reuben SS, Sklar J. Pain management in patients who undergo outpatient arthroscopic surgery of the knee. *J Bone Joint Surg Am.* 2000;82-A(12):1754–1766.

100. De Kock M, Levand'homme P, Waterloos H. Balanced analgesia: is there a place for ketamine? *Pain.* 2001;92:373.

101. Bach S, Noreng MF, Tjellden NU. Phantom limb pain in amputees during the first 12 months following limb amputation after preoperative lumbar epidural blockade. *Pain.* 1988;33:297–301.

102. Gottschalk A, Raja SN. Severing the link between acute and chronic pain: the anesthesiologists role in preventive medicine. *Anesthesiology.* 2004;101:1063–1066.

3

Patient Variables Influencing
Acute Pain Management

Joshua Wellington and Yuan-Yi Chia

Acute pain management is influenced by a number of patient variables that have been shown to affect the intensity, duration, and interpretation of pain, as well as the safety and efficacy of analgesic therapy. To develop an appropriate plan for acute pain management, factors such as patient age, race, sex, pharmacogenomics, and surgical or medical comorbidites must be considered. In general, traditional as-needed (PRN) dosing regimens have difficulty accounting for variabilities in analgesic response and interindividual differences in pain, perception, and coping skills. Patient variables also influence the safety and effectiveness of more modern and sophisticated forms of analgesic administration, such as patient-controlled analgesia (PCA), neuraxial opioids, and peripheral neural blockade (Figure 3.1).

The sections that follow identify and discuss patient-related factors known to influence analgesic dose requirement and analgesic response.

AGE

Age is among the most important patient variables influencing analgesic response.[1-4] Advancing age can alter analgesic dose response in several ways.[3,5-7] A decrease in hepatic enzymes, particularly cytochrome P450 (CYP450) microsomes and glucoronidases, as well as diminished hepatic blood flow, can reduce opioid and local anesthetic metabolism and delay drug elimination.[8] With regard to opioids, age-related reductions in plasma albumin may increase the fraction of unbound or active drug, whereas diminished pain transmission and central nervous system (CNS) activity may significantly reduce perception and subsequent processing of pain. Because of these factors, a negative correlation between age and postoperative opioid consumption is commonly observed. Age-related reduction in intravenous (IV) PCA opioid dose requirements have been observed in several clinical evaluations (Table 3.1).[3-5,7-11] Similar age-related reductions have been reported with epidural morphine (Figure 3.2).

Gagliese et al[7] observed that on the first postoperative day, young patients consumed an average of 66.6 mg of PCA with morphine, whereas older patients consumed an average of only 39.1 mg. Based on these findings, the authors suggested the following formula for determining the average morphine requirement based on patient age: Average postoperative 24-hour morphine use (mg) = 100 − age (years).

In subsequent studies, Gagliese et al[8,9] also observed that age differences in postoperative pain were scale dependent, with older patients exhibiting significantly lower scores compared with younger patients on the McGill pain questionnaire (MPQ) and present pain intensity (PPI), but not on the visual analog scale (VAS). The authors reported that VAS has insufficient sensitivity for detecting age differences in postoperative pain. Verbal descriptions of pain qualities were more sensitive in detecting these variables compared with nonverbal measures. Their studies also revealed that the decrease in opioid intake between postoperative day 1 and day 2 was greater among young patients than older patients.

It has been reported that young and elderly patients may be subjected to the same protocol for postoperative intravenous morphine titration with no significant increase in morphine-related adverse effects.[10] Moreover, it has been reported that elderly patients without cognitive deficits can attain similar levels of analgesia and were equally satisfied with pain control management as younger patients.[7]

Intact cognition is essential for optimal use of IV and epidural PCA. Several studies revealed that advancing age is associated with decreased self-administration of opioids,[2,7,10] possibly because elderly patients perceive less postoperative pain and are less willing or less able to use the PCA device. Inadequate analgesia was also previously found to be more frequent among elderly patients, findings that again may have been related to baseline cognitive deficits or acute postoperative confusional states.[11-14]

Pediatric analgesia in the acute pain setting may safely and effectively employ the use of PCA in children as young as 4 years old. This has been demonstrated in children who are experiencing acute postoperative pain as well as children with pain related to cancer and cancer treatments.[15-17] Anecdotally, if a young

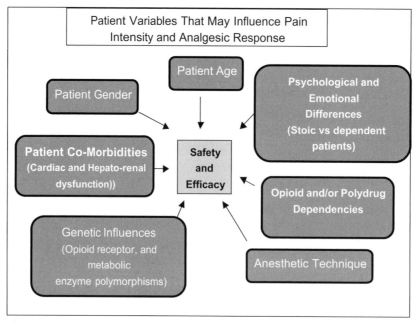

Figure 3.1: An overview of patient variables that influence pain perception, analgesic response, and analgesic safety.

child is able to play and understand the concept of video games, he or she will be able to successfully manage a PCA. PCA by proxy (ie, nurse or family member) may also be used in children with careful patient selection and education of proxy users. Serious adverse events or death may occur, especially if family members are not appropriately educated and inadvertently cause overdose by continuously administering demand doses.[18]

CULTURE OR RACE

Reaction to pain is a conditioned behavior that reflects the values of a given culture. Patients usually react in a manner related to how significant they consider the pain and how they have been taught to respond to it. Although it is impossible to make generalizations about the pain response of a specific patient group, appreciating such cultural conditioning can help health care providers assess and understand the pain experienced by a given person.[19–23] Cultural responses to pain may be classified into two major categories: the stoic, wherein patients minimize verbal expression of their discomfort, and the emotive, wherein patients are vocal in their response to pain.

Stoic patients, which include members of mainstream American culture, often behave in such a manner because of their desire to be thought of as "perfect patients" and thereby gain a sense of self-worth and self-esteem. Emotive patients, however, often verbalize their discomfort and continually ask for relief. The reasons for this behavior include fear, desire for attention, grief, and learned behavior.

With regard to the influence of cultural variables on opioid dosing, it has been noted that Asian American patients recovering from cholecystectomy required significantly less meperidine than native Hawaiians and whites.[19] In a PCA evaluation involving patients recovering from total abdominal hysterectomy, Parker et al[20] reported that African American women consumed significantly less morphine compared with age- and American Society of Anesthesiologists physical status-matched white counterparts.

Table 3.1: Intravenous Morphine Titration in Elderly Patients

Parameter	Young Patients (n = 875)	Elderly Patients (n = 175)
Age	45	76
Initial VAS (mm)	76	74
Dose IV morphine (mg)	10.8	9.5[a]
Morphine dose mg/kg	0.15	0.14[a]
Adverse events (%)	13	15

[a] Significant reduction in dose, $P < .05$; Auburn et al. Anesthesiology, 96:2002.

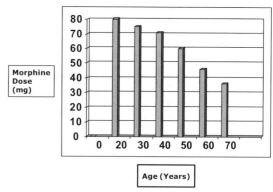

Figure 3.2: Age-related reductions in IV PCA morphine requirements in patients recovering from surgery. From: Burns JW, Hodsman NB, McLintock TT, et. al. The influence of patient characteristics on the requirements for postoperative analgesia. A reassessment using patient-controlled analgesia. *Anaesthesia.* 1989;44:2–6.[4]

Ng et al[21] observed that the patient's ethnicity has a greater impact on the amount of narcotics prescribed by the physician than on the amount of narcotics self-administered by the patient. They suggested that ethnicity itself influenced the way the physician perceived and treated pain. This disparity appears greatest in conditions wherein there are few objective findings, such as back pain, long bone fracture, and migraine.[21,22]

The effect of ethnicity on IV PCA prescribing and therapeutic response remain controversial. Some studies reported that African American and Hispanic patients are more likely to experience inadequate analgesia,[23,24] whereas other studies found no difference in opioid analgesic prescribing for African American and Hispanic children and for non-Hispanic white patients.[25-27]

SEX

The impact of sex on postoperative opioid requirements has yet to be clarified. Early investigations demonstrated gender-related differences in pain perception, morphine consumption, and effectiveness of morphine analgesia after surgery. In a study involving 4317 patients, Aubrun et al[28] concluded that women experienced more severe postoperative pain and required a greater dose (+11%) of morphine than men in the immediate postoperative period.[29] This was supported by a study by Cepeda and Carr,[29] which revealed that women require 30% more morphine to achieve a similar degree of analgesia to that of men.

Studies using models of experimental pain in mixed patient populations have presented conflicting results.[30] Olofsen et al[31] revealed that neither sex nor subject expectation (ie, placebo) contributes to the large variability in intersubject analgesic response to alfentanil. Fillingim et al[30] also found no sex-related differences in analgesic response to pentazocine. In a recent review, however, Pleym et al[32] revealed that males require 30% to 40% higher doses of opioid analgesics than females to achieve similar pain relief. In a survey of 2298 Chinese patients, Chia et al[33] also identified sex difference as the major predictor of PCA morphine consumption, with males requiring 23% to 43% more morphine than females (Table 3.2).

PSYCHOLOGICAL FACTORS

As previously stated, the response to pain is closely linked with cultural values, personality traits, and coping skills. Despite difficulties, the practitioner must resist the temptation to project his or her own cultural values and personality ideals onto others.

Early evaluations of psychological factors and their influence on acute pain revealed that highly anxious patients reported higher pain scores and required greater amounts of intramuscularly (IM) administered analgesics. Highly aggressive and angry patients also tended to consume more medication than patients whose coping styles are more passive.[34-37]

A study evaluating the importance of self-control expectancy in postoperative pain ($n = 126$) revealed that the expected emotional coping response is crucially related to the whole pain experience (intensity, latency, and duration). Self-control expectancy is associated with mastery behaviors in previous painful situations, vicarious experiences, and personality traits.[34] With regard to personality, a positive correlation between neuroticism and the ability to tolerate postoperative pain has been observed.[35] In a multivariate analysis model, preoperative neuroticism,

Table 3.2: Postoperative Measurements for Female and Male Patients

	Female	Male	Total
n (day 1)	1,444	854	2,298
VASM	4.9 ± 1.6	5.2 ± 1.3	5.2 ± 1.7
VASR	2.3 ± 1.3	2.3 ± 1.4	2.3 ± 1.5
Dose (mg)	15.3 ± 8.8	18.9 ± 8.9[a]	16.6 ± 9.0
n (day 2)	1,444	854	2,298
VASM	3.9 ± 1.4	4.7 ± 1.3[a]	4.3 ± 2.0
VASR	1.2 ± 1.1	1.6 ± 1.2	1.5 ± 1.3
Dose (mg)	23.2 ± 15.0	31.9 ± 12.4[a]	26.3 ± 13.6
n (day 3)	1,246	718	1,964
VASM	3.4 ± 1.1	4.3 ± 1.0	3.7 ± 1.6
VASR	0.9 ± 0.9	1.1 ± 1.1	0.9 ± 0.8
Dose (mg)	28.9 ± 17.3	41.4 ± 15.3[b]	32 ± 16.7

Note: Data were presented with mean ± SD or number; $n =$ case number.
[a] $P < .05$ compared with female group.
[b] $P < .01$ compared with female group.
From Chia et al. Can J Anaesth, 49 (2002), 249–255.[33]

sensitivity to cold pressure-induced pain, and age were identified as independent risk factors for early postoperative pain.[36]

Locus of control testing may be used to reveal adaptive responses to postoperative pain. The sense of control cited as a benefit for IV PCA and the overall effectiveness of self-administration dosing paradigms may be influenced by the patient's locus of control. Locus of control may be predominantly internal (within the person's control) or external (beyond the person's control).[35-38,39] Patients demonstrating an "internal" locus of control tend to be highly motivated and believe that an adverse situation can be ameliorated by active participation. In general, they do well with patient-controlled therapy that tends to restore some level of control in settings where most other aspects of care have been taken away from them. Individuals having an "external" locus of control tend to be poorly motivated and highly dependent on caregivers.[38,39] External localizers include individuals who believe in "powerful others," or that events are controlled by someone else, and those who believe in "chance," or that they have no ability to control events.[35,38] These patients may not appreciate nor achieve success with analgesic self-administration.[35,38-39]

Higher levels of internal control appear to negatively correlate with reported pain intensity scores. Thus if a patient with a predominantly internal locus of control is placed on PCA, his or her need for increased control is met, and, therefore, less anxiety and pain should be reported. For example, one study involving 76 women who underwent gynecologic surgery found that those who had an external locus of control had higher levels of pain and greater dissatisfaction with PCA. An internal locus of control was predictive of lower pain scores and increased satisfaction.[38]

A patient's ability to cope with an adverse surgical outcome also appears to influence pain scores and analgesic requirements. Patients recovering from exploratory laparotomy in which benign disease was found tended to self-administer less PCA opioids, while reporting higher satisfaction with pain therapy than age-matched individuals in which malignancy has been discovered.[39] In this setting, patients may request discontinuation of PCA in favor of IM sedation or analgesia.

SITE AND EXTENT OF SURGERY

The operative site, degree of surgical manipulation, and duration of surgery, as well as the intensity and duration of postoperative pain, may influence analgesic requirements. Surgical procedures in community hospitals are generally performed faster and with less surgical trauma than similar operations performed at training institutions. For this reason, postoperative pain scores, opioid requirements, and adverse events tend to be lower.[39]

Thoracotomies and nephrectomies are generally acknowledged as extremely painful procedures. Spinal fusion, upper abdominal surgery, and amputation also lead to severe postoperative pain.[39-41] Open procedures in orthopedic and urologic surgery result in moderate to severe pain. In contrast, patients receiving more superficial procedures such as herniorrhaphy and mastectomy generally report moderate pain and require lower doses of analgesics. It is generally assumed that endoscopic surgery minimizes tissue injury and is associated with lower postsurgical pain intensity scores than open procedures. The issue of whether an endoscopic surgery is less painful and requires lower doses of analgesics has been investigated. In one study, Soler Company et al[40] observed that open procedures are significantly more painful in orthopedic and urologic cases, whereas endoscopic procedures elicit more pain in benign gynecologic cases. The correlation of pain with the duration of the procedure is strongest for urologic surgery,[40,41] wherein severe pain rarely lasts more than 72 hours. However, consistently high pain scores were noted for more than 72 hours following thoracic surgery.[41]

A wide range of PCA opioid dose requirements has been reported in patients undergoing different orthopedic procedures.[39,41] Hip surgery patients were noted to require significantly less analgesics compared with patients who underwent total knee arthroplasty other open orthopedic procedures. The less invasive nature of hip surgery and the generally older age of patients undergoing this procedure are possible explanations.[39,41]

ANESTHETIC TECHNIQUE

Preemptive analgesia is a new concept suggesting that postoperative pain may be attenuated if pain transmission is blocked before the occurrence of noxious stimuli. Deafferentation by regional anesthesia prior to surgery, with or without general anesthesia, has been widely used to improve postoperative pain.[42-45] Numerous studies since the late 1990s have demonstrated a significant impact of preoperative epidural anesthesia or peripheral nerve blockade on decreasing postoperative pain. However, most of these studies failed to show a difference between general anesthesia and preemptive analgesia by regional blockade. This dilemma can be attributed to the definition of preemptive anesthesia as a form of treatment conducted prior to surgery, preventing the establishment of central sensitization caused by incision injury (covering only the period of surgery) and preventing the establishment of central sensitization caused by incision and inflammatory injuries (covering the period of surgery and the initial postoperative period). The result may be not significant if regional anesthesia is not continued during the postoperative period or if the effect of neural blockade is verified.[42-45]

In addition to other regional anesthesia techniques, the use of bupivacaine pain pumps may have unique utility in decreasing postoperative opioid requirements while maintaining appropriate analgesia. Cottam and colleagues[46] recently described the use of the ON-Q bupivacaine pain pump in patients undergoing laparoscopic Roux-en-Y gastric bypass. Forty patients were prospectively randomized into two groups. The first group received the ON-Q bupivacaine pain pump with catheters placed subxiphoid and radiating caudally beneath the lowest rib bilaterally. The second group did not receive the ON-Q bupivacaine pain pump. Each group was treated with meperidine PCA in the immediate postoperative period through the next morning (6 AM). The mean meperidine use by PCA was 129 mg in the ON-Q group versus 217 mg in the second group (40.5% reduction in opioid use, $P = .008$). Similar results have also been seen in patients undergoing thoracotomy,[47] inguinal hernia repair,[48] and mastectomy.[49]

PATIENT SIZE AND OPIOID PHARMACOKINETICS

Opioid analgesics are frequently administered on a milligram-per-kilogram basis; however, controversy exists regarding clinical correlations between body weight and individual dose requirement.[2,44,50-54] Of all patient variables, body weight and body surface area appear to have the least impact on opioid dose requirement and patient response.[1,2] In an early study, Tamsen and colleagues[2] found that total IV PCA was not influenced by weight or the rate of opioid elimination in age-matched patients recovering from similar surgical procedures. More recent studies have shown otherwise. Glasson et al[1] demonstrated that body weight and body surface area are significant predictors of postoperative opioid requirement. This was supported by the study of Macintyre and Jarvis,[54] which established that weight was a predictor of postoperative PCA morphine requirement. Nevertheless, both of these studies concluded that weight is a poor predictor of PCA morphine dose, and its influence is much less than that of age. Despite the lack of consistency in the above-mentioned studies, when administering opioids to obese patients, it would make sense to administer hydrophilic agents such as morphine according to their calculated lean body mass, whereas lipophilic opioids that distribute into adipose tissue may be dosed according to the patients' actual weight.

The relationship between opioid concentration and postoperative analgesia is best explained by two terms: maximum plasma concentration (MCP) associated with severe pain and minimum effective analgesic concentration (MEAC).[4,55-58] With PCA, patients at MCP can gradually increase plasma opioid concentrations and achieve MEAC. It must be recognized that the slope of the line between MCP and MEAC is quite steep. For example, a slight rise in plasma meperidine concentration by 0.05 μg/mL is all that separates effective from ineffective analgesia.[54] Self-administered opioid requirements necessary to maintain morphine and meperidine MEACs were 2.7 ± 1.1 mg/h and 26 ± 10 mg/h, respectively.[4,57] Patients utilizing PCA tend to establish and maintain MEAC, which oscillates around a mean steady-state serum concentration (C_{ss}) for each person.[4,53,57,58] Normally, the steady-state concentration reflects the ratio between drug dose and plasma clearance;

however, Tamsen et al[2,53] reported that plasma clearance and elimination rate constants were unrelated to individual hourly dose requirements among patients utilizing PCA for postoperative pain. They concluded that interindividual differences in opioid consumption could not always be explained by altered pharmacokinetics, but may reflect interindividual differences in pharmacodynamics.[53]

With regard to pharmacodynamic variability, relationships between CSF concentrations of endogenous opioids and the amount of exogenous analgesic required to maintain effective pain relief have been observed. Dahlstrom and coworkers[57] found that patients presenting with low CSF levels of β-endorphin required significantly greater amounts of PCA meperidine. These investigators observed a linear relationship between preoperative CSF concentrations of endogenous opioids and postoperative PCA demand doses and total opioid delivered.

GENE POLYMORPHISMS

As mentioned above, acute pain management is often complicated by interindividual variabilities and undesired effects of analgesics. Genetic polymorphisms are thought to play a larger role than previously realized in the interindividual variability of response to analgesics. A small, but growing, number of clinical trials have focused on the genes responsible for modulating the analgesic response to many commonly used medications.

A recent study revealed that women respond better to nalbuphine (a κ-opioid agonist) than to morphine (a μ-opioid agonist), whereas men respond better to morphine in the postoperative period,[58] suggesting the presence of sex-related differences in the opioid receptor system. Another study showed that the several single nucleotide polymorphisms (SNPs) identified in the human μ-opioid receptor gene, with the 118A>G mutation being the most common, might be associated with the clinical effects of opioid analgesics.[59,61]

In vitro, the binding of endorphin to the receptor of a homozygous G allele has been shown to be tighter by 3-fold compared with its binding to a homozygous A allele.[62] Moreover, a recent report suggested that cancer patients who were homozygous for the G118 variant required higher doses of oral morphine for long-term treatment of pain.[60] Romberg et al[63,64] studied the pharmacokinetics and pharmacodynamics of morphine-6-glucuronide (M6G), a μ-opioid agonist, and observed that A118G mutation of the human μ-opioid receptor gene also reduced analgesic responses to M6G. This genetic variation of the μ-opioid receptor was also associated with the different response of surgical pain to intravenous PCA morphine therapy. It might be warranted to extend these results to other ethnic groups.[65,66] In an recent review on the evidence for genetic modulation of analgesic response, Lötsch and Geisslinger[67] described that the 118A > G mutation of the μ-opioid receptor affected up to 17% of subjects in their response to alfentanil,[68] morphine,[69] M6G,[63,64] and levomethadone.[70]

The polymorphism of the human catechol-O-methyltransferase (COMT) gene has been found to influence the morphine requirements in cancer pain patients.[71] Dopamine, epinephrine, and norepinephrine are inactivated in the nervous system by COMT. Enzyme activity of COMT may vary 3- to 4-fold because of a common functional polymorphism (Val158Met). Patients with the Val/Val genotype needed more morphine in comparison to the Val/Met genotype and Met/Met genotype groups. Mogil and coworkers[72] found that polymorphism of the melanocortin-1-receptor (MC1R) may also affect morphine requirements in a small subset of patients. MC1R mutations may also affect pentazocine analgesic efficacy in women only.[73] Morphine requirements may also be affected by an SNP of 3435C>T in the ABCB1 (P-glycoprotein) gene.[74]

The cytochrome P450 2D6 (CYP2D6) is known to metabolize many drugs. The activity of CYP2D6 ranges from complete deficiency to ultrafast metabolism, depending on at least 16 different known alleles.[75] This may account for variation in metabolism for dextromethorphan, tramadol, and codeine, among other medications.

PATIENTS WITH HISTORIES OF SUBSTANCE ABUSE OR OPIOID DEPENDENCIES

Patients abusing heroin or diverted opioid analgesics experience the same intensity of acute postsurgical pain as nondependent individuals. Nevertheless caregivers tend to limit opioid administration in these patients. PCA is often withheld from these individuals, and neural blockade or epidural analgesic techniques are substituted because self-administered IV boluses may reinforce drug-seeking behavior.[39] More recent practice guidelines permit well-supervised PCA therapy for use by patients having a history of alcohol, cocaine, and heroin abuse. Opioid-dependent patients with a history of chronic pain and tolerance development also require increased amounts of opioids to compensate for both baseline requirements as well as that needed to control pain following surgery (see also Chapter 34, *Acute Pain Management in Patients with Opioid Dependence and Substance Abuse.*)

PATIENTS WITH ORGAN IMPAIRMENT OR FAILURE

Declines in cardiac, hepatic, and renal function are often associated with alterations in the volume of distribution, clearance, and excretion of most analgesic agents. For analgesics having high hepatic uptake and clearance, reductions in hepatic blood flow are accompanied by proportional decrements in the overall extraction rate and prolonged pharmacological effects.[76–80]

The patient with organ compromise or failure may present with unique considerations, depending on the analgesic to be administered. These patients may include those who have renal or hepatic impairment or failure or others recovering from nephrectomy and hepatic lobectomy. Analgesic efficacy may be altered not only by impaired clearance of the medication but also through the production and potential accumulation of metabolites which may be toxic. A classic example is accumulation of meperidine's renally cleared metabolite, normeperidine, which can precipitate CNS toxicity. A recent review of the impact of concurrent renal or hepatic disease on the pharmacology of the patient requiring acute pain management found specific differences in safety of the pharmacological profile among pain medications.[76,77] These differences are presented in Table 3.3. According to this table, there are a number of safer medications that can be used in patients with renal impairment as these drugs typically do not have a significantly prolonged clearance or deliver a high active metabolite load. Other medications may be used with caution wherein

Table 3.3: Pharmacological Safety Profile with Renal or Hepatic Impairment

Safest	*Require Precaution (ie, dose reduction)*	*Avoid*
	Renal impairment/failure	
Acetaminophen	Amitriptyline	Aspirin
Alfentanil	Bupivacaine	Dextropropoxyphene
Buprenorphine	Clonidine	Meperidine
Fentanyl	Gabapentin	NSAIDs
Ketamine	Hydromorphone	
Remifentanil	Levobupivacaine	
Sufentanil	Lidocaine	
	Methadone	
	Mexilitine	
	Morphine	
	Oxycodone	
	Tramadol	
	Hepatic impairment/failure	
Remifentanil	Other opioids	Amitriptyline
		Carbamazepine
		Dextropropoxyphene
		Meperidine
		Valproate

dose reduction is usually necessitated. Some drugs should not be used because of the high risk of toxicity. Although morphine remains primarily unaffected by renal failure, accumulation of morphine-6-glucuronide (an active metabolite that may induce CNS irritability) and morphine-3-glucuronide (inactive metabolite) have been reported.[78] Buprenorphine may provide analgesic efficacy in patients with renal failure requiring intermittent hemodialysis. Filitz and coworkers[79] recently found that buprenorphine and its metabolite norbuprenorphine were not elevated in plasma levels in chronic pain patients with end-stage renal disease. Additionally, hemodialysis did not affect buprenorphine plasma levels, allowing for stable analgesia.

When using pain medications in the patient with hepatic impairment, consideration must be given to the impaired clearance and increased oral bioavailability caused by a reduced first-pass metabolism. The primary metabolic pathway for most opioids is oxidation, which may be decreased in patients with hepatic cirrhosis. Morphine and buprenorphine are exceptions that primarily undergo glucuronidation. Although glucuronidation is thought to be less affected in hepatic cirrhosis, morphine clearance is still decreased and oral bioavailability increased.[80] Remifentanil is least subject to alteration because of its clearance by ester hydrolysis; however, its practicality in the acute pain setting may be limited. As fentanyl is more often used in the acute pain setting, consideration must be given for its metabolism by the P450 enzyme CYP3A4.[81] In patients with hepatic impairment or failure, elevated plasma fentanyl levels will occur. The analgesic activity of codeine is dependent on the P450 enzyme CYP2D6 to transform into the active metabolite of morphine. The analgesic efficacy of codeine will be decreased accordingly in patients with hepatic impairment.

The use of other opioids, such as hydromorphone and oxymorphone, may be considered with close patient monitoring.

As methadone has a very long half-life, it is contraindicated in patients with severe liver disease. Dextropropoxyphene has also been implicated in several cases of hepatotoxicity.[82]

To prevent cumulative increases in levels of analgesics,[82] but maintain therapeutic plasma concentrations, it is essential that the dose of drugs that undergo hepatic biotransformation or are eliminated by the kidneys be reduced. This can be accomplished by either decreasing the amount of each dose while maintaining the normal dosing schedule or by increasing the interval between doses while administering the standard size dose. Dosage adjustment is of critical importance if renal function is less than 50% of normal and the agent to be administered is to a great degree (>50%) excreted unchanged or has active metabolites that are primarily eliminated by the kidney.[39,77–79] Patients suffering congestive heart failure experience greater reductions in hepatic and renal perfusion than blood flow directed to the heart, lungs, and central nervous system. As would be expected both hepatic clearance/biotransformation and renal elimination of drug will be compromised, whereas delivery of free drug to the nervous system and heart may be increased.

CONCLUSION

Patient variables clearly influence analgesic dose requirements and analgesic response. Factors associated with the greatest reduction in analgesic requirement as well as potential toxicity include increasing patient age and hepatorenal dysfunction. Variables responsible for increased analgesic requirement and less effective pain control include opioid tolerance, more extensive surgery, and cultural influences. Cognitive deficits lead to reductions in both analgesic requirement as well as ineffective pain control. It seems likely that understanding and utilizing genetic polymorphisms that mediate receptor efficacy and drug metabolism will have clinical usefulness by either increasing analgesic sensitivity or diminishing toxicity. In the near future, oral and intravenous analgesic dosing and selection of optimal compounds may be facilitated by presurgical analysis of genetic markers. At present, elderly patients and those presenting with multiorgan failure have the most to gain from advances in neuraxial analgesic therapy and continuous neural blockade. Such therapy provides highly effective pain control and reduction in stress responses to pain, whereas at the same time reducing opioid burden and the deleterious effects of opioids on the CNS.

REFERENCES

1. Glasson JC, Sawyer WT, Lindley CM, Ginsberg B. Patient-specific factors affecting patient-controlled analgesia dosing. *J Pain Palliat Care Pharmacother.* 2002;16:5–21.
2. Tamsen A, Hartvig P, Fagerlund C, Dahlstrom B. Patient-controlled analgesic therapy. II. Individual analgesic demand and analgesic plasma concentrations of pethidine in postoperative pain. *Clin Pharmacokinet.* 1982;7:164–175.
3. Bellville JW, Forrest WH Jr, Miller E, Brown BW Jr. Influence of age on pain relief from analgesics: a study of postoperative patients. *JAMA.* 1971;217:1835–1841.
4. Burns JW, Hodsman NB, McLintock TT, et al. The influence of patient characteristics on the requirements for postoperative analgesia: a reassessment using patient-controlled analgesia. *Anaesthesia.* 1989;44:2–6.

5. Kaiko RF. Age and morphine analgesia in cancer patients with postoperative pain. *Clin Pharmacol Ther.* 1980;28:823–826.

6. Austin KL, Stapleton JV, Mather LE. Relationship between blood meperidine concentrations and analgesic response: a preliminary report. *Anesthesiology.* 1980;53:460–466.

7. Gagliese L, Jackson M, Ritvo P, et al. Age is not an impediment to effective use of patient-controlled analgesia by surgical patients. *Anesthesiology.* 2000;93:601–610.

8. Gagliese L, Weizblit N, Ellis W, Chan VW. The measurement of postoperative pain: a comparison of intensity scales in younger and older surgical patients. *Pain.* 2005;117:412–420.

9. Gagliese L, Katz J. Age differences in postoperative pain are scale dependent: a comparison of measures of pain intensity and quality in younger and older surgical patients. *Pain.* 2003;103:11–20.

10. Aubrun F, Monsel S, Langeron O, et al. Postoperative titration of intravenous morphine in the elderly patient. *Anesthesiology.* 2002;96:17–23.

11. Ready LB, Chadwick HS, Ross B. Age predicts effective epidural morphine dose after abdominal hysterectomy. *Anesth Analg.* 1987;66:1215–1218.

12. Portenoy RK, Kanner RM. Patterns of analgesic prescription and consumption in a university-affiliated community hospital. *Arch Intern Med.* 1985;145:439–441.

13. Faherty BS, Grier MR. Analgesic medication for elderly people post-surgery. *Nurs Res.* 1984;33:369–372.

14. Monk TG, Barker RK, White PF. Use of PCA in geriatric patients-effect of aging on the postoperative analgesic requirement. *Anesth Analg.* 1990;70:S272.

15. Ruggiero A, Barone G, Liotti L, et al. Safety and efficacy of fentanyl administered by patient controlled analgesia in children with cancer pain. *Support Care Cancer.* 2007;15:569–573.

16. Marchetti G, Calbi G, Vallani A. PCA in the control of acute and chronic pain in children. *Pediatr Med Chir.* 2000;22:9–13.

17. Collins JJ, Geake J, Grier He, Berde CB, et al. Patient-controlled analgesia for mucositis pain in children: a three-period crossover study comparing morphine and hydromorphone. *J Pediatr.* 1996;129:722–728.

18. Anghelescu DL, Burgoyne LL, Oakes LL, Wallace DA. The safety of patient-controlled analgesia by proxy in pediatric oncology patients. *Anesth Analg.* 2005;101:1623–1627.

19. Streltzer J, Wade TC. The influence of cultural group on the under-treatment of postoperative pain. *Psychosom Med.* 1981;43:397–403.

20. Parker RK, Perry F, Holtman B, et al. Demographic factors influencing the PCA morphine requirement. *Anesthesiology.* 1990;73:A818.

21. Ng B, Dimsdale JE, Rollnik JD, Shapiro H. The effect of ethnicity on prescriptions for patient-controlled analgesia for postoperative pain. *Pain.* 1996;66:9–12.

22. Tamayo-Sarver JH, Hinze SW, Cydulka RK, Baker DW. Racial and ethnic disparity in emergency department analgesic prescription. *Am J Public Health.* 2003;93:2067–2073.

23. Todd KH, Samaroo N, Hoffman JR. Ethnicity as a risk for inadequate emergency department analgesia. *JAMA.* 1993;269:1537–1539.

24. Todd KH, Deaton C, D'Adamo AP, Goe L. Ethnicity and analgesic practice. *Ann Emerg Med.* 2000;35:11–16.

25. Yen K, Kim M, Stremski ES, Gorelick MH. Effect of ethnicity and race on the use of pain medications in children with long bone fractures in the emergency department. *Ann Emerg Med.* 2003;42:41–47.

26. Fuentes EF, Kohn MA, Neighbor ML. Lack of association between patient ethnicity or race and fracture analgesia. *Acad Emerg Med.* 2002;9:910–915.

27. VanderBeek BL, Mehlman CT, Foad SL, et al. The use of conscious sedation for pain control during forearm fracture reduction in children: does race matter? *J Pediatr Orthop.* 2006;26:53–57.

28. Aubrun F, Salvi N, Coriat P, Riou B. Sex- and age-related differences in morphine requirements for postoperative pain relief. *Anesthesiology.* 2005;103:156–160.

29. Cepeda MS, Carr DB. Women experience more pain and require more morphine than men to achieve a similar degree of analgesia. *Anesth Analg.* 2003;97:1464–1468.

30. Fillingim RB, Ness TJ, Glover TL, et al. Experimental pain models reveal no sex differences in pentazocine analgesia in humans. *Anesthesiology.* 2004;100:1263–1270.

31. Olofsen E, Romberg R, Bijl H, et al. Alfentanil and placebo analgesia: no sex differences detected in models of experimental pain. *Anesthesiology.* 2005;103:130–139.

32. Pleym H, Spigset O, Kharasch ED, Dale O. Gender differences in drug effects: implications for anesthesiologists. *Acta Anaesthesiol Scand.* 2003;47:241–259.

33. Chia YY, Chow LH, Hung CC, et al. Gender and pain upon movement are associated with the requirements for postoperative patient-controlled iv analgesia: a prospective survey of 2,298 Chinese patients. *Can J Anaesth.* 2002;49:249–255.

34. Bachiocco V, Morselli AM, Carli G. *J Pain Symptom Manage.* 1993;8:205–214.

35. Cronin M, Redfern PA, Utting JE. Psychometry and postoperative complaints in surgical patients. *Br J Anaesth.* 1973;45:879–886.

36. Bisgaard T, Klarskov B, Rosenberg J, Kehlet H. Characteristics and prediction of early pain after laparoscopic cholecystectomy. *Pain.* 2001;90:261–269.

37. Snell CC, Fothergill-Bourbonnais F, Durocher-Hendriks S. Patient controlled analgesia and intramuscular injections: a comparison of patient pain experiences and postoperative outcomes. *J Adv Nurs.* 1997;25:681–690.

38. Johnson L, Magnani BJ, Chan V, Ferante F. Modifiers of patient-controlled analgesia efficacy: locus of control. *Pain.* 1989;39:17–22.

39. Sinatra RS, Preble L. Patient variables influencing acute pain management. In Sinatra RS, Hord A, Ginsberg B, Preble L, eds. *Acute Pain: Mechanisms and Management.* St. Louis, MO: Mosby; 1992.

40. Soler Company E, Faus Soler M, Montaner Abasolo M, et al. Factors affecting postoperative pain. *Rev Esp Anestesiol Reanim.* 2001;48:163–170.

41. Beaussier M. Frequency, intensity development and repercussions of postoperative pain as a function of the type of surgery. *Ann Fr Anesth Reanim.* 1998;17:471–493.

42. Nguyen A, Girard F, Boudreault D, et al. Scalp nerve blocks decrease the severity of pain after craniotomy. *Anesth Analg.* 2001;93:1272–1276.

43. Dunbar PJ, Visco E, Lam AM. Craniotomy procedures are associated with less analgesic requirement than other surgical procedures. *Anesth Analg.* 1990;88:335–340.

44. Egbert AM. Postoperative pain management in the frail elderly. *Clin Geriatr Med.* 1996;12:583–599.

45. Mahfouz AK, Nabawi KS. Preemptive analgesia in rhegmatogenous retinal detachment surgery: is it effective? *Retina.* 2002;22:602–606.

46. Cottam DR, Fisher B, Atkinson J, et al. A randomized trial of bupivicaine pain pumps to eliminate the need for patient controlled analgesia pumps in primary laparoscopic Roux-en-Y gastric bypass. *Obes Surg.* 2007;17:595–600.

47. Wheatley GH, Rosenbaum DH, Paul MC, et al. Improved pain management outcomes with continuous infusion of a local anesthetic after thoracotomy. *J Thorac Cardiovasc Surg.* 2005;130:464–468.

48. Sanchez B, Waxman K, Tatevossian R, et al. Local anesthetic infusion pumps improve postoperative pain after inguinal hernia repair: a randomized trial. *Am Surg.* 2004;70:1002–1006.

49. Morrison JE Jr, Jacobs VR. Reduction or elimination of postoperative pain medication after mastectomy through use of a temporarily placed local anesthetic pump vs. control group. *Zentralbl Gynakol.* 2003;125:17–22.

50. Aubrun F, Langeron O, Quesnel C, et al. Relationships between measurement of pain using visual analog score and morphine requirements during postoperative intravenous morphine titration. *Anesthesiology.* 2003;98:1415–1421.

51. Austin KL, Stapleton JV, Mather LE. Multiple intramuscular injections: a source of variability in analgesic response to meperidine. *Pain.* 1980;8:47–62.

52. Gil KM. Psychologic aspects of acute pain. *Anesthesiol Rep.* 1990;2:246–255.

53. Tamsen A, Hartvig P, Dahlstrom B, et al. PCA therapy in the early postoperative period. *Acta Anaesthesial Scand.* 1979;23:462–470.

54. Macintyre PE, Jarvis DA. Age is the best predictor of postoperative morphine requirements. *Pain.* 1995;64:357–364.

55. Rosenquist RW, Rosenberg J, United States Veterans Administration. Postoperative pain guidelines. *Reg Anesth Pain Med.* 2003;28:279–288.

56. Ferrante FM, Orav EJ, Rocco AG, Gallo J. A statistical model for pain in patient-controlled anesthesia and conventional intramuscular opioid regimens. *Anesth Analg.* 1988;67:457–461.

57. Dahlstrom B, Tamsen A, Paalzow L, et al. Patient-controlled analgesic therapy. IV. Pharmacokinetics and analgesic plasma concentrations of morphine. *Clin Pharmacokinet.* 7:266–279.

58. Gear RW, Miaskowski C, Gordon NC, et al. The kappa opioid nalbuphine produces gender- and dose-dependent analgesia and antianalgesia in patients with postoperative pain. *Pain.* 1999;83:339–345.

59. Lötsch J, Geisslinger G. Are mu-opioid receptor polymorphisms important for clinical opioid therapy? *Trends Mol Med.* 2005;11:82–89.

60. Klepstad P, Rakvag TT, Kaasa S, et al. The 118 A > G polymorphism in the human micro-opioid receptor gene may increase morphine requirements in patients with pain caused by malignant disease. *Acta Anaesthesiol Scand.* 2004;48:1232–1239.

61. Mantione KJ, Goumon Y, Esch T, Stefano GB. Morphine 6beta glucuronide: fortuitous morphine metabolite or preferred peripheral regulatory opiate? *Med Sci Monit.* 2005;11:MS43–MS46.

62. Bond C, LaForge KS, Tian M, et al. Single-nucleotide polymorphism in the human mu opioid receptor gene alters beta-endorphin binding and activity: possible implications for opiate addiction. *Proc Natl Acad Sci USA.* 1998;95:9608–9613.

63. Romberg R, Olofsen E, Sarton E, et al. Pharmacokinetic-pharmacodynamic modeling of morphine-6-glucuronide–induced analgesia in healthy volunteers: absence of sex differences. *Anesthesiology.* 2004;100:120–133.

64. Romberg RR, Olofsen E, Bijl H, et al. Polymorphism of mu-opioid receptor gene (OPRM1:118A/G) does not protect against opioid-induced respiratory depression despite reduced analgesic response. *Anesthesiology.* 2005;102:522–530.

65. Chou WY, Wang CH, Liu PH, et al. The human opioid receptor A118G polymorphism affects intravenous patient-controlled

66. Chou WY, Yang LC, Lu HF, et al. Association of mu opioid receptor gene polymorphism (A118G) with variations in morphine consumption for analgesia after total knee arthroplasty. *Acta Anaesthesiol Scand.* 2006;50:787–792.

67. Lötsch J, Geisslinger G. Current evidence for a genetic modulation of the response to analgesics. *Pain.* 2006121:1–5.

68. Caraco Y, Maroz Y, Davidson E. Variability in alfentanil analgesia may be attributed to polymorphism in the mu-opioid receptor gene. *Clin Pharmacol Ther.* 2001;69:63.

69. Skarke C, Lötsch J, Geisslinger G, et al. Analgesic effects of morphine and morphine-6-glucuronide in a transcutaneous electrical pain model in healthy volunteers. *Clin Pharmacol Ther.* 2003;73:107–121.

70. Lötsch J, Skarke C, et al. Modulation of the central nervous effects of levomethadone by genetic polymorphisms potentially affecting its metabolism, distribution, and drug action. *Clin Pharmacol Ther.* 2006;79:72–89.

71. Rakvag T, Klepstad P, Baar C, et al. The Val 158Met polymorphism of the human catechol-*O*-methyltransferase (COMT) gene may influence morphine requirements in cancer pain patients. *Pain.* 2005;116:73–78.

72. Mogil JS, Ritchie J, Smith SB, et al. Melanocortin-1-receptor gene variants affect pain and mu-opioid analgesia in mice and humans. *J Med Genet.* 2005;42:583–587.

73. Mogil JS, Wilson SG, Chesler EJ, et al. The melanocortin-1-receptor gene mediates female-specific mechanisms of analgesia in mice and humans. *Proc Natl Acad Sci USA.* 2003;100:4867–4872.

74. Baar C, Laugsand E, Rekvag T, et al. Genetic variation in the gene for P-glycoprotein: implications for the clinical efficacy of morphine. Abstract 11th World Congress of Pain. International Association for the Study of Pain. (2005) Program No. 1073-P515.

75. Sachse C, Brockmöller J, Bauer S, Roots I. Cytochrome P450 2D6 variants in a Caucasian population: allele frequencies and phenotypic consequences. *Am J Hum Genet.* 1997;60:284–295.

76. Murphy EJ. Acute pain management pharmacology for the patient with concurrent renal or hepatic disease. *Anaesth Intensive Care.* 2005;33:311–322.

77. Yogaratnam D, Miller MA, Smith BS. The effects of liver and renal dysfunction on the pharmacokinetics of sedatives and analgesics in the critically ill patient. *Crit Care Nurs Clin North Am.* 2005;17:245–250.

78. Davies G, Kingswood C, M. Street. Pharmacokinetcs of opioids in renal dysfunction. *Clin Pharmacokinet.* 1996;31:410–422.

79. Filitz J, Griessinger N, Sittl R, et al. Effects of intermittent hemodialysis on buprenorphine and norbuprenorphine plasma concentrations in chronic pain patients treated with transdermal buprenorphine. *Eur J Pain.* 2006;10:743–748.

80. Tegeder I, Lötsch J, Geisslinger G. Pharmacokinetics of opioids in liver disease. *Clin Pharmacokinet.* 1999;37:17–40.

81. Feierman DE, Lasker JM. Metabolism of fentanyl, a synthetic opioid analgesic, by human liver microsomes: role of CYP3A4. *Drug Metab Dispos.* 1996;24:932–939.

82. Bergeron L, Guy C, Ratrema M, et al. Dextropropoxyphene hepatotoxicity: four cases and literature review. *Therapie.* 2002;57:464–472.

4

Acute Pain: A Psychosocial Perspective

Francis J. Keefe

Our understanding of the psychosocial aspects of pain has advanced considerably since the early 1980s. Much has been learned about psychosocial factors that influence pain and psychosocial interventions that can enhance pain control.[1,2] Recently, there has been growing interest in applying the psychosocial perspective to enhance our understanding and ability to treat acute pain.

This chapter focuses specifically on psychosocial aspects of acute pain. The chapter is divided into four sections. The first section provides a conceptual background on psychosocial aspects of acute pain. The second section highlights research on the role of psychosocial factors in acute pain. The third summarizes the results of recent studies testing the efficacy of psychosocial interventions for acute pain. The chapter concludes with a discussion of future directions for work in this important area.

CONCEPTUAL BACKGROUND

Traditionally, acute pain has been understood using a biomedical model.[2] According to this model, acute pain is a warning signal that results from nociceptive input as a result of tissue damage or injury. In the biomedical approach, careful assessments are conducted to identify sources of tissue damage or injury that are causing pain. Medical and/or surgical interventions designed to correct or ameliorate underlying tissue damage or injury are then carried out to eliminate or reduce pain.[2] In the biomedical model, psychosocial factors play a secondary role in that they are viewed simply as responses to pain itself.

Although the biomedical model has been very influential in understanding and treating acute pain, its limitations have become increasingly clear since the late 1950s.[2] One problem with this model is that acute pain is not always proportional to the amount of tissue damage or injury. A classic study conducted by Beecher[3] at the Anzio beachhead found that 66% of wounded soldiers reported feeling no pain. Beecher reasoned that a psychological factor (e, the expectation that the wound would result in removal from the battlefield to a safe setting) tempered the experience of pain. Pain-free injuries have been noted not only in battlefield situations but also in civilian situations. In a study of 138 alert and oriented patients seen in an emergency room setting, Melzack et al[4] found that 37% reported feeling no pain at the time of injury. Delays in the onset of pain ranged from 1 to 9 hours. Taken together, the results of these studies suggest that the relationship between injury and pain is not as simple and straightforward as assumed by the traditional biomedical model.

Other limitations of the biomedical model include its failure to account for observations such as pain that returns and persists following neurosurgical lesions to pain pathways, variations in pain, or pain relief following the same treatments that occur in patients with very similar degrees of tissue pathology.[2,5] The biomedical model also fails to address the effects that psychosocial factors can have on the pain experience.

Growing recognition of the limitations of the traditional medical model, has spurred interest in alternative theories of pain. One of the most influential of these theories is Melzack and Wall's gate control theory.[6] The basic tenet of this theory is that there is a gating mechanism in the dorsal horn of the spinal cord that influences the transmission of noxious input from the periphery to the brain. Important from a psychosocial perspective is the notion that the action of the spinal gating mechanism is influenced, not only by peripheral input (ie, relative balance of large diameter and small diameter fiber input), but also by descending input from higher brain centers. The gate control theory proposes that, under certain circumstances (eg, exposure to danger, use of adaptive coping skills, or high levels of social support), neural processes in the brain can be activated in a way that closes the gate in the spinal cord and inhibits transmission of noxious signals to the brain. Under other circumstances (eg, when preoccupied with pain, depressed, or exposed to ongoing interpersonal stress), neural processes in the brain can be activated in a way that opens the gate and facilitates transmission of noxious signals to the brain. The gate control theory thus underscores that, through its influence on spinal gating mechanisms, the brain plays a crucial role in pain inhibition and facilitation.

The gate control theory was important because it provided a way of integrating psychosocial variables into our understanding and treatment of pain. In contrast to the traditional biomedical model, the gate control theory did not view psychosocial factors as simply responses to pain but rather as an integral component of pain processing.[5] The gate control theory not only stimulated laboratory and clinical research on the psychology of pain, it also led to heightened interest in the role that psychological interventions might play in managing acute and persistent clinical pain.[1]

More recently, Melzack[5,7] has proposed the neuromatrix theory of pain, a theory that builds on and extends concepts introduced in the gate control theory. Melzack had studied persons with total spinal sections who experienced phantom body pains (ie, pains that persisted despite a lack of clear-cut peripheral tissue pathology).[5] To account for such phenomena, he proposed that pain is produced by a "body-self neuromatrix," reflecting input from a network of widely distributed brain neurons. The neuromatrix consists of a network made up of neurons that loop between the thalamus and the cortex and the cortex and limbic systems. The neuromatrix theory states that the composition of the neuromatrix is initially determined by genetic background, but that it is subsequently modified by a person's sensory experiences. Although this theory recognizes sensory input as an important factor influencing pain, it maintains that sensory input represents only one of three major sources of neural inputs that affect the neuromatrix. The other two inputs reflect the activity of *cognitive-evaluative factors* (eg, tonic brain inputs resulting from learning and personality, phasic inputs resulting from attention and mood) and *motivational-affective factors* (eg, the hypothalamic-pituitary-adrenal system, immune system, and endogenous opiates). The neuromatrix theory also identifies three important neural outputs of the pain neuromatrix that can themselves influence pain. These outputs include brain programs responsible for *perception* (cognitive-evaluation, sensory-discriminative, and motivational affective dimensions of pain perception), *action* (involuntary and voluntary pain responses, coping strategies, and social communications of pain), and *stress regulation* (immune system activity, levels of cortisol, noradrenaline, cytokines, and endorphins). According to this theory, the loops of the neuromatrix network diverge (to allow parallel processing in cognitive-evaluation, sensory-discriminative, and motivational-affective inputs) and converge to allow interactions between the outputs of this parallel processing (ie, the perceptual, action, and stress-regulation programs).[7] The repetitive cyclical processing and synthesis of neural signals produces a characteristic pattern that is experienced by the individual as pain.

A major contribution of the neuromatrix theory is its emphasis on the role that stress and stress regulation systems play in the pain experience. Pain is not only a sensory phenomenon, but also a major stressor.[7] When pain is severe or prolonged it can alter homeostasis and trigger stress regulation responses designed to reinstate homeostasis (eg, release of cortisol, cytokines) that can heighten pain. Not surprisingly, the neuromatrix theory has provided a conceptual foundation for the growing emphasis on the use of skills that enhance control over stress in psychosocial protocols for managing pain.

In summary, although the biomedical model remains influential in the assessment and treatment of acute pain, there is growing recognition of its limitations. Since the mid-1960s, influential theories of pain have emerged (eg, the gate control theory and neuromatrix theory) that highlight the role that psychosocial factors can play in the acute pain experience.

PSYCHOSOCIAL FACTORS AND ACUTE PAIN

Converging lines of evidence suggest that psychosocial factors play an important role in the experience of acute pain. In this section, we consider four psychosocial factors that are among the most intensively studied in the context of acute clinical pain: anxiety, pain-related anxiety and fear, pain catastrophizing, and the social context.

Anxiety

Pain can be influenced by and, in turn, influence negative affect (eg, anxiety, depression, and anger).[1] Of the negative affects associated with acute pain, there is growing evidence that anxiety is the most important. Feeney,[8] for example, conducted a cross-sectional study examining the relationship of negative affect to acute pain in older adults. Participants in this study were 100 older patients (mean age = 79 years) who were recently (within 5 days) admitted to a rehabilitation unit after orthopedic surgery (e.g., hip or knee replacements). All participants completed a measure of pain along with five measures of negative affect (ie, measures of state anxiety, trait anxiety, depression, state anger, and trait anger). Multiple regression analysis was performed to examine the relative contribution of the five measures of negative affect in predicting pain. The results of the regression analysis revealed that state anxiety (i.e., transitory or situational anxiety) was the only variable that significantly contributed to the prediction of pain. State anxiety accounted for 27% of the variance in pain, whereas the combination of the other variables accounted for only 3.8% of the variance. Taken together, this cross-sectional study suggests that state anxiety may be the most significant contributor to acute postoperative pain in older adults recovering from orthopedic surgery.

One limitation of the Feeney study[8] was that it was cross sectional in nature (i.e., it assessed anxiety and pain at the same time). This makes it difficult to test the hypothesis that anxiety is a risk factor for acute pain. To rigorously test this hypothesis, one needs to conduct longitudinal research in which anxiety is assessed at the time of a baseline pain-free period and participants are then followed to assess their pain status after an event that is likely to cause pain (eg, surgery).

Several recent longitudinal studies have examined the relative importance of anxiety as a risk factor that might predict postoperative pain. For example, Carr et al[9] conducted a study that examined the influence of presurgical anxiety and depression on acute pain following major gynecological surgery. In this study, 85 women having gynecological surgery completed measures of anxiety and depression prior to surgery and were then followed to assess their pain status 2 days, 4 days, and 10 days following surgery. Data analyses revealed that 44.7% of the sample reported a high level of anxiety (score > 7) prior to surgery and that patients with high anxiety were significantly more likely to report high levels of pain on days 2, 4, and 10 following surgery. Only 11.8% of patients reported a high level of depression (score > 7) prior to surgery and patients with high depression were significantly more likely to report high levels of pain on only one of the postsurgical days examined (day 4). Taken together, these findings suggest that anxiety is common in patients undergoing major gynecological surgery and that anxiety measured prior to surgery shows a strong relationship to the subsequent development of postoperative pain.

Katz et al conducted a longitudinal study that examined how well presurgical anxiety and other emotional factors predicted acute pain following breast cancer surgery.[10] Prior to surgery, 109 women having breast cancer completed demographic measures and assessments of emotional functioning (state anxiety, depression, somatic preoccupation, and illness behavior). Two days after surgery measures of pain were collected. Data analyses revealed that state anxiety (ie, transitory or situational anxiety) was the only risk factor significantly ($P = .003$) associated with the risk of developing acute pain following surgery. The results of this study suggest that, when compared to other emotional factors, presurgical state anxiety is a very important risk factor for postoperative pain following breast cancer surgery.

Taken together, the studies reviewed in this section underscore the importance of anxiety in understanding acute pain. Anxiety is not only correlated with acute pain when both are assessed simultaneously but also an important risk factor for the subsequent development of acute pain. Anxiety is more strongly associated with the risk of developing acute pain than other negative affects (eg, depression or anger) or other emotional factors (eg, somatic preoccupation and illness behaviors). Finally, these studies suggest that state anxiety (ie, anxiety that is situational or transitory in nature) seems to be more important in understanding acute pain than trait anxiety (ie, anxiety that reflects a disposition or personality trait).

Pain-Related Anxiety and Fear

Given evidence of the importance of state anxiety in acute pain, it is not surprising that researchers have begun to focus on more specific aspects of anxiety that might be particularly relevant to how persons respond to acute pain. One potentially salient source of anxiety for persons at risk for acute pain is anxiety or fear about pain itself (i.e., pain-related anxiety and fear). A number of recent studies have examined the role of pain-related anxiety and fear in acute pain.

A good example of this research is a study by Aaron et al examining burn-specific pain anxiety (ie, anxiety regarding the anticipation of pain during or after medical procedures involved in the care for burns [eg, debridement]).[11] In this study, 27 patients with acute burn injuries completed a measure of burn-specific pain anxiety along with two other standard anxiety measures (a state anxiety measure and a mood measure of anxiety). All three anxiety measures were found to significantly predict total pain medication taken over 24 hours. The burn-specific pain anxiety measure, however, was clearly the best predictor of acute pain experienced during debridement procedures. Burn-specific pain anxiety also was the best predictor of physical functioning. These results suggest that anxiety measures that are specific to fears of pain may add something over and above measures of general anxiety in predicting pain and functioning in burn survivors.

To measure the range of anxiety symptoms specific to pain, McCracken, Zayfert, and Gross developed the Pain Anxiety Symptoms Scale (PASS).[12] The PASS has four subscales assessing (1) fear (fearful thoughts about pain or its consequences), (2) cognitive anxiety (cognitive symptoms related to pain such as racing thoughts or excessive preoccupation), (3) somatic anxiety (somatic symptoms such as sweating or heart speeding), and (4) escape/avoidance (overt behavioral responses such as trying to avoid all activities). The PASS mainly has been used in studies of persons with persistent pain,[12,13] where it has been found to predict higher levels of disability and interference due to pain.

A recent study by Thomas and France suggests that pain-related anxiety as measured by the PASS might be useful in understanding recovery from an acute pain experience (ie, low back injury).[14] In that study, a sample of 43 individuals who were within 3 weeks on an initial episode of low back pain completed the PASS at a baseline evaluation. At baseline and 3, 6, and 12 weeks later they also participated in an assessment session in which they completed a series of physical performance measures that involved reaching for three targets (high, middle, and low) at both high and low speeds. Data analyses revealed that participants with high levels of pain-related anxiety showed significantly smaller excursions of the lumbar spine during the reaches to all targets at 3 and 6 weeks. The authors observed that, when asked to perform reaches, participants with high pain-related anxiety adopted pain-avoidant postures that minimized motion of the lumbar spine. Their results suggest that anxiety about pain may alter movement patterns in a way that could impair recovery from an acute pain episode.

Excessive and irrational fears of movement and injury/reinjury (kinesiophobia) have been noted in persons experiencing pain.[15] In studies of persistent pain conditions (eg, chronic low back pain), kinesiophobia has been linked to increased pain, psychological distress, and physical disability.[15]

Given that acute pain often occurs in the context of an injury, kinesiophobia may also be relevant to understanding adjustment in persons with acute pain. Several recent studies have examined this possibility. In a cross-sectional study of 615 acute low back pain patients seen in primary care settings, Swinkels-Meewisse et al[16] found that individuals scoring high on a measure of kinesiophobia (the Tampa Scale of Kinesiophobia) had much higher levels of pain and physical disability. Buitenhuis et al[19] conducted a prospective study of 590 individuals who developed neck pain symptoms following a whiplash injury caused by a car crash.[17] All participants completed a measure of kinesiophobia at baseline and were followed up for assessments of their neck symptoms 6 and 12 months later. Data analyses revealed that those with higher baseline levels of kinesiophobia were much more likely to experience longer durations of neck symptoms such as pain.

Swinkels-Meewisse et al[18] also conducted a prospective study testing the predictive utility of kinesiophobia in explaining recovery from acute low back pain.[18] In this study, 555 patients with acute low back pain (pain < 4 weeks) completed a baseline measure of kinesiophobia and underwent follow-up evaluations of their pain and functional status 6 weeks and 6 months later. Data analysis showed that the baseline measure of kinesiophobia was the strongest predictor of functional disability, even stronger than baseline pain severity.

In sum, anxieties and fear about pain itself seem to be important in explaining the short- and long-term pain and disability experienced by persons having acute pain. The precise mechanisms underlying the effects of pain-related anxiety and fear on acute pain are not known. However, evidence suggests that persons with high pain-related anxiety or fear avoid movements and activities that are important to the process of recovering from acute pain[14,19] When such avoidance patterns become entrenched, they can lead to disuse, deconditioning, and high levels of physical and psychological disability, all of which can increase the risk of persistent pain.[15]

Pain Catastrophizing

Pain catastrophizing has been found to be one of the most important psychosocial predictors of pain and adjustment to pain.[20] Pain catastrophizing has been defined as the tendency to ruminate on and magnify pain sensations and to feel helpless when confronted with pain.[20] Although there is a large and growing literature on pain catastrophizing, most of the research has been conducted in studies of chronic pain and experimental pain. In these studies, higher levels of pain catastrophizing have been associated with higher levels of pain, psychological distress, analgesic intake, pain behavior, and physical disability.[20]

Is catastrophizing relevant to acute clinical pain? Two recent studies have examined the predictive utility of pain catastrophizing in persons undergoing surgery. Pavlin et al[21] tested whether pain catastrophizing could predict postsurgical pain in persons undergoing anterior cruciate ligament (ACL) repair. Participants, 48 surgical candidates, completed a pain-catastrophizing measure prior to undergoing ACL surgery. Measures of pain and analgesic intake were then collected 1, 2, and 7 days after surgery. Results demonstrated that pain catastrophizing was a significant predictor of postoperative pain. Patients who scored high on pain catastrophizing reported 33% to 74% higher levels of maximum pain and were significantly more likely to report pain on walking than those who scored low on pain catastrophizing.

Strulov et al[22] recently tested the relative importance of pain catastrophizing and responses to experimental pain stimuli in predicting pain after elective cesarean section. Participants, 47 women who were scheduled for elective cesarean sections, completed a pain catastrophizing measure and rated a series of painful experimental heat stimuli prior to surgery. Pain ratings and measures of analgesic intake were then collected from all participants on day 1 and day 2 following their surgery. Multiple regression analysis was conducted to examine the relative importance of pain catastrophizing and ratings of experimental pain in predicting postsurgical pain. These analyses revealed that preoperative ratings of experimental pain were a significant predictor of pain on day 1 after surgery and that pain catastrophizing was a significant predictor of pain on day 2 after surgery. Neither pain catastrophizing nor ratings of experimental pain predicted analgesic intake.

Like pain-related fear, pain catastrophizing may be important in explaining disability resulting from acute pain conditions such as low back pain. Swinkels-Meewisse et al[18] conducted a study of acute low back pain patients in which they examined the relative importance of pain catastrophizing and pain-related fear (kinesiophobia) in predicting physical performance and self-reported disability. Participants, 96 individuals with an acute episode of low back pain, completed a self-report measure of physical disability (the Roland Disability Questionnaire) and then were timed as they performed a dynamic lifting task (lifting a 7-kg bag from the floor to the table and then back to the floor). Regression analyses demonstrated that, even after controlling for demographic variables and pain intensity, both pain catastrophizing and pain-related fear were significant predictors of self-reported disability. Pain-related fear, however, was the only factor that was a significant predictor of actual physical performance during the lifting task.

Physical examination is an important component in any assessment of acute pain. Can catastrophizing influence the results of a clinical examination? Although this possibility has not been examined in the context of acute pain, a recent study by Turner et al[23] tested it in the context of a chronic pain condition (pain related to temporamandibular disorders [TMD]). In this study, 338 patients with TMD completed a series of measures assessing pain, pain-related activity interference, health care use, and depression and underwent a clinical examination from an oral medicine specialist. Study results showed that pain catastrophizing was not related to clinical examination measures considered to be more objective (ie, measures of maximum assisted jaw opening or jaw joint sounds). Pain catastrophizing, however, was significantly related to clinical examination measures considered to have a more subjective component (ie, extraoral muscle site palpation pain severity and joint site palpation pain severity). What makes these findings regarding the effects of pain catastrophizing on clinical examination findings particularly impressive is that they were obtained even after controlling for demographic variables, pain duration, and depression severity.

The studies reviewed above suggest that pain catastrophizing may be a risk factor for acute pain and may be related to self-reports of physical disability in persons suffering from acute pain. The findings of these studies also suggest that pain catastrophizing may show a stronger relationship to more subjective measures of adjustment to pain (eg, self-reports of pain/disability and physical exam findings based on self-report) than to more objective measures (eg, analgesic intake, physical performance, or physical exam findings that are less reliant on self-report). This raises the possibility that the effects of pain catastrophizing on acute pain may be related to the way that pain is processed, perceived, and responded to emotionally.

Brain-imaging studies provide one way of examining this intriguing hypothesis. An example of the type of imaging study that could be conducted in acute pain conditions is a functional magnetic resonance imaging (fMRI) study conducted by Gracely et al.[24] In this study, fMRI was used in 29 fibromyalgia patients to assess their brain responses to acute pain stimuli (blunt pressure stimuli). Results showed that high levels of pain catastrophizing were associated with increased activity in brain regions related to the anticipation of pain (eg, medial frontal cortex and cerebellum), attention to pain (eg, dorsal anterior cingulate cortex and dorsolateral prefrontal cortex), and emotional responses to pain (eg, claustrum and closely connected to the amygdala). These findings suggest that pain catastrophizing may alter perceptions of pain by modifying neural processes related to attention to pain, anticipation of pain, and increased emotional responding.

Social Context

Acute pain occurs in a social context that often includes family, friends, and health care providers. There is growing evidence that pain not simply has an impact on those in the social context, but that it also can be influenced by its social context.

Witnessing a loved one experiencing acute pain is a difficult and stressful experience. Facial expressions of pain, in particular, can have a powerful impact on others. Botvinick et al[25] used fMRI to study the neural responses of pain-free observers to videotapes of persons experiencing moderate pain versus no pain. They found that when participants viewed facial expressions of moderate pain, they showed increased brain activity in areas known to be involved in the actual experience of pain (eg, anterior insula and anterior cingulate cortex). Thus, witnessing pain in another can produce an increase in neural activity in cortical areas related to the first-hand experience of pain.

Saarela et al[26] conducted an fMRI study in which they had pain-free observers view photographs of faces of chronic pain patients whose pain was transiently increased. After viewing each photo, the observers were asked to estimate the amount of pain the patient experienced. Analysis of the fMRI data showed that viewing the pain faces produced increases in observers' levels of neural activity in regions of the brain involved in the pain experience (ie, the bilateral anterior insula, left anterior cingulate cortex, and left inferior parietal lobe.) In addition, the level of brain activation in the observer corresponded to their estimates of pain in the patient. Observers showed high levels of brain activation when they estimated the patients' pain intensity as high and low levels of brain activation when they estimated the patients' pain intensity as low. Finally, the observers ratings of their own emotional empathy were found to correlate with the strength of brain activations that occurred in response to viewing the pain faces (specifically in the left anterior insula and left inferior frontal gyrus).

The results of these recent fMRI studies support the notion that there are sensory neural mirroring mechanisms that may support the understanding of other's pain and suffering. From an evolutionary perspective, the ability to detect pain and respond appropriately to others in pain has survival value.[27] Clinically, acute pain may elicit a variety of responses from others, including reassurance, sympathy, or encouragement to use pain-coping strategies. These responses, in turn, may influence the pain and distress experienced by the individual having acute pain.

The vast majority of studies on the social context of acute pain have been conducted in children undergoing painful medical procedures. In these studies, child-parent or child-staff interactions have been directly observed and coded. Data analyses have then been conducted to determine how parental or staff behaviors relate to children's distress. In a study of 77 preschool children undergoing immunizations, Frank et al[28] found that maternal behaviors predicted 53% of the distress in children's behavior. Interestingly, reassurance behaviors commonly used by parents (eg, "You can do this" and "Don't worry") were associated with much higher levels of child distress. Although this finding seems counterintuitive, the link between reassurance and higher levels of child distress has been reported in a number of studies.[29] Three mechanisms have been proposed to explain the link between reassurance and increased pain/distress[29]: (1) such responses serve as a warning that orients the person to pain or distress, (2) such responses reinforce apprehension and distress behaviors, and (3) such responses release the expression of negative emotions that otherwise might not be expressed.

To date, the most rigorous observational study of the relationship of adult behavior to children's coping during a painful medical procedure has been conducted by Blount et al.[30] This study focused on 23 children (aged 5 to 13 years) having acute lymphocytic leukemia who were undergoing bone marrow aspirations and lumbar puncture procedures. Audiotapes were made during the procedures and written transcriptions made of the verbal interactions between the child and adults who were present (eg, parents, nurses, residents). These transcripts were then systematically coded by trained observers to assess both child and adult behaviors. Sequential lagged analyses were conducted to determine how behaviors exhibited by adults related to subsequent distress and coping behaviors on the part of the child. Findings showed that adults' reassurance, apologizing,

criticizing, and giving control to the child significantly increased the likelihood of childhood distress. In contrast, encouraging the child to use coping procedures, talking about unrelated topics, or directing humor to the child significantly increased the likelihood the child would engage in coping behaviors. These findings underscore the important role that adults can play in influencing children's experiences during painful medical procedures. They also highlight the fact certain parental/staff responses commonly thought to be helpful to children (eg, reassurance, giving control to the child), in fact, can increase distress, whereas other responses (eg, humor, talking about other topics) can reduce distress.

The results of a recent study by Lang et al[31] suggests that similar phenomena may occur in adults undergoing invasive procedures. In this study, videotapes were made of 159 patients undergoing potentially painful procedures (eg, administration of local anesthetic, percutaneous puncture/catheter insertion, tract or vessel dilatation, and intravascular injection of contrast medium). All statements made by health care providers during the videotapes were transcribed and coded by trained observers. The observers coded two categories of behavior: (1) warning statements that the upcoming procedure would be painful or undesirable and (2) expressions of sympathy after a potentially painful procedure. Patients also provided ratings of their own pain and anxiety during and after the procedures on scales from 0 to 10. Data analyses revealed that when health care professionals warned the patient about pain, the patient experienced significantly higher levels of pain as compared to when they did not warn. When health care professionals sympathized with patients about their pain, the patient experienced higher levels of anxiety but not pain.

Considered as a whole, the studies reviewed above reinforce the notion that, although acute pain is a private event, it does influence and is influenced by others. Witnessing acute pain in another activates empathic neural processes that likely play a key role in determining the responses of loved ones and health care providers to acute pain. Although certain empathic responses to acute pain (eg, reassurance) are common in patients' significant others, they may paradoxically increase pain and distress. In contrast, other common responses (eg, distraction or humor) may actually help decrease distress in persons experiencing acute pain.

PSYCHOLOGICAL INTERVENTIONS FOR ACUTE PAIN

Evidence that psychosocial factors can influence pain has helped spur the development of a number of psychosocial protocols for managing acute pain. In this section, we highlight studies testing the efficacy of four psychosocial interventions for managing acute pain: (1) distraction, (2) cognitive-behavioral therapy, (3) hypnosis, and (4) virtual reality.

Distraction

There is a growing consensus that distraction is one of the most important psychosocial strategies for managing pain. Distraction is believed to work because it uses up cognitive resources that otherwise might be devoted to pain.[32]

Distraction has been found to be particularly effective in children. Sparks,[33] for example, tested the efficacy of two distraction techniques on the pain experienced by children undergoing a diptheria-tetanus-pertussis injection. A sample of 105 children ranging in age from 4 to 6 years was randomly assigned to one of two distraction conditions (touch or bubble blowing) or to a standard care control condition. Children in the touch condition were given light skin stroking near the injection site just before and after the injection. Children in the bubble blowing condition were encouraged to blow bubbles during the injection. Data analyses revealed that, when compared to the standard care condition, both touch and bubble blowing produced significant decreases in pain. This study shows that distraction interventions that are inexpensive, easy to use, and well accepted by young children can produce significant reductions in injection pain.

In managing injection pain in children, are certain forms of distraction more effective than others? MacLaren and Cohen[34] compared distraction that required an overt response (interactive toy) with a passive distraction (movie watching). Participants, 88 young children (aged 1 to 7 years), were randomly assigned to one of three conditions: (1) playing with one of two age-appropriate interactive toys (eg, a toy robot that made sounds, played music, and moved when buttons were pressed), (2) watching an age-appropriate movie (eg, *Toy Story 2*, *The Little Mermaid*) on a hand-held DVD player, or (3) standard care. Distress was measured using parent and nurse reports and direct observations of children's level of distraction were made before, during, and after the injection. Results indicated that children in the passive condition not only appeared to be more distracted on observation, but also were rated as less distressed than children in the interactive condition. Children in the interactive toy condition were rated as showing no differences in distress from those in the standard care condition, although on observation they appeared to be significantly more distracted. These results are somewhat surprising in that one might expect that tasks requiring a response from a child would be more distracting and thus more effective in reducing distress during a painful procedure than those not involving such task demands. Nevertheless, this study underscores the potential of high-quality visual materials (eg, Hollywood-made movies) in distracting children from acute pain.

As noted earlier, reassurance is a common behavior exhibited by parents responding to distress in children undergoing acutely painful medical procedures. Manimala, Blount, and Cohen conducted one of the few direct experimental comparisons of reassurance and distraction in the management of acute pain in children (ages 3 to 6).[35] In this study, 82 parent-child dyads were assigned randomly to one of three conditions: reassurance, distraction, or attention control. Parents assigned to the reassurance condition were asked to provide reassurance in ways that they usually do with their child before, during, and after the injection. Parents assigned to the distraction condition were encouraged to play with their children with toys and to talk about nonmedical topics prior to the injection. They were also taught to encourage the child to use a party blower immediately before, during, and after the injection. Parents in the attention control condition spent time talking with an experimenter regarding the child's medical history and how the child usually handles painful medical procedures. Data analyses revealed a number of significant between-group differences in the treatment conditions. First, children in the distraction condition exhibited the lowest level of distress. Second, children in the reassurance group were much more likely to need to be restrained during the

procedure than children in the distraction and control groups. Finally, parents in the reassurance group were significantly more distressed after the procedure than parents in the distraction or control groups. Taken together, these findings reinforce the notion that reassurance is not a very effective strategy for managing pain during injections in children and that distraction techniques can provide benefits for both children and their parents.

How does distraction compare to the effects of topical anesthetics that are now being widely used in managing pain that occurs during injections of children? Cohen et al[36] conducted a study in which they compared the effects of a nurse-directed distraction intervention, an anesthetic (eutectic mixture of local anesthetics [EMLA]), and typical care. Participants, 39 fourth-grade children undergoing a series of immunizations were exposed to both experimental interventions using a within subjects design. The order of interventions was randomly determined. In the distraction intervention, a nurse assisted the child to select a movie to watch and encouraged the child to focus on the movie before, during, and after the immunization. Videotaped records of each immunization were taken and later coded for signs of child distress and coping behaviors. Data analyses revealed that the distraction intervention produced significant reductions in distress and increases in coping behavior. In contrast the EMLA intervention had no effects on children's distress or coping behaviors. The authors conclude that a nurse-assisted intervention can decrease child distress and increase coping behavior in children undergoing a painful medical procedure.

Overall, the findings of the distraction studies reviewed above are in line with the results of two meta-analyses that have examined the effects of distraction on pain and distress in children undergoing painful medical procedures. The first meta-analysis included studies testing the effects of distraction in a range of painful medical procedures and reported that distraction had a mean effect size of 0.62 for pain and a mean effect size of 0.33 for distress.[37] The second meta-analysis focused specifically on needle-related procedures and reported that distraction produced a mean effect size of 0.24 for pain.[38]

Cognitive-Behavioral Therapy

The term cognitive-behavioral therapy (CBT) is used to describe multicomponent psychosocial interventions. CBT interventions for acute pain are more comprehensive than simple distraction interventions and rely on combinations of techniques such as distraction, relaxation training, positive self-talk, imagery, and reinforcement. A good example of a multicomponent CBT protocol is that used in a study by Manne et al.[39] That study examined the efficacy of CBT in reducing child and parent distress during a venipuncture procedure in children having cancer who required multiple venipunctures. All children in this study had previously shown difficulty coping with acute venipuncture pain in that they had required physical restraint during a prior venipuncture. The CBT protocol tested combined four major components: distraction (slow blowing with a party blower), parental involvement, positive reinforcement (stickers of cartoon characters), and therapist coaching. Role playing with therapist coaching was used prior to the procedure and the therapist was present during the first venipuncture to systematically teach the parents and children how to best use the CBT techniques. Children in this study ($N = 23$, aged 3 to 9 years) and their parents were randomly assigned to the CBT protocol or an attention control intervention that encouraged parents to use whatever techniques they thought might help the child. Measures of child and parent distress and ratings of pain were obtained over the course of a series of three venipuncture procedures. Data analyses revealed that, when compared to attention control, the CBT protocol produced significant reductions in observations of children's distress, parents' ratings of the child's distress, and parents' ratings of their own distress. The CBT protocol also significantly reduced the use of physical restraint. The CBT protocol yielded no significant reductions in children's reports of pain, however. The authors speculated that this was possibly because the party blower was not as potent a distractor as had been used in other studies (eg, watching movies.)

Jay et al[40] compared CBT to general anesthesia in reducing distress in children with leukemia who were undergoing painful bone marrow aspiration (BMA) procedures. All children were studied over the course of two BMAs. Prior to one BMA they received CBT and prior to the other they received a short-acting mask anesthesia. The order of these treatments was randomly determined and counterbalanced across subjects. The CBT protocol involved filmed modeling of coping skills (eg, coping self-statements, use of slow breathing, and imagery), rehearsal with breathing and imagery exercises, and positive reinforcement (eg, a small trophy). The anesthesia consisted of halothane adjusted as indicated to maintain light anesthesia and prevent movement. To assess treatment effects, the investigators collected direct observations of child and parent distress during the BMAs, as well as child ratings of pain and fear and parent ratings of anxiety and coping difficulty. The results indicated that the effects of CBT and general anesthesia were quite similar. Both interventions produced reductions in childrens' ratings of pain and fear and parent ratings of their own anxiety and coping difficulties. Taken together, these results suggest that CBT and general anesthesia are both viable alternatives to managing pain and distress in children undergoing painful procedures.

Liossi and Hatira[41] conducted a study that compared the effects of CBT and hypnosis on acute pain. Participants, 30 children (aged 5 to 15 years) with leukemia who had to undergo two BMAs as part of their medical treatment protocol, were randomly assigned to receive a multicomponent CBT protocol, a hypnosis intervention, or standard treatment. At baseline and following treatment, the investigators collected measures of child reported pain and anxiety and nurse ratings of child behavioral distress. Data analyses revealed that the children who received either CBT or hypnosis reported significantly less pain and anxiety than children in the control condition. Although there were no significant differences in the effects of CBT and hypnosis on pain, hypnosis was more effective than CBT in reducing anxiety and distress. Taken together, these findings support the efficacy of CBT in managing pain and anxiety during BMA. They also suggest that, during BMA procedures, hypnosis may be even more effective than CBT in the control of anxiety and behavioral distress.

The evidence reviewed above and from a recent meta-analysis by Uman et al[38] suggest that CBT interventions for acute pain can be effective, particularly in reducing behavioral distress during BMAs. These interventions, however, are more time intensive than other psychosocial treatments (eg, simple distraction) and their effects may not be superior to those of other medical treatments (eg, general anesthesia) or psychosocial treatments (eg, hypnosis).

Hypnosis

The term *hypnosis* has been used to describe interactions in which an individual responds to suggestions from a therapist (hypnotist) in a way that alters perception, memory, or actions.[42] Although hypnosis has been used for the relief of pain for over 100 years, early reports of its effects were primarily anecdotal and uncontrolled in nature. Rigorous controlled studies of the effects of hypnosis on acute clinical pain are a relatively recent development.[42]

Lang et al[43] conducted a randomized clinical trial to test the effects of hypnosis in managing acute pain in patients undergoing percutaneous diagnostic and therapeutic vascular and renal procedures.[43] Participants, 241 persons ranging in age from 18 to 92 years, were randomly assigned to one of three conditions: structured attention, structured attention plus hypnosis, or standard care control. For patients in the structured attention condition, a therapist was present during the procedure who engaged in interventions designed to structure the patient's attention (eg, attentive listening, provision of the perception of control, encouragement, use of neutral descriptions, or avoiding negatively loaded suggestions). For patients in the structured attention and hypnosis condition, the therapist provided the same attentional structuring, but also guided the patient through a self-hypnosis script that included instructions in relaxation and imagery. The treatment protocols were well standardized and featured structured treatment manuals, systematic therapist training, and ongoing monitoring of fidelity of treatment administration. Patients in all three treatment groups had the same access to drugs that were delivered via patient-controlled analgesia (PCA). Data analyses revealed that although pain increased over the course of the procedure for patients in the structured attention and control conditions, it showed no such increase for patients in the hypnosis condition. Hypnosis also significantly reduced procedure time and drug use. Interestingly, hypnosis also significantly reduced the risk of the patient becoming hemodynamically unstable with only 1 hypnosis patient developing instability versus 10 patients in the structured attention and 12 patients in the standard care condition. All three treatments were found to reduce anxiety. These results suggest that hypnosis can produce not only reductions in acute pain during invasive medical procedures, but also reduce drug use and improve hemodynamic stability.

More recently, Lang et al[44] examined whether a similar self-hypnosis protocol could be effective in reducing pain during large core needle biopsy, a procedure that is painful and anxiety provoking for many women.[44] In this study, 236 women scheduled for breast biopsy were randomized to receive structured attention, structured attention plus hypnosis, or standard care. Treatment outcome was assessed by having patients rate their pain and anxiety every 10 minutes during the procedure. Results showed that, although pain increased significantly in all three groups, the slope of the increase was significantly less in the hypnosis and structured attention groups. Anxiety decreased significantly over the course of the procedure in the hypnosis group, whereas it increased significantly in the standard care and showed no change in the structured attention group. These findings suggest that both hypnosis and structured attention may both have benefits for patients undergoing large core breast biopsy.

Conscious sedation is becoming widely used in the management of acute pain. Can hypnosis enhance the effects of conscious sedation on pain and anxiety? This question was addressed in a controlled study conducted by Faymonville et al.[45] In this study, 60 patients scheduled for plastic surgery under local anesthesia and intravenous sedation were randomly assigned to either a hypnosis condition or a stress reduction control condition. Patients in the hypnosis condition were encouraged to focus on a pleasant life experience during the surgery and were given suggestions and relaxation training by an anesthesiologist to facilitate their ability to do so. Those in the stress reduction control condition received instruction from an anesthesiologist in deep breathing, relaxation, and distraction methods. Data analysis revealed that, when compared to the stress reduction intervention, the hypnosis intervention produced significant reductions in self-report and direct observation measures of pain and anxiety. In addition, vital signs during the operation were more stable and postoperative nausea and vomiting were significantly lower for patients in the hypnosis versus stress reduction group. Finally, patients in the hypnosis group reported significantly higher levels of intraoperative control and overall satisfaction with the procedure than patients in the stress reduction group. Overall, this study provides strong support for the efficacy of hypnosis as an adjunct to conscious sedation.

Some individuals are more susceptible to hypnosis than others and, therefore, might respond better to hypnotic interventions for acute pain. Harmon et al[46] examined the effects of hypnotic susceptibility in a rigorous study testing the effects of a hypnosis protocol for managing pain during childbirth. In this study, 63 nulliparous women (aged 18 to 35 years) completed a measure of hypnotic susceptibility. Based on their scores on this measure they were divided into high and low hypnotic susceptibility groups. All women were then randomly assigned to one of two conditions: childbirth preparation with skill mastery and childbirth preparation with skill mastery plus hypnosis. Patients in the childbirth education and skill mastery condition received six 1-hour sessions that provided information about childbirth, training in coping skills (eg, breathing techniques for different stages of labor, focal point distraction), and practice in applying learned coping skills during an ischemic pain task. Patients in the hypnosis condition received the same training, but also received a hypnotic induction focused on relaxation and analgesia prior to each training session. Data analysis revealed that patients in the hypnosis condition had overall better birth experiences in that they reported significantly less pain and had shorter labors, took less medication, had higher Apgar scores, and had more frequent spontaneous births. Patients in both conditions who were highly hypnotizable reported significantly lower levels of pain than those who were not. Those in the hypnosis group who were highly susceptible to hypnosis also reported significantly lower levels of postpartum depression. These results underscore the utility of hypnosis in managing labor pain and suggest that hypnotic susceptibility may be an important individual difference variable that contributes to heightened responsiveness to hypnotic interventions for acute pain.

Taken together the findings of the studies above coupled with those reported in a recent meta-analysis[38] and systematic review[47] suggest that hypnosis can be beneficial in managing acute pain. What makes hypnosis impressive as a psychosocial intervention is that it appears to produce benefits not only in terms of pain and distress but also in terms of other, important pain-related outcomes (eg, medication intake, surgery time).

There are a number of possible biological mechanisms by which hypnosis can affect pain, including reductions in involuntary sympathetic responses to pain, increases in endogenous opioid release, changes in brain activity (anterior cingulate cortex), and inhibition of pain at the spinal cord level.[42] As suggested by the findings of Harmon et al,[46] there are likely individual differences in hypnotic susceptibility that influence how much acute pain relief persons might expect with hypnosis. By incorporating assessments of hypnotic susceptibility into clinical practice, one might be able to select those patients who are most likely to benefit from hypnosis.

Virtual Reality

Virtual reality is the most recent psychosocial intervention to be used in the management of acute pain. Computer-based virtual reality methods provide persons with exposure to immersive, three-dimensional, interactive environments that can absorb attentional resources and potentially reduce acute pain.

Das et al[48] conducted the first study to test the effects of playing an interactive virtual reality game on pain experienced by children during burn management procedures. During the virtual reality intervention, children used a computer mouse and wore a head-mount display with a tracking system that enabled them to use head movements to move and interact with the virtual environment. The environment used game software (based on the game *Quake* by ID Software) and simulated being on a track and shooting monsters. In this pilot study ($n = 9$ children aged 5 to 16 years), a within-subjects design was used in which pain ratings were collected during burn management procedures under two conditions: (1) when the child was interacting with the virtual reality environment and (2) when the child was not doing so. All children received standard pharmacological management of their pain and the total amount of time taken during the procedure did not differ by treatment condition. Results indicated that pain ratings were significantly lower ($P < .01$) when virtual reality was provided during burn management procedures (mean = 1.3 on a scale from 0 to 10) than when it was not (mean = 4.1). Comments from nursing staff also revealed that the children were much more cooperative and distracted from the procedures when virtual reality was used.

Hoffman and his colleagues[49–53] have published a number of studies examining the effects of virtual reality in controlling acute pain in adults. These include case studies demonstrating the benefits of virtual reality in controlling acute pain during transurethral microwave thermotherapy[49] and burn wound care during hydrotherapy.[50] One of the first controlled studies conducted by this group[51] was a small within-subjects study of children ($n = 7$, aged 9 to 32 years) that compared the effects of virtual reality and a control condition in reducing pain that occurred in burn victims who were doing range-of-motion exercises as part of their physical therapy. In this study, the virtual environments included SpiderWorld, in which the participants could explore a room and pick up and touch virtual objects (eg, spiders, candy) with his/her virtual hand, and SnowWorld, in which the participant could explore a virtual canyon with a river and waterfalls and shoot snowballs at igloos and snowmen. The study was conducted over 3 days of therapy and, on each day, patients rated their pain once after undergoing range-of-motion exercises while being provided with virtual reality and again after undergoing the exercises when no virtual reality was provided. Data analyses revealed that pain ratings were significantly lower when virtual reality was used than when it was not. The virtual reality intervention yielded significant effects on all five pain measures collected (average pain, worst pain, pain unpleasantness, bothersomeness of pain, and time spent thinking of pain). Notably, significant effects were evident even among those patients who reported reporting severe to excruciating pain levels (6 of the 7 patients).

In sum, virtual reality is a relatively new intervention for managing acute pain that shows promise in early case reports and small scale, preliminary studies. Larger-scale, randomized clinical trials are needed to more definitively test the efficacy of this psychosocial intervention.

Two studies, conducted in pain-free volunteers, suggest some interesting directions for future work in this area. First, because the technology for virtual reality is developing rapidly, there is a need to determine whether older, low-technology virtual reality is just as effective as newer, high-technology virtual reality. Hoffman et al[52] conducted a study that systematically compared the effects of high-tech versus low-tech virtual reality on ratings of thermal pain in normal volunteers. The high-tech virtual reality system provided many features: shutting out reality (using helmet and headphones), providing input to multiple senses (both sight and sound), providing a panoramic/surround view rather than a more limited narrow field of view, providing more vivid/high resolution display, using head tracking to enable subjects to view different places in the virtual world by turning their head, and providing participants with the opportunity to interact with the virtual world. The low tech virtual reality environment provided exposure to a virtual environment, but none of these features. All participants were exposed to a baseline thermal pain stimulus and asked to rate its severity. They were then randomly assigned to either the high-tech or low-tech virtual reality environment and during exposure to that environment received a second presentation of the thermal pain stimulus and asked to rate it. Each participant also rated their level of presence in the virtual world (ie, how much they had the illusion of actually being in the virtual world). Data analysis showed that thermal pain ratings were significantly lower (mean = 0.1) for participants receiving the high-tech virtual reality intervention than for those receiving the low-tech virtual reality (mean = 3.1). Furthermore, across both conditions, ratings of presence in the virtual world were strongly correlated with amount of pain relief reported. Based on these findings one might expect improvements in acute clinical pain would be more likely in patients who are exposed to newer and more advanced virtual reality technologies. They also suggest that patients who report a strong sense of presence when initially exposed to virtual reality might show the best outcomes.

A second study conducted in pain-free volunteers examined the effects of an intervention that combined virtual reality with post-hypnotic suggestions.[53] Participants in this study were tested for hypnotic susceptibility, underwent a baseline thermal pain testing session, and were then randomly assigned to hypnosis or no hypnosis conditions. Half of the participants in each of these conditions was then assigned to either receive a virtual reality distraction or not during delivery of a second thermal pain testing session. Results showed that the virtual reality intervention was effective in reducing pain, regardless of participants' hypnotic susceptibility. The effects of the hypnosis intervention, however, were evident only in persons who were highly susceptible to hypnosis. Although not statistically significant, there was a trend for high hypnotizable participants who received the combination of hypnosis and virtual reality to show larger improvements in worst pain and pain unpleasantness ratings than achieved with virtual reality alone. An interesting direction for future research would be test the efficacy of a combined virtual reality/hypnosis protocol in managing acute clinical pain.

FUTURE DIRECTIONS

One of the most important future directions involves translating what is currently known about the psychosocial perspective on acute pain into clinical practice. Although we now know that psychosocial factors, such as anxiety, pain catastrophizing, and pain-related fear, can influence acute pain, these factors are rarely assessed in clinical practice. Brief instruments are available that could enable clinicians to assess such factors in practice settings.[54] Information gathered using such measures could be helpful to clinicians in several ways. First, they could increase clinicians awareness of important aspects of each patient's pain-related psychosocial functioning. Second, they could aid in identifying patients who are likely to have difficulty managing acute pain. Third, they may be useful in selecting patients who are likely to need more intensive psychosocial treatment. Finally, these instruments could be used to monitor psychosocial outcomes among patients whose acute pain is managed with conventional medical and surgical treatments.

To date, psychosocial interventions have been tested mainly in efficacy studies. Efficacy studies use carefully screened and selected patients and rely on highly standardized treatment protocols and interventionists who are usually highly trained. An important next step in this area is to conduct effectiveness studies (ie, to determine whether psychosocial interventions can show similar effects in more typical practice settings). In effectiveness studies, patient screening and selection is less rigid, interventions are not as strictly standardized, and the intervention is delivered by staff who typically work in the treatment setting and who usually have not received extensive training and ongoing supervision. If effectiveness studies demonstrate that psychosocial interventions can enhance acute pain management, then these interventions are much more likely to be disseminated into clinical practice. The likelihood that psychosocial interventions for acute pain will be fully disseminated into clinical practice is enhanced by the fact that a number of these interventions (eg, distraction techniques) require relatively little training, are easy to use, and are inexpensive.

Another important future direction is to develop and test tailored interventions that are matched to the resources and needs of patients who are experiencing acute pain. Patients who are highly susceptible to hypnosis, for example, might benefit more from a protocol that primarily focuses on teaching them to use suggestion and imagery to manage pain than a multicomponent protocol that teaches unrelated pain coping skills. Patients who are prone to high levels of pain catastrophizing might need a tailored approach that elicits their overly negative thoughts about acute pain and teaches them how to question, challenge, and restructure these thoughts. Patients who have a high level of anxiety and fear about pain may benefit from modelling, graded exposure, and mastery experiences designed to enhance their perceived efficacy in pain control and their ability to approach and master rather than avoid pain experiences. A major advantage of treatment tailoring is that it can streamline treatment, making it less costly and more readily available for those patients who need it.

One psychosocial factor that potentially can have an important effect on acute pain is the physical environment.[55] The environments in which acute pain are treated are typically quite sterile and devoid of distracting features that might divert a person from their pain. There is growing evidence that environmental stimuli, including exposure to light and natural scenes, can affect the acute pain experience.[55] Walch et al,[56] for example, found that spine surgery patients who recovered from surgery in a room with bright sunlight required significant less opioid analgesics than those who were in a dim room. In a study of myocardial infarction patients, Beauchemin and Hays[57] reported that individuals whose hospital rooms were brightly lit had significantly shorter hospital stays and tended to have lower mortality rates than those in darker rooms. Ulrich et al[58] examined the effects of randomly assigning heart surgery patients to rooms that provided views of nature as compared to views of abstract art or a control blank panel. Patients whose rooms enabled them to view nature were significantly more likely to switch from strong analgesics to weaker analgesics over the course of their hospital stay. Patients with views of nature also experienced significantly lower levels of anxiety during their hospitalization. Such findings have implications for the design of the treatment facilities in which acute pain is treated. They suggest that incorporating design elements (e.g., more window views of natural scenes and more use of light) into the design of new clinics and hospitals may provide a means of enhancing acute pain control.

Much of the research on psychosocial interventions for acute pain has been conducted in children undergoing painful procedures. Clinical observations also suggest that psychosocial interventions are more frequently used in managing acute pain in children than in adults. The underutilization of psychosocial interventions in adults is unfortunate, particularly given the evidence that these interventions can help. In particular, psychosocial interventions could be more widely used in older adults with chronic diseases who often experience episodes of acute pain as a result of their disease or its treatment. There is a clear need for additional research testing the efficacy of psychosocial interventions for acute pain in adults.

An interesting direction for future studies of adults is testing the effects of involving a partner or caregiver in psychosocial acute pain management protocols. Partners and caregivers are often interested in helping their loved one manage acute pain but uncertain what role they can play. In the acute care setting, partners and caregivers can benefit from learning how to most appropriately use pain medication and how to assist the patient in their efforts to cope with pain. Partner-assisted pain management interventions have shown promise in the treatment of chronic pain conditions such as arthritis pain, chronic lower back pain, and cancer pain.[1] Future studies need to explore the efficacy of partner- and caregiver-assisted approaches to the control of adults experiencing acute pain.

CONCLUSIONS

Advances in pain theory and research underscore the importance of psychosocial factors in understanding acute pain. Psychosocial

protocols for managing acute pain have been developed and refined and show promise in the management of many acute pain conditions. In the future, psychosocial approaches to assessing and treating pain are likely to become more fully integrated into acute pain practice settings. As psychosocial approaches become more fully disseminated, it is likely that they will be better able to prevent and reduce the pain and suffering accompanying the acute pain experience.

Preparation of this chapter was supported by grants from the National Institutes of Health (R01 CA107477-01, R01 CA100743-01, R01 CA91947-01, CA122704, CA014236, AR47218, AR049059, AR050245, and AR05462). We also Dr Verena Knowles, John P. Keefe, and Joni Duke for their assistance with this chapter.

REFERENCES

1. Keefe FJ, Rumble ME, Scipio CD, Giardano L, Perri LM. Psychological aspects of persistent pain: current state of the science. *J Pain*. 2004;5:195–211.
2. Keefe FJ, Abernethy AP, Campbell, LC. Psychological approaches to understanding and treating disease-related pain. *Ann Rev Psychol*. 2005;56:601–630.
3. Beecher HK. Measurement of Subjective Responses. New York, NY: Oxford University Press; 1959.
4. Melzack R, Wall PD, Ty TC. Acute pain in an emergency clinic: latency of onset and descriptor patterns related to different injuries. *Pain*. 1982;14:33–43.
5. Melzack R. Pain: past, present and future. *Can J Exp Psychol*. 1993;47(4):615–629.
6. Melzack R, Wall PD. Pain mechanisms: A new theory. *Science*. 1965;150(3699):971–979.
7. Melzack R. Pain and the neuromatrix in the brain. *J Dent Educ*. 2001;65(12):1378–1382.
8. Feeney SL. The relationship between pain and negative affect in older adults: anxiety as a predictor of pain. *J Anxiety Disord*. 2004;18:733–744.
9. Carr ECJ, Thomas VN, Wilson-Barnet J. Patient experiences of anxiety, depression and acute pain after surgery: a longitudinal perspective. *Int J Nurs Stud*. 2005;42:521–530.
10. Katz J, Poleshuck EL, Andrus CH, et al. Risk factors for acute pain and its persistence following breast cancer surgery. *Pain*. 2005;119:16–25.
11. Aaron LA, Patterson DR, Finch CP, Carrougher GJ, Heimbach DM. The utility of a burn specific measure of pain anxiety to prospectively predict pain and function: a comparative analysis. *Burns*. 2001;27:329–334.
12. McCracken LM, Zayfert C, Gross RT. The pain anxiety symptoms scale: development and validation of a scale to measure fear of pain. *Pain*. 1992;50:67–73.
13. Ring D, Kadzielski J, Malhotra L, Lee SG, and Jupiter JB. Psychological factors associated with idiopathic arm pain. *J. Bone Jt. Surg. (Am.)*. 2005;87(2):374–380.
14. Thomas JS, France CR. Pain-related fear is associated with avoidance of spinal motion during recovery from low back p-ain. *Spine*. 2007;32(16):E460–E466.
15. Vlaeyen JWS, Linton SJ. Fear-avoidance and its consequences in chronic musculoskeletal pain: a state of the art. *Pain*. 2000;85:317–332.
16. Swinkels-Meewisse IEJ, Roelofs J, Verbeek ALM, Oostendorp RAB, Vlaeyen JWS. Fear of movement/(re)injury, disability and participation in acute low back pain. *Pain*. 2003;105:371–379.

17. Buitenhuis J, Jaspers JPC, Fidler V. Can kinesiophobia predict the duration of neck symptoms in acute whiplash? *Clin J Pain.* 2006;22(3):272–277.

18. Swinkels-Meewissee IEJ, Roelofs J, Oostendorp RAB, Verbeek ALM, Vlaeyen JWS. Acute low back pain: pain-related fear and pain catastrophizing influence physical performance and perceived disability. *Pain.* 2006;120:36–43.

19. George SZ, Fritz JM, McNeil DW. Fear-avoidance beliefs as measured by the fear-avoidance beliefs questionnaire: change in fear-avoidance beliefs questionnaire is predictive of change in self-report of disability and pain intensity for patients with acute low back pain. *Clin J Pain.* 2006;22(2):197.

20. Sullivan MJL, Thorn B, Haythornthwaite J, et al. Theoretical perspectives on the relation between catastrophizing and pain. *J Clin Pain.* 2001;17:52–64.

21. Pavlin DJ, Sullivan MJL, Freund PR, Roesen K. Catastrophizing: a risk factor for postsurgical pain. *Clin J Pain.* 2005;21:83–90.

22. Strulov L, Zimmer EZ, Granot M, Tamir A, Jakobi P, Lowenstein L. Pain catastrophizing, response to experimental heat stimuli, and post-cesarean section pain. *J Pain.* 2007;8(3):273–279.

23. Turner JA, Brister H, Huggins K, Mancl L, Aaron LA, Truelove EL. Catastrophizing is associated with clinical examination findings, activity interference, and health care use among patients with temporomandibular disorders. *J Orofac Pain.* 2005;19(4):291–300.

24. Gracely RH, Geisser ME, Giesecke T, et al. Pain catastrophizing and neural responses to pain among persons with fibromyalgia. *Brain.* 2004;127:835–843.

25. Botvinick M, Jha AP, Bylsma LM, Fabian SA, Solomon PE, Prkachin KM. Viewing facial expressions of pain engages cortical areas involved in the direct experience of pain. *NeuroImage* 2005;25:312–319.

26. Saarela MV, Hlushchuk Y, Williams AC, Schurmann M, Kalso E, Hari R. The compassionate brain: humans detect intensity of pain from another's face. *Cereb Cortex.* 2007;17:230–237.

27. Williams AC de C. Facial expressions of pain: an evolutionary account. *Behav Brain Sci.* 2002;25:439–488.

28. Frank NC, Blount RL, Smith AJ, Manimala MR, Martin JK. Parent and staff behavior, previous child medical experience, and maternal anxiety as they relate to child procedural distress and coping. *J Pediatr Psychol.* 1995;20:277–289.

29. McMurtry CM, McGrath PJ, Chambers CT. Reassurance can hurt: parental behavior and painful medical procedures. *J Pediatr.* 2006;148(4):560–561.

30. Blount RL, Corbin SM, Sturges JW, Wolfe VV, Prater JM, James LD. The relationship between adults' behavior and child coping and distress during BMA/LP procedures: a sequential analysis. *Behav Ther.* 1989;20:585–601.

31. Lang EV, Hatsiopoulou O, Koch T, et al. Can words hurt? Patient-provider interactions during invasive procedures. [Clinical Trial. Comparative Study. Journal Article. Randomized Controlled Trial. Research Support, U.S. Gov't, P.H.S.] *Pain.* 2005;114(1–2):303–309.

32. McCaul KD, Mallot JM. Distraction and coping with pain. *Psychol Bull.* 1984;95:516–533.

33. Sparks L. Taking the "ouch" out of injections for children: using distraction to decrease pain. *Am J Matern Child Nurs.* 2001;26(2):72–78.

34. MacLaren JE, Cohen LL. A comparison of distraction strategies for venipuncture distress in children. *J Pediatr Psychol.* 2005;30(5):387–396.

35. Manimala MR, Blount RL, Cohen LL. The effects of parental reassurance versus distraction on child distress and coping during immunizations. *Child Health Care.* 2000;29(3):167–177.

36. Cohen LL, Blount RL, Cohen RJ, Schaen ER, Zaff JF Comparative study of distraction versus topical anesthesia for pediatric pain management during immunizations. *Health Psychol.* 1999;18:591–598.

37. Kleiber C, Harper DC. Effects of distraction on children's pain and distress during medical procedures: a meta-analysis. *Nurs Res.* 1999;48(1):44–49.

38. Uman LS, Chambers CT, McGrath PJ, Kisely S. Psychological interventions for needle-related procedural pain and distress in children and adolescents (review). *Cochrane Library.* 2007;3:1–77.

39. Manne SL, Redd WH, Jacobsen PB, Gorfinkle K, Schorr O. Behavioral intervention to reduce child and parent distress during venipuncture. *J Consult Clin Psychol.* 1990;58(5):565–572.

40. Jay S, Elliott CH, Fitzgibbons I, Woody P, Siegel S. A comparative study of cognitive behavior therapy versus general anesthesia for painful medical procedures in children. *Pain.* 1995;62:3–9.

41. Liossi C, Hatira P. Clinical hypnosis versus cognitive behavioral training for pain management with pediatric cancer patients undergoing bone marrow aspirations. *Int J Clin Exp Hypn.* 1999;47(2):104–116.

42. Patterson DR. Jensen MP. Hypnosis and clinical pain. *Psychol Bull.* 2003;129(4):495–521.

43. Lang EV, Benotsch EG, Fick LJ, et al. Spiegel D. Adjunctive non-pharmacological analgesia for invasive medical procedures: a randomised trial. [Clinical Trial. Journal Article. Randomized Controlled Trial. Research Support, U.S. Gov't, P.H.S.] *Lancet.* 2000;355(9214):1486–1490.

44. Lang EV, Berbaum KS, Faintuch S, et al. Adjunctive self-hypnotic relaxation for outpatients medical procedures: a prospective randomized trial with women undergoing large core breast biopsy. *Pain.* 2006;126:155–164.

45. Faymonville ME, Mambourg PH, Joris J, et al. Psychological approaches during conscious sedation Hypnosis versus stress reducing strategies: a prospective randomized study. *Pain.* 1997;73:361–367.

46. Harmon TM, Hynan MT, Tyre TE. Improved obstetric outcomes using hypnotic analgesia and skill mastery combined with childbirth education. *J Consult Clin Psychol.* 1990;58(5):525–530.

47. Neron S, Stephenson R. Effectiveness of hypnotherapy with cancer patients' trajectory: emesis, acute pain, and analgesia and anxiolysis in procedures. *Int J Clin Exp Hypn.* 2007;55(3):336–354.

48. Das DA, Grimmer KA, Sparnon AL, McRae SE, Thomas BH. The efficacy of playing a virtual reality game in modulating pain for children with acute burn injuries: a randomized controlled trial [ISRCTN87413556]. *BMC Pediatrics.* 2005;5(1):1–10.

49. Wright JL, Hoffman HG, Sweet RM. Virtual reality as an adjunctive pain control during transurethral microwave thermotherapy. *J Urol.* 2005;66(6):1320.

50. Hoffman HG, Patterson DR, Magula J, et al. Water-friendly virtual reality pain control during wound care. *J Clin Psychol.* 2004;60(2):189–195.

51. Hoffman HG, Patterson DR, Carrougher GJ, Sharar SR. Effectiveness of virtual reality-based pain control with multiple treatments. *Clin J Pain.* 2001;17:229–235.

52. Hoffman HG, Sharar SR, Coda B, et al. Manipulating presence influences the magnitude of virtual reality analgesia. *Pain.* 2004;111:162–168.

53. Patterson DR, Hoffman HG, Palacios AG, Jensen MJ. Analgesic effects of posthypnotic suggestions and virtual reality distraction on thermal pain. *J Abnorm Psychol.* 2006;115(4):834–841.

54. Jensen MP, Keefe FJ, Lefebvre JC, Romano JM, Turner JA. One- and two-item measures of pain beliefs and coping strategies. *Pain.* 2003;104:453–469.

55. Malenbaum S, Keefe FJ, Williams A, Ulrich R, Somers TJ. Pain in its environmental context: implications for designing environments to enhance pain control. *Pain.* 2008;134(3):241–244.

56. Walch JM, Rabin BS, Day R, Williams JN, Choi K, Kang JD. The effect of sunlight on postoperative analgesic medications use: a prospective study of patients undergoing spinal surgery. *Psychosom Med.* 2005;67:156–163.

57. Beauchemin KM, Hays P. Dying in the dark: sunshine, gender, and outcomes in myocardial infarction. *J R Soc Med.* 1998;91: 352–354.

58. Ulrich RS, Lunden O, Etinge JL. Effects of exposure to nature and abstract pictures on patients recovery from heart surgery. *Psychophysiology.* 1993;S1–S7.

5

Nonsteroidal Anti-Inflammatory Drugs and Acetaminophen: Pharmacology for the Future

Jon McCormack and Ian Power

The nonsteroidal anti-inflammatory drugs (NSAIDs) encompass a heterogeneous group of therapeutic agents used in a wide spectrum of analgesic and anti-inflammatory roles. From aspirin, the first NSAID commercially produced for analgesic prescription over 100 years ago, the conventional NSAIDs were derived, and had been in clinical use for many years before their mechanism of action (ie, inhibiting prostaglandin synthesis) was elucidated. Acetaminophen is an analgesic and antipyretic agent that may be classified as an NSAID by virtue of its mechanism of action on prostaglandin metabolism. The development of the highly selective coxibs has been ongoing since the mid-1990s. This chapter discusses the history, pharmacokinetic properties, perioperative use, and adverse effects of the NSAIDs.

HISTORY

The Salicylates

In the 18th century the bark of the willow tree (*Salix alba*) was noted to have analgesic properties, whereby a letter from Rev. Mr Edward Stone to the Royal Society in 1763 described "*a bark of an English tree, which I have found by experience to be a powerful astringent, and very efficacious in curing anguish and intermitting disorders.*" These properties were conferred by a glycoside of salicylic acid, named sialicin, first isolated from natural sources as yellow crystals by Buchner in 1828. German chemists also succeeded in isolating salicylic acid from Meadowsweet (*Spirea ulmaria*) but it was not until the latter part of the century, in 1860, that Kolbe synthesized salicylic acid and its sodium salt from phenol, carbon dioxide, and sodium. Following this, the availability of inexpensive synthetic salicylates encouraged their use for many clinical indications, and their analgesic, antipyretic, and anti-inflammatory effects were used to treat acute rheumatic fever, gout, and arthritis. However, even at this early stage side effects were recognized, prompting a chemist named Hoffman in 1893 to develop a salicylate that was less irritating to the stomach, a side effect displayed by his father following his sodium salicylate treatment for arthritis. Hoffman's development of acetyl salicylic acid (Figure 5.1), which he mis-

takenly believed would be less irritating to the gastric mucosa as a result of reduced acidity, was produced and launched into clinical practice by Bayer as *aspirin*, with the *a* from *acetyl*, and *spirin* from *Spirsaure*, the salicylic acid derivative of the Meadowsweet plant.

Nonsteroidal Anti-Inflammatory Drugs

The term *nonsteroidal anti-inflammatory drugs*, or NSAIDs, is a collective term for a chemically heterogeneous group of drugs synthesized since the early 1900s that have analgesic, anti-inflammatory, and antipyretic properties in common with aspirin. These nonopioid analgesics can be classified by a chemical structure that confers broadly similar characteristics within each group, these being carboxylic acids, pyrazolones, oxicams, napthylalkalones, and *p*-aminophenol derivatives, as detailed in Table 5.1.

All of the NSAIDs have similar effects within a spectrum, but those offering the greatest potential for the relief of acute pain have marked analgesic effect with relatively mild anti-inflammatory action. The higher doses of these agents required for anti-inflammatory effects tends to be associated with a higher rate of adverse events.

Coxibs

Coxib is the term applied to NSAIDs that have a preferential inhibitory action against cyclooxygenase (COX) type 2, an isoform of cyclooxygenase, which is generally undetectable in normal tissues but present in high concentrations in macrophages and is induced at the sites of acute inflammation. Some of the nonselective NSAIDs were discovered to have preferential activity against COX-2 versus COX-1, for example, meloxicam, and it was noted that the rate of gastric irritation in patients on these therapies was comparable to placebo. The quest for COX-2 inhibitors of higher selectivity led to the development of rofecoxib and celecoxib, released to the market in 1999. Sales of these COX-2 inhibitors rapidly expanded into a multibillion-dollar industry within 2 years; however, their success was short

Table 5.1: Classification of the NSAIDs Aspirin, and Acetaminophen

Chemical Structure	Examples
Carboxylic Acids	Salicylates: acetyl salicylic acid, diflusinal, salsalate
	Propionic acids: ibuprofen, naproxen, fenbufen, fenoprofen, ketoprofen, flurbiprofen
	Acetic acids: indomethacin, sulindac, etodolac, ketorolac, tolmetin, diclofenac
	Anthranilic acids: mefenamic acid
Pyrazolones	Phenylbutazone, azapropazone
Oxicams	Piroxicam, tenoxicam, meloxicam
Coxibs	Celecoxib, parecoxib, lumiracoxib
Naphthylalkalones	Nabumetone
Para-aminophenols	Acetaminophen

lived, and, by 2004, rofecoxib had been voluntarily withdrawn by the manufacturer, and valdecoxib followed in 2005. When the Food and Drug Administration released more detailed follow-up data from the original studies, it demonstrated that, including gastrointestinal side effects, the overall adverse event rate was higher with rofecoxib than traditional NSAID control, in particular, the rate of adverse ischemic myocardial events was significantly higher. Debate is ongoing as to whether this is a class effect of COX-2 inhibitors,[1] and, to date, celecoxib and newer COX-2 agents, such as lumiracoxib, continue to be marketed.

The *para*-Aminophenols

Despite having no effect on prostaglandin metabolism, acetaminophen is frequently classified and described along with NSAIDs as a nonopioid analgesic agent. Acetaminophen is only one of several *p*-aminophenol compounds synthesized in the 19th century for analgesic and antipyretic purposes. The parent compound, acetanilide, was released in 1886, but was soon found to be excessively toxic by way of methemoglobin production. In 1887, phenacetin was introduced and used for a considerable period of time until a linkage with high dosing for prolonged periods of time and the development of renal papillary necrosis was identified, this being referred to clinically as *analgesic nephropathy*. In 1949, the active ingredient of both acetanilide and phenacetin was shown to be *N-*

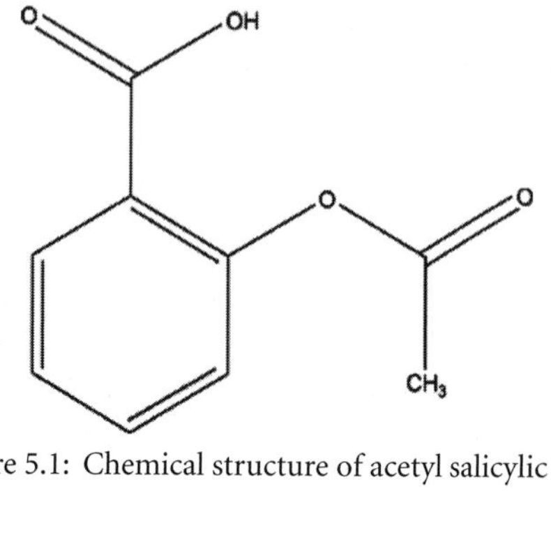

Figure 5.1: Chemical structure of acetyl salicylic acid.

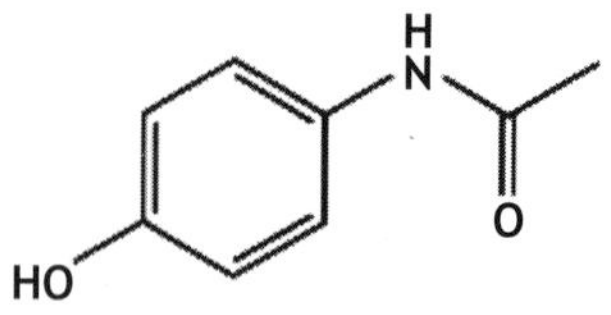

Figure 5.2: Chemical structure of acetaminophen.

(4-hydroxyphenyl) acetamide (Figure 5.2), or acetaminophen, the production of which popularized its use in clinical practice as an effective analgesic and antipyretic, though not anti-inflammatory agent. The launch of solubilized acetaminophen for intravenous (IV) injection to the European market in early 2004 has greatly influenced acetaminophen prescription, particularly in the perioperative period.

PROSTAGLANDIN PHYSIOLOGY

Prostaglandins, first isolated in 1935 by Van Euler in seminal fluid, were so named after the discovery of their high rate of release from the prostate gland. They were initially described as locally active tissue agents mediating smooth muscle tone, and although various types have been identified, they are all based on prostanoic acid (Figure 5.3). A 20-carbon chain molecule with a 5-carbon ring, with varying degrees of saturation and substitution in this ring between each prostaglandin. The nomenclature of different prostaglandins is derived from their original identification processes, with prostaglandin E first isolated in ether and prostaglandin F in phosphate (Swedish: *fosfate*). Prostglandins are members of the eicosanoid family, oxygenated metabolites of arachidonic acid, which also includes the leukotrienes.

Prostaglandin Synthesis

The basal rate of prostaglandin synthesis is low. An increase in production is triggered by stimuli including trauma, which activates tissue phospholipases to release arachidonic acid from plasma membrane phospholipids. Prostaglandin endoperoxidase synthase (PEH), a membrane bound glycoprotein with cyclooxygenase and hydroperoxidase catalytic activities, then converts arachidonic acid to the various prostaglandins (Figure 5.4).

Cyclooxygenase first inserts two oxygen molecules into the 20-carbon arachidonic acid to yield the cyclic endoperoxide PGG_2, which is then converted by hydroperoxidase to PGH_2. From these intermediates, the principal stable prostaglandin products include PGE_2, D_2, $F_{2\alpha}$, I_2 (prostacyclin), and thromboxane A_2.

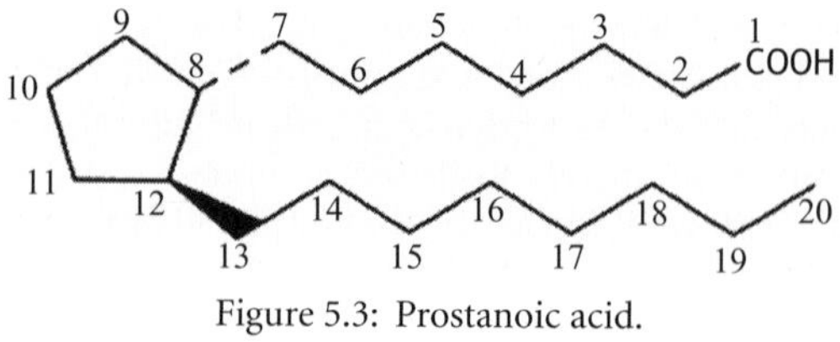

Figure 5.3: Prostanoic acid.

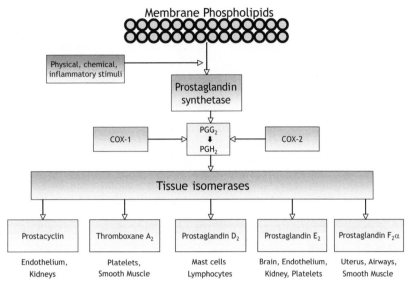

Figure 5.4: Schematic representation of prostaglandin biosynthetic pathways.

Prostaglandin Catabolism

Prostaglandins are rapidly broken down to inactive metabolites and do not circulate in the bloodstream unchanged. Specific enzymatic catabolic pathways exist, though some prostaglandins are inherently chemically unstable. For example, prostacyclin (PGI_2) undergoes rapid nonenzymatic PGH_2 hydrolysis to 6-keto-$PGF_{1\alpha}$, which is then enzymatically metabolized to 2,3-dinor-6-keto-$PGF_{1\alpha}$. Similarly, the platelet aggregator and vasoconstrictor thromboxane A_2 is very unstable and quickly degrades to thromboxane B_2. The rapid spontaneous breakdown of certain prostaglandins implies that measurement of the inactive metabolite may be the best indicator of rate of synthesis of the parent compound.[2]

Enzymatic and nonenzymatic metabolism limit the action of prostaglandins locally to the site of synthesis, hence they can be thought of as locally acting hormones, allowing tissues to react to their own immediate conditions, without necessarily having systemic effects.

MECHANISMS OF ACTION

Many of the effects of these drugs, including analgesia, can be attributed to inhibition of prostaglandin synthesis, though this may not explain all of their actions. There is evidence that these chemical substances interfere with the basic cellular processes involved in neutrophil activation triggered by inflammatory stimuli.

Inhibition of Prostaglandin Synthesis

Although salicylates have been used clinically since the 19th century, their mechanism of action was not elucidated until 1971 when Sir John Jane showed that aspirin and indomethacin inhibited prostaglandin synthesis in various tissues.[3] It is now clear that aspirin and the NSAIDs work by inhibiting the cyclooxygenase component of PGH synthase, thus locally preventing the production of all prostaglandins and thromboxanes from membrane phospholipids. The term *COX inhibitors* is often used to describe these drugs.

Aspirin irreversibly inhibits COX by binding to the protein and acetylating it at Ser350, such that new enzymes must be produced by the cell before prostaglandin synthesis can recommence. In contrast, the other NSAIDs do not acetylate the enzymes, but are reversible inhibitors that prevent cyclooxygenase activity only while there are effective plasma concentrations of the drug present. In general, NSAIDs do not inhibit the alternative lipoxygenase pathway of arachidonic acid metabolism and thus have no effect on the production of inflammatory leukotrienes. Certain NSAIDs are an exception to this, for example, ketoprofen, which may be a dual inhibitor of both cyclooxygenase and lipoxygenase enzymes, thereby interfering with the production of prostaglandins, thromboxane, and leukotrienes. Whether this confers additional clinical advantage to ketoprofen, is unclear.

Inhibition of Neutrophil Aggregation

Although prostaglandin inhibition seems to explain the analgesic and antipyretic effects of the drugs it may not fully explain their anti-inflammatory actions. Problems have persisted in explaining the anti-inflammatory action solely by an effect on prostaglandin synthesis. For example, sodium salicylate has no effect on prostaglandin synthesis in vitro, but is an effective anti-inflammatory agent in vivo. Another problem is that aspirin has anti-inflammatory effects only at doses far higher than those required to inhibit cyclooxygenase.

Some of the anti-inflammatory effects of these drugs may result from a completely different mechanism, this being inhibition of neutrophil activation by inflammatory stimuli. When exposed to certain ligands, neutrophils are activated by "twin signals" (intracellular calcium and protein kinase C), inhibition of which by NSAIDs prevents neutrophil aggregation in vivo and in vitro. This may be a chemical effect related to NSAID structure, their planar lipophilic molecules inhibiting many intracellular processes. NSAIDs even inhibit cellular aggregation in primitive

Table 5.2: Clinical and Pharmacokinetic Data for some NSAIDs

Drug	Daily Dose (mg)	Dosing Interval (h)	Time to Peak Plasma Concentration (h)	Elimination Half-Life (h)	Plasma Protein Binding (%)
Aspirin	1800–3600	4	1–2	0.25	80–90
Propionic acids					
Ibuprofen	1200–2400	6–8	0.5–1.5	2–2.5	99
Ketoprofen	00–200	6–8	1.5–2	1.5	94
Naproxen	500–750	10	1–2	12–15	99
Acetic acids					
Diclofenac	150	12	1–2	1–2	99
Indomethacin	75–150	6–12	1–2	12–15	92–99
Ketorolac	40–90	6	1	4–6	99
Anthranilic acids					
Mefenamic acid	1500	8	2–4	3–4	99
Pyrazolones					
Phenylbutazone	300–400	6–8	2	50–100	98
Oxicams					
Piroxicam	20	24	2–4	53	99
Tenoxicam	20	24	1–2.6	72	99
Coxibs					
Celecoxib	200–400	12	2–3	4–15	97
Parecoxib (IV)	40	24	0.5	8–11	98
Lumiracoxib	200–400	24	5	4	98
Naphthylalkalones					
Nabumetone	1000	24	6	24	99
p-Aminophenols					
Acetaminophen	2000–4000	6	0.5–1	2	10

marine cell cultures that do not synthesize prostaglandin, indicating that this effect is a basic chemical property common to these drugs.

Analgesic Effects

Tissue injury leads to nociception, first, by direct damage to nerve endings; second, by inflammation from the release of prostaglandins from damaged tissues; and, third, by hyperalgesia mediated by nerve fiber sprouting and invasion of phagocytes and fibroblasts.[4]

Prostaglandins are involved in the tissue reaction to injury, and PGE_2 and PGI_2 produced at the site of damage sensitize pain receptors to histamine and bradykinin, leading to hyperalgesia. It is unclear if prostaglandins produce pain themselves or if they increase the effect of other painful stimuli on nerve endings, but it is recognized that they are involved in nociceptor activation by painful stimuli. For example, PGE_2 increases the afferent input from single C fibers in response to heat and bradykinin, an effect prevented by lysine salicylate. Therefore, by preventing prostaglandin synthesis at the site of tissue damage, NSAIDs inhibit nociceptor activation and act as analgesics. As this effect is thought to occur in damaged tissue, NSAIDs have been described as "peripherally acting analgesics." Although this is the case, there is good evidence that NSAIDs diffuse into the cerebrospinal fluid where they also have an action within the CNS. For example, indomethacin, ibuprofen, and diclofenac depress the evoked response of rat thalamic neurons to peripheral nerve stimulation in a dose-dependent manner, demonstrating a central action contributing to their analgesic effect.[5] The analgesic and antipyretic effects of acet-

aminophen are thought to be entirely mediated through central prostaglandin inhibition, as the drug appears devoid of peripheral activity.

PHARMACOKINETICS OF NSAIDS

General Principles

Some details relating to NSAIDs, aspirin, and acetaminophen administration, including dose, frequency, and pharmacokinetic variables, are given in Table 5.2.

Absorption following a dose of NSAID is rapid by all routes of administration, whether enteral or by injection, and following an oral dose NSAIDs are generally rapidly absorbed through the upper small intestine, although the rate may be slowed in the presence of food. Sulindac, nabumetone, and parecoxib are prodrugs that are converted to their active forms by hepatic metabolism, and aspirin is activated by rapid hydrolysis in the plasma to salicylate. Notably, diclofenac undergoes significant first-pass hepatic metabolism when administered orally.

In general, the NSAIDs are highly protein bound and have relatively low volumes of distribution, on the order of 0.1 L/kg, the unbound fraction being biologically active. As a consequence, NSAIDs can potentiate the effects of other highly protein-bound drugs, including oral anticoagulants, oral hypoglycemics, sulfonamides, and anticonvulsants, by displacing them from plasma protein binding sites. NSAIDs may potentiate the effect of lithium by reducing its clearance and also by interference with the effects of diuretics and antihypertensive drugs, these side effects being more common in elderly patients. The dose of NSAIDs should be reduced if there is any evidence of renal impairment.

Hepatic biotransformation followed by renal excretion accounts for the majority of elimination, with only small amounts excreted unchanged. Thirty percent to 40% of the inactive metabolites of the acetic acids and oxicams are excreted in bile.

Aspirin

Acetyl salicylate has analgesic, anti-inflammatory, and antipyretic properties and should be considered the forerunner of the NSAIDs. In addition to its widespread use as a minor analgesic, aspirin has a well-established role in the prophylaxis of coronary and cerebral thromboses, and the treatment of myocardial infarction and preeclampsia.

An oral dose is rapidly absorbed and hydrolyzed in the plasma, therefore aspirin has a relatively short half-life of 15 minutes, although the resulting salicylic acid has a longer half life of 2–3 hours. Both aspirin and the salicylate contribute to the clinical effects, with the latter perhaps being most important for anti-inflammatory actions. Aspirin also has a uricosuric effect. Common side effects include dyspepsia and peptic ulceration, bleeding problems, tinnitus, and deafness. In low doses of 300–600 mg aspirin is an effective analgesic, which is used for the relief of mild to moderate pain. Higher doses of 3.6–4.2 g are given for the anti-inflammatory action required to treat rheumatoid arthritis, at which level many patients experience dyspepsia, occult gastrointestinal bleeding, and tinnitus. Severe gastrointestinal bleeding and hepatic and renal problems can rarely occur. Aspirin is contraindicated in children younger than 12 years, because of the potential for precipitating Reye's syndrome, featuring acute hepatic failure with encephalopathy.

Hypersensitivity to aspirin tends to present in two forms. In the first, sensitivity is associated with rhinitis, nasal polyps, and bronchospasm. In the second, aspirin can produce urticaria, wheals, angioneurotic oedema, and severe hypotension. Both forms may be precipitated in aspirin sensitive subjects by other NSAIDs.

Various preparations have been introduced to attempt to reduce the gastrointestinal side effects of salicylates. Choline magnesium trisilicate is a long-acting nonacetylated ester, diflusinal is a nonacetylated fluorinated salicylate, and salasalate is an aspirin ester that is hydrolyzed slowly. There is some evidence that patients tolerate these preparations better, especially when high anti-inflammatory doses are required.

Mild aspirin intoxication results in the characteristics of "salicylism," featuring deafness, tinnitus, dizziness, and headache. Severe poisoning can produce a life-threatening metabolic derangement with hyperventilation, tinnitus, deafness, hypotension, metabolic acidosis, and coma. These features develop because of uncoupling of oxidative phosphorylation, increasing metabolic rate and hydrogen ion and carbon dioxide production. Initially a respiratory alkalosis develops, because of direct stimulation of the respiratory center, but later the central nervous system (CNS) becomes depressed and the underlying severe metabolic acidosis is revealed. Treatment includes gastric decontamination, primarily with activated charcoal, but forced gastric emptying with concurrent airway protection may still be considered when presentation to the emergency department is within 1 hour of ingestion. Forced alkaline diuresis with sodium bicarbonate infusion is used if the plasma salicylate level exceeds 500 mg/L (3.6 mmol/L) in adults, as a high urinary pH promotes excretion of this weak acid.

Propionic Acids

Agents of this class are the choice for inflammatory joint disease, because although they have weaker anti-inflammatory actions than aspirin, they are much better tolerated. Of all the NSAIDs, the propionic acids are the group least associated with side effects, though dyspepsia, gastrointestinal hemorrhage, and rashes may occur.

Acetic Acids

This group contains the NSAIDs most commonly used for the relief of postoperative pain, including indomethacin, diclofenac, and ketorolac.

Indomethacin is the oldest agent and has potent anti-inflammatory, analgesic and antipyretic effects. However, it is also the agent within this class associated with a high incidence of gastrointestinal side effects and dose-related CNS problems, including headache, confusion, hallucinations, and vertigo. Rectal administration may reduce gastrointestinal side effects. Diclofenac is also often given rectally, but as a means to avoid the high rate of first-pass metabolism, rather than to avoid upper gastrointestinal side effects, which may still occur with rectal administration. A longer-acting but less potent prodrug, sulindac, is converted to an active metabolite in the liver, the sulfated active product of which is excreted in the bile and then reabsorbed through the small intestine, with this mechanism of absorption reported as having improved gastrointestinal tolerance.

Anthranilic Acids

Mefenamic acid is a relatively weak anti-inflammatory agent commonly used for osteoarthritis and rheumatoid arthritis. It is also used extensively for the relief of dysmenorrhea, because of inhibitory actions on uterine prostaglandin metabolism. Side effects include dyspepsia, rashes, gastrointestinal bleeding, and diarrhea, which may lead to dehydration and renal insufficiency in elderly patients. This NSAID has also been associated with interstitial nephritis. Of the newer NSAIDs, mefenamic acid is commonly involved in self-poisoning, which may result in convulsions that are sensitive to benzodiazepine therapy.

Pyrazolones

Phenylbutazone is a toxic, extremely potent and very long-acting anti-inflammatory agent. Widespread reactions to phenylbutazone, common and severe, include dyspepsia, peptic ulceration, gastrointestinal bleeding, mouth ulceration, renal and hepatic impairment, and a spectrum of skin rashes ranging from mild erythema to toxic epidermal necrolysis. The drug produces marked salt and water retention that can exacerbate cardiac failure. There is also a reported association with severe bone marrow depression presenting as agranulocytosis or aplastic anemia. Azapropazone is also a pyrazolone that displays less marrow toxicity though a similar gastrointestinal and fluid retention adverse effect profile.

Naphthylalkalones

The single member of this group, nabumetone, is a nonacidic, inactive prodrug. After oral administration, it undergoes extensive first-pass hepatic metabolism that results in conversion to 6-methoxy-2-naphthylacetic acid, a more potent inhibitor of prostaglandin synthesis than the parent compound. The most common side effects are gastrointestinal, and accumulation can occur with renal impairment or in the elderly.

Oxicams

Piroxicam and tenoxicam are very long-acting drugs with elimination half-lives on the order of a couple of days, hence are given as a single daily dose. They are weakly acidic agents that are extensively plasma protein bound with small volumes of distribution. Both are metabolized in the liver, the inactive breakdown products being excreted in the bile and urine, and there is no apparent accumulation in hepatic or renal impairment or in the elderly. Side effects include dyspepsia, gastrointestinal hemorrhage, and rashes. Both drugs may increase serum liver transaminase concentrations and may precipitate cardiac failure.

Coxibs

The coxibs comprise a heterogenous group of drugs, all of which have in common a selectivity for COX-2 over COX-1 to variable degrees. Rofecoxib, a coxib recently withdrawn from clinical practice, had up to 300 times greater affinity for COX-2 over COX-1, whereas celecoxib, for example, has greater affinity of approximately 30 times.[6] Analgesic efficacy over placebo is well documented, both in acute postoperative pain and in chronic arthritis, although generally coxibs provide analgesia that is as efficacious, but not superior to, conventional NSAIDs.[7,8]

In similarity to other NSAIDs, the coxibs are well absorbed from the upper small intestine and, with the exception of celecoxib, have a high bioavailability, with a generally slightly longer duration of action allowing once or twice daily dosing. Hepatic metabolism produces inactive metabolites excreted via bile and urine.

The coxibs have been demonstrated in extensive trials, notably the VIGOR study, to have a significantly lower upper gastrointestinal side-effect profile compared to traditional NSAIDs; indeed, the rate of these complications approximates that of placebo. However, gastrointestinal side effects aside, the coxibs have a similar adverse event profile to other NSAIDs. Fluid retention may occur within 2 weeks of commencing treatment with rofecoxib, resulting in accumulation of edema and significant elevations in systolic blood pressure. The coxibs also have a reduced antiplatelet activity compared to aspirin and, to a lesser degree, the nonselective NSAIDs, which may predispose to thrombotic events. The controversy surrounding this mechanism and the resultant increase in adverse myocardial events was fundamental to the voluntary worldwide withdrawal of rofecoxib by the manufacturers.

Acetaminophen

Acetaminophen is an effective analgesic and antipyretic, but has little, if any, anti-inflammatory action. It has not been shown to be a more efficacious analgesic than traditional nonsteroidal agents; however, fewer adverse events are repeatedly reported, with the incidence of gastrointestinal erosions, nephrotoxicity, and platelet dysfunction being comparable to placebo at therapeutic doses. The mechanism of action of acetaminophen has been debated over many years, and it is now

accepted that acetaminophen has effects at the peripheral, spinal cord, and brain levels. In the periphery, acetaminophen metabolism by peroxidase produces reactive compounds that inhibit bradykinin-generated impulses within nociceptive fibers.[9] In animal models, acetaminophen has been demonstrated to weakly inhibit isoform 3 of cyclooxygenase enzyme (COX-3), a splice-variant of COX-1, in the brain,[10] although the exact role of COX-3 has not yet been elucidated in humans.[11]

From this, it has been hypothesized that subsequent reductions in prostaglandin production may result in an increase in the activity of descending serotonergic pathways, so modulating nociceptive inputs.[12] At the spinal cord level, acetaminophen has been shown to antagonize neurotransmission via NMDA, substance P, and nitric oxide pathways, all of which are implicated in nociception.[13,14]

Acetaminophen is rapidly absorbed from the small intestine after oral administration, with the rate of absorption having been used as a marker of gastric emptying, and is now also available as a solubilized preparation for intravenous administration. The preparation of intravenous acetaminophen recently released in the United Kingdom and Europe (Perfalgan, Bristol-Myers Squibb, New York, USA) is dissolved in mannitol and pH buffered by disodium phosphate, with cysteine added as an antioxidant. A 100-mL solution is presented as 10 mg/mL for administration over a period of 15 minutes. Minor urticaria has been reported, particularly with rapid administration, although systemic hypersensitivity is extremely rare.[15] Acetaminophen rapidly crosses the blood-brain barrier,[16] where it is preferentially concentrated in the cerebrospinal fluid, and onset of clinical action has been demonstrated within 5–10 minutes with a peak clinical analgesic effect at 1–2 hours.[9] In comparison with the other NSAIDs, it is not highly protein bound and has a larger volume of distribution. Unlike nonsteroidal agents, acetaminophen is safe in pregnancy and children, down to neonatal ages.

At nontoxic doses, hepatic metabolism by cytochrome p450 2E1 primarily results in inactive glucuronide conjugates, 90% of which are renally excreted. Under normal conditions about 4% of the dose is metabolized by hydroxylation to N-acetyl-p-benzoquinone imine, a hepatotoxic alkylating agent. The healthy liver will rapidly detoxify this reactive intermediate by conjugation with sulfydril groups of glutathione, and subsequent excretion as mercapturic derivatives. With larger doses, the rate of formation of the metabolite exceeds the rate at which it can be conjugated with glutathione, and so it combines with the hepatocyte macromolecules resulting in cellular death. The resultant clinical picture is of acute centrilobular hepatocellular necrosis, occasionally with acute tubular necrosis in the kidneys. Specific treatment for this comprises N-acetylcysteine or methionine, synthetic alternatives to hepatic glutathione, which are conjugated to the reactive metabolite of acetaminophen preventing liver damage. In adults, a relatively small dose of 10–15 g (20–30 tablets) can produce potentially fatal hepatic, and sometimes renal, damage. Early signs of poisoning are nausea and vomiting, followed by the development of right-sided subcostal pain and tenderness 1 day later. Liver damage is maximal 3 to 4 days later after ingestion and may lead to death. Early signs may therefore be minimal even when toxic doses have been ingested, and, as the specific antidotes effectively protect the liver maximally if given up to 12–15 hours after ingestion, every overdose should be considered serious and managed accordingly. In the hospital, treatment consists of gastric emptying if the acetaminophen was ingested within 4 hours of presentation, and the administration of intravenous *N*-acetylcysteine according to the measured plasma acetaminophen concentration, which may be a useful predictor of the risk of hepatic failure if taken 4 hours following ingestion. *N*-acetylcysteine therapy should be administred if the plasma acetaminophen concentration falls above the line joining 200 mg/L (1.32 mmol/L) at 4 hours and 30 mg/L (0.2 mmol/L) at 15 hours following ingestion. *N*-acetylcysteine may be given even if the patient presents when more than 15 hours have elapsed following the overdose, but its value is then less sure. Patients receiving concomitant drugs inducing hepatic enzymes are more likely to develop hepatotoxicity and should therefore be given acetylcysteine at lower plasma acetaminophen concentrations. Outside the hospital, emesis should be induced and oral methionine given.

NSAIDS AND PERIOPERATIVE ANALGESIA

In the perioperative period, parenteral preparations of traditional NSAIDs, coxibs and intravenous acetaminophen are available to allow uninterrupted delivery of analgesics for acute perioperative pain throughout the fasting period. Rectal preparations of acetaminophen, diclofenac, and indomethacin may be used; however, side effects of indomethacin tend to preclude use in the acute perioperative phase.

Acetaminophen

The analgesic efficacy of acetaminophen has been widely studied and compared with nonsteroidal anti-inflammatory agents and opioid analgesics. Acetaminophen has been shown to have an efficacy equal to aspirin on a dose-per-dose basis.[17] It is important to note that acetaminophen has little or no anti-inflammatory properties.

Intravenous propacetamol is a prodrug that is rapidly hydrolyzed by plasma esterases to acetaminophen that has been available for over a decade; however, difficulties in solubilizing acetaminophen delayed production of an intravenous preparation of the active agent. The recent European launch of acetaminophen for intravenous injection (Perfalgan) has transformed analgesic prescription, particularly in the perioperative period. It is important to note that all of the pharmacokinetic and pharmacodynamic data presented by the manufacturer of intravenous acetaminophen relates to a different intravenous drug, propacetamol, following reference to a bioequivalence study demonstrating identical pharmacokinetic profiles between propacetamol and acetaminophen.[18]

The number needed to treat (NNT) is a marker for comparison of clinical efficacy based on pooled results from systematic reviews. The NNT relates to the number of patients needed to receive active treatment versus placebo to achieve a 50% reduction in pain scores. As a single agent for the management of moderate pain, the NNT of acetaminophen is 3.8 (95% CI, 3.4–4.4),[19] although for moderate to severe postoperative pain optimal analgesia cannot be achieved using a single agent alone, but a balanced approach in combination with nonsteroidal agents can result in up to a 40%–50% reduction in opioid requirements.[15,20–22] Intravenous acetaminophen (1 g) has been demonstrated to be as efficacious as intramuscular morphine (10 mg) following dental extractions,[23] and as effective as intramuscular ketorolac (30 mg) following lower limb arthroplasty.[24]

Although there is no therapeutic benefit conferred over the same dose of oral or rectal acetaminophen, the advantage in the perioperative period lies with the intravenous dose. With preoperative fasting regulations and impaired oral intake for periods of several hours up to several days depending on the surgical procedure, along with an avoidance of the prescription of regular rectal acetaminophen for prolonged periods, patients may have until recently been denied the analgesic benefit from perioperative acetaminophen administration that has been demonstrated in dental, gynecological, orthopedic, and general surgery.[25–29,30–33] The widespread availability of intravenous acetaminophen should now improve analgesic provision in the perioperative period, with the economic caveat that the prescription should be converted to an oral dose as soon as the patient can tolerate enteral intake. In therapeutic doses, acetaminophen is an inherently safe agent, with no statistically different differences between the reported incidence of adverse effects when comparing acetaminophen with placebo.[34]

Aspirin

Aspirin is normally considered to be an oral analgesic for the relief of mild pain, but intravenous salicylates have been compared with opioids in the presence of moderate to severe pain after surgery. In a large systematic review a single dose of aspirin 600 mg was shown to have a NNT of 4.4 (95% CI, 4.0–4.9); however, after a single dose gastric irritation and drowsiness were reported.[17] Lysine acetylsalicylate (LAS) (1.8 g IV) is equivalent to 1 g of aspirin, but a single bolus gave poor relief of severe postoperative pain compared with morphine (10 mg). Studies using continuous intravenous infusions of LAS have produced better results. After inguinal herniorraphy infusions of LAS were as effective as morphine and produced less drowsiness, nausea, and vomiting.[35]

After thoracic surgery, LAS (7.2 g) given intravenously over 24 hours gave analgesia equivalent to morphine (40 mg), although the salicylate was not as effective as the opiate in the immediate postoperative period.[36] After major gynaecological surgery, LAS was at least as good an analgesic as morphine, with less nausea, vomiting, and respiratory impairment.[37] Although such studies give a favorable view of the use of LAS infusions, the drug is seldom used in clinical practice, perhaps because of injection site problems, including venous thrombosis.

Ibuprofen

Ibuprofen has been available in both the UK and the US for over 4 decades and, in that time, has proved itself to be an efficacious and well-tolerated anti-inflammatory and analgesic agent. Oral and topical gel preparations may also be purchased over the counter, and, in addition to medical prescriptions, ibuprofen accounts for almost one-third of all NSAID use. Near complete absorption following oral administration results rapidly in a high bioavailability.

The antipyretic and analgesic effects of ibuprofen have been shown to be dependent on plasma concentrations, with ibuprofen being highly protein bound, mainly to albumin. Distribution is widespread, but of note ibuprofen is secreted at significant concentrations in synovial fluid, which is assumed to account for its anti-inflammatory effect.[38] Metabolism is primarily accounted for by hepatic biotransformation and subsequent renal excretion of glucuronide conjugates. Ibuprofen has been studied extensively in postsurgical, obstetric, and dental pain, where it is consistently found to be more efficacious than placebo, with a combined NNT of 2.7 (95% CI, 2.5–3.0) for the 400-mg oral dose and a dose-dependent improvement in the analgesic effect.[39] Ibuprofen (400 mg) has also been shown to be equivalent to diclofenac (50 mg) for postsurgical pain. As would be expected, side effects are in keeping with all other NSAIDs; however, these are uncommon and, where they do present, tend to be mild and transient. Most trials have reported a side-effect rate comparable with that of placebo.

Diclofenac

Diclofenac is available in tablet, suppository, and injectable preparations. This was the first parenteral NSAID to be marketed in the UK for the relief of postoperative pain. Additionally, diclofenac has been shown to be effective in relieving pain associated with smooth muscle spasm, including renal and biliary colic, for which it may be the analgesic of choice. Intramuscular diclofenac can be given in a dose of 75 mg up to twice per day as the total daily dose must not exceed 150 mg. Administration by deep intramuscular injection should be for no more than 2 days because of the risk of muscle damage. The advantages associated with diclofenac administration following hip arthroplasty include less cognitive impairment and a reduction in time to mobilization. The benefits of diclofenac in abdominal surgery are less apparent. After major abdominal surgery, diclofenac (75 mg) given every 12 hours reduced morphine consumption, although concern was expressed about the antiplatelet effect and increased postoperative blood loss.[40] The results with diclofenac have been more encouraging after minor day case surgery, where it is as effective as fentanyl after arthroscopic surgery and more effective than opioids after surgical removal of impacted wisdom teeth.[41] Diclofenac may also be useful in pediatric surgery, for instance, after tonsillectomy rectal diclofenac is as effective as pethidine or papaveretum and after inguinal herniornaphy is comparable in analgesic effect with caudal local anesthetic block.[42] A systematic review concluded a combined NNT for diclofenac (50 mg) of 2.3 (95% CI, 2.0–2.7) for postsurgical pain.[39]

Naproxen

Naproxen is a propionic acid derivative like ibuprofen but its higher potency and its side-effect profile limits it to a "prescription only" medicine. It has a similar pharmacokinetic profile to that of ibuprofen, with rapid and complete absorption from the small intestine with a high biovailability, 99% protein binding, and hepatic glucuronidation followed by renal excretion of inactive metabolites.

A systematic review of the efficacy of naproxen for postoperative analgesia found an NNT of 2.6 (95% CI, 2.2–3.2), with a side-effect profile similar to that of placebo, though reporting of side effects has been inconsistent.[43] Naproxen has recently been brought to public attention in two very different areas. First, naproxen was used as the NSAID comparator in the first major publication comparing the COX-2 inhibitor rofecoxib with older NSAIDs.[44] Subsequent detailed analysis of the full data provoked much controversy, with the excess in cardiovascular adverse events in the rofecoxib group being attributed to a

suggested cardioprotective effect of naproxen. Additional exploration implicated other commonly used nonselective NSAIDs, including ibuprofen and diclofenac, in having an excess adverse cardiovascular risks. Further data are awaited to provide a satisfactory conclusion to this debate, though current guidelines from the European Medicines Agency is that nonselective NSAIDs should be prescribed at the lowest dose for the shortest time, and surveillance for adverse effects will continue.

The second area in which the profile of naproxen has been raised is a potential role in delaying the progression of Alzheimers disease has been postulated. Epidemiological studies demonstrated a slowing of progression of cognitive impairment in patients treated with long-term NSAIDs, the proposed mechanism of action featuring inhibition of extracellular amyloid-β aggregation. Subsequent randomized controlled trials have as yet failed to demonstrate a conclusive benefit,[45] and the definitive ADAPT study, proposed for a 7-year period, was terminated after only 3 years because of concerns about adverse cardiovascular events in the control (naproxen) group.[46]

Ketorolac

Ketorolac was the first injectable NSAID to be marketed in the United States for the relief of acute pain. Chemically, it is a pyrroloacetic acid similar in structure to the earlier compounds tolmetin and zomepirac and is prepared as the trometamol (tromethamine in the United States) salt to increase its water solubility. In animal models, ketorolac has analgesic, antipyretic, and anti-inflammatory actions, which are attributed to prevention of prostaglandin synthesis by inhibition of cyclooxygenase. At the dose used clinically, it has a much greater analgesic than anti-inflammatory action, with the analgesic effect being 800 times greater than that of aspirin.

Many studies have assessed the value of ketorolac for postoperative analgesia. The oral form is as effective as acetaminophen and codeine after gynecological surgery.[47] After orthopedic surgery oral ketorolac compares well with acetaminophen, diflusinal, and dihydrocodeine.[48] Intramuscular ketorolac is effective after minor surgery, although the time to onset of analgesic action is greater than 30–60 minutes. Ketorolac has repeatedly been shown to be superor to placebo and opioid following oral surgery. When given prophylactically before minor operations, ketorolac and morphine reduced postoperative pain to a similar degree, but the opioid produced more sedation.

Initial studies suggested that ketorolac was as good an analgesic as opioids after major surgery, but such optimism has not been substantiated. In single-dose intramuscular studies performed on the first or second day following operation in the presence of moderate to severe pain, ketorolac was superior to morphine and had a longer duration of action. However, more recent studies have found that ketorolac alone is unsuitable for the treatment of severe pain immediately after abdominal surgery but is as effective as morphine the day after surgery when pain intensity is less.[49]

The effect of combining ketorolac with opioids has been examined after upper abdominal surgery. Continual intramuscular infusion of ketorolac at 1.5 and 3 mg/hour significantly reduced patient-controlled morphine consumption by 30% over 24 hours, improved pain scores, and, at the higher dose, reduced postoperative increases in arterial PCO_2. Ketorolac, therefore, appears to have a "morphine sparing" effect that also minimizes the respiratory depressant effects of the opioid.

PIROXICAM

Piroxicam has a long half-life, allowing once-daily oral administration. It has been repeatedly shown to be an effective postoperative analgesic agent. After hip surgery performed under spinal anesthesia, piroxicam reduced patient requirements for morphine by 50% with no significant side effects.[50] Comparing a single dose of piroxicam (20 or 40 mg) against placebo the NNT for 50% pain relief was 2.7 (95% CI, 2.1–3.8) and 1.9 (95% CI, 1.2–4.3), respectively.[51] A preemptive analgesic role has also been identified, with a dose given prophylactically before oral surgery substantially reducing the requirements for postoperative analgesia.[52]

Tenoxicam

This preferential COX-2 inhibitor has a longer half-life than piroxicam. Once-daily dosing of 20–40 mg is recommended, with a rapid and complete absorption after oral administration, being unaffected by concomitant food or antacid ingestion and reaching peak plasma concentrations within 2 hours. Despite relatively poor distribution, tenoxicam is preferentially secreted into the synovial fluid, making it an attractive agent for chronic inflammatory joint conditions. Initial studies performed in elderly patients with both rheumatoid disease and osteoarthritis demonstrated that, despite the long half-life of 49–81 hours, there was no progressive accumulation at steady-state dosing.[30] In patients with ankylosing spondylitis both the efficacy and risk of gastrointestinal blood loss is similar to that of piroxicam, seen in around 8% of patients,[53] with a susceptibility to toxicity in some individuals thought to relate to mutations in serum albumin, allowing a higher plasma concentration of unbound agent.[54] Renal toxicity is rare in patients with normal, age related, or mild to moderate renal impairment, with less than 0.1% patients demonstrating a rise in serum creatinine after 5 years of treatment.[32]

Valdecoxib

Valdecoxib is a second-generation COX-2 inhibitor with a selectivity of around 60:1 for COX-2 over COX-1. It is indicated for relief of symptoms from rheumatoid joint disease, osteoarthritis, and menstrual pain and in these situations it has been shown to be superior to placebo and at least equivalent to conventional NSAIDs. For postsurgical pain, valdecoxib was found to provide comparable analgesia to oxycodone and acetaminophen and was opioid sparing following laparoscopic cholecystecomy and lower-limb arthroplasty.[55] It is an orally administered preparation that has a high bioavailability and a half-life of 8–11 hours. Similar to the other COX-2 inhibitors, valdecoxib has a lower rate of endoscopy proven gastrointestinal adverse effects than ibuprofen, naproxen, or diclofenac (5% vs 13%),[33] and bleeding complications resulting from platelet inhibition were not reported.[56] Valdecoxib was voluntarily withdrawn from the US market after Food and Drug Administration (FDA) recommendations in light of a doubled risk of cardiac and cerebrovascular adverse events compared to placebo (OR 2.3, 95% CI, 1.1–4.7)[57]

and case reports of fatal Stevens-Johnson syndrome, these hypersensitivity reactions being triggered by the sulfonamide component of the drug.

Parecoxib

The development of an injectable form of the poorly water soluble valdecoxib led to the development of parecoxib, this being a prodrug of valdecoxib, the first COX-2 inhibitor released for parenteral administration. After intravenous or intramuscular injection it is rapidly hydrolyzed, with a half-life of 20 minutes, by hepatic cytochromes to valdecoxib, thereafter displaying the same pharmacokinetic and pharmacodynamic characteristics as valdecoxib described previously. Comparisons between the other injectable NSAIDs, primarily ketorolac, have demonstrated a comparable analgesic efficacy in postsurgical pain, with a reduced incidence of gastric side effects.[58] As with valdecoxib, this drug is contraindicated in patients with a history of sensitivity to sulfonamides because of the risk of potentially fatal skin reactions.

Celecoxib

Celecoxib was the first COX-2 inhibitor released, in 1998, for symptom control in rheumatoid disease and osteoarthritis. It is relatively highly selective, with a preference of almost 30:1 for COX-2 over COX-1. Oral bioavailability is lower than the other coxibs, at around 40%, but in common with other NSAIDs, widespread distribution and hepatic metabolism confers an attractive pharmacokinetic profile. As with valdecoxib, a sulfonamide moiety may induce serious allergic reactions.

Celecoxib was shown to have an efficacy similar to that of active NSAID comparators for symptom control in rheumatoid arthritis, with onset of analgesia within 1 hour of oral administration, no endoscopic evidence of gastric erosions after 7 days of treatment,[59] and a 71% (95% CI, 59–79%) reduction in endoscopically proven ulcers at 3 months compared with conventional NSAIDs.[60] For acute postoperative pain, celecoxib has been shown to be moderately effective with an NNT of 4.5 (95% CI, 3.3–7.2), comparable to acetaminophen or aspirin alone.[34]

The largest study comparing the long-term effects of celecoxib administration with conventional NSAIDs was the CLASS study. Over 8000 patients with arthritis were randomized to received celecoxib, ibuprofen, or diclofenac, with 57% receiving treatment for 6 months. The incidences of all upper gastrointestinal complications in the celecoxib and NSAID groups were 1.4% vs 2.9% ($P = .02$), although any benefit conferred by celecoxib was negated if aspirin was coadministered, and the difference between study groups was not significant at 12 months.[61] This study was intentionally designed to be pragmatic with regard to simulation of real-world clinical experience and, unlike patients recruited into the VIGOR study, coadministration of aspirin therapy was permitted; however, only when patients from this group were excluded did the results achieve statistical significance for reduction in gastrointestinal complications.

The role of celecoxib in chemoprevention of cancer has been extensively investigated. At present the exact mechanism is unclear, but COX-2 enzyme inhibition by NSAIDs is thought to suppress carcinogenic pathways, possibly by inducing apoptosis in proliferating cancer cells, as the elevated arachidonic acid levels that result from COX-2 inhibition induce the formation

Table 5.3: Myocardial Infarction Rate, Stroke Rate, and Composite APTC(71) Rate among Naproxen, Conventional NSAIDs, and Placebo

Drug/Class	Myocardial Infarction RR (95% CI)	Stroke RR (95% CI)	APTC Composite End Point RR (95% CI)
Naproxen	1.69 (0.82–3.48)	1.42 (0.7–2.91)	1.49 (0.94–2.36)
Non-naproxen NSAIDs	0.8 (0.28–2.25)	0.91 (0.35–2.35)	0.83 (0.46–1.51)
Placebo	1.27 (0.25–6.56)	0.59 (0.13–2.74)	1.08 (0.41–2.86)

of ceramide, a mediator of apoptosis.[62] COX-2 expression has been found to be locally elevated in colonic adenocarcinoma in 90% of malignant cases and 40% of premalignant cases, with levels being normally undetectable in healthy mucosa.[63] Celecoxib has been demonstrated, mainly experimentally, to suppress the tumor volume and growth advancement of many neoplasms, including colonic, gastric, esophageal, hepatocellular, and breast tumors,[64] and, at present, has an FDA licence for inclusion for chemoprophylaxis in patients with familial adenomatous polyposis coli.

Further investigation into cancer treatment has led to evidence of adverse cardiovascular effects of celecoxib. The APC trial, over a 33-month period, although demonstrating that celecoxib was an effective carcinoprophylactic agent, also demonstrated an increase in adverse cardiac events compared with placebo, with risk ratios of 2.6 (95% CI, 1.1–6.1) for 400 mg and 3.4 (95% CI, 1.5–7.9) for 800 mg doses.[65] On the announcement of these results, the ADAPT study, a proposed 7-year trial assessing the value of celecoxib versus naproxen and placebo in Alzheimer's disease, was halted after three years of recruitment because of investigator concerns over the cardiovascular safety of naproxen, with a 50% increase in adverse events, though at that stage there was no significant increase in risk with celecoxib.[46]

At present, the precise answer on the cardiovascular risk profile of celecoxib is awaited. Adverse events have been documented as secondary outcomes from meta-analyses or trials with effects on cancer or Alzheimer's disease as primary aims. A recent systematic review of the cardiovascular risk of celecoxib and conventional NSAIDs, demonstrating an odds ratio of myocardial infarction of 2.3 (95% CI, 1.0–5.1) compared to placebo and 1.9 (95% CI, 1.1–3.1) compared to other NSAIDs, although for composite cardiovascular end points there were no differences between agents.[66] Recruitment has recently commenced in the PRESCISION trial, a large (manufacturer sponsored) multicenter randomized study to evaluate exclusively the cardiovascular risk of celecoxib and traditional NSAIDs in 20,000 patients with arthritis (and, as such, placebo comparison would be unethical), the results of which are due to be available in 2010.

Lumiracoxib

Lumiracoxib is the most selective COX-2 inhibitor with a COX-2:COX-1 selectivity of 400:1.[6] It has a carboxylic acid group, resembling that of diclofenac, and in binding to a unique site on the enzyme is suggested it may have an improved biochemical selectivity over the other coxibs. It is also the only acidic coxib, and it has been hypothesised that this property results in accumulation in sites of inflammation, hence prolonging clinical effect. It has rapid absorption following oral administration, with a high bioavailability reaching peak plasma concentrations within 2 hours and a short half-life of 3–6 hours, although despite

this rapid action once daily dosing has been shown to provide effective analgesia in osteoarthritis and rheumatoid arthritis and following orthopedic surgery that is superior to placebo and as efficacious as diclofenac and celecoxib. As with tenoxicam, drug concentrations peak within synovial fluid from 5 hours following administration up to 24 hours postdose.[67] Endoscopic identification of gastroduodenal ulceration confirms a comparable rate to celecoxib and 3 times less than ibuprofen (0.32 versus 0.92%); however, abnormalities in liver function tests were over 4 times more common (2.57% vs 0.63%), though an increased risk of hepatitis in the clinical setting has not yet been documented.[68] Despite the high COX-2 selectivity, myocardial and cerebrovascular adverse events have been demonstrated to be equivalent to traditional NSAIDs, coxibs, and placebo (Table 5.3)[69]; however, lumiracoxib has not yet received FDA approval for launch in the United States while further data are awaited.

Other NSAIDs

Indomethacin has marked anti-inflammatory actions and is normally used in the management of chronic inflammatory diseases, including ankylosing spondylitis and gout. Early studies confirmed its efficacy as a postoperative analgesic, with evidence of impressive reductions in both pain intensity and morphine requirements; however, the lack of a parenteral preparation, and a frequently demonstrated association with bleeding complications, including wound hematoma, hematemesis, and increased surgical blood loss, has limited its use in clinical practice.

Parenteral ketoprofen use following surgery has also been studied, where intravenous administration following nasal surgery significantly reduced pain scores and requirements for further analgesia compared with patients given opioids.

SIDE EFFECTS

Unfortunately, the NSAIDs possess undesirable effects as a consequence of their mechanism of action, and they are a major cause of serious adverse reactions reported to the regulatory authorities. Prostaglandins acts as paracrine hormones and interference with them can cause disturbances in local tissue metabolism. These effects are well recognized in association with long-term aspirin or NSAID therapy. In the postoperative period, the main concerns are the possibility of peptic ulceration, interference with platelet function, and renal impairment.

Previously, the lack of investigation into the effects of NSAIDs in the postoperative period led to the following comment: "NSAID therapy should also be withheld from patients who are about to undergo surgery because of the risk of acute renal failure, as well as impaired hemostasis resulting from the effects of these agents on platelet function."[71] Increasing evidence is now available demonstrating both the benefits and risks of these valuable analgesic agents when given perioperatively, with regard to cardiovascular, gastrointestinal, platelet, and renal function. NSAID adverse events are consistently shown to be dose dependent, for all agents, and appropriate selection of dose and patient groups should minimize the risk of these events occurring.

Cardiovascular Effects

Since the late 1990s, the introduction of COX-2-specific NSAIDs and subsequent head-to-head comparisons with conventional agents, primarily for examination of analgesic or anti-inflammatory benefits, has unmasked the differing cardiovascular risk profiles between agents, leading to unanswered questions regarding cardiovascular safety stimulating reevaluation of risk not only of the coxibs, but also of the conventional NSAIDs. The mechanism of these adverse events can be explained by the effect of all NSAIDs on platelet prostaglandin metabolism. Reversible inhibition of the vasodilator prostacyclin (PGI_2) from endothelial cells, without a balanced reduction of platelet thromboxane A_2 (TXA_2), as seen with aspirin, leads to unopposed vasoconstriction and enhanced platelet aggregation, predisposing the patient to hypertension and thrombosis resulting in myocardial infarction, stroke, or cardiovascular mortality. In vitro evidence for this effect of COX-2 inhibitors had been previously documented, and confirmation of the importance of unopposed TXA_2 action in the face of PGI_2 inhibition in humans was subsequently published.[72]

Placebo-based comparisons of several coxibs have suggested this is a class-mediated effect, and all agents of this class have the same attributable risks to varying degrees. This was highlighted by the VIGOR study, post hoc analysis of which preempted the global withdrawal of rofecoxib from the market. In achieving the primary aim of demonstrating a significantly reduced rate of serious gastrointestinal adverse events compared to naproxen, a 5-fold increase in myocardial infarction was reported.[44] There may be two explanations for this not being replicated in the celecoxib CLASS trial.[61] First, participants suffered predominantly from osteoarthritis, as opposed to predominance of rheumatoid disease in the VIGOR study, with the latter being associated with a 50% higher myocardial infarction rate, and, second, 21% of patients in CLASS were on concomitant aspirin therapy and hence were exposed to conventional antiplatelet therapy. Valdecoxib was approved by the FDA on the basis of trials demonstrating gastrointestinal side effects; however, an application for licensing of its injectable prodrug parecoxib was rejected on the basis of an increase in cardiovascular events, this trial having been conducted in patients undergoing coronary artery bypass grafting. Confirmation of an adverse cardiovascular profile came with the results of the APPROVe trial, where rofecoxib was compared with placebo for chemoprophylaxis of colorectal adenocarcinomas, demonstrating a 2-fold increase in cardiovascular and cerebrovascular events.[73]

To date, controversy persists as to whether this is a class- or agent-specific effect. Rofecoxib, parecoxib/valdecoxib, and etoricoxib have all been implicated in raising cardiovascular risk but celecoxib and lumaricoxib have not, as yet, shown these adverse events with statistical significance. Following the release of details regarding termination of the ADAPT trial, an explanation for the increase risk of adverse events with naproxen was required. Suggestions of differing behavior between naproxen

Table 5.4: Relative Risk of Cardiovascular Adverse Events in Coxibs and Conventional NSAIDs

Drug	Relative Risk of Serious CVS Events	95% Confidence Interval
Rofecoxib	2.19	1.64–2.91
Celecoxib	1.06	0.91–1.23
Diclofenac	1.41	.16–1.7
Naproxen	0.97	0.87–1.07
Ibuprofen	1.07	0.97–1.18
Piroxicam	1.06	0.70–1.59

and "non-naproxen NSAIDs" cannot be explained pharmacologically, with diclofenac being the conventional NSAID that structurally most resembles a coxib (celecoxib). A retrospective population analysis of over 16,000 patients prescribed 1 of 4 conventional NSAIDs or celecoxib demonstrated no difference in cardiovascular adverse events between the five agents studied.[74] Similarly, a recent systematic review supported the results of randomized trials (Table 5.4), although diclofenac appeared to have a significantly increased risk, further suggesting an emphasis on its relative COX-2 affinity.[75] This has been reaffirmed with results from the MEDAL trial assessing long-term therapy in arthritis, suggesting that dicofenac has a similar cardiovascular risk profile as etoricoxib.[76] The most up-to-date evidence, a European systematic review, concluded that, excluding naproxen, nonselective NSAIDs may be associated with a small increase in adverse cardiac and cerebrovascular events comparable to that of the coxibs,[77] this relating to a population incidence of 3 additional adverse events per 1000 patients compared with placebo. As yet, ibuprofen at up to 1200 mg/d has not been shown to increase cardiovascular risk, which is compatible with its pharmacological profile of relatively equal potency and duration of COX-1 and COX-2 inhibition.[78]

Gastrointestinal Effects

The association of NSAID ingestion with gastric and duodenal ulcers is well recognized, with up to 20% of patients on NSAID therapy having endoscopically proven ulceration at any one time[79] and 1% to 4% developing symptomatic ulcers annually. NSAIDs have also been demonstrated to produce enteropathy.

Peptic Ulcers

Aspirin has been known to damage the human gastric mucosa for some time and many investigations have suggested that NSAIDs have similar effects. The gastric and duodenal epithelia have various protective mechanisms against acid and enzymatic attack: mucous, bicarbonate secretion, hydrophobic properties of the mucosa, rapid cellular regeneration, and an abundant blood supply. Prostaglandins are involved with many of these protective factors, the mechanisms of which can be disrupted by aspirin and NSAIDs, although the exact relationship between ulceration and these drugs has been questioned.

Prostaglandins work at various sites to maintain mucosal integrity. This knowledge led to the development of a synthetic prostaglandin analog, misoprostil, to prevent NSAID induced ulcers. NSAIDs inhibit regenerative cellular proliferation at ulcer margins, a critical mechanism for mucosal repair, and

Table 5.5: Relative Risk of Gastrointestinal Side Effects of Conventional NSAIDs

Agent	RR of GI Side Effects	95% CI
Indomethacin	2.25	1.01–5.08
Naproxen	1.83	1.25–2.68
Diclofenac	1.73	1.21–2.46
Piroxicam	1.66	1.14–2.44
Tenoxicam	1.43	0.4–5.14
Meloxicam	1.24	0.98–1.56
Ibuprofen	1.19	0.53–1.54

misoprostil has been shown to reduce this harmful effect. The gastric microvascular endothelium is known to be a major target for aspirin-mediated injury, and, in combination with the antiplatelet effect, this significantly increases the risk of upper gastrointestinal hemorrhage.

The clinical implications of this are unclear as it is not known if such effects are produced by administering NSAIDs at relatively high doses in the acute postoperative period. It could be that prolonged fasting, the stress of surgery, manipulation of the tissues at operation, and administration of other drugs may render surgical patients at greater risk of mucosal damage from NSAIDs. Even NSAID therapy of relatively short duration can produce severe peptic ulceration and bleeding. Without doubt, NSAIDs should be avoided if the patient has a history of gastric ulceration as this predisposes to further problems developing.

A comprehensive meta-analysis of randomized controlled trials assessing the risk of gastrointestinal side effects compared with NSAID nonusers demonstrated that indomethacin has the highest risk of adverse events compared to other NSAIDs (Table 5.5), with a maximal risk of events at 14 days, and ibuprofen has the lowest risk. The peak time of adverse events for other NSAIDs was 50 days, although this varied depending on increasing age, increasing dose, and underlying pathology.[80]

With regard to the coxibs, rofecoxib was shown to have a 50% relative risk reduction in adverse gastrointestinal events compared with diclofenac[44]; however, celecoxib could not be demonstrated to have a beneficial effect over ibuprofen or diclofenac for symptomatic peptic ulcer incidence.[61] A significant reduction in adverse events was demonstrated only following subgroup analysis (excluding participants on concomitant aspirin therapy) for the development of complicated and symptomatic ulcers.

Evidence regarding parenteral administration of NSAIDs is less conclusive. Early animal experimentation suggested that ketorolac had a favorable therapeutic ratio for gastrointestinal erosions but human studies have been less reassuring, with dose-dependent invasive gastric ulceration present in volunteers following intramuscular administration.

Enteropathy

NSAIDs also have effects on the lower gut, producing enteropathy. This may be a common problem, and it is estimated that 10% of cases of newly diagnosed colitis may be related to ingestion of NSAIDs. Animal studies have shown that NSAID-induced enteropathy is similar to inflammatory bowel disease

with an increase in bowel wall permeability, and indomethacin can produce intestinal lesions temporally related to inhibition of prostacyclin synthesis. The production of protective intestinal mucin is increased by prostaglandins and reduced by aspirin. Patients receiving long-term NSAID therapy for arthritis have an abnormal increase in bowel permeability affecting the small and large intestine. This enteropathy may be similar to Crohn's disease and has been shown to persist for up to 16 months following ingestion. It is thought that NSAIDs impair bowel wall integrity and allow damage from bacterial translocation by decreasing mucosal prostaglandin synthesis.

Platelet Clotting Function

Platelet cyclooxygenase is essential for the production of cyclic endoperoxidases and thromboxane A_2, important mediators of aggregation and vasoconstriction, which constitute the primary hemostatic response to vessel injury. Although it is clear that aspirin and the NSAIDs inhibit aggregation and prolong skin bleeding time in volunteers by around 30% on average, information suggests that significant perioperative bleeding results in 1% of patients treated with NSAIDs, although in the perioperative situation the hemostatic response may be altered by the physiological stress response to surgery.

Aspirin is well recognized as a factor increasing blood loss after surgery, a problem also encountered with NSAIDs. Any aspirin ingestion in the 7 days before cardiac surgery significantly increases the risk of repeat surgery for rebleeding and the requirement for platelets and other blood products and prolongs the stay of the patient in the intensive care unit and in the hospital.[81] The hemostatic effects of aspirin may last up to 14 days as it irreversibly inhibits platelet cyclooxygenase by acetylation of this enzyme. After aspirin therapy, hemostasis returns to normal only when new platelets have been made, as after being formed they cannot produce new enzymes.

In comparison, other NSAIDs are reversible inhibitors of cyclooxygenase and affect platelets only while there are effective circulating concentrations of the drug present. It is therefore likely that the duration of the antiplatelet effect of NSAIDs will be shorter than that of aspirin, although the magnitude of the effect may be the same.

Ketorolac is known to inhibit platelet function in volunteers, as does diclofenac, which can also produce severe spontaneous bruising. In patients having surgery, both ketorolac and diclofenac prolong skin bleeding time and inhibit platelet function in vitro within 1 hour of intramuscular administration, although a significant increase in operative blood loss is not apparent.[82]

Unfortunately, surgical patients are often given other agents that could potentially interact with the antiplatelet effect of NSAIDs. Warfarin, unfractionated heparin, and, more commonly, low-molecular-weight heparins are given prophylactically against deep venous thrombosis and pulmonary embolism, with interaction between these agents and NSAIDs potentially leading to increased bleeding at operation. The combination of heparin and ketorolac has been studied in volunteers with the conclusion that the interaction is probably clinically insignificant. Examination of the effect of concurrent administration of ketorolac and warfarin demonstrated that there is no interaction, although close monitoring of patients on this combination was recommended.

In certain pain states the antiplatelet effect of NSAIDs may paradoxically be beneficial. For example, ketorolac has been shown to be very useful for the relief of pain in sickle cell disease, vaso-occlusive crises, and complex regional pain syndrome.

Renal Function

The adverse renal effects are a serious and significant problem. Most studies have examined the effects of long-term oral NSAID intake for medical conditions and have found the regular consumption of nonopioid analgesics should be routinely considered as a risk factor for any noncongenital cause of chronic renal failure. However, NSAIDs are valuable adjuncts to postoperative analgesic regimes and should not be withheld as there is an absence of evidence to suggest that short-term therapy in appropriately selected patients predisposes to any chronic renal impairment.

Renal Prostaglandin Physiology

The kidney has enzymes for the synthesis of most prostaglandins, where they have various physiological roles, including the maintenance of renal blood flow and glomerular filtration rate in the presence of circulating vasoconstrictor hormones, regulation of tubular handling of electrolytes, and modulation of the actions of other renal hormones.

PGI_2 and PGE_2 are the prostaglandins produced in the kidney in greatest abundance. There is a degree of specialization of function and PGI_2 and PGE_2 are produced at different sites with distinct actions. PGI_2 is synthesized in the collecting tubules where it enhances sodium, chloride, and water excretion, and PGE_2 is synthesized in the medullary interstitial cells, producing vasodilation and natriuresis and in the glomeruli to maintain glomerular filtration rate.

Prostaglandins and Renal Blood Flow

Normally renal prostaglandins have little effect on the control of blood flow to the kidneys, but in certain circumstances their effect is greatly enhanced. Vasoconstrictor hormones, including renin, angiotensin, norepinephrine, and vasopressin, produce a compensatory increase in renal vasodilator prostaglandins by inducing the enzyme phospholipase. In clinical conditions where there are high concentrations of circulating vasoconstrictors renal blood flow may become prostaglandin dependent. In such circumstances, NSAIDs may impair renal function by abolishing the protective vasodilator action of prostaglandins, thus allowing the unopposed action of vasoconstrictors.

During and after anaesthesia and surgery, there is an increase in circulating hormones with vasoconstrictor properties, often described as a component of the metabolic response to surgical stress. It has been postulated that the anesthetized patient is particularly susceptible to the adverse renal effects of NSAIDs, as the compensatory increase in vasodilator prostaglandins is prevented. Animal work has supported this view, where the anesthetized dog having a laparotomy is much more sensitive to the adverse affects of NSAIDs than the awake animal. The risk of unexpected blood loss and acute hypotension during surgery may further increase the risks associated with NSAID administration. During experimental hemorrhage and hypotension, renal prostaglandins oppose the actions of angiotensin II to activate the specific chemoreceptors contributing to autoregulation of renal blood flow.

Prostaglandins and Renal Tubular Function

Prostaglandins are also important in regulating the handling of electrolytes by renal tubules. They inhibit reuptake of chloride ions from the ascending limb of the loop of Henle, resulting in increased excretion of salt and water. Animal experiments show that normal tubular excretion of sodium and water is dependent on prostaglandins that suppress renal medullary sodium-potassium ATP-ase, and PGE_1 stimulates chloride ion secretion in the renal epithelial cells. Fluid retention based on these mechanisms is implicated in the development of congestive cardiac failure in patients with established cardiac disease, with an odds ratio of 2.1 (95% CI, 1.2–3.3) compared to controls not taking NSAIDs prior to hospital admission.

The coxibs have also been implicated in causing fluid retention resulting in hypertension. A meta-analysis of coxibs vs placebo and coxibs vs conventional NSAIDs demonstrated a mean rise of systolic blood pressure of 3.8 mmHg and 2.8 mmHg, respectively.[83] COX-2 is widely implicated in renal prostaglandin synthesis, and at present it is not possible to attribute the proportion of adverse cardiovascular events from salt and water retention with resulting vascular congestion and hypertension from the adverse events suspected to result from unopposed TXA_2 action in platelets.[84] Additional fluid retention may be caused by rofecoxib, as this is metabolized by the same enzyme as aldostereone, cytosol reductase. An argument has been proposed that there may be direct competition for the enzyme binding site between rofecoxib and aldosterone, resulting in an increase in plasma concentrations of the latter and hence further sodium retention,[85] although this has not been proved in a randomized controlled trial. Interestingly, blood pressure does not seem to be elevated with celecoxib treatment, as celecoxib has been reported to have inhibitory properties on certain isoforms of carbonic anhydrase, possibly offsetting some of the effects of sodium and fluid retention and hence preventing the expected rise in blood pressure.

Interaction with Renin and Vasopressin

Renal prostaglandins also increase the release of renin and inhibit the effect of vasopressin on the collecting ducts. Intravenous infusions of prostacyclin increase renin release in humans and consequently affect aldosterone production and potassium excretion. Indeed, excessive renal prostaglandin production has been implicated in the hypokalemic alkalosis associated with high renin, aldosterone, and angiotensin II concentrations of Barrter's syndrome, in which platelet defects are also found. NSAIDs also potentiate vasopressin. Renal prostaglandins and vasopressin interact and modulate each other. Vasopressin enhances renal tubular production of cyclic adenosine monophosphate, thus increasing permeability and water resorption, this being prevented by prostaglandins therefore increasing water excretion. Inhibition of prostaglandin production by certain NSAIDs may increase renal water retention, such that indomethacin has been used as a treatment for nephrogenic diabetes insipidus.

NSAIDs and Renal Function

Renal prostaglandins are important in regulating renal blood flow, tubular function, renin and aldosterone release, and the action of vasopressin. Therefore, NSAIDs may reduce renal blood flow and impair excretion of water and electrolytes. The clinical significance of this depends on the age and general medical condition of the patient.

Studies examining the effect of short-term NSAID administration of renal function have shown that adverse effects can occur after only a few doses in susceptible individuals. A systematic review demonstrated that as a group, NSAIDs cause a statistically significant, but clinically unimportant, transient mean fall in creatinine clearance of 18 mL/min in healthy adults in the acute postoperative period, and there were no reported cases of postoperative renal failure requiring dialysis attributable to NSAID administration.[86] Risk factors for NSAID nephrotoxicity include age (over 60 years), atherosclerosis, diuretic therapy, existing renal impairment, and states of renal hypoperfusion, including cardiac failure, hepatic cirrhosis, and hypovolemia. Many of these factors are present in patients having general surgery, and general anesthesia and surgery may produce an additional tendency toward NSAID-induced adverse effects.

Other Renal Effects

"Analgesic nephropathy" comprising papillary necrosis or interstitial fibrosis is a recognized cause of drug-induced renal failure that has been reported with most NSAIDs. The "renal flank pain" syndrome, a sudden onset renal failure with hematuria and discomfort, has been produced by various NSAIDs, including ketorolac, even after only a few doses.

Other Side Effects of Nonsteroidal Anti-Inflammatory Drugs

Aspirin-sensitive asthma is the precipitation of bronchospasm by aspirin and is commonly seen in patients who have asthma with chronic rhinitis or allergic polyps. The effect becomes obvious soon after the ingestion of aspirin, and individuals may be sensitive to other NSAIDs. This affects about 10% of asthmatics, usually in middle age. The importance of this syndrome has been emphasized by reports of fatal bronchospasm precipitated in asthmatic patients by ingestion of proprietary preparations containing NSAIDs.

The mechanism of this is unclear but the potency of the drug as a cyclooxygenase inhibitor is important. By inhibiting cyclooxygenase, more arachidonic acid precursor may be available to lipoxygenase pathways, producing substances known to cause bronchospasm, including leukotrienes. There may be an interaction with peptide endothelin-1, which may be involved in exaggerating bronchial muscle tone in asthmatics and which increases lipoxygenase products of arachidonic acid metabolism. Other factors are certainly involved as individuals with this disorder have an abnormal platelet response to aspirin in vitro, with the release of cytotoxic mediators, a prostaglandin-dependent mechanism. The ability of an NSAID to produce this syndrome is directly related to its potency as an inhibitor of prostaglandin synthesis. It may be prudent to avoid parenteral NSAIDs, including diclofenac and ketorolac, in all asthmatic patients because of their very powerful cyclooxygenase inhibition.

Hepatotoxicity

Aspirin and the NSAIDs can have adverse effects on the liver, normally after prolonged and excessive exposure. Diclofenac may produce fatal hepatitis, which can develop within a few weeks of commencing oral therapy. The risk of precipitating liver effects as a consequence of a short course of NSAIDs is unclear, although borderline increases in serum aminotransferase concentrations may occur in almost 15% of patients.

Injection Site Damage

Intramuscular diclofenac may produce appreciable pain on injections and is associated with muscle damage and increases in serum creatinine phosphokinase. Studies have shown that intramuscular ketorolac does not produce pain or changes in serum creatinine phosphokinase. The irritant nature of parenteral diclofenac was empahsized by the observation that after-intramuscular injection diclofenac produces venous thrombosis, although this can be minimized by dilution in dextrose solution. Injection site pain is a significant problem with diclofenac and has led to the widespread use of rectal preparations.

Other Side Effects

Mild CNS effects have been reported after ketorolac, including somnolence, headache, and dizziness. Blood dyscrasias, erythema multiforme, anaphylaxis, urticaria, pancreatitis, and aseptic meningitis have been reported, although all are uncommon. In preterm infants, indomethacin reduces cerebral blood flow and oxygen delivery, potentially increasing the risk of hypoxic brain injury, although it is not known if NSAIDs do this in older children or adults. Some myocardial protection against coronary vessel occlusion can be conferred in animals by preconditioning episodes of ischemia, an effect blocked by cyclooxygenase inhbitors, suggesting a possible protective role for prostaglandins, probably prostacyclin. It is unclear if this implies that NSAIDs have any effect on the consequences of acute myocardial ischemia in humans. All NSAIDs should be used with caution during pregnancy as they may increase the length of gestation by delaying spontaneous labor and affect closure of the ductus arteriosus in the newborn.

CONCLUSION

Aspirin and the NSAIDs have been used therapeutically for analgesic and anti-inflammatory purposes for over 100 years. They have a well-established role in both acute pain management and chronic pain conditions, though the limitations of adverse events must be recognized with long-term use. Increasing the selectivity of the enzyme targets of NSAIDs has resulted in the development of the coxibs, these agents having an analgesic efficacy comparable to conventional NSAIDs, with an improved gastrointestinal side-effect profile.

Debate regarding the risk from the antiplatelet effect of both coxibs and conventional NSAIDs is ongoing; however, it is paramount that patients should not be denied effective analgesic provision from NSAID therapy. Considering the presented data, and the continued emergence of evidence of increased thrombotic risk with coxib use, optimal outcome should be achieved by careful prescribing in an appropriate group of patients with therapy tailored to the minimum effective dose and minimum duration of therapy possible for NSAIDs of any class. The requirement for long-term therapy, particularly if at high doses, should be reviewed regularly. The reformulation and European launch of solubilized acetaminophen in solution has greatly improved the delivery of this efficacious analgesic. Previously, where fasting regulations and postoperative ileus may have prevented oral administration, and with variable bioavailability from rectal absorption, one now has the facility to administer regular acetaminophen throughout the perioperative period, hence improving analgesia and reducing the potential for adverse effects as a result of its opioid-sparing effect. A switch to the less expensive oral route is recommended as soon as possible.

REFERENCES

1. Zhang J, Ding EL, Song Y. Adverse effects of cyclooxygenase 2 inhibitors on renal and arrhythmia events: metaanalysis of randomized trials. *JAMA*. 2006;296(13):1619–1632.

2. Roberts LJ. Comparative metabolism and fate of the eicosanoids. In: Willis AL, ed. *Handbook of Eicosanoids, Prostaglansins and Related Lipids*. Boca Raton, FL: CRC Press, 1987:233-244.

3. Vane JR. Inhibition of prostaglandin synthesis as a mechanism of action for aspirin-like drugs. *Nat New Biol*. 1971;231(25):232–235.

4. Cousins MJ. John J. Bonica distinguished lecture: acute pain and the injury response: immediate and prolonged effects. *Reg Anesth*. 1989;14(4):162–179.

5. Jurna I, Brune K. Central effect of the non-steroid anti-inflammatory agents, indomethacin, ibuprofen, and diclofenac, determined in C fibre-evoked activity in single neurones of the rat thalamus. *Pain*. 1990;41(1):71–80.

6. Tacconelli S, Capone ML, Patrignani P. Clinical pharmacology of novel selective COX-2 inhibitors. [Review] [112 refs] Current Pharmaceutical Design. 10(6):589–601, 2004.

7. Chen LC, Elliott RA, Ashcroft DM. Systematic review of the analgesic efficacy and tolerability of COX-2 inhibitors in post-operative pain control. [Review] [49 refs] Journal of Clinical Pharmacy & Therapeutics. 29(3):215–29, 2004 Jun.

8. Romsing J, Moiniche S. A systematic review of COX-2 inhibitors compared with traditional NSAIDs, or different COX-2 inhibitors for post-operative pain. [See comment]. [Review] [58 refs] Acta Anaesthesiologica Scandinavica. 48(5):525–46, 2004.

9. Anderson BJ, Pons G, Autret-Leca E, Allegart K, Boccard E. Pediatric intravenous paracetamol (propacetamol) pharmacokinetics: a population analysis. *Pediatr Anesthes*. 2005;15(4):282–292.

10. Hersh EV, Lally ET, Moore PA. Update on cyclooxygenase inhibitors: has a third COX isoform entered the fray?. [Review] [89 refs] Current Medical Research & Opinion. 21(8):1217–26, 2005 Aug.

11. Graham GG, Scott KF. Mechanism of action of paracetamol. [Article]. *Am J Therapeut*. 2005;12(1):46–55.

12. Pini LA, Sandrini M, Vitale G. The antinociceptive action of paracetamol is associated with changes in the serotonergic system in the rat brain. *Eur J Pharmacol*. 1996;308(1):31–40.

13. Bjorkman R. Central antinociceptive effects of non-steroidal anti-inflammatory drugs and paracetamol: experimental studies in the rat. *Acta Anaesthesiol Scand Suppl*. 1995;103:1–44.

14. Bjorkman R, Hallman KM, Hedner J, Hedner T, Henning M. Acetaminophen blocks spinal hyperalgesia induced by NMDA and substance P. *Pain*. 1994;57(3):259–264.

15. Peduto VA, Ballabio M, Stefanini S. Efficacy of propacetamol in the treatment of postoperative pain: morphine sparing effect in orthopedic surgery. Italian Collaborative Group on Propacetamol. *Acta Anaesthesiol Scand*. 1998;42(3):293–298.

16. Bannwarth B, Netter P, Lapicque F, Gillet P, Pere P, Boccard E et al. Plasma and cerebrospinal fluid concentrations of paracetamol after a single intravenous dose of propacetamol. *Br J Clin Pharmacol*. 1992;34(1):79–81.

17. Edwards JE, Oldman A, Smith L, et al. Single dose oral aspirin for acute pain. *Cochrane Database Syst Rev*. 2000;(2):CD002067.

18. Flouvat B, Leneveu A, Fitoussi S, Delhotal-Landes B, Gendron A. Bioequivalence study comparing a new paracetamol solution for injection and propacetamol after single intravenous infusion in healthy subjects. *Int J Clin Pharmacol Ther*. 2004;42(1):50–57.

19. Internet. 2007. Ref Type: Electronic Citation

20. Kehlet H, Dahl JB. The value of "multimodal" or "balanced analgesia" in postoperative pain treatment. *Anesth Analg*. 1993;77(5): 1048–1056.

21. Mimoz O, Incagnoli P, Josse C, Gillon MC, Kuhlman L, Mirand A et al. Analgesic efficacy and safety of nefopam vs. propacetamol following hepatic resection*. *Anaesthesia*. 2001;56(6):520–525.

22. Sinatra R. Role of COX-2 inhibitors in the evolution of acute pain management. [Review] [34 refs] Journal of Pain & Symptom Management. 24(1 Suppl):S18–27, 2002 Jul.

23. Van Aken H, Thys L, Veekman L, Buerkle H. Assessing analgesia in single and repeated administrations of propacetamol for post-operative pain: comparison with morphine after dental surgery. *Anesth Analg*. 2004;98(1):159–165, table.

24. Zhou TJ, Tang J, White PF. Propacetamol versus ketorolac for treatment of acute postoperative pain after total hip or knee replacement. *Anesth Analg*. 2001;92(6):1569–1575.

25. Romsing J, Moiniche S, Dahl JB. Rectal and parenteral paracetamol, and paracetamol in combination with NSAIDs, for postoperative analgesia. *Br J Anaesth*. 2002;88(2):215–226.

26. Skjelbred P, L++kken P. Paracetamol versus placebo: effects on post-operative course. *Eur J Clin Pharmacol*. 1979;15(1):27–33.

27. Cobby TF, Crighton IM, Kyriakides K, Hobbs GJ. Rectal paracetamol has a significant morphine-sparing effect after hysterectomy. *Br J Anaesth*. 1999;83(2):253–256.

28. Hernandez-Palazon J, Tortosa JA, Martinez-Lage JF, Perez-Flores D. Intravenous administration of propacetamol reduces morphine consumption after spinal fusion surgery. *Anesth Analg*. 2001;92(6):1473–1476.

29. Korpela R, Korvenoja P, Meretoja OA. Morphine-sparing effect of acetaminophen in pediatric day-case surgery. *Anesthesiology*. 1999;91(2):442–447.

30. Bird HA. Clinical experience with tenoxicam: a review. *Scand J Rheumatol Suppl*. 1987;65:102–106.

31. Gonzalez JP, Todd PA. Tenoxicam. A preliminary review of its pharmacodynamic and pharmacokinetic properties, and therapeutic efficacy. *Drugs*. 1987;34(3):289–310.

32. Heintz RC. Tenoxicam and renal function. *Drug Saf*. 1995; 12(2):110–119.

33. Edwards JE, McQuay HJ, Moore RA. Efficacy and safety of valdecoxib for treatment of osteoarthritis and rheumatoid arthritis: systematic review of randomised controlled trials. *Pain*. 2004;111(3): 286–296.

34. Barden J, Edwards JE, McQuay HJ, Moore RA. Single dose oral celecoxib for postoperative pain. *Cochrane Database Syst Rev*. 2003;(2):CD004233.

35. Cashman JN, Jones RM, Foster JM, Adams AP. Comparison of infusions of morphine and lysine acetyl salicylate for the relief of pain after surgery. *Br J Anaesth*. 1985;57(3):255–258.

36. Jones RM, Cashman JN, Foster JM, Wedley JR, Adams AP. Comparison of infusions of morphine and lysine acetyl salicylate for the relief of pain following thoracic surgery. *Br J Anaesth*. 1985;57(3):259–263.

37. Kweekel-de Vries WJ, Spierdijk J, Mattie H, Hermans JM. A new soluble acetylsalicylic acid derivative in the treatment of postoperative pain. *Br J Anaesth*. 1974;46(2):133–135.

38. Davies NM. Clinical pharmacokinetics of ibuprofen: the first 30 years. *Clin Pharmacokinet*. 1998;34(2):101–154.

39. Collins SL, Moore RA, McQuay HJ, Wiffen PJ. Oral ibuprofen and diclofenac in post-operative pain: a quantitative systematic review. *Eur J Pain*. 1998;2(4):285–291.

40. Hodsman NB, Burns J, Blyth A, Kenny GN, McArdle CS, Rotman H. The morphine sparing effects of diclofenac sodium following abdominal surgery. *Anaesthesia.* 1987;42(9):1005–1008.

41. Campbell WI, Kendrick R, Patterson C. Intravenous diclofenac sodium. Does its administration before operation suppress postoperative pain? *Anaesthesia.* 1990;45(9):763–766.

42. Moores MA, Wandless JG, Fell D. Paediatric postoperative analgesia. A comparison of rectal diclofenac with caudal bupivacaine after inguinal herniotomy. *Anaesthesia.* 1990;45(2):156–158.

43. Mason L, Edwards JE, MRMH. Single dose oral naproxen and naproxen sodium for acute postoperative pain. *Cochrane Database Syst Rev.* 2004; 4.

44. Bombardier C, Laine L, Reicin A, Shapiro D, Burgos-Vargas R, Davis B et al. Comparison of upper gastrointestinal toxicity of rofecoxib and naproxen in patients with rheumatoid arthritis. VIGOR Study Group. *N Engl J Med.* 2000;343(21):1520–8, 2.

45. Gasparini L, Ongini E, Wenk G. Non-steroidal anti-inflammatory drugs (NSAIDs) in Alzheimer's disease: old and new mechanisms of action. [Review] [141 refs] Journal of Neurochemistry. 91(3):521–36, 2004 Nov.

46. ADAPT Research Group. Cardiovascular and Cerebrovascular Events in the Randomized, Controlled Alzheimer's Disease Anti-Inflammatory Prevention Trial (ADAPT). *PLoS Clini Trials.* 2006;1(7):e33.

47. Vangen O, Doessland S, Lindbaek E. Comparative study of ketorolac and paracetamol/codeine in alleviating pain following gynaecological surgery. *J Int Med Res.* 1988;16(6):443–451.

48. McQuay HJ, Poppleton P, Carroll D, Summerfield RJ, Bullingham RE, Moore RA. Ketorolac and acetaminophen for orthopedic postoperative pain. *Clin Pharmacol Ther.* 1986;39(1):89–93.

49. Power I, Noble DW, Douglas E, Spence AA. Comparison of i.m. ketorolac trometamol and morphine sulphate for pain relief after cholecystectomy. *Br J Anaesth.* 1990;65(4):448–455.

50. Serpell MG, Thomson MF. Comparison of piroxicam with placebo in the management of pain after total hip replacement. *Br J Anaesth.* 1989;63(3):354–356.

51. Edwards JE, Loke YK, Moore RA, McQuay HJ. Single dose piroxicam for acute postoperative pain. *Cochrane Database Syst Rev.* 2000;4:CD002762.

52. Hutchison GL, Crofts SL, Gray IG. Preoperative piroxicam for postoperative analgesia in dental surgery. *Br J Anaesth.* 1990;65(4):500–503.

53. Gonzalez JP, Todd PA. Tenoxicam. A preliminary review of its pharmacodynamic and pharmacokinetic properties, and therapeutic efficacy. [erratum appears in Drugs 1988 Jan;35(1): preceding 1].

54. Albengres E, Urien S, Barre J, Nguyen P, Bree F, Jolliet P et al. Clinical pharmacology of oxicams: new insights into the mechanisms of their dose-dependent toxicity.

55. Fenton C, Keating GM, Wagstaff AJ. Valdecoxib: a review of its use in the management of osteoarthritis, rheumatoid arthritis, dysmenorrhoea and acute pain. *Drugs.* 2004;64(11):1231–1261.

56. Chavez ML, DeKorte CJ. Valdecoxib: a review. *Clin Ther.* 2003;25(3):817–851.

57. Aldington S, Shirtcliffe P, Weatherall M, Beasley R. Increased risk of cardiovascular events with parecoxib/valdecoxib: a systematic review and meta-analysis. *N Z Med J.* 2005;118(1226): U1755.

58. Jain KK. Evaluation of intravenous parecoxib for the relief of acute post-surgical pain. *Expert Opin Investig Drugs.* 2000;9(11):2717–2723.

59. Simon LS, Lanza FL, Lipsky PE, et al. Preliminary study of the safety and efficacy of SC-58635, a novel cyclooxygenase 2 inhibitor: efficacy and safety in two placebo-controlled trials in osteoarthritis and rheumatoid arthritis, and studies of gastrointestinal and platelet effects. *Arthritis Rheum.* 1998;41(9):1591–1602.

60. Deeks JJ, Smith LA, Bradley MD. Efficacy, tolerability, and upper gastrointestinal safety of celecoxib for treatment of osteoarthritis and rheumatoid arthritis: systematic review of randomised controlled trials.

61. Silverstein FE, Faich G, Goldstein JL, et al. Gastrointestinal toxicity with celecoxib vs nonsteroidal anti-inflammatory drugs for osteoarthritis and rheumatoid arthritis: the CLASS study: a randomized controlled trial. *JAMA.* 2000;284(10):1247–1255.

62. Hilmi I, Goh KL. Chemoprevention of colorectal cancer with nonsteroidal anti-inflammatory drugs.

63. Williams CS, Luongo C, Radhika A, et al. Elevated cyclo-oxygenase-2 levels in Min mouse adenomas. *Gastroenterology.* 1996;111(4):1134–1140.

64. Kismet K, Akay MT, Abbasoglu O, Ercan A. Celecoxib: a potent cyclooxygenase-2 inhibitor in cancer prevention. [Review] [168 refs] Cancer Detection & Prevention. 28(2):127–42, 2004.

65. Bertagnolli MM, Eagle CJ, Zauber AG, Redston M, Solomon SD, Kim K et al. Celecoxib for the prevention of sporadic colorectal adenomas. *N Engl J Med.* 2006;355(9):873–884.

66. Caldwell B, Aldington S, Weatherall M, Shirtcliffe P, Beasley R. Risk of cardiovascular events and celecoxib: a systematic review and meta-analysis. [See comment]. [Review] [36 refs] Journal of the Royal Society of Medicine. 99(3):132–40, 2006 Mar.

67. Rordorf CM, Choi L, Marshall P, Mangold JB. Clinical pharmacology of lumiracoxib: a selective cyclo-oxygenase-2 inhibitor. *Clin Pharmacokinet.* 2005;44(12):1247–1266.

68. Bannwarth B, Berenbaum F. Clinical pharmacology of lumiracoxib, a second-generation cyclooxygenase 2 selective inhibitor. *Expert Opin Investig Drugs.* 2005;14(4):521–533.

69. Matchaba P, Gitton X, Krammer G, et al. Cardiovascular safety of lumiracoxib: a meta-analysis of all randomized controlled trials > or =1 week and up to 1 year in duration of patients with osteoarthritis and rheumatoid arthritis. *Clin Ther.* 2005;27(8):1196–1214.

70. Collaborative overview of randomised trials of antiplatelet therapy. I. Prevention of death, myocardial infarction, and stroke by prolonged antiplatelet therapy in various categories of patients. Antiplatelet Trialists' Collaboration. *BMJ.* 1994;308(6921):81–106.

71. Clive DM, Stoff JS. Renal syndromes associated with nonsteroidal antiinflammatory drugs. *N Engl J Med.* 1984;310(9):563–572.

72. Cheng Y, Austin SC, Rocca B, et al. Role of prostacyclin in the cardiovascular response to thromboxane A2. *Science.* 2002;296(5567):539–541.

73. Bresalier RS, Sandler RS, Quan H, et al. Cardiovascular events associated with rofecoxib in a colorectal adenoma chemoprevention trial. *N Engl J Med.* 2005;352(11):1092–1102.

74. Huang WF, Hsiao FY, Wen YW, Tsai YW. Cardiovascular events associated with the use of four nonselective NSAIDs (etodolac, nabumetone, ibuprofen, or naproxen) versus a cyclooxygenase-2 inhibitor (celecoxib): a population-based analysis in Taiwanese adults. *Clin Ther.* 2006;28(11):1827–1836.

75. McGettigan P, Henry D. Cardiovascular risk and inhibition of cyclooxygenase: a systematic review of the observational studies of selective and nonselective inhibitors of cyclooxygenase 2.

76. Merck provides preliminary analyses of the completed MEDAL program for ARCOXIA (etoricoxib). www.merck.com. 2006.

77. Kearney PM, Baigent C, Godwin J, Halls H, Emberson JR, Patrono C. Do selective cyclo-oxygenase-2 inhibitors and traditional non-steroidal anti-inflammatory drugs increase the risk

of atherothrombosis? Meta-analysis of randomised trials. *BMJ.* 2006;332(7553):1302–1308.

78. Wang D, Wang M, Cheng Y, Fitzgerald GA. Cardiovascular hazard and non-steroidal anti-inflammatory drugs. [erratum appears in Curr Opin Pharmacol. 2005 Oct;5(5):556 Note: Wong, Dairong [corrected to Wang, Dairong]].

79. Hawkey CJ, Skelly MM. Gastrointestinal safety of selective COX-2 inhibitors.

80. Richy F, Bruyere O, Ethgen O, et al. Time dependent risk of gastrointestinal complications induced by non-steroidal anti-inflammatory drug use: a consensus statement using a metaanalytic approach.

81. Bashein G, Nessly ML, Rice AL, Counts RB, Misbach GA. Preoperative aspirin therapy and reoperation for bleeding after coronary artery bypass surgery. *Arch Intern Med.* 1991;151(1):89–93.

82. Power I, Chambers WA, Greer IA, Ramage D, Simon E. Platelet function after intramuscular diclofenac. *Anaesthesia.* 1990;45(11):916–919.

83. Aw TJ, Haas SJ, Liew D, Krum H. Meta-analysis of cyclooxygenase-2 inhibitors and their effects on blood pressure. *Arch Intern Med.* 2005;165(5):490–496.

84. Krum H, Aw TJ, Liew D, Haas S. Blood pressure effects of COX-2 inhibitors.

85. Aw TJ, Liew D, Tofler GH, Schneider HG, Morel-Kopp MC, Billah B et al. Can the blood pressure effects of COX-2 selective inhibitors be explained by changes in plasma aldosterone levels? *J Hypertens.* 2006;24(10):1979–1984.

86. Lee A, Cooper MC, Craig JC, Knight JF, Keneally JP. Effects of nonsteroidal anti-inflammatory drugs on postoperative renal function in adults with normal renal function. *Cochrane Database Syst Rev.* 2004;(2):CD002765.

6

Local Anesthetics in Regional Anesthesia and Acute Pain Management

John Butterworth, MD

GENERAL CONSIDERATIONS

Although the multiple medicinal properties of cocaine (including its ability to produce numbness) were appreciated by indigenous South Americans long before European explorers arrived, the birth of local and regional anesthesia is usually designated as 1884, the year when Köller and Gartner published their findings after producing topical cocaine anesthesia of frogs, rabbits, dogs, and each other's corneas.[1-5] Unhindered by drug registration agencies, regulations regarding human experimentation, or standards for safety, purity, or efficacy, physicians quickly adopted the "new" agent and used it for an expanding array of procedures. Within the same calendar year (1884) but on a distant continent the American surgeon Halsted performed mandibular nerve and brachial plexus blocks.[1] By the end of the first quarter of the 20th century, cocaine and other local anesthetics (LA) had been used for spinal, caudal, epidural, paravertebral, celiac, and intravenous regional blocks, and physicians had begun compounding local anesthetics with additives to enhance their duration and safety.

Building on this rapid early progress, the field continues to advance on multiple fronts. This chapter will focus on mechanisms of local anesthetic action, pharmacodynamics, additives, and toxicity, and, in particular, on how local anesthetics can be most effectively used in regional anesthesia (RA) and pain medicine. We will also consider how potential new formulations and new compounds might lead to improved options for the clinician.

STRUCTURE AND FUNCTIONS OF Na CHANNELS

Local anesthetics produce peripheral nerve blocks by binding and inhibiting voltage-gated Na channels in nerve membranes. Na channels are large, integral membrane proteins that contain a larger α-subunit and 1 or 2 smaller β-subunits. Ion conduction and local anesthetic binding both take place within the subunit, which contains 4 homologous domains each with 6 helical, membrane-spanning segments (Figure 6.1).[6,7] When present, subunits regulate expression, insertion into plasma membranes, voltage dependence, and kinetics of α subunits.[8,9] Humans have 10 Na channel genes, only 9 of these genes are "functional," distributed over 4 chromosomes.[7,8] Na channel forms for unmyelinated axons, nodes of Ranvier, small dorsal root ganglion nociceptors, skeletal muscle, and cardiac muscle each derive from specific genes.[8] Specific channel isoforms have differing affinities for tetrodotoxin and responses to local anesthetics.[10]

ELECTROPHYSIOLOGY OF Na$^+$ CHANNELS

Na channels exist in at least 3 native, functional conformations: "resting," "open," and "inactivated.[6,11] These three conformations were first identified in the early 1950s in experiments conducted by Professor Sir Alan Hodgkin and Professor Sir Andrew Huxley and, in some cases, with Professor Sir Bernard Katz (all three were recipients of a Nobel Prize). During action potentials Na channels "open" briefly, allowing extracellular Na ions to flow into the cell, depolarizing the plasma membrane. After a few milliseconds, Na channels "inactivate" (whereupon the Na current ceases). In lower animals (eg, squid), repolarization of nerve membranes is facilitated by a contribution from K channels with K ion flow from inside to outside the cell; this contribution is much emphasized in physiology and anesthesiology textbooks. Nevertheless, most readers of this chapter will have greater interest in human than squid neurophysiology. Mammalian myelinated fibers require no contribution from K currents for membrane repolarization; they only require that the Na channels quickly cease to conduct Na ions.[6,11] The total number of Na ions that enters the cell during a typical nerve action potential is vanishingly small relative to prevailing transmembrane gradients such that each action potential has essentially no lasting effect on the membrane potential.

Ion-selective permeability and voltage gating are both remarkable evolutionary accomplishments on the part of ion channel molecules. Of the two ion channel features, the mechanism underlying ion-selective permeability is more easily understood and multiple forms of selectively permeable glasses are

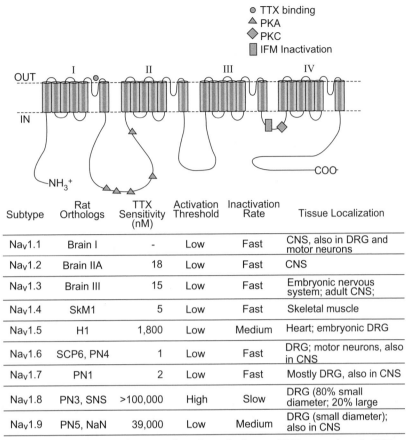

Subtype	Rat Orthologs	TTX Sensitivity (nM)	Activation Threshold	Inactivation Rate	Tissue Localization
Na$_V$1.1	Brain I	-	Low	Fast	CNS, also in DRG and motor neurons
Na$_V$1.2	Brain IIA	18	Low	Fast	CNS
Na$_V$1.3	Brain III	15	Low	Fast	Embryonic nervous system; adult CNS;
Na$_V$1.4	SkM1	5	Low	Fast	Skeletal muscle
Na$_V$1.5	H1	1,800	Low	Medium	Heart; embryonic DRG
Na$_V$1.6	SCP6, PN4	1	Low	Fast	DRG; motor neurons, also in CNS
Na$_V$1.7	PN1	2	Low	Fast	Mostly DRG, also in CNS
Na$_V$1.8	PN3, SNS	>100,000	High	Slow	DRG (80% small diameter; 20% large
Na$_V$1.9	PN5, NaN	39,000	Low	Medium	DRG (small diameter); also in CNS

Figure 6.1: Mammalian voltage-gated Na channel subtypes. TTX = tetrodotoxin, PKA = protein kinase A, PKC = protein kinase C, IFM = intracellular loop responsible for first inactivation. III S6 and IV S1 responsible for inactivation. Reprinted from: Lai J, Porreca F, Hunter J, Gold M. Voltage-gated sodium channels and hyperalgesia. *Annu Rev Pharmacol Toxicol.* 2004;44:372.[7]

produced for use as ion-selective electrodes. Recent x-ray crystallographic studies have provided us with a better appreciation for voltage-gating phenomena. Channels are likely "gated" by paddle-shaped voltage sensors (containing a dipole) that move within and out of the plasma membrane, contorting the ion conducting "pore" of voltage-gated ion channels.[12,13]

ELECTROPHARMACOLOGY OF LOCAL ANESTHESIA

Local anesthesia results when local anesthetics bind Na channels in peripheral neurons, inhibiting the increased Na permeability that underlies action potentials.[6,11] Molecular biologic techniques have permitted investigators to isolate regions of the Na channel molecule that are relevant to the production of local anesthesia. In particular, local anesthetic binding has been localized to S6 regions of α subunits.[6,7,14]

Local anesthetic inhibition of Na currents increases with repetitive depolarizations, a phenomenon often called "use dependent," "frequency dependent," or "phasic" block.[6,11] But, why does the extent of local anesthetic inhibition increase with repetitive depolarizations? Each succeeding depolarization presents a new opportunity for local anesthetics to encounter a Na channel that, not yet having bound a local anesthetic,

is "open" or "inactivated," both of which forms have greater local anesthetic affinity than "resting" channels.[6,11,15] Thus, the fraction of channels that are bound by local anesthetic progressively increases with repetitive depolarizations, resulting in a progressive decline in the magnitude of the Na current and action potential.

Many compounds other than local anesthetics will inhibit Na channels: general anesthetics, α_2 agonists, tricyclic antidepressants, and nerve toxins.[11,16–19] Perhaps one of these "nontraditional" Na channel antagonists will prove safer or more effective than traditional local anesthetics.

LOCAL ANESTHETIC ACTIONS AT SITES UNRELATED TO Na⁺ CHANNELS OR NERVE BLOCK

Local anesthetics have many actions other than those related to Na channels and nerve block, and these local anesthetic actions have been the subject of recent review articles.[20–22] Circulating local anesthetics have profound effects on coagulation, inflammation, microcirculation, immune responses to infection and malignancy, postoperative gastrointestinal function, and analgesia.[20,21] Infused local anesthetics may relieve neuropathic pain.[22]

LOCAL ANESTHETIC STRUCTURES

All local anesthetics used in clinical medicine share certain structural features that render them all amphiphilic.[2,5,19,23,24] One end of the molecule is more hydrophobic as a consequence of its containing a benzene ring, often with alkyl substituents. The other end of the molecule is more hydrophilic as a consequence of its containing a tertiary amine. The pK_a of this amine is generally >7.4; therefore, the preponderance of local anesthetic molecules found in vivo will be protonated (positively charged). These two structural elements are separated by a hydrocarbon chain or ring and by an amide or ester bond.[3,5,11,25]

Two of the currently available local anesthetics, ropivacaine and levobupivacaine, are prepared for clinical use as single S(−) enantiomers.[26] Mepivacaine, bupivacaine, etidocaine, prilocaine, and cocaine are prepared as racemic mixtures; the remaining local anesthetics have no asymmetric carbon atoms. The various local anesthetics available commercially differ markedly in their potential clinical applications and toxicity. In clinical practice, not every local anesthetic is suitable for every regional block procedure. Thus, an astute clinician will select among a restricted set of compounds for the one with the onset and duration of action most consistent with surgical needs.

A variety of other compounds other than "conventional" local anesthetics have been used in animal and human experiments to produce regional anesthesia (as well as to block the Na channels, as was previously discussed).[10,11,19,27,28] Some amphiphilic compounds share multiple structural features with local anesthetics (eg, calcium channel blockers and tricyclic antidepressants). Others (eg, the nerve toxins tetrodotoxin and saxitoxin) bear no structural similarities to conventional local anesthetics, clearly bind to a different active site, and resemble "classical" local anesthetics only by being organic compounds that inhibit Na currents.[6] Still other agents that inhibit nerve conduction, for example, the general anesthetic halothane, bind at Na channel sites yet to be specifically identified.

PHYSICOCHEMICAL PROPERTIES OF LOCAL ANESTHETICS

Local anesthetics may be characterized by their potency, delay of onset, and duration of action, and there are associations between the physicochemical properties of local and these properties. On the basis of their anesthetic profile in humans, the local anesthetics may be classified as follows:

1. Agents with relatively short durations of action and low potency, including procaine and chloroprocaine
2. Agents with intermediate durations of action and moderate potency, including lidocaine and mepivacaine, and prilocaine
3. Agents with prolonged duration of action and high potency including tetracaine, bupivacaine, levobupivacaine, ropivacaine, and etidocaine.

Chloroprocaine, lidocaine, mepivacaine, prilocaine, and etidocaine possess a relatively rapid onset of action. Tetracaine, bupivacaine, and ropivacaine have prolonged latencies of onset. In general, increasing potency associates with increasing lipid solubility, protein binding, delay of onset, and duration of action.

Physicochemical properties that have been linked to clinical local anesthetic actions include lipid solubility, plasma protein binding, and pK_a. Lipid solubility has a strong association with the potency of local anesthetic compounds, particularly among chemically similar compounds in experiments on isolated nerves in vitro. However, the correlation is less robust in human anesthesia. Chloroprocaine has a relatively low lipid solubility, with an octanol:buffer partition coefficient for the free-base, neutral form of 810 at body temperature. Chloroprocaine is administered at concentrations of 2% to 3% for epidural anesthesia. However, bupivacaine has much greater lipid solubility, with an octanol:water partition coefficient for the free-base hentral form of 3420 at body temperature.[29] Bupivacaine produces effective epidural anesthesia at concentrations between 0.50% to 0.75%, indicating that it may be (roughly) 4 times more potent than chloroprocaine.

Increasing lipid solubility also associates with increasing duration of action. Among the following pairs of related anesthetics, lidocaine and etidocaine, mepivacaine and bupivacaine, and procaine and tetracaine, the second agent in the pair has greater lipid solubility and the longer duration of action. Increased lipid solubility also associates with increased delay of onset for every drug pair just cited, save that of lidocaine vs etidocaine, where etidocaine has an onset as fast as lidocaine's. Etidocaine's anomalously rapid onset remains poorly understood.

All clinically useful compounds must have at least some minimal lipid solubility. The protonated (charged) forms of local anesthetics have much lower octanol:buffer partition coefficients than the neutral (uncharged) forms.[29] At body temperature, the charged form of bupivacaine has an octanol-water partition coefficient of 2, whereas the neutral base local anesthetic has a coefficient of 3420. Compounds that do not readily permeate membranes (eg, QX314, an obligatorily charged quaternary analog of lidocaine) will not produce conduction block if applied on the extracellular side of a nerve (as would take place during clinical regional anesthesia). Obligatorily charged local anesthetics will potently block Na currents when applied within cytoplasm, a finding that promotes many useful insights about the local anesthetic binding site.[6,11,19]

The pK_a of a compound identifies the pH at which the neutral and charged forms are present in equal concentrations. pK_a has a much-discussed but, in truth, nonexistant association with the speed of onset of local anesthesia.[30] Local anesthetics must diffuse across tissue and/or membrane to inhibit Na channels in all circumstances save when a drug is introduced directly into the cytoplasm. Therefore, in nearly all clinical circumstances, rapid onset is favored by increasing the amount of drug in the base (uncharged or neutral) form. The percentage of a specific local anesthetic that is present in the base form when injected into tissue is inversely related to the pK_a of that agent. Using these facts, many authors make a leap of faith and assert that one can predict the relative speed of onset among differing local anesthetics by comparing their pK_as.[30] Unfortunately, faith in this rule is *not* supported by the available data, despite the many examination questions that have been written on this topic. Mepivacaine, lidocaine, and etidocaine, for example, possess pK_as of 7.7, 7.8, and 7.9, respectively, at body temperature.[29] Yet, despite a greater pK_a, the onset of block with etidocaine is at least as fast as with the other two agents. Tetracaine possesses a pK_a of 8.4 at 36°C. At the same temperature, chloroprocaine has a pK_a of 9.1. Nevertheless, the onset of block with chloroprocaine for all forms of regional anesthesia is considerably faster than with tetracaine (and this holds true even when adjustments are made for their relative potencies). Die-hard, zealous devotees of the pK_a "rule" have argued that chloroprocaine is used at greater concentrations than other local anesthetics, and attribute chloroprocaine's more rapid onset of action to the larger number of molecules of this agent that are administered compared to other agents. This explanation finally collapsed when exactly the same doses of 1% chloroprocaine and 1% lidocaine were compared for spinal anesthesia,[31] and chloroprocaine had a shorter onset time than lidocaine. Thus, pK_a does not predict rate of onset.

It has long been part of the "canon" that the extent of protein binding of local anesthetics determines their duration of action.[30] There is no question that one can demonstrate a correlation among lipid solubility, protein binding, potency, and duration of action. *Nevertheless, despite the correlation, there is no direct relationship between local anesthetic protein binding and local anesthetic binding to Na channels.* For any drug, the less water soluble the compound the greater fraction of the drug will be protein bound in blood.[32] The only conceivable connection between protein binding and duration of local anesthetic action lies in the fact that local anesthetics of increased lipid solubility (by definition) are protein bound to greater extent when they reach the blood stream. For thermodynamic reasons, more lipid soluble agents will have a greater tendency than less lipid soluble agents to remain in a lipid-rich environment (eg, the plasma membrane) than to diffuse into the blood. The greater the propensity that the local anesthetic molecule has for remaining within the membrane (rather than diffusing away from the nerve towards the blood stream), the longer that the molecule has the potential to bind the Na channels contained within the membrane and produce nerve block. Once the local anesthetic molecule enters the blood stream, it is highly unlikely to reenter the nerve membrane and contribute to conduction block.

Bupivacaine is about 95% protein bound. It has an octanol: buffer partition coefficient for the free base form of 3420, great potency, and a long duration of action.[29] However, procaine is only 6% protein bound and much less potent. It has an octanol:buffer partition coefficient for the free base form of 100 and a relatively short duration of action. Mepivacaine and lidocaine are both intermediate in terms of protein binding (55% to 75%) and in terms of lipid solubility (partition coefficients for the free base forms of 130 and 366, respectively), potency, and anesthetic duration. As should be obvious, it is silly to consider the nonspecific binding of a drug to α_1-acid glycoprotein and albumin (the two serum proteins to which local anesthetics bind) as having any direct relationship to the duration of binding of that drug to its specific binding site in the Na channel, other than as an index of lipid solubility, which defines the propensity of a molecule to remain within a lipid-rich environment (eg, membrane).[33]

LOCAL ANESTHETIC PHARMACODYNAMICS

Local Anesthetic Volumes and Concentrations during Nerve Block

When 40–35 mL of 0.5% ropivacaine is injected to produce a brachial plexus block, only a very small fraction of the local anesthetic molecules will actually be bound by Na channels in the brachial plexus.[34] As is generally true during regional anesthesia, most of the injected local anesthetic will be "nonspecifically" bound by other nearby membranes and tissues and/or removed by the blood stream. As a consequence, the extent and the duration of local anesthetic effects can be only loosely correlated with local anesthetic content of nerves in animal experiments.[35-38]

To block conduction, the anesthesia must cover a sufficient length of nerve. This "critical length" exceeds 2 cm (far more than the 3 Ranvier nodes specified in textbooks) except at very increased local anesthetic concentrations.[39]

In all circumstances, the mass of drug (the total number of local anesthetic molecules) administered will influence the onset, quality, and duration of anesthesia.[30] For any agent, as the mass of drug increases, the likelihood of satisfactory anesthesia and the duration of anesthesia will increase and the latency of onset of anesthesia will decrease. In general, the dosage of local anesthetic administered can be increased by administering a larger volume of a less concentrated solution or a smaller volume of a more concentrated solution.

Clinicians and basic scientists continue to debate whether volume, concentration, or total mass (the product of volume and concentration) of drug is paramount in determining the success of blocks. For example, in laboring women, increasing the bupivacaine concentration from 0.125% to 0.5% while maintaining the same injectate volume (10 mL) decreased latency, improved the incidence of satisfactory epidural analgesia, and increased the duration of action.[40] In surgical anesthesia increasing the bupivacaine concentration from 0.5% to 0.75% (at constant volume) produced a faster onset and longer duration of sensory anesthesia and increased the likelihood of satisfactory sensory anesthesia and the degree of motor block.[41] When prilocaine was administered in the epidural space either as 30 mL of a 2% solution or 20 mL of 3% solution, there was no difference in onset, depth, or duration of anesthesia or of motor block.[41] In epidural analgesia the volume of anesthetic solution administered may influence the "spread" of anesthesia; for example, 30 mL of 1% lidocaine administered in the epidural space anesthetized 4 more dermatomes than 10 mL of 3% lidocaine.[42] However, in rat sciatic nerve blocks a smaller volume of a more concentrated local anesthetic solution produce a denser, more persistant block than a larger volume of a less concentrated solution.[36] Nevertheless, multiple clinical studies suggest that except for a consistent positive correlation between injectate volume and the dermatomal spread of epidural anesthesia, the primary qualities of regional anesthesia, namely onset, depth, and duration of blockade, are related to the mass of drug injected (ie, the product of volume times concentration) and the proximity of the local anesthetic molecules to the intended target.[43,44]

MAXIMUM DOSES

Most review articles and book chapters present a table of "maximal safe doses" of local anesthetics, despite there being no way to specify one, universal, practical, maximal "safe" dose of a local anesthetic.[45] The maximal tolerable dose depends on many factors, including the intended (and actual) site of injection, the duration of time over which the local anesthetic was injected, additives, and patient-related factors such as size and body habitus and the presence of pregnancy or disease. The same drug dose given for intercostal blocks produces greater peak local anesthetic concentrations than when given for plexus or epidural blocks.[1,30] A dose given over 24 hours may be well tolerated, but not when given over 24 seconds. Forty milliliters of local anesthetic is well tolerated when administered for

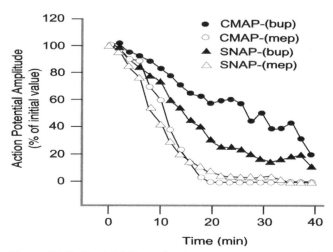

Figure 6.2: Earlier inhibition of sensory nerve action potentials improved to compound motor action potentials in volunteers receiving median nerve blocks with bupivacaine. Volunteers receiving mepivacaine showed no difference in latency of inhibition of sensory versus motor nerves. Reprinted from: Butterworth J. Clinical pharmacology of local anesthetics. Adapted from Hadzic A ed. *Textbook of Regional Anesthesia and Acute Pain Management.* New York, NY: McGraw Hill; 2007.[1]

interscalene block; 0.4 mL is poorly tolerated if injected into the nearby vertebral artery.

DIFFERENTIAL SENSORY NERVE BLOCK

In addition to the properties already described, one other important clinical consideration is the ability of local anesthetic agents to differentially inhibit sensory versus motor fibers. Physicians have long known that nerve fibers of differing sizes have differing susceptibility to local anesthetics (directly applied pressure, lack of oxygen, and lack of glucose). In general, among fibers of similar types, larger fibers are more resistant to local anesthetic block.[37] Smaller myelinated fibers (eg, Aδ fibers) are more susceptible to local anesthetics than larger myelinated fibers (eg, Aα or Aβ fibers). Larger unmyelinated fibers are less susceptible to block than smaller unmyelinated fibers.[46] The "size principle" fails when unmyelinated fibers are compared with myelinated fibers, because the (smaller) unmyelinated fibers (eg, C fibers) as a group are *less* susceptible to local anesthetics than the (generally larger) myelinated fibers.[35] As a consequence, conventional local anesthetic techniques cannot completely block all pain-transmitting Aδ and C fibers without also inhibitioning some motor fibers. In other words, local anesthetics will not produce analgesia sufficient for surgical incision without motor block.[1,3,11]

Some agents (eg, bupivacaine and ropivacaine) are relatively selective for sensory fibers.[47] These agents are often used in epidural solutions for surgical anesthesia, obstetric analgesia, and postoperative relief of pain owing to their ability to provide adequate sensory analgesia while preserving motor function, particularly at concentrations ≤0.25%. Thus, laboring parturients can be pain free yet still able to walk. Etidocaine and lidocaine, however, show little separation between sensory and motor blockade.[30] At concentrations required to achieve adequate epidural sensory anesthesia required, etidocaine and lidocaine have a rapid onset of action and, in the case of etidocaine, a prolonged duration of anesthesia; however, with both

sensory anesthesia is associated with a profound degree of motor blockade, and the motor block can sometimes outlast the sensory block during offset of anesthesia.

Differences among local anesthetics are sometimes most apparent during the onset or offset of peripheral nerve block.[47] For example, during onset of median nerve block with mepivacaine there is almost no difference in the relative inhibition of sensory nerves as assessed by the amplitude of sensory nerve action potentials (SNAPS) vs motor nerves as assessed by compound motor action potential (CMAP) amplitudes. Onset of bupivacaine was slower than with mepivacaine, but inhibition of SNAP amplitude occurred earlier than CMAP. At steady state, both agents inhibited SNAPs and CMAPs comparably and profoundly after 20 minutes of injection (Figure 6.2).[47]

As previously noted, the fact that specific genes produce the Na channels found in unmyelinated nerves, motor nerves, and dorsal root ganglia offers the tantalizing possibility that structural differences in these various channel forms might be sufficient to permit design and development of selective inhibitors.[10,48]

OTHER FACTORS INFLUENCING ACTIVITY

Many factors influence the adequacy of regional anesthesia, including the local anesthetic dose, temperature, site of administration, pregnancy, and drug additives. In general, the fastest onset and shortest duration of anesthesia occur with spinal and subcutaneous injections. Plexus blocks have a slower onset and longer duration.[1,30] For a given dose of local anesthetic, spread of neuraxial anesthesia increases during pregnancy because of decreases in thoracolumbar cerebrospinal fluid (CSF) volume and an increased neural susceptibility to local anesthetics (Figure 6.3).[49–51]

USE OF ADDITIVES WITH LOCAL ANESTHETIC SOLUTIONS

With most agents and most block procedures, onset, duration, and adequacy of anesthesia may be altered by addition of

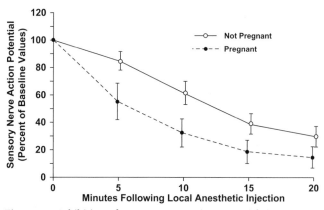

Figure 6.3: Inhibition of sensory nerve action potentials in pregnant women contrasted with women who were not pregnant. All subjects received median nerve blocks with 5 mL of 1% lidocaine. All data expressed as means ± SEM. Reprinted from: Butterworth J, Walker F, Lysak S. Pregnancy increases median nerve susceptibility to lidocaine. *Anesthesiology.* 1990;72:963.[49]

vasoconstrictors. Attempts have been made to alter the onset and duration of anesthesia by using mixtures of local anesthetics, carbonation (adding carbon dioxide), or addition of bicarbonate or any of a long list of other additives to local anesthetic solutions. Vasoconstrictors, typically epinephrine, are frequently added to local anesthetic solutions to decrease the rate of vascular absorption and allow a greater fraction of injected anesthetic molecules to reach the nerve membrane. In the end, the goal is to increase the time over which local anesthetic molecules persist near nerves, potentially increasing the depth and duration of anesthesia. In clinical anesthesia, local anesthetic solutions often contain a 1:200,000 (5 μg/mL) concentration of epinephrine.[25,30] Limited information is available regarding the optimum concentration of epinephrine with local anesthetic agents other than lidocaine or block procedures other than local infiltration.[52]

Epinephrine has differing effects on differing local anesthetics. Procaine, lidocaine, and mepivacaine are significantly prolonged by epinephrine during infiltration anesthesia, peripheral nerve blocks, or epidural anesthesia.[3,2,30,53] The effect of epinephrine on bupivacaine depend on the setting, block technique, and concentration of drug used. Bupivacaine local infiltration blocks are prolonged by epinephrine.[54] Epinephrine does not produce clinically useful prolongation of bupivacaine epidural blocks. The frequency and duration of adequate labor analgesia were improved when epinephrine 1:200,000 was added to 0.125% or 0.25% bupivacaine[40]; however, addition of epinephrine to 0.5% or 0.75% bupivacaine did not significantly improve epidural blocks for either obstetric or surgical patients.[40,55] Motor block is increased following the epidural administration of epinephrine-containing solutions of bupivacaine and etidocaine.[55] Epinephrine improves the quality of analgesia provided by dilute intrathecal solutions of bupivacaine + opioid.[56] The differing effects of epinephrine in prolonging the duration of differing local anesthetics is most apparent during spinal anesthesia. Epinephrine greatly increases the duration of tetracaine spinal anesthesia but prolongs lidocaine and bupivacaine spinal anesthesia to a lesser extent.[57–61]

Other α agonists such as clonidine and phenylephrine also have been used as additives to solutions of local anesthetics. α_2 agonists have local anesthetic properties in vitro. Clonidine and quanfacine will block both Aα and C fibers (Figure 6.4).[16] Prolongation of regional anesthesia by clonidine could be the result of pharmacodynamic prolongation of local anesthetic effects, a direct action of clonidine on nerves, a central action of clonidine, or some combination of these effects.[62] Clonidine markedly prolongs the duration of mepivcaine and lidocaine plexus blocks.[63] Either oral or intrathecal clonidine prolongs the duration tetracaine spinal anesthesia.[64,65] Intrathecal clonidine prolongs the duration of lidocaine, mepivacaine, and bupivacaine spinal anesthesia.[66,67] Clonidine, like epinephrine, has less effect on the duration of plexus blocks produced by bupivacaine or ropivacaine than on those produced by mepivacaine or lidocaine.[68]

Carbonation (addition of carbon dioxide) of local anesthetic solutions was once thought to speed the onset of action of various local anesthetics.[1,69] Carbon dioxide enhances diffusion of local anesthetics through nerve sheaths of isolated nerves and hastens inhibition of action potentials.[70,71] A double-blinded study, however, failed to demonstrate a significantly more rapid onset of action when lidocaine carbonate was compared with lidocaine hydrochloride for epidural blockade.[72] In fact, addition

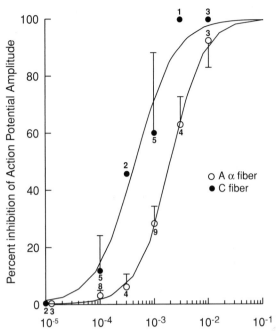

Figure 6.4: Concentration-dependent inhibition by clonidine of Aα and C fibers in rat sciatic nerves. The total number of nerves studied at each concentration is given on the figure. All data provided as means and standard derivatives. Reprinted from: Butterworth J, Strichartz G. The α_2-adrenergic agonists clonidine and guanfacine produce tonic and phasic block of conduction in rat sciatic nerve fibers. *Anesth Analg.* 1993;76:297.[16]

of NaHCO₃ to lidocaine (which would be expected to reduce the fraction of the protonated local anesthetic form) reduced the onset delay relative to the carbonated preparation.[72] Other double-blind studies failed to show benefit from carbonation of bupivacaine.[73,74] Thus, the available date show no consistent benefit to carbonation of local anesthetic solutions under clinical conditions.

Adding sodium bicarbonate to local anesthetic solutions immediately before injection inconsistently speeds the onset of conduction blockade.[72,75–77] Bicarbonate will increase the pH of the local anesthetic solution and increase the fraction of local anesthetic molecules in the uncharged base form. In theory, more local anesthetic molecules could diffuse across the nerve sheath and nerve membrane, speeding the onset of anesthesia. In vitro studies of pH adjustment suggest that the apparent potency of local anesthetics increases at more basic pH.[78] Addition of bicarbonate to lidocaine prior to median nerve block increased rate of onset of motor block without altering sensory nerve block.[77] Numerous clinical studies have been performed in which the addition of sodium bicarbonate to local anesthetic solutions has either improved or had no effect on the latency, duration, or effectiveness of local anesthesia.[79] Bicarbonate likely has its greatest benefit when added to local anesthetic solutions compounded with epinephrine by the manufacturer. Epinephrine-containing solutions have a reduced pH relative to "plain" solutions to increase the shelf life. Finally, addition of bicarbonate reduces the pain from subcutaneous injection of local anethetics.[80]

Other additive effects are specific to a particular regional block (Table 6.1).

Table 6.1: Additives in Local Anesthetic Solutions Used for Specific Regional Anesthetic Procedures

Opthalmic Blocks	Intravenous Regional Anesthesia	Minor Peripheral Blocks	Brachial Blocks Plexus	Intercostal Blocks	Epidural Anesthesia and Analgesia	Spinal Anesthesia and Analgesia
Hyaluronidase, epinephrine, bicarbonate, and clonidine improve reliability of anesthesia.[85,113]; multiple local anesthetics and multiple additives are often employed.	Clonidine and dexmedetomidine reduce discomfort during and after IVRA; ketorolac improves intraoperative and postoperative analgesia.[28,91]	Solutions containing epinephrine have been used for digital nerve blocks without ischemic sequelae.[73,129]	Epinephrine is often used to reduce blood LA concentrations and serves as a marker for accidental iv injection.[99] Clonidine improves anesthesia with lidocaine and mepivacaine, with less effect on bupivacaine or ropivacaine.[99] Bicarbonate reduces the onset time for anesthesia and may reduce duration.	Epinephrine is nearly always included to decrease local anesthetic concentrations in blood.[11,32,127]	Epinephrine reduces local anesthetic concentrations in blood and increases cardiac output.[9] Clonidine produces analgesia, sedation, and increases local anesthetic blood concentrations.[92] Epidural combinations of local anesthetics and opioids provide better analgesia to than from the agents given separately.[33] Clonidine is popular for postoperative caudal analgesia in children.[83]	Addition of dextrose or water will influence baricity, distribution of local anesthetics within the CSF, and permit patient positioning to influence dermatomal spread of spinal anesthesia.[48] Vasoconstrictors greatly prolong tetracaine spinal anesthesia.[30,68] Clonidine (intrathecal or oral) may be used to prolong spinal anesthesia.[37,102] Adding fentanyl to LA solutions improves the quality of intraoperative and postoperative analgesia without prolonging motor block, time to voiding, or recovery time.[5,74]

VASODILATOR PROPERTIES

The clinical activity of local anesthetics is modified by their vasodilator properties. Faster vascular absorption reduces the number of local anesthetic molecules available for binding to Na channels. Faster absorption into the blood stream reduces the apparent local anesthetic in vivo potency and duration of action. All local anesthetics except cocaine both constrict and dilate vascular smooth muscle, depending on the concentration.[81–83] At reduced concentrations local anesthetics inhibit nitric oxide release and cause vasoconstriction. At the much greater concentrations used for regional anesthesia these agents cause vasodilations.[83]

Local Anesthetic Blood Concentrations, Protein Binding, Metabolism, and Pharmacokinetics

As previously mentioned, in blood, all local anesthetics are partially protein bound, primarily to α_1-acid glycoprotein (AGP) and secondarily to albumin.[30,32] Affinity for AGP increases with LA hydrophobicity and decreases with protonation and acidosis.[84] Extent of protein binding is influenced by the concentration of AGP. Both protein binding and protein concentration

decline during pregnancy, but these changes have limited clinical importance.[85] During longer-term infusion of LA and LA-opioid combinations concentrations of serum binding proteins progressively increase.[84] There is considerable first-pass uptake of local anesthetics by lung.[86]

Esters undergo rapid hydrolysis in blood, catalyzed by pseudocholinesterase.[30,87] Procaine and benzocaine are metabolized to *p*-aminobenzoic acid (PABA). The amides undergo oxidative N-dealkylation in the liver (by cytochrome P450).[1,30] Amide LA clearance depends on hepatic blood flow, hepatic extraction, and enzyme function and is reduced by drugs that decrease hepatic blood flow such as β-adrenergic or H_2-receptor blockers and by heart or liver failure.[30,87]

TOXIC SIDE EFFECTS OF LOCAL ANESTHETICS

It is often assumed that all toxic side effects of local anesthetics are caused by unwanted binding of local anesthetic to Na channels in the central nervous and cardiovascular systems.[88] However, local anesthetics will inhibit many other targets aside from the Na channels, including multiple forms of voltage-gated

Table 6.2: Concentrations of Local Anesthetics that Inhibit Cardiac Function

LA	dP/dt_{max} (65%) ($\mu g/mL$)	EF (65%) ($\mu g/mL$)	FS (65%) ($\mu g/mL$)	CO (75%) ($\mu g/mL$)
BUP	2.3 (1.7–3.0)	3.2 (2.2–4.7)	2.1 (1.5–3.1)	3.6 (2.1–6.0)
LBUP	2.4 (1.9–3.1)	3.1 (1.4–2.9)	1.3 (0.9–1.8)	3.3 (2.0–5.5)
ROP	4.0 (3.1–5.2)[a]	4.2 (3.0–6.0)	3.0 (2.1–4.2)[b]	5.0 (3.1–8.3)
LID	8.0 (5.7–11.0)[c]	6.3 (4.0–9.9)[d]	5.5 (3.5–8.7)[c]	15.8 (8.3–30.2)[c]

Note: Data represented are concentration estimates and 95% confidence intervals.

Abbreviations: dP/dt_{max} (65%) = local anesthetic concentration that reduced maximal change in left-ventricular pressure over time to 65% of baseline value. EF (65%) = local anesthetic concentration that reduced left-ventricular ejection fraction to 65% of baseline value. FS (65%) = local anesthetic concentration that reduced fractional shortening to 65% of baseline value. CO (75%) = local anesthetic concentration that reduced cardiac output to 75% of baseline value. BUP = bupivacaine; LBUP = levobupivacaine; ROP = ropivacaine; LID = lidocaine.

[a] ROP > BUP, LBUP; $P < .05$.

[b] ROP > LBUP; $P < .05$.

[c] LID > BUP, LBUP, ROP; $P < .01$

[d] LID > BUP, LBUP; $P < .01$.

Reprinted from: Groban L, Deal D, Vernon, Jason, James R, Butterworth J. Does local anesthetic stereoselectivity or structure predict myocardial depression in anesthetized canines? *Reg Anesth Pain Med.* 2002;27:460–468.[102]

ion channels, enzymes, receptors, and G-protein-mediated signaling.[11,19,23,89–94] Local anesthetic binding to any or all of these sites could contribute to toxicity, spinal or epidural analgesia, or analgesia during local anesthetic infusions.[99]

CENTRAL NERVOUS SYSTEM SIDE EFFECTS

Local anesthetic central nervous system toxicity most likely results from disinhibition of inhibiting pathways, with the ultimate potential result of convulsion. Increasing LA doses produce a stereotypical sequence of signs and symptoms culminating in seizures.[1,3,5,25,30,86] Further LA dosing may lead to central nervous system (CNS) depression, possibly including respiratory arrest. More potent local anesthetics, such as bupivacaine, produce seizures at lower blood concentrations and lower doses than less potent local anesthetics, such as lidocaine. Both metabolic and respiratory acidoses decrease the convulsive dose of lidocaine in experimental amounts, and the result can likely be extrapolated to other anesthetics and to humans.[96] CNS toxicity can promote cardiac toxicity.[87] Cardiovascular signs of CNS excitation (eg, increased arterial blood pressure) appear at lower local anesthetic concentrations than those associated with cardiac depression.[97]

CARDIOVASCULAR TOXICITY

Bupivacaine binds more avidly to cardiac Na channels and, once bound, remains bound for a longer time than lidocaine.[6,11,98] Bupivacaine R(+) isomers bind cardiac Na channels more avidly than S(−) isomers (levobupivacaine and ropivacaine).[26] Local anesthetics inhibit conduction within the heart with the same

rank order of potency as they demonstrate inhibition of impulses in peripheral nerve.[98] Local anesthetics produce concentration-dependent myocardial depression. Local anesthetics bind and inhibit Ca and K channels in the heart, but only at concentrations much greater than those required for maximal binding to Na channels.[11,90] Local anesthetics bind β-adrenergic receptors and inhibit epinephrine-stimulated cyclic adenosine monophosphate (AMP) formation.[23,88]

Most local anesthetics will not produce cardiovascular toxicity in animals until blood concentration exceed 3 times those that produce seizures. Nevertheless, there are reports of simultaneous seizures and cardiac toxicity with bupivacaine in patients.[1,5,25] Supraconvulsant doses of bupivacaine more commonly produce arrhythmias in dogs than supraconvulsant doses of ropivacaine or lidocaine.[24]

In most species and in most animal models of cardiac toxicity, the rank order of local anesthetic potency appears to be bupivacaine > levobupivacaine > ropivacaine (Table 6.2).[97,99] Furthermore, arrhythmias were more common in dogs receiving toxic doses of bupivacaine or levobupivacaine than those receiving lidocaine or ropivacaine.[100–102] There were notable differences among local anesthetics in the responses to attempted resuscitation. Dogs given lidocaine could be resuscitated, but required continuing infusion of epinephrine to maintain an adequate blood pressure. Conversely, many dogs receiving bupivacaine or levobupivacaine could not be resuscitated using standard drugs and techniques. Those dogs receiving bupivacaine, levobupivacaine, or ropivacaine that could be defibrillated often required no other therapy.[100–102] Similar differences were observed in pigs: Bupivacaine had a greater propensity for arrhythmias than lidocaine. Bupivacaine was 4 times more potent than lidocaine at producing myocardial depression but 16 times more potent at producing arrhythmias in pigs.[105] As noted earlier, it is often assumed that all LA cardiovascular toxicity arises from one, common fundamental mechanism. Given that bupivacaine seems much more prone to arrhythmias than lidocaine, and that the response to resuscitation drugs and techniques differ among these drugs, it seems likely that the mechanism of cardiovascular toxicity may also differ between these two agents.

METHEMOGLOBINEMIA

Generations of anesthesia textbooks have focused on the unique metabolism of prilocaine to *o*-toluidine, and the resulting (and allegedly predictable) production of methemogloblinemia in adults with prilocaine doses >600 mg.[30] A recent study demonstrates the unpredictability of the prilocaine dose that will result in clinically important methemogloblinemia in adults.[104] More importantly, perioperative methemogloblinemia more commonly arises in North America from use of the topical local anesthetic benzocaine, dehydration, or treatment of infections with dapsone than from use of prilocaine in any form.[105]

ALLERGY

Textbooks state that there is an increased incidence of allergy to ester local anesthetics metabolized to *p*-aminobenzoic acid (procaine and benzocaine) and a greater incidence of allergy to ester than amide local anesthetics.[30] If there are convincing data confirming these assertions I cannot find them. Evidence for allergic cross reactions between methylparaben and *p*-aminobenzoic acid is also sparse, despite this being a frequent topic of questions on certification examinations. The most important fact about local anesthetic allergy is that it is rare. Multiple studies show that when patients with apparent "allergic" or even anaphylactoid reactions to local anesthetics are subjected to standard testing, almost none will have immune responses to preservative-free local anesthetics.[106,107]

TREATMENT OF LOCAL ANESTHETIC TOXICITY

Treatment of adverse local anesthetic reactions should be guided by their severity. Serious degrees of methemoglobinemia are treated with intravenous (IV) oxygen and methylene blue (1 mg/kg). Anaphylactoid reactions may require epinephrine, corticosteroids, and fluid resuscitation. Minor degrees of central nervous system excitation can be allowed to terminate spontaneously. Even when local anesthetics produce seizures, the only requirement is that one maintain the airway and provide oxygen. Seizures may be terminated with intravenous thiopental (1–2 mg/kg), midazolam (0.05–0.10 mg/kg), or propofol (0.5–1 mg/kg). In the event of local anesthetic-induced cardiovascular depression, milder degrees of hypotension may be treated by infusion of intravenous fluids and vasopressors (phenylephrine, 0.5–5 mcg/kg/min, norepinephrine, 0.02–0.2 mcg/kg/min, or vasopressin, 2–20 units IV). If contractile failure is evident, epinephrine (1–15 mcg/kg IV bolus) may be required. Unfortunately, a recent survey of academic anesthesia departments confirmed a lack of consensus regarding resuscitation drugs for local anesthetic cardiovascular toxicity.[108,109] I suggest that the

Guidelines for Advanced Cardiac Life Support be followed with a few substitutions.[109] I suggest that amiodarone and vasopressin be substituted for lidocaine and epinephrine, respectively.[110–112] Once advanced cardiac life support begins, intravenous lipid should be considered. Animal experiments demonstrate the remarkable ability of lipid infusion to resuscitate animals from bupivacaine overdosage, even after unsuccessful attempts of "conventional" resuscitative techniques and drugs.[113,114] The mechanism remains controversial, but may involve the lipid serving as a "sponge" for the local anesthetic, facilitating its removal from heart and brain.[115,116] A growing number of case reports (see http://www.lipidrescue.org/) provide evidence that lipid infusion may also be effective in humans.[117,118] In the case of a continuing lack of response to resuscitation efforts, consideration should be given to placing the patient on cardiopulmonary bypass with the hope of supporting the circulation long enough to permit the liver to clear the local anesthetic.[119]

REFERENCES

1. Butterworth J. Clinical pharmacology of local anesthetics. In: Hadzic A, ed. *Textbook of Regional Anesthesia and Acute Pain Management.* New York, NY: McGraw-Hill; 2007.
2. Calatayud J, González A. History of the development and evolution of local anesthesia since the coca leaf. *Anesthesiology.* 2003;98:1503–1508.
3. de Jong RH. *Local Anesthetics.* St. Louis, MO: Mosby, Inc.; 1994.
4. Keys TE. *The History of Surgical Anesthesia.* Park Ridge, IL: American Society of Anesthesiologists Wood Library; 1996.
5. Strichartz GR, ed. *Handbook of Experimental Pharmacology: Local Anesthetics.* Vol. 81. New York, NY: Springer-Verlag; 1987.
6. Hille B. *Ion Channels of Excitable Membranes.* 3rd ed. Sunderland, MA: Sinauer Associates, Inc.; 2001.
7. Lai J, Porreca, F, Hunter J, et al. Voltage-gated sodium channels and hyperalgesia. *Annu Rev Pharmacol Toxicol.* 2004;44:372.
8. Chahine M, Ziane R, Vijayaragavan K, Okamura Y. Regulation of Na_v channels in sensory neurons. *Trends Phamacol Sci.* 2005;26:496–502.
9. Lopez-Santiago LF, Pertin M, Morisod X, et al. Sodium channel beta2 subunits regulate tetrodotoxin-sensitive sodium channels in small dorsal root ganglion neurons and modulate the response to pain. *J Neurosci.* 2006;26:7984–7994.
10. Leffler A, Reiprich A, Mohapatra DP, et al. Use-dependent block by lidocaine but not amitriptyline is more pronounced in tetrodotoxin (TTX)-Resistant Na_v1.8 than in TTX-sensitive Na^+ channels. *J Pharmacol Exp Ther.* 2007;320:354–364.
11. Butterworth JF, Strichartz GR. Molecular mechanisms of local anesthesia: a review. *Anesthesiology.* 1990;72:711–734.
12. Jiang Y, Lee A, Chen J, et al. X-ray structure of a voltage-dependent K+ channel. *Nature.* 2003;423:33–41.
13. Jiang Y, Ruta V, Chen J, et al. The principle of gating charge movement in a voltage-dependent K+ channel. *Nature.* 2003;423:42–48.
14. Godwin SA, Cox JR, Wright SN. Modeling of benzocaine analog interactions with the D4S6 segment of Na_v4.1 voltage-gated sodium channels. *Biophys Chem.* 2005;113:1–7.
15. Hanck DA, Makielski JC, Sheets MF. Kinetic effects of quaternary lidocaine block of cardiac sodium channels: a gating current study. *J Gen Physiol.* 1994;103:19–43.
16. Butterworth JF, Strichartz GR. The alpha 2-adrenergic agonists clonidine and guanfacine produce tonic and phasic block of conduction in rat sciatic nerve fibers. *Anesth Analg.* 1993;76:295–301.

17. Kohane DS, Lu NT, Gokgol-Kline AC, et al. The local anesthetic properties and toxicity of saxitonin homologues for rat sciatic nerve block in vivo. *Reg Anesth Pain Med*. 2000;25:52–59.

18. Sudoh Y, Cahoon EE, Gerner P, et al. Tricyclic antidepressants as long-acting local anesthetics. *Pain*. 2003;103:49–55.

19. Yanagidate F, Strichartz G. Local anesthetics. *Handb Exp Pharmacol*. 2007;177:95–127.

20. Cassuto J, Sinclair R, Bonderovic M. Anti-inflammatory properties of local anesthetics and their present and potential clinical implications. *Acta Anaesthesiol Scand*. 2006;50:265–282.

21. Hahnenkamp K, Theilmeier G, Van Aken H, et al. The effects of local anesthetics on perioperative coagulation, inflammation, and microcirculation. *Anesth Analg*. 2002;94:1441–1447.

22. Tremont-Lukats IW, Challapalli V, McNicol ED, et al. Systemic administration of local anesthetics to relieve neuropathic pain: a systematic review and meta-analysis. *Anesth Analg*. 2005;101:1738–1749.

23. Butterworth J, James RL, Grimes J. Structure-affinity relationships and stereospecificity of several homologous series of local anesthetics for the beta2-adrenergic receptor. *Anesth Analg*. 1997;85:336–342.

24. Feldman HS, Arthur GR, Covino BG. Comparative systemic toxicity of convulsant and supraconvulsant doses of intravenous ropivacaine, bupivacaine, and lidocaine in the conscious dog. *Anesth Analg*. 1989;69:794–801.

25. Tetzlaff J. *Clinical Pharmacology of Local Anesthetics*. Woburn, MA: Butterworth-Heinemann; 2000.

26. Nau C, Strichartz GR. Drug chirality in anesthesia. *Anesthesiology*. 2002;97:495–502.

27. Garrido R, Lagos N, Lattes K, et al. Gonyautoxin: new treatment for healing acute and chronic anal fissures. *Dis Colon Rectum*. 2005;48:335–340.

28. Rodrriguez-Navarro AJ, Lagos N, Lagos M et al. Neosaxitoxin as a local anesthetic: preliminary observations from a first human trial. *Anesthesiology*. 2007;106:339–345.

29. Strichartz GR, Sanchez V, Arthur GR, et al. Fundamental properties of local anesthetics. II. Measured octanol:buffer partition coefficients and pKa values of clinically used drugs. *Anesth Analg*. 1990;71:158–170.

30. Covino BG, Vasallo HG. *Local Anesthetics: Mechanisms of Action and Clinical Use*. New York, NY: Grune & Stratton; 1976.

31. Kouri ME, Kopacz DJ. Spinal 2-chloroprocaine: a comparison with lidocaine in volunteers. *Anesth Analg*. 2004;98:75–80.

32. Taheri S, Cogswell LP, Gent A, et al. Hydrophobic and ionic factors in the binding of local anesthetics to the major variant of human alpha1-acid glycoprotein. *J Pharmacol Exp Ther*. 2003;304:71–80.

33. Lipkind GM, Fozzard HA. Molecular modeling of local anesthetic drug binding by voltage-gated sodium channels. *Mol Pharmacol*. 2005;68:1611–1622.

34. Popitz-Bergez FA, Leeson S, Strichartz GR, et al. Relation between functional deficity and intraneural local anesthetic during peripheral nerve block; a study in the rat sciatic nerve. *Anesthesiology*. 1995;83:583–592.

35. Huang JH, Thalhammer JG, Raymond SA, et al. Susceptibility to lidocaine of impulses in different somatosensory afferent fibers of rat sciatic nerve. *J Pharmacol Exp Ther*. 1997;282:802–811.

36. Nakamura T, Popitz-Bergez F, Birknes J, et al. The critical role of concentration for lidocaine block of peripheral nerve in vivo: studies of function and drug uptake in the rat. *Anesthesiology*. 2003;99:1189–1197.

37. Raymond SA, Gissen AJ. Mechanisms of differential nerve block. In: Strichartz GR, eds. *Handbook of Experimental Pharmacology: Local Anesthetics*. Vol. 81. New York, NY: Springer-Verlag; 1987.

38. Sinnott CJ, Cogswell III LP, Johnson A, et al. On the mechanism by which epinephrine potentiates lidocaine's peripheral nerve block. *Anesthesiology*. 2003;98:181–188.

39. Raymond SA, Steffensen SC, Gugino LD, et al. The role of length of nerve exposed to local anesthetics in impulse blocking action. *Anesth Analg*. 1989;68:563–570.

40. Littlewood DG, Buckley P, Covino BG, et al. Comparative study of various local anesthetic solutions in extradural block in labour. *Br J Anaesth*. 1979;51:47.

41. Scott DB, McClure JH, Giasi RM, et al. Effects of concentration of local anaesthetic drugs in extradural block. *Br J Anaesth*. 1980;52:1033.

42. Erdimir HA, Soper LE, Sweet RB. Studies of factors affecting peridural anesthesia. *Anesth Analg*. 1965;44:400.

43. Krenn H, Deusch E, Balogh B, et al. Increasing the injection volume by dilution improves the onset of motor blockade, but not sensory blockade of ropivacaine for brachial plexus block. *Eur J Anaesthesiol*. 2003;20:21–25.

44. Liu SS, Ware PD, Rajendran S. Effects of concentration and volume of 2-chloroprocaine on epidural anesthesia in volunteers. *Anesthesiology*. 1997;86:1288–1293.

45. Rosenberg PH, Veering BT, Urmey WF. Maximum recommended doses of local anesthetics: a multifactorial concept. *Reg Anesth Pain Med*. 2004;29:564–575.

46. Gissen AJ, Covino BG, Gregus J. Differential sensitivities of mammalian nerve fibers to local anesthetic agents. *Anesthesiology*. 1980;53:467–474.

47. Butterworth J, Ririe DG, Thompson RB, et al. Differential onset of median nerve block: randomized, double-blind comparison of mepivacaine and bupivacaine in healthy volunteers. *Br J Anaesth*. 1998;81:515–521.

48. Amir R, Argoff CE, Bennett GJ, et al. The role of sodium channels in chronic inflammatory and neuropathic pain. *J Pain*. 2006;7:S1–S29.

49. Butterworth JF, Walker FO, Lysak SZ. Pregnancy increases median nerve susceptibility to lidocaine. *Anesthesiology*. 1990;72:962–965.

50. Fagraeus L, Urban BJ, Bromage PR. Spread of epidural analgesia in early pregnancy. *Anesthesiology*. 1983;58:184–187.

51. Popitz-Bergez FA, Leeson S, Thalhammer JG, et al. Intraneural lidocaine uptake compared with analgesic differences between pregnant and nonpregnant rats. *Reg Anesth*. 1997;22:363–371.

52. Harwood TN, Butterworth JF, Colonna DM, et al. Plasma bupivacaine concentrations and effects of epinephrine after superficial cervical plexus blockade in patients undergoing carotid endarterectomy. *J Cardiothorac Vasc Anesth*. 1999;13:703–706.

53. Liu S, Carpenter RL, Chiu AA, et al. Epinephrine prolongs duration of subcutaneous infiltration of local anesthesia in a dose-related manner: correlation with magnitude of vasoconstriction. *Reg Anesth*. 1995;20:378–384.

54. Swerdlow M, Jones R. The duration of action of bupivacaine, prilocaine, and lignocaine. *Br J Anaesth*. 1970;42:335.

55. Sinclair CJ, Scott DB. Comparison of bupivacaine and etidocaine in extradural blockade. *Br J Anaesth*. 1984;56:147.

56. Soetens FM. Levobupivacaine-sufentanil with or without epinephrine during epidural labor analgesia. *Anesth Analg*. 2006;103:182–186.

57. Armstrong IR, Littlewood DG, Chambers WA. Spinal anesthesia with tetracaine – effect of added vasoconstrictor. *Anesth Analg*. 1983;62:793.

58. Chambers WA, Littlewood DG, Logan MR, et al. Effect of added epinephrine on spinal anesthesia with lidocaine. *Anesth Analg*. 1981;60:417.

59. Chambers WA, Littlewood DG, Scott DB. Spinal anesthesia with hyperbaric bupivacaine: effect of added vasoconstrictors. *Anesth Analg.* 1982;61:49.

60. Concepcion M, Maddi R, Francis D, et al. Vasoconstrictors in spinal anesthesia with tetracaine: a comparison of epinephrine and phenylephrine. *Anesth Analg.* 1984;63:134.

61. Moore J M, Liu SS, Pollock JE, et al. The effect of epinephrine on small-dose hyperbaric bupivacaine spinal anesthesia: clinical implications for ambulatory surgery. *Anesth Analg.* 1998;86:973–977.

62. Gaumann DM, Brunet PC, Jirounek P. Clonidine enhances the effects of lidocaine on C-fiber action potential. *Anesth Analg.* 1992;74:719–725.

63. Ohom G, Machmachi A, Diarra DP, et al. The effects of clonidine added to mepivacaine for paronychia surgery under axillary brachial plexus block. *Anesth Analg.* 2005;100:1179–1183.

64. Larsen B, Dorscheid E, Macher-Hanselmann F, et al. Does intrathecal clonidine prolong the effect of spinal anesthesia with hyperbaric mepivacaine? A randomized double-blind study. *Anaesthesist.* 1998;47:741–746.

65. Ota K, Namiki A, Iwasaki H, et al. Dose-related prolongation of tetracaine spinal anesthesia by oral clonidine in humans. *Anesth Analg.* 1994;79:1121–1125.

66. Dobrydnjov I, Samarutel J. Enhancement of intrathecal lidocaine by addition of local and systemic clonidine. *Acta Anaesthesiol Scand.* 1999;43:556–562.

67. Racle JP, Benkhadra A, Poy JY, et al. Prolongation of isobaric bupivacaine spinal anesthesia with epinephrine and clonidine for hip surgery in the elderly. *Anesth Analg.* 1987;66:442–446.

68. Ilfeld BM, Morey TE, Thannikary LJ, et al. Clonidine added to a continuous interscalene ropivacaine perineural infusion to improve postoperative analgesia: a randomized, double-blind, controlled study. *Anesth Analg.* 2005;100:1172–1178.

69. Morrison DH. A double-blind comparison of carbonated lidocaine and lidocaine hydrochloride in epidural anaesthesia. *Can Anaesth Soc J.* 1981;28:387.

70. Catchlove RF. The influence of CO_2 and pH on local anesthetic action. *J Pharmacol Exp Ther.* 1972;181:298–309.

71. Gissen AJ, Covino BG, Gregus J. Differential sensitivity of fast and slow fibers in mammalian nerve. IV. Effect of carbonation of local anesthetics. *Reg Anaesth.* 1985;10:68.

72. Curatolo M, Petersen-Felix S, Arendt-Nielse L, et al. Adding sodium bicarbonate to lidocaine enhances the depth of epidural blockade. *Anesth Analg.* 1998;86:341–347.

73. Brown DT, Morrison DH, Covino BG, et al. Comparison of carbonated bupivacaine and bupivacaine hydrochloride for extradural anaesthesia. *Br J Anaesth.* 1980;52:419.

74. McClure JH, Scott DB. Comparison of bupivicaine hydrochloride and carbonated bupivacaine in brachial plexus block by the interscalene technique. *Br J Anaesth.* 1981;53:523.

75. Arakawa M, Aoyama Y, Ohe Y. Block of the sacral segments in lumbar epidural anaesthesia. *Br J Anaesth.* 2003;90:173–178.

76. Candido KD, Winnie AP, Covino BG, et al. Addition of bicarbonate to plain bupivacaine does not significantly alter the onset or duration of plexus anesthesia. *Reg Anesth.* 1995;20:133–138.

77. Ririe DG, Walker FO, James RL, et al. Effect of alkalinization of lidocaine on median nerve block. *Br J Anaesth.* 2000;84:163–168.

78. Butterworth JF, Lief PA, Strichartz GR. The pH-dependent local anesthetic activity of diethylaminoethanol, a procaine metabolite. *Anesthesiology.* 1988;68:501–506.

79. Hilgier M. Alkalinization of bupivacaine for brachial plexus block. *Reg Anaesth.* 1985;10:59.

80. Davies RJ. Buffering the pain of local anaesthetics: a systematic review. *Emerg Med.* 2003;15:81–88.

81. Benzaquen BS, Cohen V, Eisenberg MJ. Effects of cocaine on the coronary arteries. *Am Heart J.* 2001;142:402–410.

82. Blair MR. Cardiovascular pharmacology of local anaesthetics. *Br J Anaesth.* 1975;47:247.

83. Johns RA, DiFazio CA, Longnecker DE. Lidocaine constricts or dilates rat arterioles in a dose dependent manner. *Anesthesiology.* 1985;62:141–144.

84. Thomas JM, Schug SA. Recent advances in the pharmacokinetics of local anaesthetics. Long-acting amide enantiomers and continuous infusions. *Clin Pharmacokinet.* 1999;36:67–83.

85. Fragneto RY, Bader AM, Rosinia F, et al. Measurements of protein binding of lidocaine throughout pregnancy. *Anesth Analg.* 1994;79:295–297.

86. Rothstein P, Arthur GR, Feldman HS, et al. Bupivacaine for intercostal nerve blocks in children: blood concentrations and pharmacokinetics. *Anesth Analg.* 1986;65:625–632.

87. Mather LE, Copeland SE, Ladd LA. Acute toxicity of local anesthetics: underlying pharmacokinetic and pharmacodynamic concepts. *Reg Anesth Pain Med.* 2005;30:553–566.

88. Butterworth J, Cole L, Marlow G. Inhibition of brain cell excitability by lidocaine, QX314, and tetrodotoxin: a mechanism for analgesia from infused local anesthetics? *Acta Anaesthesiol Scand.* 1993;37:516–523.

89. Butterworth JF, Brownlow RC, Leith JP, et al. Bupivacaine inhibits cyclic-3',5'-adenosine monophosphate production: a possible contributing factor to cardiovascular toxicity. *Anesthesiology.* 1993;79:88–95.

90. Hirota K, Browne T, Appadu BL, et al. Do local anaesthetics interact with dihydropyridine binding sites on neuronal L-type Ca2+ channels? *Br J Anaesth.* 1997;78:185–188.

91. McCaslin PP, Butterworth J. Bupivacaine suppresses [Ca(2+)](i) oscillations in neonatal rat cardiomyocytes with increased extracellular K+ and is reversed with increased extracellular Mg(2+). *Anesth Analg.* 2000;91:82–88.

92. Olschewski A, Olschewski H, Bräu ME, et al. Effect of bupivacaine on ATP-dependent potassium channels in rat cardiomyocytes. *Br J Anaesth.* 1999;82:435–438.

93. Siebrands CC, Friederich P. Structural requirements of human ether-a-go-go related gene channels for block by bupivacaine. *Anesthesiology.* 2007;106:523–531.

94. Ueta K, Sugimoto M, Suzuki T, et al. In vitro antagonism of recombinant ligand-gated ion-channel receptors by stereospecific enantiomers of bupivacaine. *Reg Anesth Pain Med.* 2006;31:19–25.

95. McClean G. Intravenous lidocaine: an outdated or underutilized treatment for pain? *J Palliat Med.* 2007;10:798–805.

96. Englesson S, Grevsten S. The influence of acid-base changes on central nervous system toxicity of local anaesthetic agents. II. *Acta Anaesthesiol Scand.* 1974;18:88–103.

97. Ohmura S, Kawada M, Ohta T, et al. Systemic toxicity and resuscitation in bupivacaine-, levobupivacaine-, or ropivacaine-infused rats. *Anesth Analg.* 2001;93:743–748.

98. Heavner JE. Cardiac toxicity of local anesthetics in the intact isolated heart model: a review. *Reg Anesth Pain Med.* 2002;27:545–555.

99. Chang DH, Ladd LA, Copeland S, et al. Direct cardiac effects of intracoronary bupivacaine, levobupivacaine and ropivacaine in the sheep. *Br J Pharmacol.* 2001;132:649–658.

100. Groban L, Deal DD, Vernon JC, et al. Ventricular arrhythmias with or without programmed electrical stimulation after incremental overdosage with lidocaine, bupivacaine, levobupivacaine, and ropivacaine. *Anesth Analg.* 2000;91:1103–1111.

101. Groban L, Deal DD, Vernon JC, et al. Cardiac resuscitation after incremental overdosage with lidocaine, bupivacaine,

levobupivacaine, and ropivacaine in anesthetized dogs. *Anesth Analg.* 2001;92:37–43.

102. Groban L, Deal DD, Vernon JC, et al. Does local anesthetic stereoselectivity or structure predict myocardial depression in anesthetized canines? *Reg Anesth Pain Med.* 2002;27:460–468.

103. Nath S, Häggmark S, Johansson G, Reiz S. Differential depressant and electrophysiologic cardiotoxicity of local anesthetics: an experimental study with special reference to lidocaine and bupivacaine. *Anesth Analg.* 1986;65:1263–1270.

104. Vasters FG, Eberhart LH, Koch T, et al. Risk factors for prilocaine-induced methaemoglobinaemia following peripheral regional anaesthesia. *Eur J Anaesthesiol.* 2006;23:760–765.

105. Ash-Bernal R, Wise R, Wright SM. Acquired methemoglobinemia: a retrospective series of 138 cases at 2 teaching hospitals. *Medicine.* 2004;83:265–273.

106. Berkun Y, Ben-Zvi A, Levy Y, et al. Evaluation of adverse reactions to local anesthetics: experience with 236 patients. *Ann Allergy Asthma Immunol.* 2003;91:342–345.

107. Jacobsen RB, Borch JE, Bindslev-Jensen C. Hypersensitivity to local anaesthetics. *Allergy.* 2005;60:262–264.

108. Corcoran W, Butterworth J, Weller RC, et al. Local anesthetic-induced cardiac toxicity: a survey of contemporary practice strategies among academic anesthesiology departments. *Anesth Analg.* 2006;103:1322–1326.

109. Guidelines 2000 for cardiopulmonary resuscitation. *Circulation.* 2000;102(Suppl 1):I-1-I-384.

110. Krismer AC, Hogan QH, Wenzel V, et al. The efficacy of epinephrine or vasopressin for resuscitation during epidural anesthesia. *Anesth Analg.* 2001;93:734–742.

111. Mayr VD, Raedler C, Wenzel V, et al. A comparison of epinephrine and vasopressin in a porcine model of cardiac arrest after rapid intravenous injection of bupivacaine. *Anesth Analg.* 2004;98:1426–1431.

112. Simon L, Kariya N, Pelle-Lancien E, et al. Bupivacaine-induced QRS prolongation is enhanced by lidocaine and by phenytoin in rabbit hearts. *Anesth Analg.* 2002;94:203–207.

113. Weinberg GL, Ripper R, Feinstein D, et al. Lipid emulsion infusion rescues dogs from bupivacaine-induced cardiac toxicity. *Reg Anesth Pain Med.* 2003;28:198–202.

114. Weinberg GL, VadeBoncouer T, Ramaraju, GA, et al. Pretreatment or resuscitation with a lipid infusion shifts the dose-response to bupivacaine-induced asystole in rats. *Anesthesiology.* 1998;88:1071–1075.

115. Stehr SN, Ziegeler JC, Pexa A, et al. The effects of lipid infusion on myocardial function and bioenergetics in I-bupivacaine toxicity in the isolated rat heart. *Anesth Analg.* 2007;104:186–192.

116. Weinberg GL, Ripper R, Murphy P, et al. Lipid infusion accelerates removal of bupivacaine and recovery from bupivacaine toxicity in the isolated rat heart. *Reg Anesth Pain Med.* 2006;31:296–303.

117. Litz RJ, Popp M, Stehr SN, et al. Successful resuscitation of a patient with ropivacaine-induced asystole after axillary plexus block using lipid infusion. *Anaesthesia.* 2006;61:800–801.

118. Rosenblatt MA, Abel M, Fischer GW, et al. Successful use of a 20% lipid emulsion to resuscitate a patient after a presumed bupivacaine-related cardiac arrest. *Anesthesiology.* 2006;105:217–218.

119. Soltesz EG, van Pelt F, Byrne JG. Emergent cardiopulmonary bypass for bupivacaine cardiotoxicity. *J Cardiothorac Vasc Anesth.* 2003;17:357–358.

7

Pharmacology of Novel Non-NSAID Analgesics

P. M. Lavand'homme and M. F. De Kock

Although many patients undergo surgery on a daily basis, perioperative and more specifically postoperative pain still remain underevaluated and poorly treated.[1]

There is now growing recognition that poorly relieved acute pain increases the occurrence of cognitive dysfunction, immune suppression, and chronic postsurgical pain. Consequently, perioperative treatments may have long-term implications on patient outcome and quality of life.[2] Unfortunately, commonly used analgesics such as opioids and nonsteroideal anti-inflammatory drugs (NSAIDs) are not devoid of side effects that interfere with early rehabilitation and may impair patient outcome.[3] A recent consensus on acute postsurgical pain management supports the use of *multimodal analgesia* (a combination of two or more analgesic agents or analgesic modalities with different mechanisms of action) to improve perioperative pain control and to reduce analgesia-related adverse effects.[4] Adjuvant drugs such as α_2-adrenoceptor agonists, *N*-methyl-D-aspartate (NMDA) receptor antagonists, and gabapentin present with interesting properties to improve perioperative pain control. Specifically, these classes of compounds are more effective to relieve pain in states where the central nervous system is sensitized, as it is the case after tissue incision and display interesting antihyperalgesic properties. In combination with opioids, use of these adjuvant drugs result in relevant opioid sparing effect. Thus, reducing opioid-related adverse effects such as nausea and vomiting, sedation, and opioid-induced hyperalgesia that contributes to further sensitization of the central nervous system (CNS). When studying the mechanism of action of drugs that modulate pain sensation, it is important to consider not exclusively their interactions with the nervous system, but also their *effects on components of the immune reaction*. This is readily apparent for drugs directly related with the course of the inflammatory process (ie, NSAIDs). An immune mechanism may also account for the pain modulation obtained with drugs such as clonidine, ketamine, gabapentin and pregabalin. Reasons underlying this assertion are found in the close interrelation between the nervous and immune systems. Drugs acting on the nervous system interfere directly or indirectly with the immune function and results in the therapeutic effect. An ideal drug in the perioperative setting would be the one that does not negatively affect, but rather helps to maintain immune homeostasis by preventing any excessive systemic pro- or anti-inflammatory reaction.

This chapter reviews the basic knowledge concerning the use of α_2-adrenoceptor agonists (clonidine), NMDA receptor antagonists (ketamine), and gabapentin as analgesic adjuvants.

For each class of drug, our approach considers the following:

- Receptors involved and underlying mechanisms
- Pharmacology of analgesia under different pain conditions
- Pharmacology of the drug and related side effects
- Interaction with other analgesics, specifically, opioids
- Immune modulatory effects

CLONIDINE AND α_2-ADRENOCEPTOR AGONISTS

α_2-Adrenergic Receptors and Pain Modulation

Adrenergic receptors, α and β receptors, form the interface between the endogenous catecholaminergic system and the target cells that mediate the biological effects of the sympathetic nervous system in the body. Among the adrenergic receptors, α_2-adrenergic receptors (α_2-AR) mediate several physiological functions and have a great therapeutic potential in the field of pain control.[5] Although three major subtypes of α_2-AR have been defined (α_{2A}, α_{2B}, α_{2C}), no significant subtype-selective ligands are clinically available to date.[6] The descending noradrenergic system has an inhibitory effect on nociceptive processing at both supraspinal and spinal levels. Furthermore, a peripheral expression of α_2-AR also seems to participate in the control of pain processing.

Noradrenergic innervation of the spinal cord arises from the locus coeruleus (A5 and A6) and subcoeruleus (A7) nuclei located in the brainstem. Like electrical stimulation of these noradrenergic nuclei, local injection of α_2-agonist will activate the descending noradrenergic system and release norepinephrine (NE), which in turn activates adrenoceptors in the spinal cord and produces analgesia.[7] NE-containing terminals are distributed in the laminae of the dorsal horn. This includes superficial laminae, substantial gelatinosa, where primary nociceptive afferents terminate, and the intermediolateral column, which comprises sympathetic preganglionic neurons.

In contrast to opioids, the major site of α_2-agonists analgesic effect is the spinal cord, where these drugs have shown an efficacy and potency similar to that of opioids in both animal models and humans. The α_2-adrenoceptors belong to G-protein-coupled receptor family (Gi/o), which inhibitory effects rely on the increase of potassium channels conductance and the depression of calcium conductance, resulting in either membrane hyperpolarization or decrease in transmitter release.[7] Mimicking the action of endogenous NE, antinociceptive effects of α_2-AR agonists are mediated by spinal modulation of pain transmission at both pre- and postsynaptic sites on small afferent fibers. The postsynaptic inhibition of dorsal horn neurons results from the ability of α_2 agonists to hyperpolarize dorsal horn neurons and to decrease neuronal excitation mostly by activation of postsynaptic G-protein-coupled inwardly rectifying potassium channels (GIRKs).[8] Presynaptic binding to α_2-adrenoceptors in the spinal cord leads to the reduction of excitatory neurotransmitters release. Both Aδ and C primary afferent transmission are depressed, yielding a reduction of the release of excitatory transmitters like substance P, calcitonin gene-related peptide (CGRP), and glutamate.[9,10] This modulatory effect of α_2-AR agonists on excitatory neurotransmitter release is due to activation of the α_2A-receptor subtype because glutamate release is inhibited by adrenergic agonists with a relative potency of clonidine = dexmedetomidine > norepinephrine > ST91 $\gg$ phenylephrine = 0.

In addition to the aforementioned mechanisms, the antinociceptive effect of spinal norepinephrine and therefore α_2-AR agonists is also mediated through a local release of inhibitory neurotransmitters like acetylcholine (ACh) and subsequent nitric oxide (NO) release, γ-aminobutyric acid (GABA), and perhaps NE and endogenous opioid peptide.

Several experimental studies suggest a cholinergic interaction in α_2-AR-mediated antinociception at the level of the spinal cord. In the rat, spinal injection of muscarinic antagonist attenuates the analgesic effect of intrathecal clonidine, whereas intrathecal administration of cholinesterase inhibitor is potentiated. In a larger animal model, with a spinal cord size closer to that of humans, the antinociceptive effect of spinal clonidine is enhanced by cholinesterase inhibitor neostigmine and associated to ACh release in cerebrospinal fluid (CSF).[11] These observations are consistent with the fact that ACh release plays an important role in the antinociceptive effect of spinally administered α_2-AR agonists. The mechanism of α_2-AR-mediated release of ACh is not fully understood but might rely on a postsynaptic activation of α_2-AR on intrinsic spinal inhibitory interneurons that in turn release ACh (for schematic representation of possible neuronal circuits in the dorsal horn, see Detweiler et al).[11] In human volunteers, epidural administration of clonidine increases CSF concentrations of ACh inhibitory neurotransmitter[12] and under intraoperative conditions, analgesic doses of intrathecal but not intravenous clonidine increase ACh in CSF of patients.[13] These observations indicate that the analgesic effects observed after intravenous

clonidine administration are not mediated by a cholinergic mechanism at the spinal level and support the combination of α_2-AR agonists with a cholinesterase inhibitor to enhance neuraxial analgesia. Finally, it is worth noting that, according to different binding to spinal α_2-AR, specifically dexmedetomidine being more α_2 selective than clonidine, dexmedetomidine induces a greater ACh release than clonidine after intrathecal administration.

Adrenergic receptors located on either supraspinal or peripheral noradrenergic terminals act in an autoinhibitory manner to diminish further NE release. At the spinal cord level, similar autoinhibitory α_2-adrenoceptors exist, probably of the α_{2A} subtype. However, the regulation of NE release in the spinal cord is complex because experimental studies have implicated a local release of NE in the antinociceptive effect of spinal α_2-AR agonists. This local NE release must occur from indirect actions because of activation of a spinal circuit, perhaps following ACh and subsequent NO release.[14]

Finally, an important contribution to the spinal mechanisms that underlie norepinephrine antinociceptive action is mediated through GABA and glycine inhibitory neurotransmitter release following presynaptic activation of α_1-adrenoceptors.[15] This effect certainly contributes to analgesic and antihyperalgesic effects of clonidine because the drug is a mixed α_2-/α_1-AR agonist.

Progress in molecular biology and immunochemistry has facilitated the mapping of α_2-adrenergic receptors in normal and pathophysiologic conditions in animal species and in humans. Effectively, α_2-AR subtype expression and function seems to be species specific. In rodents, there is a strong expression of α_{2A}-AR in brain and supraspinal adrenergic nuclei. At the spinal level, α_{2A}-AR are predominant and found in the terminals of peptide-containing primary afferents, which supports their role in the presynaptic inhibition of substance P and CGRP release. Whereas, the α_{2C}-AR subtype appears to be expressed on local spinal neurons where they mediate adrenergic agonists-induced hyperpolarization.[16] In human spinal cord, α_2-AR are present in the gray matter only, in dorsal horn laminae with expression sacral > cervical > thoracic = lumbar. In addition, adrenoceptors are found in thoracic and the lumbar intermediolateral cell column and also in the ventral horn lamina IX.[17] These findings support the mediated effects of α_2-agonists on nociception, autonomic function, and motor tone. The α_{2A} and α_{2B} subtypes are predominant, whereas the α_{2C}-AR is virtually absent, restricted to the lumbar area. The α_2-adrenoceptors expressed in human dorsal root ganglia represent another possible site of action for adrenergic agonists (for example, after epidural administration) and contribute to 20% of the α_2-AR found in the dorsal horn after being trafficked centrally. In human dorsal root ganglia, α_{2B} and α_{2C} subtypes are found at all spinal levels.[17] To date, clinically available drugs are not selective for a particular α_2 subtype. However, whether α_2-AR agonists may be an attractive analgesic alternative because they are devoid of respiratory depressant effect and addictive liability. Some of their related side effects, namely sedation and hypotension, are currently hindering the clinical use of nonselective α_2-agonists for pain management.[6] Experimental studies have shown that α_{2A}-AR activation accounts for analgesic, hemodynamic and sedative effects of α_2-adrenoceptor agonists. Whereas, activation of α_{2C}-AR, a subtype predominant in humans, also produces analgesia without major side effects.[18] All these findings might support

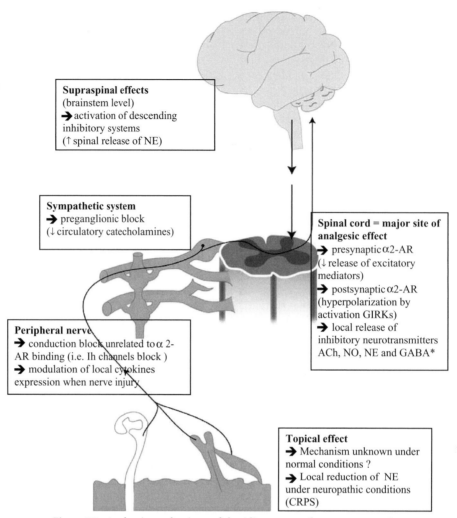

Figure 7.1: Analgesic mechanisms of clonidine, an α_2-adrenoceptor agonist.

the future development of subtype selective drugs to improve clinical practice (Figure 7.1).

Pharmacology of Analgesia under Different Pain Conditions

Both clinical and experimental observations have clearly highlighted the fact that α_2-AR agonists are more effective to relieve pain in pathological states where central sensitization is present.[19] In addition, α_2-AR agonists, and specifically clonidine, which is commonly used in clinical practice, demonstrate greater analgesic effects after spinal than systemic administration, favoring the neuraxial route of injection.[20] Early observations have revealed the considerable potential of spinal α_2-AR agonists to alleviate neuropathic pain poorly responsive to opioids both in animal models and in humans.[21,22] In animals following nerve injury, spinal adrenoceptor agonists relieve mechanical allodynia and thermal hyperalgesia. These are features of neuropathic pain, an effect mediated locally in the vicinity of the spinal cord and the intermediolateral cell column. In patients suffering intractable cancer pain, epidural clonidine reduces pain scores in those with a neuropathic pain component (56% success vs 16% success when pain is from somatic or

visceral origin).[21] Among the possible explanations, the fact that α_2-AR agonists inhibit sympathetic outflow in the intermediolateral cell column of the dorsal horn might contribute to their efficacy in neuropathic pain states involving a sympathetic component. Moreover, and perhaps more importantly, animal studies have pointed out the fact that nerve injury strongly modifies CNS mechanisms underlying the α_2-AR antinociceptive effect. In normal animals, clonidine effect mostly relies on binding to α_{2A}- and α_2-nonA-adrenoceptors. Under neuropathic pain conditions, the antiallodynic effect of clonidine depends primarily on its interaction with α_2-nonA-adrenoceptors, probably α_{2C}-AR.[23] The plasticity of spinal α_2-AR subtypes after nerve injury has been demonstrated in animal models. Not only an ipsilateral decrease of immunoreactivity for the α_{2A} subtype located on C fiber terminals occurs, but also a significant increase for the α_{2C} subtype immunoreactivity ipsilateral to the injury is present.[24] The fact that α_{2C}-AR are located in the deep dorsal horn close to the normal terminations of large-diameter fibers involved in the processing of mechanical inputs may support the efficacy of spinal clonidine against mechanical allodynia and hyperalgesia. Finally, the spinal α_2-adrenergic-cholinergic interaction for analgesia is also modified following nerve injury whereby clonidine antiallodynic effects are mediated by activation of spinal inhibitory cholinergic interneurons.[25] A subsequent local release of NO seems also to play an important role in the antihyperalgesic effect of spinal clonidine under neuropathic conditions.

Postoperative Pain Condition

Postoperative pain also represents a state of central hypersensitivity but presents with specific features and underlying mechanisms clearly distinct from those that result from inflammatory or neuropathic pain.[1] The extent of postoperative mechanical hyperalgesia surrounding the wound seems to correlate to the degree of CNS sensitization and can be modulated by intrathecal administration of clonidine in both an animal model of paw incision[26] and postoperative patients.[27] Experimental observations have shown that descending noradrenergic inhibitory systems are activated in the postoperative period. The potency of intrathecal clonidine against mechanical hypersensitivity in a postincisional pain model is similar to that observed in animals subjected to acute noxious stimuli, mostly limited by side effects such as sedation and diuresis.[26] In contrast, ST-91 (the diethyl derivative of clonidine, a hydrophilic and mostly α_2-nonA-adrenergic agonist) shows a greater efficacy than clonidine in the incisional pain model. By consequence, postoperative hypersensitivity most resembles nerve injury-induced hypersensitivity and clonidine antihyperalgesic effect is mediated through both α_{2A}- and α_2-nonA-adrenoceptors activation. Further, subsequent spinal cholinergic activation underlies the effect of clonidine but not that of ST-91 (and spinal muscarinic as well as nicotinic receptors are involved in the antihyperalgesic action of clonidine after incision.[26])

These experimental findings have allowed a better understanding of clinical observations related to the potency and the efficacy of α_2-AR agonists under different conditions. In summary, neuraxial but not systemic administration of clonidine reduces experimental pain and hyperalgesia.[20] Clinical trials have shown that the doses of neuraxial clonidine, either spinal or epidural, needed to relieve neuropathic pain are less than 25% of those needed to treat postoperative pain. In acute pain conditions, the potency ratio of intrathecal:epidural clonidine is >6:1; whereas in neuropathic conditions or experimental conditions involving a state of mechanical hypersensitivity such as peri-incisional mechanical hyperalgesia, the ratio is <2:1.[19]

Peripheral Use of α_2-AR Agonist Clonidine

Whether a central location of α_2-adrenergic receptors is clearly demonstrated, the presence of α_2-AR on peripheral nerves and nociceptive afferent fibers has been subject to debate. However, in perioperative conditions, the addition of clonidine to local anesthetics in peripheral nerve blocks clearly enhances the efficacy and the duration of the sensory block with little impact on motor block.[28] Among the possible mechanisms of action, a direct "local anesthetic like" effect on the peripheral nerve seems more likely than some vasoconstrictive effect or centrally mediated analgesic effect. In vitro, clonidine shows a concentration-dependent block of conduction in rat sciatic nerve fibers, with a greater inhibition of C-fiber than A-fiber action potential,[29] which explains why sensory and analgesic effects of perineural clonidine outlast the effects on motor block. This experimental local anesthetic effect is observed only with high doses of clonidine alone (500 μM = 134 μg/mL), doses that are irrelevant to the doses used in clinical practice (10 μg/mL = 34 μM) to extend the duration of action of local anesthetics. Moreover, this local effect is not inhibited by perineural coadministration of α_2-AR antagonists. By consequence, several experimental studies are in agreement with the fact that a clonidine conduction block on nonmyelinated nerve fibers is not mediated by α_2-adrenoceptors but rather relies on a different mechanism, for example, by blocing Ih channels or hyperpolarization-activated cation currents.[30] Recently, clinical concentrations of clonidine (<100 μM) have demonstrated a partial inhibition of voltage-gated sodium and potassium channels in spinal dorsal horn neurons, an effect that might contribute to the analgesic effect of the drug during intrathecal administration where CSF concentrations of clonidine range from 6 to 100 μM.[31] Finally, although perineural clonidine alone is not analgesic in postoperative patients at clinically usable doses,[28] intra-articular administration of these doses (1–2 μg/kg) has shown an analgesic effect comparable to that of morphine,[32] and the addition of clonidine to intravenous regional anesthesia with lidocaine improves postoperative analgesia.[33] Experimental data seem to support the antinociceptive effects of topical clonidine mediated through activation of α_2-AR expressed on peripheral terminals of cutaneous nociceptors, although the precise mechanisms remain unclear but do not involve endogenous local opioid peptides.[34] Nevertheless, repeated topical clonidine application results in the development of antinociceptive tolerance just like repeated administration of topical morphine does.[34]

In contrast to physiologic conditions, α_2-AR can be expressed abnormally in primary sensory afferent fibers following nerve injury. Topical application of clonidine relieves hyperalgesia in patients suffering chronic regional pain syndromes, specifically in those where pain is sympathetically maintained.[35] Because clonidine effects seem to be confined to the vicinity of the patch, the site of action is likely peripheral and might involve the activation of presynaptic α_2-AR, α_2-autoreceptors, which locally inhibits the release of norepinephrine and prevent its α_1-mediated hyperalgesic effect.[35] Futhermore, application of clonidine at the site of nerve injury reduces the development of neuropathic pain and hyperalgesia in animals.[36,37] The underlying mechanism of action involves a local modulation of proinflammatory cytokines expression, specifically a reduction of local tumor necrosis factor α (TNF-α) by macrophages and immune cells recruited at the site of the lesion during the Wallerian degeneration process. The effect of clonidine is mediated mostly through the α_{2A} subtype located on macrophages and lympocytes. The stimulation of α_2-adrenoceptor transforms cytokine gene expression in leukocytes and thereby clonidine reduces the changes in ion channel expression in DRG cells, which leads to neuronal hyperexcitability and neuropathic hypersensitivity.

Pharmacology of Clinically Available Adrenergic Agonists as Analgesics: Clonidine and Dexmedetomidine

Among the α_2-AR agonists available in clinical practice, clonidine is the most widely used and has received approval for systemic and neuraxial use,[38,39] whereas dexmedetomidine is currently available for systemic use only.

Clonidine was developed in the mid-1950s as an antihypertensive medication. The drug is a selective agonist for α_2-AR

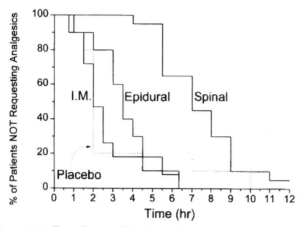

Figure 7.2 Effect of route of administration on duration of analgesia from a small dose of clonidine. Duration of analgesia, defined as median time until other analgesic medication is required, is similar for 150 μg clonidine by intramuscular (I.M.) or epidural injection and placebo but is longer for spinal clonidine injection. From Eisenach et al, *Anesthesiology* 1996;85:55–76 (with permission).

with a ratio of 200:1 (α_2:α_1 ratio) but for α_2-AR, the drug is not subtype selective (binding with α_{2A}-, α_{2B}-, and α_{2C}-AR). Clonidine is a high-lipid-soluble drug with a high volume of distribution. After oral administration, clonidine is rapidly and almost completely absorbed, with a peak plasma concentration occurring within 3 hours. The drug is partly (50%) metabolized in the liver to inactive metabolites and partly excreted as unchanged drug in the urine.[40] The elimination half-life ranges from between 9 to 12 hours, extending up to 40 hours in patients with renal impairment. Clonidine is absorbed through the skin and therapeutic plasma concentrations are achieved 48 to 72 hours after application of transdermal delivery system, roughly equivalent to concentrations resulting from oral intake.[41] However, the preferred route of administration for α_2-AR agonists is the neuraxial route and countless clinical trials as well as complete toxicologic assessment support the safety of intraspinal use of the drug.[39] Clonidine produces postoperative analgesia that is more profound and longer lasting after spinal than after epidural and systemic injection (Figure 7.2).

Further, clonidine's analgesic effect is directly related to CSF concentrations of the drug both in volunteers and in postoperative patients, which implies that the major site of action for analgesia is located in the spinal cord (Figure 7.3).

In contrast, there is a poor correlation between plasma concentration and analgesia, whereas such systemic absorption accounts for most of the drug's side effects. Early experimental studies in sheep have demonstrated that plasma and CSF clonidine concentrations differ among the routes of administration. The bioavailability of clonidine in plasma following intrathecal and epidural injection 85 ± 20% and 105 ± 15% of that following intravenous (IV) injection, respectively. CSF bioavailability of clonidine following epidural and intravenous administration is 14% ± 2% and 0.02% ± 0.007% of that following intrathecal injection, respectively.[42] In volunteers, an epidural bolus of clonidine 700 μg shows a rapid absorption into systemic circulation with a time of peak concentration of 12 minutes.[43] The time for CSF peak concentration is around 31 minutes with a β half-life of 79 ± 11 min. Clonidine elimination half-life from CSF correlates with the duration of its analgesic effect and this effect is short lasting, although a dose-dependent increase in duration

but not in intensity has been observed for intrathecal dose range over 150–450 μg in the postoperative setting.[44] Epidural administration of clonidine produces postoperative analgesia at doses greater than 3 μg/kg, mainly between 300 and 800 μg,[45] but this effect is short lasting (between 2 and 5 hours) and the use of a continuous infusion is usually needed. To maintain an analgesic effect, the effective dose range for epidural clonidine infusion lies between 10 to 40 μg/h, resulting in CSF concentrations of 12–45 ng/mL.[45] In perioperative conditions, epidural clonidine 4 μg/kg bolus dose followed by continuous infusion of 2 μg/kg/h reduces postoperative pain scores and early analgesic requirements with a greater extent than the same dose administered by intravenous route does.[46] However, during the continuous infusion, an important systemic absorption occurs that finally results to similar plasma concentrations of the drug for both routes.[46] In summary, experimental studies in volunteers and clinical trials in postoperative patients suggest that the minimum effective CSF concentration of clonidine for pain relief situates around 76 ± 15 ng/mL. Furthermore, plasma clonidine concentrations over 2 ng/mL have also been associated to an analgesic effect of the drug (Table 7.1).[47]

Dexmedetomidine (MPV-1440) is the pharmacologically active D isomer of medetomidine, a specific α_2-AR agonist widely used in veterinarian medicine. The drug shares the same anesthetic and analgesic properties as clonidine. However, dexmedetomidine has a considerably higher α_2:α_1-AR selectivity ratio than clonidine: 1620:1 versus 220:1 (ie, at least 4 times more selective for α_2-AR than clonidine). The drug also has higher lipophilicity (3.5 times greater than that of clonidine) and higher protein binding (94%). The duration of action is short, with a mean elimination half-life of 2.3 hours compared to 7.7 hours for clonidine (ie, its half-life is 4-fold shorter than clonidine's half-life). Systemic use has been investigated in human

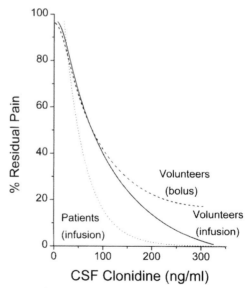

Figure 7.3 Correlation between measured (volunteers) or calculated (patients) cerebrospinal fluid (CSF) concentrations of clonidine and percent of pain. Pain was determined by pain report to noxious thermal stimulation in volunteers receiving epidural clonidine bolus (dashed line), or by amount of patient-controlled analgesia (PCA) morphine use in postoperative patients receiving epidural clonidine infusions (dotted line). From Eisenach et al, *Anesthesiology* 1996;85:655–76 (with permission).

Table 7.1: Pharmacokinetics of Clonidine Administration in Human Volunteers and Patients

Doses and Routes of Administration	Plasma Concentrations	CSF Concentrations
Oral – transcutaneous		
3 μg/kg	± 0.55 ng/mL[41]	
4.5–6 μg/kg	1.7 ± 0.4 ng/mL[41]	
Intravenous		
Bolus 4–5 μg/kg	**1.5 – 2.0 ng/mL**[a47]	0.6 ± 0.2 ng/mL[13]
1 μg/kg/h	0.25 ± 0.1 ng/mL[49]	
4 μg/kg/h	2.0 ± 0.9 ng/mL[49]	
Epidural		
Bolus 150 μg	0.56 ± 0.1 ng/mL[22]	228 ± 60 ng/mL[22]
Bolus 750 μg	3.8 ± 0.6 ng/mL[43]	390 ± 78 ng/mL[43]
4 μg/kg + 2 μg/kg/h	4.5 ± 2.0 ng/mL[46]	**> 150 ng/mL**[a,45]
Intrathecal		
Bolus 1 μg/kg		1600 ± 200 ng/mL[13]

[a] Concentrations in bold have been associated with an analgesic effect of clonidine in human volunteers and patients.

volunteers and is currently assessed, specifically for sedation, in postoperative and intensive care patients.[48] The doses usually involve a bolus dose of 0.5–1.0 μg/ kg followed or not by a continuous infusion ranging from 0.2 to 0.7 μg/kg/h.[49] In volunteers, dexmedetomidine produces analgesia but carries a high rate of side effects such as sedation, amnesia and immediate memory impairment, hypotension, and bradycardia in a dose-dependent fashion.[49–51] The sympatholytic effects of dexmedetomidine similarly to that of other α_2-AR agonists involve a decrease of plasma catecholamines, epinephrine and norepinephrine, by 72% (range 40–90%).[52,53] In postoperative patients, however, the analgesic and potent opioid-sparing effect of dexmedetomidine goes along with a lesser magnitude in the suppression of sympathetic tone, plasma catecholamines decrease, degree of hypotension, and bradycardia.[52,53] In contrast, all the studies (experimental and clinical ones) support unaffected respiratory rate and blood oxygen saturation.[49,53,54] Finally, dexmedetomidine seems to possess neuroprotective effects,[55] as well as beneficial effects, on glomerular filtration associated to increased diuresis.[56]

Although the drug is not labeled for neuraxial administration, the pharmacokinetics and pharmacodynamics of spinal drug injection have been studied in sheep.[54] Single intrathecal or epidural bolus of dexmedetomidine (100 μg), a dose comparable to clonidine (300 μg), results in very low – almost undetectable – plasma concentrations. In contrast, CSF concentrations after epidural injection reaches 22% of the dose, a higher bioavailability than that of clonidine, related to the greater lipophilicity of dexmedetomidine.[54] Similarly to clonidine, dexmedetomidine analgesic effect is mediated by spinal α_2-AR binding and partly relies on ACh release in the dorsal horn: greater concentrations of ACh are released after intrathecal injection of dexmedetomidine than clonidine in sheep.[57] The drug might therefore represent an interesting alternative to clonidine for neuraxial analgesia. In postoperative patients, an epidural bolus dose of 2 μg/kg provides 4–6 hours of analgesia and reduces postoper-

ative analgesic requirements during the first 24 hours by 70%. Blood pressure and heart rate are, respectively, decreased by 20% and 25%.

Nonanalgesic Effects Resulting from Clonidine and α_2-AR Agonist Administration

Although α_2-AR agonists, and specifically clonidine in the clinical setting, are an attractive alternative to opioids because they are devoid of respiratory depressant effects and are non-addictive, their use still remains hindered by two major side effects (ie, hemodynamic depression and sedation). There is a close relationship between the plasma levels of the drug and the importance of the side effects observed, meaning that systemic absorption accounts for most of these side effects.

CARDIOVASCULAR AND HEMODYNAMIC EFFECTS

α_2-AR are involved in the control of blood pressure homeostasis at several locations[58] and α_2-AR agonists affect blood pressure in a complex fashion because of opposing actions at multiple sites.[39] After intravenous administration, nonselective activation of α_2-AR leads to a biphasic blood pressure response: a short hypertensive phase mediated by peripheral vascular α_{2B}-AR that is usually followed by a longer-lasting fall in the blood pressure below baseline level, mediated by central α_{2A}-AR.[58] After oral administration, the hypotensive action prevails, which explains the clinical development of these compounds as antihypertensive drugs. After neuraxial administration, the mechanisms underlying α_2-AR agonists hemodynamic effects are even more complex and also involve a spinal local action on sympathetic preganglionic neurons in the the intermediolateral cell column.

Clonidine, because of lipophilic properties, will undergo a rapid and extensive systemic resorption after neuraxial administration. Binding of the drug to postsynaptic α_{2A}-AR in the nucleus tractus solitarius and locus coeruleus of the brainstem reduce sympathetic drive. Further, clonidine is not a pure α_2-AR agonist and also activates central nonadrenergic imidazoline receptors in the lateral reticular nucleus, which results in hypotension and antiarrythmogenic effect. In the periphery, in a dose-related manner, clonidine, which is a α_2/α_1 adrenoceptor agonist, produces a vasoconstrictive effect by direct activation of α_1-AR on peripheral blood vessels. Moreover, binding to presynaptic α_{2A}-AR at sympathetic terminals will reduce norepinephrine release. Epidural administration of clonidine, either bolus dose or continuous infusion, results in decreased plasma levels of norepinephrine but does not affect epinephrine or dopamine levels.[43] In summary, the dose response for clonidine after either systemic or neuraxial administration is U-shaped.[39] In addition to supraspinal and peripheral effects, neuraxial administration of clonidine directly inhibits sympathetic preganglionic neurons in the intermediolateral cell column of the spinal cord. Regarding the location of these cells, the hypotension resulting from spinal clonidine is more profound after thoracic than cervical or lumbar injection.[39] Finally, it is worth noting that the hypotensive effect of clonidine is of greater magnitude in hypertensive than in normotensive subjects.[58] Hemodynamic effects of clonidine begin within 30 minutes and last approximately 6–8 hours after a single injection. α_2-AR agonists reduce heart rate partly by inhibition of norepinephrine release and by a vagomimetic effect. The resulting reduction in the myocardial oxygen demand partly accounts for the cardioprotective effects of clonidine and related compounds.

SEDATION, ANXIOLYSIS, AND ANESTHESIA

Noradrenergic neurons are involved in the regulation of a range of behaviors, including the sleep/wake cycle, feeding, thermoregulation, attention, and motor activity and development.[59] Sedation commonly follows the use of α_2-AR agonists, an effect mediated by their action on α_{2A}-AR located in the locus coeruleus.[59,60] The sedative effect is most likely from systemic absorption of the drug with vascular redistribution to higher centers rather than a cephalad migration in CSF, because a delayed onset has not been observed from epidural or spinal injection nor has delayed hypotension.[39] Sedation is dose dependent with a rapid onset (<20 minutes) and a duration of 4–6 hours. Furthermore, among α_2-AR agonists, the more α_2 selective, such as dexmedetomidine, exert not only greater sedative but also anxiolytic effects, a tranquilizing effect comparable to that of benzodiazepine compounds.[59,60] Clonidine exerts a biphasic effect, being anxiolytic at low α_2 range concentrations and inducing anxiogenic behavior at the higher doses by α_1 action.

The sedative and anxiolytic effects observed with α_2-AR agonists are consistent with the well-known anesthetic-sparing effect associated to their perioperative use. Further, the aforementioned properties are not accompanied by respiratory depression.

RESPIRATORY EFFECTS

Clonidine and other α_2-AR agonists alone do not induce profound respiratory depression even after an overdose and they do not potentiate the respiratory depression from opioids. Experimental data in both human volunteers and patients have shown a stable hemoglobin oxygen saturation over the time following clonidine and dexmedetomidine administration.[59]

OTHER EFFECTS

α_2-AR agonists demonstrate a potent sympatholytic effect and in stress situations, they reduce but do not suppress neurohormonal secretions induced by the activation of the sympathoadrenal system.[59] The drugs also enhance growth hormone release by an effect on hypophyseal cells and can inhibit insulin release by direct action on the pancreatic cells. Both effects of α_2-AR agonists are short lasting and are not relevant for clinical practice even for long-lasting administration, in contrast to the hormonal effects that result from a chronic exposure to opioids. Other common side effects from clonidine and α_2-AR agonists involve dry mouth and dizziness, but no urinary retention nor constipation.[59]

Interactions with Other Analgesics

The α_2-adrenergic agonists exert their analgesic effect essentially at the level of the spinal cord through mechanisms independent of those underlying opioid analgesia. Preclinical studies with spinal α_2-AR agonists have demonstrated that their analgesic effect may be enhanced synergistically in the presence of other spinal analgesics such as local anesthetics, opioids, and cholinergic agonists. Both intrathecal clonidine and local anesthetic significantly suppress the formalin-induced nociceptive response and their combination displays a synergistic antinociceptive effect in animals.[61] Clonidine, the most widely used α_2 agonist in clinical practice, intensifies and prolongs sensory anesthesia and analgesia from intrathecal and epidural local anes-

thetics.[39] Coadministration of clonidine with neuraxial local anesthetics also provides an interesting local anesthetic-sparing effect during continuous infusion and hence reduces the risk for motor impairment associated with the use of high doses of local anesthetic. The mechanisms by which clonidine enhances local anesthetic-induced spinal analgesia are still unclear, but might involve a modulatory effect of the drug on voltage-gated sodium channels as recently demonstrated.[31]

The interactions between α_2-agonists and opioid analgesics have been extensively studied in experimental models because both drugs share a common mechanism of action (ie, activation of descending adrenergic inhibitory pathways). Effectively, systemic administration of opioids stimulates the spinal release of norepinephrine.[62] Most of the animal data reveal systemic additivity and spinal supraadditivity (ie, synergy) for the antinociceptive effect of α_2 agonists associated with opioids,[63,64] the degree of synergism varying with the opioid chosen. Unlike these animal studies, clinical trials have failed to show a synergistic interaction between spinal clonidine and opioid agonists, although the combination can be successfully used to manage pain, and the dose of both components can be reduced by 60%.[65] Furthermore, it is worth noting that, whether experimental studies show synergistic antinociceptive effect when adrenergic agonists and opioids are combined, side effects such as sedation show only additivity, which is of major interest for clinical use (Figure 7.4).

The combination of both drugs also presents some interest during long-term administration of opioids that inevitably leads to the development of some degree of tolerance. Because α_2-agonists and opioids exert their analgesic effects via different receptors and pathways, there is a strong rationale for using α_2-agonists either as a "drug holiday" or in combination with opioids to reduce the development of tolerance to the latter. Animal studies have explored tolerance and cross-tolerance between these agents and suggest that cross-tolerance is minor.[66] Clinical observations showing the analgesic efficacy of epidural clonidine in cancer patients receiving high doses of opioids support these experimental data,[21] as well as the maintenance of an intrathecal clonidine analgesic effect during long-lasting continuous infusion in chronic pain patients. In addition, experimental studies have also found that dexmedetomidine, which possesses a greater intrinsic activity at the α_2-AR and, therefore, a larger receptor reserve during continuous administration, is subject to a lesser

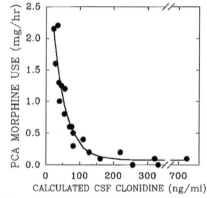

Figure 7.4 PCA morphine use, in milligrams per hour, as a function of calculated CSF clonidine concentrations, in nanograms per milliliter. From Mendez et al, *Anesthesiology* 1990;73:848–52 (with permission).

degree of tolerance development than clonidine.[67] In contrast to spinal use, systemic α_2-agonists administration induces tolerance to the hypnotic effects, but minimally to the analgesic and sympatholytic effects of the drugs.

Immunologic Effects of α_2-AR Agonists

Under stress conditions (eg, trauma, infection), overactivity of the sympathetic nervous system (SNS) is reported. This suppresses cellular-mediated immunity by reducing the macrophage and lymphocyte cells production of proinflammatory cytokines and by stimulating the release of immunosuppressive (ie, anti-inflammatory) factors.[68] It is generally accepted that the SNS exercises a tonic inhibitory control on the inflammatory reaction. In other words, NE possesses local and systemic anti-inflammatory properties. α_2-adrenoceptors are present on human lymphocytes.[69] The total number of yohimbine sites is 19.9 ± 5.3 fmol/107 lymphocytes. However, the α_2-AR-mediated effects on NE-induced anti-inflammatory properties are less clear than these mediated by the β_2-adrenoceptors.[68,70] Clonidine seems to have global immune protective properties in clinical situations of marked SNS hyperactivity, such as during opioid withdrawal. Numerous experimental studies indicate that opioids have direct and indirect immunomodulatory properties. West and coworkers[71] have demonstrated that clonidine is able to completely reverse the immunodepressant effects related to opioid withdrawal in rats. The mechanism involved is probably the presynaptic regulation of NE spillover and activation of the hypothalamic-pituitary-adrenal (HPA) axis.

The perioperative period is another situation where sustained activity of the SNS and depression of cellular immunity exist. Von Dossow and coworkers[72] reported that clonidine changes the ratio of T-lymphocyte subpopulations in peripheral blood of patients undergoing cardiac surgery in favor of a proinflammatory response. These results indicates that clonidine, by reducing the release of norepinephrine (presynaptic inhibitory effect), may modulate the tonic inhibitory control exercised by the sympathetic nervous system on the cellular immunity. Therefore, this effect may be favorable for maintaining immune balance after major surgery. In addition, α_2-adrenoceptor agonists exert a direct immune effect at the site of the tissue lesion, as demonstrated after peripheral nerve injury.

Administration of clonidine directly at the injury site modulates the local production of inflammatory cytokines and promotes the release of anti-inflammatory cytokines.[36] This contrasts with previous experimentations indicating that α_2-AR stimulation increases TNF-α production by lipopolysaccharide-(LPS) challenged macrophages that would promote rather than reduce inflammation.[73] Furthermore, clonidine also recruits anti-inflammatory pathways. Effectively, perineural administration of clonidine, acting on α_{2A}-adrenoceptors, prevents both increase in leukocytes number and cytokines production induced by an inflammatory reaction.[74] A possible mechanism underlying these observations is the inhibition by clonidine of a sensory neurons protein kinase (P-38 mitogen activated) involved in the development and maintenance of inflammatory-induced modifications of nociception. Moreover, clonidine, by reducing the activity of the Na^+/H^+ exchangers, may interfere with the endothelial production of interleukin 8 (IL-8) chemokine and reduce the number of neutrophils attracted at the site of inflammation.

KETAMINE AND NMDA RECEPTORS ANTAGONISTS

NMDA Receptors and Pain Modulation

Ketamine is a clinically available noncompetitive antagonist at the ionotropic glutamate NMDA receptor. This type of receptor participates in the excitatory neurotransmission of the CNS along with other excitatory aminoacid receptors (ie, the ionotropic α-amino-3-hydroxy-5-methyl-4-isoxazol-propionic acid (AMPA)/kainate receptors and the G-protein-coupled metabotropic receptors).[75] Glutamate excitatory neurotransmission is a sophisticated neurotransmission implicating summation and cotransmission. Moreover, the biologic activity of the receptors is also strongly influenced by the efficiency of the active transporters that clear the excitatory synaptic cleft from its agonist glutamate. At the cellular level, excitatory neurotransmission controls the permeability of calcium in the CNS. Therefore, excitatory neurotransmission not only determines immediate actions in the CNS, but also has long-term influence on neuronal circuitry, also called *synaptic plasticity*. Synaptic plasticity is fundamental to many neurobiological functions and excitatory neurotransmission. Hence it governs highly specific functions such as learning and memories, of which underlying mechanisms share striking similarities with those involved in pain processing.[75] By consequence, the use of NMDA antagonists is often limited by major side effects, such as memory impairment, psychomimetic side effects, ataxia, and motor incoordination. Among the various excitatory amino acid receptors subtypes, the NMDA receptor site appears more specifically linked to long-term changes in neurons as its activation leads to calcium entry into the postsynaptic neuron and in sequence to a cascade of biochemical events, including G-protein activation and c-Fos transcription. In relation to its prominent role, the NMDA receptor displays unique properties and differs from other ligand-gated ion channels. First, the receptor controls a cation channel highly permeable to calcium. Second, simultaneous binding of glutamate and glycine, the coagonist, is required to activate NMDA receptor. Third, at resting membrane potential, the NMDA receptor channel is blocked by extracellular magnesium.[75] Finally, the NMDA receptor becomes activated only when pain stimulus is sustained and intense and, hence, when sufficient quantities of glutamate are released. These conditions usually correlate with tissue injury and NMDA activation facilitates pain processing in the CNS, inducing "pathological pain," which in clinical expression is called *hyperalgesia*. According to the aforementioned physiological findings, NMDA-mediated excitatory neurotransmission is incriminated in both mediate (hyperalgesia) and probably long-term modifications (persistent pain) of perception following tissue injury.

Morphologic studies in animals have identified the presence of NMDA receptors at different levels of the CNS. Peripheral receptors are located on both unmyelinated and myelinated axons in peripheral somatic tissues and the expression of these receptors is enhanced by inflammation, therefore contributing to peripheral sensitization under that condition.[76] Further, peripheral administration of noncompetitive NMDA antagonists, either MK801 or ketamine, produces a local anesthetic-like effect. However, most of the effects of NMDA antagonists rely on their binding with central, either spinal or supraspinal, receptors.[75,77] Most of the small-diameter primary afferent fibers

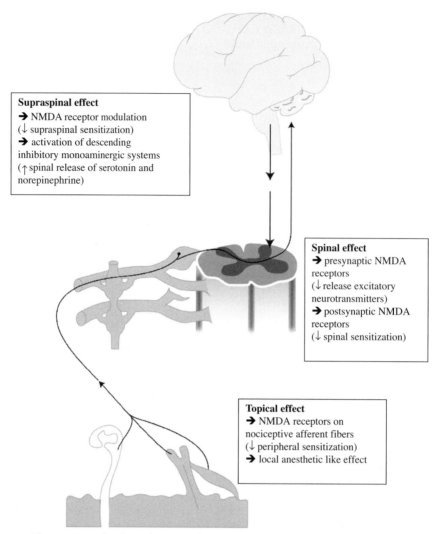

Figure 7.5: Analgesic mechanisms of ketamine, a nonselective NMDA antagonist.

in the dorsal horn express NMDA receptors and activation of these presynaptic receptors leads to the release of substance P and also to enhanced release of glutamate in response to subsequent stimuli. Postsynaptic NMDA receptors mediate central sensitization of dorsal horn neurons through calcium-dependent pathway. At a higher level, NMDA receptors located in the brainstem play a role in mediating supraspinal sensitization and their expression is upregulated under inflammatory conditions, underlying supraspinal neuronal hyperexcitability (Figure 7.5).

Pharmacology under Different Pain States

The above-mentioned findings have prompted the assessement of NMDA receptor antagonists in various experimental and clinical pain conditions. It is worth noting that ketamine, the most clinically used among available NMDA receptors antagonists, presents with different mechanisms of action, some of them being unrelated to NMDA receptor binding. For ketamine, these other mechanisms include binding to opioid receptors with a preference for μ-receptors.[78] However, the affinity of ketamine for these receptors is 10 times less than that for the NMDA receptor and, in humans, naloxone does not reverse the analgesic effect of ketamine. Ketamine also interacts with muscarinic

cholinergic receptors[79] and inhibits neuronal nicotinic receptors in a clinically relevant concentration range.[80] The drug produces anticholinergic symptoms (eg, tachycardia, bronchodilatation, salivation) and ketamine anesthesia can be reversed by cholinesterase inhibitors. Additionally, ketamine is able to block sodium channels and hence displays a local anesthetic-like effect as demonstrated in humans.

To date, opinions still differ regarding the drug's mechanisms of action and it is highly possible that mechanisms that underlie the effect of ketamine differ from one pain condition to another one. In animal models, selective NMDA antagonists (eg, MK801) inhibit the hyperexcitability of spinal cord nociceptive neurons and remove hyperalgesia without affecting baseline responses.[81,82] In contrast, a nonselective NMDA antagonist (ie, ketamine) displays analgesic properties in acute pain conditions. However, after intrathecal administration, the analgesic effect observed is weak, subject to controversy according to different experimental reports, and dose escalation is limited by side effects such as motor impairment (analgesic effect:motor dysfunction ratio <2).[81] The preclinical findings are in agreement with clinical data that demonstrate only weak analgesic effect following neuraxial administration of ketamine, as well as potential neurotoxicity linked to long-term continuous spinal administration.[38] In addition, after systemic administration under acute pain conditions, ketamine produces its antinociceptive effect by a mechanism unrelated to NMDA receptor binding (ie, by supraspinal activation of the descending inhibitory monoaminergic system).[82] Transection of lower thoracic spinal cord abolishes the analgesic effect of ketamine in rats and spinal administration of either adrenergic antagonists (yohimbine) or serotonin antagonist (methysergide) block the antinociceptive effect of systemic ketamine.[82] Systemic administration of ketamine increases the local concentrations of norepinephrine and serotonin in lumbar CSF under acute pain conditions.[82] In contrast to acute pain conditions, after tissue injury resulting in CNS sensitization, NMDA antagonists and ketamine exert an antihyperalgesic effect locally mediated at the spinal cord level by blocking NMDA receptors.[81,82] These experimental findings in animal models of inflammatory and neuropathic pain have been reproduced in clinical trials. In human volunteers, ketamine reduces the magnitude of both primary and secondary hyperalgesia from capsaicin injection or burn injury. As well, in patients suffering neuropathic pain, ketamine alleviates abnormal pain associated with CNS sensitization.[83]

Postoperative Pain Conditions

Although postoperative pain is a very common acute pain condition, incisional pain presents with unique characteristics that differ from pure inflammatory or neuropathic pain conditions. Plantar incision in rat yields to a transitory (approximately lasting for 1 hour) segmental increase of excitatory amino acids (glutamate and aspartate) in the spinal cord that is driven by input from primary afferent fibers from the site of injury.[84] That increase of excitatory amino acids accounts for the enhanced responsiveness of dorsal horn neurons, a phenomenon that relies on an NMDA-independent spinal mechanism.[85] Effectively, intrathecal competitive and noncompetitive (eg, MK801) NMDA antagonists are ineffective to alleviate postoperative pain behaviors and mechanical hyperalgesia. Rather, intrathecal injection of non-NMDA AMPA/kainate receptor antagonist alleviates mechanical hyperalgesia after plantar incision and, moreover, spinal mechanisms underlying secondary hyperalgesia require calcium-permeable AMPA/kainate receptor activation.[86,87]

Following experimental plantar incision, systemic, but not intrathecal, ketamine alleviates mechanical hyperalgesia and the effect of the drug is reversed by spinal administration of either adrenergic (yohimbine) or serotoninergic (methysergide) antagonist.[88] These findings suggest that ketamine activates monoaminergic descending inhibitory pathways at the supraspinal sites to reduce hypersensitivity in this model. Although the exact supraspinal mechanism underlying ketamine effect remains unknown, activation of κ-opioid receptors rather than μ-opioid receptors might be involved. Experimental results in animal models support clinical observations showing that systemic administration of low doses of ketamine significantly reduces the area of hyperalgesia for punctate mechanical stimuli surrounding the incision.[89] Further, ketamine suppression of central sensitization secondary to surgical injury is obtained only after systemic, but not after epidural, administration of the drug.[90] Beyond the supraspinal activation of the monoaminergic descending inhibitory system,[82,88] ketamine also possesses interesting anti-inflammatory properties. Interactions with the purinergic system have been demonstrated with adenosine release secondary to ketamine administration,[91] as well as a mod-

ulation of proinflammatory cytokines production secondary to surgical trauma. Ketamine regulates the inflammatory reaction and specifically suppress the production of the proinflammatory cytokines: TNF-α, interleukin 6 (IL-6), and interferon-γ (IFN-γ).[92,93] Ketamine also exerts direct anti-inflammatory effects on central macrophages and peripheral leucocytes stimulated with lipopolysaccharide.[94,95] Finally, systemic ketamine might also mediate its postoperative antihyperalgesic effects via peripheral mechanism.

Peripheral Use of Noncompetititve NMDA Antagonist Ketamine

Some of the same mechanisms described in the CNS may also operate in the periphery, in particular, the mechanisms underlying central sensitization may also underlie peripheral sensitization that accounts for the development of primary hyperalgesia after tissue injury and contributes to induce and maintain central sensitization. All cells in dorsal root ganglia (DRG) express NMDA receptors and experimental studies in animal have demonstrated bidirectional transport of NMDA receptors to both spinal cord dorsal horn and to nociceptive afferent terminals.[76] In rat and in human, ionotropic glutamate receptors (ie, NMDA, AMPA, and kainite) are localized on unmyelinated axons at the dermal-epidermal junction.[76] A considerable population of myelinated axons, including Aδ and Aβ fibers, also express glutamate receptors. Activation of these peripheral receptors by local injection of glutamate or glutamate agonists results in nociceptive behavior in animals. The expression of these receptors is enhanced by inflammation, therefore contributing to peripheral sensitization of nociceptors under that condition as demonstrated in synovial fluid of patients with arthritis.[96] Therefore, local administration of NMDA antagonists alleviates pain behaviors in animal models of peripheral inflammation consecutive to formalin or carrageenan injection.[76] In humans, results from peripheral administration of clinically available ketamine are mixed. In volunteers, it reduces the development of hyperalgesia consecutive to experimental burn injury,[97] but fails to inhibit capsaicin-induced hyperalgesia.[98] In postoperative patients, ketamine enhances the local anesthetic and analgesic action of bupivacaine during wound infiltration postherniorrhaphy[99] but not after cesarean section.[100]

Pharmacology of Ketamine and S(+)Ketamine

Ketamine is a phencyclidine derivative that produces "dissociative anesthesia," characterized by electroencephalogram evidence of dissociation between the thalamocortical and limbic systems. Its potential as an adjuvant analgesic were first reported in 1965. Ketamine must be considered a drug that is vulnerable to abuse and precautions against unauthorized use should be taken. The drug is available as a racemic mixture containing equal amounts of the two optical isomers. However, the enantiomer S(+) ketamine has recently become clinically available in some countries. S(+) ketamine shows a 4-fold greater affinity for NMDA receptors and therefore displays a clinical analgesic potency approximately 2 times greater than that of racemic ketamine, allowing a 70% reduction of the dose when continuously administered.[101,102] S(+) ketamine also displays a shorter duration of action than racemic ketamine and induces less cognitive impairment than racemic ketamine at an equianalgesic low dose.[102]

In perioperative conditions, ketamine has been administered by several routes, including intravenous, intramuscular, subcutaneous, oral, intranasal, intrarectal, and neuraxial (epidural, caudal, and intrathecal). Nonetheless, intravenous administration remains the most used, although, after epidural or caudal administration, ketamine rapidly accesses the systemic circulation with high bioavailability. Neuraxial administration should not be favored for two reasons: first, the neurotoxicity of spinal ketamine remains largely unknown in humans and previous reports of neuropathologic findings after continuous administration of either ketamine[103] or S(+) ketamine[104] in cancer patients allow only the clinical epidural use of preservative-free ketamine in low doses and within the setting of clinical trials.[101] Second, as previously discussed, the analgesic and antihyperalgesic benefits of a perioperative neuraxial administration of ketamine are controversial.[90,105]

Ketamine, with its high lipid solubility, has a rapid onset of action and a relatively short duration of action with an elimination half-life of 1–2.5 hours. The drug is not significantly bound to plasma proteins and leaves the blood rapidly to be redistributed into the tissues and highly perfused tissues, such as the brain, where the peak concentration may be 4 to 5 times that present in plasma. Further, the high lipid solubility of ketamine ensures a rapid transfer across the blood-brain barrier. Ketamine is extensively metabolized by hepatic microsomal enzymes and an important pathway of metabolism involves demethylation of ketamine by cytochrome P450 enzymes to form the active metabolite norketamine, which is one-fifth to one-third as potent as ketamine, and accounts for the prolonged central effects of the drug (beyond 6 hours). Norketamine is eliminated by the kidneys. Following systemic administration, less than 4% of the dose of ketamine is found unchanged in the urine and fecal excretion accounts for less than 5% of the dose.

After oral administration, ketamine undergoes an extensive first-pass metabolism that results in small ketamine concentrations but high large norketamine concentrations in blood and tissues.[106] Chronic administration of ketamine stimulates the activity of the enzymes responsible for its metabolism and resulting accelerated metabolism secondary to enzyme induction may contribute to observed tolerance to the analgesic effect of the drug.

In clinical conditions, low doses of ketamine are usually used for their analgesic and antihyperalgesic properties. An effective analgesia can be achieved with the use of subanesthetic doses of ketamine (ie, systemic administration of 0.2 to 0.5 mg/kg) and ketamine is more potent to alleviate somatic than visceral pain. In general, low doses are defined as a bolus dose of less than 1 mg/kg and an infusion rate of less than 20 μg/kg/min (1.2 mg/kg/h).[107] The effect of these low doses or subanesthetic doses corresponds to inhibiting action on NMDA receptor-mediated pain facilitation, although other mechanisms of action may exist. Effectively, ketamine exerts its clinical effects at concentrations from 0.1- to 9.0 μM, which is identical to its NMDA receptor occupancy range.[108] Therapeutic plasma concentrations of ketamine are within micromolar range (0.3–1.04 μM) following low-dose administration, whereas IC_{50} values for inhibiting cloned human NMDA receptor-induced Ca^{2+} influx or electrophysiological response situate between 1.6 and 6.2 μM.[109]

Finally, it is worth noting that, as demonstrated in animals, another dose range than the low doses previously reported exists

in which ketamine has no effect on its own but yields an opioid-sparing effect and potentiates opioid agonists. Recently, Tucker et al[110] identified dosing regimens capable of eliciting a clinical benefit in the coadministration of ketamine with opioids. In human volunteers, they demonstrated that very low doses of ketamine (ie, serum concentrations of 30–120 ng/mL), although devoid of any antinociceptive effect, potentiates the antinociceptive effect of fentanyl without increasing sedation. However, in clinical practice and perioperative settings, administration of doses lower than 0.15 mg/kg failed to show any postoperative benefit.[101]

Other Effects Than Analgesic Effects

Both experimental and clinical experiences have demonstrated that NMDA antagonists effects go along with a narrow therapeutic window, which is not surprising given the abundance of NMDA receptors in the CNS and their crucial role in functions such as memory and motor tone. Hemodynamic and respiratory side effects of ketamine are very limited, as well as sedation, which is lower than observed after opioid administration. Futhermore, low doses of ketamine, as recommended in clinical practice, do not appear to enhance opioid-induced sedation or nausea and vomiting.[107] In summary, the majority of clinical trials and meta-analysis to date acknowledge that subanesthetic dose of ketamine are a safe and useful adjuvant to standard-practice opioid analgesia. However, the major concern remains the risk of psychomimetic side effects, such as hallucinations, vivid dreams, and nightmares. Experiments in volunteers have shown that the psychodysleptic effects of ketamine are dose related and plasma concentrations as small as 50 ng/mL and higher interfere with memory function and impair cognitive function tasks.[107] In patients, the incidence of these disturbing reactions varies from 5% to more than 30%[107] and the highest risk is found in sedated patients who do not receive benzodiazepine, whereas in patients undergoing general anesthesia, the incidence is really low and independent of benzodiazepine premedication.[111] In addition, clinical experience has also demonstrated that anxious and apprehensive patients are more likely to exhibit psychomimetic side effects.[83] Among other adverse effects associated with ketamine administration, dizziness, blurred vision and troubles of proprioception are also commonly reported.[83,107]

Interaction with Other Analgesics

The mechanism of action of NMDA receptor antagonists differs from that of classic analgesics such as opioids. Indeed, NMDA antagonists demonstrate an antihyperalgesic effect because they reduce central hyperexcitability (ie, facilitated response to sensory inputs) without affecting basal nociceptive threshold. Therefore, their association with classical analgesics seems particularly useful to improve postoperative pain management where such sensitization is present. The potentiation of opioids analgesic effect by NMDA receptor antagonists, even at very low doses, was observed in various animal studies as well as in experimental pain in human volunteers.[110] In postoperative conditions, the combination of both drugs results to a postoperative reduction of either intravenous or epidural opioids after intraoperative ketamine.[105,112] A median dose of intravenous ketamine of 0.4 mg/kg (range from 0.1 to 1.6 mg/kg) administered during anesthesia significantly decreases cumulative 24-hour morphine consumption by 27%–47%.[111] Although the association yields in a significant opioid-sparing effect, the reduction of well-known postoperative opioid adverse effects, such as nausea and vomiting, is controversial. In contrast, another adverse effect resulting from perioperative opioid use has recently gained attention: the "paradoxical hyperalgesic effect" of opioid drugs, which results in the enhancement of postoperative pain and on the development of a pseudotolerance to the analgesic effect of opioids.[113] Even a single opioid administration induces a short-lasting analgesic effect followed by a delayed antianalgesic or hyperalgesic effect. The exaggeration of postoperative pain and hyperalgesia was clearly demonstrated in animals[114] and in humans.[115] The acute tolerance to the analgesic effect of postoperative opioids results from a process of pain sensitization rather than a decrease in opioid effectiveness. The mechanisms underlying this physiological phenomenon involve simultaneous activation of both pain inhibitory and pain facilitatory systems in which NMDA receptors play a prominent role because systemic administration of NMDA receptor antagonists prevents opioid-induced hyperalgesia in both animals and humans.[116,117] Intravenous administration of low doses of ketamine currently is an interesting tool that can be used to improve postoperative pain relief and to prevent escalating opioid needs, particularly in patients in whom postoperative pain is difficult to control (patients who are opioid addicts or who are taking opioid treatment for chronic pain).

Immunomodulatory Effects

Ketamine is characterized by its ability to interact with numerous neurotransmitter systems (eg, NMDA, monoaminergic, opiates, cholinergic, and adenosine). Therefore, it is not surprising that the drug interferes with immune function. In fact, the beneficial effects of ketamine treatment in patients suffering major inflammatory stress (septic shock) have been long suspected. Septic shock patients sedated with ketamine show improved cardiovascular stability and experimental studies have extended the benefits to improved survival.[118,119] Ketamine modulates the production of cytokines and promotes an inhibition of the inflammatory response. The release of proinflalmmatory cytokines (TNF-α, IL-1) is significantly reduced.[120] In humans, three studies considering ketamine in patients undergoing major surgery (cardiac surgery and orthotopic liver transplantation) deserve attention.[92,93] Extracorporal circulation is a potent activator of the inflammatory cascade. In this situation, a single preoperative subanesthetic dose of ketamine (0.25–0.5 mg/kg) significantly reduces the circulating levels of IL-6, an effect measured immediately after discontinuation of the cardiopulmonary bypass but also at the 7th postoperative day. By consequence, a single preoperative dose of ketamine has a prolonged systemic anti-inflammatory effect. Similarly, in patients undergoing liver transplantation, one dose of ketamine reduced the postoperative release of TNF-α and IL-6 without affecting IL-10. The mechanisms underlying ketamine effect on the production of proinflammatory cytokines by the immune competent cells may rely on the reduction of nuclear inductible transcription factor (Nf-κb) expression, which is responsible for the increased production of inflammatory cytokines in monocytes and macrophages. The same mechanism accounts for the repression of proinflammatory cytokine release of NE acting on β2-adrenoceptors. Here, it is worth noting that part of the pharmacologic action of ketamine is mediated by the recruitment of the descending noradrenergic system.[82,88]

Ketamine also inhibits the action of neutrophils and interferes with adhesion and chemotaxy of these leukocytes by reducing the amount of adhesion molecules expressed, hence limiting their progression to the inflammatory site.[121] Ketamine also impairs the bactericidal properties of neutrophils by reducing their superoxide production.[122] Interesting to point out are the interactions between ketamine and the adenosine pathway.[91] Adenosine possesses immunomodulatory properties and some of the anti-inflammatory effects of ketamine (inhibition of chemotaxy and reduction of superoxyde production) are blocked by the concomitant administration of A2-adenosine receptor antagonist. Ketamine also interacts with NO production. The drug inhibits both endothelial nitric oxide synthase and inducible nitric oxide synthase in a dose-related effect, totally independent of its NMDA receptor antagonist properties. Finally, ketamine is a potent stimulator of the HPA axis, a system that promotes potent anti-inflammatory properties. This effect on the HPA axis is not NMDA mediated because two other NMDA-receptor antagonists (ie, memantine and MK-801) do not affect cortisol production. Once again, an interaction with the sympathetic system or the production of prostaglandin E2 are the suspected mechanisms.

Ketamine-induced systemic anti-inflammatory effects have been reported to promote survival in several rodent animal models of septic shock or burn injury,[119] but in humans there is no study to confirm or inform these observations. The immune properties of ketamine might be involved in the beneficial effects on the reduction of both postoperative hyperalgesia and residual pain development observed in patients after major abdominal surgery.[90] It is generally confirmed that immunomodulation is the mechanism underlying the antihyperalgesic effects of the drug after traumatic injury in humans. Effectively, the doses necessary for the anti-inflammatory effect are in the same range as the doses required for the antihyperalgesic effect of the drug. Further, as for antihyperalgesic effects, anti-inflammatory effects persist long after ketamine has disappeared from the organism.

GABAPENTIN AND PREGABALIN

Anticonvulsants and Voltage-Gated Calcium Channels for Pain Modulation

Gabapentin, an alkylated GABA analog, was synthetized in 1977 and developed as a clinical anticonvulsant. Recent experimental and clinical observations suggest that the drug may also be useful to treat other neurologic and psychiatric conditions such as spasticity, anxiety, and pain. Specifically, gabapentin seems to be a "large specter" analgesic or, more precisely, a "large spectre" antihyperalgesic drug working in different conditions where sensitization is present.[123]

Gabapentin and its derivative compound pregabalin (ie, S(+)-3-isobutyl-gaba) are structural analogs of GABA but, unlike GABA, they cross the blood-brain barrier and do not bind to GABAA or GABAB receptors. Futhermore, the fact that gabapentin might increase neuronal GABA levels is also subject to controversy. Finally, unlike other antiepileptic drugs, gabapentin and pregabalin do not interact with sodium channels. Both drugs belong to a unique class of compounds characterized by a high-affinity binding to the α2-δ protein, an auxiliary subunit of the voltage-gated calcium channels (VGCC) in neuronal tissue.[124,125] Although the exact mechanisms of action remain largely unknown, studies in genetically modified mice have demonstrated that selective binding to the α_2-δ subunit of calcium channels is necessary for gabapentin- and pregabalin-induced antinociceptive, anticonvulsant, and anxiolytic effects.[126]

All excitable cells express plasma membrane VGCCs that tranduce electrical activity into intracellular biochemical events. The depolarization of cellular membrane triggers the opening of VGCCs to allow a rapid influx of extracellular calcium.[127] Intracellular pools of free ionized calcium play a major role in cellular functions, and the intracellular calcium increase contributes to depolarize membranes and to initiate transmitter release, transcription through kinase activation, and phosphorylation of membranes proteins that will activate a variety of intracellular enzymes.[128] Calcium ions can enter into the cell through different gateways, mostly through the opening of membrane VGCCs that are specifically voltage-activated and also through receptors-gated channels, such as the NMDA and the calcium-permeable AMPA ionophores. Although the major role of the latter type has been emphasized for acute and chronic nociceptive processing, the role of the former type (ie, VGCCs) in pain modulation has been to date mainly examined in chronic pain states, specifically as a target for the treatment of neuropathic pain.[128] VGCCs are large multiprotein complexes with a pore-forming α_1 subunit as the center, surrounded by auxiliary α_2-δ, β, and subunits.[127] These auxiliary VGCC subunits play an important role for the regulation of channel function, regulating its biophysical properties, rate of channel activation or inactivation, as well as expression and trafficking of the channel.[129] Finally, the association of different auxiliary subunits with different pore-forming channels define the principal families of high-voltage activated calcium channels such as L-, N-, P/Q- or R-type channels.

The α_2-δ *site of N-type VGCC*, which is a target for gabapentin and related compounds, is densely expressed in the superficial dorsal horn, substantia gelatinosa, of the spinal cord where primary afferents synapse as well as in DRG neurons and in the forebrain.[128,129] Further, several experimental studies suggest that actions of α_2-δ ligands are primarily restricted to presynaptic VGCC because they result in a reduction of excessive neurotransmitter release.[128,129] The drugs provoke a subtle inhibitory modulation of monoamine (ie, norepinephrine, epinephrine, and dopamine) release in the cortex, an effect that accounts for the anxiolytic and antidepressive effects of gabapentin and pregabalin.[124] They also reduce the release of excitatory neurotransmitters, such as substance P, CGRP, and glutamate in the spinal cord.[124,125] However, it is paramount to note that "sensitized" conditions are a prerequisite to the effects of α_2-δ ligands on neurotransmission; in other words, α_2-δ ligands have minimal effects on physiological transmitter release, whereas they significantly inhibit "abnormal sensitized" release.[129] Under hyperexcitable or pathological conditions (eg, tissue damages secondary to inflammation and nerve injury), an excessive influx of calcium from sustained VGCCs opening leads to an important release of excitatory neurotransmitters. The binding of α_2-δ ligands to the auxiliary subunit allosterically modulates VGCCs to reduce the excessive influx of calcium and its subsequent neurotransmitters release (Figure 7.6).[129]

Potency and Mechanisms of Action under Different Pain Conditions

Both the location of the α_2-δ subunit and the fact that gabapentin and pregabalin easily cross the blood-brain barrier argue in favor of a major central site of action. Furthermore, whether systemic and spinal administration of gabapentin are effective in modulating nociceptive processing, the doses needed for an intrathecal effect are considerabily lower than those needed for a systemic effect.[130,131] However, even by spinal delivery, gabapentin, like other drugs acting on VGCCs, fail to alter the response to an acute nociceptive stimulus at doses that do not produce a significant motor dysfunction,[128] whereas these drugs effectively alleviate hypersensitivity consecutive to tissue injury in different experimental models. It is well established that hyperalgesia represents the clinical expression of central neuronal excitability and sensitization and gabapentin's ability to modulate the phenomenon traduces an important centrally mediated effect of the drug.

Therefore, gabapentin relieves hypersensitivity in inflammatory conditions and affects NMDA-mediated currents in spinal neurons from rats with experimental arthritis but not from normal rats.[132] Gabapentin has no effect on pain behaviors during phase 1 of rat formalin test, a brief phase that reflects physiologic pain, but strongly modulates the phase 2 of the test, a long-lasting phase that correlates with central sensitization induced by a continuous low level of small afferent input following formalin injection into the paw.[133,134] The drug dose dependently inhibits the nociceptive behavior in phase 2 and a pretreatment is more effective than a posttreatment.[134] Posttreatment administration of spinal gabapentin is one-third as potent as pretreatment but that decreased antinociceptive efficacy still distinguishes gabapentin from NMDA-receptor antagonists that are ineffective when administered after formalin injection and constitutes an indirect evidence that gabapentin does not directly interact with NMDA receptor.[134] The same study also demonstrated that gabapentin effects are highly stimulus dependent and, hence, preferential for conditions in which there will be a greater induction of central sensitization.

In human volunteers, oral gabapentin at a dose of 1200 mg shows no effect on pain transmission in normal skin, but significantly reduces hyperalgesia induced by experimental thermal injury[135] or capsaicin injection.[136] Central nervous system plasticity at different levels underlies both the development and the maintenance of neuropathic pain, a pathophysiological condition that is particularly sensitive to gabapentin administration, both in animal models and in humans.[137] Experimental models of neuropathic pain have revealed that upregulation of α_2-δ subunit expression in both the spinal cord and the dorsal root ganglia correlates with the development of mechanical allodynia.[138,139] This phenomenon certainly does explain the efficacy of both systemic and intrathecal gabapentin in neuropathic pain conditions.[140] A recent study reports the antihyperalgesic and antiallodynic effects of the drug after intracerebroventricular administration in animals with peripheral nerve injury, suggesting that the drug also acts at a supraspinal level. The supraspinal effect of gabapentin seems to be mediated by the descending noradrenergic system, resulting in the activation of spinal α_2 adrenoceptors and hence cholinergic muscarinic activation and NO cascade.[141]

Postoperative Pain Condition

Tissue lesions secondary to surgical incision and postoperative pain also result in central sensitization that is clinically expressed as spontaneous pain and mechanical hyperalgesia surrounding the wound.[1] Regarding the antihyperalgesic properties of gabapentin in a wide range of pain states produced by central sensitization, the drug has also been evaluated in various experimental models of incisional pain.[130,131,142] Single dose of

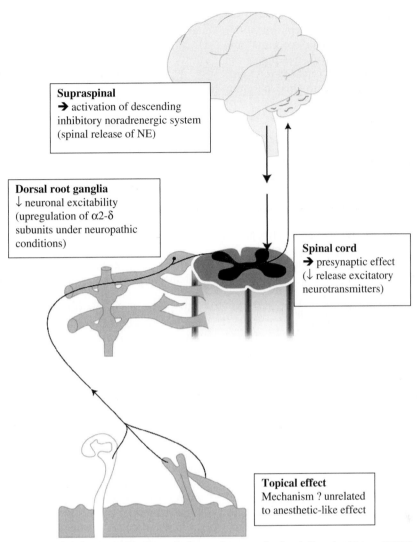

Suprasinal
➔ activation of descending inhibitory noradrenergic system (spinal release of NE)

Dorsal root ganglia
↓ neuronal excitability (upregulation of α2-δ subunits under neuropathic conditions)

Spinal cord
➔ presynaptic effect (↓ release excitatory neurotransmitters)

Topical effect
Mechanism ? unrelated to anesthetic-like effect

Figure 7.6: Analgesic mechanisms of gabapentin, an α_2-δ subunit ligand at N-type VGCC (voltage gated calcium channel).

subcutaneous gabapentin (3–30 mg/kg) administered 1 hour before surgery blocks the postoperative development of heat hyperalgesia and tactile allodynia for several hours in a dose-dependent manner.[131] When the drug is administered 1 hour after surgery, an antihyperalgesic effect was still observed but only for a short duration. The results of gabapentin contrasted with those observed after subcutaneous morphine administration that was shorter lasting and more effective against thermal hyperalgesia. There are several clinical implications resulting from these experimental findings. First, gabapentin seems more effective than morphine to alleviate postoperative mechanical hyperalgesia and, hence, evoked pain associated with movement.[123] Second, this class of compounds are capable of blocking the induction and the maintenance of dorsal horn neurons sensitization and their effect, when administered before the lesion, outlasts the pharmacological half-life of the drug.[123] Intrathecal gabapentin at much lower doses (10–100 μg) also reduced postoperative punctate mechanical hyperalgesia after paw incision in a dose-related manner.[130,142] These later studies highlighted the increased potency of the spinal route of administration, supporting a central mechanism of action for the drug. Furthermore, spinal injection does

not necessitate the entry of gabapentin into cells or nerve terminals via the L-amino acid transporter (a mechanism that facilitates intestinal absorption)[130] that is consistent with an action of gabapentin on extracellular sites such as the α_2-δ subunit of voltage-sensitive calcium channels on dorsal horn neurons. A subsequent study recently confirmed that the antiallodynic effect of intrathecal gabapentin after tissue incision involves spinal N-type VGCCs.[143] However, although the efficacy of gabapentin depends on its binding to the α_2-δ auxiliary subunit of VGCCs, the analgesic mechanisms underlying the drug action still remain unknown. Because systemic gabapentin is also very effective in relieving postoperative hypersensitivity, the effect of a supraspinal administration (ie, intracerebroventricular injection) was evaluated in an incisional pain model.[144] Results from this study showed that, by that route, gabapentin activates the descending noradrenergic system and induces spinal norepinephrine release, which produces analgesia via spinal α_2-AR stimulation, followed by activation of GIRKs. In contrast with neuraxial analgesia from α_2-adrenoceptor agonists, analgesia from gabapentin did not involve a cholinergic mediation at spinal level. In addition to the animal study, the authors also validated their hypothesis in humans.[144]

Preoperative administration of oral gabapentin (1200 mg) significantly enhanced the CSF levels of norepinephrine within 2 hours in patients undergoing orthopedic or urogenital procedures. In the gabapentin group of patients, norepinephrine concentrations were 461 (400–864) pg/mL (median, interquartile range) versus 329 (238–432) pg/mL in the placebo group ($P < .005$).[144]

Peripheral Use of Gabapentin

All experimental data support a central site of action for gabapentin and pregabalin. The effects related to local administration of the drugs are scarce. However, intraplantar administration of gabapentin and S(+)-3-isobutylgaba significantly reduces nociceptive behaviors during both phase 1 and phase 2 in the formalin test.[145] These results contrast with that of spinal administration that alleviates only the nociceptive effects observed during phase 2.[136] Further, the peripheral mechanism of action of the drug cannot be attributed to a local anesthetic effect.[145]

Pharmacology of Gabapentin and Pregabalin

Both gabapentin and pregabalin (second generation of compounds binding to α_2-δ subunit) are small molecules nonmetabolizable branched-chain amino acids. For clinical use, both drugs exist only as an oral form (capsules or tablets) and undergo intestinal absorption throughout the small intestine and the colon via a L-transporter family system (large amino acid transport [LAT], including phenylalanine, isoleucine, leucine, and valine). The transporter and its capacities facilitate the passage of gabapentin and pregabalin from the intestinal lumen to the systemic circulation.[125] For a single oral dose of gabapentin (300 mg), the plasmatic peak of concentration (2.7 μg/mL) is reached after 3 hours. At therapeutic doses, gabapentin absorption usually occurs within a T_{max} of 3 to 4 hours, whereas pregabalin is more rapidly absorbed, with T_{max} occurring 0.5 to 1 hour postdose. However, the amount of gabapentin absorbed is dose dependent, and the fraction of dose absorbed decreases from 74% to 62% to 27% over the dose range of 100 mg to 300 mg and then to a 1600-mg single dose (saturation of L-transporter system). In contrast, the amount of pregabalin absorbed is independent of the dose administered and the fraction of dose absorbed remains constant (ie, >90% over the dose range of 10 to 300 mg for a single dose). Gabapentin and pregabalin do not bind to plasma proteins (<5% protein binding). The drugs easily cross the blood-brain barrier and very high concentrations are found in the CNS. At steady state, CSF levels of gabapentin are 5%–35% of plasma levels but cerebral levels are 80% of those found in plasma. Both drugs undergo negligible metabolism in humans and do not inhibit cytochrome P450 enzymes that mediate the metabolism of several drugs, therefore adjustment of dosage in patients with liver disease is not necessary and interactions with other drugs are unlikely. Gabapentin and pregabalin are predominately eliminated by renal excretion, necessitating dosage adjustment in patients with impaired renal function secondary to kidney disease or to the effects of aging. In subjects with normal renal function, elimination half-life for both drugs is approximately 5–7 hours and is unrelated to the dose. In summary, both drugs have the advantage of a negligible metabolism and interaction with other drugs in humans. However, pregabalin has a nonsaturable absorption at clinically relevant doses, resulting in linear pharmacokinetics and,

Table 7.2: Side-Effect Profile of Gabapentin in Chronic Pain and Postoperative Patients

	Chronic Pain (%)		Perioperative Use (%)	
	Placebo	*Treatment*	*Placebo*	*Treatment*
Sedation	9.8	20.2 %[a,139]	9.7–10.3	19–21[a,153,154]
Dizziness	7.8	17.9[a]	16	17.6[153]
Fatigue	4.9	11.1		
Ataxia	5.2	13.2		
Headache	9.1	8.7		
Nausea	7.5	6	17–25	19–21[153]

[a] Significant difference in the occurrence of the side effect between placebo group and patients receiving gabapentin.

therefore, a greater efficacious response than that observed for gabapentin.

Nonanalgesic Effects: Side-Effect Profile

Several clinical trials have demonstrated the safety of gabapentin administration, even for chronic use.[137] Overdose (up to 50 g) seems to cause no or minimal toxicity in humans. Observations made in symptomatic patients following overdose have reported effects of drowsiness (66%), dizziness (33%), nausea/vomiting (22%), and tachycardia and hypotension (<20%).[146] Gabapentin and pregabalin do not show hemodynamic impairment in animal models or in humans, even after spinal administration in animals,[147] which contrasts with the major cardiovascular side effects observed spinal administration of selective N-type VGCC blockers such as SNX-111.[127] Respiratory depression also does not seem to be a concern after overdose of gabapentin alone: with plasma levels of 62 μg/mL, patients were lethargic but remained easily arousable.[148]

Similarly, very few and relatively mild side effects have been reported after perioperative administration and, to date, some consider gabapentin and pregabalin a reliable alternative to ketamine and NMDA antagonists in the treatment of postoperative pain and the prevention of central sensitization (Table 7.2).[149]

Synergy with Other Analgesics

Gabapentin enhances the antinociceptive effects of opioids in different experimental models ranging from acute to chronic pain as well as in human volunteers. Further, coadministration of gabapentin also inhibits the development of antinociceptive tolerance to systemic[150] and spinal morphine administration. This attenuation of morphine tolerance by intrathecal gabapentin is associated with a suppression of morphine-evoked spinal release of excitatory aminoacids such as gluatamate and aspartate. To maintain this effect, gabapentin needs to be continued during morphine administration because tolerance to morphine becomes apparent within the 48 hours of discontinuing gabapentin.[150] Gabapentin seems also capable of partially restoring opioid efficacy when tolerance is already present.[150] In the postoperative setting, these findings found their expression in the opioid sparing effect that results from gabapentin administration.[123,151–153] Because opioids induce several adverse effects and also because they lack effectiveness to relieve pain evoked by movement, the beneficial combination of gabapentin or pregabalin with opioids is of paramount interest in perioperative patients. Furthermore, these drugs might be useful to manage acute pain in opioid-dependent patients.

Gabapentin and pregabalin share similar antihyperalgesic effect to NSAIDs because these compounds do not alter the nociceptive threshold in uninjured conditions but normalize the lowered nociceptive threshold induced by tissue injury. Coadministration of gabapentin or pregabalin with NSAIDs demonstrates either an additive or a synergistic effect in reducing hypersensitivity in experimental models.[154,155] Finally, gabapentin also potentiates the antihyperalgesic effect of spinal clonidine and spinal neostigmine in animal models of formalin test[156] and incisional pain.[130]

Immunomodulatory Effects

At the present time, no study can be found in the literature that specifically address the gabapentin/pregabalin interaction with immune function. The VGCCs mediate a well-characterized calcium influx pathway that is most exclusively identified in excitable neuronal cells. Recently, this type of calcium channel has been identified on nonexcitable cells, specifically on lymphocytes, mainly on T_H2 lymphocytes.[157] Calcium influx into these cells is essential for activation, differentiation and effector function. By binding to α_2-δ subunit of VGCCs, gabapentin and related compounds may modulate excessive calcium influx in these immune cells cells and probably affect the inflammatory process.

REFERENCES

1. Brennan TJ, Zahn PK, Pogatzki-Zahn EM. Mechanisms of incisional pain. *Anesthesiol Clin North Am* 2005;23:1–20.

2. Lavand'homme P. Perioperative pain. *Curr Opin Anaesthesiol.* 2006;19:556–561.

3. Kehlet H. Postoperative opioid sparing to hasten recovery: what are the issues? *Anesthesiology.* 2005;102:1083–1085.

4. Rathmell JP, Wu CL, Sinatra RS, et al. Acute post-surgical pain management: a critical appraisal of current practice, December 2–4, 2005. *Reg Anesth Pain Med.* 2006;31:1–42.

5. Yaksh TL, Reddy SV. Studies in the primate on the analgetic effects associated with intrathecal actions of opiates, alpha-adrenergic agonists and baclofen. *Anesthesiology.* 1981;54:451–467.

6. Maze M. Alpha2-Adrenoceptors in pain modulation. Which subtype should be targeted to produce analgesia? *Anesthesiology.* 2000;92:934–936.

7. Yoshimura M, Furue H. Mechanisms for the anti-nociceptive actions of the descending noradrenergic and serotonergic systems in the spinal cord. *J Pharmacol Sci.* 2006;101:107–117.

8. Mitrovic I, Margeta-Mitrovic M, Bader S, Stoffel M, Jan LY, Basbaum AI. Contribution of GIRK2-mediated postsynaptic signaling to opiate and alpha 2-adrenergic analgesia and analgesic sex differences. *Proc Natl Acad Sci USA.* 2003;100: 271–276.

9. Kawasaki Y, Kumamoto E, Furue H, Yoshimura M. Alpha 2 adrenoceptor-mediated presynaptic inhibition of primary afferent glutamatergic transmission in rat substantia gelatinosa neurons. *Anesthesiology.* 2003;98:682–689.

10. Li X, Eisenach JC. Alpha2a-adrenoceptor stimulation reduces capsaicin-induced glutamate release from spinal cord synaptosomes. *J Pharmacol Exp Ther.* 2001;299:939–944.

11. Detweiler DJ, Eisenach JC, Tong C, Jackson C. A cholinergic interaction in alpha 2 adrenoceptor-mediated antinociception in sheep. *J Pharmacol Exp Ther.* 1993;265:536–542.

12. Hood DD, Mallak KA, Eisenach JC, Tong C. Interaction between intrathecal neostigmine and epidural clonidine in human volunteers. *Anesthesiology.* 1996;85:315–325.

13. De Kock M, Eisenach JC, Tong C, Schmitz AL, Scholtes JL. Analgesic doses of intrathecal but not intravenous clonidine increase acetylcholine in cerebrospinal fluid in humans. *Anesth Analg.* 1997;84:800–803.

14. Li X, Zhao Z, Pan HL, Eisenach JC, Paqueron X. Norepinephrine release from spinal synaptosomes: auto-alpha2 -adrenergic receptor modulation. *Anesthesiology.* 2000;93:164–172.

15. Baba H, Shimoji K, Yoshimura M. Norepinephrine facilitates inhibitory transmission in substantia gelatinosa of adult rat spinal cord (part 1): effects on axon terminals of GABAergic and glycinergic neurons. *Anesthesiology.* 2000;92:473–484.

16. Stone LS, Broberger C, Vulchanova L, et al. Differential distribution of alpha2A and alpha2C adrenergic receptor immunoreactivity in the rat spinal cord. *J Neurosci.* 1998;18:5928–5937.

17. Ongioco RR, Richardson CD, Rudner XL, Stafford-Smith M, Schwinn D. Alpha2-adrenergic receptors in human dorsal root ganglia: predominance of alpha2b and alpha2c subtype mRNAs. *Anesthesiology.* 2000;92:968–976.

18. Stone LS, Fairbanks CA, Wilcox GL. Moxonidine, a mixed alpha(2)-adrenergic and imidazoline receptor agonist, identifies a novel adrenergic target for spinal analgesia. *Ann N Y Acad Sci.* 2003;1009:378–385.

19. Eisenach JC, Hood DD, Curry R. Relative potency of epidural to intrathecal clonidine differs between acute thermal pain and capsaicin-induced allodynia. *Pain.* 2000;84:57–64.

20. Eisenach JC, Hood DD, Curry R. Intrathecal, but not intravenous, clonidine reduces experimental thermal or capsaicin-induced pain and hyperalgesia in normal volunteers. *Anesth Analg.* 1998;87:591–596.

21. Eisenach JC, DuPen S, Dubois M, Miguel R, Allin D. Epidural clonidine analgesia for intractable cancer pain. The Epidural Clonidine Study Group. *Pain.* 1995;61:391–399.

22. Glynn CJ, Jamous MA, Teddy PJ. Cerebrospinal fluid kinetics of epidural clonidine in man. *Pain.* 1992;49:361–367.

23. Duflo F, Li X, Bantel C, Pancaro C, Vincler M, Eisenach JC. Peripheral nerve injury alters the alpha2 adrenoceptor subtype activated by clonidine for analgesia. *Anesthesiology.* 2002;97:636–641.

24. Stone LS, Vulchanova L, Riedl MS, et al. Effects of peripheral nerve injury on alpha-2A and alpha-2C adrenergic receptor immunoreactivity in the rat spinal cord. *Neuroscience.* 1999;93:1399–1407.

25. Paqueron X, Li X, Bantel C, Tobin JR, Voytko ML, Eisenach JC. An obligatory role for spinal cholinergic neurons in the antiallodynic effects of clonidine after peripheral nerve injury. *Anesthesiology.* 2001;94:1074–1081.

26. Duflo F, Conklin D, Li X, Eisenach JC. Spinal adrenergic and cholinergic receptor interactions activated by clonidine in postincisional pain. *Anesthesiology.* 2003;98:1237–1242.

27. De Kock M, Lavand'homme P, Waterloos H. The short-lasting analgesia and long-term antihyperalgesic effect of intrathecal clonidine in patients undergoing colonic surgery. *Anesth Analg.* 2005;101:566–572.

28. Brummett CM, Wagner DS. The use of alpha-2 agonists in peripheral nerve blocks: a review of history of clonidine and a look at a possible future for dexmedetomidine. *Semin Anesth, Perioperative Med Pain.* 2006;25:84–92.

29. Butterworth JF, Strichartz GR. The alpha2-adrenergic agonists clonidine and guanfacine produce tonic and phasic block of conduction in rat sciatic nerve fibers. *Anesth Analg.* 1993;76:295–301.

30. Kroin JS, Buvanendran A, Beck DR, Topic JE, Watts DE, Tuman KJ. Clonidine prolongation of lidocaine analgesia after sciatic nerve block in rats Is mediated via the hyperpolarization-activated cation current, not by alpha-adrenoreceptors. *Anesthesiology.* 2004;101:488–494.

31. Wolff M, Heugel P, Hempelmann G, Scholz A, Mühling J, Olschewski A. Clonidine reduces the excitability of spinal dorsal horn neurones. *Br J Anaesth.* 2007;98:353–361.

32. Gentili M, Juhel A, Bonnet F. Peripheral analgesic effect of intra-articular clonidine. *Pain.* 1996;64:593–596.

33. Reuben SS, Steinberg RB, Klatt JL, Klatt ML. Intravenous regional anesthesia using lidocaine and clonidine. *Anesthesiology.* 1999;91:654–658.

34. Dogrul A, Uzbay IT. Topical clonidine antinociception. *Pain.* 2004;111:385–391.

35. Davis KD, Treede RD, Raja SN, Meyer RA, Campbell JN. Topical application of clonidine relieves hyperalgesia in patients with sympathetically maintained pain. *Pain.* 1991;47:309–317.

36. Lavand'homme PM, Eisenach JC. Perioperative administration of the alpha2-adrenoceptor agonist clonidine at the site of nerve injury reduces the development of mechanical hypersensitivity and modulates local cytokine expression. *Pain.* 2003;105:247–254.

37. Lavand'homme PM, Ma W, De Kock M, Eisenach JC. Perineural alpha(2A)-adrenoceptor activation inhibits spinal cord neuroplasticity and tactile allodynia after nerve injury. *Anesthesiology.* 2002;97:972–980.

38. Hodgson PS, Neal JM, Pollock JE, Liu SS. The neurotoxicity of drugs given intrathecally (Spinal). *Anesth Analg.* 1999;88:797–809.

39. Eisenach JC, De Kock M, Klimscha W. alpha(2)-adrenergic agonists for regional anesthesia. A clinical review of clonidine (1984–1995). *Anesthesiology.* 1996;85:655–674.

40. Davies DS, Wing LMH, Reid JL, Neill E, Tippett P, Dollery CT. Pharmacokinetics and concentration-effect relationships of intravenous and oral clonidine. *Clin Pharmacol Ther.* 1976;21:593–601.

41. Segal IS, Jarvis DJ, Duncan SR, White PF, Maze M. Clinical efficacy of oral-transdermal clonidine combinations during the perioperative period. *Anesthesiology.* 1991;74:220–225.

42. Castro MI, Eisenach JC. Pharmacokinetics and dynamics of intravenous, intrathecal and epidural clonidine in sheep. *Anesthesiology.* 1989;71:418–425.

43. Eisenach J, Detweiler D, Hood D. Hemodynamic and analgesic actions of epidurally administered clonidine. *Anesthesiology.* 1993;78:277–287.

44. Filos KS, Goudas LC, Patroni O, Polyzou V. Hemodynamic and analgesic profile after intrathecal clonidine in humans: a dose-response study. *Anesthesiology.* 1994;81:591–601; discussion 527A–528A.

45. Mendez R, Eisenach JC, Kashtan K. Epidural clonidine analgesia after cesarean section. *Anesthesiology.* 1990;73:848–852.

46. De Kock M, Crochet B, Morimont C, Scholtes JL. Intravenous or epidural clonidine for intra- and postoperative analgesia. *Anesthesiology.* 1993;79:525–531.

47. Bernard JM, Kick O, Bonnet F. Comparison of intravenous and epidural clonidine for postoperative patient-controlled analgesia. *Anesth Analg.* 1995;81:706–712.

48. Maze M, Scarfini C, Cavaliere F. New agents for sedation in the intensive care unit. *Crit Care Clin.* 2001;17:881–897.

49. Hall JE, Uhrich TD, Barney JA, Arain SR, Ebert TJ. Sedative, amnestic, and analgesic properties of small-dose dexmedetomidine infusions. *Anesth Analg.* 2000;90:699–705.

50. Belleville JP, Ward DS, Bloor BC, Maze M. Effects of intravenous dexmedetomidine in humans. I. Sedation, ventilation, and metabolic rate. *Anesthesiology.* 1992;77:1125–1133.

51. Bloor BC, Ward DS, Belleville JP, Maze M. Effects of intravenous dexmedetomidine in humans. II. Hemodynamic changes. *Anesthesiology* 1992;77:1134–1142.

52. Talke P, Richardson CA, Scheinin M, Fisher DM. Postoperative pharmacokinetics and sympatholytic effects of dexmedetomidine. *Anesth Analg.* 1997;85:1136–1142.

53. Ebert TJ, Hall JE, Barney JA, Uhrich TD, Colinco MD. The effects of increasing plasma concentrations of dexmedetomidine in humans. *Anesthesiology.* 2000;93:382–394.

54. Eisenach JC, Shafer SL, Bucklin BA, Jackson C, Kallio A. Pharmacokinetics and pharmacodynamics of intraspinal dexmedetomidine in sheep. *Anesthesiology.* 1994;80:1349–1359.

55. Ma D, Rajakumaraswamy N, Maze M. alpha2-Adrenoceptor agonists: shedding light on neuroprotection? *Br Med Bull.* 2004;71:77–92.

56. Frumento RJ, Logginidou HG, Wahlander S, Wagener G, Playford HR, Sladen RN. Dexmedetomidine infusion is associated with enhanced renal function after thoracic surgery. *J Clin Anesth.* 2006;18:422–426.

57. Bouaziz H, Hewitt C, Eisenach JC. Subarachnoid neostigmine potentiation of alpha 2-adrenergic agonist analgesia: dexmedetomidine versus clonidine. *Reg Anesth.* 1995;20:121–127.

58. Philipp M, Brede M, Hein L. Physiological significance of alpha2-adrenergic receptor subtype diversity: one receptor is not enough. *Am J Physiol Regulatory Integrative Comp Physiol.* 2002;283:R287–R295.

59. Maze M, Tranquilli W. Alpha-2 adrenoceptor agonists: defining the role in clinical anesthesia. *Anesthesiology.* 1991;74:581–605.

60. Maze M, Regan JW. Role of signal transduction in anesthetic action. Alpha 2 adrenergic agonists. *Ann N Y Acad Sci.* 1991;625:409–422.

61. Nishiyama T, Hanaoka K. Intrathecal clonidine and bupivacaine have synergistic analgesia for acute thermally or inflammatory-induced pain in rats. *Anesth Analg.* 2004;98:1056–1061, table of contents.

62. Bouaziz H, Tong C, Yoon Y, Hood DD, Eisenach JC. Intravenous opioids stimulate norepinephrine and acetylcholine release in spinal cord dorsal horn: systematic studies in sheep and an observation in a human. *Anesthesiology.* 1996;84:143–154.

63. Ossipov MH, Harris S, Lloyd P, Messineo E, Lin BS, Bagley J. Antinociceptive interaction between opioids and medetomidine: systemic additivity and spinal synergy. *Anesthesiology.* 1990;73:1227–1235.

64. Ossipov MH, Harris S, Lloyd P, Messineo E. An isobolographic analysis of the antinociceptive effect of systemically and intrathecally administered combinations of clonidine and opiates. *J Pharmacol Exp Ther.* 1990;255:1107–1116.

65. Eisenach JC, D'Angelo R, Taylor C, Hood DD. An isobolographic study of epidural clonidine and fentanyl after cesarean section. *Anesth Analg.* 1994;79:285–290.

66. Martin TJ, Kim SA, Eisenach JC. Clonidine maintains intrathecal self-administration in rats following spinal nerve ligation. *Pain.* 2006;125:257–263.

67. Hayashi Y, Guo TZ, Maze M. Desensitization to the behavioral effects of alpha 2-adrenergic agonists in rats. *Anesthesiology.* 1995;82:954–962.

68. Maes M, Lin A, Kenis G, Egyed B, Bosmans E. The effects of noradrenaline and alpha-2 adrenoceptor agents on the production of monocytic products. *Psychiatry Res.* 2000;96:245–253.

69. Titinchi S, Clark B. Alpha 2-adrenoceptors in human lymphocytes: direct characterisation by [3H]yohimbine binding. *Biochem Biophys Res Commun.* 1984;121:1–7.

70. Szelenyi J, Kiss JP, Puskas E, Szelenyi M, Vizi ES. Contribution of differently localized alpha 2- and beta-adrenoceptors in the

modulation of TNF-alpha and IL-10 production in endotoxemic mice. *Ann N Y Acad Sci.* 2000;917:145–153.

71. West JP, Dykstra LA, Lysle DT. Immunomodulatory effects of morphine withdrawal in the rat are time dependent and reversible by clonidine. *Psychopharmacology (Berl).* 1999;146:320–327.

72. von Dossow V, Baehr N, Moshirzadeh M, et al. Clonidine attenuated early proinflammatory response in T-cell subsets after cardiac surgery. *Anesth Analg.* 2006;103:809–814.

73. Spengler RN, Sud R, Knight PR, Ignatowski TA. Antinociception mediated by alpha(2)-adrenergic activation involves increasing tumor necrosis factor alpha (TNFalpha) expression and restoring TNFalpha and alpha(2)-adrenergic inhibition of norepinephrine release. *Neuropharmacology.* 2007;52:576–589.

74. Romero-Sandoval EA, McCall C, Eisenach JC. Alpha2-adrenoceptor stimulation transforms immune responses in neuritis and blocks neuritis-induced pain. *J Neurosci.* 2005.25;8988–8994.

75. Petrenko AB, Yamakura T, Baba H, Shimoji K. The role of N-Methyl-D-Aspartate (NMDA) receptors in pain: a review. *Anesth Analg.* 2003;97:1108–1116.

76. Carlton SM. Peripheral excitatory amino acids. *Curr Opin Pharmacol.* 2001;1:52–56.

77. Gordh T, Karlsten R, Kristensen J. Intervention with spinal NMDA, adenosine, and NO systems for pain modulation. *Ann Med.* 1995;27:229–234.

78. Hustveit O, Maurset A, Oye I. Interaction of the chiral forms of ketamine with opioid, phencyclidine, sigma and muscarinic receptors. *Pharmacol Toxicol.* 1995;77:355–359.

79. Durieux M. Inhibition by ketamine of muscarinic acetylcholine receptor function. *Anesth Analg.* 1995;81:57–62.

80. Abelson KS, Goldkuhl RR, Nylund A, Hoglund AU. The effect of ketamine on intraspinal acetylcholine release: involvement of spinal nicotinic receptors. *Eur J Pharmacol.* 2006;534:122–128.

81. Chaplan SR, Malmberg AB, Yaksh TL. Efficacy of spinal NMDA receptor antagonism in formalin hyperalgesia and nerve injury evoked allodynia in the rat. *J Pharmacol Exp Ther.* 1997;280:829–838.

82. Kawamata T, Omote K, Sonoda H, Kawamata M, Namiki A. Analgesic mechanisms of ketamine in the presence and absence of peripheral inflammation. *Anesthesiology.* 2000,;93:520–528.

83. Hocking G, Cousins MJ. Ketamine in chronic pain management: an evidence-based review. *Anesth Analg.* 2003;97:1730–1739.

84. Zahn PK, Sluka KA, Brennan TJ. Excitatory amino acid release in the spinal cord caused by plantar incision in the rat. *Pain.* 2002;100:65–76.

85. Zahn PK, Pogatzki-Zahn EM, Brennan TJ. Spinal administration of MK-801 and NBQX demonstrates NMDA-independent dorsal horn sensitization in incisional pain. *Pain.* 2005;114:499–510.

86. Zahn PK, Umali E, Brennan TJ. Intrathecal non-NMDA excitatory amino acid receptor antagonists inhibit pain behaviors in a rat model of postoperative pain. *Pain.* 1998;74:213–223.

87. Pogatzki EM, Niemeier JS, Sorkin LS, Brennan TJ. Spinal glutamate receptor antagonists differentiate primary and secondary mechanical hyperalgesia caused by incision. *Pain.* 2003;105:97–107.

88. Koizuka S, Obata H, Sasaki M, Saito S, Goto F. Systemic ketamine inhibits hypersensitivity after surgery via descending inhibitory pathways in rats. *Can J Anaesth.* 2005;52:498–505.

89. Stubhaug A, Breivik H, Eide PK, Kreunen M, Foss A. Mapping of punctuate hyperalgesia around a surgical incision demonstrates that ketamine is a powerful suppressor of central sensitization to pain following surgery. *Acta Anaesthesiol Scand.* 1997;41:1124–1132.

90. De Kock M, Lavand'homme P, Waterloos H. 'Balanced analgesia' in the perioperative period: is there a place for ketamine? *Pain.* 2001;92:373–380.

91. Mazar J, Rogachev B, Shaked G, et al. Involvement of adenosine in the antiinflammatory action of ketamine. *Anesthesiology.* 2005;102:1174–1181.

92. Bartoc C, Frumento RJ, Jalbout M, Bennett-Guerrero E, Du E, Nishanian E. A randomized, double-blind, placebo-controlled study assessing the anti-inflammatory effects of ketamine in cardiac surgical patients. *J Cardiothorac Vasc Anesth.* 2006;20:217–222.

93. Hill GE, Anderson JL, Lyden ER. Ketamine inhibits the proinflammatory cytokine-induced reduction of cardiac intracellular cAMP accumulation. *Anesth Analg.* 1998;87:1015–1019.

94. Shibakawa YS, Sasaki Y, Goshima Y, Echigo N, Kamiya Y, Kurahashi K, Yamada Y, Andoh T. Effects of ketamine and propofol on inflammatory responses of primary glial cell cultures stimulated with lipopolysaccharide. *Br J Anaesth.* 2005;95:803–810.

95. Hofbauer R, Kaye AD, Kapiotis S, Frass M. The immune system and the effects of non-volatile anesthetics on neutrophil transmigration through endothelial cell monolayers. *Curr Pharm Des.* 1999;5:1015–1027.

96. McNearney T, Baethge BA, Cao S, Alam R, Lisse JR, Westlund KN. Excitatory amino acids, TNF-alpha, and chemokine levels in synovial fluids of patients with active arthropathies. *Clin Exp Immunol.* 2004;137:621–627.

97. Warncke T, Jorum H, Stubhaug A. Local treatment with the N-methyl-D-aspartate receptor antagonist ketamine, inhibit development of secondary hyperalgesia in man by a peripheral action. *Neurosci Lett.* 1997;227:1–4.

98. Gottrup H, Bach FW, Jensen TS. Differential effects of peripheral ketamine and lidocaine on skin flux and hyperalgesia induced by intradermal capsaicin in humans. *Clin Physiol Funct Imaging.* 2004;24:103–108.

99. Tverskoy M, Oren M, Vaskovich M, Dashkovsky I, Kissin I:.Ketamine enhances local anesthetic and analgesic effects of bupivacaine by peripheral mechanism: a study in postoperative patients. *Neurosci Lett.* 1996;215:5–8.

100. Zohar E, Luban I, Zunser I, Shapiro A, Jedeikin R, Fredman B. Patient-controlled bupivacaine wound instillation following cesarean section: the lack of efficacy of adjuvant ketamine. *J Clin Anesth.* 2002;14:505–511.

101. Himmelseher S, Durieux ME. Ketamine for perioperative pain management. *Anesthesiology.* 2005;102:211–220.

102. Pfenninger EG, Durieux ME, Himmelseher S. Cognitive impairment after small-dose ketamine isomers in comparison to equianalgesic racemic ketamine in human volunteers. *Anesthesiology.* 2002;96:357–366.

103. Karpinski N, Dunn J, Hansen L, Masliah E. Subpial vacuolar myelopathy after intrathecal ketamine: report of a case. *Pain.* 1997;73:103–105.

104. Vranken JH, Troost D, Wegener JT, Kruis MR, Van Der Vegt MH. Neuropathological findings after continuous intrathecal administration of S(+) ketamine for the management of neuropathic cancer pain. *Pain.* 2005;117:231–235.

105. Bell R, Dahl JB, Moore R, Kalso E. Peri-operative ketamine for acute post-operative pain: a quantitative and qualitative systematic review (Cochrane review). *Acta Anaesthesiol Scand.* 2005; 49:1405–1428.

106. Grant IS, Nimmo WS, Clements JA. Pharmacokinetics and analgesic effect of i.m. and oral ketamine. *Br J Anaesth.* 1981;53:805–810.

107. Schmid R, Sandler A, Katz J. Use and efficacy of low-dose ketamine in the management of acute postoperative pain: a

review of current techniques and outcomes. *Pain*. 1999;82:111–125.

108. Oye I, Paulson O, Maurset A. Effects of ketamine on sensory perception: evidence for a role of N-methyl-D-aspartate receptors. *J Pharmacol Exp Ther*. 1992;260:1209–1213.

109. Fisher K, Coderre TJ, Hagen NA. Targeting the N-methyl-D-aspartate receptor for chronic pain management: preclinical animal studies, recent clinical experience and future research directions. *J Pain Symptom Manage*. 2000;20:358–373.

110. Tucker A, Kim Y, Nadeson R, Goodchild CS. Investigation of the potentiation of the analgesic effects of fentanyl by ketamine in humans: a double-blinded, randomised, placebo controlled, crossover study of experimental pain. *BMC Anesthesiol*. 2005;5:2–14.

111. Elia N, Tramer MR. Ketamine and postoperative pain – a quantitative systematic review of randomised trials. *Pain*. 2005;113:61–70.

112. Subramaniam K, Subramaniam B, Steinbrook RA. Ketamine as an adjuvant analgesic to opioids: a quantitative and qualitative systematic review. *Anesth Analg*. 2004;99:482–495.

113. Simonnet G, Rivat C. Opioid-induced hyperalgesia: abnormal or normal pain? *NeuroReport*. 2003;14:1–7.

114. Richebe P, Rivat C, Laulin JP, Maurette P, Simonnet G. Ketamine improves the management of exaggerated postoperative pain observed in perioperative fentanyl-treated rats. *Anesthesiology*. 2005;102:421–428.

115. Joly V, Richebe P, Guignard B, Fletcher D, Maurette P, Sessler DI, Chauvin M. Remifentanil-induced postoperative hyperalgesia and its prevention with small-dose ketamine. *Anesthesiology*. 2005;103:147–155.

116. Angst MS, Clark DJ. Opioid-induced hyperalgesia: a qualitative systematic review. *Anesthesiology*. 2006;104:570–587.

117. Carroll IR, Angst MS, Clark DJ. Management of perioperative pain in patients chronically consuming opioids. *Reg Anesth Pain Med*. 2004;29:576–591.

118. Takenaka I, Ogata M, Koga K, Matsumoto T, Shigematsu A. Ketamine suppresses endotoxin-induced tumor necrosis factor alpha production in mice. *Anesthesiology*. 1994;80:402–408.

119. Taniguchi T, Takemoto Y, Kanakura H, Kidani Y, Yamamoto K. The dose-related effects of ketamine on mortality and cytokine responses to endotoxin-induced shock in rats. *Anesth Analg*. 2003;97:1769–1772.

120. Kawasaki C, Kawasaki T, Ogata M, Nandate K, Shigematsu A. Ketamine isomers suppress superantigen-induced proinflammatory cytokine production in human whole blood. *Can J Anaesth*. 2001;48:819–823.

121. Weigand MA, Schmidt H, Zhao Q, Plaschke K, Martin E, Bardenheuer HJ. Ketamine modulates the stimulated adhesion molecule expression on human neutrophils in vitro. *Anesth Analg*. 2000;90:206–212.

122. Zilberstein G, Levy R, Rachinsky M, et al. Ketamine attenuates neutrophil activation after cardiopulmonary bypass. *Anesth Analg* 2002;95:531–536, table of contents.

123. Gilron I. Review article: The role of anticonvulsant drugs in postoperative pain management: a bench-to-bedside perspective. *Can J Anaesth*. 2006;53:562–571.

124. Taylor CP, Gee NS, Su TZ, et al. A summary of mechanistic hypotheses of gabapentin pharmacology. *Epilepsy Res*. 1998;29:233–249.

125. Taylor CP, Angelotti T, Fauman E. Pharmacology and mechanisms of action of pregabalin: the calcium channel alpha2-delta subunit as a target for antiepileptic drug discovery. *Epilepsy Res*. 2007;73:137–150.

126. Li CY, Zhang XL, Matthews EA, et al. Calcium channel alpha2delta1 subunit mediates spinal hyperexcitability in pain modulation. *Pain*. 2006;125:20–34.

127. Cao YQ. Voltage-gated calcium channels and pain. *Pain*. 2006;126:5–9.

128. Yaksh TL. Calcium channels as therapeutic targets in neuropathic pain. *J Pain*. 2006;7:S13–S30.

129. Dooley DJ, Taylor CP, Donevan S, Feltner D. Ca2+ channel alpha2delta ligands: novel modulators of neurotransmission. *Trends Pharmacol Sci*. 2007;28:75–82.

130. Cheng JK, Pan HL, Eisenach JC. Antiallodynic effect of intrathecal gabapentin and its interaction with clonidine in a rat model of postoperative pain. *Anesthesiology*. 2000;92:1126–1131.

131. Field MJ, Holloman EF, McCleary S, Hughes J, Singh L. Evaluation of gabapentin and S-(+)-3-isobutylgaba in a rat model of postoperative pain. *J Pharmacol Exp Ther*. 1997;282:1242–1246.

132. Stanfa LC, Singh L, Williams RG, Dickenson AH. Gabapentin, ineffective in normal rats, markedly reduces C-fibre evoked responses after inflammation. *NeuroReport*. 1997;8:587–590.

133. Shimoyama N, Shimoyama M, Davis AM, Inturrisi CE, Elliott KJ. Spinal gabapentin is antinociceptive in the rat formalin test. *Neurosci Lett*. 1997;222:65–67.

134. Kaneko M, Mestre C, Sanchez EH, Hammond DL. Intrathecally administered gabapentin inhibits formalin-evoked nociception and the expression of Fos-like immunoreactivity in the spinal cord of the rat. *J Pharmacol Exp Ther*. 2000.292;743–751.

135. Werner MU, Perkins FM, Holte K, Pedersen JL, Kehlet H. Effects of gabapentin in acute inflammatory pain in humans. *Reg Anesth Pain Med*. 2001;26:322–328.

136. Dirks J, Petersen KL, Rowbotham MC, Dahl JB. Gabapentin suppresses cutaneous hyperalgesia following heat-capsaicin sensitization. *Anesthesiology*. 2002;97:102–107.

137. Gilron I, Flatters SJ. Gabapentin and pregabalin for the treatment of neuropathic pain: A review of laboratory and clinical evidence. *Pain Res Manag*. 2006;11(suppl A):16A–29A.

138. Abe M, Kurihara T, Han W, Shinomiya K, Tanabe T. Changes in expression of voltage-dependent ion channel subunits in dorsal root ganglia of rats with radicular injury and pain. *Spine*. 2002;27:1517–1524; discussion 1525.

139. Li CY, Song YH, Higuera ES, Luo ZD. Spinal dorsal horn calcium channel alpha2delta-1 subunit upregulation contributes to peripheral nerve injury-induced tactile allodynia. *J Neurosci*. 2004;24:8494–8499.

140. Luo ZD, Calcutt NA, Higuera ES, et al. Injury type-specific calcium channel alpha 2 delta-1 subunit up-regulation in rat neuropathic pain models correlates with antiallodynic effects of gabapentin. *J Pharmacol Exp Ther*. 2002;303:1199–1205.

141. Takeuchi Y, Takasu K, Honda M, Ono H, Tanabe M. Neurochemical evidence that supraspinally administered gabapentin activates the descending noradrenergic system after peripheral nerve injury. *Eur J Pharmacol*. 2007;556:69–74.

142. Buvanendran A, Kroin JS, Kerns JM, Nagalla SN, Tuman KJ. Characterization of a new animal model for evaluation of persistent postthoracotomy pain. *Anesth Analg*. 2004;99:1453–1460; table of contents.

143. Cheng JK, Chen CC, Yang JR, Chiou LC. The antiallodynic action target of intrathecal gabapentin: Ca2+ channels, KATP channels or N-methyl-d-aspartic acid receptors? *Anesth Analg*. 2006;102:182–187.

144. Hayashida K, DeGoes S, Curry R, Eisenach JC. Gabapentin activates spinal noradrenergic activity in rats and humans and reduces hypersensitivity after surgery. *Anesthesiology*. 2007;106:557–562.

145. Carlton SM, Zhou S. Attenuation of formalin-induced nociceptive behaviors following local peripheral injection of gabapentin. *Pain.* 1998;76:201–207.

146. Klein-Schwartz W, Shepherd JG, Gorman S, Dahl B. Characterization of gabapentin overdose using a poison center case series. *J Toxicol Clin Toxicol.* 2003;41:11–15.

147. Yoon MH, Yaksh TL. The effect of intrathecal gabapentin on pain behavior and hemodynamics on the formalin test in the rat. *Anesth Analg.* 1999;89:434–439.

148. Fischer J, Barr A, Rogers S, Fischer P, Trudeau V. Lack of serious toxicity following gabapentin overdose. *Neurology* 1994;44:982–983.

149. Dahl JB, Mathiesen O, Moiniche S. 'Protective premedication': an option with gabapentin and related drugs? A review of gabapentin and pregabalin in in the treatment of post-operative pain. *Acta Anaesthesiol Scand.* 2004;48:1130–1136.

150. Gilron I, Biederman J, Jhamandas K, Hong M. Gabapentin blocks and reverses antinociceptive morphine tolerance in the rat paw-pressure and tail-flick tests. *Anesthesiology.* 2003;98:1288–1292.

151. Ho KY, Gan TJ, Habib AS. Gabapentin and postoperative pain – a systematic review of randomized controlled trials. *Pain* 2006;126:91–101.

152. Hurley RW, Cohen SP, Williams KA, Rowlingson AJ, Wu CL. The analgesic effects of perioperative gabapentin on postoperative pain: a meta-analysis. *Reg Anesth Pain Med.* 2006;31:237–247.

153. Seib RK, Paul JE. Preoperative gabapentin for postoperative analgesia: a meta-analysis. *Can J Anaesth.* 2006;53:461–469.

154. Hurley RW, Chatterjea D, Rose Feng M, Taylor CP, Hammond DL. Gabapentin and pregabalin can interact synergistically with naproxen to produce antihyperalgesia. *Anesthesiology.* 2002;97:1263–1273.

155. Yoon MH, Yaksh TL. Evaluation of interaction between gabapentin and ibuprofen on the formalin test in rats. *Anesthesiology.* 1999;91:1006–1013.

156. Yoon MH, Choi JI, Kwak SH. Characteristic of interactions between intrathecal gabapentin and either clonidine or neostigmine in the formalin test. *Anesth Analg.* 2004;98:1374–1379, table of contents.

157. Gomes B, Savignac M, Moreau M, Leclerc C, Lory P, Guery JC, Pelletier L. Lymphocyte calcium signaling involves dihydropyridine-sensitive L-type calcium channels: facts and controversies. *Crit Rev Immunol.* 2004;24:425–447.

8

Pharmacokinetics of Epidural Opioids

Bradley Urie and Oscar A. de Leon-Casasola

In a healthy individual, pain is a complex sensory experience associated with actual or potential tissue damage.[1] Noxious inputs stimulate the unspecialized, peripheral nerve fibers (C and Aδ nociceptors). Both nerve types transmit signals to the dorsal horn; unmyelinated, small C fibers conduct electrical pulses induced by thermal, pressure, and chemical stimuli generally at a rate <1 m/s, whereas the myelinated, medium Aδ nociceptors transmit a quicker message (5 to 30 m/s) when activated by mechanical pressure and temperature.[1] At the molecular level, pain stimulates the release of many mediators from the keratinocytes and blood vessels in the dermis, including prostaglandins (PGEs), substance P, and calcitonin gene-related peptide (CGRP).[1] These neurotransmitters bind to receptors on the nociceptive fibers and cause depolarization and the subsequent transmission of signals to the central nervous system (CNS), as well as the release of neurotransmitters from the nerve itself into the periphery. This phenomenon, called axon reflex, causes vasodilation and inflammation and results in a positive feedback loop that begins to recruit silent nociceptors, pain fibers in close proximity to the initially activated nerve.[1] As nociceptive fibers and mast cells have opioid receptors, this is the first site of action of opioids. Opioid receptors can inhibit the release of CGRP and substance P from nerves, thereby preventing the feed-forward mechanism of pain that typically results in sensitization local to the injury site.[2] These injury-induced neuromodifications can be perceived as allodynia or hyperalgesia. Moreover, peripheral sensitization drives the repeated release of molecular mediators at the dorsal horn, causing secondary hyperalgesia. The pain fibers synapse with their secondary fibers at the superficial laminae (I and II) of the dorsal horn. Depolarization of the first-order neuron induces the opening of voltage-gated calcium channels at the body of this cell, allowing the influx of calcium into it. Calcium binds to vesicles containing neurotransmitters and stimulates their release. The neurotransmitters bind to their corresponding receptors on the postsynaptic or secondary neurons and induce an excitatory event there. Secondary fibers cross the spinal cord and carry their impulses via the spinothalamic tract to the thalamus on the contralateral side to where the information originated. Opioid receptors and their ligands are present on the superficial dorsal horn, particularly on Rexed's lamina II, also known as substantia gelatinosa. At the spinal level, opioid pharmacotherapy blocks voltage-gated calcium channels and opens potassium channels at the presynaptic level. In contrast, opioid receptor activation results in the opening of potassium channels at the postsynaptic level and potassium efflux. These events lead to a hyperpolarization of the first- and second-order neurons, which inhibits the conduction of pain signals to the central nervous system.[1]

Descending pathways from the somatosensory cortex also modulate the perception of pain. The activation of cells within the periaqueductal gray (PAG) and rostral ventromedial medulla (RVM) stimulate descending fibers to release serotonin and norepinephrine at the level of the spinal cord.[3] This event modulates spinal nociceptive conduction.[3] Opioids exerting their effect at the supraspinal level promote descending pain modulation by promoting the release of an inhibitory neurotransmitter in the brain (γ-aminobutyric acid or GABA).[4] In this mechanism, called *opioid disinhibition*, opioids release GABA from the PAG, RVM, and others and activate the descending inhibitory pathways, increasing the concentrations of serotonin and norepinephrine at the presynaptic level and in this way modulating pain signals at the spinal cord. This may be the fundamental reason underlying better analgesic effects after intraspinal administrations of opioids when compared to parenteral opioids.

Epidural opioid therapy is considered the gold standard for postoperative pain management.[5] There is a large evidence base available that details the potent efficacy of opioids administered epidurally for the management of postoperative pain. In addition to effective analgesia, reduced side effects may be achieved by targeting spinal μ-opioid receptors. After epidural administration, morphine has been demonstrated to primarily produce analgesia by targeting the dorsal horn of the spinal cord, whereas the site of action of other congeners with higher lipid solubility is more controversial. Opioids that preferentially redistribute systemically when injected in the epidural space may be better administered via a different route, to avoid the increased invasiveness of epidural catheters and needles.

Table 8.1: Lipophilicity and Permeability Values for Selected Epidural Opioids[2]

Opioid Agent	Octanol:Buffer Coefficient	Meningeal Permeability Coefficient
Morphine	1	0.6
Alfentanil	129	2.3
Fentanyl	955	0.9
Sufentanil	1737	0.75

CRITICAL STUDIES AND CLINICAL TRIALS

Pharmacokinetics of Epidurally Administered Opioids

The physical and chemical properties of each opioid determine their lipid solubility and ultimately, the effectiveness of the analgesia produced.[2] The octanol:buffer partition coefficient is a measure of the lipid solubility and correlates with the degree of penetration into the spinal cord after epidural administration; however, lipophilicity correlates with meningeal permeability in a nonlinear fashion.[2] For example, despite a significant difference between the octanol:buffer partition coefficients of morphine and sufentanil, their meningeal permeability coefficients are comparable (see Table 8.1), and essentially, the arachnoid membrane treats them in a similar manner. The optimal octanol:buffer coefficient range that results in maximal meningeal permeability appears to be between 129 (the value for alfentanil) and 560 (the coefficient of bupivacaine). Based only on physical and chemical characteristics, the ideal agents for administration in the epidural space theoretically are meperidine, hydromorphone, and alfentanil. Agents with intermediate lipophilicity migrate more readily past the lipid and aqueous zones of the primary barrier (the arachnoid membrane) and correspondingly have higher meningeal permeability coefficients. The amount of opioid that progresses to the supraspinal level is determined by the vascular permeability of the agent, whereas the concentration of opioid in the spinal cord following epidural administration is affected by vascular and meningeal permeability and fat sequestration.[2]

The majority of studies that consider the pharmacokinetic behavior of opioids in the epidural space rely on inferences from measurements of plasma and, occasionally, cerebrospinal fluid (CSF). A pioneer study by Bernards et al[24] simultaneously sampled opioid concentrations in the epidural, intrathecal, and plasma spaces to characterize the pharmacokinetics of epidurally administered opioids. Moreover, epidural fat concentrations around the epidural catheter were also sampled. Following epidural injection, drug concentrations of individually administered morphine, fentanyl, alfentanil, and sufentanil in each of these compartments of pigs were sampled by microdialysis techniques or fat tissue biopsies.

Statistical analyses were used to calculate the areas under the curve (AUC) of the drug concentration relative to the time since administration for each compartment, the mean residence time (MRT) of each opioid, and the elimination half-lives. The resulting data set suggested pharmacokinetic differences between the opioids that correlated to the physiochemical properties of the structure of each drug. Significantly, the hydrophobicity of each individual opioid directly correlated to the observed MRT in the extracellular fluid of the lumbar epidural space ($P < .0001$) (Figure 8.1) and in the central venous plasma compartment

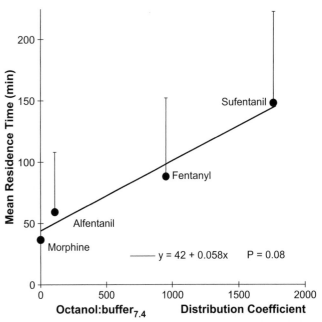

Figure 8.1: Opioid mean epidural residence time after epidural administration by bolus injection. Relationship between the octanol: buffer distribution coefficients of the opioids and their mean residence time in the extracellular fluid of the lumbar epidural space. ($P = .0001$)

($P = .0004$) (Figure 8.2). For example, the shortest MRT was seen for morphine, the opioid with the lowest octanol:buffer partition coefficient, followed by increasingly larger values for alfentanil, fentanyl, and sufentanil. Moreover, the terminal elimination half-lives in the lumbar epidural space were linearly related to the lipophilicity of the opioid as well. These resulted in

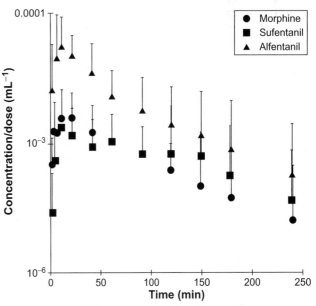

Figure 8.2: Opioid plasma concentrations in central compartment after epidural administration by bolus injection. Dose-normalized concentration-time plots for morphine, alfentanil, and sufentanil in central venous plasma after administration into the lumbar epidural space. There are no data for fentanyl because too few of the concentrations were within the measurable range.

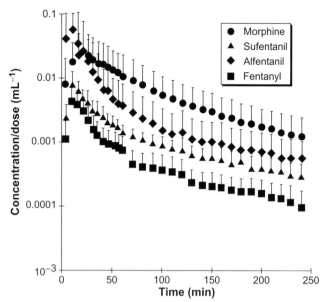

Figure 8.3: CSF opioid concentrations after epidural administration by bolus injection. Dose-normalized concentrations of morphine, alfentanil, fentanyl, and sufentanil in the cerebrospinal fluid of the lumbar intrathecal space opposite the lumbar epidural site of administration.

significant higher drug concentrations in the CSF for morphine when compared to either fentanyl or sufentanil (Figure 8.3). Thus, if the MRT in the epidural space was longer for fentanyl and sufentanil, plasma concentrations of fentanyl were absent after 4 hours of administration, and the CSF concentrations of this drug were significantly lower than morphine, where did the drug go? Likely, the fat in the epidural space sequesters hydrophobic compounds (fentanyl and sufentanil) more readily, resulting in longer MRTs and elimination half-lives (Figure 8.4). Possibly, then, hydrophobic opioids (fentanyl and sufentanil) have less bioavailability to the spinal cord, as suggested by multiple postoperative, human studies that have shown that epidurally injected alfentanil, fentanyl, and sufentanil induce negligible analgesic effects through a spinal mechanism.[6–9]

Another interesting question is how opioids migrate to the brainstem area after epidural administration in the lumbar area. As the cardiac cycle induces the movement of the CSF, it is not dilution but rather bulk movements generated by the systole and diastole of the heart that influence how epidurally injected agents – including opioids – travel in the CSF.[10,11] Cardiac cycles induce the expansion and contraction of the brain and spinal cord and result in a heterogeneous motion of the CSF. As the rate of simple diffusion is too slow to account for the movement of CSF, the cephalic spread of epidurally injected opiates should be primarily because of motions induced by cardiac cycles, hence, approximately the same for all opiates. Supraspinal migration of an agent will predominately vary based on the rate of CSF clearance.

Little evidence has suggested whether the observed supraspinal action of opioids is because of intrathecal rostral spread or significant uptake in the systemic circulation and redistribution to the brain. Two short-duration studies gave initial insight into the cephalic migration of morphine. First, a trial by Nordberg and colleagues[12] considered the localization of morphine following epidural administration and found that the concentration of morphine in the CSF was between 45 and 250 times higher

than in the plasma, varying with time from administration, yet the elimination half-life of the opioid was similar between the blood and CSF. Also, a 6-hour time-course analysis of both blood and CSF concentrations of morphine epidurally administered in the lumbar region found that the blood concentration attained peak levels between 2 and 10 minutes after injection.[13] Morphine levels in the plasma then rapidly declined to below minimum effective concentration (MEC) for morphine by 120 minutes, suggesting that analgesia and side effects experienced after 2 hours could not be attributed to a systemic effect of the agent.[13]

A clinical study by Angst and colleagues[25] examined the rostral spread of epidurally administered morphine by assessing the analgesic effects of the opioid on heat and electrical pain over a 24-hour period. During this double-blinded, placebo-controlled, crossover investigation, 9 healthy volunteers had 5 mg morphine or saline injected into the lumbar epidural space in a randomized fashion. Fluoroscopy confirmed the correct needle placement, and on each analgesic evaluation, plasma samples were drawn to assess morphine concentrations by gas chromatography and mass spectroscopy. Nociceptive heat and electrical stimuli were applied to the lumbar (L4), thoracic (T10), cervical (C2), and trigeminal (V2) dermatomes and both the lowest temperature and current that evoked pain (pain threshold) and highest temperature and current tolerated (pain tolerance) were measured.

The AUCs for the difference in heat pain threshold at L4 and T10 from baseline versus time after epidural injection were significantly different between morphine and saline ($P < .017$), whereas the AUCs describing the same data gathered for heat pain tolerance suggested significant differences for all the dermatomes tested ($P < .017$). Similar data analyses of electrical pain tolerance found that AUCs describing the percentage change from baseline versus time was significantly different between epidurally injected morphine and saline at L4 and

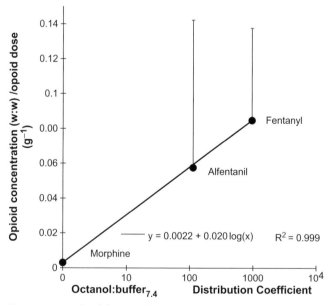

Figure 8.4: Epidural fat opioid concentrations after epidural administration by bolus injection. Relationship between the octanol: buffer distribution coefficients of the opioids and their dose-normalized concentrations in fat taken from the lumbar epidural space at the conclusion of the experiment.

T10 ($P < .017$). Overall, significant supraspinal analgesic effects were recorded as long as 10 hours after injection and persisted as a trend throughout the 24-hour observation period.

The average plasma morphine concentration was highest at the first measurement taken (2 hours), but was still approximately half of the plasma MEC necessary to produce analgesia from morphine. In 8 participants, the morphine concentration in the blood declined below the detection limit of 1 ng/mL by 10 hours. This suggests that the extended analgesic effects produced by morphine were likely induced by distribution through a spinal mechanism rather than uptake into the blood before redistribution to the brain.

Selected Epidural Alfentanil Clinical Trials

As mentioned previously, alfentanil has an octanol:buffer coefficient in the optimal range, suggesting that the lipophilicity of the opioid may be superior to other congeners when administered epidurally for postoperative pain control. This has been supported by a pharmacokinetic study that found that the uptake of epidural alfentanil into the general circulation was a slow process when measured by a stable isotope method.[14] Perhaps consequently, peak plasma levels remained low after epidural administration of alfentanil (<10 ng/mL).[14]

A study by Chauvin and colleagues[26] compared the efficacy of analgesia and frequency of oxygen desaturation when alfentanil was administered epidurally and intravenously. Thirty-two randomized, postoperative patients received intermittent 250-μg boluses of either epidural alfentanil or intravenous (IV) alfentanil with 10-minute and 5-minute lockout intervals, respectively. The resulting pain scores and sedation scores of the 2 study groups did not significantly differ. The time to maximum analgesia was shorter for the participants treated intravenously ($P < .03$), whereas the mean total consumption of alfentanil was 39% lower for the group administered the agent epidurally. The authors concluded that because epidural administration of alfentanil induces the same incidence of hypoxemic events, epidurally injecting alfentanil offered no clinical advantage over intravenous administration.

Similarly, another comparative study[27] found IV infusion of alfentanil to be equally effective as epidural infusion for postoperative pain. The study included 20 participants randomly allocated to receive an epidural loading dose of 0.75 mg of alfentanil and an infusion of 0.36 mg/h of alfentanil, epidurally or intravenously. Similar and subanalgesic mean plasma concentrations of alfentanil were obtained for both groups (<20 ng/mL). Likewise, the total morphine consumption and pain scores were statistically insignificant between the 2 groups. The incidence of side effects were comparable, as well; dyspepsia was reported by 11 of 15 of the epidural group and 12 of 17 of the IV group, and emesis was observed in 6 of 15 patients of the epidural group and 4 of 17 patients in the IV group. Hence, this study, as well as a later study of alfentanil as an adjuvant to epidural bupivacaine,[15] indicated that a similar efficacy for treating postoperative pain is achieved by either epidural or intravenous infusion of alfentanil. This suggests that analgesia by alfentanil is not due to a spinal mechanism of action.

Selected Epidural Fentanyl Clinical Trials[6,7,16]

Fentanyl is one of the most commonly used opioid analgesics and has a high octanol:buffer coefficient and a rapid onset of action.

A prospective study of 1030 surgical patients given fentanyl patient-controlled epidural analgesia (PCEA) reported a low incidence of side effects: 16.7% pruritus, 14.8% nausea, 13.2% sedation, 6.8% hypotension, 2% motor block, and 0.3% respiratory depression (respiratory rate <8 breaths/min).[17] However, the value of utilizing fentanyl for epidural analgesia is controversial. A randomized, double-blinded study by Scott et al[16] found that epidural infusion of 2 mg/mL ropivacaine and 4 μg/mL fentanyl was effective at providing pain relief with a low degree of motor block for patients undergoing major abdominal surgery. Yet, 2 randomized, double-blinded studies that considered the value of IV compared to epidural administration of fentanyl for knee arthroplasty[7] or thoracoabdomial esophagectomy[18] concluded that there was no clinical advantage to epidurally administering fentanyl, as plasma concentrations[7,18] and the incidences of side effects[7] were similar.

Furthermore, a randomized, double-blinded comparison of IV and epidural fentanyl infusions for postthoracotomy pain relief by Sandler and colleagues[28] found that both routes utilized systemic absorption to achieve similar levels of analgesia. Twenty-nine participants were given infusions of 10 μg/mL fentanyl, by either position-verified lumbar epidural catheter or IV catheter, and then administered the equivalent volume of saline by the alternate route. Both fentanyl infusions rates and plasma concentrations stabilized for the study groups approximately 8 hours following surgery, and mean plasma levels of 1.8 ± 0.5 ng/mL (for the epidural cohort) and 1.6 ± 0.6 ng/mL (for the IV cohort) were observed. Participants in the epidural group required significantly larger fentanyl infusion doses than those administered fentanyl intravenously (1.95 ± 0.45 μg/kg/h and 1.56 ± 0.36 μg/kg/h, respectively; $P = .0002$), in contrast to reports from other studies that integrated PCEA pumps and found higher doses necessitated by patients administered fentanyl intravenously. Ten-centimeter visual analog scale (VAS) scores between the study groups were not significantly different at any point during the entire postoperative data collection period and analgesia of <3 on a scale of 10 were achieved by all patients. Similarly, there were no significant differences in the incidences of nausea, vomiting, or pruritus for the 2 study groups, and all observed side effects were classified as mild. Overall, the comparable results for the study groups suggest that the mechanism of analgesia for both IV and epidural administration of fentanyl is similar and likely by systemic absorption.

Another trial of 50 randomly assigned patients prospectively compared fentanyl analgesia administered epidurally to IV administration.[18] Postoperatively, 5-μg/mL infusions of fentanyl at the lumbar or thoracic epidural space or radial artery were started and adjustments to the dose were made by the addition of 15 μg/kg fentanyl boluses to maintain a VAS score of ≤30/100 at rest. In contrast to the study by Sandler and colleagues, this trial found that the patients in the IV group required larger fentanyl boluses during the first 6 hours (lumbar = 104 ± 24 μg, thoracic = 93 ± 19 μg, IV = 137 ± 71 μg; $P = .02$) and needed more frequent boluses throughout the study (lumbar = 3 ± 9, thoracic = 4 ± 8, IV = 6 ± 12; $P = .04$). Similar to previous studies, there were no significant differences between the IV and epidural groups in the analgesia achieved at rest and after coughing or the number of patients requiring treatment for pruritus (lumbar = 2, thoracic = 1, IV = 0). Patients administered fentanyl intravenously experienced a significantly higher incidence of nausea (lumbar = 1, thoracic = 2, IV = 8; $P = .009$) and longer average postoperative stays (lumbar = 14.4 ± 5.6 days, thoracic = 11.1 ± 2.5 days, IV = 15.6 ± 5.3; $P = .02$). Yet, the authors concluded that equivalent analgesia was achieved by all 3 routes of administration using similar doses of fentanyl regardless of the site of epidural catheter insertion (lumbar versus thoracic).[18]

Selected Sufentanil Epidural Therapy Clinical Trials

Sufentanil has a structure that confers strong lipophilicity; however, the meningeal permeability coefficient of the opioid is between the values for morphine and fentanyl. Similar to fentanyl, the analgesia produced by epidurally administering sufentanil seemingly is a result of both spinal and supraspinal effects. Various studies have reported signs that sufentanil is absorbed systemically, yet the observed incidences of side effects[8] and dose requirements[19] of the opioid have suggested a spinal site of action as well. For example, a randomized, double-blinded study of 40 patients who were given bupivacaine and sufentanil by PCEA or IV PCA found comparable pain scores, extension of sensory block, and incidences of side effects between the 2 study groups; however, the IV group consumed twice as much sufentanil (48 hours postsurgery: 207 ± 100 μg used by the IV group, 107 ± 57 μg used by the epidural group; $P < .05$).[19] The authors concluded that a spinal mechanism of action contributed to the analgesia produced by epidural administration of sufentanil with a local anesthetic.[19] Although a study by Menigaux et al[20] reported results that primarily indicated that sufentanil analgesia is produced through systemic absorption and recirculation supraspinally, as did the following authors.

Miguel and colleagues[29] implemented a double-blinded, prospective design to investigate the site of action of epidurally administered sufentanil. Fifty patients who underwent intra-abdominal operations were randomized to the epidural group (who received 1 μg/mL sufentanil infusion epidurally and an IV saline infusion) or the IV group (who received 1 μg/mL sufentanil infusion intravenously and an epidural saline infusion). Pain levels assessed by VAS scores were comparable for both study groups for patients at rest and while coughing. Furthermore, a similar amount of supplemental bolus or PCA morphine was required by the 2 study groups to maintain a VAS score ≤30/100. The concentrations of sufentanil in the plasma, the incidences and severities of pruritus, and the nausea scores were also comparable between the 2 study groups. However, the IV group required significantly more numbers of lower dose adjustments due to excessive sedation or respiratory depression (IV group = 6, epidural group = 1; $P < .05$). The authors concluded that minor clinical differences result from administering sufentanil by epidural or IV. This suggests that both routes of sufentanil induce analgesia through a similar, systemic mechanism.

Selected Immediate and Extended Epidural Morphine Clinical Trials

Morphine was the first opioid approved for intraspinal use and, concomitantly, has been the most comprehensively studied.

A large, randomized, double-blinded trial compared the efficacy of analgesia and side-effect profiles for groups administered 0.1 mg/kg morphine epidurally or intramuscularly to a group given saline placebo.[30] Following orthopedic surgery, 174 patients were monitored for pain and given pentazocine, piritramide, or metamizol as requested. Postoperatively, the frequency with which patients experienced no surgical site pain was

significantly greater within the epidural group (epidural = 64% of patients, intramuscular = 27% of patients; $P = .05$). Also, the percentage of patients requiring further analgesics (epidural group = 19%, intramuscular group = 61%, saline group = 64%; $P < .05$) and the percentage of patients who experienced poor sleep during the first night following surgery (epidural group = 14%, intramuscular group = 42%; $P < .05$) were significantly lower for the epidural group. The incidences of nausea, vomiting, and headache were comparable among the 3 study groups, but the frequency of pruritus and disturbances in micturition were significantly higher for the patients administered morphine epidurally. The authors concluded that epidurally administered morphine had a spinal mechanism of action because of the significant clinical differences and extended duration of analgesia when compared to systemically released morphine.

To lengthen the duration of analgesia beyond the 24-hour maximum typically observed following epidural injection of morphine,[21] a new, lipid-based delivery system that encapsulates morphine was developed.[22] This extended-release epidural morphine (EREM) provides analgesia up to 48 hours following a single injection and, as an indwelling catheter is not required, concerns related to anticoagulation and other complications may be obviated.[22] Sentinel trials demonstrated the efficacy of EREM for postoperative pain relief following hip arthroplasty[22] and elective cesarean delivery,[23] and recent pharmacokinetic data described the effective use of EREM following injection of an epidural anesthetic.[21] Gambling and colleagues[31] designed a controlled, dose-ranging study of 541 patients administered EREM for analgesia after lower abdominal surgery. Patients were randomized to a standard epidural morphine group (5 mg) or one of 5 study groups of EREM (doses: 5, 10, 15, 20, or 25 mg). Postoperatively, all patients were given access to 10–20 μg of fentanyl delivered by IV PCA with 6-minute lockout intervals. Significantly fewer patients within the EREM study groups required no additional fentanyl analgesia throughout the first 48 hours following EREM administration ($P < .01$). Furthermore, patients given 15, 20, or 25 mg of EREM reported significantly lower pain intensity scores than patients in the standard morphine cohort ($P = .0107, .0056, .0004$, respectively). All groups experienced classic opioid-related adverse events; the only significant differences between the EREM groups and the standard morphine group were with the incidences of pruritus ($P < .05$) and urinary retention ($P < .05$). The authors observed that the best analgesia with the fewest side effects was achieved by administration of 15 mg of EREM and recommended that a multimodal pain management approach – such as the addition of a nonsteroidal antiinflammatory drug to the regimen – could further reduce the dose required to provide effective analgesia and, concomitantly, the occurrence of side effects. Another double-blinded trial, by Hartrick et al,[32] randomized 168 patients to 3 groups (administered either 20 or 30 mg of EREM or sham epidural injection) to consider the efficacy and safety of EREM following knee arthroplasty. On request for further postoperative analgesia, patients in the EREM groups received an IV bolus of 0.2 mg/mL hydromorphone and then saline IV PCA, whereas patients in the sham epidural group received an IV bolus of 1 mg/mL morphine, followed by morphine via IV PCA pump. The pain intensity recall scores from 4 through 30 hours after epidural injection were significantly improved in the groups treated with EREM compared to the group administered IV PCA ($P \leq .038$). Also, the mean total opioid consumption was significantly lower for the patients treated with

EREM relative to those given IV PCA analgesia ($P < .001$), and the EREM groups had a significantly longer period before additional analgesia was required ($P = .001$). EREM-administered patients tolerated physical therapy on days 2 and 3 significantly better than those that received IV PCA morphine ($P = .01$ for both days). Almost all patients reported mild to moderate side effects that were consistent with epidural opioid administration. The EREM treatment groups had significantly higher prevalences of pyrexia and pruritus, primarily within the group given 30 mg EREM. Although the incidences of respiratory depression among the EREM study groups were not significantly greater, the 9 patients who experienced respiratory events were at least 65 years of age and the authors suggested that lower dose studies (10 or 15 mg) were warranted for older patients.

CONCLUSIONS

Despite ample pharmacokinetic evidence suggesting that lipid-soluble opioids have a weak intraspinal effect after epidural administration; these medications continue to be used for postoperative epidural administration. The underlying reason may be the lower cephalad migration when compared to hydrophilic opioids and, thus, the lower incidence of respiratory depression after a bolus administration. However, continuous infusion administration may not be associated with such a high degree of cephalad migration and makes drugs as hydromorphone and morphine ideal for postoperative epidural administration.

REFERENCES

1. Basbaum AI, Jessell TM. The Perception of Pain. In: Kandel ER, Schwartz JH, Jessell TM, eds. *Principles of Neural Science*. 4th ed. New York, NY: McGraw-Hill; 2000:472–479.

2. Leon-Casasola OA, Lema MJ. Postoperative epidural opioid analgesia: what are the choices? *Anesth Analg*. 1996;83:867–875.

3. Robinson DA, Calejesan AA, Wei F, Gebhart GF, Zhuo M. Endogenous facilitation: from molecular mechanisms to persistent pain. *Curr Neurovasc Res*. 2004;1:11–20.

4. Jensen TS. Opioids in the brain: supraspinal mechanisms in pain control. *Acta Anaesthesiol Scand*. 1997;41:123–132.

5. Ready LB. Acute pain: lessons learned from 25,000 patients. *Reg Anesth Pain Med*. 1999;24:499–505.

6. Guinard JP, Mavrocordatos P, Chiolero R, Carpenter RL. A randomized comparison of intravenous versus lumbar and thoracic epidural fentanyl for analgesia after thoracotomy. *Anesthesiology*. 1992;77:1108–1115.

7. Loper KA, Ready LB, Downey M, et al. Epidural and intravenous fentanyl infusions are clinically equivalent after knee surgery. *Anesth Analg*. 1990;70:72–75.

8. Miguel R, Barlow I, Morrell M, et al. A prospective, randomized, double-blind comparison of epidural and intravenous sufentanil infusions. *Anesthesiology*. 1994;81:346–352.

9. Coda BA, Brown MC, Risler L, Syrjala K, Shen DD. Equivalent analgesia and side effects during epidural and pharmacokinetically tailored intravenous infusion with matching plasma alfentanil concentration. *Anesthesiology*. 1999;90:98–108.

10. Quencer RM, Post MJ, Hinks RS. Cine MR in the evaluation of normal and abnormal CSF flow: intracranial and intraspinal studies. *Neuroradiology*. 1990;32:371–391.

11. Enzmann DR, Pelc NJ. Normal flow patterns of intracranial and spinal cerebrospinal fluid defined with phase-contrast cine MR imaging. *Radiology*. 1991;178:467–474.

12. Nordberg G, Hedner T, Mellstrand T, Dahlstrom B. Pharmacokinetic aspects of epidural morphine analgesia. *Anesthesiology*. 1983;58:545–551.

13. Gourlay GK, Cherry DA, Cousins MJ. Cephalad migration of morphine in CSF following lumbar epidural administration in patients with cancer pain. *Pain*. 1985;23:317–326.

14. Burm AG, Haak-van der Lely F, van Kleef JW, et al. Pharmacokinetics of alfentanil after epidural administration: investigation of systemic absorption kinetics with a stable isotope method. *Anesthesiology*. 1994;81:308–315.

15. van den Nieuwenhuyzen MC, Stienstra R, Burm AG, Vletter AA, van Kleef JW. Alfentanil as an adjuvant to epidural bupivacaine in the management of postoperative pain after laparotomies: lack of evidence of spinal action. *Anesth Analg*. 1998;86:574–578.

16. Scott DA, Blake D, Buckland M, et al. A comparison of epidural ropivacaine infusion alone and in combination with 1, 2, and 4 microg/mL fentanyl for seventy-two hours of postoperative analgesia after major abdominal surgery. *Anesth Analg*. 1999;88:857–864.

17. Liu SS, Allen HW, Olsson GL. Patient-controlled epidural analgesia with bupivacaine and fentanyl on hospital wards: prospective experience with 1,030 surgical patients. *Anesthesiology*. 1998;88:688–695.

18. Guinard JP, Carpenter RL, Chassot PG. Epidural and intravenous fentanyl produce equivalent effects during major surgery. *Anesthesiology*. 1995;82:377–382.

19. Joris JL, Jacob EA, Sessler DI, et al. Spinal mechanisms contribute to analgesia produced by epidural sufentanil combined with bupivacaine for postoperative analgesia. *Anesth Analg*. 2003;97:1446–1451.

20. Menigaux C, Guignard B, Fletcher D, et al. More epidural than intravenous sufentanil is required to provide comparable postoperative pain relief. *Anesth Analg*. 2001;93:472–476, 474th contents page.

21. Gambling D, Hughes T, Gould EM, Manvelian G. A pharmacokinetic and phamacodynamic study of a single dose of epidural DepoDur following epidural bupivacaine: a randomized controlled trial in patients undergoing lower abdominal surgery. Paper presented at: American Society of Regional Anesthesia and Pain Medicine, 2006; Rancho Mirage, CA.

22. Viscusi ER, Martin G, Hartrick CT, Singla N, Manvelian G. Forty-eight hours of postoperative pain relief after total hip arthroplasty with a novel, extended-release epidural morphine formulation. *Anesthesiology*. 2005;102:1014–1022.

23. Carvalho B, Riley E, Cohen SE, et al. Single-dose, sustained-release epidural morphine in the management of postoperative pain after elective cesarean delivery: results of a multicenter randomized controlled study. *Anesth Analg*. 2005;100:1150–1158.

24. Bernards CM, Shen DD, Sterling ES, et al. Epidural, cerebrospinal fluid, and plasma pharmacokinetics of epidural opioids (part 1): differences among opioids. *Anesthesiology*. 2003;99:455–465.

25. Angst MS, Ramaswamy B, Riley ET, Stanski DR. Lumbar epidural morphine in humans and supraspinal analgesia to experimental heat pain. *Anesthesiology*. 2000;92:312–324.

26. Chauvin M, Hongnat JM, Mourgeon E, et al. Equivalence of postoperative analgesia with patient-controlled intravenous or epidural alfentanil. *Anesth Analg*. 1993;76:1251–1258.

27. van den Nieuwenhuyzen MC, Burm AG, Vletter AA, Stienstra R, van Kleef JW. Epidural vs. intravenous infusion of alfentanil in the management of postoperative pain following laparotomies. *Acta Anaesthesiol Scand*. 1996;40:1112–1118.

28. Sandler AN, Stringer D, Panos L, et al. A randomized, double-blind comparison of lumbar epidural and intravenous fentanyl

infusions for postthoracotomy pain relief. Analgesic, pharma-cokinetic, and respiratory effects. *Anesthesiology.* 1992;77:626–634.

29. Miguel R, Barlow I, Morrell M, et al. A prospective, randomized, double-blind comparison of epidural and intravenous sufentanil infusions. *Anesthesiology.* 1994;81:346–352.

30. Lanz E, Theiss D, Riess W, Sommer U. Epidural morphine for postoperative analgesia: a double-blind study. *Anesth Analg.* 1982;61:236–240.

31. Gambling D, Hughes T, Martin G, Horton W, Manvelian G. A comparison of Depodur, a novel, single-dose extended-release epidural morphine, with standard epidural morphine for pain relief after lower abdominal surgery. *Anesth Analg.* 2005; 100:1065–1074.

32. Hartrick CT, Martin G, Kantor G, Koncelik J, Manvelian G. Evaluation of a single-dose, extended-release epidural morphine formulation for pain after knee arthroplasty. *J Bone Joint Surg Am.* 2006;88:273–281.

9

Transitions from Acute to Chronic Pain

Frederick M. Perkins

Pain is defined as an unpleasant sensory and emotional experience,[1] and pain is something that most people would like to avoid. A commonly accepted definition of chronic pain is pain that lasts more than 3 months. Since the late 1990s, there has been a realization that certain surgical procedures are associated with a significant incidence of chronic pain. In particular there appear to be certain surgical procedures where the preoperative prevalence of chronic pain is low, and then the postoperative prevalence of chronic pain is significantly higher. The purpose of this chapter is to (1) review the literature that documents the prevalence of chronic pain following certain surgical procedures, (2) review the progression of acute postoperative pain to chronic pain, (3) summarize some proposed mechanisms that facilitate the development of chronic pain, and (4) review interventions that have either been shown to decrease the incidence of chronic pain or that have been proposed to decrease the incidence of chronic pain following surgery.

EVIDENCE OF PERSISTENT POSTSURGICAL PAIN

There have been a number of reviews since the late 1990s that document a significant prevalence of chronic pain following surgery.[2–4] These reviews have identified particular surgical procedures with a low prevalence of preoperative pain that then have a significant increase in prevalence of chronic pain. Table 9.1 lists surgical procedures that have been associated with an increased prevalence of chronic pain. Examples of surgical procedures not associated with an increased prevalence of pain are also included. Surgical procedures associated with a significantly increased prevalence of chronic pain include inguinal hernia repair,[5] thoracotomy,[6] breast surgery,[7] and lower extremity amputation.[8] Of note is the observation that the prevalence of pain following surgery tends to decrease from 3 to 6 months and to 12 months but then appears to stabilize. This has been noted following inguinal hernia repair,[9] thoracotomy,[10] breast surgery,[11] and lower extremity amputation.[8]

A number of predictors of the persistence of pain following surgery have been identified. One of the most robust is increased severity of acute postoperative pain,[3] and as a surrogate the

amount of opioid consumed in the acute postoperative period. Younger patients, female gender, and the existence of preoperative chronic pain are also risk factors for persistent postoperative pain.[4]

PROGRESSION FROM ACUTE TO CHRONIC PAIN

Pain is not chronic initially. Although this is an axiomatic statement, it is surprising how often clinicians are not cognizant of it in their daily practice. Acute pain is initiated by stimulation of nociceptors, usually in conjunction with tissue damage in the case of surgery. These nociceptors are mostly high-threshold peripheral sensory neurons. Information is transmitted to the dorsal horn of the spinal cord by these neurons, and then to the brain. The signals that arrive to the brain allow the individual to perceive the location, intensity, and duration of the noxious stimulus, and these data can be interpreted as pain.

Almost immediately after the surgical injury, the manner in which the information is transferred is modified. In the periphery there is release of prostaglandins, bradykinins, and other mediators that by and large decrease the amount of stimulus needed to cause depolarization of the nociceptive neuron (peripheral sensitization). In the dorsal horn, two separate but probably related phenomena can be observed. The first has the catchy name of *wind-up* and was first put forth by Mendell and Wall in 1965[26] to describe rate-dependent amplification of transmission to the brain. This is when the frequency of nociceptor simulation increases to more than 2 Hz, and then the rate of transmission of information to the brain is no longer linear but exponential. The second phenomenon is central sensitization. Again, this results in amplification of information transmission to the brain from the dorsal horn. Both phenomena involve activation of *N*-methyl-D-aspartic acid (NMDA) receptors in the dorsal horn, but wind-up is a short-lived response that rapidly reverts to baseline, whereas sensitization is a longer-lived phenomenon. Over a period of hours following a surgical injury there is altered gene transcription in both sensory neurons and in the dorsal horn. These result in increased release of excitatory neurotransmitters and decreased release of inhibitory

Table 9.1: Prevalence of Persistent Postoperative Pain

Surgical Procedure	Prevalence of Chronic Pain (%)	Prevalence of Preoperative Pain (%)
Amputation	Stump pain, 62	Very common if
Lower extremity[3]	Phantom pain, 70	ischemic disease
Thoracotomy[3]		
Posterolateral	50	Uncommon
VATS	31	Uncommon
Mastectomy[3]	30	Uncommon
+ axillary dissection	50	Uncommon
Prostatectomy		
Radical[22]	32	Uncommon
Sternotomy		
CABG[23]	30	Common (angina)
Valve[24]	32	Uncommon
Colectomy[16]	28	Uncommon
Mammoplasty		
Augmentation[20]	20	Uncommon
Vasectomy[25]	15	Uncommon
Hernia repair,		
inguinal[5]	12	Common, incident pain
Cesarean section[14]	6	>95 (labor pain)
Pelvic fracture		
Open fixation[21]	48	>99
Lumbar spine,		
Discectomy[19]	44	Common
Hysterectomy[18]	32	62
Cholecystectomy[15]	23	Common
Arthroplasty, hip[12]	20	99
Dental,		
Root canal[17]	12	Common
Cataract extraction,	<1	<1
With lens implant[13]		

neurotransmitters. With peripheral and spinal sensitization, the pain threshold is rapidly decreased following injury. There are good detailed reviews of these phenomena.[4,27]

An even longer-lived sensitization occurs with injury to nerves. This long-lived sensitization has a number of similarities to memory.[28] There are other observed changes that may alter pain perception if there is nerve injury. Incorporation of tetrodotoxin-resistant sodium channels in nociceptive neurons in the dorsal root ganglion is observed, and there is upregulation of voltage-gated calcium channels. Altered input to wide dynamic range cell bodies in the dorsal horn is noted, and there can be significant anatomic remodeling of the dorsal horn on the microscopic level.[29] With persistent pain there are data that there is brain atrophy and that the extent of atrophy is related to the duration of pain in years.[30]

PREDICTORS OF ACUTE AND CHRONIC PAIN

All of the above statements and observations are generalities. The human race is not homogeneous, and the extent to which any one individual displays the above may be highly variable. Bennett developed and described the first animal model of chronic

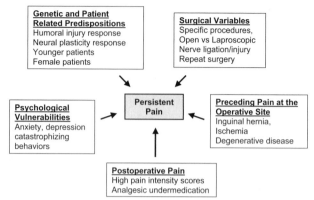

Figure 9.1: Perioperative risk factors for persistent pain following surgery. Summarized from data presented in references 3, 4, 18, 37, 38, 39.

neuropathic pain in a strain of Wistar rats.[31] He has noted that his model is less successful in other strains of Wistar rats and does not reliably produce pain behaviors in Sprague-Dawley rats. There is little reason to expect humans to be uniform in their reactions to tissue and nerve damage. In the early 1950s, Lasagna and Beecher[32] documented difficulty in finding "an optimal" dose of morphine. Subsequent studies by Lasagna and colleagues documented both under treatment of pain in a significant portion of patients following surgery and variability of patient response to opioids. The patient's pain experience did not correlate with the patient's stated pain threshold or tolerance. Subsequent studies have documented that pain threshold as measured by pressure algometry does not predict the extent of postoperative pain.[33] Recently, there have been studies that show a correlation between the extent of pain in an experimental first-degree burn and the extent of pain with anterior cruciate ligament repair.[34] There is also a correlation between heat pain threshold and the extent of acute pain following cesarean section.[35] This is of interest because the severity of postoperative pain is one of the most robust predictors of progression to chronic pain.[3,4] It is therefore not surprising that genetic predictors of pain have been identified.[36] It has also been observed that younger patients and female patients experience more acute pain and are more likely to develop persistent pain following surgery.[4]

Another predictor of persistent postsurgical pain has been evidence of nerve damage. Benedetti et al[37] observed that following thoracotomy, patients who demonstrated intercostal nerve dysfunction, as evidenced by loss of the superficial abdominal reflex, had more acute pain and were more likely to have persistent pain. Rogers et al[38] were able to demonstrate intercostal nerve dysfunction related to use of a rib spreader. Inguinal hernia repair and breast surgery with axillary dissection both place nerves at risk for damage.

There are also some psychological predictors of acute pain, including anxiety and possibly neuroticism and narcissism.[3] Chronic phantom limb pain following lower limb amputation is more likely in patients who display catastrophizing (Figure 9.1).[39]

INTERVENTIONS TO DECREASE PERSISTENT POSTSURGICAL PAIN

Because the intensity of acute pain and the probability of nerve damage both are predictors of chronic pain, the surgical approaches that minimize these risks should be of benefit. A number of surgical techniques have been documented to decrease the prevalence of persistent postsurgical pain.

For inguinal hernia repair there are a number of surgical approaches that can be considered. There are open repairs either with or without mesh. There are laparoscopic repairs that may or may not include the use of staples. The effect of these different approaches has been looked at in a number of studies. A systematic review of nerve preservation compared to sectioning found three randomized controlled trials and four cohort trials.[40] Intentional sectioning of the ilioinguinal and iliohypogastric nerves did not alter the probability of persistent pain following hernia repair at 6 months (21% prevalence of pain for nerve sectioning and 23% prevalence for nerve preservation), but nerve dysfunction was common in both groups. An early systematic review comparing open hernia repair to laparoscopic repair[41] noted that few studies reported the prevalence of chronic pain, and there were no significant differences. Two more recent reviews of the same topic[42,43] found a significant decrease in risk of chronic pain with laparoscopic repair (8% prevalence) compared to open mesh repair (13% prevalence). A review of open hernia repair using mesh versus not using mesh found a lower prevalence of persistent pain and a lower hernia recurrence rate with mesh repairs.[44] These findings are similar to the findings from a Cochrane Database Review[45] in which cumulative data revealed a prevalence of 6% for chronic pain following mesh repairs and 10% for open repairs. There have been a number of recent randomized controlled studies comparing lightweight mesh to standard mesh,[46,47] but there has not been a rigorous meta-analysis or systematic review. The combined prevalence of chronic pain with lightweight mesh was 27%, whereas with standard mesh it was 33%.

For breast surgery, the use of sentinel node biopsy has been found to decrease the prevalence of chronic pain. In one randomized controlled study[48] women were randomized to a sentinel node study arm or an axillary dissection study arm. Women in the sentinel node arm where cancer was found in a sentinel node also underwent an axillary dissection. Women who did not have cancer in the sentinel node were less likely to receive adjuvant cancer therapy and were significantly less likely to develop persistent axillary pain (8% at 24 months) compared to those who had a primary axillary dissection and adjuvant therapy (39% at 24 months). Women with negative nodes on a sentinel node biopsy are significantly less likely to develop arm pain and other arm symptoms. Women who undergo a secondary axillary node dissection were as likely or more likely to develop chronic pain as those who underwent a primary axillary node dissection.[49] At least one group of researchers have noted a decreasing prevalence of arm pain and symptoms following axillary dissection related to surgeons being more aware of the problem.[50] Simple mastectomy appears to be associated with less persistent pain that lumpectomy.[3]

A number of studies suggested that the incision type is of importance regarding the prevalence of postthoracotomy chronic pain[3] in that a posterolateral, muscle-splitting incision is associated with more pain than an anterior or muscle-sparing incision. Recently, a report from Ochroch et al[51] using data from their 2002 study[52] looked at the effect of surgical incision type and found that patients who underwent posterolateral thoracotomy were more limited in their physical activity than those who had muscle-sparing incisions, despite no significant differences in pain prevalence or pain intensity between the groups. This is an area that needs further investigation.

There are reports that handling of intercostals nerves at closure following posterolateral thoracotomy can alter the prevalence of persistent pain. When patients were randomized to having the intercostal nerves protected by an intercostal muscle harvest, the average intensity of postoperative pain was decreased acutely and for the 12 weeks of follow-up.[53] Total pain prevalence at 12 weeks was not reported, but the prevalence of moderate to severe pain at 12 weeks was 22% for the nerve protected group and 28% for the control group (not significant). In a case series ($n = 280$), closure with sutures placed through the lower rib rather than under it (where the intercostals nerve could be compressed) resulted in significantly less intense pain through 3 months of follow-up, and patients from the control group were more likely to use neuropathic pain descriptors on the short form of the McGill Pain Questionnaire.[54] Pain prevalence data were not reported.

If acute pain in and of itself causes persistent pain, then interventions that decease acute pain may decrease the prevalence and severity of chronic pain. Thus far, there are no data indicating that the type of anesthesia or analgesia alters the prevalence of pain following inguinal hernia repair.

There have been two randomized controlled studies that looked at the influence of perioperative paravertebral blockade on persistent pain following breast surgery. Both found a significantly lower prevalence of chronic pain in women who had the block. One was a follow-up study of 60 women who had participated in an acute perioperative pain study.[50,55] In this study, the prevalence of pain at both 6 and 12 months was significantly lower among the women who had received a block (17% vs. 40% at 6 months and 7% vs. 33% at 12 months). The second study was smaller (29 subjects) and involved the placement of a paravertebral catheter preoperatively in the patients in the treatment arm.[56] This was dosed with 10 mL of 0.25% bupivacaine prior to surgery and reinjected every 12 hours for 48 hours with the same dose. A telephone follow-up inquired about pain 3 months following surgery ("Do you have chronic pain as a result of your breast surgery?"). The paravertebral block group had significantly lower pain prevalence at 3 months (0% vs. 80%). If the 6-month data from the first study are combined with the 3-month data from the second study then the calculated odds ratio of persistent pain in the paravertebral block groups is 0.05 (OR 0.02–0.11), and this is highly significant.

In both of these studies the severity of acute pain in the paravertebral block groups was less than in the control groups. A recent study[57] using a multiple injection technique for paravertebral block found less pain in the treatment group only while in the postanesthesia care unit, but they did not have a benefit on postoperative days 1 or 2. Long-term follow-up data were not reported. Thus, there may be important differences in how paravertebral block is performed that will need to be investigated in the future.

For thoracotomy, there are two randomized controlled trials that demonstrated a decreased prevalence of chronic pain when epidural analgesia was used intraoperatively and postoperatively[58,59] and a subsequent study that did not find a difference in pain intensity.[52] Ochroch et al[52] did not find a significant effect of intra- and postoperative epidural local anesthetic versus postoperative only on a mixed surgical population (32% posterolateral thoracotomy and 68% muscle-sparing thoracotomy) followed for 48 weeks. The studies where epidural analgesia made a difference included only patients undergoing posterolateral thoracotomy and used a higher concentration of local anesthetic postoperatively than the negative study by

Ochroch et al.[52] Additionally Ochroch et al[52] did not report pain prevalence data, and their study was probably underpowered for the analysis that they used.

There are also some data that adjuvant treatments to decrease acute pain may decrease the prevalence of chronic pain. Most of these studies are in women undergoing breast surgery. Fassoulaki and colleagues published two randomized controlled studies of perioperative gabapentin.[60,61] In the first study, women received gabapentin (1200 mg/d; 400 mg 3 times per day) starting the evening before surgery, mexiletine (600 mg/d; 200 mg 3 times per day), or placebo 3 times per day.[60] There were no significant differences in pain prevalence or pain intensity, or in analgesic requirement at 3 months follow-up, although the character of the pain in the control group tended to be burning rather than throbbing, aching, or stabbing. In the second study women undergoing breast cancer surgery received a combination of gabapentin (1600 mg/d; 400 mg 4 times a day) for 10 days starting the evening before surgery, plus EMLA cream (20 g) for 3 days starting the day of surgery plus intraoperative irrigation of the brachial plexus with 10 mL of 0.75% ropivacaine.[61] The control group underwent placebo administration of each of the interventions. This study found significantly decreased pain prevalence at both 3- and 6-month follow-up in the intervention group (30% versus 57% at 6 months). The calculated odds ratio for pain at 6 months is 0.32 (OR 0.18–0.62). Whether gabapentin or local anesthetics or the combination can alter long-term pain following breast surgery is not clear, and follow-up at 12 months and longer is needed. Reuben et al[62] randomized women scheduled for breast cancer surgery to receive either venlafaxine (75 mg for 2 weeks starting the night before surgery) or placebo. Persistent pain at 6-month follow-up was significantly less in the venlafaxine group (29%) compared to the control group (72%). Clearly there is a need for follow-up studies to confirm these findings on perioperative interventions aimed at reducing persistent pain after breast surgery, but early results suggest utility for these interventions.

SUMMARY AND CONCLUSIONS

The data cited above clearly indicate that certain surgical procedures are associated with a significant prevalence of chronic pain. Surgical techniques that are associated with less acute pain appear to be associated with less chronic pain. Paravertebral block and epidural analgesia with significant doses of local anesthetic appear to decrease both acute pain intensity and the prevalence of chronic pain. Neither the dose of local anesthetic necessary nor the extent of neuroblockade needed has been defined. Finally, the perioperative use of adjuvant medications, such as gabapentin or venlafaxine, may decrease the prevalence of chronic pain, but these studies need to be confirmed.

REFERENCES

1. Merskey H, Bogduk N. *Classification of Chronic Pain. Descriptions of Chronic Pain Syndromes and Definitions of Pain Terms.* 2nd ed. Seattle, WA: IASP Press; 1994.
2. Macrae WA. Chronic pain after surgery. *Br J Anaesth.* 2001;87:88–98.
3. Perkins FM, Kehlet H. Chronic pain as an outcome of surgery. *Anesthesiology.* 2000;93:1123–1133.
4. Kehlet H, Jensen TS, Woolf CJ. Persistent postsurgical pain: risk factors and prevention. *Lancet.* 2006;367:1618–1625.
5. Aasvang E, Kehlet H. Chronic postoperative pain: the case of inguinal herniorrhaphy. *Br J Anaesth.* 2005;95:69–76.
6. Gottschalk A, Cohen SP, Yang S, Ochroch EA. Preventing and treating pain after thoracic surgery. *Anesthesiology.* 2006;104:594–600.
7. Jung BF, Ahrendt GM, Oaklander AL, Dworkin RH. Neuropathic pain following breast cancer surgery: proposed classification and research update. *Pain.* 2003;104:1–13.
8. Jensen TS, Krebs B, Nielsen J, Rasmussen P. Immediate and long-term phantom limb pain in amputees: incidence, clinical characteristics and relationship to pre-amputation limb pain. *Pain.* 1985;21:267–278.
9. Callesen T, Bech K, Kehlet H. Chronic pain after inguinal hernia repair: a prospective study after 500 operations. *Br J Surg.* 1999;86:1528–1531.
10. Landreneau RJ, Mack MJ, Hazelrigg SR, et al. Prevalence of chronic pain after pulmonary resection by thoracotomy or video-assisted thoracic surgery. *J Thorac Cardiovasc Surg.* 1994;107:1079–1085.
11. Tasmuth T, Kataja M, Blomqvist C, von Smitten K, Kalso E. Treatment-related factors predisposing to chronic pain in patients with breast cancer: a multivariate approach. *Acta Oncol.* 1997;36:625–630.
12. Nikolajsen L, Brandsborg B, Jensen TS, Kehlet H. Chronic pain following total hip arthroplasty: a nationwide questionnaire study. *Acta Anaesthesiol Scand.* 2006;50:495–500.
13. Snellingen T, Evans JR, Ravilla T, Foster A. Surgical interventions for age-related cataract. *Cochrane Database Syst Rev.* 2006;1:1–28.
14. Nikolajsen L, Sorensen HC, Jensen TS, Kehlet H. Chronic pain following caesaran section. *Acta Anaesthesiol Scand.* 2004;48:111–116.
15. Bisgaard T, Rosenberg J, Kehlet H. From acute to chronic pain after laparoscopic cholecystectomy: a prospective follow-up analysis. *Scand J Gastroenterol.* 2005;40:1358–1364.
16. Lavand'homme P, De Kock M, Waterloos H. Intraoperative epidural analgesia combined with ketamine provides effective preventive analgesia in patients undergoing major digestive surgery. *Anesthesiology.* 2005;103:813–820.
17. Polycarpou N, Ng YL, Canavan D, Moles DR, Gulabivala K. Prevalence of persistent pain after endodontic treatment and factors affecting its occurrence in cases with complete radiographic healing. *Int Endodont J.* 2005;38:169–178.
18. Brandsborg B, Nikolajsen L, Hansen CT, Kehlet H, Jensen TS. Risk factors for chronic pain after hysterectomy. *Anesthesiology.* 2007;106:1003–1012.
19. Atlas SJ, Keller RB, Wu YA, Deyo RA, Singer DE. Long-term outcomes of surgical and nonsurgical management of sciatica secondary to a lumbar disc herniation: 10 year results from the Maine lumbar spine study. *Spine.* 2005;30:927–935.
20. Romundstad L, Breivik H, Roald H, Romundstad PR, Stubhaug A. Chronic pain and sensory changes after augmentation mammoplasty: long term effects of preincisional administration of methylprednisolone. *Pain.* 2006;124:92–99.
21. Meyhoff CS, Thomsen CH, Rasmussen LS, Nielsen PR. High incidence of chronic pain following surgery for pelvic fracture. *Clin J Pain.* 2006;22:167–172.
22. Gottschalk A, Smith DS, Jobes DR, et al. Preemptive epidural analgesia and recovery from radical prostatectomy. *JAMA.* 1998;279:1076–1082.
23. Bruce J, Drury N, Poobalan AS, Jeffrey RR, Smith WC, Chambers WA. The prevalence of chronic chest and leg pain following cardiac surgery: a historical cohort study. *Pain.* 2003;104:265–273.
24. Jensen MK, Andersen C. Can chronic poststernotomy pain after cardiac valve replacement be reduced using thoracic epidural analgesia? *Acta Anaesthesiol Scand.* 2004;48:871–874.

25. Awsare NS, Krishnan J, Boustead GB, Hanbury DC, McNicholas TA. Complications of vasectomy. *Ann R Coll Surg Engl.* 2005; 87:406–410.

26. Mendell LM, Wall PD. Responses of single dorsal cord cells to peripheral cutaneous unmyelinated fibres. *Nature.* 1965;206: 97–99.

27. Woolf CJ. Dissecting out mechanisms responsible for peripheral neuropathic pain: implications for diagnosis and therapy. *Life Sci.* 2004;74:2605–2610.

28. Ru-Rong J, Kohno T, Moore KA, Woolf CJ. Central sensitization and LTP: do pain and memory share similar mechanisms? *Trends Neurosci.* 2003;26:696–705.

29. Woolf CJ, Shortland P, Reynolds M, Ridings J, Doubell T, Coggeshall RE. Reorganization of central terminals of myelinated primary afferents in the rat dorsal horn following peripheral axotomy. *J Comp Neurol.* 1995;360:121–134.

30. Apkarian AV, Sosa Y, Sonty S, et al. Chronic pain is associated with decreased prefrontal and thalamic gray matter. *J Neurosci.* 2004;24:10410–10415.

31. Bennett GJ, Xie Y-K. A peripheral mononeuropathy in rat that produces disorders of pain sensation like those seen in man. *Pain.* 1988;33:87–107.

32. Lasagna L, Beecher HK. The optimal dose of morphine. *JAMA.* 1954;156:230–234.

33. Katz J, Kavanagh BP, Sandler AN, et al. Preemptive analgesia: clinical evidence of neuroplasticity contributing to postoperative pain. *Anesthesiology.* 1992;77:439–446.

34. Werner MU, Duun P, Kehlet H. Prediction of postoperative pain by preoperative nociceptive responses to heat stimuli. *Anesthesiology.* 2004;100:115–119.

35. Pan PH, Coghill R, Houle TT, et al. Multifactorial preoperative predictors of postcesarean section pain and analgesic requirements. *Anesthesiology.* 2006;104:417–425.

36. Diatchenko L, Nackley AG, Slade GD, Fillingim RB, Maixner W. Idiopathic pain disorders: pathways of vulnerability. *Pain.* 2006;123:226–230.

37. Benedetti F, Amanzio M, Casadio C, et al. Control of postoperative pain by transcutaneous electrical nerve stimulation after thoracic operations. *Ann Thorac Surg.* 1997;63:773–776.

38. Rogers ML, Henderson L, Mahajan RP, Duffy JP. Preliminary findings in the neurophysiological assessment of intercostal nerve injury during thoracotomy. *Eur J Cardio-thorac Surg.* 2002;21:298–301.

39. Hanley MA, Jensen MP, Ehde DM, Hoffman AJ, Patterson DR, Robinson LR. Psychosocial predictors of long-term adjustment to lower-limb amputation and phantom limb pain. *Disabil Rehabil.* 2004;26:882–893.

40. Wijsmuller AR, van Veen RN, Bosch JL, Lange JF, Kleinrensink GJ, Lange JF. Nerve management during open hernia review. *Br J Surg.* 2007;94:17–22.

41. Collaboration EH. Laparoscopic compared with open methods of groin hernia repair: systematic review of randomised controlled trials. *Br J Surg.* 2000;87:860–867.

42. Schmedt CG, Sauerland S, Bittner R. Comparison of endoscopic procedures vs Lichtenstein and other open mesh techniques for inguinal hernia repair: a meta-analysis of randomized trials. *Surg Endosc.* 2005;19:188–199.

43. McCormack K, Wake B, Perez J, et al. Laparoscopic surgery for inguinal hernia repair; systematic review of effectiveness and economic evaluation. *Health Technol Assess.* 2005;9:1–203.

44. Grant AM. Open mesh versus non-mesh repair of groin hernia: meta-analysis of randomised trials based on individual patient data. *Hernia.* 2002;6:130–136.

45. McCormack K, Scott NW, Go PMNYH, Grant AM. EU hernia trialists: laparoscopic techniques versus open techniques for inguinal hernia repair. *Cochrane Database Syst Rev.* 2005;12:4.

46. Bringman S, Wollert S, Osterberg J, Smedberg S, Granlund H, Heikkinen T-J. Three-year results of a randomized clinical trial of lightweight or standard polypropylene mesh in Lichtenstein repair of primary inguinal hernia. *Br J Surg.* 2006;93:1056–1059.

47. O'dwyer PJ, Kingsnorth AN, Molloy RG, Small PK, Lammers B, Horeyseck G. Randomized clinical trial assessing impact of a lightweight or heavyweight mesh on chronic pain after inguinal hernia repair. *Br J Surg.* 2005;92:166–170.

48. Veronesi U, Paganelli G, Viale G, et al. A randomized comparison of sentinel-node biopsy with routine axillary dissection in breast cancer. *New Engl J Med.* 2003;349:546–553.

49. Husen M, Paaschburg B, Flyger HL. Two-step axillary operation increases risks of arm morbidity in breast cancer patients. *Breast.* 2006;15:620–628.

50. Kairaluoma PM, Bachman MS, Rosenberg PH, Pere PJ. Preincisional paravertebral block reduces the prevalence of chronic pain after breast surgery. *Anesth Analg.* 2006;103:703–708.

51. Ochroch EA, Gottschalk A, Augoustides JG, Aukburg SJ, Kaiser LR, Shrager JB. Pain and physical function are similar following axillary, muscle-sparing vs posterolateral thoracotomy. *Chest.* 2005;128:2664–2670.

52. Ochroch EA, Gottschalk A, Augostides J, et al. Long-term pain and activity during recovery from major thoracotomy using thoracic epidural analgesia. *Anesthesiology.* 2002;97:1234–1244.

53. Cerfolio RJ, Bryant AS, Patel B, Bartolucci AA. Intercostal muscle flap reduces the pain of thoracotomy: a prospective randomized trial. *J Thorac Cardiovasc Surg.* 2005;130:987–993.

54. Cerfolio RJ, Price TN, Bryant AS, Bass CS, Bartolucci AA. Intracosal sutures decrease the pain of thoracotomy. *Ann Thorac Surg.* 2003;76:407–412.

55. Kairaluoma PM, Bachman MS, Korpinen AK, Rosenberg PH, Pere PJ. Single-injection paravertebral block before general anesthesia enhances analgesia after breast cancer surgery with and without associated lymph node biopsy. *Anesth Analg.* 2004;99:1837–1843.

56. Iohom G, Abdalla H, O'Brien J, et al. The associations between severity of early postoperative pain, chronic postsurgical pain and plasma concentration of stable nitric oxide products after breast surgery. *Anesth Analg.* 2006;103:995–1000.

57. Moller JF, Nikolajsen L, Rodt SA, Ronning H, Carlsson PS. Thoracic paravertebral block for breast cancer surgery: a randomized double-blind study. *Anesthesiology.* 2007;105:1848–1851.

58. Obata H, Saito S, Fujita N, Fuse Y, Ishizaki K, Goto F. Epidural block with mepivacaine before surgery reduces long-term postthoracotomy pain. *Can J Anaesth.* 1999;46:1127–1132.

59. Senturk M, Ozcan PE, Talu GK, et al. The effects of three different analgesia techniques on long-term postthoracotomy pain. *Anesth Analg.* 2002;94:11–15.

60. Fassoulaki A, Patris K, Sarantopoulos C, Hogan Q. The analgesic effect of gabapentin and mexiletine after breast surgery. *Anesth Analg.* 2002;95:985–991.

61. Fassoulaki A, Triga A, Melemeni A, Sarantopoulos C. Multimodal analgesia with gabapentin and local anesthetics prevents acute and chronic pain after breast surgery for cancer. *Anesth. Analg.* 2005;101:1427–1432.

62. Reuben SS, Makari-Judson G, Lurie SD. Evaluation of efficacy of the perioperative administration of venlafaxine XR in the prevention of postmastectomy pain syndrome. *J Pain Sympt Manag.* 2004;27:133–139.

10

Molecular Basis and Clinical Implications of Opioid Tolerance and Opioid-Induced Hyperalgesia

Larry F. Chu, David Clark, and Martin S. Angst

Opioids were first cultivated around 3400 BC by the Sumerians in the Tigris-Euphrates river systems of lower Mesopotamia.[1] Named from the ideograms *hul* and *gil*, the word for poppy translates to the "joy plant." Ancient Sumerian writings found on clay tablets from Nippur show that opioid medications were used to treat pain and to "ease the harshness of life."[2] These medications have most commonly been used for the treatment of acute and cancer-related pain.[3] However, recent evidence suggests that opioid medications may also be useful for the treatment of chronic nonmalignant pain, at least for short periods of time.[4–15]

Increasing Use of Opioid Medications

Pain management has recently gained prominence and priority among patients, physicians, and health care providers for a variety of reasons. Since the late 1990s, pharmaceutical manufacturers introduced heavy marketing of drugs such as Oxycontin and cyclooxygenase 2 (COX-2) inhibitors to consumers and physicians.[16,17] In August 1999, the Joint Commission on Accreditation of Health Care Organizations (JCAHO) issued transformative new pain management standards to improve assessment of pain as "the fifth vital sign."[18] In late 2000, the US congress passed into law a provision declaring the 10-year period from January 1, 2001, as the Decade of Pain Control and Research.[19] Recently, national and international medical and political organizations have joined a growing movement to establish pain management as a fundamental human right,[20,21] and individual states have even passed legislation mandating continuing medical education for pain management and end-of-life issues.[22]

Perhaps because of these events, opioid medications have been increasingly prescribed by primary care physicians and other health care providers for acute and chronic painful conditions.[23,24] A study of Australian opioid prescribing trends from 1986 to 1996 by Bell[25] found an almost 5-fold increase in the amount of oral morphine use during this period, as well as dramatic increases in opioid prescribing for noncancer pain. Long-term use and opioid dose escalation was associated with one-third of these cases. More recently, Olsen et al[23] studied opioid prescribing patterns by US primary care physicians from 1992 to 2001 and found a 54% increase in the incidence of opioid prescribing at its peak in 1999 (41 per 1000 visits in 1992–1993 compared to 63 per 1000 visits in 1998–1999).[23] The trend stabilized in 2001, the latest year for which data were analyzed in the study. Opioids are now among the most common medications prescribed by physicians in the United States[26] and accounted for 235 million prescriptions in 2004.[27]

Clinical Implications of Growing Opioid Use

The growing prevalence of opioid use in the general medical population has led to new concerns about the clinical implications of this exposure over time. Common concerns stemming from chronic opioid use include iatrogenic opioid dependence or addiction and adverse side effects. The need for dose escalation in some patients because of apparent loss of efficacy with chronic use is another problem that is typically ascribed to the development of opioid tolerance. Recent evidence suggests that opioids are responsible for yet another problem that may potentially limit their usefulness over time, opioid-induced hyperalgesia (OIH).[28–31] OIH is a unique, definable, and characteristic increased sensitivity to pain that is distinct from the patient's underlying original painful condition, which may explain loss of opioid efficacy in some cases.

Treatment of acute pain in the presence of analgesic tolerance and/or opioid-induced hyperalgesia can present a challenge for the clinician. Many of these patients suffer from inadequately treated postoperative pain because clinicians are unsure how to best treat their acute pain management needs. Unfortunately, there is a dearth of quality prospective clinical evidence that directly addresses factors that may influence the efficacy of opioids in treating pain after prolonged opioid exposure. The focus of this chapter is to highlight important aspects of our current understanding of opioid tolerance and opioid-induced hyperalgesia with respect to their mechanistic underpinnings and clinical ramifications. Our goal is to provide a framework to understand and treat acute pain in patients after prolonged opioid use.

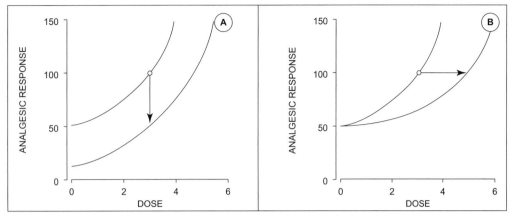

Figure 10.1: Alterations in the opioid dose-response relationship with chronic opioid administration. We present a hypothetical diagram showing changes in analgesic response (such as cold pressor tolerance time) as a function of analgesic dose (such as target plasma remifentanil concentration) after chronic opioid administration. Opioid-naïve patients are shown as black lines. (A) In opioid-induced hyperalgesia, the dose-response curve of the chronic opioid user is shifted downward and the patient experiences increased pain to noxious stimuli at baseline (shown as decreased analgesic response when analgesic dose is zero). (B) In analgesic tolerance, the slope of the dose-response curve of the chronic opioid user becomes attenuated and rightward shifted; however, there is no significant change in pain sensitivity at baseline (shown as an identical analgesic response in opioid naïve and chronic opioid users when analgesic dose is zero).

ADAPTATION TO PROLONGED OPIOID EXPOSURE: TOLERANCE VERSUS HYPERALGESIA

Adaptation to Opioid Therapy

Experience tells us that individual patients can respond quite differently to opioid medications. Some patients require only a small amount of opioid medication for effective pain control, whereas others require larger amounts over time to maintain the same level of analgesia. After a period of dose escalation, many patients plateau and some can be maintained on stable dosing for long periods of time. The need for dose escalation and the putative loss of effectiveness over time reflects the body's physiologic adaptation to chronic opioid exposure and the etiology is both complex and multifactorial in nature.

Mechanisms of Observed Adaptations

Physiologic changes that may occur with chronic opioid exposure include physical dependence, opioid tolerance, and OIH. These adaptations can occur fairly quickly after the initial opioid exposure. Studies have shown that signs of tolerance can occur in patients who received opioids as little as 2 weeks before surgery, leading to increased perioperative opioid requirements.[32] A recent prospective observational study by Chu et al[33] showed that increased sensitivity to pain, OIH, can occur after only 4 weeks of chronic opioid therapy.

Although tolerance and opioid-induced hyperalgesia are the principal mechanisms involved in physiologic adaptation to opioids over time, other changes may also occur. Opioids can induce euphoria by indirectly enhancing dopamine release in the nucleus accumbens, leading to psychological dependence in some individuals.[34] Addiction and or drug-seeking behavior has been associated with high psychiatric morbidity according to self-reported symptoms of anxiety and depression, history of sexual or physical abuse, and history of psychologic adjustment.[35] The astute clinician must be cognizant that these psychological factors may present yet another reason for

observed need for increasing opioid doses over time in some individuals.[36]

Definition of Opioid-Induced Hyperalgesia

OIH is most broadly defined as a state of nociceptive sensitization caused by exposure to opioids. It is characterized by a paradoxical response whereby a patient receiving opioids for the treatment of pain may actually become more sensitive to pain over time. This increased sensitivity to pain is a new, unique entity that is distinct from the patient's original underlying painful condition. In clinical settings, OIH may represent one of many reasons for declining levels of analgesia while receiving opioids. Another manifestation might be the experience of excessive pain after an otherwise straightforward surgical procedure. This phenomenon is thought to result from neuroplastic changes in the central and peripheral nervous systems leading to sensitization of pronociceptive pathways. OIH can exist in a wide variety of settings that are described in further detail in later sections of this chapter.

Differentiation of Opioid Tolerance and Opioid-Induced Hyperalgesia

A common clinical observation in patients receiving opioid medication for the treatment of pain is the need to increase the dose over time in some patients to maintain adequate analgesia. This observation is typically ascribed to the development of tolerance to the analgesic effects of opioid medications. However, the loss of analgesic efficacy can also be caused by opioid-induced hyperalgesia. It is important to note that OIH and analgesic tolerance are two distinct pharmacologic phenomena that can result in similar net effects on opioid dose requirements.

For illustrative purposes, we have constructed a theoretical diagram showing changes that may occur after chronic opioid use that are indicative of analgesic tolerance and OIH (Figure 10.1). Figure 10.1(A) describes changes associated with opioid-induced hyperalgesia. In this scenario, a patient with OIH experiences increased pain or enhanced pain sensitivity even in the setting of low serum opioid levels. This is reflected by a downward shift in the opioid dose-analgesic response curve. These patients have uniquely increased sensitivity to pain (y-axis) at baseline (eg, in the absence of opioid analgesia), compared to opioid-naïve individuals. This figure suggests that OIH might be most evident between doses of opioids or during periods of abstinence when serum opioid levels nadir and may unmask underlying opioid-induced hyperalgesia. This observation is consistent with a central or peripheral sensitization of pronociceptive pathways that is thought to underlie the mechanism of OIH.

In contrast, Figure 10.1(B) represents changes associated with the development of analgesic tolerance. These changes are uniquely characterized by a rightward shift of the opioid dose-analgesic response curve that is consistent with habituation or desensitization of antinociceptive pathways mediated by opioid medications. It is important to note that both OIH and analgesic tolerance result in an observed decrease in opioid effectiveness for a given dose of medication. It could therefore be difficult in some clinical settings to determine if a patient were developing OIH, tolerance, or both, to opioids. Carefully documenting baseline pain and analgesic sensitivity using quantitative sensory testing before and after initiating chronic opioid therapy may help elucidate this diagnostic dilemma.

Analgesic Paradox of Dose Escalation

The observation that two pharmacologically distinct mechanisms may have similar net effects on opioid dose escalation over time has important clinical implications. In the case of analgesic tolerance, *desensitization of opioid antinociceptive* pathways over time can be addressed by simply increasing the opioid dose. However, patients with OIH suffer from *sensitization of pronociceptive pathways* and this same maneuver will paradoxically aggravate the problem and worsen the patient's pain. Patients with OIH will require other means of acute pain management that do not involve dose escalation of opioid medications.

In clinical practice, it may be difficult to distinguish these two phenomena because the observed dose escalation may be a manifestation of pharmacologically distinct and dimorphic etiologies involving desensitization of antinociceptive and/or sensitization of pronociceptive pathways. Further complicating the picture is the fact that even chronic forms of pain will naturally wax and wane and the underlying disease causing the chronic pain may progress over time. A clear understanding of the molecular mechanisms and clinical presentation of opioid tolerance and OIH will help the clinician correctly diagnose and determine the best approach to treat acute pain in these patients.

ANALGESIC TOLERANCE

Introduction to Tolerance

The term *tolerance* as defined in the preceding sections refers to the waning analgesic effect of opioids when administered chronically. It is important to note that this term is often used freely to describe any loss in analgesia, but providers must be very wary of alternative explanations. It is important not to invoke this explanation for declining treatment effects if advancing nociceptive stimulation or disease is the true root cause. For example, loss of treatment effect in a patient being treated for pain related to a malignancy might result from advancing disease or the effects of

chemotherapy or radiation. In such a situation, reevaluation of disease status should be completed promptly. When dealing with a patient experiencing pain of nonmalignant etiology, advancing underlying disease like progressive arthritic changes, disk degeneration, or nerve damage might explain the requirement for increasing doses of opioids to maintain a specified level of relief. In this case, objective documentation of advancing disease may be inconclusive as little relationship exists between x-rays, MRI scans, findings on physical exam, and so on, and reported pain levels. Advancing pain because of central and peripheral nerve damage is particularly problematic as it is often very unclear what the specific mechanism of pain generation might be. Even though neuropathic pain may be properly thought of as chronic in many situations, this is not to say that a stable course is expected. The nature and intensity of neuropathic pain of many common etiologies, including postherpetic neuralgia, diabetic neuropathy, amputation, spinal cord injury, and thalamic stroke, can all wax and wane over time. Alternative mechanisms explaining escalating opioid requirements need not be limited to physical issues, especially when dealing with chronic nonmalignant pain. For example, depression, anxiety, legal issues, and psychosocial stressors all play a role in the success of a pain management program.

In acute and subacute settings, for example, when treating postoperative pain or pain from trauma, it is particularly important to be aware of alternative explanations to tolerance when opioid requirements escalate. Perioperatively the causes of enhanced pain from the surgical area could involve a range of etiologies, including infection, bleeding, ischemia, failure of an element of the surgical procedure, rapidly advancing primary disease, new injury, and so on. Alternative explanations need to be considered and pursued at the same time that the patient's need for comfort is addressed; these are not mutually exclusive goals. Thus, in clinical settings, assignment of the diagnosis of opioid tolerance is often clouded by uncertainty surrounding the underlying cause of the pain.

Acute Opioid Tolerance

What, then, is the human evidence for opioid analgesic tolerance? Though the published data are quite limited at this point, several studies are worthy of mention. Beginning at the acute end of the treatment duration spectrum, investigators have infused human volunteers with opioids for a period of hours while following opioid analgesia in the subjects. This type of paradigm is perhaps closest in a clinical sense to how drugs might be administered perioperatively. Unfortunately, the data are somewhat mixed. An early study using the cold pressor model of pain involving immersion of the hand and arm in ice water showed an apparent fading of analgesia after about 90 minutes of remifentanil infusion.[37] This was interpreted as showing an acute tolerance and raised the question as to whether it was possible, even during the course of opioid infusion used as part of an anesthetic plan, that patients would accommodate to the ongoing presence of these drugs and show less effect. A subsequent study probably more rigorous in design suggests that at least for remifentanil used at clinically relevant infusion rates, we may not have much about which to be concerned.[38] This follow-up study used heat and electrical models of pain in human volunteers and demonstrated stable levels of analgesia with remifentanil infusion for 3 hours. The incorporation of a control group into the study paradigm makes the data particularly compelling.

Other clinical data approach the issue of acute tolerance from a different angle. Several studies have been constructed to randomize patients to either high or low doses of intraoperative opioids and have followed postoperative opioid consumption and pain as indices of opioid sensitivity and tolerance. These studies have the feature of using opioid administration protocols within the range of what are actually used in a relevant clinical setting and follow endpoints that help us address our actual clinical concern. The majority of this work has shown somewhat higher rates of opioid consumption in patients receiving larger intraoperative opioid doses than those receiving smaller total doses,[39–42] although not all studies have reached this conclusion.[38,43] These results may seem paradoxical given the lingering belief that aggressive intraoperative analgesia might actually reduce postoperative pain and analgesic requirements. Somewhat reassuringly, the amount of increase in postoperative opioids was found to be relatively small and generally within the range of what would otherwise be available to the patient by using a patient-controlled analgesia (PCA) device. Not resolved at this point is whether modest to moderate differences in postoperative opioid consumption potentially resulting from limited acute opioid tolerance lead to poorer pain control, greater frequency of opioid side effects, poorer surgical outcomes, and so on. Furthermore, it is unclear whether other aspects of the anesthetic plan (eg, concomitantly administered agents) might be able to mitigate any tolerance occurring acutely. Finally, it should be noted that these types of clinical data provide only indirect evidence for the development of tolerance and an alternative explanation (ie, OIH may explain observed differences in postoperative opioid consumption and pain).

The issue of opioid tolerance occurring in the setting of acute and self-limited pain can also be approached from the aspect of clinical experience. After all, a tremendous collective experience in the management of postoperative pain and pain related to minor and major injuries is available. It is most often observed, whether the source of the pain is surgical or from some other traumatic injury expected to heal without sequelae, that most patients consume relatively large amounts of analgesics for the first few days, but then requirements taper rapidly. In fact, virtually all studies following postoperative PCA opioid consumption demonstrate a peak of use during the first 24 hours followed by rapidly tapering requirements depending on the type of surgery or trauma. This is not to say that all patients can be made comfortable immediately using systemic opioids or that there is not substantial variation in opioid requirements between patients, because there are.[44] However, a pattern of steadily increasing postoperative or posttraumatic opioid requirement should be cause for reevaluation of the source of the pain and reasons for the increasing discomfort. Seldom will practitioners arrive at the conclusion that some form of opioid adaptation like tolerance is responsible for escalating early postoperative analgesic requirements.

Although often vaguely described, tolerance to fentanyl, remifentanil, and similar opioids has been reported in the literature pertaining to sedation, such as occurs in intensive care units, particularly in pediatric intensive care units (see Delvaux et al).[45] Generally these reports involve sedation during mechanical ventilation using near-anesthetic infusion rates of opioids for several days. Dose escalation is often reported and seems to be commonplace in the intensive care setting. In one particularly elegant report, Tobias et al[46] used monitoring of the bispectral processed electroencephalogram index to document escalating opioid requirements in an intensive care unit (ICU) patient receiving opioids. Although dose increases or the inclusion of additional sedatives generally allows ongoing sedation of these ICU patients, opioid withdrawal can be problematic and may require slow weaning of the opioids in the extubation and recovery process. The particular prevalence of tolerance and dependence in the pediatric setting seems to parallel observations made in rodent model systems in which young animals acquire tolerance more rapidly than older ones.[47]

Tolerance after Chronic Administration

The case for opioid tolerance with chronic opioid administration is quite different. Ideally, we would hope to address the issue of tolerance by prospectively following a group of patients initiated and maintained on opioids with similar pain etiologies in blinded placebo-controlled fashion. This type of study is unavailable. One study using a reasonable, but nonoptimal structure prospectively followed back pain patients given morphine.[33] In this study, opioid analgesic dose responsiveness was assessed using experimental pain paradigms and computer-targeted infusions both before and at 1 and 6 months after the initiation of treatment. Significant changes were noted in opioid potency even after 1 month of treatment. Inter-subject variability was, however, high. For no subject was tolerance complete, however.

Observational evidence collected from postoperative patients demonstrates that chronically opioid-consuming patients often require substantial increases in opioid administration to achieve pain control. In a sentinel study, de Leon-Casasola et al[48] measured the postoperative opioid requirements for chronically opioid-consuming patients versus opioid-naïve controls. The chronically opioid-consuming patients were on average consuming 183 mg of oral morphine equivalent per day. Postoperative pain was managed with epidural morphine and local anesthetic mixtures. The previously opioid-consuming patients required approximately 3 times as much epidural morphine to maintain a level of comfort similar to the previously opioid-naïve patients. The chronically opioid-consuming patients also required approximately 4 times as much breakthrough intravenous morphine. In a separate case-controlled study by Rapp et al,[49] postoperative PCA morphine requirements were compared for 180 chronic opioid-consuming and 180 control patients having major surgeries. Distinct from the patients followed in the epidural study, these opioid-consuming patients were using only about a 40-mg morphine oral equivalent. In this study, PCA morphine requirements were also about 3 times as large for previously opioid-consuming patients as drug naïve controls. It is concerning that the chronic opioid-consuming patients did not achieve the same level of pain relief and had higher levels of side effects, including sedation, despite their augmented opioid dosing. Thus, using postoperative pain as the model in which to study tolerance, chronically opioid-consuming patients seem to require several times the total opioid dose to control pain in the postoperative period, and may be more prone to serious side effects. It needs to be emphasized that, although we may be able to conclude that tolerance was observed in a cross-sectional sense, the requirements for individual patients was quite variable. Thus, it was not concluded that a reliable and safe prediction of postoperative opioid requirements could be made from preoperative data alone. Moreover, there are many patient variables that have been linked to opioid requirements like sex, age, depression, anxiety, neuroticism, and

Table 10.1: Factors Tending to Promote Increasing Use of Opioids versus Those Tending to Limit Dose Increases; Note That Analgesic Tolerance Is Only One of Many Factors Affecting Opioid Dosing

Factors Limiting Dose Increases	Factors Promoting Dose Increases
Fear of dependence or addiction	Analgesic tolerance
Side effects	Advancing underlying disease
Lack of efficacy of preceding dose increases	Exacerbation of depression, anxiety or other psychosocial factors
Costs	Addiction or diversion
Physician attitudes	Opioid-induced hyperalgesia

preexisting pain conditions, in addition to the preoperative use of opioids.[50–54] It is noteworthy that some of the psychological factors like depression are independently associated with an increased likelihood to consume opioids and to suffer from aggravated perioperative pain.[55]

Other clinical evidence is available from various sources indicating that for many patients with relatively stable pain conditions, opioid dose requirements rise over time at a variable rate. Following the amount of drug prescribed to or consumed by patients is often taken as a measurement of opioid requirement to reach a certain level of pain control. Thus, some would conclude that changes in the quantity of opioid prescribed or consumed can be used as an index of opioid potency and, therefore, constitute a valid index of tolerance. Before proceeding to studies that for the most part rely on this methodology, we need to consider some of the pitfalls associated with this approach. As listed in Table 10.1, many factors other than changes in the intrinsic pharmacological potency of the opioid may influence opioid prescription and consumption. Thus, studies failing to objectively measure opioid potency have significant limitations in power.

Accepting the limitations of the factors listed in Table 10.1, we can proceed to a discussion of typical patterns for opioid dose escalations in patients treated for chronic forms of pain. At this point, a significant number of studies exist showing opioid consumption over time. The stability can be highly variable, although the reader is directed to the reports of Milligan, Galer, Portenoy, and Buntin-Mushock as examples of studies following dose escalation in different settings.[15,47,56,57] The data presented in these studies generally involved substantial sample sizes followed closely for a several-months to 3-year time course. The studies were completed both prospectively as components of analgesic trials, as part of an opioid patient registry effort, and as a retrospective analysis of a single large academic clinic's experience. Although diverse in their structure, the studies reached similar conclusions with respect to the rates of dose escalation. In general, the collective experience involves a period of relatively rapid dose escalation lasting several weeks to a few months in which, if the patients are given the flexibility, doses of opioids seem to increase in a manner paralleling improvement in pain control followed by a period of up to 3 years duration in which doses tend to increase at a slower rate in the setting of stable pain scores. Many patients discontinue opioid use during the first several months of treatment, and this factor does further confound interpretation of the dosing patterns. However, looking at opioid

consumption rates within the confines of what was allowed in these divergent settings, consumption was not observed to spiral upward and out of control. In other words, human tolerance was not judged to advance at a rapid or therapy-limiting rate after the period of initial dose titration. Differences in metabolism of opioids over time have not emerged as able to explain changing dose requirements. As was discussed earlier, however, none of the patients in the studies cited here had formal evaluation of opioid potency against a standardized painful stimulus followed over time. Thus we cannot make any definitive conclusions concerning the long-term rate of tolerance.

Mechanisms of Tolerance

The study of opioid analgesic tolerance has been ongoing since the late 1970s. The vast majority of the work has been pursued in rodent models or in cell lines; little mechanistic information is available from studies using human volunteer or patient populations. Although the use of models has been necessary for progress to be made in terms of understanding tolerance, there are several areas of concern regarding interpretation of most of the available studies. First, the doses of opioids used in rats and mice are far higher than the majority of human patients would ever receive. It is not uncommon, for example, for laboratory mice or rats to receive escalating morphine doses to reach 40–50 mg/kg/d. This is the human equivalent of several grams of drug per day, a relatively uncommon occurrence. Second, the period of exposure to opioids in animal studies is often very acute (single or a few doses), which, as presented before, does not mimic the clinical scenarios where tolerance issues seem to be most problematic. So-called "chronic" dosing in animals often consists of 3–7 days of administration that in human clinical terms is still acute treatment. The reasons for use of these animal dosing strategies are generally that profound tolerance in rodents is often seen after short-term exposure, and there are significant logistic and cost-related difficulties associated with long-term opioid administration. However, the effects studied by investigators are generally very robust and lend themselves to rigorous experimental investigation. So, although human confirmation of even basic mechanistic findings in rodents is generally lacking, we do have a very good understanding at this point of what some of the more likely mechanisms of tolerance might be.

Opioid Receptor Desensitization and Trafficking

One of the most fundamental ways an organism can reduce sensitivity to an agent acting through a receptor is to alter receptor expression and function. These sorts of mechanisms have been demonstrated to apply to opioid receptor signaling. Most of this work has been done on μ-opioid receptor systems as this receptor is likely the most relevant to the overall effects of most commonly used opioids in humans. Reports can be identified demonstrating that under some conditions a reduction in receptor protein or μ-opioid receptor ligand binding can be observed.[58] However, the majority of the work that has been done in rodents using a number of natural and synthetic opioids has failed to find substantial differences in μ-opioid receptor expression in various regions of the brain and spinal cord.[59–62] Although it is possible that in subregions of the brain there are, in fact, relevant changes, we cannot ascribe opioid tolerance to a simple global downregulation of receptors for the commonly used opioids. Thus, attention has turned to the issues of receptor trafficking and receptor-effector coupling.

As opposed to the largely negative data surrounding opioid effects on overall expression levels, a great deal of work has suggested that the μ-opioid receptor (as well as the δ-opioid receptor) are functionally uncoupled from second-messenger systems after acute and chronic opioid exposure. One of the first events in this uncoupling involves phosphorylation. Excellent reviews on the topic of opioid receptor phosphorylation and desensitization are available.[63–65] The rate and degree of phosphorylation are highly dependent on the agonist with more rapid phosphorylation observed for high-potency agonists than for morphine itself.[66–69] The sites of phosphorylation are many, but most work has focused on the cytoplasmic tail with particular attention given to phosphorylation of key serine residues like Ser[375] of the rat μ-opioid receptor.[70] Many protein kinases have predicted or demonstrated phosphorylation sites on the μ-opioid receptor, and, although not the only site of functionally important phosphorylation, Ser[375] seems to be the target for the GRK2 and GRK3 receptor kinases. This phosphorylation is believed to take place within minutes of agonist exposure. Receptor phosphorylation is reversible through the action of intracellular phosphatase enzymes. Phosphorylation of the receptor is felt to interfere with receptor-guanosine triphosphate (GTP) binding protein coupling or with subsequent binding of arrestin molecules and removal of the receptor from the cell surface.

The removal of phosphorylated opioid receptors from the cell surface via clathrin-dependent internalization, the dephosphorylation of the receptors, and, finally, their degradation or recycling to the cell surface have been studied in some detail as well. The β-arrestins are key proteins initiating this process. It has been shown, for example, that μ-opioid receptor activation is rapidly followed by the interaction of this receptor with both β-arrestin 1 and β-arrestin 2.[71,72] The interaction of receptor with arrestin molecules functionally desensitizes the μ-opioid receptors. This interaction is, again, dependent on the agonist used, with much greater β-arrestin interaction initiated by use of selective high-potency agonists as opposed to morphine.[73] Differences in the strength of interaction of opioid receptors with β-arrestins and subsequent internalization and recycling have been implicated in the differences in the rapidity and degree of tolerance observed in response to exposure to opioid ligands.

The actual process of internalization and recycling is probably common to a large degree with other GTP binding protein-coupled receptors (see Claing et al for a review).[74] The general steps are (1) aggregation of β-arrestin or AP-2 adapter protein-associated receptors on the cell surface membrane (oligomerization), (2) activation of clathrin and dynamin under the plasma membrane, and (3) internalization of the receptors for further processing. This internalization can be, for high-affinity agonists, a rapid process taking only minutes to be initiated. The ultimate fate of the receptor in terms of degradation or return to the cell surface membrane depends on the specific agonist molecule used, the state of phosphorylation, the association of β-arrestin, interactions with additional proteins, and the period of exposure of cells to the opioid agonist.

Alterations in GTP Binding Protein Coupling

The step after opioid-receptor interaction in the classical receptor signaling cascade is interaction of receptors with GTP binding proteins and the subsequent interaction of those proteins with additional signaling molecules or effectors such as ion channels. Tolerance to opioids probably involves alterations

in these interactions as well. The types of basic changes that have been noted are as follows: (1) alterations in expression of GTP binding protein subunits and (2) alterations in the coupling of the activated subunits to effector molecules. The details of alterations in coupling to GTP binding proteins was reviewed recently.[75] Functionally we might suspect a fundamental alteration in GTP coupling as chronic exposure to morphine has in some systems been linked to the stimulation as compared with the usual inhibition of adenylate cyclase (AC) activity seen after acute morphine exposure.[76,77]

Several studies have demonstrated the upregulation of G_s in the brain tissue of animals exposed to morphine.[78–80] Recently, it was demonstrated that after chronic morphine administration using a coimmunoprecipitation that μ-opioid receptors were associated with G_s protein.[81] Other data from the same group suggest that a second stimulatory mechanism is operative. In this case the GTP binding protein subunits seem to act under conditions of chronic morphine exposure as stimulatory to AC.[82,83] Although paradoxically opposite effects on the modulation of all opioid coupled effectors has not been demonstrated, these effects on AC show that not only declining, but even opposite opioid effects can result from chronic exposure and explain tolerance.

Protein Kinase Activation

Although several dozen individual protein molecules have been implicated in supporting opioid analgesic tolerance, it is unlikely that all of these molecules are activated independently of one another. One point in signaling pathways where large numbers of downstream molecules can be activated in response to the increased activity of a single protein is when a protein kinase is involved. In the area of opioid tolerance, several kinases have been explored in some detail as to their ability to control a range of downstream molecules functional in the tolerance process. The roles for various protein kinases has been reviewed recently.[84]

Protein kinase C (PKC) is probably the best investigated of the protein kinases relevant to opioid tolerance. One of the first reports of PKC activation during chronic morphine exposure was in 1995 by Mayer et al[85] using autoradiography. These investigators found evidence of PKC translocation in the superficial layers of the spinal cord. Other investigators used enzyme assays to show enhanced PKC activity in CNS tissue from animals chronically exposed to opioids.[86,87] Still other groups used pharmacological inhibitors of varying degrees of specificity to demonstrate that PKC activity may be important for the full manifestation of opioid tolerance.[87,88] The later availability of knockout mice led to conflicting reports of the role of the specific PKC isoform PKC-γ.[89,90] Thus, although there is some uncertainty as to the specific isoforms involved, overall spinal PKC activity is likely related to the development of opioid tolerance.

Calcium/calmodulin-dependent kinase type 2 (CaMKII) is a kinase widely distributed in the central nervous system (CNS) that has been linked to opioid tolerance, learning, and some aspects of chronic pain. This enzyme is upregulated at the mRNA and protein levels in the spinal cords of opioid-tolerant mice and rats.[91,92] Inhibitors of the enzyme can reverse opioid tolerance.[93] In an elegant series of nonpharmacological experiments, Koch et al[94] showed that a constitutively active form of CaMKII could enhance desensitization of μ-opioid receptors in transfected HEK293 cells, whereas transfection with an opioid receptor with mutated CaMKII phosphorylation binding sites (S261A/S266A) showed less desensitization. Although CaMKII has many potential targets in CNS and peripheral neurons, the μ-opioid receptor itself may be one of the more relevant proteins for promoting opioid tolerance.

Several additional kinases in addition to those discussed above have received at least some attention by investigators interested in opioid tolerance. For example, several laboratories have described the involvement of the monoxide signaling systems heme oxygenase and nitric oxide synthase in morphine tolerance.[95–98] The monoxide signaling molecules produce carbon monoxide (CO) and nitric oxide (NO), respectively, and activate guanylate cyclase in a synergistic manner, thus increasing cGMP levels in the CNS,[99,100] The cGMP thus produced can activate protein kinase G (PKG), which goes on to phosphorylate many intracellular targets. In fact, the cGMP signaling system is upregulated at many points after morphine exposure.[98] Likewise, protein kinase A (PKA) is activated by the excess cyclic adenosine monophosphate produced in cells in response to chronic morphine exposure (see previous). Investigators have addressed the issue as to whether PKA inhibitors reduce opioid tolerance, with the results generally suggesting CNS PKA activity is required for ongoing opioid tolerance.[101–104]

N-methyl-D-aspartate Receptor

The *N*-methyl-D-aspartate (NMDA) receptor is one of the principal excitatory receptors and is expressed throughout the CNS. The association between this receptor and opioid tolerance was first reported in 1991 in a series of studies in which morphine was administered systemically along with the noncompetitive NMDA antagonist MK-801.[105] This report was rapidly followed by others showing that the tolerance-reducing effects could be obtained using the intrathecal injection of MK-801.[106,107] It has also been observed that dextromethorphan and several other NMDA antagonists of varying degrees of selectivity can reduce or eliminate opioid tolerance. Later, it was observed that, in the brain and spinal cord, morphine could enhance the expression of NMDA receptor subunits when given in single or multiple daily doses.[97,108,109]

The mechanism whereby activation of the NMDA receptor leads to opioid tolerance has been the subject of a number of investigations.[110–112] The emerging model is that morphine exposure leads to NMDA receptor activation that subsequently opens the NMDA channel pore to admit calcium ion. The increase in calcium ion concentration then activates PKC, which goes on to activate a number of additional proteins, ultimately causing tolerance. The simultaneous activation of glucocorticoid receptors in spinal tissue as a consequence of morphine exposure leading to the upregulation of both PKC and NMDA receptors further supports this process,[113] The authors of the work supporting this mechanism have carefully pointed out that this mechanism is similar to that proposed to support at least some forms of neuropathic pain. Thus, tolerance and some forms of chronic pain may to a degree share mechanistic components. This may also explain the relatively refractory nature of neuropathic pain to treatment with opioids.

The simultaneous administration of an NMDA receptor antagonist, dextromethorphan, and morphine has been used in attempts to reduce opioid tolerance in humans. Galer et al[56] provided data from large-scale clinical trials showing no difference in pain control or opioid consumption in populations of patients with arthritic pain given morphine alone versus morphine plus dextromethorphan. There was no difference in pain control or the amount of morphine consumed between these groups. Reasons for the study's failure include the very limited amount of tolerance seen in the control (morphine) group, inadequate dose of dextromethorphan, or a fundamental difference in human versus rodent physiology.

Ion Channels

Ion channels are some of the final effector molecules involved in tolerance. Regardless of the cellular mechanisms involved, conduction of a nociceptive nerve impulse is ultimately determined by whether a neuron fires or remains quiescent. Because it is the properties of a neuron's ion channels that ultimately govern the probability of firing, ion channels are the final arbiters of analgesia, hyperalgesia, and opioid tolerance. Chronic opioid exposure effects on second-messenger systems were already presented. The activities of both potassium and calcium ion channels are both modulated by some of the same second-messenger systems known to be affected by chronic opioid exposure.

Calcium ion channels were first associated with opioid tolerance when it was noted that calcium ion channel expression increased after chronic opioid exposure.[114] The inflow of calcium ion both participates in the depolarization of excitable cells and supports subsequent calcium-dependent elements of plasticity in those cells. Several other groups provided complementary results with reports of increases in N-type channel binding activity,[115] but no changes in L-type binding[58] after morphine exposure in brain preparations. Using pharmacological tools, evidence has been provided suggesting that activity in N-type,[116] T-type,[116] R-type,[117] and L-type[118] calcium ion channels expressed in the brain and spinal cord support opioid tolerance. In fact, as a general principal calcium ion tends to support tolerance in CNS neurons. Thus intracerebroventricular injections of calcium chelators and ion channel antagonists both reduce morphine tolerance if this opioid is simultaneously administered.[119]

The situation pertaining to the expression and regulation of potassium ion channels is more complex. Reports have provided data generally demonstrating increases in various types of potassium ion channels, including Kv1.5 and 1.6,[120] and ATP-sensitive channels[121] after chronic opioid exposure. Some investigators found little evidence for alterations in functional coupling between opioid receptors and potassium ion channels.[123] Chen et al,[123] however, found that chronic morphine exposure markedly diminished opioid gating of potassium ion channels in amygdala neurons. Furthermore, chronic exposure of dorsal root ganglion neurons to opioid agonists leads to alterations in action potential duration, suggesting diminished potassium channel modulation by opioids.[124,125]

Cytokines and Innate Immunity

Since the late 1990s, the field of pain research has witnessed a rapidly advancing awareness of the roles members of the innate immune system have in controlling pain in various settings. Cytokines in particular have been studied to determine their roles in various types of inflammatory and neuropathic pain (see Watkins et al[126] for a review). It has already been mentioned in this chapter that tolerance and neuropathic pain seem to share some common mechanistic components (ie, the activation of NMDA channels and PKC).[85] Because of the pronociceptive nature of many cytokines produced in glial cells in the CNS, and because opioid tolerance is often associated with the enhancement of nociceptive sensitivity, concerted efforts have been made to identify roles for cytokines in opioid tolerance.

Some of the first steps taken were to determine if chronically administered opioids could activate glia in the spinal cord, and whether these activated glia produce cytokines. Investigators were rapidly able to demonstrate the activation of both microglia and astrocytes in rodent models of tolerance.[127,128] Although activated glia can perform many functions, one is to produce inflammatory mediators such as cytokines. Again, investigators showed that spinal levels of IL-1, IL-2, and IL-6, commonly studied cytokines with many roles in nociception, were increased in abundance after chronic opioid exposure.[129–131] Levels of the same cytokines are not necessarily expressed in greater amounts in skin and peripheral tissue under similar conditions. Broad-spectrum inhibitors of cytokine production, such as interferons, propentofylline, and selective agents like IL-1 receptor antagonist (IL-1ra) can reduce tolerance.[129,132,133] At this point in time we still have a limited knowledge of the range of cytokines produced in response to chronic opioid administration and the functions of each alone or as a group.

Genetic Approaches to Opioid Tolerance

Biomedical science is increasingly turning to the genome to provide clues as to the mechanisms of disease and drug action. One of the many advantages of genomic-based research is that the process for nomination of genes to be investigated in particular phenomena (eg, opioid tolerance) can be objective and independent of the bias of constructing a hypothesis based on existing data. Thus investigators can use naturally occurring variations in DNA sequence and the resulting differences in function to gain insight into complex physiological phenomena.

Differences in the degree of tolerance developing in inbred strains of mice have been investigated for some time.[134,135] The differences can be profound in these models and range from manyfold shifts in opioid dose-response curves to no discernable change in sensitivity for other strains treated with opioids in an identical manner. Using a haplotype-based technique for genomic analysis, Liang and colleagues[136,137] recently identified two genes found to modulate opioid hyperalgesia, physical dependence, and tolerance. The first association to be described using this approach was with the gene coding for the β_2-adrenergic receptor. Antagonists of this receptor were in the same series of experiments found to reduce morphine tolerance. The same result was obtained when comparing wild-type to β_2-adrenergic knockout mice.[136,137] Given the roles in tolerance already demonstrated for changes resulting in the activation of the AC system, this association may be viewed as highly plausible.

A second report from the same team of investigators linked variants of the gene coding for the P-glycoprotein drug transporter to tolerance.[138] In this case it was determined that adequate efflux of opioid from the CNS was required for tolerance to be fully manifest. These results were in line with an earlier report that found that pharmacological blockade of opioid efflux from the CNS could reduce tolerance.[139] It has not yet been determined why opioid efflux from the CNS is required for the full manifestation of tolerance.

Mechanistic Distinction of Tolerance and OIH

Analgesic tolerance and OIH generally occur under similar circumstances. In fact, when a panel of 16 strains of inbred mice were compared with respect to their propensity to develop tolerance versus their propensity to develop OIH, the correlation was high.[138] However, the correlation was not exact. Where examined, most maneuvers that limit opioid tolerance also reduce OIH. These similarities have led some investigators to conclude that opioid tolerance and OIH are really different manifestations of the same underlying physiological changes.[140] In fact, it seems very likely that many opioid-induced phenomena, especially those tending to sensitize nociceptive circuitry, contribute to both phenomena. Moreover, at the bedside, it is often very difficult to separate loss of treatment effect because of tolerance from what might be because of OIH.

There are, however, a few reports suggesting that the two phenomena can be distinguished under at least some conditions. For example, Dunbar and Karamian[141] showed that repeated opioid abstinence during intrathecal opioid infusion could enhance OIH independently of any effect on tolerance. Later studies showed that the intrathecal administration of ketorolac along with morphine could reduce OIH but did not effect tolerance.[142] Thus we might conclude that OIH and tolerance are phenomena with significant but perhaps not complete overlap. As such, it is possible that strategies could emerge that would be more effective in treating one over the other phenomenon.

OPIOID-INDUCED HYPERALGESIA

OIH versus Opioid Dosage

It is perhaps useful from a clinical, if not mechanistic, standpoint to consider OIH in three different settings. As reviewed in detail elsewhere, OIH is seen in both humans and in animal models in the settings of very low-dose opioid administration, during maintenance dosing, and when doses are extremely high.[28] The vast majority of experimental and clinical data concerns the situation where opioid doses are relatively stable or are oscillating in a manner consistent with standard therapeutic approaches. We, therefore, focus our discussion on the human and animal data related to these scenarios. We refrain from discussing OIH in the setting of very low-dose opioid administration as the clinical relevance of this phenomena has yet to be established and been discussed elsewhere.[28] Finally, we briefly discuss OIH when opioid doses are extremely high.

OIH Occurrence under Common Therapeutic Conditions: Human Evidence

Clinical reports of hyperalgesia associated with opioid use span more than 100 years, as noted by Rossbach in 1880, "[W]hen dependence on opioids finally becomes an illness of itself, opposite effects like restlessness, sleep disturbance, hyperesthesia, neuralgia and irritability become manifest."[143] Over the past decade, observational, cross sectional, and prospective controlled trials have began to characterize the expression and potential clinical significance of OIH in humans. These studies have been conducted using several distinct cohorts and methodologies: (1) former opioid addicts on methadone maintenance therapy, (2) perioperative exposure to opioids in patients undergoing surgery, (3) healthy human volunteers after acute opioid exposure using human experimental pain testing, and, more recently, (4) a prospective observational study in opioid-naïve pain patients undergoing initiation of chronic opioid therapy.

Former Opioid Addicts on Methadone Maintenance Therapy

A number of studies have examined pain sensitivity in opioid addicts maintained on methadone using cold pressor, electrical, and pressure pain models.[144–150] These studies show a modality-specific hyperalgesia to cold pressor pain in these patients compared to matched or healthy controls.[144–148] In contrast, hyperalgesia was weak or absent in electrically and mechanically evoked pain models.[144,148–150] Studies of healthy human volunteers were also unable to detect development of OIH in thermal pain models.[152,153] These results suggest that OIH develops differently for various types of pain.[144,148,149]

Recently Pud et al[153] conducted a study of cold pressor testing in a cohort of opioid addicts (OA) presenting for a 4-week inpatient detoxification program. Cold pressor pain measurements were taken on admission and 7 and 28 days thereafter. In contrast to previous studies, the authors found increased latency to the onset of pain and decreased VAS pain scores for peak pain in the OA group compared to healthy controls. However, they did resolve a significant decrease (~50%) in cold pressor tolerance in the OA group compared to controls that is consistent with earlier findings by other investigators.[144–148] The authors could not readily explain the mixed finding of increased cold pressor latency and hypoalgesia in the setting of decreased cold pressor tolerance and putative hyperalgesia in the OA group. They postulate that pain avoidance behavior[154,155] and markedly low frustration levels[156] may cause addicts to initially deny the feeling of pain. However, when denial becomes impossible, their tendency to overreact[157] causes them to very quickly terminate the stimulus. Therefore, it may not be so much the intensity of pain as it may be the aversive character and/or unpleasantness of pain that becomes exaggerated in these patients. This may also explain why OIH is much more prominent in the cold pressor test than in models of acute heat and electrical pain. The latter pain models cause significantly less pronounced negative affect than the cold pressor test at similar levels of pain intensity.[158]

The Pud study also offers some insight into the reversibility of OIH in this population. The authors did not see a significant change in pain sensitivity over time during the 4 weeks of opioid abstinence. This is in contrast to work by Compton[145] and Hay et al,[159] who found higher pain tolerance and decreased pain sensitivity in opioid addicts who were abstinent for 6 months to 1 year compared to current opioid users or controls. These results suggest that OIH in this patient population may be reversible to some extent but requires a long period of opioid abstinence.

Taken as a whole, these studies provide observations that are compatible with the hypothesis that OIH is caused by chronic opioid exposure. It is important to understand the limitations of these studies. The cross-sectional or retrospective nature of these studies (ie, the cohort was already chronically exposed to opioids) precludes establishing a firm causal relationship between opioid use and development of OIH. In addition, unique properties of the OA population may confound pain measurements in these patients. Finally, another limitation of these studies is the possibility that increased pain sensitivity may intrinsically predispose people to become opioid addicts and require methadone to prevent relapse after detoxification. This hypothesis is supported by the observation that current users of opioid or cocaine are more sensitive to cold pressor pain than former users of either drug.[145]

Perioperative Exposure to Opioids

A small number of clinical studies have looked at OIH in the setting of acute perioperative opioid exposure. Two prospective controlled clinical studies reported increased postoperative pain despite increased postoperative opioid use in patients who received high doses of intraoperative opioids.[39,42] A separate study of women undergoing cesarean section found intraoperative exposure to intrathecal fentanyl also leads to a similar finding of increased postoperative opioid consumption without improved analgesia compared to women who received placebo intrathecal saline injections.[40] More recently, a study by Joly et al[160] directly measured the development of secondary wound hyperalgesia after acute intraoperative opioid exposure. The authors found that high-dose intraoperative exposure to the potent, ultrashort-acting μ-opioid agonist remifentanil increased peri-incisional wound allodynia and hyperalgesia measured by von Frey hairs compared to low-dose intraoperative remifentanil in patients undergoing major abdominal surgery.

In contrast, other studies showed no effect of intraoperative opioid dose on postoperative pain sensitivity. Cortinez et al found neither increased pain nor postoperative opioid consumption after high-dose intraoperative remifentanil exposure in patients undergoing elective gynecologic surgery.[43] A more recent study by Lee et al[161] also failed to see a significant difference in postoperative pain or opioid consumption in patients who received intraoperative remifentanil compared to 70% nitrous oxide after colorectal surgery. Finally, Hansen et al[162] also failed to see a sustained significant difference in postoperative pain or opioid consumption in patients who received intraoperative remifentanil compared to saline infusion after major abdominal surgery. Although the authors of this study did find a significant increase in VAS score in the remifentanil group compared to placebo during the immediate postoperative period that is suggestive of OIH, this difference was no longer significant 2 hours after surgery or during the remainder of the 24-hour observation period. The failure to observe an effect of intraoperative opioid exposure on postoperative pain and opioid consumption in these studies may be because of lower total intraoperative opioid exposure in the cases of the Cortinez and Lee studies when compared to the positive results of Guignard et al,[42] suggesting a dose-dependent effect of opioids on the development of OIH.

These observations provide mixed support for a hypothesis of development of OIH after acute perioperative opioid exposure. Importantly, these observations provide only indirect evidence in support of this phenomenon. As noted previously in this chapter, the need for dose escalation to maintain analgesia can be because of the development of analgesic tolerance, opioid-induced hyperalgesia, or simultaneous expression of both phenomena. No causal relationship between acute perioperative opioid exposure and development of OIH can be established without direct measurement of pain sensitivity. Although Joly et al[160] have successfully implemented quantitative assessment of pain into a clinical study of OIH and postoperative pain, further work incorporating these methodologies into high-quality prospective trials will be needed to further characterize the expression and clinical significance of OIH after acute opioid exposure in the perioperative setting.

Acute Opioid Exposure in Healthy Volunteers using Experimental Pain Methods

Several studies have examined the development of OIH in humans after acute short-term exposure to opioids. Multiple

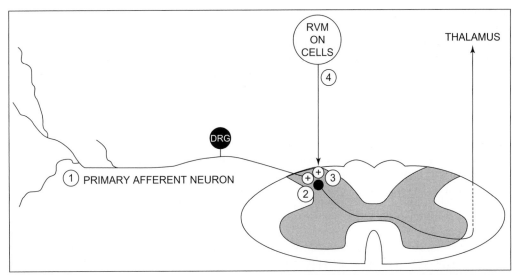

Figure 10.2: Possible molecular mechanisms for opioid-induced hyperalgesia. Some mechanisms that have been studied include (1) sensitization of primary afferent neurons, (2) enhanced production and release of excitatory neurotransmitters as well as diminished reuptake of neurotransmitters, (3) sensitization of second-order neurons to excitatory neurotransmitters, and (4) neuroplastic changes in the rostral ventromedial medulla that may increase descending facilitation via "on-cells" leading to upregulation of spinal dynorphin and enhanced primary afferent neurotransmitter release and pain.

studies have found aggravation of experimentally induced hyperalgesic skin lesions after short-term infusion of remifentanil. Angst et al[157] and Koppert et al[163–165] found significant enlargement of the area of mechanical hyperalgesia induced by transdermal electrical stimulation after 30 to 90 minutes of exposure to remifentanil. Using the heat-capsaicin-rekindling model, Hood et al[151] found a similar aggravation of hyperalgesia after 60- to 100-minute remifentanil infusions. This hyperalgesia was observed up to 4 hours after remifentanil exposure was discontinued and was absent when assessed on the following day. Aggravation of pressure-evoked pain after short-term remifentanil infusion in a single study of healthy volunteers has also been reported, although unequal nociceptive input during remifentanil and control infusions may account for the observed postinfusion hyperalgesia.[166] Finally, Compton et al[167,168] found increased sensitivity to cold pressor pain in a small cohort of healthy human volunteers following precipitated opioid withdrawal after induction of acute physical opioid dependence. Taken together, these findings provide direct evidence for development of OIH in humans using models of secondary hyperalgesia and cold pressor pain.

Prospective Observational Study in Chronic Pain Patients

Although the studies cited above provide useful information, they are somewhat limited by their cross-sectional rather than prospective study design, failure to distinguish tolerance from hyperalgesia, or use of short-term rather than the long-term opioid exposure that is typical when opioids are used for the treatment of chronic pain. Recently, Chu et al[33] attempted to overcome some of these shortcomings by conducting the first prospective observational study documenting the development of opioid-induced hyperalgesia in opioid-naïve chronic pain patients.

Patients with moderate to severe chronic low back pain were prospectively assessed for both analgesic tolerance and hyperalgesia after 1 month of oral morphine therapy using tonic cold (cold pressor) and phasic heat experimental pain models. The study found significant hyperalgesia and analgesic tolerance in the cold but not heat pain models. This modality-specific response suggests that certain types of pain are more likely to be aggravated by OIH than others. Indeed, human experimental pain studies by Doverty et al[148] showed more pronounced hyperalgesia in the cold pressor model than a model of electrical pain in methadone maintenance patients compared to matched controls. Angst et al[152] and Hood et al[151] also failed to show hyperalgesia to heat pain in the setting of aggravated mechanical hyperalgesia after cessation of acute remifentanil infusion in healthy human volunteers. There are, however, several limitations of this study. The study cohort reflects a very small sample size, and there was no placebo group or blinding of subjects and the investigators to the treatment. Despite these limitations, this preliminary study is the first to prospectively document development of OIH in opioid-naïve chronic pain patients and suggests that the phenomenon can occur within 4 weeks after exposure to moderate doses (median dose 75 mg/d) of morphine.

Mechanisms of OIH

More than 90 publications have described and characterized OIH in various animal models. The majority of these have been tabulated and presented in a recent publication.[28] These studies suggest a model for OIH that considers this process to be neurobiologically multifactorial. It appears that, in general, neurobiological systems that respond to opioids acutely to provide analgesia may change over time in such a way as to enhance nociception, especially in the setting of declining opioid doses. A diagram of several of the best investigated sites of such plasticity is provided in Figure 10.2. The mechanisms relevant to each site are probably unique.

Peripheral Effects of OIH

The terminals of primary afferent neurons were the first site of plasticity contributing to OIH that was evaluated in animals.

Because it was recognized that μ-opioid receptors are expressed on both the central and peripheral terminals of primary afferent neurons, it was considered possible that the peripheral injection of selective opioid agonists could cause functional changes in the neurons. In a series of studies, the selective μ-opioid agonist DAMGO was injected in microliter volumes into the skin of the hind paws of rats.[169–173] These injections were acutely associated with antinociception, repeated injection was associated with tolerance, and mechanical hyperalgesia was interpreted as a sign of "local" physical dependence. This ability to cause tolerance and hyperalgesia was not limited to opioid receptors as α_1-adenosine and α_2-adenosine agonists lead to similar findings.[172] Subsequent studies revealed roles for PKC and AC in modulating this phenomenon.[170,171] CNS penetration is therefore not required for some degree of hyperalgesia to emerge from repeated drug administration.

A series of studies by Liang et al[136] later used contemporary genetic mapping techniques to associate the β_2-adrenergic receptor (β_2-AR) with OIH after repeated morphine administration to mice. It was observed that the local hind paw administration of selective β_2-AR antagonists reduced the thermal and mechanical manifestations of OIH, whereas the local administration of β_2-AR agonists actually enhanced nociceptive sensitization.

Spinal Effects of OIH

Plasticity underlying OIH has been observed in the spinal cord after intraspinal and systemic opioid administration. One of the first studies in this area involved the daily bolus administration of intrathecal morphine to rats for more than 1 week.[174] The animals displayed thermal hyperalgesia at both 8 and 10 days after initiation of treatment. Later observations, largely confirmed by subsequent investigators, showed that NMDA and non-NMDA excitatory amino acid receptors as well as PKC mediate this phenomenon. Dunbar and Pulai[175] added to these early observations by showing that if intrathecal morphine was infused in a continuous manner, then the degree of OIH that developed was smaller than if bolus administration with intermittent abstinence was employed. Spinal blockade of the NMDA receptor again reduced OIH.

Other groups have shown that the same systems operate to support OIH after systemic opioid administration. For example, the administration of the NMDA receptor blockers MK-801 or ketamine reduce or reverse OIH because of the chronic (days) systemic administration of opioids to rats and mice.[176–183] Likewise, animals lacking the gene for PKC-γ did not develop OIH normally after systemic opioid administration.[184] The PKC observations were further supported by the work of Sweitzer et al,[185] who used primarily pharmacological tools to show PKC isoforms participated in OIH as studies in rat pups.

Since the time of the early observations, more spinal receptor systems have been explored in the setting of OIH. For example, the enhanced production and release of spinal dynorphin seems to support OIH.[186] Likewise, spinal cyclooxyganase has been implicated in intrathecal injection of ibuprofen reduces OIH.[187] Spinal cytokines like IL-1 and chemokines like fractalkine have been implicated as well.[129] The latter observations connect OIH with the emerging appreciation of spinal inflammation as participating in many abnormal pain syndromes. More recently Vera-Portocarrero et al[188] provided an elegant series of studies in which substance P (sP) conjugated to saporin was used as an intrathecal neurotoxin to ablate neurokinin 1 receptor expressing cells in the spinal cord. This maneuver prevented the normally observed morphine-induced sensitization in rats. These investigators also discovered that the serotonin 5-HT3 receptor that participates in a spinal-supraspinal-spinal loop to maintain nociceptive sensitization, needed to be active for expression of OIH.

Regardless of the pharmacological basis for spinal sensitization by opioids, additional biochemical and behavioral observations suggest that the dorsal horn of the spinal cord is central to many of the mechanisms converging to support OIH. The intrathecal injection of sP or glutamate lead to greatly enhanced nociceptive behaviors when compared with saline treated OIH-induced mice.[189] In addition, neuronal activation in the spinal cord dorsal horn (as shown by Fos expression) was far greater in the morphine-treated animals after intrathecal SP or glutamate injection. This evidence suggests that spinal cord neurons are sensitized to nociceptive neurotransmitters after chronic morphine treatment.[189] It is important to note that chronic morphine treatment causes the increased expression of the nociceptive neurotransmitters sP and calcitonin gene-related peptide (CGRP).[190] Moreover, chronic opioid administration leads to decreased expression of the spinal glutamate transporters excitatory amino-acid carrier 1 and glutamate/aspartate transporter. Thus, once released, excitatory amino acids linger in the synapse for a sustained period.[191]

Supraspinal Effects of OIH

Although the majority of the work done in exploring the mechanistic basis of OIH has involved the spinal cord and peripheral neurons, there is growing appreciation that higher CNS centers may participate in supporting this and other forms of abnormal pain sensitivity through enhanced descending facilitation to the spinal cord dorsal horn. The focus of this work has been the rostral ventromedial medulla (RVM). Microinjection of local anesthetic to stop neuronal discharge from this structure or lesioning of the dorsolateral funiculus which carries descending nerve fibers from the RVM prevents or reverses not only OIH but also tolerance to opioids.[140,192] Work pursuant to these observations suggests that cholecystokinin released in the RVM and acting through cholecystokinin 2 receptors might activate the RVM and support the descending influences.[193]

Opioid Distribution

The OIH mechanisms that have been presented thus far involve pharmacodynamic etiologies. Indeed, little evidence has emerged over the years for pharmacokinetic factors governing phenomena such as opioid tolerance or hyperalgesia. Recent results have caused us to reappraise this situation. Liang et al[138] used an in silico haplotypic genetic mapping strategy to identify genes linked to the thermal OIH trait after measuring the degree of thermal sensitization developing after 4 days of morphine treatment in 16 inbred strains of mice. The most strongly linked gene was that coding for the P-glycoprotein drug transporter. This relatively nonselective drug transporter was known to be able to control brain levels of opioids, including morphine, by mediating the efflux of the drug across the blood-brain barrier.[194] Additional studies showed that inhibition of P-glycoprotein eliminated OIH as did genetic deletion of the *abcb1a/b* genes coding for P-glycoprotein transporters in mice. Finally, brain levels of morphine were inversely statistically correlated with the development of OIH in the inbred strains. This evidence suggests that drug distribution as well as pharmacodynamic issues need to be considered in understanding OIH.

OIH: Very High Opioid Doses

OIH has also been observed when very large doses of opioids are provided or the doses of opioids are rapidly escalated. Although there is a dearth of high-quality prospective clinical evidence to characterize very high dose OIH, many case reports or series exist (Table 10.2). Most of these reports involve the systemic or intrathecal administration of morphine, raising the possibility that metabolites such as morphine-3-glucuronide, which is known to cause neuroexcitation, could contribute to hyperalgesia.[195–197] In this setting many patients develop both increased pain at the sites of ongoing pain as well as allodynia or even myoclonus.[198–200] Opioid rotation or substitution of a different opioid generally reduced the symptoms sharply.[199,201–204]

Animal studies have replicated these findings. Several studies using rats demonstrated that the intrathecal injection of opioids at doses 10 times or more those typically employed in analgesic studies evoked segmental nocifensive behaviors.[205–207] In contrast to the low-dose OIH phenomenon, high-dose OIH does not appear to be mediated by opioid receptors.[205–209] Two of the key pieces of information leading to this conclusion are that opioid antagonists do not efficiently reduce this type of OIH, and the stereospecificity of high-dose OIH does not fit the specificity for binding to opioid receptors.

Two nonopioid receptor systems may contribute to these effects. The first is glycine. The intrathecal injection of glycine dose dependently reversed the allodynia caused by the intrathecal administration of high doses of morphine.[209] These effects were compatible with the excitatory and allodynia producing effects of intrathecal strychnine.[207] It is not clear whether these effects are mediated through the glycine binding site on the NMDA receptor or perhaps some other site.[209] Other studies have focused on the spinal cord NMDA receptor system for mediating the hyperalgesia and allodynic effects of large doses of morphine. For example, the NMDA receptor antagonist MK-801 reduced the allodynia caused by the intrathecal injection of morphine in rats.[208]

High-dose opioid OIH is an uncommon but problematic clinical phenomenon. Clinical situations do not always suggest OIH is the only possible cause of the accelerating pain symptoms. Considerable clinical confidence is required to reduce opioid doses in patients experiencing large amounts of pain. For this reason, one of the maneuvers commonly recommended when faced with this uncertain situation is to rotate the opioid.[28,201,203,204,210] In fact, methadone seems to have particular efficacy in reducing high-dose opioid OIH.[199,203,210] This may be due to methadone's weak NMDA receptor blocking properties.[211]

Modulation of OIH with Multimodal Therapies

The precise molecular mechanisms responsible for the development of OIH are just beginning to be understood. Preclinical models implicate the glutaminergic system and pathological activation of NMDA receptors in the development of central sensitization. Clinical work in attenuating or preventing the expression of OIH has primarily focused on manipulation of the glutaminergic system, either through direct or indirect modulation of the NMDA receptor (Table 10.3). Although few studies

have looked directly at modulation of OIH in humans, growing preclinical and clinical evidence suggest a role for biochemical modulation of OIH with adjuvant therapies, specifically NMDA receptor antagonists, α_2 agonists, and COX-2 inhibitors (Table 10.4). Evidence in support of these drug targets are discussed in the subsequent sections. However, the clinical efficacy and significance of these approaches still need to be studied in large, prospective clinical trials.

Human Evidence for NMDA Receptor Modulation of OIH

The NMDA receptor is composed of several different subunits (NR1, NR2A-D, and sometimes NR3A/B) that are variably expressed in different regions of the brain and during development.[212] The subunit expression of individual NMDA receptors can affect their function and binding sensitivity to neuromodulators.[213] Splicing variants of these subunits further diversifies receptor expression.[214] The varied and ubiquitous expression of NMDA receptors throughout the CNS can create challenges in targeting pathological activation of NMDA receptors while still permitting normal physiologic activation to occur. Indeed, side effects associated with first-generation NMDA receptor antagonists, such as ketamine and dextromethorphan, have limited their clinical utility in some patients precisely because of this reason.

Ketamine Modulation of OIH

Ketamine is well known as a dissociative anesthetic developed for clinical use in the 1960s. It uniquely provides rapid hypnosis and analgesia while maintaining cardiovascular function with minimal depression of respiratory drive and airway muscle activity and tone.[215,216] A relatively high incidence of psychotomimetic effects, especially when used as a sole anesthetic agent, have limited its clinical use as an anesthetic agent in recent times.[217]

Ketamine is known to be an uncompetitive antagonist of the phencyclidine binding site of the NMDA receptor, where its primary anesthetic effects are thought to occur.[218] Several recent studies have examined the use of ketamine in low subanesthetic doses in conjunction with opioid medications in an attempt to attenuate the expression of OIH and/or analgesic tolerance, largely because of its NMDA receptor antagonist properties.

Meta-analysis of studies examining perioperative low-dose ketamine in conjunction with opioid administration found small improvements in postoperative pain scores and delayed time to first analgesic request, but these outcomes were not clinically significant.[219] However, perioperative ketamine did reduce postoperative opioid consumption by 30%, but did not reduce opioid-associated side effects except for nausea and vomiting[220] and was not found to be a significant adjuvant to opioid administered by PCA devices.[221] Despite these findings, two studies have shown marked reduction in postoperative wound hyperalgesia with perioperative ketamine administration, consistent with attenuation of central sensitization.[222,223] Although the effect of ketamine on postoperative wound hyperalgesia is not related to OIH *per se*, it suggests a role for ketamine in attenuating the expression other conditions associated with central sensitization, such as OIH.

Where ketamine has found significant utility is in patients who require large amounts of opioid medications or exhibit some degree of opioid tolerance.[225–227] Human experimental pain studies have directly shown that administration

Table 10.2: Case Reports Documenting High-Dose, Opioid-induced Allodynia/Hyperalgesia

Reference	Opioid	Route	Dose	Hyperalgesia (n)	Remarks
Sjogren et al (1994)[199]	M	PO, IM, IV	60–300 mg/d PO; 150–960 mg/d IM; 20 g/d IV	Generalized allodynia, myocloni (1)	N = 4; cancer pain; substituting morphine with methadone, sufentanil, or ketobemidone reversed allodynia
Sjogren et al (1993)[198]	M	IV	175–200 mg/h	Generalized allodynia (5), aggravated neuralgia (3), myocloni (4)	N = 8; cancer pain (described in detail, n = 2), dose escalation aggravated allodynia
Wilson et al (2003)[200]	M	IT	37.5 mg/h	Spontaneous pain, allodynia not reported	n = 1; cancer pain, 50-fold reduction of IT morphine resolved pain aggravation.
De Conno et al (1991)[201]	M	IT	80 mg/d	Spontaneous pain and allodynia in dermatomes S5-T5, myocloni	N = 1; cancer pain, primary pain T4-T7, dose reduction to 50 mg/d reduced allodynia
Lawlor et al (1997)[210]	M	IV	600 mg/h	Generalized allodynia, myocloni	N = 1; cancer pain, substituting morphine with methadone reversed allodynia
Sjogren et al (1998)[203]	M	PO, IT	400 mg/d IV; 48 mg/d IT	Generalized or lumbosacral segmental allodynia, myocloni (1)	N = 3; cancer and nonmalignant pain (described in detail, n = 2), dose reduction or substituting morphine with sufentanil, gentanyl, or methadone reversed allodynia
Heger et al (1999)[204]	M	IV	105 mg/h	Generalized allodynia	N = 1; cancer pain in infant, reduction of morphine resolved allodynia
Parisod et al (2003)[313]	M	IT	0.2 and 0.5 mg bolus	Allodynia in dermatomes T6-T7	N = 1; central pain after spinal injury, administration of naloxone did not reverse hyperalgesia
Mercadante et al (2003)[232]	M/MET	IV/PO	200/75 mg/d; 90/90 mg/d	Generalized allodynia	N = 2; cancer pain, switching second patient to methadone did not reverse hyperalgesia
Devulder (1997)[314]	SF	IT	25–50 mg/d	Generalized allodynia of the lower body	N = 1; left lumbosciatic pain after failed back surgery, cessation of sufentanil resolved allodynia
Mercadante et al (2005)[228]	F	TD	12 mg/d (5 patches, 100 mcg/h)	Generalized allodynia, myocloni	N = 1; cancer pain, switching to methadone resolved allodynia
Guntz et al (2007)[315]	F/RF	TD/IV	1.8 mg/d fentanyl (1 patch, 75 mcg/h) and 6.3 mg remifentanil intraoperatively over 5 hours	Severe postoperative pain. Aggravation of pain with morphine bolus.	N = 1; postoperative pain, administration of ketamine and removal of fentanyl patch dramatically reduced pain
Axelrod et al (2007)[229]	F/HM	TD/IV	12 mg/d fentanyl (5 patches, 100 mcg/h), hydromorphone 24 mg/h	Spontaneous pain	N = 1; cancer pain, switching to methadone resulted in adequate pain control
Ackerman (2006)[308]	M/HM	IT	18 mg/d morphine[321]	Pain poorly controlled on high doses IT opioid, no myocloni or allodynia[321]	N = 1; lumbar back pain, tapering of IT opioid and substitution with anticonvulsant, TCA and NSAIDS improved pain control
Chung et al (2004)[230]	HM	IV	1,890 mg/d	Aggravation of pain, myocloni, confusion, hallucinations	N = 1; cancer pain, switching to methadone resulted in resolution of myocloni and resolution of pain

Abbreviations: F = fentanyl; HM = hydromorphone; IT = intrathecal; IV = intravenous, M = morphine, MET = methadone; NSAIDS = nonsteroidal anti-inflammatory drugs; PO = per oral; RF = remifentanil; SF = sufentanil; TCA = tricyclic antidepressants; TD = transdermal.

Table 10.3: Selected Studies Investigating Pharmacologic Modulation of Opioid-Induced Hyperalgesia and/or Analgesic Tolerance in Human

Reference	Model	Drug	Route	Target	Outcome Measure	Remarks
Dudgeon et al (2007)[317]	Cancer pain treated with morphine	DM	PO	NMDA	PS, OC	N = 65; no effect detected.
Galer et al (2005)[56]	Chronic nonmalignant pain treated with morphine	DM	PO	NMDA	PS, OC	N = 829; no effect detected.
Joly et al (2005)[160]	Remifentanil-induced postoperative hyperalgesia	K	IV	NMDA	PPH, OC	N = 75; small dose ketamine prevents remifentanil-induced postoperative hyperalgesia.
Angst et al (2003)[152]	Remifentanil-induced postinfusion aggravation of hyperalgesia (IDES model)	K	IV	NMDA	PPH	N = 10; ketamine abolished remifentanil-induced aggravation of preexisting hyperalgesia.
Koppert et al (2003)[165]	Remifentanil-induced postinfusion aggravation of hyperalgesia (IDES model)	K, C	IV	NMDA	PPH	N = 13; ketamine abolished and clonidine significantly attenuated remifentanil-induced aggravation of preexisting hyperalgesia.
Luginbuhl et al (2003)[166]	Remifentanil-induced hyperalgesia	K	IV	NMDA	EP, PP	N = 14; no effect detected.
Troster et al (2006)[163]	Remifentanil-induced post-infusion aggravation of hyperalgesia (IDES model)	PC	PO	COX2	PPH	N = 15; preventative administration of parecoxib reduced postinfusion hyperalgesia.
Singler et al (2007)[238]	Remifentanil-induced aggravation of hyperalgesia (IDES model)	PR	IV	?NMDA[323–325]	PPH	N=15; propofol attenuates and delays development of postinfusion antianalgesia, but aggravates hyperalgesia.

Abbreviations: C = clonidine; COX2 = cyclooxygenase 2 enzyme; DM = dextromethorphan; EP = electrical pain; K = ketamine; IDES = intradermal electrical stimulation; OC = opioid consumption; PC = parecoxib; PP = pressure pain; PPH = pin-prick hyperalgesia assessed by von Frey hair; PR = propofol; PS = self-reported pain score

of (S)-ketamine abolishes remifentanil-induced aggravation of hyperalgesia induced by intradermal electrical stimulation.[152,165] Joly et al[160] have recently corroborated these findings in the postsurgical patient population.

In summary, there is some evidence to show that perioperative administration of low-dose ketamine may modulate the expression of OIH or analgesic tolerance and that it reduces postoperative wound hyperalgesia after acute intraoperative opioid exposure. These findings support the hypothesis that its NMDA receptor antagonism modulates changes in antinociceptive and pronociceptive systems. However, the clinical significance of these benefits still needs to be proven in larger prospective studies.

Methadone and Opioid Switching for Modulation of OIH

Methadone has been shown to have weak NMDA receptor antagonism.[211] Many case reports show that clinicians choose to switch patients to this opioid when OIH is suspected, such as when high doses of other opioid agents fail to improve or even aggravate chronic pain. Six published reports in the literature show that opioid rotation to methadone significantly improved or resolved suspected OIH.[199,203,210,228–230]

Methadone provides unique advantages for opioid switching or rotation, including incomplete cross-tolerance with opioid

receptors and NMDA receptor antagonism.[229,231] The conversion to methadone from other opioids is complex and careful use of lower conversion ratios may be indicated when patients are on high opioid doses. Vigilance for signs of methadone toxicity, including Torsades de Points, is indicated when high doses are administered.

Despite its use in opioid rotation for modulation of OIH, it should be noted that methadone exposure has been linked to increased pain states in observational and cross-sectional studies of former opioid addicts maintained on methadone.[144–148] Therefore, opioid switching to methadone should be undertaken with the understanding that it may have an instrinsic ability to activate pronociceptive pathways, despite its NMDA receptor antagonist properties. Indeed, one case report has shown aggravation of OIH with methadone and failure of methadone to reverse OIH.[232] However, these observations may have been confounded by development of renal failure and accumulation of morphine-3-glucuronide metabolites. These metabolites have been shown to produce neuroexcitatory and antianalgesic effects in some studies.[233,234] It should also be noted that methadone rotation has been used to treat cases of OIH induced by high opioid doses, and it may not be valid to generalize that this benefit would also apply to OIH with lower opioid dose exposure typical of maintenance therapies.

Table 10.4: Possible Drugs for Modulation of Opioid-Induced Hyperalgesia in Humans

Drug Class	Site of Action	Prototype Drugs
High-affinity noncompetitive NMDA receptor antagonists	NMDA receptor	MK-801[212]
		Phencyclidine[212]
Low-moderate-affinity, open-channel noncompetitive NMDA receptor antagonists	NMDA receptor	Amantidine[321,322]
		CHF3381[323–325]
		Dextromethorphan[56,326]
		Ketamine[165,166,180–182,223,226,327,328]
		Memantine[212]
		Neramexane[329,330]
		Zenvia[331]
NR2B antagonists	NMDA receptor, NR2B subunit	Ifenprodil[332]
		Traxoprodil Mesylate[333,334]
		RGH-896[335]
COX-2 inhibitors	Cyclooxygenase 2 enzyme	Parecoxib[163]
Opioid agonist and NMDA receptor antagonist	NMDA receptor	Methadone[211,229]
		Ketobemidone[199]

Dextromethorphan for Modulation of OIH

Dextromethorphan is a noncompetitive NMDA receptor antagonist typically used as a cough suppressant. Numerous studies have indirectly examined the ability of dextromethorphan to attenuate or prevent expression of OIH and/or analgesic tolerance in patients on opioid therapy. Although these studies will not be reviewed here in their entirety, one recent study bears mentioning. In perhaps the largest clinical study of dextromethorphan and opioids to date, Galer et al conducted three large randomized, double-blinded, placebo-controlled multicenter trials of morphidex (morphine and dextromethorphan mixture in a 1:1 ratio) in 829 patients with chronic nonmalignant pain. Various indirect measures of opioid tolerance and/or hyperalgesia were taken over a 3-month observation period, including mean change in average daily pain intensity from baseline to last 7 days on treatment and percentage change in daily morphine use from baseline to last 30 days on treatment. Theoretically, any analgesic superiority of morphidex or reduced morphine requirements needed to treat pain when coadministered with dextromethorphan might result from modulation of OIH and/or tolerance. The study did not find any significant difference between morphidex and morphine alone in these outcome measures. The lack of treatment effect is discordant with results in some animal studies and early clinical trials[235–237] and as previously mentioned, may be the result of insufficient dextromethorphan dose and/or the limited degree of tolerance observed in the untreated (morphine without dextromethorphan) group. Further clinical studies will need to be conducted to elucidate these findings.

MANAGEMENT OF PATIENTS CHRONICALLY CONSUMING OPIOIDS

Patients on chronic opioid therapy have increased analgesic requirements and experience poorer pain control in the postoperative period.[48,49,52] High levels of postoperative pain are associated with an increased risk for pulmonary and cardiovascular complications, are the most common reason for delayed discharge or unexpected hospital admission after ambulatory surgery, and are responsible for prolonged recovery time after inpatient surgery.[250–253] The intensity of postoperative pain is correlated with the risk of developing chronic postsurgical pain, a condition estimated to affect 5%–10% of the surgical population.[254] Although the aggressive treatment of postoperative pain is imperative in all patients, it may be especially relevant in patients on chronic opioid therapy. This patient population may be particularly vulnerable to develop chronic pain conditions, including persistent postoperative pain.

Perioperative Considerations

The adequate management of perioperative pain in patients on chronic opioid therapy is complex. For example, patients on an average daily dose of morphine (180 mg) before surgery required 3–4 times higher opioid doses for a period 3 times longer than that required in opioid-naïve patients.[48] Despite the use of increased opioid doses, postoperative pain was more difficult to control.[49] Special considerations regarding the preoperative, intraoperative, and postoperative pain management are necessary when providing care to patients on chronic opioid therapy.

Preoperative Considerations

Patients on chronic opioid therapy represent a particular patient population with respect to pain management. Proper identification of these patients is the responsibility of the surgical team, the perioperative clinical staff, and the anesthesia team assigned to the case. Although there is some indication that the daily preoperative opioid dose correlates with increased postoperative opioid requirements, such correlation is moderate and the minimum daily opioid dose that significantly increases postoperative opioid requirements is not known.[49] All patients on chronic opioid therapy should be informed that their postoperative course may be complicated by aggravated pain and a need for opioid doses in excess of those required in opioid-naïve patients. Patients should also be educated about the potential for developing opioid withdrawal if they mistakenly omit their daily opioid dose before surgery. Such omission may occur because intake of food and liquids is discouraged.

Preoperative efforts should focus on formulating a perioperative pain management plan (Table 10.5). Important elements of such a plan include educating patients about the need to take their daily opioid dose before surgery, and the availability of alternative analgesic techniques that complement opioid therapy in the postoperative period. If patients abstain from their oral opioid dose on the day of surgery because oral intake of fluids and medication is not allowed, plans should be made to administer opioids by an alternative route.

Intraoperative Considerations

During surgery the required opioid dose is composed of the dose taken chronically before surgery and the dose made necessary by

Table 10.5: Considerations for Pain Management in Patients on Chronic Opioid Therapy[a]

Time Interval	Considerations
Preoperative	Determine precise preoperative opioid use (dose, type, etc)
	Emphasize importance of continuing preoperative opioid regimen up to the day of surgery (prevent withdrawal)
	Educate about possibility of exaggerated pain and increased opioid requirements postoperatively and explore patient's experiences with previous surgeries to identify effective/ineffective pain management strategies
	Educate about alternative analgesic strategies (eg, regional techniques)
	Establish a perioperative pain management plan
	Start adjuvant analgesic therapies according to perioperative pain management plan (eg, acetaminophen 1000 mg and/or 600–1200 mg gabapentin before surgery)
Intraoperative	Administer opioids to meet the following requirements: chronic daily dose, suppression of pain in response to surgical stimulation, suppression of pain because of tissue injury
	Consider titrating long-acting opioids to a spontaneous respiratory rate of 14–16 per minute at the end of surgery
	Administer adjuvant analgesic medications according to the perioperative pain management plan (eg, ketamine 0.5 mg/kg intravenous bolus followed by 4 µg/kg/min infusion, 1000 mg acetaminophen per rectum, and/or ketorolac 30 mg IV bolus)
	Institute appropriate regional techniques according to the perioperative pain management plan (continuous techniques are preferred, eg, continuous femoral nerve block for total knee arthroplasty)
Postoperative (acute)	Expect increased postoperative opioid requirements (2- to 4-fold range as an initial assumption) that vary significantly among patients on chronic opioid therapy
	Aggressive titration to individual needs for achieving adequate pain control is required in the postoperative care unit
	Start opioid patient controlled analgesia either for breakthrough pain if oral route is available for administering 1.5 times the preoperative dose or as a sole technique if oral route is not available (consider basal rate in opioid-dependent patients)
	If patients are treated with regional techniques, plan to administer at least half of the preoperative opioid requirement via the systemic route
	Consider continuation of acetaminophen 1000 mg every 6 hours and/or cyclooxygenase inhibitors for several days with attention to possible side effects (eg, bleeding, renal failure)
	Consider continuation of ketamine if started in the operating room or initiation of a ketamine postoperatively if pain proves refractory to other measures
	Regularly monitor patients for signs of opioid withdrawal or overdosing. Patients on chronic opioid therapy are at greater risk for respiratory depression than opioid-naïve patients
Postoperative (transition)	Use the daily intravenous opioid dose to calculate oral opioid equivalents
	Administer 2/3 of the oral opioid equivalent as a long-acting opioid and allow the remaining 1/3 to be administered as a short-acting opioid for breakthrough pain
	Consider continuing adjuvant analgesics (eg, acetaminophen, cyclooxygenase inhibitors)
	Plan tapering for postoperative opioid doses toward the preoperative dose and discuss tapering strategy with patient and health care providers; determine the need for specialty follow-up if regimen is complex

[a] Adapted from Carroll et al.[336]

surgical stimulation and tissue injury. Long-acting opioids seem best suited to substitute for the opioid dose taken chronically because relatively stable plasma concentrations are provided for a prolonged period of time. Short-acting opioids are a suitable choice for alleviating pain because of surgical stimulation. However, short-acting opioids may not provide adequate coverage for pain resulting from tissue injury because such pain outlasts the duration of surgery. The type of surgery allows predicting to what extent such pain may be present in the postoperative period. Initiating therapy with long-acting opioids intraoperatively for effective control of postoperative pain associated with tissue injury is particularly valuable if aggressive opioid titra-

tion in the immediate postoperative period is difficult. Such difficulties can arise because resources to obtain and administer opioids quickly at the bedside are limited or reluctance of the recovery room staff to administer sufficiently large opioid doses expediently.

If regional anesthesia techniques are chosen, either as the sole anesthetic technique or as a component of a more comprehensive anesthetic plan, a patient will still need systemic opioids. On one hand, the chronic daily opioid dose has to be substituted to prevent withdrawal. On the other hand, a patient may be on chronic opioid therapy for a pain condition that is not affected by the surgery or the regional technique. For example, a patient undergoing hip arthroplasty under epidural anesthesia may take opioids for chronic low back pain. Effective treatment strategies for both the pain at the site of surgery and the chronic low back pain are required postoperatively. In this case the postoperative surgical pain is controlled with epidural techniques. However, systemic opioids are likely necessary to prevent withdrawal and exacerbation of this patient's chronic low back pain. Several reports document opioid withdrawal in patients on chronic opioid therapy receiving opioids only via the intrathecal or epidural route in the postoperative period.[255] However, the use of opioids and a local anesthetic (bupivacaine 0.1%) via the epidural route and systemic opioids for break through pain was sufficient for preventing withdrawal.[48,256] In our one experience, daily systemic administration of at least half of the preoperative opioid dose is sufficient to prevent withdrawal when using regional anesthetic techniques.

Postoperative Considerations

Patients on chronic opioid therapy will require higher postoperative opioid doses for a prolonged period of time compared with opioid naïve patients.[49,257] Switching patients from an intravenous or epidural to an oral opioid regimen requires special attention. No broadly accepted guidelines facilitating this process are available. An approach that has worked well in our institution is to convert the daily postoperative intravenous opioid dose to an oral dose equivalent. Two-thirds of the oral dose equivalent are administered in the form of a long-acting opioid and one-third is administered in the form of a short-acting opioid on an as-needed basis. The long-acting opioid provides a steady baseline control of pain, whereas the short-acting opioid allows alleviation of breakthrough pain. As the surgical pain subsides, cutting back on the breakthrough medication is a simple way by which patients can reduce the total daily opioid dose. Conversion guidelines have recently been described in some detail and are summarized in Table 10.6.

Transition to an oral regimen should overlap with intravenous or epidural/intrathecal opioid administration because time is required to reach steady-state plasma concentrations of orally administered drugs. This is particularly true for long-acting opioids with a long elimination half-life such as methadone. Overlapping oral and intravenous or epidural/intrathecal opioid administration bears the risk of overdosing and patients should be monitored for signs of sedation of respiratory depression.

If the oral route is available throughout the postoperative period, providing 1.5 times the preoperative opioid dose by this route, and offering intravenous opioids via PCA for breakthrough pain until surgical pain is resolving, has worked well for a majority of our patients. Alternatively, intravenous opioids could be offered via PCA during the first few days after surgery during which pain is most prominent. After this period, the total daily intravenous opioid dose could be converted to oral opioid equivalents as discussed above.

Patients on chronic opioid therapy typically require prolonged opioid administration for adequate control of postoperative pain. Attempting to discharge these patients on their preoperative opioid dose often results in inadequate pain control. It is a reasonable goal to taper patients toward their preoperative dose over the course of 2 to 4 weeks. Clarifying these expectations with patients and participating health care providers

Table 10.6: Equianalgesic Parenteral and Oral Opioid Doses[a]

Opioid[b]	Parenteral	Oral
Morphine	10.0	30.0
Hydromorphone	1.5	7.5
Oxymorphone	1.0	10
Oxycodone	–	25.0
Hydrocodone	–	30.0
Fentanyl[c]	0.1	–
Meperidine	75	300.0
Methadone[d]	5	7.5
Levorphanol	2	4.0
Codeine	130	200.0

[a] Adapted from Gammaitoni et al.[337]

[b] Conversion tables are guidelines for approximating dosage equivalence. Substantial interpatient differences should be expected.

[c] The dose of transdermal fentanyl in μg/h is about half the 24-hour dose of oral morphine (eg, 100 μg/h transdermal fentanyl = 200 mg/d oral morphine)

[d] Methadone can be significantly more potent than typically assumed when rotating patients from another opioid to methadone. This may partially result from the NMDA antagonist properties of methadone. In this setting the conversion ratio may well exceed 10:1.

improves the likelihood of providing adequate postoperative pain control. Patients on particularly high preoperative opioid doses may require longer than 4 weeks for tapering toward their preoperative dose. Plans should be made to ascertain that patients will be able to obtain the necessary opioid prescription. This is important if larger than preoperative doses are required for a prolonged period of time because an outside physician may be hesitant to issue such a prescription. Scheduling follow-up visits at a pain clinic may facilitate this process.

A surgical procedure may reduce the source of chronic pain requiring chronic opioid therapy. In this scenario, it is quite possible that a patient will be tapered to a lower daily opioid dose than required before the surgery.

Adjuvant Medications

The concept of using a multimodal or balanced approach to treat postoperative pain more effectively has gained wide acceptance.[258] Combing various classes of drugs with different mechanism of action to optimize pain control while reducing the potential for side effects seems particularly pertinent to the management of postoperative pain in patients on chronic opioid therapy. However, studies specifically examining the usefulness of multimodal analgesic regimens in patients on chronic opioid therapy are lacking. Similarly, relatively few studies have examined to what extent different combinations of adjuvant analgesics offer proved advantage compared with the use of a single adjuvant analgesic. However, available data suggests that combining different adjuvant analgesics can provide at least additive effects.[259,260]

The utility of an increasing number of agents as part of a multimodal regimen has been explored. However, cyclooxygenase inhibitors and paracetamol, NMDA receptor antagonists, and, lately, the anticonvulsant gabapentin have received most attention and, therefore, their coadministration with opioids will be discussed here. More detailed information about the pharmacology and clinical utility of these drugs as well as alternative adjuvant analgesics drugs and strategies not discussed here are provided in special chapters throughout this book.

Cyclooxygenase Inhibitors and Paracetamol/ Acetaminophen

Nonselective and selective cyclooxygenase inhibitors as well as paracetamol play an important role as adjuvant analgesics supplementing opioids for the treatment of postoperative pain.[258] Different drugs are available for parenteral, oral, and/or rectal administration. A major mechanism underlying the analgesic and anti-inflammatory actions of COX inhibitors is the decreased formation of prostaglandins in peripheral tissue and the CNS. The mechanism underlying the analgesic action of paracetamol remains uncertain.

The analgesic efficacy of COX inhibitors and paracetamol has been documented after various surgeries and several reviews and meta-analysis support their role in reducing postoperative pain and opioid requirements.[258,261–263] Nonselective COX inhibitors and selective COX-2-inhibitors provide equipotent analgesic effects, whereas paracetamol is less efficacious.[264] Adding a COX inhibitor to an opioid regimen reduces opioid requirements by about 30%, whereas paracetamol reduces the requirement by about 20%.[265,266] Studies mainly conducted in patients undergoing orthopedic procedures reported a 20%–50% reduction in postoperative pain in addition to opioid-sparing effects.[267–270] However, the opioid-sparing effects provided by COX inhibitors and paracetamol may not be associated with a clinically relevant reduction of opioid side effects.[265,266] Some evidence suggests that combining COX inhibitors with acetaminophen provides superior postoperative pain control than either class of drug when given alone.[263]

COX inhibitors are often omitted from a perioperative analgesic regimen based on concerns that their use could cause serious adverse outcomes. Nonselective COX inhibitors such as ketorolac, diclofenac, and ibuprofen can cause gastrointestinal ulceration, impaired renal function, diminished platelet aggregation, and thromboembolic cardiovascular events.

The short-term use (days) of nonselective COX inhibitors in the elderly population resulted in a gastrointestinal ulceration rate of 20%–40%.[271,272] The elderly population may be at particular risk for developing gastrointestinal bleeding complications as a consequence of such ulceration.

Prostaglandins regulate renal blood flow and glomerular filtration rate. They are particularly important for maintaining these functions in ischemic or diseased kidneys. For this reason, nonselective and selective COX inhibitors should be avoided in patients suffering from hypovolemia, low cardiac output, or impaired renal function resulting from a disease such as diabetes or the use of a nephrotoxic drug such as an aminoglycoside.[273] However, a recent meta-analysis suggests that the perioperative use of COX inhibitors should not be discouraged in patients with normal renal function.[274]

Nonselective COX inhibitors impair the aggregation of blood platelets and their use has been associated with an increased perioperative blood loss.[275,276] It is not clear under what circumstances such inhibition of platelet aggregation becomes clinically relevant. However, it seems prudent to avoid nons-

elective COX inhibitors in patients with preexisting bleeding disorders, patients undergoing surgeries with significant bleeding potential and patients undergoing surgeries at sites particularly vulnerable to bleeding complications (eg, craniotomy).

Longer-term use of nonselective and selective COX inhibitors is associated with an increased risk for thromboembolic cardiovascular complications.[277,278] In the perioperative setting, administration of COX inhibitors to patients undergoing coronary bypass grafting also increased the number of thromboembolic cardiovascular complications.[279] However, in patients not requiring extracorporeal circulation during surgery, the short-term administration of COX inhibitors is unlikely to increase such risks and their use should not be discouraged.[280]

The side-effect profile of selective COX-2 inhibitors does not include the risk for gastrointestinal ulceration and platelet inhibition.[271,272,276] However, COX-2 inhibitors have a similar risk as nonselective COX inhibitors for causing renal impairment and cardiovascular thromboembolic complications.[273,278] In contrast, paracetamol offers a very safe side-effect profile when used within its therapeutic range. Safety concerns relate mainly to its hepatotoxic effects when used in excess of the daily recommended dose.[281]

NMDA Receptor Antagonists

This class of drugs includes ketamine, dextromethorphan, and amantadine. NMDA receptors play a key role in nociceptive signal transmission as well as in the development of opioid tolerance and/or opioid-induced hyperalgesia. The choice of an NMDA receptor antagonist may be particularly attractive in patients on chronic opioid therapy because its use may not only attenuate nociceptive signaling but also alleviate preexisting opioid tolerance and/or opioid-induced hyperalgesia.[226,227,282] Among the various NMDA receptor antagonists, ketamine has received most attention and is discussed in some detail.

Several meta-analyses and reviews document opioid-sparing and analgesic effects when administering subhypnotic doses of ketamine by the parenteral route during various types of surgery.[219–221] Most commonly ketamine has been given intravenously or epidurally as a bolus, a continuous infusion, or as a combined bolus/infusion regimen. Administration of ketamine has safely and effectively been extended into the postoperative period, in some instances by directly combing it with an opioid for administration via PCA.[283,284] Ketamine provides opioid-sparing effects in the range of 30%–50% and likely reduces the incidence of opioid-related side effects such as nausea and vomiting.[220] To what degree coadministration of ketamine reduces, not only opioid requirements, but also postoperative pain compared with the sole administration of an opioid is harder to quantify. Current evidence suggests that such additional analgesic effects do exist but may be modest.[221] Overall, coadministration of ketamine appears to be most beneficial in surgeries associated with moderate to severe postoperative pain.[221] At this point, the optimal dose of ketamine and the most advantageous form for its administration remain unresolved issues. Analysis of available data suggests that a dose in excess of 30 mg/d is unlikely to further reduce postoperative opioid requirements.[220]

A study of particular interest reported a decreased incidence of chronic postsurgical pain when ketamine was administered during surgery.[223] Patients on chronic opioid therapy may represent a population that is quite vulnerable for developing chronic pain conditions. In this context, coadministration of ketamine for the prevention of chronic postsurgical pain may be particularly beneficial.

The widespread clinical use of ketamine as an adjuvant analgesic has been limited by its psychomimetic side effects, including hallucination and bad dreams. However, the risk for the occurrence of such side effects appears to be low in patients undergoing general anesthesia.[219–221] Coadministration of ketamine causes sedation and diplopia in some patients but such side effects rarely forced its discontinuation.[221]

Alternative antagonists at the NMDA receptor include dextromethorphan and amantadine. Dextromethorphan has been studied in some detail and a recent meta-analyses provide some insight into its effectiveness as an adjuvant analgesic.[285] In contrast, reports on amantadine are sparse. Dextromethorphan given by the intravenous route provides opioid-sparing effects and reduces opioid-related side effects.[285] Dextromethorphan is less effective when given by the oral route before surgery. Although some reports suggest that intravenous dextromethorphan may lower opioid requirements to a similar extent as ketamine, the relative effectiveness of these two drugs as adjuvant analgesic remains to be determined.

Gabapentin

Gabapentin was developed as an anticonvulsive but, lately, it has received most attention for its analgesic and antihyperalgesic action that are pertinent for the treatment of postoperative and neuropathic pain. Gabapentin and the more recently introduced Pregabalin, act via inhibition of the $\alpha_2\delta$ subunit of a voltage-sensitive calcium channel.[286] Recent reviews document clear opioid-sparing and analgesic effects when administering 600–1200 mg of oral gabapentin before surgery.[287,288] Gabapentin also reduces the incidence of opioid-related side effects such a nausea, vomiting, and pruritus.[288] Studies in patients mainly undergoing orthopedic and abdominal surgeries reported an opioid-sparing effect in the range of 30%–50%. In most of these studies, coadministration of gabapentin decreased postoperative pain by an additional 30%–50%, in addition to the opioid-sparing effect. At this point it remains unclear whether extending a multidose regiment of gabapentin into the postoperative period adds any additional benefit.

Gabapentin attenuates sensitization of central neuronal mechanisms that facilitate pain signaling after tissue trauma and are likely involved in the development of persistent postsurgical pain. One study documented that the perioperative administration of gabapentin lowered the incidence and severity of pain 1 month after surgery.[289] Future studies need to corroborate that the perioperative administration of gabapentin can prevent the development of chronic postsurgical pain.

Administration of gabapentin before surgery is associated with increased sedation in the immediate postoperative period.[288] Available data suggest that pronounced sedation occurs only in a small fraction of patients.[290] However, the sedative action of gabapentin and pregabalin should be considered in vulnerable patients (eg, concomitant medications and risk of falling).

Regional Anesthetic Techniques

Regional anesthesia is an attractive choice in patients on chronic opioid therapy because superior analgesia can be provided to patients at risk for developing aggravated postoperative pain.

Local anesthetics are the primary class of drugs used for regional techniques, although adjuvant drugs such as opioids, α_2-adrenergic agonists, and COX inhibitors are coadministered. Only a few studies have specifically examined the clinical utility of regional anesthesia techniques in patients on chronic opioid therapy. However, the efficacy of these techniques can be inferred from studies in opioid-naïve patients. Several chapters throughout this book provide detailed discussion of different regional techniques. The following paragraphs are intended to provide an overview and discuss aspects specific to patients on chronic opioid therapy.

Infiltration and Wound Lavage

Direct administration of local anesthetics into the surgical wound can reduce postoperative opioid requirements. This technique should be considered when other regional techniques are not applicable. The success of techniques used for administering local anesthetics into surgical wounds depends on the (1) type of surgery; (2) type, amount, and concentration of local anesthetic; and (3) particular techniques used for administering the drug. Accordingly, results of studies examining the clinical utility of this technique have been mixed. Direct injection of local anesthetics into wounds provides a relatively short-lived analgesic effect for the first few hours after surgery. For abdominal surgeries subfascial as opposed to epifascial or subcutaneous injection seems critical for achieving optimal analgesic results.[258]

The relatively short-lived benefit of administering local anesthetics into wounds has led to the development of catheter-based techniques for continuous drug administration. Such techniques have successfully been implemented to reduce postoperative pain and opioid requirements for up to 5 days in patients undergoing inguinal hernia repair, sternotomy, and spinal fusion.[291–293] However, other studies using this technique have reported negative results.[294]

Local anesthetics have been administered into the pleural and peritoneal cavity and some studies in patients undergoing abdominal surgeries reported significant, but short-lasting, analgesic and opioid-sparing effects.[295,296] However, the effectiveness and safety of intracavitary instillation of local anesthetics for postoperative pain control remains controversial.[258]

The intra-articular injection of local anesthetics and other adjuvant analgesics, including opioids, is a common practice in patients undergoing surgery of the joints. Although the sole administration of a local anesthetic or an opioid provides some short-lived pain relief and opioid-sparing effects, the overall clinical significance of this practice has been questioned.[297,298] However, more recent studies, using a multimodal pharmacological approach for intra-articular injections, reported more impressive results. For example, the combined injection of a local anesthetic, a nonsteroidal anti-inflammatory drug (NSAID), and epinephrine not only provided relevant and sustained pain relief, but also allowed for earlier discharge and improved joint function 1 week after surgery.[299,300]

Peripheral Nerve Blockade

Peripheral nerve blockade, including such techniques as the axillary, interscalene, paravertebral, femoral, and sciatic block, are very effective for postoperative pain control and significantly reduce postoperative opioid consumption. Single bolus injection techniques are familiar to a majority of anesthesiologists and are most effective during the first 24 hours after surgery. However, the use of catheter-based techniques has become more popular and allows for prolonged drug administration and pain control. Direct comparison of such techniques with PCA opioid administration is favorable and suggests that at least comparable pain control and opioid-sparing effects but also possibly greater patient satisfaction can be achieved.[301–303]

Epidural Blockade

In contrast to the regional techniques described above, special efforts have been made to examine the clinical utility of epidural techniques for postoperative pain control in patients on chronic opioid therapy. As discussed previously, epidural opioid requirements for providing postoperative pain control and epidural or systemic opioid requirements for alleviating breakthrough pain are higher in patients on chronic opioid therapy than in opioid-naïve patients.[49,257]

Considering the use of very potent opioid in patients on chronic opioid therapy merits special considerations. Highly potent, lipophilic opioids such as sufentanil may be more efficacious in these than less potent hydrophilic opioids such as morphine. For example, deLeon-Casasola and Lema[304] reported that a patient on high preoperative methadone doses was refractory to high doses of epidural morphine, but responded well to sufentanil. This differential efficacy may result from the fact that opioids with higher potency elicit analgesic effects at a lower receptor occupancy. In a prospective follow-up study in cancer patients on chronic opioid therapy, the author confirmed that epidural sufentanil provided superior postoperative pain control compared with morphine.[256] This finding was echoed by a study documenting superior postoperative pain control in patients on chronic opioid therapy who received epidural fentanyl rather than epidural morphine.[49] Administration of an epidural opioid, particularly a very potent lipophilic compound, in combination with a local anesthetic, is an attractive approach for effectively treating postoperative pain for a prolonged postoperative period.

Adjuvant analgesics have been administered by the epidural route for further improving postoperative pain control in patients on chronic opioid therapy. The use of clonidine or low-dose epinephrine, both agonists at the α_2-adrenergic receptor, has been advocated.[257] For example, superior postoperative pain control was demonstrated when coadministering epinephrine with epidural fentanyl and bupivacaine.[305]

MANAGEMENT CONSIDERATIONS OF PERIOPERATIVE OPIOID THERAPY IN OPIOID-NAÏVE PATIENTS

Balanced Anesthesia: Limiting Perioperative Opioid Exposure

Opioid analgesic medications are commonly used to treat pain in the perioperative setting. Yet, these medications are fraught with side effects that include postoperative nausea and vomiting, urinary retention, pruritus, constipation, and other problems that limit their potential usefulness. Modern anesthetic practice has evolved over time to embrace the concept of "balanced anesthesia."[306] This practice encourages the use of multiple approaches to analgesia to limit the dose of opioid medication administered in the perioperative period. Many of these

techniques have already been described in the preceding section of this chapter. Techniques for acute pain management in the perioperative setting have also been described in detail by the American Society for Anesthesiology's task force on acute pain management.[307] Please refer to Chapter 12: The role of preventive multimodal analgesia and impact on patient outcome.

Despite these practices, very large doses of opioid medication are occasionally administered in the perioperative setting when other analgesic methods are not practical or desirable. These situations may include coagulopathy or other conditions that preclude neuraxial anesthetic techniques, surgeon or patient preference, and allergy or intolerance of other analgesic medications.

Treating Suspected OIH

The consequences of very large doses of perioperative opioid administration vis-à-vis opioid tolerance and OIH have already been discussed earlier in this chapter. The first goal in treatment should be to determine if postoperative analgesia is adequate in this clinical setting. If the patient reports adequate postoperative analgesia, diligent postoperative evaluation of pain and careful tapering of opioid medication may be all that is required to successfully manage postoperative pain. However, if the patient reports unsatisfactory postoperative analgesia, especially in the setting of escalating opioid dosing, opioid-induced hyperalgesia should be considered.

There is a dearth of high-quality clinical evidence to guide treatment of iatrogenic OIH. Current evidence for treatment of suspected OIH comes mainly from individual clinical case reports or small case series. One such report suggests that opioid switching to methadone, sufentanil, or ketobemidone may significantly improve or resolve suspected OIH.[199,203,210,228–230] Initiation of adjuvant analgesic therapies with concomitant opioid weaning should also be considered. Administration of an NMDA receptor antagonist such as ketamine has been shown to dramatically improve postoperative analgesia in a case of suspected iatrogenic OIH.[249] Treatment of OIH with weaning of opioids and substitution with an anticonvulsant, tricyclic antidepressants (TCA), and NSAIDS improved pain control in another recent case report.[308] Evidence from human experimental pain studies suggest that the α_2 agonist clonidine may also help attenuate the effects of OIH.[165]

In the absence of high-quality clinical evidence, treatment of suspected iatrogenic OIH that develops in opioid-naïve patients in the perioperative setting should be tailored to the specific needs and responses of the individual patient. When OIH is suspected, the clinician should first consider opioid switching and/or tapering and initiation of adjuvant analgesic therapies, as tolerated by the patient. These treatments include NSAIDS; COX-2 inhibitors; NMDA receptor antagonists; α_2 agonists, such as clonidine; and regional or neuraxial anesthetic techniques, where appropriate.

FUTURE CHALLENGES

A Dearth of High-Quality Clinical Evidence

Management of acute pain after prolonged opioid exposure is a challenging problem for clinicians. The molecular mechanisms of opioid tolerance and OIH continue to be rapidly elucidated through animal models. At the same time, advances in this area of clinical pain management are hindered by a dearth of high-quality prospective clinical evidence from which to guide clinical practice.

Optimal Use of Adjuvants in This Population

As previously discussed, patients with chronic opioid exposure undergo physiologic changes over time that limit the efficacy of opioid medications for the treatment of acute pain. Therefore, use of other analgesic medications and adjuvant therapies are the principal method of acute pain management in these patients. Yet, high-quality clinical evidence for the optimal use of adjuvants in this population is lacking.

Most clinical data on modulation of opioid tolerance and OIH come from human experimental pain studies on healthy volunteers. Efficacy and effectiveness of adjuvant therapies such as NMDA receptor antagonists, COX-2 inhibitors, and $\alpha_2\delta$ ligands (eg, gabapentin and pregabalin) in acute pain management for chronic opioid users remains to be fully characterized.

Usefulness of Preoperative Detoxification

There are few data available about the reversibility of physiologic adapatation to prolonged opioid exposure. However, it seems reasonable to consider reversibility of opioid tolerance and opioid-induced hyperalgesia in the preoperative management of patients on chronic opioid therapy. Detoxification from opioid therapy may be a useful preoperative maneuver if these adaptations can be acutely reversed in the perioperative period.

Currently available evidence on reversibility of OIH stems mainly from the opioid addict population. In these patients, data suggest that OIH may indeed be reversible to some extent, but it appears to require periods of abstinence longer than 4 weeks.[145,159] These observations must be qualified by the unique psychological factors of this patient population that may influence their pain behavior, such as avoidance behavior, markedly low frustration levels, and their tendency to overreact. Therefore, these observations may not be entirely generalizable to nonaddicted, opioid-dependent patients. Further work is needed to characterize the reversal of opioid tolerance and OIH in the chronic pain population.

Impact on Chronic Persistent Pain after Surgery

The incidence of the development of chronic persistent pain after surgery is not well characterized and may be underestimated and underreported.[309,310] Although the incidence varies depending on the type of surgery, estimates for selected procedures range from 50% for thoracotomy, 30%–81% for limb amputation, 50% for breast surgery, and 3%–56% for gallbladder surgery.[311] A review of predictive factors of chronic pain after surgery by Perkins et al[311] has shown that the intensity of acute postoperative pain directly predicts the development of chronic persistent pain.[316] It is therefore reasonable to hypothesize that patients who have been chronically exposed to opioids, and who are more likely to have increased postoperative pain may also be at increased risk for the development of chronic persistent pain after surgery.

Already, there is evidence to suggest that perioperative acute pain interventions may have a long-term postoperative impact on the development of chronic pain after surgery. For instance, a retrospective cohort study in 100 patients with a history of resolved complex regional pain syndrome by Reuben et al[312]

found that perioperative regional anesthesia reduced the incidence of postoperative recurrence of chronic regional pain syndrome after upper extremity surgery from to 72% in the control group (36 of 50 patients who did not receive regional anesthesia) to 10% in the treated group (5 of 50 patients who received stellate ganglion block; $P < .01$). More work needs to be done to study the impact of acute pain management on the development of persistent pain after surgery, particularly in patients with a history of chronic opioid exposure.

In conclusion, our understanding of acute pain management in opioid-dependent patients is just beginning. Future research will hopefully lead to high-quality prospective clinical studies that will provide evidence-based treatment plans to help more effectively guide clinical care.

The authors thank Chris Stave, M.L.S., Lane Medical Library, Stanford University Medical Center, Stanford, California, for his advice and expertise with literature search. The authors also thank Erin Reiland, who provided administrative support for this review. Dr. Chu's work is supported by a career development award from the National Institute of General Medical Sciences of the National Institutes of Health, 5K23GM071400-04.

REFERENCES

1. Booth M. *Opium: A History*. New York, NY: St. Martin's Press; 1998.
2. Krjtikos P, Papadaki, SP. The history of poppy and of opium and their expansion in antiquity. *Bull Narc*. 1967;3:17–38.
3. WHO. *Achieving Balance in National Opioids Control Policy: Guidelines for Assessment*. Geneva, Switzerland: World Health Organization; 2000.
4. Gimbel JS, Richards P, Portenoy RK. Controlled-release oxycodone for pain in diabetic neuropathy: a randomized controlled trial. *Neurology*. 2003;60(6):927–934.
5. Raja SN, Haythornthwaite JA, Pappagallo M, et al. Opioids versus antidepressants in postherpetic neuralgia: a randomized, placebo-controlled trial. *Neurology*. 2002;59(7):1015–1021.
6. Rowbotham MC, Twilling L, Davies PS, Reisner L, Taylor K, Mohr D. Oral opioid therapy for chronic peripheral and central neuropathic pain. *N Engl J Med*. 2003;348(13):1223–1232.
7. Watson CP, Moulin D, Watt-Watson J, Gordon A, Eisenhoffer J. Controlled-release oxycodone relieves neuropathic pain: a randomized controlled trial in painful diabetic neuropathy. *Pain*. 2003;105(1–2):71–78.
8. Dellemijn PL, Vanneste JA. Randomised double-blind active-placebo-controlled crossover trial of intravenous fentanyl in neuropathic pain. *Lancet*. 1997;349(9054):753–758.
9. Caldwell JR, Hale ME, Boyd RE, et al. Treatment of osteoarthritis pain with controlled release oxycodone or fixed combination oxycodone plus acetaminophen added to nonsteroidal antiinflammatory drugs: a double blind, randomized, multicenter, placebo controlled trial. *J Rheumatol*. 1999;26(4):862–869.
10. Roth SH, Fleischmann RM, Burch FX, et al. Around-the-clock, controlled-release oxycodone therapy for osteoarthritis-related pain: placebo-controlled trial and long-term evaluation. *Arch Intern Med*. 2000;160(6):853–860.
11. Moulin DE, Iezzi A, Amireh R, Sharpe WK, Boyd D, Merskey H. Randomised trial of oral morphine for chronic non-cancer pain. *Lancet*. 1996;347(8995):143–147.
12. Arkinstall W, Sandler A, Goughnour B, Babul N, Harsanyi Z, Darke AC. Efficacy of controlled-release codeine in chronic non-malignant pain: a randomized, placebo-controlled clinical trial. *Pain*. 1995;62(2):169–178.

13. Kalso E, Edwards JE, Moore RA, McQuay HJ. Opioids in chronic non-cancer pain: systematic review of efficacy and safety. *Pain.* 2004;112(3):372–380.

14. Katz N. Methodological issues in clinical trials of opioids for chronic pain. *Neurology.* 2005;65(12 suppl 4):32–49.

15. Portenoy RK, Farrar JT, Backonja MM, et al. Long-term use of controlled-release oxycodone for noncancer pain: results of a 3-year registry study. *Clin J Pain.* 2007;23(4):287–299.

16. Meier B. Sales of painkiller grew rapidly, but success brought a high cost. *New York Times.* March 5, 2001.

17. Adams C. Painkiller's sales far exceeded levels anticipated by maker. *Wall Street Journal.* May 16, 2002.

18. Yadgood MC, Miller PJ, Mathews PA. Relieving the agony of the new pain management standards. *Am J Hosp Palliat Care.* 2000;17(5):333–341.

19. Lippe PM. The decade of pain control and research. *Pain Med.* 2000;1(4):286.

20. Brennan F, Carr DB, Cousins M. Pain management: a fundamental human right. *Anesth Analg.* 2007;105(1):205–221.

21. Cousins MJ, Brennan F, Carr DB. Pain relief: a universal human right. *Pain.* Nov 2004;112(1–2):1–4.

22. Thomson H. A new law to improve pain management and end-of-life care: learning how to treat patients in pain and near death must become a priority. *West J Med.* 2001;174(3):161–162.

23. Olsen Y, Daumit GL, Ford DE. Opioid prescriptions by U.S. primary care physicians from 1992 to 2001. *J Pain.* 2006;7(4):225–235.

24. Clark JD. Chronic pain prevalence and analgesic prescribing in a general medical population. *J Pain Symptom Manage.* 2002;23(2):131–137.

25. Bell JR. Australian trends in opioid prescribing for chronic non-cancer pain, 1986–1996. *Med J Aust.* 1997;167(1):26–29.

26. RxList: The Internet Drug index. The Top 300 Prescriptions for 2005 by Number of US Prescriptions Dispensed. http://www.rxlist.como/top200.htm. Accessed May 7, 2007.

27. Rowbotham MC, Lindsey CD. How effective is long-term opioid therapy for chronic noncancer pain? *Clin J Pain.* 2007;23(4):300–302.

28. Angst MS, Clark JD. Opioid-induced hyperalgesia: a qualitative systematic review. *Anesthesiology.* 2006;104(3):570–587.

29. Mao J. Opioid-induced abnormal pain sensitivity. *Curr Pain Headache Rep.* 2006;10(1):67–70.

30. Ossipov MH, Lai J, King T, Vanderah TW, Porreca F. Underlying mechanisms of pronociceptive consequences of prolonged morphine exposure. *Biopolymers.* 2005;80(2–3):319–324.

31. Simonnet G, Rivat C. Opioid-induced hyperalgesia: abnormal or normal pain? *NeuroReport.* 2003;14(1):1–7.

32. Twycross RG. Choice of strong analgesic in terminal cancer: diamorphine or morphine? *Pain.* 1977;3(2):93–104.

33. Chu LF, Clark DJ, Angst MS. Opioid tolerance and hyperalgesia in chronic pain patients after one month of oral morphine therapy: a preliminary prospective study. *J Pain.* 2006;7(1):43–48.

34. Marsden CA. Dopamine: the rewarding years. *Br J Pharmacol.* 2006;147(suppl 1):136–144.

35. Wasan AD, Butler SF, Budman SH, Benoit C, Fernandez K, Jamison RN. Psychiatric history and psychologic adjustment as risk factors for aberrant drug-related behavior among patients with chronic pain. *Clin J Pain.* 2007;23(4):307–315.

36. Stein DJ, van Honk J, Ipser J, Solms M, Panksepp J. Opioids: from physical pain to the pain of social isolation. *CNS Spectr.* 2007;12(9):669–670, 672–674.

37. Vinik HR, Kissin I. Rapid development of tolerance to analgesia during remifentanil infusion in humans. *Anesth Analg.* 1998;86(6):1307–1311.

38. Gustorff B, Nahlik G, Hoerauf KH, Kress HG. The absence of acute tolerance during remifentanil infusion in volunteers. *Anesth Analg.* 2002;94(5):1223–1228, table of contents.

39. Chia YY, Liu K, Wang JJ, Kuo MC, Ho ST. Intraoperative high dose fentanyl induces postoperative fentanyl tolerance. *Can J Anaesth.* 1999;46(9):872–877.

40. Cooper DW, Lindsay SL, Ryall DM, Kokri MS, Eldabe SS, Lear GA. Does intrathecal fentanyl produce acute cross-tolerance to i.v. morphine? *Br J Anaesth.* 1997;78(3):311–313.

41. Crawford MW, Hickey C, Zaarour C, Howard A, Naser B. Development of acute opioid tolerance during infusion of remifentanil for pediatric scoliosis surgery. *Anesth Analg.* 2006;102(6):1662–1667.

42. Guignard B, Bossard AE, Coste C, et al. Acute opioid tolerance: intraoperative remifentanil increases postoperative pain and morphine requirement. *Anesthesiology.* 2000;93(2):409–417.

43. Cortinez LI, Brandes V, Munoz HR, Guerrero ME, Mur M. No clinical evidence of acute opioid tolerance after remifentanil-based anaesthesia. *Br J Anaesth.* 2001;87(6):866–869.

44. Aubrun F, Langeron O, Quesnel C, Coriat P, Riou B. Relationships between measurement of pain using visual analog score and morphine requirements during postoperative intravenous morphine titration. *Anesthesiology.* 2003;98(6):1415–1421.

45. Delvaux B, Ryckwaert Y, Van Boven M, De Kock M, Capdevila X. Remifentanil in the intensive care unit: tolerance and acute withdrawal syndrome after prolonged sedation. *Anesthesiology.* 2005;102(6):1281–1282.

46. Tobias JD, Berkenbosch JW. Tolerance during sedation in a pediatric ICU patient: effects on the BIS monitor. *J Clin Anesth.* 2001;13(2):122–124.

47. Buntin-Mushock C, Phillip L, Moriyama K, Palmer PP. Age-dependent opioid escalation in chronic pain patients. *Anesth Analg.* 2005;100(6):1740–1745.

48. de Leon-Casasola OA, Myers DP, Donaparthi S, et al. A comparison of postoperative epidural analgesia between patients with chronic cancer taking high doses of oral opioids versus opioid-naive patients. *Anesth Analg.* 1993;76(2):302–307.

49. Rapp SE, Ready LB, Nessly ML. Acute pain management in patients with prior opioid consumption: a case-controlled retrospective review. *Pain.* 1995;61(2):195–201.

50. Joels CS, Mostafa G, Matthews BD, et al. Factors affecting intravenous analgesic requirements after colectomy. *J Am Coll Surg.* 2003;197(5):780–785.

51. Kain ZN, Sevarino F, Alexander GM, Pincus S, Mayes LC. Preoperative anxiety and postoperative pain in women undergoing hysterectomy: a repeated-measures design. *J Psychosom Res.* 2000;49(6):417–422.

52. Kalkman CJ, Visser K, Moen J, Bonsel GJ, Grobbee DE, Moons KG. Preoperative prediction of severe postoperative pain. *Pain.* 2003;105(3):415–423.

53. Riley TR, 3rd. Predictors of pain medication use after percutaneous liver biopsy. *Dig Dis Sci.* 2002;47(10):2151–2153.

54. Thomas T, Robinson C, Champion D, McKell M, Pell M. Prediction and assessment of the severity of post-operative pain and of satisfaction with management. *Pain.* 1998;75(2–3):177–185.

55. Breckenridge J, Clark JD. Patient characteristics associated with opioid versus nonsteroidal anti-inflammatory drug management of chronic low back pain. *J Pain.* 2003;4(6):344–350.

56. Galer BS, Lee D, Ma T, Nagle B, Schlagheck TG. MorphiDex (morphine sulfate/dextromethorphan hydrobromide combination) in the treatment of chronic pain: three multicenter, randomized, double-blind, controlled clinical trials fail to demonstrate enhanced opioid analgesia or reduction in tolerance. *Pain.* 2005;115(3):284–295.

57. Milligan K, Lanteri-Minet M, Borchert K, et al. Evaluation of long-term efficacy and safety of transdermal fentanyl in the treatment of chronic noncancer pain. *J Pain.* 2001;2(4):197–204.

58. Bernstein MA, Welch SP. mu-Opioid receptor down-regulation and cAMP-dependent protein kinase phosphorylation in a mouse model of chronic morphine tolerance. *Brain Res Mol Brain Res.* 1998;55(2):237–242.

59. Ben Y, Smith AP, Schiller PW, Lee NM. Tolerance develops in spinal cord, but not in brain with chronic [Dmt1]DALDA treatment. *Br J Pharmacol.* 2004;143(8):987–993.

60. Buzas B, Rosenberger J, Cox BM. Mu and delta opioid receptor gene expression after chronic treatment with opioid agonist. *NeuroReport.* 1996;7(9):1505–1508.

61. Ray SB, Gupta YK, Wadhwa S. Expression of opioid receptor-like 1 (ORL1) & mu opioid receptors in the spinal cord of morphine tolerant mice. *Indian J Med Res.* 2005;121(3):194–202.

62. Ronnekleiv OK, Bosch MA, Cunningham MJ, Wagner EJ, Grandy DK, Kelly MJ. Downregulation of mu-opioid receptor mRNA in the mediobasal hypothalamus of the female guinea pig following morphine treatment. *Neurosci Lett.* 1996;216(2):129–132.

63. Johnson EE, Christie MJ, Connor M. The role of opioid receptor phosphorylation and trafficking in adaptations to persistent opioid treatment. *Neurosignals.* 2005;14(6):290–302.

64. Marie N, Aguila B, Allouche S. Tracking the opioid receptors on the way of desensitization. *Cell Signal.* 2006;18(11):1815–1833.

65. Zuo Z. The role of opioid receptor internalization and beta-arrestins in the development of opioid tolerance. *Anesth Analg.* 2005;101(3):728–734, table of contents.

66. Arden JR, Segredo V, Wang Z, Lameh J, Sadee W. Phosphorylation and agonist-specific intracellular trafficking of an epitope-tagged mu-opioid receptor expressed in HEK 293 cells. *J Neurochem.* 1995;65(4):1636–1645.

67. Deng HB, Yu Y, Pak Y, et al. Role for the C-terminus in agonist-induced mu opioid receptor phosphorylation and desensitization. *Biochemistry.* 2000;39(18):5492–5499.

68. Deng HB, Yu Y, Wang H, Guang W, Wang JB. Agonist-induced mu opioid receptor phosphorylation and functional desensitization in rat thalamus. *Brain Res.* 2001;898(2):204–214.

69. Zhang L, Yu Y, Mackin S, Weight FF, Uhl GR, Wang JB. Differential mu opiate receptor phosphorylation and desensitization induced by agonists and phorbol esters. *J Biol Chem.* 1996;271(19):11449–11454.

70. Schulz S, Mayer D, Pfeiffer M, Stumm R, Koch T, Hollt V. Morphine induces terminal micro-opioid receptor desensitization by sustained phosphorylation of serine-375. *Embo J.* 2004;23(16):3282–3289.

71. Bohn LM, Dykstra LA, Lefkowitz RJ, Caron MG, Barak LS. Relative opioid efficacy is determined by the complements of the G protein-coupled receptor desensitization machinery. *Mol Pharmacol.* 2004;66(1):106–112.

72. Bohn LM, Gainetdinov RR, Caron MG. G protein-coupled receptor kinase/beta-arrestin systems and drugs of abuse: psychostimulant and opiate studies in knockout mice. *Neuromolecular Med.* 2004;5(1):41–50.

73. Whistler JL, von Zastrow M. Morphine-activated opioid receptors elude desensitization by beta-arrestin. *Proc Natl Acad Sci U S A.* 1998;95(17):9914–9919.

74. Claing A, Laporte SA, Caron MG, Lefkowitz RJ. Endocytosis of G protein-coupled receptors: roles of G protein-coupled receptor kinases and beta-arrestin proteins. *Prog Neurobiol.* 2002;66(2):61–79.

75. Gintzler AR, Chakrabarti S. Post-opioid receptor adaptations to chronic morphine; altered functionality and associations of signaling molecules. *Life Sci.* 2006;79(8):717–722.

76. Wang L, Gintzler AR. Morphine tolerance and physical dependence: reversal of opioid inhibition to enhancement of cyclic AMP formation. *J Neurochem.* 1995;64(3):1102–1106.

77. Wang L, Gintzler AR. Altered mu-opiate receptor-G protein signal transduction following chronic morphine exposure. *J Neurochem.* 1997;68(1):248–254.

78. Basheer R, Tempel A. Morphine-induced reciprocal alterations in G alpha s and opioid peptide mRNA levels in discrete brain regions. *J Neurosci Res.* 1993;36(5):551–557.

79. Parolaro D, Rubino T, Gori E, et al. In situ hybridization reveals specific increases in G alpha s and G alpha o mRNA in discrete brain regions of morphine-tolerant rats. *Eur J Pharmacol.* 1993;244(3):211–222.

80. Rubino T, Parenti M, Patrini G, Massi P, Parolaro D. Morphine withdrawal syndrome and G protein expression: a study of the time course in the rat central nervous system. *Eur J Neurosci.* 1995;7(11):2334–2340.

81. Chakrabarti S, Regec A, Gintzler AR. Biochemical demonstration of mu-opioid receptor association with Gsalpha: enhancement following morphine exposure. *Brain Res Mol Brain Res.* Apr 27 2005;135(1–2):217–224.

82. Chakrabarti S, Rivera M, Yan SZ, Tang WJ, Gintzler AR. Chronic morphine augments G(beta)(gamma)/Gs(alpha) stimulation of adenylyl cyclase: relevance to opioid tolerance. *Mol Pharmacol.* 1998;54(4):655–662.

83. Chakrabarti S, Wang L, Tang WJ, Gintzler AR. Chronic morphine augments adenylyl cyclase phosphorylation: relevance to altered signaling during tolerance/dependence. *Mol Pharmacol.* 1998;54(6):949–953.

84. Wang ZJ, Wang LX. Phosphorylation: a molecular switch in opioid tolerance. *Life Sci.* 2006;79(18):1681–1691.

85. Mayer DJ, Mao J, Price DD. The development of morphine tolerance and dependence is associated with translocation of protein kinase C. *Pain.* Jun 1995;61(3):365–374.

86. Li Y, Roerig SC. Alteration of spinal protein kinase C expression and kinetics in morphine, but not clonidine, tolerance. *Biochem Pharmacol.* 1999;58(3):493–501.

87. Narita M, Makimura M, Feng Y, Hoskins B, Ho IK. Influence of chronic morphine treatment on protein kinase C activity: comparison with butorphanol and implication for opioid tolerance. *Brain Res.* 1994;650(1):175–179.

88. Bilsky EJ, Inturrisi CE, Sadee W, Hruby VJ, Porreca F. Competitive and non-competitive NMDA antagonists block the development of antinociceptive tolerance to morphine, but not to selective mu or delta opioid agonists in mice. *Pain.* 1996;68(2–3):229–237.

89. Yukhananov RY, Kissin I. Comment on Zeitz, K.P., et al., Reduced development of tolerance to the analgesic effects of morphine and clonidine in PKC mutant mice, PAIN 94 (2002) 245–253. *Pain.* Apr 2003;102(3):309–310; author reply 310–301.

90. Zeitz KP, Malmberg AB, Gilbert H, Basbaum AI. Reduced development of tolerance to the analgesic effects of morphine and clonidine in PKC gamma mutant mice. *Pain.* 2001;94(3):245–253.

91. Liang D, Li X, Clark JD. Increased expression of Ca2+/calmodulin-dependent protein kinase II alpha during chronic morphine exposure. *Neuroscience.* 2004;123(3):769–775.

92. Lou L, Zhou T, Wang P, Pei G. Modulation of Ca2+/calmodulin-dependent protein kinase II activity by acute and chronic morphine administration in rat hippocampus: differential regulation of alpha and beta isoforms. *Mol Pharmacol.* 1999;55(3):557–563.

93. Wang ZJ, Tang L, Xin L. Reversal of morphine antinociceptive tolerance by acute spinal inhibition of Ca(2+)/calmodulin-dependent protein kinase II. *Eur J Pharmacol.* 2003;465(1–2):199–200.

94. Koch T, Kroslak T, Mayer P, Raulf E, Hollt V. Site mutation in the rat mu-opioid receptor demonstrates the involvement of calcium/calmodulin-dependent protein kinase II in agonist-mediated desensitization. *J Neurochem.* 1997;69(4):1767–1770.

95. Bhargava HN, Cao YJ, Zhao GM. Effect of 7-nitroindazole on tolerance to morphine, U-50,488H and [D-Pen2, D-Pen5] enkephalin in mice. *Peptides.* 1997;18(6):797–800.

96. Kolesnikov YA, Pan YX, Babey AM, Jain S, Wilson R, Pasternak GW. Functionally differentiating two neuronal nitric oxide synthase isoforms through antisense mapping: evidence for opposing NO actions on morphine analgesia and tolerance. *Proc Natl Acad Sci U S A.* 1997;94(15):8220–8225.

97. Liang D, Li X, Lighthall G, Clark JD. Heme oxygenase type 2 modulates behavioral and molecular changes during chronic exposure to morphine. *Neuroscience.* 2003;121(4):999–1005.

98. Liang DY, Clark JD. Modulation of the NO/CO-cGMP signaling cascade during chronic morphine exposure in mice. *Neurosci Lett.* 2004;365(1):73–77.

99. Minneman KP, Iversen IL. Enkephalin and opiate narcotics increase cyclic GMP accumulation in slices of rat neostriatum. *Nature.* 1976;262(5566):313–314.

100. Racagni G, Zsilla G, Guidotti A, Costa E. Accumulation of cGMP in striatum of rats injected with narcotic analgesics: antagonism by naltrexone. *J Pharm Pharmacol.* 1976;28(3):258–260.

101. Lim G, Wang S, Lim JA, Mao J. Activity of adenylyl cyclase and protein kinase A contributes to morphine-induced spinal apoptosis. *Neurosci Lett.* 2005;389(2):104–108.

102. Smith FL, Javed RR, Elzey MJ, Dewey WL. The expression of a high level of morphine antinociceptive tolerance in mice involves both PKC and PKA. *Brain Res.* 2003;985(1):78–88.

103. Smith FL, Javed RR, Smith PA, Dewey WL, Gabra BH. PKC and PKA inhibitors reinstate morphine-induced behaviors in morphine tolerant mice. *Pharmacol Res.* 2006;54(6):474–480.

104. Wagner EJ, Ronnekleiv OK, Kelly MJ. Protein kinase A maintains cellular tolerance to mu opioid receptor agonists in hypothalamic neurosecretory cells with chronic morphine treatment: convergence on a common pathway with estrogen in modulating mu opioid receptor/effector coupling. *J Pharmacol Exp Ther.* 1998;285(3):1266–1273.

105. Trujillo KA, Akil H. Inhibition of morphine tolerance and dependence by the NMDA receptor antagonist MK-801. *Science.* 1991;251(4989):85–87.

106. Gutstein HB, Trujillo KA. MK-801 inhibits the development of morphine tolerance at spinal sites. *Brain Res.* 1993;626(1–2):332–334.

107. Kest B, Mogil JS, Shamgar BE, Kao B, Liebeskind JC, Marek P. The NMDA receptor antagonist MK-801 protects against the development of morphine tolerance after intrathecal administration. *Proc West Pharmacol Soc.* 1993;36:307–310.

108. Fitzgerald LW, Ortiz J, Hamedani AG, Nestler EJ. Drugs of abuse and stress increase the expression of GluR1 and NMDAR1 glutamate receptor subunits in the rat ventral tegmental area: common adaptations among cross-sensitizing agents. *J Neurosci.* 1996;16(1):274–282.

109. Zhu H, Jang CG, Ma T, Oh S, Rockhold RW, Ho IK. Region specific expression of NMDA receptor NR1 subunit mRNA in hypothalamus and pons following chronic morphine treatment. *Eur J Pharmacol.* 1999;365(1):47–54.

110. Manning BH, Mao J, Frenk H, Price DD, Mayer DJ. Continuous co-administration of dextromethorphan or MK-801 with morphine: attenuation of morphine dependence and naloxone-reversible attenuation of morphine tolerance. *Pain.* 1996;67(1):79–88.

111. Mao J, Mayer DJ. Spinal cord neuroplasticity following repeated opioid exposure and its relation to pathological pain. *Ann N Y Acad Sci.* 2001;933:175–184.

112. Price DD, Mayer DJ, Mao J, Caruso FS. NMDA-receptor antagonists and opioid receptor interactions as related to analgesia and tolerance. *J Pain Symptom Manage.* 2000;19(1 Suppl): S7–S11.

113. Lim G, Wang S, Zeng Q, Sung B, Yang L, Mao J. Expression of spinal NMDA receptor and PKCgamma after chronic morphine is regulated by spinal glucocorticoid receptor. *J Neurosci.* 2005;25(48):11145–11154.

114. Ramkumar V, El-Fakahany EE. Increase in [3H]nitrendipine binding sites in the brain in morphine-tolerant mice. *Eur J Pharmacol.* 1984;102(2):371–372.

115. Suematsu M, Ohnishi T, Shinno E, et al. Effect of prolonged administration of clonidine on [3H]PN 200–110 and [125I]omega-conotoxin binding in mouse brain. *Neurosci Lett.* 1993;163(2):193–196.

116. Wang YX, Gao D, Pettus M, Phillips C, Bowersox SS. Interactions of intrathecally administered ziconotide, a selective blocker of neuronal N-type voltage-sensitive calcium channels, with morphine on nociception in rats. *Pain.* 2000;84(2–3):271–281.

117. Yokoyama K, Kurihara T, Saegusa H, Zong S, Makita K, Tanabe T. Blocking the R-type (Cav2.3) Ca2+ channel enhanced morphine analgesia and reduced morphine tolerance. *Eur J Neurosci.* 2004;20(12):3516–3519.

118. Dogrul A, Bilsky EJ, Ossipov MH, Lai J, Porreca F. Spinal L-type calcium channel blockade abolishes opioid-induced sensory hypersensitivity and antinociceptive tolerance. *Anesth Analg.* 2005;101(6):1730–1735.

119. Smith FL, Dombrowski DS, Dewey WL. Involvement of intracellular calcium in morphine tolerance in mice. *Pharmacol Biochem Behav.* 1999;62(2):381–388.

120. Matus-Leibovitch N, Vogel Z, Ezra-Macabee V, Etkin S, Nevo I, Attali B. Chronic morphine administration enhances the expression of Kv1.5 and Kv1.6 voltage-gated K+ channels in rat spinal cord. *Brain Res Mol Brain Res.* 1996;40(2):261–270.

121. Campbell VC, Dewey WL, Welch SP. Comparison of [(3)H] Glyburide binding with opiate analgesia, tolerance, and dependence in ICR and Swiss-Webster mice. *J Pharmacol Exp Ther.* 2000;295(3):1112–1119.

122. Chiou LC, Yeh GC, Fan SH, How CH, Chuang KC, Tao PL. Prenatal morphine exposure decreases analgesia but not K+ channel activation. *NeuroReport.* 2003;14(2):239–242.

123. Chen X, Marrero HG, Murphy R, Lin YJ, Freedman JE. Altered gating of opiate receptor-modulated K+ channels on amygdala neurons of morphine-dependent rats. *Proc Natl Acad Sci U S A.* 2000;97(26):14692–14696.

124. Crain SM, Shen KF, Chalazonitis A. Opioids excite rather than inhibit sensory neurons after chronic opioid exposure of spinal cord-ganglion cultures. *Brain Res.* 1988;455(1):99–109.

125. Shen KF, Crain SM. Dual opioid modulation of the action potential duration of mouse dorsal root ganglion neurons in culture. *Brain Res.* 1989;491(2):227–242.

126. Watkins LR, Hutchinson MR, Ledeboer A, Wieseler-Frank J, Milligan ED, Maier SF. Norman Cousins Lecture. Glia as the "bad guys": implications for improving clinical pain control and the clinical utility of opioids. *Brain Behav Immun.* 2007;21(2):131–146.

127. Cui Y, Chen Y, Zhi JL, Guo RX, Feng JQ, Chen PX. Activation of p38 mitogen-activated protein kinase in spinal microglia mediates morphine antinociceptive tolerance. *Brain Res.* 2006; 1069(1):235–243.

128. Tai YH, Wang YH, Wang JJ, Tao PL, Tung CS, Wong CS. Amitriptyline suppresses neuroinflammation and up-regulates glutamate transporters in morphine-tolerant rats. *Pain.* 2006; 124(1–2):77–86.

129. Johnston IN, Milligan ED, Wieseler-Frank J, et al. A role for proinflammatory cytokines and fractalkine in analgesia, tolerance, and subsequent pain facilitation induced by chronic intrathecal morphine. *J Neurosci.* 2004;24(33):7353–7365.

130. Raghavendra V, Rutkowski MD, DeLeo JA. The role of spinal neuroimmune activation in morphine tolerance/hyperalgesia in neuropathic and sham-operated rats. *J Neurosci.* 2002;22(22):9980–9989.

131. Song P, Liu XY, Zhao ZQ. Interleukin-2-induced antinociception in morphine-insensitive rats. *Acta Pharmacol Sin.* 2002; 23(11):981–984.

132. Dougherty PM, Harper C, Dafny N. The effect of alpha-interferon, cyclosporine A, and radiation-induced immune suppression on morphine-induced hypothermia and tolerance. *Life Sci.* 1986;39(23):2191–2197.

133. Raghavendra V, Tanga FY, DeLeo JA. Attenuation of morphine tolerance, withdrawal-induced hyperalgesia, and associated spinal inflammatory immune responses by propentofylline in rats. *Neuropsychopharmacology.* 2004;29(2):327–334.

134. Kest B, Hopkins E, Palmese CA, Adler M, Mogil JS. Genetic variation in morphine analgesic tolerance: a survey of 11 inbred mouse strains. *Pharmacol Biochem Behav.* 2002;73(4):821–828.

135. Liang DY, Guo T, Liao G, Kingery WS, Peltz G, Clark JD. Chronic pain and genetic background interact and influence opioid analgesia, tolerance, and physical dependence. *Pain.* 2006;121(3):232–240.

136. Liang DY, Liao G, Wang J, et al. A genetic analysis of opioid-induced hyperalgesia in mice. *Anesthesiology.* 2006;104(5):1054–1062.

137. Liang DY, Shi X, Li X, Li J, Clark JD. The beta2 adrenergic receptor regulates morphine tolerance and physical dependence. *Behav Brain Res.* 2007;181(1):118–126.

138. Liang DY, Liao G, Lighthall GK, Peltz G, Clark DJ. Genetic variants of the P-glycoprotein gene Abcb1b modulate opioid-induced hyperalgesia, tolerance and dependence. *Pharmacogenet Genomics.* 2006;16(11):825–835.

139. King M, Su W, Chang A, Zuckerman A, Pasternak GW. Transport of opioids from the brain to the periphery by P-glycoprotein: peripheral actions of central drugs. *Nat Neurosci.* 2001;4(3):268–274.

140. Ossipov MH, Lai J, King T, et al. Antinociceptive and nociceptive actions of opioids. *J Neurobiol.* 2004;61(1):126–148.

141. Dunbar SA, Karamian IG. Periodic abstinence enhances nociception without significantly altering the antinociceptive efficacy of spinal morphine in the rat. *Neurosci Lett.* 2003;344(3):145–148.

142. Dunbar SA, Karamian I, Zhang J. Ketorolac prevents recurrent withdrawal induced hyperalgesia but does not inhibit tolerance to spinal morphine in the rat. *Eur J Pain.* 2007;11(1):1–6.

143. Rossbach M. Ueber die Gewoehnung an Gifte. *Pflugers Archieve Gesamte Physiologie des Menschen.* 1880;21:213–225.

144. Doverty M, Somogyi AA, White JM, et al. Methadone maintenance patients are cross-tolerant to the antinociceptive effects of morphine. *Pain.* 2001;93(2):155–163.

145. Compton MA. Cold-pressor pain tolerance in opiate and cocaine abusers: correlates of drug type and use status. *J Pain Symptom Manage.* 1994;9(7):462–473.

146. Compton P, Charuvastra VC, Ling W. Pain intolerance in opioid-maintained former opiate addicts: effect of long-acting maintenance agent. *Drug Alcohol Depend.* 2001;63(2):139–146.

147. Compton P, Charuvastra VC, Kintaudi K, Ling W. Pain responses in methadone-maintained opioid abusers. *J Pain Symptom Manage.* 2000;20(4):237–245.

148. Doverty M, White JM, Somogyi AA, Bochner F, Ali R, Ling W. Hyperalgesic responses in methadone maintenance patients. *Pain.* 2001;90(1–2):91–96.

149. Dyer KR, Foster DJ, White JM, Somogyi AA, Menelaou A, Bochner F. Steady-state pharmacokinetics and pharmacodynamics in methadone maintenance patients: comparison of those who do and do not experience withdrawal and concentration-effect relationships. *Clin Pharmacol Ther.* 1999;65(6):685–694.

150. Schall U, Katta T, Pries E, Kloppel A, Gastpar M. Pain perception of intravenous heroin users on maintenance therapy with levomethadone. *Pharmacopsychiatry.* 1996;29(5):176–179.

151. Hood DD, Curry R, Eisenach JC. Intravenous remifentanil produces withdrawal hyperalgesia in volunteers with capsaicin-induced hyperalgesia. *Anesth Analg.* 2003;97(3):810–815.

152. Angst MS, Koppert W, Pahl I, Clark DJ, Schmelz M. Short-term infusion of the mu-opioid agonist remifentanil in humans causes hyperalgesia during withdrawal. *Pain.* 2003;106(1–2):49–57.

153. Pud D, Cohen D, Lawental E, Eisenberg E. Opioids and abnormal pain perception: new evidence from a study of chronic opioid addicts and healthy subjects. *Drug Alcohol Depend.* 2006;82(3):218–223.

154. Khantzian EJ. The self-medication hypothesis of addictive disorders: focus on heroin and cocaine dependence. *Am J Psychiatry.* 1985;142(11):1259–1264.

155. Khantzian EJ. The self-medication hypothesis of substance use disorders: a reconsideration and recent applications. *Harv Rev Psychiatry.* 1997;4(5):231–244.

156. Beck TA, Wright DF, Newman FC, Liese SB. *Cognitive Therapy of Substance Abuse.* New York, NY: The Guilford Press; 1993.

157. Martin WR, Jasinski DR, Haertzen CA, et al. Methadone – a reevaluation. *Arch Gen Psychiatry.* 1973;28(2):286–295.

158. Rainville P, Feine JS, Bushnell MC, Duncan GH. A psychophysical comparison of sensory and affective responses to four modalities of experimental pain. *Somatosens Mot Res.* 1992;9(4):265–277.

159. Hay JL, White JM, Somogyi AA, Bochner F, Rounsefell B, Semple T. Clinical evidence for opioid-induced hyperalgesia. *Proceedings of the Australasian Society of Clinical and Experimental Pharmacologists and Toxicologists.* 2003;10:4.

160. Joly V, Richebe P, Guignard B, et al. Remifentanil-induced postoperative hyperalgesia and its prevention with small-dose ketamine. *Anesthesiology.* 2005;103(1):147–155.

161. Lee LH, Irwin MG, Lui SK. Intraoperative remifentanil infusion does not increase postoperative opioid consumption compared with 70% nitrous oxide. *Anesthesiology.* 2005;102(2):398–402.

162. Hansen EG, Duedahl TH, Romsing J, Hilsted KL, Dahl JB. Intraoperative remifentanil might influence pain levels in the immediate post-operative period after major abdominal surgery. *Acta Anaesthesiol Scand.* 2005;49(10):1464–1470.

163. Troster A, Sittl R, Singler B, Schmelz M, Schuttler J, Koppert W. Modulation of remifentanil-induced analgesia and postinfusion hyperalgesia by parecoxib in humans. *Anesthesiology.* 2006;105(5):1016–1023.

164. Koppert W, Dern SK, Sittl R, Albrecht S, Schuttler J, Schmelz M. A new model of electrically evoked pain and hyperalgesia in human skin: the effects of intravenous alfentanil, S(+)-ketamine, and lidocaine. *Anesthesiology.* 2001;95(2):395–402.

165. Koppert W, Sittl R, Scheuber K, Alsheimer M, Schmelz M, Schuttler J. Differential modulation of remifentanil-induced analgesia and postinfusion hyperalgesia by S-ketamine and clonidine in humans. *Anesthesiology.* 2003;99(1):152–159.

166. Luginbuhl M, Gerber A, Schnider TW, Petersen-Felix S, Arendt-Nielsen L, Curatolo M. Modulation of remifentanil-induced analgesia, hyperalgesia, and tolerance by small-dose ketamine in humans. *Anesth Analg.* 2003;96(3):726–732.

167. Compton P, Miotto K, Elashoff D. Precipitated opioid withdrawal across acute physical dependence induction methods. *Pharmacol Biochem Behav.* 2004;77(2):263–268.

168. Compton P, Athanasos P, Elashoff D. Withdrawal hyperalgesia after acute opioid physical dependence in nonaddicted humans: a preliminary study. *J Pain.* 2003;4(9):511–519.

169. Aley KO, Green PG, Levine JD. Opioid and adenosine peripheral antinociception are subject to tolerance and withdrawal. *J Neurosci.* 1995;15(12):8031–8038.

170. Aley KO, Levine JD. Different mechanisms mediate development and expression of tolerance and dependence for peripheral mu-opioid antinociception in rat. *J Neurosci.* 1997;17(20):8018–8023.

171. Aley KO, Levine JD. Dissociation of tolerance and dependence for opioid peripheral antinociception in rats. *J Neurosci.* 1997;17(10):3907–3912.

172. Aley KO, Levine JD. Multiple receptors involved in peripheral alpha 2, mu, and A1 antinociception, tolerance, and withdrawal. *J Neurosci.* 1997;17(2):735–744.

173. Arts KS, Holmes BB, Fujimoto JM. Differential contribution of descending serotonergic and noradrenergic systems to central Tyr-D-Ala2-Gly-NMePhe4-Gly-ol5 (DAMGO) and morphine-induced antinociception in mice. *J Pharmacol Exp Ther.* 1991;256(3):890–896.

174. Mao J, Price DD, Mayer DJ. Thermal hyperalgesia in association with the development of morphine tolerance in rats: roles of excitatory amino acid receptors and protein kinase C. *J Neurosci.* 1994;14(4):2301–2312.

175. Dunbar SA, Pulai IJ. Repetitive opioid abstinence causes progressive hyperalgesia sensitive to N-methyl-D-aspartate receptor blockade in the rat. *J Pharmacol Exp Ther.* 1998;284(2):678–686.

176. Celerier E, Laulin JP, Corcuff JB, Le Moal M, Simonnet G. Progressive enhancement of delayed hyperalgesia induced by repeated heroin administration: a sensitization process. *J Neurosci.* 2001;21(11):4074–4080.

177. Celerier E, Laulin J, Larcher A, Le Moal M, Simonnet G. Evidence for opiate-activated NMDA processes masking opiate analgesia in rats. *Brain Res.* 1999;847(1):18–25.

178. Laulin JP, Celerier E, Larcher A, Le Moal M, Simonnet G. Opiate tolerance to daily heroin administration: an apparent phenomenon associated with enhanced pain sensitivity. *Neuroscience.* 1999;89:631–636.

179. Laulin JP, Larcher A, Celerier E, Le Moal M, Simonnet G. Long-lasting increased pain sensitivity in rat following exposure to heroin for the first time. *Eur J Neurosci.* 1998;10(2):782–785.

180. Rivat C, Laulin JP, Corcuff JB, Celerier E, Pain L, Simonnet G. Fentanyl enhancement of carrageenan-induced long-lasting hyperalgesia in rats: prevention by the N-methyl-D-aspartate receptor antagonist ketamine. *Anesthesiology.* 2002;96(2):381–391.

181. Laulin JP, Maurette P, Corcuff JB, Rivat C, Chauvin M, Simonnet G. The role of ketamine in preventing fentanyl-induced hyperalgesia and subsequent acute morphine tolerance. *Anesth Analg.* 2002;94(5):1263–1269.

182. Celerier E, Rivat C, Jun Y, et al. Long-lasting hyperalgesia induced by fentanyl in rats: preventive effect of ketamine. *Anesthesiology.* 2000;92(2):465–472.

183. Li X, Angst MS, Clark JD. A murine model of opioid-induced hyperalgesia. *Brain Res.Mol.Brain Res.* 2001;86:56–62.

184. Celerier E, Simonnet G, Maldonado R. Prevention of fentanyl-induced delayed pronociceptive effects in mice lacking the protein kinase C gamma gene. *Neuropharmacology.* 2004;46(2):264–272.

185. Sweitzer SM, Wong SM, Tjolsen A, Allen CP, Mochly-Rosen D, Kendig JJ. Exaggerated nociceptive responses on morphine withdrawal: roles of protein kinase C epsilon and gamma. *Pain.* 2004;110(1–2):281–289.

186. Vanderah TW, Gardell LR, Burgess SE, et al. Dynorphin promotes abnormal pain and spinal opioid antinociceptive tolerance. *J Neurosci.* 2000;20(18):7074–7079.

187. Dunbar SA, Karamov IG, Buerkle H. The effect of spinal ibuprofen on opioid withdrawal in the rat. *Anesth Analg.* 2000;91(2):417–422.

188. Vera-Portocarrero LP, Zhang ET, King T, et al. Spinal NK-1 receptor expressing neurons mediate opioid-induced hyperalgesia and antinociceptive tolerance via activation of descending pathways. *Pain.* 2007;129(1–2):35–45.

189. Li X, Clark JD. Hyperalgesia during opioid abstinence: mediation by glutamate and substance p. *Anesth Analg.* 2002;95(4):979–984.

190. Belanger S, Ma W, Chabot JG, Quirion R. Expression of calcitonin gene-related peptide, substance P and protein kinase C in cultured dorsal root ganglion neurons following chronic exposure to mu, delta and kappa opiates. *Neuroscience.* 2002;115(2):441–453.

191. Mao J, Sung B, Ji RR, Lim G. Chronic morphine induces downregulation of spinal glutamate transporters: implications in morphine tolerance and abnormal pain sensitivity. *J Neurosci.* 2002;22(18):8312–8323.

192. Vanderah TW, Suenaga NM, Ossipov MH, Malan TP, Jr., Lai J, Porreca F. Tonic descending facilitation from the rostral ventromedial medulla mediates opioid-induced abnormal pain and antinociceptive tolerance. *J Neurosci.* 2001;21(1):279–286.

193. Xie JY, Herman DS, Stiller CO, et al. Cholecystokinin in the rostral ventromedial medulla mediates opioid-induced hyperalgesia and antinociceptive tolerance. *J Neurosci.* 2005;25(2):409–416.

194. Schinkel AH, Wagenaar E, van Deemter L, Mol CA, Borst P. Absence of the mdr1a P-Glycoprotein in mice affects tissue distribution and pharmacokinetics of dexamethasone, digoxin, and cyclosporin A. *J Clin Invest.* 1995;96(4):1698–1705.

195. Hemstapat K, Monteith GR, Smith D, Smith MT. Morphine-3-glucuronide's neuro-excitatory effects are mediated via indirect activation of N-methyl-D-aspartic acid receptors: mechanistic studies in embryonic cultured hippocampal neurones. *Anesth Analg.* 2003;97(2):494–505, table of contents.

196. Smith MT. Neuroexcitatory effects of morphine and hydromorphone: evidence implicating the 3-glucuronide metabolites. *Clin Exp Pharmacol Physiol.* 2000;27(7):524–528.

197. Wright AW, Mather LE, Smith MT. Hydromorphone-3-glucuronide: a more potent neuro-excitant than its structural analogue, morphine-3-glucuronide. *Life Sci.* 2001;69(4):409–420.

198. Sjogren P, Jonsson T, Jensen NH, Drenck NE, Jensen TS. Hyperalgesia and myoclonus in terminal cancer patients treated with continuous intravenous morphine. *Pain.* 1993;55(1):93–97.

199. Sjogren P, Jensen NH, Jensen TS. Disappearance of morphine-induced hyperalgesia after discontinuing or substituting morphine with other opioid agonists. *Pain.* 1994;59(2):313–316.

200. Wilson GR, Reisfield GM. Morphine hyperalgesia: a case report. *Am J Hosp Palliat Care.* 2003;20(6):459–461.

201. De Conno F, Caraceni A, Martini C, Spoldi E, Salvetti M, Ventafridda V. Hyperalgesia and myoclonus with intrathecal infusion of high-dose morphine. *Pain.* 1991;47(3):337–339.

202. Lawlor P, Turner K, Hanson J, Bruera E. Dose ratio between morphine and hydromorphone in patients with cancer pain: a retrospective study. *Pain.* 1997;72:79–85.

203. Sjogren P, Thunedborg LP, Christrup L, Hansen SH, Franks J. Is development of hyperalgesia, allodynia and myoclonus related to morphine metabolism during long-term administration? Six case histories. *Acta Anaesthesiol Scand.* 1998;42(9):1070–1075.

204. Heger S, Maier C, Otter K, Helwig U, Suttorp M. Morphine induced allodynia in a child with brain tumour. *Bmj.* 1999; 319(7210):627–629.

205. Woolf CJ. Intrathecal high dose morphine produces hyperalgesia in the rat. *Brain Res.* 1981;209(2):491–495.

206. Yaksh TL, Harty GJ. Pharmacology of the allodynia in rats evoked by high dose intrathecal morphine. *J Pharmacol Exp Ther.* 1988;244(2):501–507.

207. Yaksh TL, Harty GJ, Onofrio BM. High dose of spinal morphine produce a nonopiate receptor-mediated hyperesthesia: clinical and theoretic implications. *Anesthesiology.* 1986;64(5):590–597.

208. Sakurada T, Watanabe C, Okuda K, et al. Intrathecal high-dose morphine induces spinally-mediated behavioral responses through NMDA receptors. *Brain Res Mol Brain Res.* 2002;98(1–2):111–118.

209. Hara N, Minami T, Okuda-Ashitaka E, et al. Characterization of nociceptin hyperalgesia and allodynia in conscious mice. *Br J Pharmacol.* 1997;121(3):401–408.

210. Lawlor P, Walker P, Bruera E, Mitchell S. Severe opioid toxicity and somatization of psychosocial distress in a cancer patient with a background of chemical dependence. *J Pain Symptom Manage.* 1997;13(6):356–361.

211. Callahan RJ, Au JD, Paul M, Liu C, Yost CS. Functional inhibition by methadone of N-methyl-D-aspartate receptors expressed in Xenopus oocytes: stereospecific and subunit effects. *Anesth Analg.* 2004;98(3):653–659, table of contents.

212. Chen HS, Lipton SA. The chemical biology of clinically tolerated NMDA receptor antagonists. *J Neurochem.* 2006;97(6):1611–1626.

213. Goebel DJ, Poosch MS. NMDA receptor subunit gene expression in the rat brain: a quantitative analysis of endogenous mRNA levels of NR1Com, NR2A, NR2B, NR2C, NR2D and NR3A. *Brain Res Mol Brain Res.* 1999;69(2):164–170.

214. Zukin RS, Bennett MV. Alternatively spliced isoforms of the NMDARI receptor subunit. *Trends Neurosci.* 1995;18(7):306–313.

215. White JM, Ryan CF. Pharmacological properties of ketamine. *Drug Alcohol Rev.* 1996;15(2):145–155.

216. Reich DL, Silvay G. Ketamine: an update on the first twenty-five years of clinical experience. *Can J Anaesth.* 1989;36(2):186–197.

217. Annetta MG, Iemma D, Garisto C, Tafani C, Proietti R. Ketamine: new indications for an old drug. *Curr Drug Targets.* 2005; 6(7):789–794.

218. Sloan TB. Anesthetics and the brain. *Anesthesiol Clin North America.* 2002;20(2):265–292.

219. Elia N, Tramer MR. Ketamine and postoperative pain – a quantitative systematic review of randomised trials. *Pain.* 2005;113(1–2):61–70.

220. Bell RF, Dahl JB, Moore RA, Kalso E. Perioperative ketamine for acute postoperative pain. *Cochrane Database Syst Rev.* 2006(1): CD004603.

221. Subramaniam K, Subramaniam B, Steinbrook RA. Ketamine as adjuvant analgesic to opioids: a quantitative and qualitative systematic review. *Anesth Analg.* 2004;99(2):482–495, table of contents.

222. Stubhaug A, Breivik H, Eide PK, Kreunen M, Foss A. Mapping of punctuate hyperalgesia around a surgical incision demonstrates that ketamine is a powerful suppressor of central sensitization to pain following surgery. *Acta Anaesthesiol Scand.* 1997; 41(9):1124–1132.

223. De Kock M, Lavand'homme P, Waterloos H. 'Balanced analgesia' in the perioperative period: is there a place for ketamine? *Pain.* 2001;92(3):373–380.

224. Bell RF, Eccleston C, Kalso E. Ketamine as adjuvant to opioids for cancer pain. A qualitative systematic review. *J Pain Symptom Manage.* 2003;26(3):867–875.

225. Weinbroum AA. A single small dose of postoperative ketamine provides rapid and sustained improvement in morphine analgesia in the presence of morphine-resistant pain. *Anesth Analg.* 2003;96(3):789–795, table of contents.

226. Bell RF. Low-dose subcutaneous ketamine infusion and morphine tolerance. *Pain.* 1999;83(1):101–103.

227. Eilers H, Philip LA, Bickler PE, McKay WR, Schumacher MA. The reversal of fentanyl-induced tolerance by administration of "small-dose" ketamine. *Anesth Analg.* 2001;93(1):213–214.

228. Mercadante S, Arcuri E. Hyperalgesia and opioid switching. *Am J Hosp Palliat Care.* 2005;22(4):291–294.

229. Axelrod DJ, Reville B. Using methadone to treat opioid-induced hyperalgesia and refractory pain. *J Opioid Manag.* 2007;3(2):113–114.

230. Chung KS, Carson S, Glassman D, Vadivelu N. Successful treatment of hydromorphone-induced neurotoxicity and hyperalgesia. *Conn Med.* 2004;68(9):547–549.

231. Zimmermann C, Seccareccia D, Booth CM, Cottrell W. Rotation to methadone after opioid dose escalation: how should individualization of dosing occur? *J Pain Palliat Care Pharmacother.* 2005;19(2):25–31.

232. Mercadante S, Ferrera P, Villari P, Arcuri E. Hyperalgesia: an emerging iatrogenic syndrome. *J Pain Symptom Manage.* 2003; 26(2):769–775.

233. Bowsher D. Paradoxical pain. *BMJ.* 1993;306(6876):473–474.

234. Skarke C, Geisslinger G, Lotsch J. Is morphine-3-glucuronide of therapeutic relevance? *Pain.* 2005;116(3):177–180.

235. Katz NP. MorphiDex (MS:DM) double-blind, multiple-dose studies in chronic pain patients. *J Pain Symptom Manage.* 2000;19(1 Suppl):S37–S41.

236. Caruso FS. MorphiDex pharmacokinetic studies and single-dose analgesic efficacy studies in patients with postoperative pain. *J Pain Symptom Manage.* 2000;19(1 Suppl):S31–S36.

237. Chevlen E. Morphine with dextromethorphan: conversion from other opioid analgesics. *J Pain Symptom Manage.* 2000;19(1 Suppl):S42–S49.

238. Singler B, Troster A, Manering N, Schuttler J, Koppert W. Modulation of remifentanil-induced postinfusion hyperalgesia by propofol. *Anesth Analg.* 2007;104(6):1397–1403, table of contents.

239. Wang QY, Cao JL, Zeng YM, Dai TJ. GABAA receptor partially mediated propofol-induced hyperalgesia at supraspinal level and analgesia at spinal cord level in rats. *Acta Pharmacol Sin.* 2004;25(12):1619–1625.

240. Baba H, Kohno T, Moore KA, Woolf CJ. Direct activation of rat spinal dorsal horn neurons by prostaglandin E2. *J Neurosci.* 2001;21(5):1750–1756.

241. O'Rielly DD, Loomis CW. Increased expression of cyclooxygenase and nitric oxide isoforms, and exaggerated sensitivity to prostaglandin E2, in the rat lumbar spinal cord 3 days after L5-L6 spinal nerve ligation. *Anesthesiology.* 2006;104(2):328–337.

242. Malmberg AB, Yaksh TL. Hyperalgesia mediated by spinal glutamate or substance P receptor blocked by spinal cyclooxygenase inhibition. *Science.* 1992;257(5074):1276–1279.

243. Yaksh TL, Malmberg AB. Spinal actions of NSAIDS in blocking spinally mediated hyperalgesia: the role of cyclooxygenase products. *Agents Actions Suppl.* 1993;41:89–100.

244. Powell KJ, Hosokawa A, Bell A, et al. Comparative effects of cyclo-oxygenase and nitric oxide synthase inhibition on the development and reversal of spinal opioid tolerance. *Br J Pharmacol.* 1999;127(3):631–644.

245. Wong CS, Hsu MM, Chou R, Chou YY, Tung CS. Intrathecal cyclooxygenase inhibitor administration attenuates morphine antinociceptive tolerance in rats. *Br J Anaesth.* 2000;85(5):747–751.

246. Quartilho A, Mata HP, Ibrahim MM, et al. Production of paradoxical sensory hypersensitivity by alpha 2-adrenoreceptor agonists. *Anesthesiology.* 2004;100(6):1538–1544.

247. Davies MF, Haimor F, Lighthall G, Clark JD. Dexmedetomidine fails to cause hyperalgesia after cessation of chronic administration. *Anesth Analg.* 2003;96(1):195–200, table of contents.

248. De Kock M, Lavand'homme P, Waterloos H. The short-lasting analgesia and long-term antihyperalgesic effect of intrathecal clonidine in patients undergoing colonic surgery. *Anesth Analg.* 2005;101(2):566–572, table of contents.

249. Dumont H, Guntz E, Sosnowski M, Talla G, Roman A, Segers B. Opioid-induced hyperalgesia. *Eur J Anaesthesiol.* 2007;24(2):205–207.

250. Pavlin DJ, Chen C, Penaloza DA, Polissar NL, Buckley FP. Pain as a factor complicating recovery and discharge after ambulatory surgery. *Anesth Analg.* 2002;95(3):627–634, table of contents.

251. Capdevila X, Barthelet Y, Biboulet P, Ryckwaert Y, Rubenovitch J, d'Athis F. Effects of perioperative analgesic technique on the surgical outcome and duration of rehabilitation after major knee surgery. *Anesthesiology.* 1999;91(1):8–15.

252. Shea RA, Brooks JA, Dayhoff NE, Keck J. Pain intensity and postoperative pulmonary complications among the elderly after abdominal surgery. *Heart Lung.* 2002;31(6):440–449.

253. Tsui SL, Law S, Fok M, et al. Postoperative analgesia reduces mortality and morbidity after esophagectomy. *Am J Surg.* 1997;173(6):472–478.

254. Kehlet H, Jensen TS, Woolf CJ. Persistent postsurgical pain: risk factors and prevention. *Lancet.* 2006;367(9522):1618–1625.

255. Cousins MJ, Mather LE. Intrathecal and epidural administration of opioids. *Anesthesiology.* 1984;61:276–310.

256. de Leon-Casasola OA, Lema MJ. Epidural bupivacaine/sufentanil therapy for postoperative pain control in patients tolerant to opioid and unresponsive to epidural bupivacaine/morphine. *Anesthesiology.* 1994;80(2):303–309.

257. de Leon-Casasola OA. Postoperative pain management in opioid-tolerant patients. *Reg.Anesth.* 1996;21:114–116.

258. White PF. The changing role of non-opioid analgesic techniques in the management of postoperative pain. *Anesth Analg.* 2005;101(5 Suppl):S5–S22.

259. Turan A, White PF, Karamanlioglu B, et al. Gabapentin: an alternative to the cyclooxygenase-2 inhibitors for perioperative pain management. *Anesth Analg.* 2006;102(1):175–181.

260. Gilron I, Orr E, Tu D, O'Neill JP, Zamora JE, Bell AC. A placebo-controlled randomized clinical trial of perioperative administration of gabapentin, rofecoxib and their combination for spontaneous and movement-evoked pain after abdominal hysterectomy. *Pain.* 2005;113(1–2):191–200.

261. Barden J, Edwards JE, McQuay HJ, Moore RA. Oral valdecoxib and injected parecoxib for acute postoperative pain: a quantitative systematic review. *BMC Anesthesiol.* 2003;3(1):1.

262. McCrory CR, Lindahl SG. Cyclooxygenase inhibition for postoperative analgesia. *Anesth Analg.* 2002;95(1):169–176.

263. Hyllested M, Jones S, Pedersen JL, Kehlet H. Comparative effect of paracetamol, NSAIDs or their combination in postoperative pain management: a qualitative review. *Br J Anaesth.* 2002;88(2):199–214.

264. Romsing J, Moiniche S. A systematic review of COX-2 inhibitors compared with traditional NSAIDs, or different COX-2 inhibitors for post-operative pain. *Acta Anaesthesiol Scand.* 2004;48(5):525–546.

265. Romsing J, Moiniche S, Mathiesen O, Dahl JB. Reduction of opioid-related adverse events using opioid-sparing analgesia with COX-2 inhibitors lacks documentation: a systematic review. *Acta Anaesthesiol Scand.* 2005;49(2):133–142.

266. Remy C, Marret E, Bonnet F. Effects of acetaminophen on morphine side-effects and consumption after major surgery: meta-analysis of randomized controlled trials. *Br J Anaesth.* 2005;94(4):505–513.

267. Reicin A, Brown J, Jove M, et al. Efficacy of single-dose and multidose rofecoxib in the treatment of post-orthopedic surgery pain. *Am J Orthop.* 2001;30(1):40–48.

268. Reuben SS, Connelly NR. Postoperative analgesic effects of celecoxib or rofecoxib after spinal fusion surgery. *Anesth Analg.* 2000;91(5):1221–1225.

269. Hubbard RC, Naumann TM, Traylor L, Dhadda S. Parecoxib sodium has opioid-sparing effects in patients undergoing total knee arthroplasty under spinal anaesthesia. *Br J Anaesth.* Feb 2003;90(2):166–172.

270. Ng A, Smith G, Davidson AC. Analgesic effects of parecoxib following total abdominal hysterectomy. *Br J Anaesth.* 2003;90(6):746–749.

271. Harris SI, Kuss M, Hubbard RC, Goldstein JL. Upper gastrointestinal safety evaluation of parecoxib sodium, a new cyclooxygenase-2-specific inhibitor, compared with ketorolac, naproxen, and placebo. *Clin Ther.* 2001;23(9):1422–1428.

272. Stoltz RR, Harris SI, Kuss ME, et al. Upper GI mucosal effects of parecoxib sodium in healthy elderly subjects. *Am J Gastroenterol.* 2002;97(1):65–71.

273. Cheng HF, Harris RC. Renal effects of non-steroidal anti-inflammatory drugs and selective cyclooxygenase-2 inhibitors. *Curr Pharm Des.* 2005;11(14):1795–1804.

274. Lee A, Cooper MG, Craig JC, Knight JF, Keneally JP. Effects of nonsteroidal anti-inflammatory drugs on postoperative renal function in adults with normal renal function. *Cochrane Database Syst Rev.* 2007(2):CD002765.

275. Moiniche S, Romsing J, Dahl JB, Tramer MR. Nonsteroidal anti-inflammatory drugs and the risk of operative site bleeding after tonsillectomy: a quantitative systematic review. *Anesth Analg.* 2003;96(1):68–77, table of contents.

276. Hegi TR, Bombeli T, Seifert B, et al. Effect of rofecoxib on platelet aggregation and blood loss in gynaecological and breast surgery compared with diclofenac. *Br J Anaesth.* 2004;92(4):523–531.

277. Kearney PM, Baigent C, Godwin J, Halls H, Emberson JR, Patrono C. Do selective cyclo-oxygenase-2 inhibitors and traditional non-steroidal anti-inflammatory drugs increase the risk of atherothrombosis? Meta-analysis of randomised trials. *BMJ.* 2006;332(7553):1302–1308.

278. Graham DJ, Campen D, Hui R, et al. Risk of acute myocardial infarction and sudden cardiac death in patients treated with cyclo-oxygenase 2 selective and non-selective non-steroidal anti-inflammatory drugs: nested case-control study. *Lancet.* 2005;365(9458):475–481.

279. Nussmeier NA, Whelton AA, Brown MT, et al. Complications of the COX-2 inhibitors parecoxib and valdecoxib after cardiac surgery. *N Engl J Med.* 2005;352(11):1081–1091.

280. Nussmeier NA, Whelton AA, Brown MT, et al. Safety and efficacy of the cyclooxygenase-2 inhibitors parecoxib and valdecoxib after noncardiac surgery. *Anesthesiology.* 2006;104(3):518–526.

281. Graham GG, Scott KF, Day RO. Tolerability of paracetamol. *Drug Saf.* 2005;28(3):227–240.

282. Haller G, Waeber JL, Infante NK, Clergue F. Ketamine combined with morphine for the management of pain in an opioid addict. *Anesthesiology.* 2002;96(5):1265–1266.

283. Sveticic G, Gentilini A, Eichenberger U, Luginbuhl M, Curatolo M. Combinations of morphine with ketamine for patient-controlled analgesia: a new optimization method. *Anesthesiology.* 2003;98(5):1195–1205.

284. Sveticic G, Eichenberger U, Curatolo M. Safety of mixture of morphine with ketamine for postoperative patient-controlled analgesia: an audit with 1026 patients. *Acta Anaesthesiol Scand.* 2005;49(6):870–875.

285. Duedahl TH, Romsing J, Moiniche S, Dahl JB. A qualitative systematic review of peri-operative dextromethorphan in postoperative pain. *Acta Anaesthesiol Scand.* 2006;50(1):1–13.

286. Gee NS, Brown JP, Dissanayake VU, Offord J, Thurlow R, Woodruff GN. The novel anticonvulsant drug, gabapentin (Neurontin), binds to the alpha2delta subunit of a calcium channel. *J Biol Chem.* 1996;271(10):5768–5776.

287. Seib RK, Paul JE. Preoperative gabapentin for postoperative analgesia: a meta-analysis. *Can J Anaesth.* 2006;53(5):461–469.

288. Ho KY, Gan TJ, Habib AS. Gabapentin and postoperative pain – a systematic review of randomized controlled trials. *Pain.* 2006; 126(1–3):91–101.

289. Fassoulaki A, Stamatakis E, Petropoulos G, Siafaka I, Hassiakos D, Sarantopoulos C. Gabapentin attenuates late but not acute pain after abdominal hysterectomy. *Eur J Anaesthesiol.* 2006;23(2):136–141.

290. Tiippana EM, Hamunen K, Kontinen VK, Kalso E. Do surgical patients benefit from perioperative gabapentin/pregabalin? A systematic review of efficacy and safety. *Anesth Analg.* 2007;104(6):1545–1556, table of contents.

291. LeBlanc KA, Bellanger D, Rhynes VK, Hausmann M. Evaluation of continuous infusion of 0.5% bupivacaine by elastomeric pump for postoperative pain management after open inguinal hernia repair. *J Am Coll Surg.* 2005;200(2):198–202.

292. White PF, Rawal S, Latham P, et al. Use of a continuous local anesthetic infusion for pain management after median sternotomy. *Anesthesiology.* 2003;99(4):918–923.

293. Bianconi M, Ferraro L, Ricci R, et al. The pharmacokinetics and efficacy of ropivacaine continuous wound instillation after spine fusion surgery. *Anesth Analg.* 2004;98(1):166–172, table of contents.

294. Wu CL, Partin AW, Rowlingson AJ, Kalish MA, Walsh PC, Fleisher LA. Efficacy of continuous local anesthetic infusion for postoperative pain after radical retropubic prostatectomy. *Urology.* 2005;66(2):366–370.

295. Goldstein A, Grimault P, Henique A, Keller M, Fortin A, Darai E. Preventing postoperative pain by local anesthetic instillation after laparoscopic gynecologic surgery: a placebo-controlled comparison of bupivacaine and ropivacaine. *Anesth Analg.* 2000;91(2):403–407.

296. Ng A, Swami A, Smith G, Davidson AC, Emembolu J. The analgesic effects of intraperitoneal and incisional bupivacaine with epinephrine after total abdominal hysterectomy. *Anesth Analg.* 2002;95(1):158–162, table of contents.

297. Kalso E, Tramer MR, Carroll D, McQuay HJ, Moore RA. Pain relief from intra-articular morphine after knee surgery: a qualitative systematic review. *Pain.* 1997;71(2):127–134.

298. Moiniche S, Mikkelsen S, Wetterslev J, Dahl JB. A systematic review of intra-articular local anesthesia for postoperative pain relief after arthroscopic knee surgery. *Reg Anesth Pain Med.* 1999;24(5):430–437.

299. Andersen LJ, Poulsen T, Krogh B, Nielsen T. Postoperative analgesia in total hip arthroplasty: a randomized double-blinded, placebo-controlled study on peroperative and postoperative ropivacaine, ketorolac, and adrenaline wound infiltration. *Acta Orthop.* 2007;78(2):187–192.

300. Andersen KV, Pfeiffer-Jensen M, Haraldsted V, Soballe K. Reduced hospital stay and narcotic consumption, and improved mobilization with local and intraarticular infiltration after hip arthroplasty: a randomized clinical trial of an intraarticular technique versus epidural infusion in 80 patients. *Acta Orthop.* 2007;78(2):180–186.

301. Borgeat A, Schappi B, Biasca N, Gerber C. Patient-controlled analgesia after major shoulder surgery: patient-controlled interscalene analgesia versus patient-controlled analgesia. *Anesthesiology.* Dec 1997;87(6):1343–1347.

302. Lehtipalo S, Koskinen LO, Johansson G, Kolmodin J, Biber B. Continuous interscalene brachial plexus block for postoperative analgesia following shoulder surgery. *Acta Anaesthesiol Scand.* 1999;43(3):258–264.

303. Singelyn FJ, Ferrant T, Malisse MF, Joris D. Effects of intravenous patient-controlled analgesia with morphine, continuous epidural analgesia, and continuous femoral nerve sheath block on rehabilitation after unilateral total-hip arthroplasty. *Reg Anesth Pain Med.* 2005;30(5):452–457.

304. de Leon-Casasola OA, Lema MJ. Epidural sufentanil for acute pain control in a patient with extreme opioid dependency. *Anesthesiology.* 1992;76(5):853–856.

305. Niemi G, Breivik H. The minimally effective concentration of adrenaline in a low-concentration thoracic epidural analgesic infusion of bupivacaine, fentanyl and adrenaline after major surgery. A randomized, double-blind, dose-finding study. *Acta Anaesthesiol Scand.* 2003;47(4):439–450.

306. Tonner PH. Balanced anaesthesia today. *Best Pract Res Clin Anaesthesiol.* 2005;19(3):475–484.

307. Practice guidelines for acute pain management in the perioperative setting: an updated report by the American Society of Anesthesiologists Task Force on Acute Pain Management. *Anesthesiology.* 2004;100(6):1573–1581.

308. Ackerman WE, 3rd. Paroxysmal opioid-induced pain and hyperalgesia. *J Ky Med Assoc.* 2006;104(9):419–423.

309. Reuben SS. Preventing the development of complex regional pain syndrome after surgery. *Anesthesiology.* 2004;101(5):1215–1224.

310. Reuben SS, Buvanendran A. Preventing the development of chronic pain after orthopaedic surgery with preventive multimodal analgesic techniques. *J Bone Joint Surg Am.* 2007;89(6):1343–1358.

311. Perkins FM, Kehlet H. Chronic pain as an outcome of surgery. A review of predictive factors. *Anesthesiology.* 2000;93(4):1123–1133.

312. Reuben SS, Rosenthal EA, Steinberg RB. Surgery on the affected upper extremity of patients with a history of complex regional pain syndrome: a retrospective study of 100 patients. *J Hand Surg [Am].* 2000;25(6):1147–1151.

313. Parisod E, Siddall PJ, Viney M, McClelland JM, Cousins MJ. Allodynia after acute intrathecal morphine administration in a patient with neuropathic pain after spinal cord injury. *Anesth Analg.* 2003;97(1):183–186, table of contents.

314. Devulder J. Hyperalgesia induced by high-dose intrathecal sufentanil in neuropathic pain. *J Neurosurg Anesthesiol.* 1997;9(2):146–148.

315. Guntz E, Talla G, Roman A, Dumont H, Segers B, Sosnowski M. Opioid-induced hyperalgesia. *Eur J Anaesthesiol.* 2007;24(2):205–207.

316. Ackerman WE, 3rd. Personal communication regarding dosage of IT morphine and associated side effects in case report published

in Journal of the Kentucky Medical Association. In: Chu L, ed; 2007.

317. Dudgeon DJ, Bruera E, Gagnon B, et al. A phase III randomized, double-blind, placebo-controlled study evaluating dextromethorphan plus slow-release morphine for chronic cancer pain relief in terminally ill patients. *J Pain Symptom Manage.* 2007;33(4):365–371.

318. Orser BA, Bertlik M, Wang LY, MacDonald JF. Inhibition by propofol (2,6 di-isopropylphenol) of the N-methyl-D-aspartate subtype of glutamate receptor in cultured hippocampal neurones. *Br J Pharmacol.* 1995;116(2):1761–1768.

319. Grasshoff C, Gillessen T. Effects of propofol on N-methyl-D-aspartate receptor-mediated calcium increase in cultured rat cerebrocortical neurons. *Eur J Anaesthesiol.* 2005;22(6):467–470.

320. Kingston S, Mao L, Yang L, Arora A, Fibuch EE, Wang JQ. Propofol inhibits phosphorylation of N-methyl-D-aspartate receptor NR1 subunits in neurons. *Anesthesiology.* 2006;104(4):763–769.

321. Snijdelaar DG, Koren G, Katz J. Effects of perioperative oral amantadine on postoperative pain and morphine consumption in patients after radical prostatectomy: results of a preliminary study. *Anesthesiology.* 2004;100(1):134–141.

322. Sang CN. NMDA-receptor antagonists in neuropathic pain: experimental methods to clinical trials. *J Pain Symptom Manage.* 2000;19(1 Suppl):S21–S25.

323. Mathiesen O, Imbimbo BP, Hilsted KL, Fabbri L, Dahl JB. CHF3381, a N-methyl-D-aspartate receptor antagonist and monoamine oxidase-A inhibitor, attenuates secondary hyperalgesia in a human pain model. *J Pain.* 2006;7(8):565–574.

324. Bassani F, Bergamaschi M, Tonino Bolzoni P, Villetti G. CHF3381, a novel antinociceptive agent, attenuates capsaicin-induced pain in rats. *Eur J Pharmacol.* 2005;519(3):231–236.

325. Astruc B, Tarral A, Dostert P, Mariotti F, Fabbri L, Imbimbo BP. Steady-state pharmacokinetics and pharmacodynamics of CHF3381, a novel antineuropathic pain agent, in healthy subjects. *Br J Clin Pharmacol.* 2005;59(4):405–414.

326. Heiskanen T, Hartel B, Dahl ML, Seppala T, Kalso E. Analgesic effects of dextromethorphan and morphine in patients with chronic pain. *Pain.* 2002;96(3):261–267.

327. Tverskoy M, Oz Y, Isakson A, Finger J, Bradley EL, Jr, Kissin I. Preemptive effect of fentanyl and ketamine on postoperative pain and wound hyperalgesia. *Anesth.Analg.* 1994;78:205–209.

328. Ilkjaer S, Petersen KL, Brennum J, Wernberg M, Dahl JB. Effect of systemic N-methyl-D-aspartate receptor antagonist (ketamine) on primary and secondary hyperalgesia in humans. *Br J Anaesth.* 1996;76(6):829–834.

329. Klein T, Magerl W, Hanschmann A, Althaus M, Treede RD. Antihyperalgesic and analgesic properties of the N-methyl-d-aspartate (NMDA) receptor antagonist neramexane in a human surrogate model of neurogenic hyperalgesia. *Eur J Pain.* 2007.

330. Rammes G, Schierloh A. Neramexane (merz pharmaceuticals/forest laboratories). *IDrugs.* 2006;9(2):128–135.

331. Thisted RA, Klaff L, Schwartz SL, et al. Dextromethorphan and quinidine in adult patients with uncontrolled painful diabetic peripheral neuropathy: a 29-day, multicenter, open-label, dose-escalation study. *Clin Ther.* 2006;28(10):1607–1618.

332. Williams K. Ifenprodil, a novel NMDA receptor antagonist: site and mechanism of action. *Curr Drug Targets.* 2001;2(3):285–298.

333. Taniguchi K, Shinjo K, Mizutani M, et al. Antinociceptive activity of CP-101,606, an NMDA receptor NR2B subunit antagonist. *Br J Pharmacol.* 1997;122(5):809–812.

334. Boyce S, Wyatt A, Webb JK, et al. Selective NMDA NR2B antagonists induce antinociception without motor dysfunction: correlation with restricted localisation of NR2B subunit in dorsal horn. *Neuropharmacology.* 1999;38(5):611–623.

335. Gedeon Richter and Forest Laboratories Expand Relationship with Two New Collaborations for CNS Compounds. http://www.frx.com/news/PressRelease.aspx?ID=790577. Accessed May 27, 2007.

336. Carroll IR, Angst MS, Clark JD. Management of perioperative pain in patients chronically consuming opioids. *Reg Anesth Pain Med.* 2004;29(6):576–591.

337. Gammaitoni AR, Fine P, Alvarez N, McPherson ML, Bergmark S. Clinical application of opioid equianalgesic data. *Clin J Pain.* 2003;19(5):286–297.

SECTION II

Clinical Analgesia

11

Qualitative and Quantitative Assessment
of Pain

Cynthia M. Welchek, Lisa Mastrangelo, Raymond S. Sinatra, and
Richard Martinez

Pain is a prevalent medical complaint and is one of the primary reasons for which patients seek medical attention in the United States.[1] According to the American Pain Society, 50 million Americans are partially or totally disabled by pain, and 45% of all Americans seek care for persistent pain at some point in their lives.[2] It has been estimated that 50% to 80% of hospitalized patients experience considerable pain regardless of the reason for admission.[3] Despite the introduction of novel analgesics and advances in analgesic delivery systems, pain continues to be an undertreated event in a large proportion of hospitalized patients.[4] Up to 90% of individuals with pain associated with cancer or other terminal illnesses and 50% of patients with acute pain are undertreated.[4–6]

Surveys taken in postoperative settings have found that patients continue to experience moderate to very severe acute pain following both in- and outpatient surgeries.[7] Effective management of acute pain, in particular postoperative pain, is essential because it negatively affects emotions, quality of life, functionality, and recovery.[1,2,6,8–10] Poorly controlled or unrelieved pain has serious immediate and long-term consequences, including respiratory, renal, and cardiac dysfunction, immune suppression, postoperative delirium, functional impairments, and development of long-term chronic pain.[5,6] Effective pain management promotes earlier mobilization, improved sleep, and reductions in hospital stay, complications, and costs.

With the understanding that pain was much more than "harmless discomfort" that patients had to tolerate following surgery, multiple disciplines have developed guidelines to improve its assessment and management. Few health care providers would argue that without accurate pain assessment it is difficult to provide optimal pain relief. In fact, some would contend that continual assessment is perhaps the most important aspect of care necessary to provide optimal levels of analgesia. Before an adequate treatment plan can be implemented, the health care provider must establish a working diagnosis of the noxious stimulus as well as an assessment of its character and intensity.

Pain is a purely subjective experience; its assessment is an essential, yet challenging, component of patient examination. There are no existing objective measures that can serve as satisfactory assessment tools. Pain is also multidimensional and includes nociception, perception, and expression. For this reason, multiple aspects of the pain experience must be considered, including sensory, affective, and cognitive dimensions. There is no single approach to pain assessment that is appropriate for all patients or in all settings because the nature of the assessment is affected by multiple factors, including the purpose of the assessment, the setting within which the assessment occurs, the patient population, and the clinician.[11]

HISTORY OF PAIN ASSESSMENT

Created in 1986, the World Health Organization's (WHO) 3-step analgesic ladder for cancer pain represents an attempt to base pain treatment on the intensity of the pain (Figure 11.1). The WHO ladder classified cancer pain into 3 levels of severity: mild, moderate, and severe.[12] Though simplistic in nature, the WHO analgesic ladder was widely viewed as successful because it attempted to provide an organized approach to pain assessment on a global scale. Yale-New Haven Hospital's Pain Management Service employs a 4-step approach modeled after the WHO's 3-step ladder (Figure 11.2). The fourth step comprises interventional pain management techniques, including implantable devices, regional, and neuraxial analgesic techniques.

With the same intent, the Agency for Health Care Policy and Research (AHCPR), now known as the Agency for Healthcare Research and Quality (AHRQ), published clinical practice guidelines for acute pain management in 1992.[13] However, unlike previous endeavors, the AHRQ guidelines emphasized an interdisciplinary approach based on published scientific literature to create an evidence-based approach to pain assessment.

Currently implemented as a pain assessment strategy in many hospitals across the country, "Pain as the 5th Vital Sign"

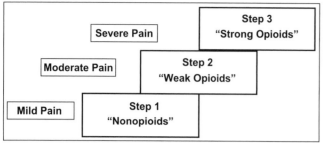

Figure 11.1: The World Health Organization (WHO) stepwise approach to pain management. Although developed to better control cancer pain, this approach can also be employed for acute and convalescent pain. Patients with a pain complaint are started at the lowest step and are treated with nonopioid analgesics. If pain increases in intensity, patients are advanced to the second step (weak to moderate strength opioids) and eventually to the final step (potent opioids). It is understood that adjuvant analgesic and nonpharmacological therapy can be employed at every step to further optimize pain relief and to reduce opioid burden. With new advances in pain medicine a fourth step (interventional pain management) may be considered for patients unable to tolerate dose escalation of strong opioids.[12]

was a slogan originally created by the American Pain Society (APS). Former APS president Dr. James Campbell stated:

> Vital Signs are taken seriously. If pain were assessed with the same zeal as other vital signs are, it would have a much better chance of being treated properly. We need to train doctors and nurses to treat pain as a vital sign. Quality care means that pain is measured and treated.[14]

This slogan has gone on to become a powerful transforming force in the pain assessment movement. In February 1999, the Veterans Hospital Administration began implementation of the Fifth Vital Sign strategy within their hospital system nationwide. Its stated intent was to reduce suffering from preventable pain and assure that pain assessment would be performed in a consistent manner.[14] The Veterans Hospital Administration's plan involves nurses utilizing a numerical pain scale for every patient encounter and documenting the result within the medical record alongside the vital signs (Figure 11.3).[14]

In 2001, the Joint Commission on Accreditation of Health Care Organizations (JCAHO) mandated evaluation of pain

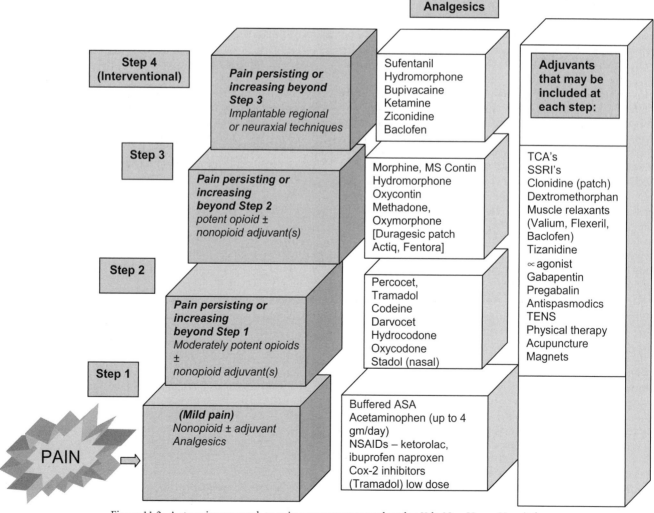

Figure 11.2: A stepwise approach to pain management employed at Yale-New Haven Hospital.

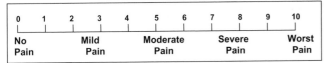

Figure 11.3: The Numerical Rating Scale. This version employs word descriptors.

scores for all patients.[3,15] The ultimate goal of this mandate was to establish a uniform approach to pain assessment and to make hospital personnel accountable for pain management. Furthermore, the JCAHO mandate established pain relief as a patient right, thereby making inadequate pain control unethical.[3] It also increased the importance of pain as a quality-of-life domain and reinforced the idea of pain relief as an indicator for quality medical care. The principle elements of JCAHO's pain management standards, found in Table 11.1, provide the foundation for an effective pain assessment and management program.

Similar attempts to improve pain assessment can be found throughout many fields of the health care industry. From 2002 to 2006, the American Society for Pain Management Nursing (ASPMN) released recommendations in the form of position statements that establish a philosophy of care and provide guidance for clinical practice in specific patient populations.[16–24] These include patients receiving analgesia via catheter techniques or requiring "PCA by proxy," those who are nonverbal, and others suffering with addictive disease, requiring "as-needed" range orders, or who are at the end of life. The ASPMN also authored position statements regarding balancing the promotion of pain relief while preventing abuse of analgesics and their view on the use of placebos in pain management. An overview of these position statements as they relate to the content of this chapter is in the Appendix.

The U.S. government has also become involved in attempting to address the challenge of acute pain. The U.S. Congress designated the period of 2001 to 2010 as the "Decade of Pain Control and Research" with the goal of increasing the visibility of pain and emphasizing the importance of pain management.[15] Since the late 1980s, there has been a significant shift in the pain assessment paradigm away from a poorly controlled, non–evidence-based approach toward one that emphasizes the following: (1) a systematic assessment of pain focusing on the patient's history, physical exam, and context or situation in which pain is occurring; (2) a focus on both the qualitative and quantitative aspects of pain (utilizing various scales and descriptors); and (3) a recognition that adequate pain control is a patient's right. Ultimately, the expectation is that achieving better assessment of pain will enable health care providers to better manage pain.

TYPES OF PAIN

Pain is a complex universal human experience, the definition of which has evolved over the years. In 1968, Margo McCaffery published a clinical definition of pain that has become the cornerstone of pain assessment: "Pain is whatever the experiencing person says it is, existing whenever he/she says it does."[25] This phrase has provided the basis for the reliability and acceptance of the "patient's self-report" of pain.[3,13,25] It was the International Association for the Study of Pain (IASP) that developed the com-

Table 11.1: JCAHO Pain Management Standards[a]

Patients have the right to appropriate assessment and management of pain.

Initial assessments and ongoing reassessments shall identify individuals with pain, and its nature and intensity.

The organization shall develop procedures for pain assessment, for recording assessment results, and for ongoing reassessment and follow-up.

The organization ensures staff competency in pain assessment and management.

The organization incorporates training on pain assessment and management in orientation of all new clinical staff.

The organization establishes policies and procedures that support appropriate prescribing or ordering of pain medications.

Patients and their families shall be educated about the importance of pain management as a component of the overall treatment strategy.

Pain relief should be included as a component of discharge planning.

The organization should consider the appropriateness and effectiveness of its pain management program by incorporating it into its performance measurement and improvement program.

[a] From Joint Commission on Accreditation of Health Care Organizations (2000).[3]

monly utilized definition of pain as "an unpleasant sensory and emotional experience which we primarily associate with tissue damage or describe in terms of such damage, or both."[26] This definition recognized pain as a combined sensory, emotional, and cognitive phenomenon for which physical pathology does not need to be present.[27] Furthermore, this definition addressed the complex nature of pain, moving away from the earlier dualistic idea that pain is of either purely psychogenic or purely somatogenic origin.

The contemporary view of pain characterizes its multidimensionality with simultaneous involvement of noxious, emotional, cognitive (thoughts), and belief components. Conceptually, pain can be thought of as being composed of 3 hierarchical levels: a sensory-discriminative component (eg, location, intensity, quality), a motivational-affective component (eg, depression, anxiety), and a cognitive-evaluative component (eg, thoughts concerning the cause and significance of the pain) (Figure 11.4).

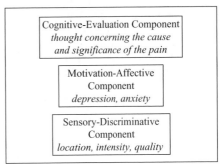

Figure 11.4: The hierachical levels of pain (modified from McCaffery M, Pasero C. *Pain: Clinical Manual.* 2nd ed. St. Louis, MO: Mosby; 1999).[25]

Table 11.2: Pain Characteristics

Types of Pain	Mechanism	Examples	Descriptors
Nociceptive	Peripheral nociceptor activation secondary to tissue damage.	Bruise, cut, bone fracture, burn, tissue damage, arthritis	Aching, sharp, throbbing, pressure, stiffness
Neuropathic	Direct injury to the sensory axons in the central or peripheral nervous system.	Postherpetic neuralgia, phantom limb, radiculopathy, pinched nerve	Burning, tingling, crushing, stabbing, electric shock
Psychogenic	Mechanism not well understood. Pain secondary to underlying psychiatric disorder.	Headache, muscle pain, back pain, abdominal pain, fibromyalgia	Complaints of pain that do not always match symptoms.
Mixed	Containing characteristics of neuropathic and nociceptive pain	Chronic headaches, low back pain	
Idiopathic	Pain with unknown mechanism		

There are 5 accepted classifications of pain: nociceptive, neuropathic, mixed, psychogenic, and idiopathic. Based on the clinical characteristics of the pain described by patients, one can speculate on the type of mechanism sustaining it. Nociceptive pain can be defined as an unpleasant sensation secondary to the activation of peripheral nociceptors located in tissues other than the peripheral and central nervous systems. Nociceptive pain can be further subdivided into somatic and visceral types. Nociceptive pain is usually time limited and resolves once the initial damage heals.[2,9,26]

Neuropathic pain represents a paradoxical form of pain secondary to trauma or dysfunction of a sensory nerve of the central or peripheral nervous system. Although neuropathic pain can be influenced by ongoing tissue injury, the maintenance of pain eventually becomes stimulus independent. Following neural injury, sensory transmission is lost and patients commonly complain of "numbness." In addition, neuropathic pain may be associated with hyperalgesia leading to allodynia and hyperpathia within the injured/denervated region, and spontaneous generation of paraesthesias, dysesthesias, or burning pain.[2,9,26]

Mixed pain refers to pain originating from multiple mechanisms or displaying characteristics of different pain types. This pain syndrome may exhibit symptoms of both neuropathic and somatic disorders. Mixed pain is commonly observed in patients with end-stage disease processes.

Psychogenic pain is a term that refers to real physical pain that originates from a psychological problem. This diagnosis requires that organic causes of pain be ruled out. A person with a psychogenic pain disorder will complain of pain that does not match his or her symptoms. It can manifest in various forms such as headaches, muscle pains, back pain, and stomach pains. Idiopathic pain is a label given to pain for which no sustainable physical or mental mechanism can be inferred. It is usually considered a diagnosis of exclusion. To avoid mislabeling a true pain condition as idiopathic, a comprehensive investigation should be performed by a pain specialist to rule out any underlying pathology. Table 11.2 provides an overview of different pain classifications.

PROCESS OF PAIN ASSESSMENT

Despite being a universal experience, pain has been historically difficult to manage because of the difficulties caregivers have in understanding individual perception and emotional responses to the noxious stimulus. As discussed above, inadequate pain assessment often results in inadequate treatment. The process of pain assessment and reassessment is essential to analyze the nature, intensity, and merit of the pain complaint.[27,28] It is this process that guides therapeutic interventions and monitors the efficacy of treatment. Assessment and documentation allow the patient's pain problem and level of discomfort to become highly visible to all members of a health care team and facilitate communication of the management plan across the continuum of care.[28]

As with any medical disease state, a detailed history and examination are key to understanding the patient's complaint and developing a treatment plan. The initial interview and examination attempts to find answers to the following questions: Where is your pain? What does it feel like? When did your pain begin? How severe is your pain? How often do you experience pain? and What improves or worsens your pain? The examination must include assessment scales and other tools designed to characterize the quality and intensity of the pain complaint.[27,28] Objective or quantitative information includes pain intensity at baseline, resting, and on effort. A diagnostic physical examination should always be performed to identify the underlying cause of the pain, to check for exacerbating factors, and to identify neuromuscular, neurological, and behavioral abnormalities. Subjective, qualitative information regarding pain should include its character (sharp vs dull vs shocking), its location and radiation, its onset and duration, and exacerbating and relieving factors.

Observer Pain Scores

Although generalizations can be made with respect to typical pain intensity and analgesic requirements following a variety of procedures, these estimations represent only a starting point from which initial therapy may be formulated. Thereafter, therapy is continually modified, depending on patient response.[27] Physicians and nurses caring for acute and chronic pain patients often employ observer scores to estimate pain intensity, need to treat, and the amount of analgesic required. Observer scores are highly objective, based primarily on behavioral and autonomic signs as well as caregiver experiences of pain. Although these scores are easily obtained, such information often reflects potentially biased and unreliable approximations of pain intensity. Observer scoring should be restricted for assessments in nonverbal and cognitively impaired patients.[27,29,30] Whenever possible, standardized pain assessment scales and patient self-reporting should be employed. "Without reproducible biologic markers or precise diagnostic tests that measure pain,"[29] the self-report remains the most reliable and accurate indicator of pain and its intensity.[13,29]

Self-Report Scales

Theoretically, acute pain like chronic pain should be evaluated in its multiple dimensions, which include intensity, location, and physical and emotional consequences. However, scales developed to evaluate these dimensions are too complex for practical use in most surgical patients. Simple methods for assessing pain intensity are more practical for use on busy care units.[27] Self-report measurement tools are classified as unidimensional or multidimensional according to the number of dimensions measured. They are best applied in patients who remain verbal and have minimal cognitive deficits. Behavioral/observational assessment tools should be used to assess pain in the nonverbal patient. It is worth noting that the scale chosen to assess a patient's initial pain complaint should be employed throughout that patient's course of treatment to provide a consistent frame of reference to determine response to therapy.

Pain is a complex, highly subjective, perceptual experience.[30] Nevertheless, the idea that "pain is what the patient says it is" helps to guide assessment and management strategies.[31] When patients report pain, they are reporting much more than intensity. However, because of its effect on quality of life and functioning, intensity has been demonstrated to be the most important contributor to the pain experience.[32] Although the intensity and location of discomfort can be assessed objectively, the experience of pain can be communicated only in a subjective way. When evaluating a patient's pain experience it is important to remain aware that "different pains with different causes feel different."[33]

ASSESSMENT TOOLS

Standardized and reproducible methods for assessing pain intensity are essential to the pain assessment and management processes. A number of tools have been developed to assess pain intensity. These instruments may be employed to quantitate pain intensity, develop a rational therapeutic regimen, and evaluate and document the efficacy of an intervention. Ideally, only validated instruments that are sensitive enough to measure change should be used. Integral to the assessment process is selection of the most patient-appropriate tool(s) that must take into consideration the patient's age, cognitive function, and previous patient experience with the tool. It is recommended that the tool(s) selected to assess pain intensity be consistently and systematically applied. Finally, it should be remembered that using a single assessment tool, particularly a unidimensional pain rating scale (UPRS), cannot facilitate an adequate assessment of the subjective and highly nuanced aspects of the pain complaint.

There are four main UPRSs used in clinical practice for objective pain assessments. These include the Numeric Rating scale (NRS), the Verbal Descriptor scale (VDS), the Visual Analog scale (VAS), and the Faces Pain scale (FPS). Each of these scales is a valid and reliable measure of pain intensity. The Iowa Pain Thermometer (IPT) is another UPRS used in

clinical practice. More subjective multidimensional pain assessment tools such as the McGill Pain Questionnaire (MPQ) and the Brief Pain Inventory are also valid measures of acute and chronic pain. Descriptions of the pain assessment tools follow. Key attributes of the commonly used unidimensional and multidimensional pain assessment tools are outlined in Tables 11.3 and 11.4.

Unidimensional Pain Rating Scales

Unidimensional pain rating scales are tools used primarily for rapid assessment and objective quantification. They allow patients to self-report a single dimension of their pain experience, the pain intensity level. These tools are most useful for assessing pain with an obvious cause such as postoperative pain and acute trauma but may oversimplify assessment of more complicated pain syndromes.[11,27]

Numeric Rating Scale

The NRS is a simple-to-use linear scale that is commonly used to quantify pain intensity in clinical settings. The NRS is typically an 11-point scale where the end points represent the extremes of pain (Figure 11.3). The NRS is a line marked with the numbers 0 to 10 at equal intervals where 0 indicates *no pain*, 5 indicates *moderate pain*, and 10 indicates *the worst pain imaginable.*

The NRS is usually presented to the patient verbally, but may be presented visually. When presented visually, the NRS may be displayed in a horizontal or vertical orientation. Patients are asked either to verbally indicate or to circle the number that best represents their current level of pain intensity. This tool has demonstrated sensitivity to treatment-induced changes in pain intensity and is useful for differentiating pain intensity at rest and during activity. The NRS can be used for analgesic research as well as for clinical pain assessment. Evidence supports the validity and reliability of the NRS in younger and older patients.[34] Pain assessment in elderly and mildly cognitively impaired patients may be better facilitated using NRSs that include greater numbers of numerical and word descriptor cues.

Verbal Rating Scale

The VRS, VDS, and Simple Descriptive scale (SDS) are interchangeable terms for a group of simple-to-use and easily understood pain intensity tools used in clinical practice. The VRS is an ordinal scale typically delineated using four to six adjectives to describe increasing levels of pain intensity. The most commonly used words are *no pain*, anchoring the left end of the scale, followed by *mild, moderate (discomforting), severe (distressing), very severe (horrible)*, and the *worst possible (excruciating) pain imaginable*, anchoring the right end of the scale. Using this scale, the patient is asked to select the word that describes his or her current level of pain. A VRS consisting of 4 pain intensity descriptors that describe pain as *none, mild, moderate*, and *severe*, each word linked to increasingly higher number scores (0, 1, 2, and 3), is commonly employed. The patient is asked what number (score) best describes his or her present level of discomfort. Verbal rating scales may either be read by the patient or spoken out loud by the caregiver, followed by a patient answer. The latter method is easily understood by noncognitively impaired patients and rapidly performed; however, it lacks accuracy and sensitivity.[33,34]

Table 11.3: Unidimensional Pain Scales

Scale	*Advantages*	*Disadvantages*	*Comments*
Numeric Rating Scale (NRS)	Historically proven validity, reliability, and sensitivity; been used in clinical practice for 20 years Reproducible results Demonstrated sensitivity for acute, chronic, noncancer, and cancer pain Simple to describe, easy to use and understand High rate of patient acceptance and adherence Requires less cognitive energy and is less likely to produce frustration Reliable for repeated use in same patient Flexible administration (including by telephone)	Not reflective of multidimensional aspects of complex pain scenarios May be less reliable for some patients (eg, elderly, and those with visual, hearing, or severe cognitive impairment)	Most commonly used method of assessing pain intensity Patient must be able to understand pain grading concept May be used in the horizontal or vertical orientation Patient may select a verbal version or draw a circle around a visual, written version to indicate the number that best describes their pain intensity level May be reliable to use for patients with mild to moderate cognitive impairment
Verbal Rating Scale (VRS) Verbal Descriptive Scale (VDS) Simple Descriptive Scale	Historically proven validity, reliability, and appropriateness in clinical practice Simple to describe Easy to use; simple word descriptors easy to understand, particularly for elderly	Limited selection of word descriptors Subjective to patient biases Lacks sensitivity to changes in pain intensity that can result in over- or underestimation of pain changes	Selection of descriptors requires basic linguistic skills and ability to identify descriptor best matching pain intensity level
Visual Analog Scale (VAS)	Documented validity, reliability, and appropriateness in clinical practice Valid and sensitive for patients with acute, chronic, and cancer pain. Reliable for repeated use in same patient	Time consuming to administer and score Description and use of scale may cause patient confusion Elderly experience difficulty understanding and completing the scale Less reliable in immediate postoperative patient with cognitive impairment Poor reproducibility with cognitive impairment Must be administered on paper or electronically	Can be used in a horizontal or vertical orientation Scale orientation may impact statistical distribution of data Ratings require quantification of pain intensity and abstract reasoning to determine length of line that corresponds to pain intensity Repeated photocopying may result in a change in the true scale length, thereby impacting accuracy of the rating measurement
Faces Pain Scale (FPS) Faces Pain Scale-Revised (FPS-R)	Documented validity, reliability, and appropriateness in clinical practice Easy to use and understand Easy to administer Correlates well with NRS Not subject to culture, sex, or ethnicity influences Useful for individuals with communication barriers (eg, elderly, cognitively impaired, or have limited language fluency or education, and children) May be perceived as easier to use compared to NRS, VAS	Must be presented in printed form Potential for distorted assessment (ie, tendency to point to the center of such scales) May be difficult to determine whether pain or mood is being measured	Good alternative for patients with communication barriers For visually impaired, enlarged photocopy may be required Looking at the facial representations may make it difficult to distinguish between pain and emotional state for some patients
Iowa Pain Thermometer (IPT)	Simple to describe Easy to use Simple word descriptors easier for elderly to understand	Must be presented in printed form	Vertical orientation used Appropriateness of use depends on visual acuity Scale enlargement may be required for visually impaired patients

Sources: Berry et al (2006),[11] Gagliase et al (2005),[34] Williamson et al (2005),[35] Ware et al (2006).[86]

Table 11.4: Multidimensional Pain Assessment Tools

Scale	Advantages	Disadvantages	Comments
Brief Pain Inventory (BPI)	Quantifies pain intensity and disability Reliable for use in a variety of clinical settings Used across cultures and languages		Administered visually Used in clinical and research settings Takes 5–15 minutes to complete
Initial Pain Assessment Inventory (IPAI)	May be completed by patient or clinician, Includes diagram for site(s) of pain		Administered visually and verbally
McGill Pain Questionnaire (MPQ)	Extensively tested and widely used in research and clinical practice Studies support validity, reliability, and sensitivity with younger adults Growing evidence of validity and reliability for elderly people with chronic pain Assesses sensory, affective, and evaluative dimensions of pain Short form takes 2–3 minutes to complete	Lengthy and complex Long form takes 5–15 minutes to complete Patient frustration with process Frequent assessments not feasible Patients may have difficulty understanding directions for use of the tool Patient may be confused by the vocabulary Repeated testing, unrelated events may result in inaccurate responses	Administered verbally in person or via telephone by caregiver, interviewer, or proxy, or patient self-administered Important to maintain consistency in administration procedure to achieve accurate results Choosing adjective descriptors requires subtle differentiation of the qualities of the pain experience Total score, not individual scale scores, is considered valid measure of pain intensity

Sources: McCaffery et al (1999),[25] Gagliase et al (2005),[34] Melzack (1975),[41] Melzack (1987).[42]

The VRS scale is not as sensitive as the NRS to treatment-induced changes in pain intensity, because only a limited number of descriptors are used. As such, a much greater change in pain intensity must exist for patients to select a higher or lower descriptor. The lack of sensitivity can lead to over- or underestimation of pain changes.[35] Evidence supports the validity and reliability of VRSs for younger patients, with supportive evidence growing for older people.[34]

Visual Analog Scale

The VAS is an efficient measure of pain intensity that has been used widely in research and clinical settings. The most common VAS is a 10-cm line, usually presented in the horizontal orientation, but it may be presented vertically, labeled at the end points with the word anchors *no pain* and *worst pain imaginable* (Figure 11.5). The patient is required to mark the line with a pencil slash at the point that corresponds best to the present level of pain intensity. Some visual analog scales are manufactured as slide rules, in which a movable line can be positioned by the patient along the 100-mm line. The length of the line from the end identified as *no pain* to the mark made by the patient is measured by the observer and recorded in millimeters on a scoring sheet, giving 101 possible scores for pain intensity. The tool should be presented with minimal verbal cues and no finger pointing by the observer.[36] It should be introduced with an appropriate standardized statement: "Please mark on the line the intensity of the pain you are experiencing at this moment." Ideally the line should be marked for pain at rest as well as pain during movement. The relative absence of descriptor cues and line markers with the VAS is believed to provide greater scientific validity, but can be confusing for both very young and elderly patients.[34,35] To minimize confusion, the patient should be instructed preoperatively as to what the line end points mean and how to mark them.

Although the VAS is easy to administer, it can be more time-consuming because the pencil mark location must be measured. The scale has a high degree of sensitivity because slight changes in pain intensity can be detected. When compared with the VRS, scores of approximately 30 mm on the 100-mm VAS corresponded to moderate pain, and a score of 54 mm or more correlated to severe pain.[35,36] One study conducted in adult emergency department patients admitted with acute pain sought to define the minimum clinically important difference in pain severity for the VAS. They demonstrated that "a mean reduction in the VAS measurement of 30 mm represents a clinically important difference in pain severity that corresponds to patients' perception of adequate pain control."[36] Studies have shown that accuracy of the VAS depends on using it in an orientation (horizontal versus vertical) consistent with the reading pattern of the population in which it is used. The vertical orientation has been associated with less user error in Chinese patients, whereas English speakers demonstrated a lower error rate when used in the horizontal orientation.[35] Studies, predominantly in young subjects, have supported the sensitivity, validity, and reliability of the VAS as a measure of pain intensity.[35,36] Use in the elderly is less certain.[34]

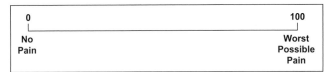

Figure 11.5: The Visual Analog Scale.

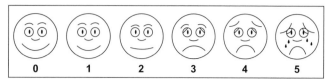

Figure 11.6: The Original Wong-Baker FACES Rating Scale. From Hockenberry MJ, Wilson D, Winkelstein ML: *Wong's Essentials of Pediatric Nursing*, ed. 7, St. Louis, 2005, p. 1259. Used with permission. Copyright, Mosby.

Faces Pain Scale

Historically, FPSs that consist of a series of six to seven faces ranging from a happy, smiling face at one end to a sad, teary face at the opposite end have been used to assess pain in the pediatric population. Several versions of FPSs have been used in clinical practice. They are intended to measure how the patient feels. Each displays facial expressions shown to be associated with pain, including brow lowering, lip tightening/cheek raising, nose wrinkling/lip raising, and eye closure. The original Wong-Baker FACES Rating Scale is the most widely recognized and is commonly used in pediatric settings (Figure 11.6).

The most up-to-date version of the FPS is the Faces Pain Scale–Revised (FPS-R). The FPS-R presents pictures of six line-drawn faces presented in a horizontal orientation. Patients are instructed to point to the face that best reflects the intensity of their pain. The facial expressions represented on the FPS-R appear less childlike compared to other FPSs (Figure 11.7). The absence of tears avoids potential cultural bias about pain expression. A rating of *no pain* is represented by a neutral face instead of a happy face at the far left of the scale. The faces show more and more pain as the scale proceeds to the right, with the face at the far right showing an expression associated with extreme pain. The FPS has displaced the OUCHER scale, which employs photographs of children rather that cartoon faces, and has become the most widely applied observational tool for pediatric patients aged 4–14 years.[38]

Although the FPSs were designed for use in the pediatric population, more recent studies have evaluated utility in the adult population, particularly the nonverbal, cognitively impaired. For some severely cognitively impaired patients, when employing an FPS as part of the pain assessment process, the health care provider may need to select the face that correlates best to the patient's observed facial expressions. The FPSs may also be useful for assessment of patients with language barriers.

IOWA PAIN THERMOMETER

The IPT is a diagram of a well-recognized thermometer reflecting an increasing level of pain intensity with word descriptors including *no pain, slight, moderate, severe, very severe*, and *the most intense pain imaginable* (Figure 11.8). The patient is

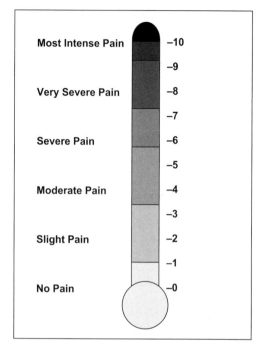

Figure 11.8: The Pain Thermometer. Modified from Herr et al. Evaluation of the Iowa Pain Thermometer and other pain intensity scales. *Pain Med.* 2007;8(7):585–600.

asked to mark beside the word that best represents the intensity or severity of his or her present pain. Cues associated with the scale include the fact that discomfort associated with increasing intensity is analogous to discomfort associated with increasing temperature displayed on a thermometer. The tool is a verbal descriptive scale used with the older adult population.

Multidimensional Pain Assessment Tools

Multidimensional pain assessment tools provide important information about the characteristics of the patient's pain and its effects on the patient's daily life. These tools were designed to facilitate the patient's self-report; however, a clinician may guide the process and assist the patient.

Initial Pain Assessment Tool

The Initial Pain Assessment tool was developed for use during initial patient evaluations (Figure 11.9). It guides the clinician in collecting information related to characteristics of the patient's pain, the patient's manner of expressing pain, factors that relieve or increase the pain, and the effects of pain on function and quality of life. A human figure diagram is provided on which the patient may indicate pain location(s). A space is provided to indicate the unidimensional pain scale used and to document the present pain intensity level, the intensity of pain at its worst and best, and the level of pain considered acceptable to the patient. A space is also provided for documenting additional comments and management plans. The tool can be used for acute and chronic pain assessment, and is useful for detecting changes in pain symptoms following a therapeutic intervention.

The OLD CART Acronym

Another tool that can be employed as an assessment guide is known by the acronym OLD CART (Figure 11.10). This tool provides an approach to questioning of the patient by the health

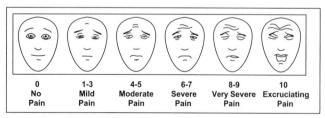

Figure 11.7: Revised FACES Scale that utilizes color gradation. This scale is used by the Yale Pain Management Service for assessing pain severity in elderly and cognitively impaired patients.

FORM 3.1

Date _____

Patient's Name _____ Age _____ Room _____

Diagnosis _____ Physician _____

Nurse _____

1. LOCATION: Patient or nurse mark drawing.

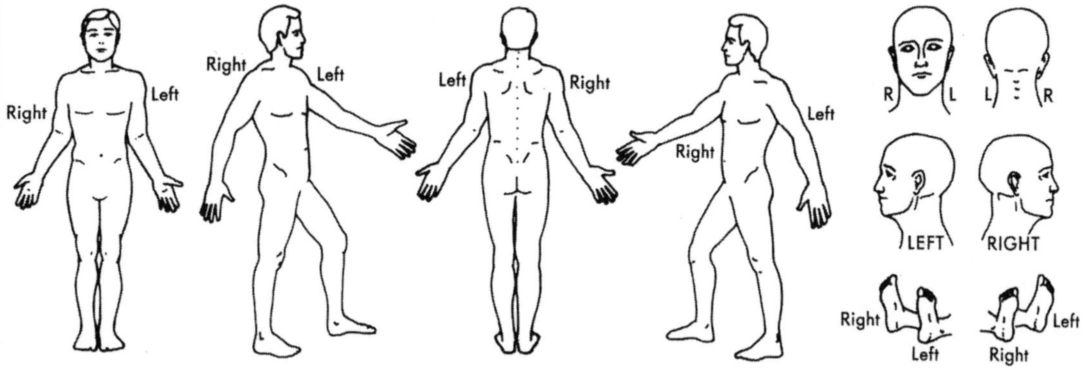

2. INTENSITY: Patient rates the pain. Scale used _____

Present: _____
Worst pain gets: _____
Best pain gets: _____
Acceptable level of pain: _____

3. QUALITY: (Use patient's own words, e.g., prick, ache, burn, throb, pull, sharp) _____

4. ONSET, DURATION, VARIATIONS, RHYTHMS: _____

5. MANNER OF EXPRESSING PAIN: _____

6. WHAT RELIEVES THE PAIN? _____

7. WHAT CAUSES OR INCREASES THE PAIN? _____

8. EFFECTS OF PAIN: (Note decreased function, decreased quality of life.)
Accompanying symptoms (e.g., nausea) _____
Sleep _____
Appetite _____
Physical activity _____
Relationship with others (e.g., irritability) _____
Emotions (e.g., anger, suicidal, crying) _____
Concentration _____
Other _____

9. OTHER COMMENTS: _____

10. PLAN: _____

May be duplicated for use in clinical practice. From McCaffery M, Pasero C: *Pain: Clinical manual,* p. 60. Copyright © 1999, Mosby, Inc.

Figure 11.9: Initial Pain Assessment Tool. From McCaffery M, Pasero C. *Pain Clinical Manual.* 2nd Ed. St Louis, MO: Mosby; 1999, with permission.[25]

"OLDCART" is an acronym that can be used as a simple pain assessment guide together with a pain intensity scale.

O: **O**nset (new or chronic pain)
L: **L**ocation (one or more sites)
D: **D**uration (intermittent or persistent)
C: **C**haracteristics (somatic – sharp, dull or aching)
      (visceral – cramping, squeezing)
      (neuropathic – shooting, burning, electrical, tingling numbness)
A: **A**ggravating factors (what makes the pain worse)
R: **R**elieving factors (what makes the pain better)
T: **T**reatment (pharmacological / nonpharmacological)
      (past or present)

Figure 11.10: The OLD CART method of pain assessment. "OLD-CART" initially published by Bates 1995 for assessing chest pain.

care provider to quickly determine onset, location, duration, and characteristics of the pain complaint, as well as factors that aggravate and relieve the pain. This process also involves retrieval of information regarding treatment received by the patient for a previous pain complaint and a discussion of the treatment plan for the current complaint. The OLD CART tool must be used in combination with an appropriate pain intensity scale. This assessment scale can be employed at the bedside and is useful in elderly and cognitively impaired patients who have difficulty with lists of questions yet can easily provide answers to caregiver presented questions.

McGill Pain Questionnaire

The McGill Pain Questionnaire (MPQ), originally conceived by Melzack and Torgerson, is one of the oldest and most extensively tested multidimensional pain assessment tools (Figure 11.11).[30,39,41] It was initially developed for general assessment of chronic pain, but it has also been validated for acute pain,[39,40] particularly postoperative pain.[40] This tool has compared to the VRS and VAS in sensitivity to changes in postoperative pain following administration of oral analgesics.[40]

Clinicians have long recognized the existence of qualitatively different aspects of pain and descriptors used to describe various forms of discomfort. "Throbbing headache," "crushing chest pain," and "heartburn" are well-recognized phrases. The MPQ employs 78 word descriptors to assess the sensory, affective, and evaluative dimensions of pain and to measure both the

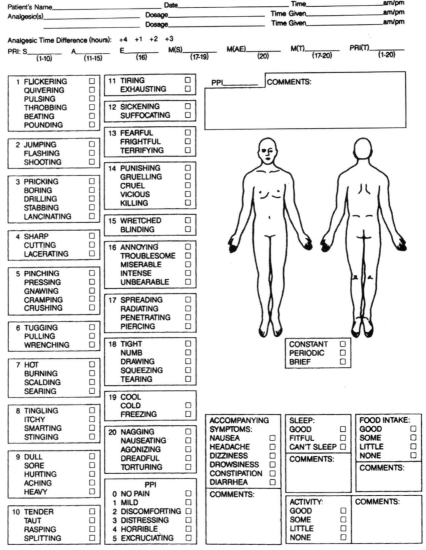

Figure 11.11: The McGill Pain Questionaire developed by Ronald Melzack MD, McGill University, Montreal, Canada. From Melzack and Torgerson. Used with permission.

subjective quality and the quantity of a patient's pain experience. The sensory dimension reflects perception of pain by the senses. The affective dimension reflects the emotional aspect of the pain experience. The evaluative dimension reflects the intensity of a patient's pain experience. The information obtained from the MPQ produces three indices, including the Pain Rating index (PRI), the Present Pain Intensity (PPI) index, and the Number of Words Chosen (NWC).

The MPQ is composed of 20 categories of adjectives that describe the qualities of pain. Within each category the adjective descriptors are arranged in order of implied pain intensity and assigned a rank value from 1 for the least painful to 5 for the most painful. Patients are asked to select one word from each category that best describes their pain and associated feelings and sensations at that particular moment in time. The rank values of the selected words are summed to obtain a Total Pain Rating Index (PRI-T) and separate scores for the sensory (PRI-S), affective (PRI-A), evaluative (PRI-E), and miscellaneous (PRI-M) subscales. The PPI index is determined by asking the patient to complete a categorical present pain intensity scale using word descriptors from *no pain* through *excruciating pain* with assigned rank values of 0 through 5.[41]

The NWC is another pain rating scale in which the net change in the number of descriptors selected is calculated. Melzack observed that significant changes in pain intensity or relief were not associated with a decrease in the NWC.[41] Patients experiencing improved analgesia tended to select one word per subclass that described a lower level of pain intensity rather than not including the subclass. One disadvantage of the MPQ is that many immigrants illiterate, and cognitively impaired individuals may not recognize some or many of the adjectives included in the questionnaire. Words may be selected without full appreciation of their meaning or not chosen because of their complexity (ie, lancinating, suffocating, etc).

Short-Form McGill Pain Questionnaire

The Short Form McGill Pain Questionnaire (SF-MPQ), originally developed for use in the research setting, has been shown to correlate with the PRI of the longer MPQ form and to be sensitive to clinical changes in pain as the result of pain management interventions.[42] The questionnaire is divided into four sections, including the PRI, the PPI-VAS, the overall PPI evaluative, and the scoring sections. The PRI section consists of 15 adjectives selected from the most commonly used words on the original MPQ that describe qualities of pain, divided into two categories for sensory and affective components of pain. Each of the 15 descriptors is ranked by the patient on a pain intensity scale of 0 (*no pain*) to 3 (*severe pain*). The PPI-VAS is marked by the patient at the point that best rates their intensity of pain at the present moment. The PPI section is used to rate the overall intensity of the pain experience and is recorded as a number from 0 (*no pain*) to 5 (*excruciating pain*).

Brief Pain Inventory

The Brief Pain Inventory (BPI) is a self-report instrument that has been employed in research and a variety of clinical settings, has been translated into several languages, and has reasonable validity and reliability.[25] This tool was developed to provide a quick and easy-to-use method to quantify pain intensity and associated disability.[43] The BPI consists of a series of 11 pain-related questions that address aspects of the pain experienced over the previous 24-hour period, such as pain location and intensity, impact on the patient's life, and type and effectiveness

Table 11.5: Keys to Assessing Pain in the Nonverbal Elderly Patient with Dementia

Anticipate and assume presence of pain based on pathology (ie, disease, injury, procedure, surgery)

Observe for behaviors at rest and during activity. Establish a baseline behavior and monitor regularly using a comprehensive list of behavioral indicators.

Observe for typical/obvious and atypical/less obvious nonverbal indicators of pain and behavioral changes.

An analgesic trial may be attempted if the presence of pain is uncertain. Assume pain is present and continue the intervention if it appears to have provided pain relief.

Source: Herr et al (2006).[64]

of treatments. Four of the questions focus on pain intensity and seven questions focus on pain's interference with function. A diagram is provided on which the patient can indicate pain location(s). The tool, a copy of which can be found in McCaffery and Pasero (1999),[25] generally takes 5 to 15 minutes to complete. Test-retest correlations, reliability in surgical populations, and validity in different groups of patients experiencing acute pain have been demonstrated.[44]

Behavioral/Observational Pain Assessment Tools

Pain assessment in the nonverbal patient or the elderly with severe dementia who are unable to communicate their pain experience with standard self-report tools presents a major challenge for health care providers. Basic steps for assessing pain in this patient population are outlined in Table 11.5 and further elucidated under *Assessment Challenges in Special Populations* in this chapter. Equally as challenging is pain assessment in the nonverbal, critically ill patient. Several behavioral/observational pain assessment tools are available to assess pain in nonverbal, cognitively impaired patients and critically ill patients, including the Pain Assessment in Advanced Dementia Scale (PAINAD) (Figure 11.12), the Face, Legs, Activity, Cry and Consolability (FLACC) (Figure 11.13), the Critical Care Pain Observation

Items*	0	1	2	Score
Breathing independent of vocalization	Normal	Occasional labored breathing. Short period of hyperventilation.	Noisy labored breathing. Long period of hyperventilation. Cheyne-Stokes respirations	
Negative vocalization	None	Occasional moan or groan. Low-level speech with a negative or disapproving quality.	Repeated troubled calling out. Loud moaning or groaning. Crying.	
Facial expression	Smiling or inexpressive	Sad. Frightened. Frown.	Facial grimacing.	
Body language	Relaxed	Tense. Distressed pacing. Fidgeting.	Rigid. Fists clenched. Knees pulled up. Pulling or pushing away. Striking out.	
Consolability	No need to console	Distracted or reassured by voice or touch.	Unable to console, distract or reassure.	
			Total**	

Figure 11.12: The Pain Assessment in Advanced Dementia scale (PAINAD). Warden V, Hurley AC, Volicer L. Development and psychometric evaluation of the Pain Assessment in Advanced Dementia (PAINAD) scale. *J Am Med Dir Assoc.* 2003;4(1):9–15.

	0	1	2
Face	No particular expression or smile	Occasional grimace or frown, withdrawn, disinterested	Frequent to constant frown, clenched jaw, quivering chin
Legs	Normal position Or Relaxed	Uneasy, restless, tense	Kicking, Or Legs drawn up
Activity	Lying quietly Normal position Moves easily	Squirming Shifting back/forth Tense	Arched Rigid Or Jerking
Cry	No cry (Awake or asleep)	Moans or whimpers Occasional complaint	Crying steadily Screams or sobs Frequent complaints
Consolability	Content Relaxed	Reassured by occasional touching, hugging, or "talking to." Distractible	Difficult to console or comfort

The **FLACC** is a behavior pain assessment scale for use in non-verbal patients unable to provide reports of pain.

Instructions: Rate the patient's score for each of the five measurement categories, add together, document total pain score

Figure 11.13: The FLACC scale (Face, Legs, Activity, Cry, Consolability scale). Originally developed to assess pain in neonates, it is now advocated for use in patients with cognitive impairments and advanced dementia. Merkel SI, Voepel-Lewis T, Shayevitz JR, Malviya S (1997) at C.S. Mott Children's Hospital, University of Michigam Health System, Ann Arbor, MI.

tool (CPOT) (Figure 11.14), and the Behavioral Pain scale (BPS) (Figure 11.15). The use of these tools are discussed under Pain Assessment Considerations in Critically Ill Patients and *Pain Assesment Considerations in Patients with Addictive Disorders*.

One approach to evaluating the presence of pain and providing treatment in the elderly with severe cognitive impairment includes forms of behavioral assessment that were initially outlined by Herr and Decker[44] and Herr and colleagues.[64] When health care providers observe behaviors indicative of pain, a determination of the etiology of the behavior should be pursued to guide the treatment plan. If the pain behavior continues after

Indicator	Description and Score
Facial expression	No muscular tension observed: **Relaxed, neutral: 0** Presence of frowning, brow lowering, orbit tightening, and levator contraction: **Tense: 1** All of the above facial movements plus eyelids tightly closed: **Grimacing: 2**
Body movement	Does not move at all (does not necessarily mean the absence of pain): **Absence of movements: 0** Slow, cautious movements, touching or rubbing the pain site, seeking attention through movements: **Protection: 1** Pulling at tube, attempting to sit up, moving limbs or thrashing, not following commands, striking at staff, trying to climb out of bed: **Restlessness: 2**
Muscle tension (evaluation by passive flexion and extension of arms)	No resistance to passive movements: **Relaxed: 0** Resistance to passive movements: **Tense, rigid: 1** Strong resistance to passive movements, inability to complete tem: **Very tense or rigid: 2**
Compliance with ventilator (for intubated patients) Or	Alarms not activated, easy ventilation: **Tolerating ventilation or movement: 0** Alarms stop spontaneously: **Coughing but tolerating ventilator: 1** Asynchrony: blocking ventilation, alarms frequently activated: **Fighting ventilator: 2**
Vocalization (for extubated patients)	Talking in normal tone or no sound: **0** Sighing, moaning: **1** Crying out, sobbing: **2**
Total possible score (range)	0 to 8

Figure 11.14: Critical Care Pain Observation tool. *Source:* Pun et al (2007).[67]

Item	Description	Score
Facial Expression	Relaxed	1
	Partially tightened (e.g. brow lowering)	2
	Fully tightened (e.g. eyelid closing)	3
	Grimacing	4
Upper Limbs	No movement	1
	Partially bent	2
	Fully bent with finger flexion	3
	Permanently retracted	4
Compliance with Verification	Tolerating movement	1
	Coughing but tolerating ventilation for most of the time	2
	Fighting ventilator	3
	Unable to control ventilation	4

Figure 11.15: The Behavioral Pain scale. From: Payen JF et al., *Criti Care Med.* 2001;29(12):2258–2263.[73]

ruling out or treating the possible causes, an empiric trial administration of an analgesic followed by assessment is warranted.[44] If the analgesic trial appears to result in pain relief, it can be assumed that pain was the probable cause of the observed behaviors and the pharmacologic and/or nonpharmacologic interventions should continue. It the analgesic trial does not appear to result in pain relief, other causes of the observed behaviors should be considered with treatment focused on other possible causes.

When employing behavioral/observational pain assessment tools in clinical practice, it should be understood that they cannot be used to quantify pain intensity. The number score obtained when using such tools is a behavior score, not a pain intensity rating.[45] As such, these tools provide for a general assessment of a patient's pain experience based on health care provider observation of patient behaviors in an effort to diagnose presence of pain and to determine efficacy of therapeutic interventions. Behavioral/observational ratings have been shown to correlate only moderately with patient self-assessment pain scores and often underestimate pain intensity.[46,47,48] Utilization of behavioral/observational ratings should be reserved for patients who have demonstrated an inability to self-report their experience.

There are disadvantages associated with the use of behavioral/observational tools. These tools do not include less obvious or atypical behavioral manifestations, thereby reducing their utility as comprehensive pain assessment methods. Also, pain behavior checklists cannot be used for patients who are unresponsive, heavily sedated, or pharmacologically paralyzed, and therefore cannot respond behaviorally to pain.[45] For behavioral/observational tools to be useful in the pain assessment process, the patient must demonstrate some of the listed behaviors.

Adjunctive Pain Assessment Tools

The use of adjunctive pain assessment tools may be indicated in certain circumstances. An example of one such tool is the Neuropathic Pain scale (NPS), a multidimensional measure of neuropathic pain found in Figure 11.16. The NPS is brief, easy for most patients to learn, requires about 5 minutes to complete, is comprehensive, and is sensitive to effects of treatment.[25] The tool employs rating scales from 0 to 10 to measure different qualities of neuropathic pain using the descriptors of *intensity, sharpness* (eg, kniflike, jabbing, jolts), and *hot* (eg, burning,

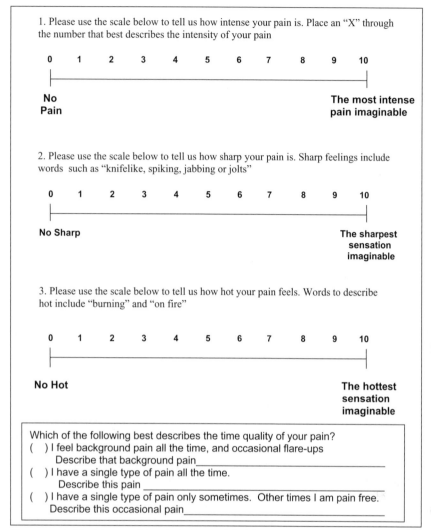

1. Please use the scale below to tell us how intense your pain is. Place an "X" through the number that best describes the intensity of your pain

0   1   2   3   4   5   6   7   8   9   10

**No
Pain**   **The most intense
pain imaginable**

2. Please use the scale below to tell us how sharp your pain is. Sharp feelings include words such as "knifelike, spiking, jabbing or jolts"

0   1   2   3   4   5   6   7   8   9   10

No Sharp   **The sharpest
sensation
imaginable**

3. Please use the scale below to tell us how hot your pain feels. Words to describe hot include "burning" and "on fire"

0   1   2   3   4   5   6   7   8   9   10

No Hot   **The hottest
sensation
imaginable**

Which of the following best describes the time quality of your pain?
(   ) I feel background pain all the time, and occasional flare-ups
        Describe that background pain_____
(   ) I have a single type of pain all the time.
        Describe this pain _____
(   ) I have a single type of pain only sometimes. Other times I am pain free.
        Describe this occasional pain_____

Figure 11.16: The Neuropathic Pain Scale. Modified from Galer B, Jensen M. Development and preliminary validation of a pain measure specific to neuropathic pain: The Neuropathic Pain Scale. *Neurology*. 1997;48:332–338.

on fire).[25] One study in 159 subjects with diabetes-related foot pain validated the use of the NPS for characterizing the complex nature of the neuropathic pain experience and for detecting the effects of analgesic therapy on different sensations and qualities of neuropathic pain.[49]

Another tool that has reportedly been found useful in the diagnosis of neuropathic pain is the Leeds Assessment of Neuropathic Symptoms and Signs (LANSS) pain scale.[50,51] A modified version of the LANSS pain scale is the S-LANSS or self-report LANSS pain scale. The LANSS pain scale has 7 items consisting of 5 symptom and 2 examination items. The purpose of this scale is to assess whether the experienced pain is predominantly because of nerve damage. Both scales are scored based on a possible 24 points. A score of 12 or more is strongly suggestive of neuropathic pain.

Assessing Patient Satisfaction and Comfort

Pain is an inherently subjective symptom, the experience of which is conveyed primarily by patients' verbal reports.[52] There is no objective measurement for the pain experience.[52,53]

Change in pain intensity and relief is measurable using continuous or ordinal instruments; however, assessing the quantitative intrinsic meaning of such change has not been clearly defined.[53,54] Caregivers can employ a simple 11-unit numerical scale to assess satisfaction with pain control or satisfaction with a particular form of analgesic therapy. Such "satisfaction scales" are usually anchored with 0 indicating no satisfaction with analgesic therapy and 10 indicating complete satisfaction with therapy. It should be recognized, however, that satisfaction with therapy represents a composite of analgesic effectiveness as well as adverse events associated with therapy. Because of a high incidence of nausea, vomiting, and other annoying side effects, satisfaction scores with opioid analgesic therapy may be low despite providing adequate pain relief.

Evaluating clinically meaningful changes in patient-reported pain intensity has become increasingly more important when interpreting data from the clinical care or research settings. Use of standard pain intensity measurement scales to quantify therapeutic intervention-associated levels of change that represent useful and clinically important improvements, particularly from the patient's perspective, has become a key area of interest.

Although the findings of available research may not generalize to all patients with acute pain, they do offer a frame of reference on which future studies may be based. The minimum clinically significant improvement in acute pain intensity measured on a 100-mm VAS has been reported to be a 13-mm reduction in the VAS score,[54,55] which corresponds to a 1.3-unit decrease on a 10-unit NRS.[56] In patients with severe acute pain, a single category improvement on a standard ordinal 5-point Likert pain relief scale (*no relief, a little, moderate, a lot,* or *complete relief*) corresponds to the minimum clinically significant reduction in pain intensity of greater than 1.3 on a 10-unit NRS.[56] Farrar et al[52,53] determined that the minimum clinically important improvement on standard pain intensity scales for patients being treated for acute breakthrough cancer pain episodes was a 33% change in both percentage pain intensity difference (using a scale of 0%–100%) and percentage of maximum total pain relief, a 2-point difference in absolute pain intensity on a 10-unit NRS, or a pain relief rating of 2 (*moderate relief*) on a 5-point standard Likert scale.[52–54]

Although minimal clinically meaningful changes in pain intensity scores are important response criteria, there is a growing need on the part of health care providers and investigators for information regarding truly meaningful improvements in pain from the individual patient's perspective.[57,58] Because the ultimate goal of pain management is to attain adequate pain relief, achieving a patient acceptable symptom state, or a satisfactory state beyond which the patient considers him or herself well, is an important patient care goal.[57,58]

Patient-perceived satisfactory improvement (PPSI), a new outcome measure for within-person improvement in pain intensity, is assessed using patients' judgments of satisfactory change.[57] The PPSI is a clinically relevant and stable concept that can be used to assess true meaningful change in pain from the patient's perspective.[57] In one prospective study of 181 arthritis patients treated with a local corticosteroid injection, PPSI was associated with a minimal reduction of 30 mm or 55% on a 100-mm VAS for pain intensity, with a 5-point categorical rating scale used as an anchor to assess PPSI.[57]

An accurate picture of the patient's actual pain experience cannot be obtained by relying solely on pain intensity measurements. "Observed reductions in pain intensity may suggest to the nurses that the patient is experiencing less pain, whereas such nurse-perceived improvements may be of no meaningful significance from the patient's perspective."[58] Instead, caregivers should strive to reduce postoperative pain to levels necessary to maximize functional capacity and for patients to perceive that they are receiving attentive analgesic care.[58]

ASSESSMENT CHALLENGES IN SPECIAL POPULATIONS

Unique challenges presented by distinct patient populations affect the health care team's ability to effectively and accurately implement a pain management plan. The challenging patient populations are outlined in Table 11.6. An awareness of these barriers and the development of assessment strategies that overcome them are essential to the careful and fair assessment of the patient's pain complaint in an effort to provide the best chance of achieving satisfactory pain relief. A pain assessment, management, and reassessment approach that openly acknowledges and addresses the concerns unique to individual patients is essential.

Table 11.6: Challenging Patient Populations

Racial and ethnic minorities

Elderly individuals

Cognitively or emotionally impaired individuals

Nonverbal patients (eg, heavily sedated, intubated)

Critically ill patients

Persons with known or suspected addictive disorders

Individuals with linguistic, cultural, or educational barriers to communication

Individuals with sickle cell disease

Individuals with HIV/AIDS

Neonates and younger pediatric patients

Pain Assessment Considerations in Racial and Ethnic Minorities

Despite guidelines, educational interventions, and standards aimed at optimizing pain management, the literature continues to report the undertreatment of pain, particularly among patients who are racial and ethnic minorities.[59] The Institute of Medicine (IOM) of the National Academy of Sciences was charged by the US Congress, in 1999, to evaluate the contribution of health care inequities to disparities in health care services delivery among racial and ethnic minorities. The IOM Study Committee report reviewed pain management as one of the clinical areas in which disparities exist.[59]

Disparities in pain care among racial and ethnic minorities receiving treatment for a variety of conditions in a variety of treatment settings is being increasingly documented in the literature. Disparities have been acknowledged in the emergency department setting, acute postoperative and cancer pain management settings, and for individuals receiving care for chronic nonmalignant pain, sickle cell disease, HIV/AIDS, and workers compensation-related conditions. It has been reported that African American and Hispanic patients are more likely than whites to be undertreated for pain.[56,59,60,61]

In a review of the literature regarding pain management disparities, Green et al[59] found that the use of analgesics in a variety of health care settings is influenced by race and ethnicity. Following is a brief synopsis of their review. Todd et al,[55] in a 1996 retrospective study, reported that Hispanics with isolated long-bone fractures were twice as likely as non-Hispanic whites to receive no pain medication during their emergency department visit. This disparity could not be explained on the basis of gender, language, insurance status, severity of the fracture, or the likelihood of associated alcohol or drug intoxication. Undertreatment of pain in the African American group could not be accounted for by significant differences in assessment of pain between the groups. It was concluded that the disparity likely occurred with the decision to administer analgesics.

Health care providers should also be aware that the terminology used by patients to describe their pain varies with ethnicity. In one study of six ethnic groups conducted in New England, surrounding culture had an impact on pain responses within an ethnic group.[15] For example, most Chinese describe tooth drilling as "sourish," whereas Americans rarely used this term, and, although whites often describe muscle pain as "deep," only half of the Mandarin Chinese used this descriptor.[15]

It must also be recognized that pain-related behaviors may vary between patients of different cultural and ethnic backgrounds. As a result of unfamiliarity of health care providers with such behavioral nuances, patients in various minority populations may be perceived as requiring less aggressive pain management because their behavior when experiencing pain may not be perceived as pain-related behavior. Judging pain only by clinician observation of patients' behavior may result in underestimation of its severity. It is, therefore, imperative that health care clinicians be aware of the unique needs and circumstances of patients from various ethnic and cultural backgrounds when assessing and managing pain. Employing pain assessment tools appropriate for patients' specific cultural and linguistic needs is critical to optimizing assessment and management.

Pain Assessment Considerations in the Elderly

Older persons often have multiple medical problems and many potential sources of chronic discomfort, making it difficult to diagnose and treat pain in this patient population. The elderly represent a particularly vulnerable and challenging patient population in whom pain is often inadequately recognized and undertreated. As the population continues to age, the number of elderly surgical patients will increase. As such, competency of health care providers in pain assessment and management in the elderly population is essential.

There exists a misconception that cognitively impaired older persons do not experience pain as severely as persons who are cognitively intact.[44] Although some studies have suggested that elderly patients report lower pain intensity than younger patients, other studies have not demonstrated age differences.[34] It was noted in one study that the proportion of patients reporting pain did not change with the degree of dementia.[46] It was also noted in the same study that about 25% of the patients reporting pain were not receiving analgesics. Pain assessment in the elderly may be complicated by concurrent illness, underreporting of symptoms, decline in cognitive function, and age-related physiologic changes.

A review of the pain management literature by Gibson and Helme[60] uncovered age-related differences underlying neurochemical, neuroanatomical, and neurophysiological mechanisms of pain. Older persons may experience altered pain sensitivity, a muted and delayed clinical pain perception, and altered quality of pain sensation when compared to younger adults.[60] It has been suggested by several studies that a lower intensity of postoperative or procedural pain is reported by older compared to younger adults.[57] Elderly persons have demonstrated lower ratings of sensory and affective dimensions of pain in McGill Pain Questionnaire reports.[46,60] Evaluating the pain experience of the elderly patient may be further complicated by differences in pain symptom manifestation when compared to younger patients. Reactions of the cognitively impaired person to painful stimuli may differ from the typical response of a cognitively intact older person. For example, pathologic conditions that produce clear pain symptoms in younger patients may manifest as confusion, restlessness, aggression, or fatigue in the elderly, resulting in misdiagnosis and delays in treatment.[59,61–63]

Poor pain management in the cognitively impaired patient population has been attributed to many factors, the most concerning of which is a failure of health care providers to recognize pain in those who are not able to communicate their pain experience.[44–46] The severely cognitively impaired, as a result of the loss of language skills, are unable to communicate their pain experience in a way that is easily understood and may be unable to assist health care providers in identifying pain etiologies. Studies have shown that cognitively impaired elderly individuals receive fewer analgesics than cognitively intact patients, although they are as likely to experience pain.[46,61–63] Until there is scientific evidence that patients with dementia actually experience less pain, "we should assume that any condition that is painful to a cognitively intact person would also be painful to those with advanced dementia who cannot express themselves."[44]

Selecting a pain rating scale for use in the elderly and cognitively impaired population has presented challenges for health care providers, although several recent studies have offered some clarity on this issue through evaluation of the feasibility, reliability, and validity of UPRSs. In two studies, Pautex and colleagues evaluated the VRS, VAS, and FPS and concluded that the majority of hospitalized elderly patients with mild or moderate dementia, and many with severe dementia, can appropriately use at least one of the scales to reliably self-report their pain experience.[46,48] Patients with severe dementia demonstrated better comprehension for the VRS and FPS.[44,48] Gagliese and colleagues[34] evaluated the NRS, VDS, VAS, and MPQ for assessing pain intensity in younger and older (18 to 86 years of age) postsurgical, cognitively intact patients.[34] In the study group, the NRS was selected most frequently as the easiest and most preferred pain intensity scale, whereas the VAS was rated as the least accurate and least preferred for future use.[34]

Several behavioral/observational pain assessment tools have been developed to interpret the expression of pain by focusing on behavior in nonverbal older adults with more severe dementia.[62–64] Because patients with dementia often present with unique behavioral profiles that would typically not be suggestive of pain in the cognitively intact person, it is important to select an observational pain tool that is comprehensive and assesses a broad range of possible pain behaviors.[64] Based on the critique by Herr and colleagues,[64] only one behavioral observation tool, the Checklist of Nonverbal Pain Indicators (CNPI), has been tested with older adults in the acute care setting and can be recommended for use in that clinical practice setting. The CNPI is an itemized list of six behavioral pain indicators commonly observed in cognitively impaired older adults, including nonverbal vocal complaints, facial grimacing or wincing, bracing, restlessness, rubbing, and verbal vocal complaints. Each item is scored both at rest and on movement. A score of 1 or 0 indicates the behavior is present or not present, respectively. The possible range of scores at rest and with movement is 0 to 6, with a possible total score of 12.

Other similar scales include the Pain Assessment in Advanced Dementia scale (PAINAD) (Figure 11.12) and the Face, Leg, Activity, Cry and Consolability Pain Assessment Tool (FLACC) (Figure 11.13) that was originally developed for neonates. These scales also incorporate lists of behavioral pain indicators commonly observed in cognitively impaired older adults. Total scores are ranked from 0, which indicates no pain-related behavior, to 10, which indicates severe pain behavior. The method of administration and scoring of these tools are simple and time efficient. One disadvantage to the use of the PAINAD, FLACC, and similar tools is that pain behavior checklists cannot be used with patients who are unresponsive, heavily sedated, or receiving neuromuscular agents.

Pain Assessment Considerations in Critically Ill Patients

Optimizing the care of postoperative, critically ill patients requires effective treatment of pain following surgery. It has been reported that 22% to 70% of intensive care unit (ICU) patients recalled having moderate to severe pain during their ICU stay.[64–65] "One of the primary causes of inadequate pain management in the ICU is the lack of appropriate pain assessment."[65] Pain is considered a major physiologic and psychological stressor among patients in the ICU setting. However, as reported by Graf and colleagues, there are "no valid or reliable physiologic or biochemical measures of pain appropriate for the ICU setting, but pain associated behaviors often indicate the presence and causes of pain."[65] Assessing pain in the ICU setting is particularly challenging because of the complexity of the issues involved in critical care.

Hemodynamic instability, delirium, anxiety, agitation, sedation, anesthesia, cognitive impairment, particularly in the elderly, and comorbidities complicate the assessment of critically ill individuals. Also, patients in the ICU setting routinely undergo procedures and treatments associated with discomfort and pain such as turning, endotracheal or nasogastric suctioning, phlebotomy, chest tubes, endotracheal tubes, wound care, dressing changes, and insertion and removal of invasive lines.[65–66] Studies have shown that turning is the most painful procedure and is closely followed by suctioning.[65] Untreated or intractable pain experienced by patients can result in anxiety and agitation that may cause breathing difficulty, patient-ventilator dyssynchrony, elevated heart rate and blood pressure, combative behavior, and posttraumatic stress disorder.[67]

Communication with critically ill patients is often further compromised by factors such as use of sedative and analgesic agents, neuromuscular blockade, mechanical ventilation, restraints, confusion, and changes in the level of consciousness.[69,70] The health care provider must be able to recognize, prioritize, and treat these issues via pharmacologic and medical interventions while balancing efficacy and patient safety. The Society of Critical Care Medicine (SCCM) together with the American Society of Health-System Pharmacists in 2002 issued updated recommendations in its clinical practice guidelines for the sustained use of sedatives and analgesics in adults to which the reader is referred for a comprehensive overview.[67,71] Included in these guidelines are the following recommendations regarding pain assessment[67,71]:

1 Critically ill patients that are agitated should be sedated only after providing adequate analgesia.
2 Pain assessment and treatment should be done regularly, using the appropriate scale.
3 The self report should be used whenever possible.
4 Nonverbal patients should be assessed through subjective observations and physiological indicators.

Sedatives and analgesics are the most popular pharmacological interventions in clinical practice. It is important to recognize that pain, delirium, anxiety, and agitation can similarly manifest; however, they have different causes and require different treatments.[67] Therefore, the use of tools that have demonstrated good reliability and validity in the ICU setting is recommended to evaluate sedation and to differentiate among pain, delirium, anxiety, and agitation.[67]

Score	Term	Description	
+4	Combative	Overtly combative, violent, immediate danger to staff	
+3	Very agitated	Pulls or removes tube(s) or catheter(s); aggressive	
+2	Agitated	Frequent nonpurposeful movement, fights ventilator	
+1	Restless	Anxious, but movements are not aggressive or vigorous	
0	Alert and calm		
-1	Drowsy	Not fully alert, but has sustained awakening (eye opening and eye contact) to voice (≥ 10 seconds)	
-2	Light sedation	Briefly awakens with eye contact to voice (< 10 seconds)	
-3	Moderate sedation	Movement or eye opening to voice (but no eye contact)	Verbal stimulation
-4	Deep sedation	No response to voice, but has movement or eye opening to physical stimulation	
-5	Unarousable	No response to voice or physical stimulation	Physical stimulation

Figure 11.17: The Richmond Agitation Sedation Scale (RASS). Modified from Sessler, et al., *Am J Repir Crit Care Med.* 2002;166:1338–1344.

Subjective sedation assessment scales include the Riker Sedation-Agitation Scale, the Motor Activity Assessment Scale, the Vancouver Interaction and Calmness Scale, and the Richmond Agitation-Sedation Scale (Figure 11.17).[67,68] Two tools to monitor delirium are the Intensive Care Delirium Screening Checklist and the Confusion Assessment Method for the ICU (CAM-ICU).[72] In accordance with the CAM-ICU, acute onset or a fluctuating course of mental status changes and the presence of patient inattention and disorganized thinking or an altered level of consciousness is indicative of delirium.[73,74]

Unrelieved acute pain, particularly in the ICU setting, is associated with an increase of stress hormone and catecholamine levels that may cause tachycardia, hypertension, and increased oxygen consumption.[74] As such, changes in physiologic variables, including heart rate, blood pressure, respiration rate, pupil size, and diaphoresis, should be included in the pain assessment process, but should not be relied on as primary indicators of the presence or absence of pain due to a lack of sensitivity and specificity to the nociceptive response.[73–75]

A routine, comprehensive reassessment of the patient's pain experience is required to optimize patient care, particularly with respect to pain management, and to prevent adverse pathologic or pharmacologic events. Pain intensity scores or behavioral/observational ratings should be obtained both at rest and after movement. It is recommended that pain be reassessed on a regular basis, including within 15 to 30 minutes after a parenteral analgesic intervention,[65] and more promptly following a patient or caregiver report of pain or change in behavior.

For those critically ill patients who are able to verbalize their pain experience, the standard unidimensional and multidimensional pain assessment tools should be employed when appropriate. The American College of Critical Care Medicine recommended in their 2002 clinical practice guidelines that the NRS and the VAS be used in the assessment of pain for ICU patients who can self-report their pain.[65]

For critically ill patients who are mechanically ventilated and unable to verbalize, yet are conscious, a basic patient self-report of pain can be sought by health care providers. In such circumstances, the patient may be asked to respond to questions regarding existence, intensity, and location of pain via simple gestures such as a yes or no nod of the head, blink of an eye, raising of an eyebrow, or hand gestures. For such patients, it is possible for the health care provider to ascertain a pain intensity level. For example, this can be accomplished by verbally describing the NRS and asking the patient to gesture when the number that correlates to their present level of pain is spoken.

When critically ill patients are unable to self report, clinicians must observe the patient for behaviors that are suggestive of the presence of pain. Important to the care of critically ill patients is to assume that pain is present if conditions, procedures, or behaviors that normally cause or indicate pain are present. Two behavioral assessment tools available to evaluate pain in nonverbal, critically ill patient are the Behavioral Pain scale (BPS)[73,74] and the Critical Care Pain Observation Tool (CPOT).[75] The validity and reliability of the BPS was demonstrated in the unconscious sedated patient. The BPS (Figure 11.15) assesses three categories of behavior, including facial expression, upper limbs, and compliance with ventilation.[69] The total score ranges from 3 (no pain) to 12 (highest pain score). The CPOT demonstrated acceptable validity and reliability in critically ill cardiac surgery patients.[70] Use of the CPOT has not been evaluated in other critical care populations. The CPOT (Figure 11.14) assesses four categories of behavior, including facial expression, body movement, muscle tension, and either compliance with the ventilator for intubated patients or vocalization for extubated patients. The total score ranges from 0 to 8 with a higher total score reflecting a greater degree of pain.[70]

Inadequate pain control and analgesic undermedication are particular concerns for the nonverbal patient who must rely entirely on their health care provider(s) to appropriately assess their pain experience using behavioral/observational assessment tools. In one study,[76] nurses responded comfortably when pain was described as incisional or nociceptive in origin. However, pain or discomfort associated with other etiologies such as procedures or treatments routinely conducted in a postsurgical patient were either ignored or not fully assessed until prompting from the patient occurred. With this in mind, health care providers must be aware of the intricacies in the process of pain assessment and must place emphasis on making an appropriate assessment. Toward this end, health care providers must use appropriate tools and apply sound clinical judgement, especially for patients who are unable to self-report pain. No single objective assessment strategy is sufficient in itself. A systematic approach is encouraged for those critically ill patients who are intubated, heavily sedated, cognitively impaired, delirious, and difficult to assess overall. Some key clinical recommendations are provided in the American Society for Pain Management Nurses position statement on pain assessment in the nonverbal patient as outlined in the Appendix of this chapter.

Pain Assesment Considerations in Patients with Addictive Disorders

A past or present history of drug abuse presents physical and psychosocial issues that can undermine pain management therapy. It is estimated that one-third of the population in the United States has used illicit drugs, and 6% to 15% have some form of a substance abuse disorder.[77] Treatment of pain in persons with addictive disorders is challenging because of caregiver suspicions that analgesics are either being diverted or abused. Because of these fears, and restrictions in opioid dosing, this patient population is particularly vulnerable to inadequate assessment and undertreatment of pain.

One study evaluated 73 patients with HIV-related pain and a history of substance abuse and 100 patients with cancer pain and no history of substance abuse.[77] The results of the study suggested that patients with substance abuse histories were more likely to be undermedicated with opioids, experience greater pain-related interference in daily functioning, and demonstrate more aberrant drug-related behaviors than patients with cancer pain. The investigators concluded that "treatment of substance abusers with pain requires skills that complement best practices in opioid prescribing."

Lack of clarity regarding terms describing dependency and addiction contribute to misunderstandings regarding pain assessment and the use of opioid analgesics to manage acute pain. Consequences of this lack of clarity include inadequate treatment of pain, unnecessary suffering, increased health care costs, and adverse physical, psychological, and social outcomes. Optimizing management of pain in patients with addictive disorders or substance abuse issues requires an understanding of the concepts of addiction, pseudoaddiction, tolerance, and physical dependence, the definitions of which are described in Chapter 34, *Acute Pain Management in Patients with Opioid Dependence and Substance Abuse*. The reader is also referred to the Appendix for the American Society for Pain Management Nursing position statement on and recommendations for managing pain in patients with addictive disease.

Pain Assessment in Pediatric Patients

Historically, pain in pediatric patients was inappropriately managed because of fears of overmedication and lack of effective assessment tools. Children are capable of expressing their pain but may require patience and understanding by their caregivers. There are a number of tools that can be used to assess pain in children; however, before employing a particular tool, caregivers must always take into account the child's age, cognitive abilities, and communication skills. The NRS may be used in elementary school patients who can grasp the meaning of increasingly higher consecutive numbers reflecting a higher value or score. In most settings, however, the OUCHER scale[37,38] and various forms of the previously described FACES scale are the primary pain assessment tools employed in pediatric care units. The OUCHER scale that employs photographs of children ranging from quiet to sobbing to screaming can be distressing to younger children; however, the photographs can be customized to include younger and older patients and patients from different racial and ethnic groups. The child selects the face that best represents him- or herself at the present time. The sad crying face, or number 5, is selected by the child having the greatest pain, whereas selection of the happy face, or 0, indicates he or she has no pain. The FACES scale can be used in all verbal children, from 3 year olds to adolescents.

For younger children, a body outline diagram can be employed to localize pain and its intensity. The tool is a representation of the front and back of a child's body, and they are instructed to use a crayon to color the area on the diagram where they hurt. They can use any color; however, they can be instructed that very bad pain can be depicted with a red crayon and mild pain with an orange one.

Pain assessment in neonates and nonverbal children requires the use of behavioral scores similar to those employed in uncommunicative adults. Although physiological changes in blood pressure, heart rate, and respiratory rate are associated with

Table 11.7: Barriers to Optimal Pain Management

Patient/family barriers

Reluctance to self-report pain and to take analgesics

Cognitive impairment; inability to communicate pain experience in an easily understood manner

Feeling of disempowerment because of health care structure and existing pain management practices within the structure

Unfamiliarity with the health care setting, personal situation, and the severity of pain experienced may encourage passivity and may translate to fear of speaking with health care providers about need for pain relief

Uncertainty about how to dialog with health care providers regarding pain management decisions.

Belief in stoicism; desire to be a good patient

False expectations for pain control

Health care provider barriers

Inadequate pain assessment

Inadequate staff knowledge regarding pain assessment and management

Exaggerated concerns about opioid tolerance, physical dependence, addiction, and adverse effects

Fear of polypharmacy and opiophobia

Inadequate understanding of correlation between pain behavior and pain intensity

Overestimation of low levels of pain and underestimation of high levels of pain by health care providers

More focus placed on curing the underlying disease than on treating pain

Lack of adequate knowledge regarding analgesic pharmacology and pain therapy (eg, analgesics given at frequencies not consistent with the drug's pharmacokinetic properties, prescribed in inadequate dosages or administered in doses lower than those prescribed)

Underuse of nonpharmacologic methods for pain management

Lack of education, awareness, and/or empathy of health care professionals regarding the importance of addressing patients' particular pain management needs

Discrepancy between the patient's and health care provider's assessment of the extent to which pain is interfering with daily activities.

Exaggerated concern about regulatory oversight

Health care systems barriers

Poor pain assessment practices

Absence of clearly articulated practice standards

Failure to make pain relief an organizational priority

Lack of accountability for pain management practices

Difficulty obtaining support from health care providers in authority positions who have responsibility for translating pain policy into practice

Failure to adopt standard pain assessment tool(s) and patient population-specific tool(s)

Failure to provide staff sufficient time or chart space to document pain-related information

Sources: Joint Commission on Accreditation of Health Care Organizations (2000),[3] Ferrell (2005),[4] Berry et al (2006),[11] Herr and Decker (2004),[44] Green et al (2003),[59] Hansson, Fridlund, and Hallstrom (2006),[80] American Geriatrics Society (AGS) Panel on Persistent Pain in Older Persons (2002).[89]

increases in pain intensity, behavioral changes such as crying, posturing, and level of agitation are more reliable indicators. The Children's Hospital of Eastern Ontario Pain scale (CHEOPS), and the Pain Discomfort scale were among the earliest behavioral observation scales used in pediatric settings. In addition to crying, the CHEOPS assigned numerical scores to facial expressions, torso turning, verbalizations, and response to touch. In recent years, the previously described FLACC scale has become the behavioral pain assessment scale utilized at many pediatric care and neonatal units.

BARRIERS TO PAIN CONTROL

Inadequate pain management is a complex problem. Correcting this problem requires knowledge of management strategies, appropriate pain assessment and reassessment, and a treatment plan tailored to meet the physical and psychological needs of the patient.[79] Numerous barriers (Table 11.7) must be overcome to effectively assess and optimally treat patients' pain. Existing barriers include concerns of the patients, their family members, health care providers, and health care systems (Figure 11.18).[80]

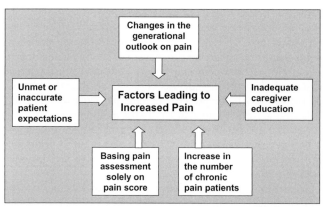

Figure 11.18: Factors responsible for increased complaints of pain. Despite improvements in pain assessment, analgesics, and analgesic delivery systems, patient complaints of acute pain severity have not decreased since the late 1990s. Factors responsible for this lack of improvement are displayed.

Patient Barriers

Effective communication between health care providers and patients is essential to a comprehensive pain assessment and treatment strategy. The presence of dementia is one important barrier to pain assessment. It has been demonstrated in a number of studies that cognitively impaired patients receive fewer analgesics compared to cognitively intact patients with similar pathology.[46] Patients with serious medical illnesses may underreport pain and pain severity. Reluctance to report pain may be associated with a variety of patient misconceptions, including the feeling that analgesics do not influence pain, a fear of becoming addicted to analgesics, an idea that good patients do not talk about pain, or a feeling that it is preferable to suffer from pain than from analgesic-associated side effects.[3,34–37] Some patients feel that complaints about pain may distract the physician from treating the real problem or that analgesics should be administered only when pain is unbearable.[81,82]

In the United States, pain is often regarded as an inevitable part of life. Many individuals believe that it is a sign of weakness to admit pain.[79,80,82] For example, it has been identified that patients with cancer often do not want to be labeled as complainers, do not want to distract their physicians from treating their cancer, or are afraid that pain means that their cancer is progressing.[59] Also, some individuals believe that pain must be accepted as part of having cancer and choose to remain stoic.

The fear of addiction, developing tolerance to, or experiencing intolerable side effects to opioids may also have a negative impact on communication between patients and clinicians. Patients are often uncomfortable talking to their health care providers about their pain and may be reluctant to participate in treatment decisions because they feel inferior to their health care provider. Additionally, ethnicity-related differences between patients and their physicians have been cited as one reason for patient unwillingness to communicate about their pain.[83] Patients may find it difficult to express themselves in terms the health care provider can understand because of demographic, language, and cultural discordance between them.[83,84]

Finally, the impact of psychological alterations such as anxiety, depression, and pain perception is noteworthy. Increased anxiety associated with hospital admission and the prospect of surgery results in behavioral and cognitive sequelae that can have a negative impact on recovery.[43] A study conducted by Carr and colleagues[43] explored the impact of anxiety and depression on postoperative pain experience in 85 women having major gynecological surgery. This study demonstrated that preoperative anxiety and depression scores correlated with postoperative pain and satisfaction scores. Findings of this study suggested, that by postoperative day 4, anxiety and depression scores increased as pain increased. It was suggested that patients' expectations about their pain and concerns about its continuation or effect on their lives contributed to the degree of anxiety and depression. Significantly higher pain scores were observed in anxious patients compared to patients who were less anxious and changes in anxiety were significantly related to changes in pain. It has also been demonstrated that younger patients with depression are more likely to experience moderate to severe postoperative pain.[68]

Health Care Provider Barriers

Health care providers have suggested poor pain assessment, patient reluctance to report pain, inadequate staff knowledge regarding pain management, and lack of staff time as major barriers to optimal pain management.[59] Additional barriers to effective assessment and optimal management of pain include incomplete knowledge of pain management modalities, differing physician attitudes about pain management, misperceptions regarding the adverse effects of opioid analgesics, and concern regarding regulatory scrutiny of medical decision making.[84,85]

Physicians and other health care providers may consider pain an accepted part of life or be influenced by patient culture, ethnicity, gender, or age biases.[79–83] Ethnic or cultural disease models and their interrelationship with patients' approach to expressing and dealing with pain may not be well understood.[79] Health care providers may have a perception or a stereotype of the patient's race and ethnicity that may influence their interpretation of patients' symptoms and behaviors, as well as their clinical decision-making process.[80,84] This may be a particular issue in the emergency department where health care providers and patients have no previously established relationship.[80,84,86]

Another factor that may play a significant role in pain assessment and management is the health care providers' level of fluency in the patient's primary language because of its impact on effective clinician/patient communication.[79] Also noteworthy, is that pain intensity as assessed by physicians and other health care providers may not be consistent with the patient's assessment. Nurses' assessments have reportedly been influenced by patient age and type and stage of illness, with less physiologic and physical suffering inferred in older patients and less intense pain assessed in both patients with no sign of pathology and those with chronic pain.[86] The experience and personality of the nurse may also influence assessment of patients' pain.[86]

Continuing deficiencies in physician education also contribute to the high incidence of poorly controlled pain. There exists no mandate or regulation dictating how much time should be spent teaching students or residents how to accurately assess and manage pain. Outside of the subspecialties of anesthesiology and pain management, physicians receive little, if any, formal training in treating pain. Yet, the majority of physicians who practice in a surgical and primary care specialties will encounter a significant number of patients experiencing moderate to severe pain. Armed solely with knowledge gained from a medical school pharmacology lecture and dosing recommendations advocated by attendings and senior residents, junior staff are generally ill equipped to adequately manage their patients' pain. The system allows for the propagation of biased and often incorrect views of pain intensity, analgesic pharmacology, and analgesic prescription with each subsequent generation of physicians.

Finally, health care system barriers, including a lack of accountability for pain management, a historical absence of clearly articulated practice standards, and a failure to make pain relief a priority, are directly responsible for inadequacies in assessment and analgesic administration.[11] System barriers include the failure of a health care organization to adopt a standard pain assessment tool(s) for the general patient population and specialized tools for the challenging patient populations.[86–90] Additionally, fragmented patient care increases the risk of poor coordination of care across treatment settings.[79]

Patient Expectations

Since the late 1970s there has been a significant rise in the level of patients' expectations in regard to the health care they receive. Through the use of various forms of media such as the Internet, patients have become more self-informed than ever before. They expect top-notch care along with successful outcomes. Some of these patients may also develop false expectations, such as that minimally invasive surgeries are not painful or that new analgesic/analgesic techniques will result in a pain free recovery. Although there are some antianxiety benefits, in telling patients that they will minimal to no pain following a surgical intervention, studies show that false patient expectations can lead to patient dissatisfaction.[7,84] Despite a good surgical outcome with appropriate pain intervention intraoperatively and postoperatively, patients may feel unsatisfied with the care they have received. A key to resolving this issue will be increasing the communication between the health care practitioner and the patient with the conversation focusing on the patient's expectations, goals of the consultations, and things to be expected in the postsurgical period.[7,84,86] This conversation allows for patients to gain some sense of control over their health situation and empowers them to assist with the formulation of their treatment plan.

Increasing Number of Chronic Pain Patients

According to the National Pain Foundation, about 75 million Americans suffer from chronic pain. Compare this number to the previous estimate of 49 million described in 1995. As the population increases, the number patients suffering degenerative diseases and persistent pain are increasing. These individuals also represent a larger proportion of those patients undergoing surgery or requiring hospitalization. As such, they present new issues for health care professionals. For many chronic pain patients, the use of COX-2 inhibitors and NSAIDs has been discontinued because of cardiac morbidity concerns and opioid analgesics substituted. Continued opioid exposure predisposes these individuals to tolerance development and dose escalation. The fact that elderly and ill opioid-dependent patients often require high doses of IV PCA morphine and oral opioids to achieve adequate postoperative pain control may be worrisome to many non–pain specialists.[89] Concerns about oversedation and risks of respiratory depression ultimately lead physicians to undermedicate these patients despite complaints of moderate to severe pain.

Overcoming the Barriers

Awareness of barriers that interfere with effective pain assessment and management is important in developing treatment plans that promote effective management and patient comfort. Because unrelieved pain may have significant adverse physical and psychological consequences, clinicians should encourage all patients to report the presence of pain, particularly in individuals who are often reluctant to discuss pain or who deny that excessive pain is present.[11] Health care providers must be aware of any personal biases they have that may interfere with clinical judgment, and they must apply knowledge in a rational, scientific manner.

Correcting educational deficits may require mandatory rotations or blocks within pain management for residents of all specialties, along with integration of pain lectures into the medical school curriculum nationwide. However, these solutions will be difficult to perform as both the medical school and residency curriculum are currently maximized in terms of available teaching time. Despite this difficulty, Yale Medical School students are required to spend 2 days of the surgical/anesthesiology rotation rounding with the pain management service. At other institutions, revaluation of the existing curricula may be necessary to determine if any topics can be deleted or minimized to allow increase exposure to pain management.

Implementing organizational protocols, policies, and procedures to guide the processes of pain assessment and management is essential.[88–90] The culture of health care organizations must be such that effective pain assessment and optimal pain management are given priority status and are recognized as essential components of quality health care.[3,88,89] Additionally, all health care providers involved in the process of pain management must be appropriately educated in the nuances of communicating with patients about their pain experience and must understand cultural differences and the impact thereof. An understanding of the available treatment modalities and the adverse effect profiles of opioid analgesics is also essential. Last, and as important, is a rational understanding of legal and regulatory considerations.[85]

CONCLUSIONS

It is well understood that unrelieved pain leads to unnecessary suffering and delays in recovery and adds to the overall cost of health care. It is also recognized that continual assessment and optimal management has positive impact on the quality of health care services and the quality of patients' lives.

Pain is a highly complex experience with several quantifiable features, including intensity, time, course, quality, impact, and personal meaning.[13] Many factors influence interindividual variability in pain sensitivity, perception, and response to analgesics. Among these factors are physiology of pain mechanisms, psychological and environmental factors, genetics, gender, ethnicity, temperament,[90] and emotional issues such as fear, anxiety, and depression.[43,67,69] Frequent and accurate assessment of pain intensity and associated qualitative variables is an essential clinical responsibility necessary to provide optimal pain management and to appreciate the effectiveness of therapy. To state that one particular method of pain assessment is best is as incorrect as saying that all patients experience the same degree of pain following similar operative procedures. The patient's self-report of his or her pain experience remains the gold standard of communication. Unidimensional NRS and VRS tools provide rapid, reliable, and objective measurement of acute pain intensity and localization. Multidimensional assessment scales and questionnaires are generally reserved for more detailed examination and management of more complex pain syndromes and persistent pain. Ultimately, it is the patient's cognitive and communicative abilities that determine which assessment tool should be employed. To avoid biases, health care providers must also appreciate nuances of assessment in a variety of patient populations, including racial and ethnic minorities, critically ill and cognitively impaired patients, those with addictive disorders, and pediatric patients.

APPENDIX

American Society for Pain Management Nursing (ASPMN) Position Statements

Position Statement	Clinical Practice Recommendations	Source: ASPMN Position Statement
"It is within the scope of nursing practice for a registered nurse (RN) to administer analgesia to patients when indicated. The ASPMN supports the role of the RN in the management and care of patients receiving analgesia by catheter techniques, including but not limited to analgesia by the epidural, intrathecal, intrapleural, and perineural routes of administration, in patients of all ages and in all care settings."	The institution's/health care facility's policies, procedures and guidelines, and the state board of nursing regulations shall define: ▪ Education and training required for involved RNs. ▪ Education needs for patients and families. ▪ RN's roles in management and monitoring of analgesia by catheter technique, including comprehensive assessment of the patient's physiological and emotional care needs and response to analgesia (ie, assessment of pain, side effects, complications) ▪ Licensed independent practitioners (LIPs) who are trained and authorized in catheter placement for analgesia by catheter techniques, test dose administration and establishment of analgesic dosage parameters. ▪ Communication between RN and LIP regarding patient status or changes in status during therapy. ▪ Record keeping requirements. ▪ Quality improvement program.	Registered Nurse Management and Monitoring by Catheter Techniques (2006)[16]
"The ASPMN recognizes the need for prompt, safe, and effective pain relief for all and supports the use of Authorized Agent Controlled Analgesia (AACA) for the patient who is unable to self administer analgesics using an analgesic infusion pump, due to cognitive or physical limitations. The ASPMN does not support the use of 'PCA by Proxy' in which an unauthorized person activates the dosing mechanism of an analgesic infusion pump and delivers analgesic medication to the patient, thereby increasing the risk for potential patient harm."	The health care institution must have clear policies, procedures, and guidelines that: ▪ Outline conditions under which AACA practice may be implemented, and a mechanism for communicating to all health care providers that a patient is receiving AACA. ▪ Outline monitoring procedures (assessment, management, reassessment, and documentation) ▪ Stipulate frequency of sedation and respiratory checks during therapy. ▪ Provide for an AACA-specific prescribing mechanism that includes drug, dosage, monitoring, and when not to activate the dosing button. ▪ Provides for education of each authorized agent, patient, family members, and other visitors regarding principles of AACA. ▪ Provides for ongoing outcomes evaluation and QI activities.	Authorized and Unauthorized ("PCA by Proxy") Dosing of Analgesic Infusion Pumps (2006)[17]
"The inability of nonverbal patients, including elders with advanced dementia, infants and preverbal toddlers, and intubated and/or unconscious patients, to communicate pain and discomfort because of developmental or physiologic issues is a major barrier for them being adequately assessed for pain and achieving adequate pain management interventions."	1. Use the Hierarchy of Pain Assessment Techniques established by McCaffery and Pasero (1999) ▪ Attempt patient self-report whenever possible. ▪ Search for etiologies of the pain. Assume pain is present (APP). ▪ Observe patient behaviors (baseline and ongoing) as indicators of pain. Recognize that the behaviors may be due to causes other than pain. ▪ Obtain report of patient's pain and changes in behavior or activity from family members or caregivers. ▪ Attempt analgesic trial after estimating pain intensity (APP), and titrate to effect. 2. Establish a procedure for assessing presence of pain and response to therapy. 3. Use behavioral pain assessment tools/scales as appropriate for the individual patient. 4. Apply physiologic indicators (changes in heart rate, blood pressure, and respiratory rate) of pain when appropriate. 5. Reassess and document at regular intervals following intervention.	Pain Assessment in the Nonverbal Patient: Position Statement with Clinical Practice Recommendations (2006)[18]
"Patients with addictive disease and pain have the right to be treated with dignity, respect, and the same quality of pain assessment and management as all other patients. This includes maintaining a balance between provision of pain relief and protection against inappropriate use of prescribed medications. Nurses are well positioned and obligated to advocate for pain management across all treatment settings for patients actively using alcohol or other drugs, patients in recovery, or those receiving methadone for opioid dependence."	Recommendations for managing pain in patients with addictive disease include: ▪ Diagnose and treat addiction, symptoms of withdrawal, and pain. ▪ Encourage patient use of external support systems. ▪ Involve patient, family and significant others in pain management planning. ▪ Ensure that implementation of plan is consistent among all involved in care. ▪ Education regarding differences between addiction, physical dependence, and tolerance. ▪ Education regarding medication options.	Pain Management in Patients with Addictive Disease (2002)[19]

(continued)

Position Statement	*Clinical Practice Recommendations*	*Source: ASPMN Position Statement*
	▪ Selection and titration of analgesics based on pain assessment, side effects, function, sleep, and mood. Be aware that higher than usual opioid doses may be required. Utilize adjunctive therapy when appropriate. ▪ Utilize the route of administration, dosage form and frequency appropriate for the individual patient. ▪ Identify, record, and discuss with the patient any behavior that suggests inappropriate medication use or patient's own acknowledgement of misuse. ▪ Minimize withdrawal symptoms by tapering opioids, benzodiazepines, or other medications with a potential for physical dependence when treatment is no longer needed. ▪ For patients who are actively using define pseudoaddiction versus addiction, assess and treat symptoms of withdrawal from alcohol and other drugs, discuss patient-acknowledged inappropriate use of medications, assess for and treat psychiatric comorbidities, avoid use of opioid agonist-antagonist agents, provide information on treatment options for addictive disease. ▪ For patients in recovery, discuss risks of unrelieved pain, concerns about relapse, and use of opioids and/or nonopioids as part of treatment plan. ▪ For patients on methadone maintenance (MM) treatment include MM provider, and either increase the daily dose and frequency of the methadone for analgesia or initiate a new opioid agent in addition to the daily MM dose.	
"Placebos should not be used by any route of administration in the assessment and/or management of pain in any individual regardless of age or diagnosis. ASPMN supports the use of placebos only in Institutional Review Board (IRB) – approved clinical trials."	▪ Implement institutional policies to ensure that the use of placebo agents to manage pain are prohibited in clinical practice unless in the context of an approved IRB-approved clinical trial.	Position Statement on Use of Placebos in Pain Management (2004)[20]
"Effective pain management requires careful individual titration of analgesics that is based on valid and reliable assessment of pain and pain relief. A registered nurse, who is competent in pain assessment and analgesic administration, can safely interpret and implement properly written "as-needed" or "PRN" range orders for analgesic medications. The ASPMN and the American Pain Society support safe medication practice and the appropriate use of PRN range orders for opioid analgesics in the management of pain."	Institutional policies shall: ▪ Define the processes required to ensure LIP competency in writing PRN opioid dosage range orders with a fixed time intervals in accordance with evidence-based clinical practice guidelines and nurse competency in interpreting and implementing these orders. A comprehensive patient history and a valid and reliable assessment of pain and pain relief, and understanding of opioid pharmacokinetics and side effect profiles are essential to safe and effective implementation of PRN range orders. ▪ Provide for dosage ranges that are large enough to permit appropriate and safe dose titration. The maximum dose within the range must be specified and may not exceed four times the minimum dose. ▪ Evaluate and document patient response to dose and interval. ▪ Ensure patient comfort and adherence to safe medication practices.	A Position Statement on the Use of "As-Needed" Range Orders for Opioid Analgesics in the Management of Acute Pain: A Consensus Statement of the American Society of Pain Management Nurses and the American Pain Society (2006)[21]
"As representatives of the health care community and law enforcement, we are working together to prevent abuse of prescription pain medications while ensuring that they remain available for patients in need."	▪ Although pharmaceutical manufacturers and distributors, and health care professionals must respect that opioid analgesics have an inherent abuse potential, the legitimate use of these drugs when medically indicated must also be respected.	A Position Statement on Promoting Pain Relief and Preventing Abuse of Pain Medications: a Critical Balancing Act (2003)[22]
"The ASPMN supports the position statements by the American Nurses' Association (ANA) on active euthanasia and assisted suicide that "Nurses individually and collectively have an obligation to provide comprehensive and compassionate end of life care which includes the promotion of comfort and the relief of pain, and at times, foregoing life-sustaining treatments." The ASPMN opposes nurse participation in assisted suicide or active euthanasia."	▪ Improved access for appropriate pain care that allows patients to die with dignity and adequate relief of pain.	ASPMN Position Statement on Assisted Suicide[23]
"The ASPMN believes that it is an ethical obligation for pain management nurses to advocate and provide for effective pain relief and symptom management to alleviate suffering for the patient receiving end of life care."	▪ Advocate for improved access to ethical and effective pain management services and other reliable treatment modalities that will benefit patients with end stage disease, fostering humane and dignified care.	ASPMN Position Statement on Pain Management at the End of Life (2002)[24]

REFERENCES

1. American Medical Association. *An American Medical Association Continuing Medical Education Program for Primary Care Physicians. Pain Management Part 2, Assessing and Treating Pain in Special Populations.* Chicago, IL: American Medical Association; June 2003.

2. Cousins MJ, Power I, Smith G. Pain: a persistent problem. *Reg Anesth Pain Med.* 2000;25:1,6–21.

3. Joint Commission on Accreditation of Health Care Organizations. *Pain Assessment and Management, an Organizational Approach.* Library of Congress Catalog No. 00-102701. 2000.

4. Ferrell B. Ethical perspectives on pain and suffering. *Pain Manag Nurs.* 2005;6(3):83–90.

5. Visser JE. Chronic post surgical pain: epidemiology and clinical implications for acute pain management. *Acute Pain.* 2006;8:73–81.

6. Kehlet H, Jensen TS, Woolf CJ. Persistent postsurgical pain: risk factors and prevention. *Lancet.* 2006; 367:1618–1625.

7. Apfelbaum JL, Chen C, Mehta SS, Gan TJ. Postoperative pain experience: results for a national survey suggest postoperative pain continues to be undermanaged. *Anesth Analg.* 2003;97:534–540.

8. Cross SA. Pathophysiology of pain. *Mayo Clin Proc.* 1994;69(4): 375–383.

9. Sinatra RS, Bigham M. The anatomy and pathophysiology of acute pain. In: Grass JA, ed. *Problems in Anesthesiology.* Vol. 10. Philadelphia, PA: *Lippincott-Raven;* 1997:8–22.

10. Desborough JP. The stress response to trauma and surgery. *Br J Anaesth.* 2000;85:109–117.

11. Berry PH, Covington EC, Dahl JL, et al. *Pain: Current Understanding of Assessment, Management, and Treatments.* Reston, VA: National Pharmaceutical Council and the Joint Commission on Accreditation of Health Care Organizations; 2006:21–29.

12. Foley KM. 2006. Appraising the WHO Analgesic Ladder on Its 20th Anniversary. Vol 19(1) Retrieved April 4, 2008 from http://www.whocancerpain.bcg.wisc.edu/?q=node/86old_site/eng/19_1/Interview.html.

13. Acute Pain Management Guideline Panel. *Acute Pain Management: Operative or Medical Procedures and Trauma. Clinical Practice Guideline.* AHCPR Pub. No. 92-0032. Rockville, MD: Agency for Health Care Policy and Research, Public Health Service, U.S. Department of Health and Human Services; February 1992.

14. Boos J, Drake A, et al. *Pain as the 5th Vital Sign Toolkit.* 1st ed. Washington, DC: American Pain Society; 2000:1–53.

15. American Nurses Association and American Society for Pain Management Nursing. 2005. *Pain Management Nursing: Scope and Standards of Practice.* Silver Spring, MD: nursesbooks.org.

16. American Society for Pain Management Nursing. Position statement: Registered nurse management and monitoring of analgesia by catheter techniques. http://www.aspmn.org/Organization/position_papers.htm.

17. American Society for Pain Management Nursing. Position statement: Authorized and unauthorized ("PCA by proxy") dosing of analgesic infusion pumps. June 2006. http://www.aspmn.org/Organization/position_papers.htm.

18. Herr K, Coyne PJ, Key T, et al. Pain assessment in the nonverbal patient: position statement with clinical practice recommendations. *Pain Manag Nurs.* 2006;7(2):44–52.

19. American Society for Pain Management Nursing. Position statement: Pain management in patients with addictive disease. September 2002. http://www.aspmn.org/Organization/position_papers.htm.

20. American Society for Pain Management Nursing. Position statement on use of placebos in pain management. July 2004. http://www.aspmn.org/Organization/position_papers.htm.

21. American Society for Pain Management Nursing. A position statement on the use of "as-needed" range orders for opioid analgesics in the management of acute pain. A consensus statement of the American Society of Pain Management Nurses and the American Pain Society. http://www.aspmn.org/Organization/position_papers.htm.

22. American Society for Pain Management Nursing. A position statement on promoting pain relief and preventing abuse of pain medications: a critical balancing act. October 2003. http://www.aspmn.org/Organization/position_papers.htm.

23. American Society for Pain Management Nursing. A position statement on assisted suicide. http://www.aspmn.org/Organization/position_papers.htm.

24. American Society for Pain Management Nursing. A position statement on pain management at the end of life. http://www.aspmn.org/Organization/position_papers.htm.

25. McCaffery M, Pasero C. *Pain Clinical Manual.* 2nd ed. St. Louis, MO: Mosby; 1999:40, 62.

26. The International Association for the Study of Pain (IASP) Task Force on Taxonomy Classification of Chronic Pain. Part III: Pain terms, a current list with definitions and notes on usage. In: Merskey H, Bogduk N, eds. *Classification of Chronic Pain.* 2nd ed. Seattle, WA: IASP Press; 1994:209–214.

27. McGuire DB. Comprehensive and multidimensional assessment and measurement of pain. *J Pain Symptom Manage.* 1992; 7(5):312–319.

28. American Pain Society (APS) Quality of Care Committee. Quality improvement guidelines for the treatment of acute pain and cancer pain. *J Am Med Assoc.* 1995;274:1874–1880.

29. Hanks-Bell M, Halvey K, Paice J. Pain assessment and management in aging. *Online J Issues Nurs.* 2004;9(3):8

30. Melzack R, Torgerson WS. On the language of pain. *Anesthesiology.* 1971;34(1):50–59.

31. McCaffrey M, Beebe A. Giving narcotics for pain. *Nursing.* 1989;19(10):161–165.

32. Caraceni A. Evaluation and assessment of cancer pain and cancer pain treatment. *Acta Anaesthesiol Scand.* 2001;45(9):1067–1075.

33. Closs SJ, Briggs M. Patients' verbal descriptions of pain and discomfort following orthopaedic surgery. *Int J Nurs Stud.* 2002;39(5):563–572.

34. Gagliese L, Weizblit N, Ellis W, et al. The measurement of postoperative pain: a comparison of intensity scales in younger and older surgical patients. *Pain.* 2005;117(3):412–420.

35. Williamson A, Hoggart B. Pain: a review of three commonly used pain rating scales. *J Clin Nurs.* 2005;14(7):798–804.

36. Lee JS, Hobden E, Stiell IG, et al. Clinically important change in the visual analog scale after adequate pain control. *Acad Emerg Med.* 2003;10(10):1128–1130.

37. Gagliese L, Katz J. Age differences in postoperative pain are scale dependent: a comparison of measures of pain intensity and quality in younger and older surgical patients. *Pain.* 2003;103(1–2):11–20.

38. Whaley L. Wong D. *Nursing Care of Infants and Children.* 4th ed. St Louis, MO: Mosby; 1991:1148.

39. Reading AE. A comparison of the McGill pain questionnaire in chronic and acute pain. *Pain.* 1982;13:185–192.

40. Jenkinson C, Carroll D, Egerton M, et al. Comparison of the sensitivity to change of long and short form pain measures. *Quality Life Res.* 1995;4:353–357.

41. Melzack R. The McGill pain questionnaire: major properties and scoring methods. *Pain.* 1975;1:277–299.

42. Melzack R. The short-form McGill pain questionnaire. *Pain.* 1987;30:191–197.

43. Carr ECJ, Thomas VN, Wilson-Barnet J. Patient experiences of anxiety, depression and acute pain after surgery: a longitudinal perspective. *Int J Nurs Stud.* 2005;42(5):521–530.

44. Herr K, Decker S. Older adults with severe cognitive impairment: assessment of pain. *Ann Long-Term Care.* 2004;12(4):46–52.

45. Pasero C, McCaffery M. No self-report means no pain-intensity rating. *J Adv Nurs.* 2005;105(10):50–53.

46. Pautex S, Herrmann F, Le Lous P, et al. Feasibility and reliability of four pain self-assessment scales and correlation with an observational rating scale in hospitalized elderly demented patients. *J Gerontol A Biol Sci Med Sci* 2005;60(4):524–529.

47. Sloman R, Rosen G, Rom M, et al. Nurses' assessment of pain in surgical patients. *J Adv Nurs.* 2005;52(2):125–132.

48. Pautex S, Michon A, Guedira M, et al. Pain in severe dementia: self-assessment or observational scales? *J Am Geriatr Soc.* 2006;54(7):1040–1045.

49. Jensen MP, Friedman M, Bonzo D, et al. The validity of the neuropathic pain scale for assessing diabetic neuropathic pain in a clinical trial. *Clin J Pain.* 2006;22(1):97–103.

50. Kaki AM, El-Yaski AZ, Youseif E. Identifying neuropathic pain among patients with chronic low-back pain: use of the leeds assessment of neuropathic symptoms and signs pain scale. *Reg Anesth Pain Med.* 2005;30(5):422–428.

51. Perez C, Galvez R, Insausti J, et al. Linguistic adaptation and Spanish validation of the LANSS (leeds assessment of neuropathic symptoms and signs) scale for the diagnosis of neuropathic pain. *Med Clin (Barc).* 2006;127(13):485–491.

52. Farrar JT, Berlin JA, Strom BL. Clinically important changes in acute pain outcome measures: a validation study. *J Pain Symptom Manage.* 2003;25(5):406–411.

53. Farrar JT, Portenoy RK, Berlin JA, et al. Defining the clinically important difference in pain outcome measures. *Pain.* 2000;88(3):287–294.

54. Gallagher EJ, Liebman M, Bijur PE. Prospective validation of clinically important changes in pain severity measured on a visual analog scale. *Ann Emerg Med.* 2001;38(6):633–638.

55. Todd KH, Funk KG, Funk JP, et al. Clinical significance of reported changes in pain severity. *Ann Emerg Med.* 1996;27(4):485–489.

56. Bernstein SL, Bijur PE, Gallagher EJ. Relationship between intensity and relief in patients with acute severe pain. *Am J Emerg Med.* 2006;24(2):162–166.

57. ten Klooster PM, Drossaers-Bakker KW, Taal E, et al. Patient-perceived satisfactory improvement (PPSI): interpreting meaningful change in pain from the patient's perspective. *Pain.* 2006; 121(1–2):151–157.

58. Sloman R, Wruble AW, Rosen G, et al. Determination of clinically meaningful levels of pain reduction in patients experiencing acute postoperative pain. *Pain Manag Nurs.* 2006;7(4):153–158.

59. Green CR, Anderson KO, Baker TA et al. The unequal burden of pain: confronting racial and ethnic disparities in pain. *Pain Med.* 2003;4(3):277–294.

60. Gibson SJ, Helme RD. Age-related differences in pain perception and report. *Clin Geriatr Med.* 2001;17:433–456.

61. Cunningham C. Managing pain in patients with dementia in hospital. *Nurs Stand.* 2006;20(46):54–58.

62. Morrison RS, Siu AL. A comparison of pain and its treatment in advanced dementia and cognitively intact patients with hip fracture. *J Pain Symptom Manage.* 2000;19:240–248.

63. Won AB, Lapane KL, Vallow S, et al. Persistent nonmalignant pain and analgesic prescribing patterns in elderly nursing home residents. *J Am Geriatr Soc.* 2004;52(6):867–874.

64. Herr K, Bjoro K, Decker S. Tools for assessment of pain innon-verbal older adults with dementia: a state-of-the-science review. *J Pain Symptom Manage.* 2006;31(2):170–192.

65. Graf C, Puntillo K. Pain in the older adult in the intensive care unit. *Crit Care Clin.* 2003;19:749–770.

66. Siffleet J, Young J, Nikoletti S, et al. Patients' self-report of procedural pain in the intensive care unit. *J Clin Nurs.* 2007;16(11):2142–2148.

67. Pun BT, Dunn J. The sedation of critically ill adults: Part 1: assessment. *J Adv Nurs.* 2007;107(7):40–48.

68. Gillies ML, Smith LN, Parry-Jones WL. Post-operative pain assessment and management in adolescents. *Pain.* 1999;70:207–215.

69. Young J, Siffleet J, Nikoletti S, et al. Use of a behavioural pain scale to assess pain in ventilated, unconscious and/or sedated patients. *Intensive Crit Care Nurs.* 2006;22(1):32–39.

70. Gelinas C, Fillion L, Puntillo KA, et al. Validation of the critical-care pain observation tool in adult patients. *Am J Crit Care.* 2006;15(4):402–407.

71. Jacobi J, Fraser GL, Coursin DB. Clinical practice guidelines for the sustained use of sedatives and analgesics in the critically ill adult. *Crit Care Med.* 2002;30(1):119–141.

72. Pun B. CEU article Part 2: Assessment and treatment of delirium in the ICU. 2005. Managing Pain, Delirium and Sedation. CEU article Part 2: Assessment and treatment of delirium in the ICU. Critical Care Nurse/Supplement Feb. 2007.

73. Payen JF, Bru O, Bosson JL, et al. Assessing pain in critically ill sedated patients by using a behavioral pain scale. *Crit Care Med.* 2001;29(12):2258–2263.

74. Aissaoui Y, Zeggwagh AA, Zekraoui A, et al. Validation of a behavioral pain scale in critically ill, sedated, and mechanically ventilated patients. *Anesth Analg.* 2005;101(5):1470–1476.

75. Gelinas C, Fillion L, Puntillo KA, et al. Validation of the critical-care pain observation tool in adult patients. *Am J Crit Care.* 2006;15(4):420–427.

76. Manias E, Botti M, Bucknall T. Observation of pain assessment and management – the complexities of clinical practice. *J Clin Nurs.* 2002;11(6):724–733.

77. Passik SD, Kirsh KL. Managing pain in patients with drug seeking behaviors. *J Supportive Oncology.* 2005;3(1):1–5.

78. Passik SD, Kirsh KL, Donaghy KB, et al. Pain and aberrant drug-related behaviors in medically ill patients with and without histories of substance abuse. *Clin J Pain.* 2006;22(2):173–181.

79. American Medical Association. An American Medical Association Continuing Medical Education Program for Primary Care Physicians. Pain Management Part 1, Overview of Physiology, Assessment, and Treatment. Chicago, IL: American Medical Association; June 2003.

80. Hansson E, Fridlund B, Hallstrom I. Effects of a quality improvement program in acute care evaluated by patients, nurses, and physicians. *Pain Manag Nurs.* 2006;7(3):93–108.

81. Stalnikowicz R, Mahamid R, Kaspi S, et al. Under-treatment of acute pain in the emergency department: a challenge. *Int J Qual Health Care.* 2005;17(2):173–176.

82. Cooper-Patrick L, Gallo JJ, Gonzales JJ, et al. Race, gender, and partnership in the patient-physician relationship. *JAMA.* 1999;282:583–589.

83. Miner J, Biros MH, Trainor A, et al. Patient and physician perceptions as risk factors for oligoanalgesia: a prospective observational study of the relief of pain in the emergency department. *Acad Emerg Med.* 2006;13(2):140–146.

84. Green CR, Wheeler JRC, Marchant B, et al. Analysis of the physician variable in pain management. *Pain Med.* 2001;2(4):317–327.

85. Bonham VL. Race, ethnicity, and pain treatment: striving to understand the causes and solutions to the disparities in pain treatment. *J Law Med Ethics.* 2001;29:52–68.

86. Hall-Lord ML, Larsson BW. Registered nurses' and student nurses' assessment of pain and distress related to specific patient and nurse characteristics. *Nurse Educ Today.* 2006;26(5):377–387.

87. Ware LJ, Epps CD, Herr K, et al. Evaluation of the revised faces pain scale, verbal descriptor scale, numeric rating scale, and Iowa pain thermometer in older minority adults. *Pain Manag Nurs.* 2006;7(3):117–125.

88. Fink R. Pain assessment: the cornerstone to optimal pain management. *BUMC Proc.* 2000;13:236–239.

89. American Geriatrics Society (AGS) Panel on Persistent Pain in Older Persons. The management of persistent pain in older persons. *J Am Geriatr Soc.* 2002;50:S205–S224.

90. Dionne RA, Bartoshuk L, Mogil J, et al. Individual responder analyses for pain: does one pain scale fit all ? *Trends Pharmacol Sci.* 2005;26(3):125–130.

12

The Role of Preventive Multimodal Analgesia and Impact on Patient Outcome

Scott S. Reuben and Asokumar Buvanendran

The primary goal of postoperative pain relief is to provide subjective comfort, inhibit trauma-induced afferent pain transmission, and blunt the autonomic and somatic reflex responses to pain. By accomplishing this, we should enhance restoration of function by allowing the patient to breath, cough, and ambulate more easily. Subsequently, these effects should improve overall postoperative outcome. Despite our increased knowledge since the late 1990s of the pathophysiology and pharmacology of nociception, acute postoperative pain still remains a major problem.[1] Patients continue to report that their primary concern before surgery is the severity of postoperative pain.[1,2] This is justified, because a recent survey has revealed that 31% of patients suffered from severe pain and another 47% from moderate pain.[1]

Unrelieved postoperative pain may result not only in suffering and discomfort but may also lead to multiple physiological and psychological consequences that can contribute to adverse perioperative outcomes (Figure 12.1).[3] These are primarily related to the surgical stress response to pain that is characterized by profound endocrine and metabolic changes resulting in increased sympathetic activity and catabolic demands.[4] General anesthesia is used to inhibit cortical responses to tissue injury, and neuromuscular blocking agents prevent muscle spasm during surgery. However, the sympathetic neuroendocrine and biochemical responses to surgical trauma are not effectively attenuated by general anesthesia alone.[4] This can potentially contribute to a higher incidence of myocardial ischemia and impaired wound healing[4,5] and delay gastrointestinal motility, resulting in prolonged postoperative ileus.[6] Further, unrelieved acute pain leads to poor respiratory effort and splinting that can result in atelectasis, hypercarbia, and hypoxemia, contributing to a higher incidence of postoperative pneumonia.[3] Additional adverse effects include psychological distress and anxiety, leading to sleeplessness and helplessness, and impaired postoperative rehabilitation that may potentially have long-term psychological consequences.[7] Finally, it has recently been recognized that unrelieved acute pain may contribute to a higher incidence of chronic postsurgical pain.[8] Therefore, strategies aimed at reducing acute pain may not only provide subjective comfort for our patients but also may result in improved postoperative outcomes and a reduction in health care expenditures.

PHYSIOLOGY OF PERIPHERAL AND CENTRAL SENSITIZATION

Tissue injury leads to pain transmission by direct mechanical and thermal damage to nerve endings, as well as the release of inflammatory mediators. The inflammatory mediators include prostaglandins that sensitize peripheral nerve endings, resulting in hyperalgesia and thus facilitating pain transmission. The perception of pain is not a hard-wired mechanism, wherein stimuli are always transmitted and processed in an identical manner each time as originally hypothesized in the 1640s by the French philosopher Rene Descartes.[9] In fact the central nervous system (CNS) exhibits a great deal of plasticity.[10] The processing of pain signals is now recognized to be a complex physiological cascade that involves dozens of different neurotransmitters and chemical substrates at several different anatomical locations. Operative procedures produce an initial afferent barrage of pain signals and generate a secondary inflammatory response, both of which contribute substantially to postoperative pain. The signals have the capacity to initiate prolonged changes in both the peripheral and CNS, leading to the amplification and prolongation of postoperative pain. Peripheral sensitization, a reduction in the threshold of nociceptor afferent peripheral terminals, is a result of inflammation at the site of surgical trauma.[11] As a result of this peripheral sensitization, low-intensity stimuli that normally would not cause a painful response prior to sensitization now become perceived as pain, an effect termed *allodynia* (Figure 12.2). In addition, patients develop *hyperalgesia*, which contributes to an exaggerated pain response following nociceptive stimuli (Figure 12.2). Central sensitization, an activity-dependent increase in the excitability of spinal neurons, is a result of persistent exposure to nociceptive afferent input from the peripheral neurons.[12] Taken together, these two processes (peripheral and central sensitization) contribute to the postoperative hypersensitivity state ("spinal wind-up") that is responsible for a decrease in the pain threshold, both at the site of injury (primary

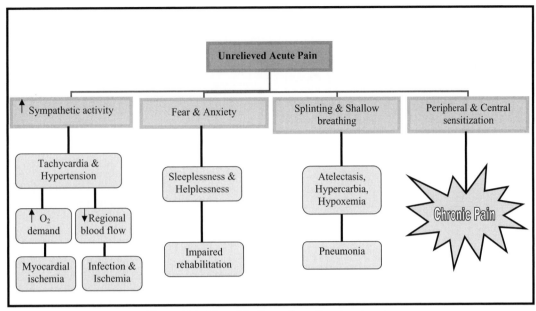

Figure 12.1: Harmful effects of unrelieved acute pain.

hyperalgesia), and in the surrounding uninjured tissue (secondary hyperalgesia) (Figure 12.3).[13] A more in-depth review of peripheral and central sensitization is presented in Chapter 1 (*Pain Pathways and Acute Pain Processing*).

Prolonged central sensitization has the capacity to lead to permanent alterations in the CNS that contribute to chronic pain long after the acute stimulus has been withdrawn. Sustained input from peripheral neurons can result in the death of inhibitory neurons, replacement with new afferent excitatory neurons, and the establishment of aberrant excitatory synaptic connections.[14] These alterations result in a prolonged state of sensitization, resulting in intractable postsurgical pain that is unresponsive to many analgesics.[15] The use of preemptive

multimodal analgesic techniques may be beneficial in reducing postoperative pain and improving clinical outcomes following operative procedures.

PREEMPTIVE ANALGESIA

Preemptive analgesia as a concept began in the early 1920s, when Crile[16] and Lower proposed that blocking noxious signals prior

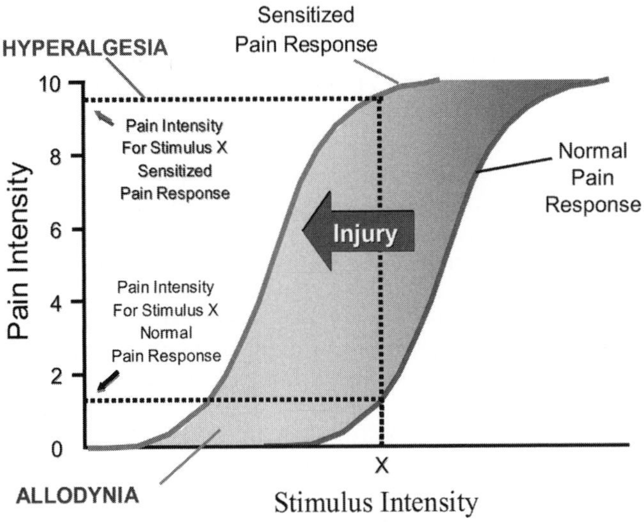

Figure 12.2: Nociceptive afferent input from trauma can sensitize the nervous system to subsequent stimuli. The normal pain response as a function of stimulus intensity is depicted by the curve on the right. Following trauma, the pain response curve is shifted to the left. As a result, noxious stimuli become more painful (hyperalgesia) and nonpainful stimuli (yellow shaded region) now become painful (allodynia).

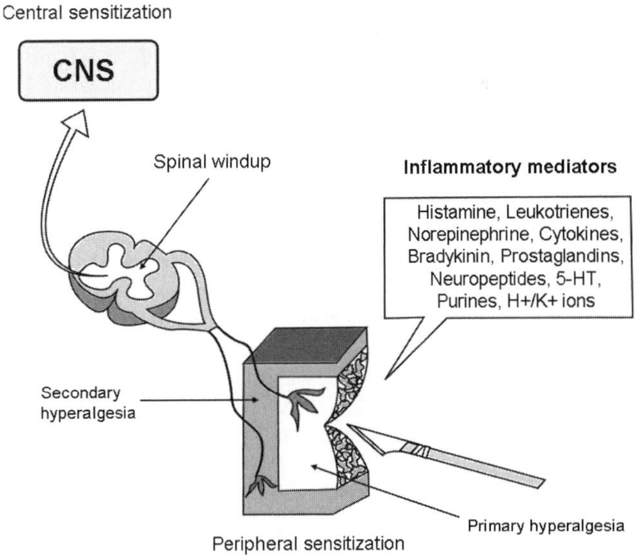

Figure 12.3: Surgical trauma leads to the release of inflammatory mediators at the site of injury, resulting in a reduction in the pain threshold at the site of injury (primary hyperalgesia) and in the surrounding uninjured tissue (secondary hyperalgesia). Peripheral sensitization results from a reduction in the threshold of nociceptor afferent terminals secondary to surgical trauma. Central sensitization is an activity-dependent increase in the excitability of spinal neurons (spinal wind-up) as a result of persistent exposure to afferent input from peripheral neurons. CNS = central nervous system, 5-HT = serotonin.

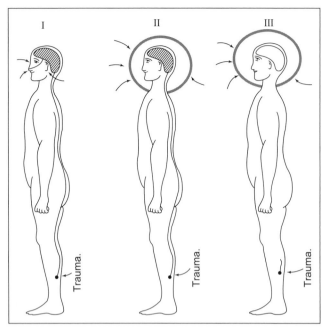

Figure 12.4: The Anoci-association theory of Crile was the first description of preventative analgesia. According to this theory: (I) Surgical trauma pain transmission and perception incites postoperative hyperactivity in the central nervous system leading to hemodymamic and metabolic instability. (II) General anesthesia attenuates pain perception during surgery; however, CNS hyperactivity is still observed. (III) Presurgical neural blockade prior to general anesthesia and surgical trauma attenuates pain perception and prevents postsurgical CNS hyperactivity. Crile GW. The kinetic theory of shock and its prevention through anoci association (shockless operation). *Lancet*. 1913;185:7–16.[16]

to a surgical incision may lead to some degree of CNS protection against postoperative pain, although at that time the mechanism remained unclear.[16]

Crile[16] believed that a combination of local-regional blocks and general anesthesia favorably influenced the postoperative recovery compared to general anesthesia alone, especially when the blocks were performed in advance of the painful stimulus. He concluded that "patients given inhalational anesthesia still need to be protected by regional anesthesia otherwise they might incur persistent CNS changes and enhanced postoperative pain" (Figure 12.4). The notion that the CNS "modulates" afferent pain signals before being perceived by the individual was further elucidated in 1965, when Melzack and Wall[10] proposed their gate theory. This landmark article suggested that incoming pain signals are subject to inhibition by either competing nonpainful afferent input at the same spinal level or from supraspinal descending pathways. For example, rubbing one's foot after stubbing the toe lessens the perception of pain because of the "closure" of a theoretical gate in the substantia gelatinosa that allows for only one type of afferent impulse to be transmitted to the CNS. However, this theory did not incorporate long-term changes in the CNS following nociceptive input and to other external factors that impinge on the individual. It is now recognized that nociceptor function is dynamic, and may be altered by tissue injury. Repetitive stimulation of small-diameter primary afferent fibers generates a progressive increase in action potential discharge and increased excitability of both peripheral and CNS neurons, an event termed *sensitization* or *wind-up*. This

is the mechanism by which pain may be prolonged beyond the duration normally expected with an acute insult. Further, this increased excitability in the CNS has the capacity to permanently alter spinal cord function, leading to the development of chronic pain following an acute injury. Preemptive analgesia has been proposed as a method of decreasing postoperative pain by the prevention or attenuation of this wind-up phenomenon.

In 1988, Wall[17] suggested that "we should consider the possibility that pre-emptive pre-operative analgesia has prolonged effects which long outlast the presence of drugs." Some of the earliest experimental evidence supporting this theory noted that a painful stimulus in rats resulted in a distinct biphasic excitatory response in dorsal horn neurons – an immediate acute peak (at 0–10 minutes) and a subsequent, prolonged tonic phase lasting 20–65 minutes.[18] The study concluded that intrathecal opiates administered prior to the first-phase response but reversed with naloxone before the expected onset of the second-phase response were capable of preventing this latter stage. However, if the opiates were administered after the painful stimulus, the inhibitory effect on the second-phase pain response in the dorsal horn was greatly diminished. This experimental model was also used to investigate the role of local anesthetics in the dorsal horn response to pain. Coderre et al[19] showed that local anesthetics applied either at the site of injury or intrathecally prior (but not subsequent) to a subcutaneous formalin injection abolished the expression of the second tonic phase of the pain response in dorsal horn neurons.

Based on this scientific evidence, investigators[13,17] hypothesized that preemptive treatment will prevent the establishment of central sensitization, decrease the incidence of hyperalgesia, and subsequently decrease the severity of postoperative pain. Since the late 1980s, hundreds of studies of varied quality have been published relating to the efficacy and utility of preemptive analgesic strategies. Unfortunately, many of these earlier studies choose a methodology whereby a preincisional strategy was compared with a placebo treatment (eg, local infiltration into the wound site before incision versus no infiltration). This study design does little to address the question of whether "pre versus post" makes a difference. Preemptive analgesia is defined when the administration of an antinociceptive intervention before a surgical incision is more effective than the same intervention administered after surgery.[20] The focus on demonstrating that pretreatment is more effective than the same treatment administered after incision or surgery has sidetracked progress because inclusion of a control group (eg, placebo administered before and after incision) has been ignored.[21] Two group studies that failed to demonstrate a superiority of the preincisional over the postincisional analgesic treatment intervention are inherently flawed, because it is not known whether the absence of an effect reflects the relative efficacy of the postoperative blockade or the inefficacy of preoperative blockade in reducing central sensitization.[21]

Despite elegant demonstrations of the effect of preemptive analgesia in many animal models, there still exists some degree of controversy regarding its validity in the clinical setting. The consensus is far from clear, with different reviewers reaching fundamentally dissimilar conclusions depending on the particular intervention used, the choice of control, the outcome measures, and the surgical model. This discrepancy has been documented by two recent systematic reviews of the literature evaluating the value of preemptive analgesia for postoperative pain relief.[22,23] Moiniche et al[22] reviewed the literature on

Table 12.1: The Efficacy of Preemptive Analgesia

Analgesic	Number of Trials (No of Patients)	Pain Intensity	Time to First Analgesic	Supplemental Analgesic Use
Epidural	19 ($n = 905$)	+	+	+
Local anesthesia	15 ($n = 671$)	?	+	+
NMDA antagonists	7 ($n = 418$)	0	?	?
NSAIDs	16 ($n = 875$)	?	+	+
Opioids	8 ($n = 392$)	0	?	?

Abbreviations: + = positive effect; 0 = no effect; ? = equivocal evidence.
NSAIDs = nonsteroidal anti-inflammatory drugs; NMDA = N-methyl-D-aspartic acid.

preemptive analgesia, including 80 randomized controlled trials (RCTs) representing 3761 patients published from 1983 to 2000. These authors analyzed the preemptive analgesic effects of nonsteroidal anti-inflammatory drugs (NSAIDs), epidural analgesics, local anesthetic wound infiltration, opioids, and N-methyl-D-aspartic acid (NMDA) antagonists on pain scores within 24 hours of surgery. Only RCTs evaluating the preoperative versus postoperative administration of these analgesic interventions were included in this quantitative and qualitative systematic review. The authors concluded that the timing of these analgesics had no effect on the quality of pain control, indicating that preemptive analgesia is no more effective than a postincisional treatment.

In contrast, a more recent meta-analysis by Ong et al[23] on the efficacy of preemptive analgesia for acute pain challenged the findings by Moniche et al.[22] Ong et al[23] analyzed 66 RCTs on preemptive analgesia for postoperative pain that were published between 1987 and 2003 and consisted of data on 3261 patients (Table 12.1). The preemptive analgesic effect of NSAIDs, epidural analgesics, local anesthetic wound infiltration, opioids, and NMDA antagonists were evaluated on three outcome variables: pain intensity scores during the first 24–48 hours of the postoperative period, time to first rescue analgesic, and total supplemental analgesic use. Based on this analysis, preemptive epidural analgesia resulted in consistent improvements in all three outcome variables. Preemptive local anesthetic wound infiltration and NSAIDs administration improved analgesic consumption and time to first analgesic request, but not postoperative pain scores. The preemptive administration of NMDA antagonists and systemic opioids provided equivocal findings.

PREVENTIVE ANALGESIA

Currently, the concept of preemptive analgesia has evolved beyond the importance of only reducing the nociceptive afferent input brought about by surgical incision. The term *preventive analgesia*[24] was introduced to emphasize the fact that central neuroplasticity is induced by pre-, intra-, and postoperative nociceptive inputs. The goal of preventive analgesia is to reduce central sensitization that arises from noxious inputs arising throughout the entire perioperative period, and not just from those occurring during the surgical incision. Thus, preventive analgesia is a broader definition of preemptive analgesia and includes any perioperative analgesic regimen able to

control the process of surgical-induced sensitization. Katz and McCartney[25] analyzed 27 clinical studies evaluating preemptive or preventive analgesia and reported a benefit with preventive analgesia, but equivocal or no benefit from preemptive treatment. These findings highlight the importance of administering treatment modalities not only for the surgical incision, but also for extending the analgesic effect into the postoperative period. Adequate preventive analgesia should include multimodal analgesic techniques aimed at attenuating peripheral and central sensitization with a sufficient duration of treatment. Effective preventive multimodal analgesic techniques may be useful in reducing, not only acute pain, but also chronic postsurgical pain and disability.[26,27]

MULTIMODAL ANALGESIA

Sufficient pain relief that allows normal function has been difficult to achieve following major surgical procedures without the risk of side effects. Although opioids still play a major role in the management of pain following surgery, they may contribute to increased hospital morbidity and health care costs.[28] Adverse events associated with the use of opioids in the postoperative setting include postoperative nausea and vomiting, ileus, respiratory depression, sedation, pruritus, urinary retention, and sleep disturbances.[29] In July 2000 the Joint Commission for Accreditation of Health Care Organizations (JCAHO) introduced a new standard for pain management, declaring pain level to be the "fifth vital sign."[30] The Commission concluded that acute and chronic pain were major causes of patient dissatisfaction in the US health care system, leading to slower recovery times, creating a burden for patients and their families, and increasing medical costs.[30] However, the increased efforts aimed at reducing patients' postoperative pain scores may have further increased the risk of adverse effects when health care providers attempted to achieve sufficient analgesia by opioids alone.[31–33]

The concept of multimodal analgesia was introduced more than a decade ago as a technique to improve analgesia and reduce the incidence of opioid-related adverse events.[34] The rationale for this strategy is the achievement of sufficient analgesia by the additive or synergistic effects between different analgesics. This allows for a reduction in the doses of these drugs, thus lowering the incidence of adverse effects. Unfortunately, most of the existing studies in acute pain management have utilized single analgesic techniques. Such treatment cannot be expected

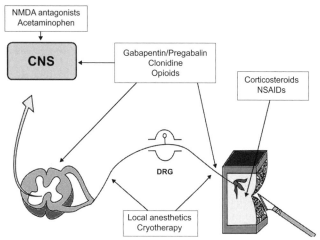

Figure 12.5: Analgesic agents and sites used to provide analgesia and attenuate nociceptive pathways. CNS = central nervous system, DRG = dorsal root ganglion, NSAIDs = nonsteroidal anti-inflammatory drugs, NMDA = *N*-methyl-D-aspartate.

to provide sufficient pain relief allowing normal function without the risk of adverse effects.[34,35] Most of the pain literature fails to address the issue of pain during daily function (eg, cough, ambulation, physical therapy). In addition to a lower incidence of adverse effects and improved analgesia, it has been demonstrated that multimodal analgesia techniques may provide for shorter hospitalization times, improved recovery and function, and decreased health care costs following surgery.[36–39] Currently, the American Society of Anesthesiologists Task Force on Acute Pain Management[40] and the Agency for Health Care Research and Quality[41] advocate the use of a multimodal analgesic approach for the management of acute pain. Because pain in the perioperative period represents several nociceptive mechanisms, a rational approach to acute pain is to combine different treatment modalities operating on different pain mechanisms to improve analgesia and reduce side effects. Currently, a variety of multimodal analgesics, including NSAIDs, opioids, local anesthetics, NMDA receptor antagonists, α_2 agonists (clonidine and dexmetomidine), and $\alpha_2\delta$ agonists (gabapentin and pregabalin), are being utilized in an attempt to target the sensitization process at one or more anatomical sites along the nociceptive pathway, including the site of injury, peripheral nerve axon, dorsal horn of the spinal cord, and cerebral cortex (Figure 12.5).

PREVENTIVE MULTIMODAL ANALGESICS

α_2 Agonists (Clonidine, Dexmedetomidine)

Experimental research in animals supports analgesic actions of α_2-adrenergic agonists at the peripheral, spinal, and brainstem sites. This is evidenced by the detection of α_2 adrenoceptors located on primary afferent terminals, on neurons in the superficial laminae of the spinal cord, and within several brainstem nuclei.[42] The precise mechanism by which clonidine exerts its analgesic effect remains unknown. Clonidine enhances peripheral nerve blocks of local anesthetics by selectively blocking conduction of A-δ and C fibers.[43–45] Clonidine causes local vasoconstriction, thereby reducing the vascular uptake of local anesthetics.[46] This last mechanism, however, is controversial. A previous study evaluating peak plasma concentrations of lidocaine revealed significantly higher levels when clonidine was used compared with epinephrine, leading the authors to conclude that clonidine lacks a local vasoconstrictor effect.[47] Recently, animal studies using clonidine for peripheral nerve blocks point the mechanism of action to be mediated via the hyperpolarization-activated cation current (Ih) and not via the α_2 adrenoceptors.[48] Clonidine may also produce an analgesic effect by releasing enkephalin-like substances.[49] In addition, because sympathetic neural activity may increase both somatic[50] and sympathetically maintained pain,[27] clonidine can reduce nociceptive pathways by inhibiting the release of norepinephrine from prejunctional α_2 adrenoceptors. α_2 adrenergic mechanisms of analgesia have been utilized for over a century. Cocaine, the first spinal anesthetic, produces analgesia primarily by its local anesthetic action, but it also inhibits norepinephrine reuptake and produces analgesia, in part, by enhancing noradrenergic stimulation of α_2 adrenoceptors.[51]

When administered via the oral, intravenous, or transdermal route, clonidine may reduce opioid requirement and improve analgesia in the postoperative setting.[52,53] Compared with clonidine, dexmedetomidine is more selective for the α_2 receptor and has a shorter duration of action.[52] The perioperative administration of dexmedetomidine (loading dose of 1 μ/kg over 10 minutes followed by 0.4 followed by 0.4 μg/kg/h for 4 hours) reduces morphine use by 66% in the early postoperative period following major inpatient surgical procedures.[54] Despite their potent sedative effects, the perioperative administration of α_2 agonists for postoperative pain management has not been associated with respiratory depression.

The addition of α_2 agonists to the local anesthetic solution for neuraxial or peripheral nerve block may also enhance and prolong analgesia.[51] Central neuraxial block with local anesthetic and clonidine improves the quality of analgesia for total joint arthroplasty.[55–58] The combination of intrathecal clonidine and morphine provided superior analgesia compared with intrathecal morphine alone following total knee arthroplasty.[55] Administration of clonidine with an epidural infusion of local anesthetic and fentanyl improved analgesia and reduced the need for rescue opioid medication following total knee arthroplasty.[56] Clonidine also results in improved postoperative analgesia when added to local anesthetic epidural infusions[57] and for combined spinal-epidural anesthesia for total hip arthroplasty.[58]

Clonidine has been shown to enhance peripheral nerve block when added to a variety of local anesthetics.[51] The addition of clonidine (1 μg/kg) to lidocaine 0.5% for intravenous regional anesthesia (IVRA) has been shown to significantly improve postoperative analgesia during the first day after upper extremity hand surgery.[59] The addition of 1 μg/kg of clonidine was well tolerated and exhibited no adverse effects (bradycardia, hypotension, hypoxemia, and/or sedation). In addition, the use of IVRA clonidine has been shown to delay the onset time of tourniquet pain in healthy, unsedated volunteers.[60] The analgesic effect of IVRA clonidine appears to be peripherally mediated and not by central redistribution, as the same dose administered parenterally provided no further analgesia.[59] Further, concentrations of clonidine in plasma (0.12 ng/mL) obtained after tourniquet deflation[60] were considerably lower than those required for a central analgesic effect (1.5–2 ng/mL) when clonidine was administered via the parenteral route to manage postoperative pain.[53]

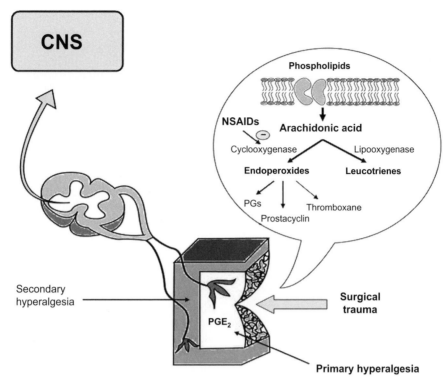

Figure 12.6: Surgical trauma leads to initiation of a biochemical cascade in which membrane phospholipids are converted to arachidonic acid and then to prostaglandins through the action of the cyclooxygenase enzyme. NSAIDs are thought to reduce postoperative pain by suppressing cyclooxygenase-mediated production of PGE_2. Prostaglandins, including PGE_2, are responsible for reducing the pain threshold at the site of injury (primary hyperalgesia), resulting in central sensitization and a lower pain threshold in the surrounding uninjured tissue (secondary hyperalgesia). CNS = central nervous system, NSAIDs = nonsteroidal anti-inflammatory drugs, PGE_2 = Prostaglandin E_2.

In addition to its effects when administered with local anesthetics, clonidine when administered alone showed analgesic effects when given via the intra-articular route.[61] Furthermore, the addition of intraarticular clonidine to morphine and bupivacaine enhanced the analgesic efficacy of both analgesics.[62] Peripheral administration of clonidine is a useful nonopioid analgesic method that is currently playing an important role in the multimodal management of acute postoperative pain.

Preemptive Analgesia with α_2 Agonists

Currently, no studies have evaluated the efficacy of administering preemptive α_2 agonists alone for the management of postoperative pain.

Nonsteroidal Anti-Inflammatory Drugs and Acetaminophen

Tissue injury leads to pain transmission by direct mechanical and thermal damage to nerve endings, as well as the release of inflammatory mediators.[63] These inflammatory mediators include arachidonic cascade metabolites that sensitize peripheral nerve endings, resulting in hyperalgesia and thus facilitating pain transmission (Figure 12.6). Prostaglandins, including prostaglandin (PG) E_2, are responsible for reducing the pain threshold at the site of injury (primary hyperalgesia), resulting in central sensitization and a lower pain threshold in the surrounding uninjured tissue (secondary hyperalgesia).[11] Traditionally, the primary site of action of NSAIDs have been attributed to their inhibition of prostaglandin synthesis in the periphery, although recent research indicates that central inhibition of cyclooxygenase 2 (COX-2) may also play an important role in modulating nociception.[64]

NSAIDs inhibit the synthesis of prostaglandins both in the spinal cord and at the periphery, thus diminishing the hyperalgesic state after surgical trauma.[64] NSAIDs are useful as the sole analgesic after minor surgical procedures[65] and may have a significant opioid-sparing effect after major surgery.[66] The use of NSAIDs has become increasingly popular because of the concern over opioid-related side effects. All NSAIDs have a ceiling effect for analgesia, but they do not demonstrate a ceiling effect with regard to side effects.[67] It is currently recommended that NSAIDs be used in the multimodal analgesic approach for the management of perioperative pain.[40,41] The recent practice guidelines for acute pain management in the perioperative setting specifically state that "unless contraindicated, all patients should receive an around-the-clock regimen of NSAIDs, Coxibs, or acetaminophen."[40]

Acetaminophen is a *p*-aminophenol derivative with analgesic and antipyretic properties similar to those of aspirin. The mechanism of action of acetaminophen is still poorly defined. Recent evidence has suggested that it may selectively act as an inhibitor of central prostaglandin synthesis in the CNS rather than in the periphery.[68] The theory that acetaminophen acts via the COX-3 receptor[69] has not been supported by recent studies.[70]

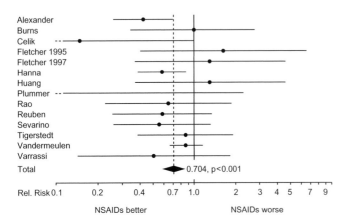

Figure 12.7: Effect of administration of nonsteroidal antiinflammatory drugs (NSAIDs) in addition to patient-controlled analgesia intravenous morphine after surgery on the relative risk of postoperative nausea and vomiting. From Marret E, et al. *Anesthesiology.* 2005;102(6):1249–1260.

In addition, there is evidence that serotonergic mechanisms are involved in the antinociceptive activity of acetaminophen.[71] A metaanalysis of randomized controlled trials of acetaminophen for postoperative pain revealed that this analgesic induced a morphine sparing effect of 20% (9 mg) over the first 24 hours postoperatively (95% CI, −15 to −3 mg), but did not reduce the incidence of morphine-related adverse effects.[72] A recent qualitative review of acetaminophen, NSAIDs, and their combination concluded that acetaminophen may provide analgesic efficacy similar to other NSAIDs following major orthopedic surgery.[73] It was concluded that acetaminophen can be a viable alternative to NSAIDs in high-risk patients because of the lower incidence of adverse effects.[73] Further, it may be appropriate to administer acetaminophen with NSAIDs or COX-2 inhibitors because the combination can have additive or synergistic effects and improve analgesia.[74] Injectable forms of acetaminophen (propacetamol and paracetamol) have been available in Europe for several decades. Compared with oral formulations, parenteral acetaminophen has a more predictable onset and duration of action.[75]

A recent metaanalysis examined whether there is any advantage of multimodal analgesia with acetaminophen, NSAIDs, or COX-2 inhibitors when added to patient-controlled analgesia (PCA) morphine.[76] The results suggested that all of the analgesic agents provided an opioid-sparing effect; however, the decrease in morphine use did not consistently result in a decrease in opioid-related adverse effects. The use of NSAIDs was associated with a decrease in the incidence of postoperative nausea and vomiting and sedation (Figure 12.7). However, the use of COX-2 inhibitors or acetaminophen did not decrease the incidence of opioid-related adverse events when compared to placebo.

A systematic review of COX-2 inhibitors versus traditional NSAIDs for postoperative pain concluded that these two analgesics demonstrate equipotent analgesic efficacy after minor and major surgical procedures.[77] However, COX-2 NSAIDs may be a viable alternative to traditional NSAIDs in the perioperative management of pain. Because COX-2 inhibitors are associated with reduced gastrointestinal side effects and an absence of

antiplatelet activity, they can be safely administered to surgical patients without the added risk of increased perioperative bleeding, which has been reported with conventional NSAIDs.[74]

Preemptive NSAID Administration

The preemptive analgesic effect of NSAIDs has been studied for a wide variety of surgical procedures and demonstrated equivocal results.[13,22,23,78] Unfortunately, many methodological problems were encountered in these studies.[20]) Reuben et al[79] were the first investigators to examine the analgesic effects of administering the same dose of NSAID either before or after arthroscopic knee surgery. The results of this study demonstrated that preoperative NSAID administration produced a significantly longer duration of postoperative analgesia, less 24 hour opioid use, and lower incidental pain scores compared with administering the same drug in the postoperative period. A review of 18 randomized, single- or double-blinded studies that used a NSAID as the target intervention revealed that only 6 studies (33%) demonstrated a preemptive analgesic effect.[78] Furthermore, the beneficial effects of preemptive NSAIDs observed in most studies were minimal. The review by Moniche et al[22] included 20 clinical trials comparing preincisional with postincisional NSAID using a parallel or crossover design. The authors concluded that some aspects of postoperative pain were improved by preemptive treatment in 4 of the 20 trials. Overall, the data demonstrated preemptive NSAIDs to be of no analgesic benefit when compared with postincisional administration of these drugs. In contrast, Ong et al's[23] review of 16 randomized controlled trials with preemptive NSAIDs concluded that these drugs improved analgesic consumption and time to first analgesic request, but not postoperative pain scores.

NMDA Receptor Antagonists (Ketamine, Dextromethorphan, Magnesium)

Nociceptive inputs from primary afferents are primarily mediated at fast glutamatergic synapses onto second-order neurons in the dorsal horn of the spinal cord through activation of the NMDA receptor.[80] Because enhancement of excitatory synaptic transmission in nociceptive pathways plays a central role in the development of hyperalgesia and is a key neural substrate underlying chronic pain,[80,81] analgesics aimed at blocking the NMDA receptor should play a pivotal role in perioperative pain management. In particular, many drugs or compounds that reduce central glutamate excitation are antagonists of the NMDA subtype of glutamate receptor. There are multiple binding sites for NMDA antagonists, and differences in pharmacological effect of each drug are related to binding sites and receptor affinity.[82]

Ketamine

Ketamine has been used as a general anesthetic and analgesic since the late 1970s. Although high doses (>2 mg/kg) of ketamine have been implicated in psychomimetic effects (eg, excessive sedation, cognitive dysfunction, hallucinations, nightmares), subanesthetic or low doses (<1 mg/kg) of ketamine have demonstrated significant analgesic efficacy without these side effects.[83,84] Further, there is no evidence to indicate that low-dose ketamine exerts any adverse pharmacological effect on respiration, cardiovascular function, nausea, vomiting, urinary retention, and constipation/prolonged adynamic postoperative ileus.[83] Recent systematic reviews have concluded that low-dose ketamine, when used as the sole analgesic agent, reduces pain following administration by the intravenous, intramuscular, or subcutaneous routes.[83,84] In contrast, there is little evidence to support low-dose epidural ketamine by itself for postoperative analgesia.[83] There is a growing body of evidence that low-dose ketamine may have an important role in postoperative pain management when used as an adjunct to opioids, local anesthetics, and other analgesic agents.[83,84] Ketamine in combination with parenteral or epidural opioids not only reduces postoperative opioid consumption but also prolongs and improves analgesia.[83,84] However, despite the opioid-sparing effect, no reduction in opioid-related side effects were observed.[83,84] Ketamine when added to local anesthetic solutions for wound infiltration can result in improved analgesia, which is mediated *via* a peripheral mechanism.[85] Ketamine is being used more frequently in the management of postorthopedic surgical pain. A single intraoperative injection of ketamine (0.15 mg/kg) improved analgesia and passive knee mobilization 24 hours after arthroscopic anterior cruciate ligament surgery[86] and improved postoperative functional outcome after outpatient knee arthroscopy.[87] Low-dose ketamine also increases postoperative pain relief for total knee arthroplasty when used in conjunction with either epidural[88] or continuous femoral nerve block.[89] Patients receiving perioperative ketamine for total knee arthroplasty also achieved an earlier improvement in knee function.[89]

Dextromethorphan

The antitussive dextromethorphan, and its metabolite, dextrorphan, have been shown to antagonize NMDA receptors in brain slices.[90] Although dextromethorphan is an open-channel blocker similar to ketamine, it produces fewer psychotomimetic effects, probably because of its lower affinity for the NMDA receptor.[91] However, results of clinical trials evaluating the analgesic efficacy of dextromethorphan have been contradictory. A recent, qualitative systematic review analyzed 28 randomized, double-blind, clinical studies of perioperative dextromethorphan in postoperative pain.[92] It was concluded that this drug has the potential to be a safe adjuvant to opioids in postoperative pain therapy, but the consistency of the potential opioid-sparing and pain-reducing effects was questionable. Consequently, the authors did not recommend the clinical use of dextromethorphan routinely for postoperative pain.[92]

Magnesium

Magnesium has been shown to be an antagonist of the NMDA receptor and in vitro data indicate that extracellular magnesium protects cerebellar neurons against the toxicity of the NMDA agonist glutamate.[93] Tramer et al[94] were the first clinicians to examine the role of magnesium sulfate in postoperative analgesia. Their studies revealed that a perioperative infusion of magnesium resulted in reduced analgesic requirements, less discomfort, and better quality of sleep without adverse effects on the postoperative management of patients undergoing lower abdominal surgery. Subsequent studies evaluating perioperative magnesium have given conflicting results with some demonstrating a beneficial effect,[95–99] whereas others showing no analgesic efficacy following surgery.[100–102] These differences may in part be related to the administration of different doses of magnesium in the perioperative period. Because the ability of peripherally administered magnesium to penetrate the blood-brain barrier is limited in the normal brain,[103] the dose used may play a key role in antinociception. In fact, it has been demonstrated that an inverse correlation exists between cerebral spinal fluid magnesium concentration and cumulative postoperative analgesic use following surgery.[101]

NMDA Antagonists and Preemptive Analgesia

NMDA receptor antagonists in preemptive analgesia have yielded equivocal analgesic efficacy. The systematic review by Moniche et al[22] examined 8 trials comparing preincisional with postincisional ketamine or dextromethorphan in a variety of surgical procedures. It was concluded that there was no improvement with preemptive ketamine and the data on dextromethorphan was too sparse to reach a definitive conclusion. In the meta-analysis by Ong et al,[23] 7 trials comparing the analgesic effect of preincisional versus postincisional systemic NMDA antagonists were included for analysis. The authors concluded that preemptive NMDA antagonists failed to yield analgesic effects consistent enough to draw conclusions regarding clinical utility. A qualitative systematic review of the role of NMDA receptor antagonists in preventive analgesia included 40 clinical trials evaluating ketamine ($n = 24$), dextromethorphan ($n = 12$), or magnesium ($n = 4$) for analysis.[104] The authors concluded that the evidence in favor of preventive analgesia was strongest for dextromethorphan and ketamine, with 67% and 58%, respectively, of studies demonstrating a reduction in pain or analgesic consumption or both. In contrast, none of the 4 studies examining magnesium demonstrated preventive analgesia.

Local Anesthetics/Regional Analgesia

The use of regional anesthetic techniques for the perioperative management of pain is not a new concept. Crile[16] believed that a combination of local regional blocks and general anesthesia favorably influenced postoperative recovery compared to general anesthesia alone, especially when the blocks were performed in advance of the painful stimulus.[16] In 1913, Crile[16] concluded that "patients given inhalational anesthesia still need to be protected by regional anesthesia otherwise they might incur persistent central nervous system changes and enhanced postoperative pain."

Wound Infiltration

Infiltrating local anesthetics into the skin and subcutaneous tissue prior to making an incision may be the simplest approach to preemptive analgesia. It is a safe procedure with few side effects and low risk for toxicity. Although the benefit of local wound infiltration has been documented, controversy exists as to the appropriate timing of administering local anesthesia for surgery. In a meta-analysis by Moiniche et al,[22] 14 randomized trials (736 patients) that compared pre- versus postincisional wound infiltration for a variety of surgical procedures demonstrated no difference in analgesic efficacy between the two techniques. In contrast, Ong et al[23] reviewed 15 randomized trials (671 patients) that compared preemptive local infiltration with postincisional infiltration and concluded that the former technique improved analgesic consumption and time to first analgesic request, but it did not achieve statistical significance with respect to reducing pain intensity. It remains unclear from these data whether local anesthetic infiltration into the wound provides long-term prevention of chronic incisional pain. Most of the studies terminated their assessment of effect at 24–48 hours, well before the abatement of the acute postoperative pain. With the recent technologic improvements in nonelectric disposable infusion pumps,[105] continuous local anesthetic wound infusion techniques are increasing in popularity for both hospitalized and outpatient surgeries.[106] However, some concerns about local anesthetic infusion include the possibility of local anesthetic toxicity, myotoxicity, chondrotoxicity, and infection.[107–110] In a study evaluating the efficacy of continuous infusions of bupivacaine for hand surgery, the investigators reported that 2 of 100 (2%) subjects developed infections at the cannula insertion site after 1 week.[109] Further, recent data from animal studies show that infusion of bupivacaine for 48 hours can lead to profound histopathologic and metabolic changes in articular cartilage.[110] These investigators concluded that caution against the use of continuous infusion devices in smaller joints is warranted. Future large-scale studies in humans are needed to address the efficacy and safety of continuous local anesthetic wound infiltration before this technique becomes widely applicable for managing postsurgical pain.

Peripheral Nerve Block

Peripheral nerve blocks are an attractive method of providing postoperative analgesia for many surgical procedures. Peripheral nerve blocks provide superior pain relief with movement (incidental pain) and may reduce surgical stress and improve rehabilitation.[106,111] Because these techniques provide for site-specific analgesia, they are associated with fewer side effects compared with other analgesic techniques.[111] The use of peripheral nerve blocks for orthopedic anesthesia has been associated with superior same-day recovery and decreased hospital readmission compared with general anesthesia.[106] Although single-injection regional anesthesia provides early analgesic efficacy, it does not provide long-term benefit compared with general anesthesia.[112] In contrast, continuous regional anesthetic techniques may prolong the benefits, thus providing for long-term efficacy following surgery. A recent meta-analysis[113] showed that continuous peripheral analgesic techniques provided superior analgesia, reduced opioid consumption, and reduced opioid-related side effects (nausea/vomiting, sedation, pruritus). However, several unresolved issues remain concerning this technique.[114] Insufficient number of subjects in these studies do not allow a proper evaluation of the safety of these techniques. The general applicability of these techniques is uncertain because of the required level of technical skill and infrastructure necessary to manage the catheters, especially on an outpatient basis. Current randomized trials are relatively small and heterogeneous, making conclusions about optimal technique for individual surgical procedures more difficult. Finally, there is insufficient evidence to determine the effectiveness of continuous peripheral analgesic techniques on long-term functional outcomes.

Epidural Block

Similar to peripheral neural blockade, epidural analgesia provides for significant incidental pain relief and reduces the neuroendocrine stress response that follows surgery that can contribute to adverse perioperative outcomes.[4] In contrast, parenteral opioids do not result in an adequate reduction in this stress response following surgery[115] and provides inferior analgesia when compared to epidural techniques for the management of postoperative pain.[116] Epidural analgesia is superior to either peripheral nerve block or PCA in blunting the surgical stress response following orthopedic surgery.[115] As a result, epidural analgesia may result in several benefits, including accelerated recovery, decreased complications, and improved patient-oriented outcomes such as quality of life and satisfaction.[116]

Further, appropriately administered epidural analgesia can improve many clinically oriented outcomes, such as reduction in the incidence of pulmonary complications, myocardial infarction, deep venous thrombosis, and pulmonary embolism.[116] However, some meta-analyses and systematic reviews[117] have reported conflicting results. These controversial findings may be a result of poorly designed studies that used ineffective epidural analgesic techniques. Optimal epidural analgesia includes catheter placement appropriate to the dermatomal incision site (eg, thoracic epidural for thoracic and upper abdominal surgery), utilization of a predominantly local anesthetic-based rather than opioid-based epidural solution, and the postoperative administration of epidural analgesics for more than 24 hours.

It is now recognized that the inflammatory response to surgical trauma may not be effectively modified by neuraxial or peripheral neural blockade alone.[118] Peripheral inflammation has been shown also to induce a widespread increase in COX-2 and PGE synthase expression in the CNS.[119] The proinflammatory cytokine interleukin 1β (IL-Iβ) is upregulated at the site of inflammation and plays a major role in inducing COX-2 in local inflammatory cells by activating the transcription factor nuclear factor-κB.[120] IL-1β is also responsible for the induction of COX-2 in the CNS in response to peripheral inflammation. Interestingly, these events are not the consequence of either neural activity arising from the sensory fibers innervating the inflamed tissue or of systemic IL-Iβ in the plasma. Instead, peripheral inflammation produces some other signal molecule that enters the circulation, crosses the blood-brain barrier, and acts to elevate IL-Iβ, leading to COX-2 expression in neuronal and non-neuronal cells throughout the CNS.[121] Thus, there appear to be two forms of input from peripheral inflamed tissue to the CNS (Figure 12.8). The first is mediated by electrical activity in sensitized nerve fibers innervating the inflamed area, which signals the location of the inflamed tissue as well as the onset, duration, and nature of stimuli applied to this tissue.[121] This input is sensitive to peripherally acting COX-2 inhibitors and to neural blockade with local anesthetics, as with epidural or spinal anesthesia.[122] The second is a humoral signal originating from the inflamed tissue, which acts to produce a widespread induction of COX-2 in the CNS. This input is not affected by regional anesthesia and will be blocked only by centrally acting COX-2 inhibitors.[118,121] One implication of this is that patients who receive neuraxial anesthesia for surgery might also need a centrally acting COX-2 inhibitor to optimally reduce postoperative pain and the postoperative stress response. Although IL-Iβ has been implicated as the main mediator of central COX-2 upregulation, it is based on animal studies. In postoperative pain, it is believed that IL-6 is probably the main mediator for upregulation of COX-2 in the CNS.[122] This was evident in a recent study that demonstrated that central PGE_2 concentrations were more likely to be reduced with the administration of parecoxib, a centrally acting COX-2 inhibitor, compared to ketorolac, a peripherally acting COX-2 inhibitor.[118] Whether this finding has any implications in the future management of acute pain is yet to be determined.

Preemptive Analgesia with Local Anesthetics

Moniche et al[22] studied the analgesic efficacy of 18 trials that evaluated presurgically versus postsurgically initiated epidural analgesic regimens. These could be divided into trials of single-dose analgesic regimens and trials of continuous analgesic regimens extending 24–72 hours into the postoperative period.

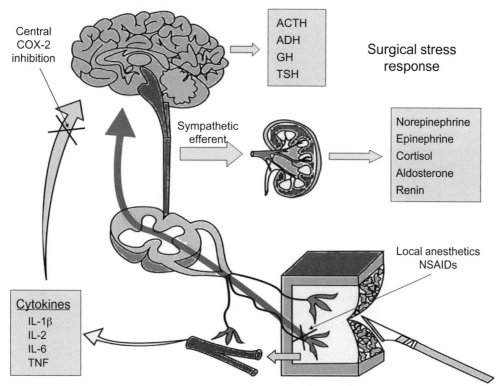

Figure 12.8: Surgical trauma induces nociceptive pathways leading to activation of the neuroendocrine stress response, which can contribute to adverse perioperative outcomes. There appears to be two forms of input from peripheral inflamed tissue to the CNS. The first is mediated by electrical activity in sensitized nerve fibers innervating the inflamed area (red arrow). This input is sensitive to peripherally-acting COX-2 inhibitors and to neural blockade with local anesthetics. The second is a humoral signal originating from the inflamed tissue (yellow arrows), which lead to the induction of cytokines that produce a widespread induction of COX-2 in the CNS. This input is not affected by regional anesthesia and will only be blocked by centrally-acting COX-2 inhibitors. COX = cyclooxygenase, NSAIDs = nonsteroidal anti-inflammatory drugs, ACTH = adrenocorticotropic hormone, antidiuretic hormone, growth hormone, thyroid stimulating hormone, IL = interleukin, TNF = tumor necrosis factor.

Neither preemptive epidural analgesic regimen demonstrated overall improvement in postoperative pain relief. In contrast, after reviewing 13 trials comparing preincisional versus postincisional epidural analgesia, Ong et al[23] concluded that preemptive epidural analgesia resulted in consistent improvements in pain intensity, supplemental postoperative analgesic requirements, and time to first rescue analgesic. Moniche et al[22] also evaluated 20 trials comparing preemptive with postincisional application of peripheral local anesthetics (wound infiltration, peripheral nerve block, and intraperitoneal infiltration). None of these 3 regimens demonstrated improved pain relief when administered preemptively for a wide variety of surgical procedures. Ong et al[23] reviewed 11 trials comparing preincisional versus postincisional peripheral local anesthetic wound infiltration. A meta-analysis of this data revealed that preemptive local anesthetic wound infiltration improved analgesic consumption and time to first analgesic request but not postoperative pain scores.

Opioids (Peripheral and Central)

Although opioids are effective for moderate to severe pain, their use is limited by dose-related adverse effects, including nausea and vomiting, ileus, respiratory depression, sedation, pruritus, urinary retention, and sleep disturbances, all of which may contribute to a delayed recovery.[29] Although opioids administered via an intravenous PCA system improve patient satisfaction, they do not reduce hospital stay or improve postoperative morbidity.[123] The inability of opioids to reduce the perioperative neuroendocrine stress response that follows surgical trauma[115] may be a contributing factor for the lack of improved outcomes observed with postoperative opioid therapy alone. This may also explain the observation that preemptive administration of systemic opioids fails to result in improved postoperative pain control.[22,23]

Another concern regarding the perioperative use of opioids is the development of tolerance[124–126] and opioid-induced hyperalgesia.[127,128] In fact, clinically relevant tolerance can occur within hours of opioid use, resulting in a reduction in their analgesic efficacy.[124–126] Further, the larger the intraoperative opioid dose, the greater the postoperative opioid requirement.[124] Therefore, the clinician should be aware that an apparent decrease in the analgesic efficacy of postoperative opioid therapy may be related to a decrease in its efficacy (pharmacological tolerance) or from an enhancement in pain sensitivity (opioid-induced hyperalgesia). If this is the case, a reduction in opioid therapy or a switch to an alternative opioid (opioid rotation) may be more beneficial. Further, the use of multimodal adjuvant drugs may not only contribute to an opioid-sparing effect but also may potentially result in a reduction in opioid-induced hyperalgesia. Experimental and clinical studies suggest that opioids activate both NMDA[126] and COX[129] pronociceptive systems, leading to hyperalgesia. Therefore, the perioperative administration of NMDA antagonists and NSAIDs is not only useful in multimodal analgesia for postoperative pain, but also may contribute to a reduction in the incidence of opioid-induced tolerance and hyperalgesia. Further, an adequate timing seems to be of particular importance for the antihyperalgesic effect of COX-2 inhibitors. Opioid-induced hyperalgesia was reduced only with the preemptive but not the simultaneous administration of a COX-2 inhibitor and an opioid.[130] This additional data further supports the importance of administering NSAIDs before rather than at the completion of surgery.

The administration of opioids via the peripheral route may represent an effective analgesic technique that avoids many of the adverse side effects reported with conventional opioid therapy. Recent studies have revealed that under conditions of inflammation, these analgesics can produce significant antinociception through peripheral mechanisms.[131] This has led to a growing number of clinical studies examining the analgesic efficacy of opioids applied locally through intraarticular, interpleural, intraperitoneal, perineural (ankle, axillary, dental), intravenous regional, or intravesicular routes.[132,133] The most consistent clinical results in humans concerning the analgesic efficacy of peripherally applied opioids have come from studies involving the intra-articular administration of morphine during arthroscopic knee surgery.[133,134]

Preemptive Opioid Administration

The preemptive administration of systemic opioids are ineffective in improving pain.[22,23] Although the preemptive peripheral administration of opioids have demonstrated analgesic efficacy in both animal[135] and human[136,137] surgical models, the data are too sparse to reach a definitive conclusion.

α₂-δ Ligands (Gabapentin, Pregabalin)

Both gabapentin and pregabalin are alkylated-aminobutyric acid analogs that were first developed clinically as anticonvulsants. These drugs bind to the α_2-δ subunit of voltage-gated calcium channels, thus preventing the release of nociceptive neurotransmitters, including glutamate, substance P, and noradrenaline.[138] Putative sites of action include peripheral neuron, primary afferent neuron, spinal neuron, and supraspinal sites.[139] These anticonvulsants can enhance the analgesic effect of morphine,[140] NSAIDs,[141] and selective COX-2 inhibitors.[142] In addition to being effective analgesics for neuropathic and chronic pain syndromes, recent evidence suggests that these anticonvulsants also provide effective postsurgical analgesia when they are administered preemptively before surgery.[143–145] The role of certain neural changes common to both neuropathic and postsurgical pain may explain these recent observations.[11,12] Further, because these drugs can interact synergistically with NSAIDs to produce antihyperalgesia,[141,142] the use of NSAIDs and α_2-δ ligands together may provide for more effective analgesia. The combination of pregabalin and celecoxib was recently shown to be superior to either single agent for postoperative pain following spinal fusion surgery.[146] This was evidenced by a significant reduction

in pain scores, morphine use, and fewer side effects during the first 24 postoperative hours with the perioperative administration of both celecoxib and pregabalin. Similar to analgesic studies with gabapentin,[143–145] pregabalin was found to be more effective than morphine in reducing movement-related pain.

The most common side effect reported with gabapentin and pregabalin are somnolence and dizziness. A meta-analysis of perioperative gabapentin treatment indicated that gabapentin was only associated with a modest increase in sedation.[144] Although sedation can be interpreted as a negative outcome of gabapentin use, its occurrence in the perioperative setting may be beneficial in contributing to anxiolysis.[147] Future large-scale studies are necessary to determine the optimal timing, duration, dosages, and impact on chronic persistent pain following a variety of surgical procedures.

Preemptive α₂-δ Ligand Administration

Although there are studies[143–145] evaluating the analgesic efficacy of preoperative gabapentin or pregabalin, there are no reports comparing the effects of preincisional with postincisional administration of these analgesics.

MULTIMODAL ANALGESIA AND CLINICAL OUTCOMES

The ideal multimodal analgesic technique should reduce the perioperative surgical stress response, decrease movement-related or dynamic pain, enhance postoperative convalescence, and improve clinical outcomes while reducing adverse analgesic-related side effects.

Although improvements in postoperative analgesia have been reported with the use of multimodal analgesic techniques, recent literature reviews have failed to document a concomitant reduction in analgesic-related adverse effects.[114,148–150] One criticism of these findings is that many of the studies relied exclusively on spontaneous reports of patients' adverse events, which may be less than rates obtained through direct assessment.[151] The use of an opioid-related symptom distress scale is a valuable instrument for the evaluation of symptom frequency, severity, and distress following surgery.[152] Utilizing this scale for patients receiving COX-2 inhibitors following laparoscopic cholecystectomy,[153] it became evident that a linear relationship exists between opioid dose and clinically meaningful opioid-related adverse events.[152] Analysis of available data suggests that once a threshold 24-hour morphine dose is reached, every additional 3- to 4-mg increase in morphine requirement is associated with one more clinically meaningful opioid-related symptom. This linear correlation identifies for the first time a connection between opioid-sparing effects and reduction of adverse effects. Further, many of the studies assessing opioid-related adverse effects used methodology that does not accurately reflect conditions in actual clinical practice. Adjuvant analgesic drugs, including NSAIDs, are more likely to be used in multiple doses, rather than single doses, for the management of postoperative pain. In addition, a more comprehensive multimodal approach (eg, combinations of regional analgesic techniques, NSAIDs, other adjuvant analgesics, and opioids), rather than bimodal therapy, is probably needed to demonstrate a reduction in opioid-related adverse events and improvement in functional outcomes.

The importance of utilizing a multimodal rather than a bimodal approach for postoperative pain management was recently demonstrated for spinal fusion surgery.[146] This study revealed that the administration singly of either celecoxib or pregabalin reduced morphine use, without a concomitant reduction in opioid-related side effects. However, the combination of these two analgesics provided both a reduction in morphine use and opioid-related side effects. The use of an opioid-related symptom distress scale for these patients confirmed the beneficial effect of utilizing both rather than one of these analgesics for spinal fusion surgery.[154] This study also revealed a significant reduction in both the incidence and severity of opioid-related side effects with the combination of celecoxib and pregabalin. Further, unlike patients receiving either drug alone, no patients receiving a combination of the two analgesics reported symptoms that were categorized as moderate or severe in nature.

The beneficial effects of utilizing preventive multimodal analgesia also have been demonstrated for major knee surgery.[37–39] In a randomized, placebo-controlled, double-blinded trial, Buvanendran et al[37] evaluated the effect of regional anesthesia/analgesia combined with a preoperative and 13-day postoperative course of a COX-2 inhibitor on opioid consumption and outcomes following total knee arthroplasty. The study reported a reduction in epidural analgesic use, in-hospital opioid consumption, pain scores, postoperative vomiting and sleep disturbance, and an increase in patient satisfaction in patients administered COX-2 inhibitors compared to placebo. In addition, improved knee range of motion was observed both at discharge and 1 month after surgery in the group receiving sustained perioperative COX-2 inhibition.

Although preventive multimodal analgesic techniques are effective in blunting the perioperative surgical stress response and decreasing movement-related pain, an additional prerequisite to improving surgical outcome and convalescence is through the implementation of "accelerated recovery programs."[36] Such programs require collaboration among the patient, surgeon, anesthesiologist, surgical nurse, and physiotherapist. The efficacy of utilizing a preventive multimodal analgesic technique in conjunction with an accelerated recovery program has recently been demonstrated for anterior cruciate ligament surgery.[38] Patients, who were administered a regimen of perioperative acetaminophen, rofecoxib, intraarticular analgesics (bupivacaine/clonidine/morphine), femoral nerve block, and postoperative cryotherapy in conjunction with an accelerated rehabilitation protocol, demonstrated a reduction in the incidence of pain, opioid use, postoperative nausea and vomiting, recovery room length of stay, and unplanned admission to the hospital. In addition, this multimodal regimen was effective in reducing the incidence of long-term patellofemoral complications, including anterior knee pain, flexion contracture, quadriceps weakness, and complex regional pain syndrome.[39]

In addition to orthopedic surgery, preventive multimodal analgesic techniques in conjunction with accelerated rehabilitation protocols are also beneficial in major abdominal, vascular, and urological surgeries.[36] These "fast track" programs emphasize the optimal use of regional anesthetic techniques and balanced analgesia, opioid-free or opioid-reduced analgesia, and the avoidance of drains, tubes, catheters, and restriction.[155] Patients enrolled in these clinical pathways have demonstrated improved pain control, reduced hospital length of stay, decreased postoperative morbidity and mortality, and a shorter time of convalescence.[36,155]

The authors thank Rebecca Reuben of the Massachusetts College of Art for creating the illustrations utilized in this chapter.

REFERENCES

1. Apfelbaum JL, Chen C, Mehta SS, Gan TJ. Postoperative pain experience: results from a national survey suggest postoperative pain continues to be undermanaged. *Anesth Analg.* 2003;97:534–540.
2. Warfield CA, Kahn CH. Acute pain management: programs in U.S. hospitals and experiences and attitudes among U.S. adults. *Anesthesiology.* 1995;83:1090–1094.
3. Kehlet H, Dahl JB. Anaesthesia, surgery, and challenges in postoperative recovery. *Lancet.* 2003;362:1921–1928.
4. Desborough JP. The stress response to trauma and surgery. *Br J Anaesth.* 2000;85:109–117.
5. Wilmore DW. From Cuthbertson to fast-track surgery: 70 years of progress in reducing stress in surgical patients. *Ann Surg.* 2002;236:643–648.
6. Holte K, Kehlet H. Postoperative ileus: a preventable event. *Br J Surg.* 2000;87:1480–1493.
7. Closs SJ. Patients' night-time pain, analgesic provision and sleep after surgery. *Int J Nurs Stud.* 1992;29:381–392.
8. Perkins FM, Kehlet H. Chronic pain as an outcome of surgery: a review of predictive factors. *Anesthesiology.* 2000;93:1123–1133.
9. Descartes R. The passions of the soul. In Descartes R, ed. *Key Philosophical Readings.* Hertordshire, UK: Wordsworth Editions Limited; 1997:358–383.
10. Melzack R, Wall PD. Pain mechanisms: a new theory. *Science.* 1965;150:971–979.
11. Raja SN, Meyer RA, Campbell JN. Peripheral mechanisms of somatic pain. *Anesthesiology.* 1988;68:571–590.
12. Woolf CJ. Evidence for a central component of post-injury pain hypersensitivity. *Nature.* 1983;303:686–688.
13. Woolf CJ, Chong MS. Preemptive analgesia – treating postoperative pain by preventing the establishment of central sensitization. *Anesth Analg.* 1993;77:362–379.
14. Coderre TJ, Katz J, Vaccarino AL, Melzack R. Contribution of central neuroplasticity to pathological pain: review of clinical and experimental evidence. *Pain.* 1993;52:259–285.
15. Woolf CJ, Salter MW. Neuronal plasticity: increasing the gain in pain. *Science.* 2000;288:1765–1768.
16. Crile GW. The kinetic theory of shock and its prevention through anoci association (shockless operation). *Lancet.* 1913;185:7–16.
17. Wall PD. The prevention of postoperative pain. *Pain.* 1988;33:289–290.
18. Dickenson AH, Sullivan AF: Subcutaneous formalin-induced activity of dorsal horn neurons in the rat: differential response to an intrathecal opiate administered pre or post formalin. *Pain.* 1987;30:349–360.
19. Coderre TJ, Vaccarino AL, Melzack R. Central nervous system plasticity in the tonic pain response to subcutaneous formalin injection. *Brain Res.* 1990;535:155–158.
20. Kissin I. Preemptive analgesia. Why its effect is not always obvious. *Anesthesiology.* 1996;84:1015–1019.
21. Katz J. Pre-emptive analgesia: evidence, current status and future directions. *Eur J Anaesthesiol.* 1995;12:8–13.
22. Moiniche S, Kehlet H, Dahl J. A qualitative and quantitative systematic review of preemptive analgesia for postoperative pain relief-the role of timing of analgesia. *Anesthesiology.* 2002;96:725–741.
23. Ong CK, Lirk P, Seymour RA, Jenkins BJ. The efficacy of preemptive analgesia for acute postoperative pain management: a meta-analysis. *Anesth Analg.* 2005;100:757–773.

24. Kissin I. Preemptive analgesia: terminology and clinical relevance. *Anesth Analg.* 1994;79:809–810. [letter]

25. Katz J, McCartney CJ. Current status of preemptive analgesia. *Curr Opin Anaesthesiol.* 2002;15:435–441.

26. Katz J, Cohen L. Preventative analgesia is associated with reduced pain disability 3 weeks but not 6 months after major gynecologic surgery by laparotomy. *Anesthesiology.* 2004;101:169–174.

27. Reuben SS. Preventing the development of complex regional pain syndrome after surgery. *Anesthesiology.* 2004;101:1215–1224.

28. Phillip BK, Reese PR, Burch SP. The economic impact of opioids on postoperative pain management. *J Clin Anesth.* 2002;14:354–364.

29. Wheeler M, Oderda GM, Ashburn MA, Lipman AG. Adverse events associated with postoperative analgesia: a systematic review. *Clin J Pain.* 2002;3:159–180.

30. Phillips DM. JCAHO pain management standards are unveiled. *JAMA.* 2000;284:4–5.

31. Kehlet H. Postoperative opioid sparing to hasten recovery. What are the issues? *Anesthesiology.* 2005;102:1083–1085.

32. Taylor S, Voytovich AE, Kozol RA. Has the pendulum swung too far in postoperative pain control? *Am J Surg.* 2003;186:472–475.

33. Vila H, Smith RA, Augustyniak MJ, et al. The efficacy and safety of pain management before and after implementation of hospital-wide pain management standards: Is patient safety compromised by treatment based solely on numerical pain ratings? *Anesth Analg.* 2005;101:474–480.

34. Kehlet H, Dahl JB. The value of "multimodal" or "balanced analgesia" in postoperative pain treatment. *Anesth Analg.* 1993;77:1048–1056.

35. Dahl JB, Rosenberg J, Dirkes WE, Morgensen T, Kehlet H. Prevention of postoperative pain by balanced analgesia. *Br J Anaesth.* 1990;64:518–520.

36. Kehlet H, Wilmore DW. Multimodal strategies to improve surgical outcome. *Am J Surg.* 2002;183:630–641.

37. Buvanendran A, Kroin JS, Tuman KJ, et al. Effects of perioperative administration of a selective cyclooxygenase 2 inhibitor of pain management and recovery of function after knee replacement. *JAMA.* 2003;290:2411–2418.

38. Reuben SS, Gutta SB, Maciolek H, Sklar J. Effect of initiating a multimodal analgesic regimen upon patient outcomes after anterior cruciate ligament reconstruction for same-day surgery: a 1200-patient case series. *Acute Pain.* 2004;6:87–93.

39. Reuben SS, Gutta SB, Maciolek H, Sklar J, Redford J. Effect of initiating a preventative multimodal analgesic regimen upon long-term patient outcomes after anterior cruciate ligament reconstruction for same-day surgery: A 1200-patient case series. *Acute Pain.* 2005;7:65–73.

40. Ashburn MA, Caplan RA, Carr DB, et al. Practice guidelines for acute pain management in the perioperative setting: an updated report by the American Society of Anesthesiologists task force on acute pain management. *Anesthesiology.* 2004;100:1573–1581.

41. United States Acute Pain Management Guideline Panel. *Acute Pain Management: Operative or Medical Procedures and Trauma.* Pub. no. 92-0032. Rockville, MD:, United States Department of Health and Human Services, Public Health Service Agency for Health Care Policy and Research, 1992.

42. Unnerstall JR, Kopajtic TA, Kuhar MJ. Distribution of alpha 2 agonist binding sites in the rat and human central nervous system: Analysis of some functional, anatomic correlates of the pharmacologic effects of clonidine and related adrenergic agents. *Brain Res Rev.* 1984;7:69–101.

43. Gaumann DM, Brunet PC, Jirounek P. Clonidine enhances the effects of lidocaine on C-fiber action potential. *Anesth Analg.* 1992;74:719–725.

44. Butterworth JF, Strichartz GR. The α_2-adrenergic agonists clonidine and guanfacine produce tonic and phasic block of conduction in rat sciatic nerve fibers. *Anesth Analg.* 1993;76:295–301.

45. Gaumann DM, Brunet PC, Jirounek P. Hyperpolarizing after potentials in C fibers and and local anesthetic effects of clonidine and lidocaine. *Pharmacology.* 1994;48:21–29.

46. Langer SZ, Duval N, Masingham R. Pharmacologic and therapeutic significance of alpha-adrenoceptor subtypes. *J Cardiovasc Pharmacol.* 1985;7:1–8.

47. Gaumann D, Forster A, Griessen M, Habre W, Poinsot O, Della Santa D. Comparison between clonidine and epinephrine admixture to lidocaine in brachial plexus block. *Anesth Analg.* 1992;75:69–74.

48. Kroin JS, Buvanendran A, Beck DR, Topic JE, Watts TE, Tuman KJ. Clonidine prolongation of lidocaine analgesia after sciatic nerve block in rats is mediated via the hyperpolarization-activated cation current (Ih) not by alpha2-adrenoreceptors. *Anesthesiology.* 2004;101:488–494.

49. Nakamura M, Ferreira SH. Peripheral analgesic action of clonidine: mediation by release of endogenous enkephaln-like substances. *Eur J Pharmacol.* 1988;146:223–228.

50. Reuben SS. Stellate ganglion blockade for acute postoperative upper extremity pain. *Anesthesiology.* 2005;102:288–289.

51. Eisenach JC, DeKock M, Klimscha W. α-2 adrenergic agonists for regional anesthesia. A clinical review of clonidine (1984–1995). *Anesthesiology.* 1996;85:655–674.

52. Smith H, Elliott J. Alpha2 receptors and agonists in pain management. *Curr Opin Anaesthesiol.* 2001;14:513–518.

53. Bernard JM, Hommeril JL, Passuti N, Pinaud M. Postoperative analgesia by intravenous clonidine. *Anesthesiology.* 1991;75:577–582.

54. Arain SR, Ruehlow RM, Uhrich TD, Ebert TJ. The efficacy of dexmedetomidine versus morphine for postoperative analgesia after major inpatient surgery. *Anesth Analg.* 2004;98:153–158.

55. Sites BD, Beach M, Biggs R, et al. Intrathecal clonidine added to a bupivacaine-morphine spinal anesthetic improves postoperative analgesia for total knee arthroplasty. *Anesth Analg.* 2003;96:1083–1088.

56. Forster JG, Rosenberg PH. Small dose of clonidine mixed with low-dose ropivacaine and fentanyl for epidural analgesia after total knee arthroplasty. *Br J Anaesth.* 2004;93:670–677.

57. Milligan KR, Convery PN, Weir P, Quinn P, Connolly D. The efficacy and safety of epidural infusions of levobupivacaine with and without clonidine for postoperative pain relief in patients undergoing total hip replacement. *Anesth Analg.* 2000;91:393–397.

58. Dobrydnjov I, Axelsson K, Gupta A, Lundon A, Holmstrom B, Granath B. Improved analgesia with clonidine when added to local anesthetic during combined spinal-epidural anesthesia for hip arthroplasty: a double-blind, randomized and placebo-controlled study. *Acta Anaesthesiol Scand.* 2005;49:538–545.

59. Reuben SS, Steinberg RB, Klatt JL, Klatt ML. Intravenous regional anesthesia using lidocaine and clonidine. *Anesthesiology.* 1999;91:654–658.

60. Lurie SD, Reuben SS, Gibson CS, DeLuca PA, Maciolek HA. Effect of clonidine on upper extremity tourniquet pain in healthy volunteers. *Reg Anesth Pain Med.* 2000;25:502–505.

61. Reuben SS, Connelly NR. Postoperative analgesia for outpatient arthroscopic knee surgery with intraarticular clonidine. *Anesth Analg.* 1999;88:729–733.

62. Joshi W, Reuben SS, Kilaru PK, Sklar J, Maciolek H. Postoperative analgesia for outpatient arthroscopic knee surgery with intraarticular clonidine and/or morphine. *Anesth Analg.* 2000;90:1102–1116.

63. Cousins MJ. Acute pain and the injury response: immediate and prolonged effects. *Reg Anesth.* 1989;14:162–179.

64. McCormack K. Non-steroidal anti-inflammatory drugs and spinal nociceptive processing. *Pain.* 1994;59:9–43.

65. Souter AJ, Fredman B, White PF. Controversies in the perioperative use of nonsteroidal anti-inflammatory drugs. *Anesth Analg.* 1994;79:1178–1190.

66. Dahl JB, Kehlet H. Non-steroidal anti-inflammatory drugs: rationale for use in severe postoperative pain. *Br J Anaesth.* 1991;66:703–712.

67. Reuben SS, Connelly NR, Lurie SD, Klatt ML, Gibson C. Dose-response of ketorolac as an adjunct to patient-controlled analgesia morphine in patients after spinal fusion surgery. *Anesth Analg.* 1998;87:98–102.

68. Muth-Selbach US, Tegeder I, Brune K, Geisslinger G. Acetaminophen inhibits spinal prostaglandin E2 release after peripheral noxious stimulation. *Anesthesiology.* 1999;91:231–239.

69. Chandrasekharan NV, Dai H, Roos KL, et al. COX-3, a cyclooxygenase-1 variant inhibited by acetaminophen and other analgesic/antipyretic drugs: cloning, structure, and expression. *Proc Natl Acad Sci USA.* 2002;99:13926–13931.

70. Hersh EV, Lally ET, Moore PA. Update on cyclooxygenase inhibitors: has a third COX isoform entered the fray? *Curr Med Res Opin.* 2005;21(8):1217–1226.

71. Pickering G, Loriot MA, Libert F, Eschalier A, Beaune P, Dubray C. Analgesic effect of acetaminophen in humans: first evidence of a central serotonergic mechanism. *Clin Pharmacol Ther.* 2006;79:371–378.

72. Remy C, Marret E, Bonnet F. Effects of acetaminophen on morphine side-effects and consumption after major surgery: meta-analysis of randomized controlled trials. *Br J Anaesth.* 2005;94:505–513.

73. Hyllested M, Jones S, Pedersen JL, Kehlet H. Comparative effect of paracetamol, NSAIDs, or their combination in postoperative pain management: a qualitative review. *Br J Anaesth.* 2002;88:199–214.

74. Sinatra R. Role of COX-2 inhibitors in the evolution of acute pain management. *J Pain Symptom Manage.* 2002;24:S18–S27.

75. Holmer PP, Owall A, Jakobsson J. Early bioavailability of paracetamol after oral or intravenous administration. *Acta Anaesthesiol Scand.* 2004;48:867–870.

76. Elia N, Lysakowski C, Tramer MR. Does multimodal analgesia with acetaminophen, nonsteroidal anti-inflammatory drugs, or selective cyclooxygenase-2 inhibitors and patient-controlled analgesia morphine offer advantages over morphine alone? *Anesthesiology.* 2005;1296–1304.

77. Romsing J, Moniche S. A review of COX-2 inhibitors compared with traditional NSAIDs, or different COX-2 inhibitors for postoperative pain. *Acta Anaesthesiol Scand.* 2004;48:525–546.

78. Katz J. Pre-emptive analgesia: importance of timing. *Can J Anaesth.* 2001;48:105–114.

79. Reuben SS, Bhopatkar S, Maciolek H, et al. The preemptive analgesic effect of rofecoxib after ambulatory arthroscopic knee surgery. *Anesth Analg.* 2002;94:55–59.

80. Salter MW. Cellular signaling pathways of spinal pain neuroplasticity as targets for analgesic development. *Curr Top Med Chem.* 2005;5:557–567.

81. Woolf CJ, Thompson SW. The induction and maintenance of central sensitization is dependent on N-methyl-D-aspartate acid receptor activation: implication for the treatment of post-injury pain hypersensitivity states. *Pain.* 1991;44:293–299.

82. Foster AC, Fagg GE. Neurobiology. Taking apart NMDA receptors. *Nature.* 1987;329:395–396.

83. Schmid RL, Sandler AN, Katz J. Use and efficacy of low-dose ketamine in the management of acute postoperative pain: a review of current techniques and outcomes. *Pain.* 1999;82:111–125.

84. Subramaniam K, Subramaniam B, Steinbrook RA. Ketamine as adjuvant analgesic to opioids: a quantitative and qualitative systematic review. *Anesth Analg.* 2004;99:482–495.

85. Tverskoy M, Oren M, Vaskovich M, Dashkovsky I, Kissin I. Ketamine enhances local anesthetic and analgesic effects of bupivacaine by peripheral mechanism: a study in postoperative patients. *Neurosci Lett.* 1996;215:5–8.

86. Menigaux C, Guignard B, Fletcher D, Dupont X, Guirimand F, Chauvin M. The benefits of intraoperative small-dose ketamine on postoperative pain after anterior cruciate ligament repair. *Anesth Analg.* 2000;90:129–135.

87. Menigaux C, Guignard B, Fletcher D, Sessler DI, Dupont X, Chauvin M. Intraoperative small-dose ketamine enhances analgesia after outpatient knee arthroscopy. *Anesth Analg.* 2001;93:606–612.

88. Himmelseher S, Ziegler-Pithamitsis D, Agiriadou H, Martin Jjelen-Esselborn S, Koch E. Small-dose S(+) ketamine reduces postoperative pain when applied with ropivacaine in epidural anesthesia for total knee arthroplasty. *Anesth Analg.* 2001;92:1290–1295.

89. Adam F, Chauvin M, Du Manoir B, Langlois M, Sessler DI, Fletcher D. Small-dose ketamine infusion improves postoperative analgesia and rehabilitation after total knee arthroplasty. *Anesth Analg.* 2005;100:475–480.

90. Wong BY, Coulter DA, Choi DW, Prince DA. Dextrorphan and dextromethorphan, common antitussives, are antieleptic and antagonize N-methyl-D-aspartate in brain slices. *Neurosci Lett.* 1988;85:261–266.

91. LePage KT, Ishmael JT, Low CM, et al. Differential binding properties of [3H] dextrorphan and [3H] MK-801 in heterologously expressed NMDA receptors. *Neuropharmacology.* 2005;49:1–16.

92. Duedahl TH, Romsing J, Moniche S, Dahl JB. A qualitative systematic review of peri-operative dextromethorphan in postoperative pain. *Acta Anaesthesiol Scand.* 2006;50:1–13.

93. Cox JA, Lysko PG, Henneberry RC. Excitatory amino acid neurotoxicity at the N-methyl-D-aspartate receptor in cultured neurons: role of the voltage-dependent magnesium block. *Brain Res.* 1989;499:267–272.

94. Tramer MR, Schneider J, Mart RA, Rifat K. Role of magnesium sulfate in postoperative analgesia. *Anesthesiology.* 1996;84:340–347.

95. Konig H, Wallner T, Marhofer P, et al. Magnesium sulfate reduces intra- and postoperative analgesic requirements. *Anesth Analg.* 1998;87:206–210.

96. Kara H, Sahin N, Ulusan V, Aydogdu T. Magnesium infusion reduces postoperative pain. *Eur J Anaesthesiol.* 2002;19:52–56.

97. Levaux CH, Bonhomme V, Dewandre PY, et al. Effect of intra-operative magnesium sulfate on pain relief and patient comfort after major lumbar orthopaedic surgery. *Anaesthesia.* 2003;58:131–135.

98. Bhatia A, Kashyap L, Pawar DK, Trikha A. Effect of intraoperative magnesium infusion on perioperative analgesia in open cholecystectomy. *J Clin Anesth.* 2004;16:262–265.

99. Sehan TO, Tugrul M, Sungur MO, et al. Effects of three different dose regimens of magnesium on propofol requirements, haemodynamic variables and postoperative pain relief in gynaecological surgery. *Br J Anaesth.* 2006;96.

100. Wilder-Smith CH, Knopfli R, Wilder-Smith OH. Perioperative magnesium infusion and postoperative pain. *Acta Anesthesiol Scand.* 1997;41:1023–1027.

101. Ko SH, Lim HR, Kim DC, et al. Magnesium sulfate does not reduce postoperative analgesic requirements. *Anesthesiology.* 2001;95:640–646.

102. Paech MJ, Magann EF, Doherty DA, et al. Does magnesium sulfate reduce the short- and long-term requirements for pain

relief after caesarean delivery? A double-blind placebo-controlled trial. *Am J Obstet Gynecol.* 2006;194:1596–1602.

103. McKee JA, Brewer RP, Macy GE, et al. Analysis of the brain bioavailability of peripherally administered magnesium sulfate: a study in humans with acute brain injury undergoing prolonged induced hypermagnesemia. *Crit Care Med.* 2005;33:661–666.

104. McCartney CJ, Sinha A, Katz J. A qualitative systematic review of the role of N-methyl-D-aspartate receptor antagonists in preventive analgesia. *Anesth Analg.* 2004;98:1385–1400.

105. Skryabina EA, Dunn TS. Disposable infusion pumps. *Am J Health Syst Pharm.* 2006;63:1260–1268.

106. Chelly JE, Ben-David B, Williams BA, Kentor ML. Anesthesia and postoperative analgesia: outcomes following orthopedic surgery. *Orthopedics.* 2003;26:S865–S871.

107. Zink W, Graf BM. Local anesthetic myotoxicity. *Reg Anesth Pain Med.* 2004;29:333–340.

108. Kreitzer JM, Reuben SS. Central nervous system toxicity in a patient receiving continuous intrapleural bupivacaine. *J Clin Anesth.* 1996;8:666–668.

109. Kulkarni M, Elliot D. Local anaesthetic infusion for postoperative pain. *J Hand Surg.* 2003;28:300–306.

110. Gomoll AH, Kang RW, Williams JM, Bach BR, Cole BJ. Chondrolysis after continuous intra-articular bupivacaine infusion: an experimental model investigating chondrotoxicity in the rabbit shoulder. *Arthroscopy.* 2006;22:813–819.

111. Capdevilla X, Barthelet Y, Biboulet P, Ryckwaert Y, Rubenovitch J, d'Athis F. Effects of perioperative analgesic technique on the surgical outcome and duration of rehabilitation after major knee surgery. *Anesthesiology.* 1999;91:8–15.

112. McCartney CJL, Brull R, Chan VS, et al. Early but no long-term benefit of regional compared with general anesthesia for ambulatory hand surgery. *Anesthesiology.* 2004;101:461–467.

113. Richman JM, Liu SS, Courpas G, et al. Does continuous peripheral nerve block provide superior pain control to opioids? A meta-analysis. *Anesth Analg.* 2006;102:248–257.

114. Rathmell JP, Wu CL, Sinatra RS, et al. Acute post-surgical pain management: a critical appraisal of current practice. *Reg Anesth Pain Med.* 2006;31:1–42.

115. Adams HA, Saatweber P, Schmitz CS, Hecker H. Postoperative pain management in orthopedic patients: no differences in pain score, but improved stress control by epidural anaesthesia. *Eur J Anaesthesiol.* 2002;19:658–665.

116. Block BM, Liu SS, Rowlingson AJ, Cowan AR, Cowan JA, Wu CL. Efficacy of postoperative epidural analgesia: a meta-analysis. *JAMA.* 2003;290:2455–2463.

117. De Leon-Casasola OA. When it comes to outcome, we need to define what a perioperative epidural technique is. *Anesth Analg.* 2003;96:315–318.

118. Reuben SS, Buvanendran A, Kroin JS, et al. Postoperative modulation of central nervous system prostaglandins E2 by cyclooxygenase inhibitors after vascular surgery. *Anesthesiology.* 2006;104:411–416.

119. Kroin JS, Buvanendran A, McCarthy RJ, et al. Cyclooyxgenase-2 (COX-2) inhibitor potentiates morphine antinociception at the spinal level in a post-operative pain model. *Reg Anesth Pain Med.* 2002;27:451–455.

120. Dai YQ, Jin DZ, Zhu XZ, et al. Triptolide inhibits COX-2 expression via NF-kappa B pathway in astrocytes. *Neuroscience.* 2006;55:154–160.

121. Samad TA, Sapirstein A, Woolf CJ. Prostanoids and pain: unraveling mechanisms and revealing therapeutic targets. *Trends Mol Med.* 2002;8:390–396.

122. Buvanendran A, Kroin JS, Berger RA, et al. Up-regulation of prostaglandin E2 and interleukins in the central nervous sys-

tem and peripheral tissue during and after surgery in humans. *Anesthesiology.* 2006;104:403–410.

123. Walder B, Schafer M, Henzi I, et al. Efficacy and safety of patient-controlled opioid analgesia for acute postoperative pain: a quantitative systematic review. *Acta Anaesthesiol Scand.* 2001;45:795–804.

124. Chia YT, Liu K, Wang JJ, Kuo MC, Ho ST. Intraoperative high dose fentanyl induces postoperative fentanyl tolerance. *Can J Anaesth.* 1999;48:872–877.

125. Guignard B, Bossard AE, Coste C, et al. Acute opioid tolerance: intraoperative remifentanil increases postoperative pain and morphine requirement. *Anesthesiology.* 2000;93:409–417.

126. Larcher A, Laulin JP, Celerier E, Le Moal M, Simmonnet G. Acute tolerance associated with a single opiate administration: involvement of N-methyl-D-aspartate-dependent pain facilatory systems. *Neuroscience.* 1998;84:583–589.

127. Mao J. Opioid-induced abnormal pain sensitivity: implications in clinical opioid therapy. *Pain.* 2002;100:213–217.

128. Angst MS, Clark DJ. Opioid-induced hyperalgesia: a qualitative systematic review. *Anesthesiology.* 2006;104:570–587.

129. Powell KJ, Hosokawa A, Bell A, et al. Comparative effects of cyclo-oxygenase and nitrous oxide synthase inhibition on the development and reversal of spinal opioid tolerance. *Br J Pharmacol.* 1999;127:631–634.

130. Troster A, Sittl R, Singler B, et al. Modulation of remifentanil-induced analgesia and postinfusion hyperalgesia by parecoxib in humans. *Anesthesiology.* 2006;105:1016–1023.

131. Stein C. Peripheral mechanisms of opioid analgesia. *Anesth Analg.* 1993;76:182–191.

132. Picard PP Tramer MR, McQuay HJ, Moore RA. Analgesic efficacy of peripheral opioids (all except intra-articular): a qualitative systematic review of randomized controlled trials. *Pain.* 1997;72:309–318.

133. Kalso E, Smith L, McQuay HJ, Moore RA. No pain, no gain: clinical excellence and scientific rigour-lessons learned from IA morphine. *Pain.* 2002;98:269–275.

134. Reuben SS, Sklar J. Postoperative pain management for outpatient arthroscopic knee surgery. *Current Concepts Review. J Bone Joint Surg.* 2000;82:1754–1766.

135. Reichart JA, Daughters RS, Rivard R, Simone DA. Peripheral and preemptive opioid antinociception in a mouse visceral pain model. *Pain.* 2001;89:221–227.

136. Denti M, Randelli P, Bigoni M, Arino MR, Fraschini N. Pre- and postoperative intra-articular analgesia for arthroscopic surgery of the knee and arthroscopic-assisted anterior cruciate ligament reconstruction. A double-blind randomized prospective study. *Knee Surg Sports Traumatol Arthrosc.* 1997;5:206–212.

137. Reuben SS, Sklar J, El-Mansouri M. The preemptive analgesic effect of intraarticular bupivacaine and morphine after ambulatory arthroscopic knee surgery. *Anesth Analg.* 2001;92:923–926.

138. Qin N, Yagel S, Momplaisir ML, Codd EE, D'Andrea MR. Molecular cloning and characterization of the human voltage-gated calcium channel $\alpha 2\delta$-4 subunit. *Mol Pharmacol.* 2002;62:485–496.

139. Gilron I. Is gabapentin a "broad-spectrum" analgesic? *Anesthesiology.* 2002; 97:537–539.

140. Eckhardt K, Ammon S, Hofmann U, Riebe A, Gugeler N, Mikus G. Gabapentin enhances the analgesic effect of morphine in healthy volunteers. *Anesth Analg.* 2000;91:185–191.

141. Hurley RW, Chatterjea D, Rose Feng M, Taylor CP, Hammond DL. Gabapentin and pregabalin can interact synergistically with naproxen to produce antihyperalgesia. *Anesthesiology.* 2002; 97:1263–1273.

142. Gilron I, Orr E, Tu D, O'Neill JP, Zamora JE, Bell AC. A placebo-controlled randomized clinical trial of perioperative administration of gabapentin, rofecoxib and their combination for spontaneous and movement-evoked pain after abdominal hysterectomy. *Pain.* 2005;113:191–200.

143. Dahl JB, Mathiesen O, Moniche S. "Protective premedication": an option with gabapentin and related drugs? A review of gabapentin and pregabalin in the treatment of post-operative pain. *Acta Anaesthesiol Scand.* 2004;48:1130–1136.

144. Hurley RW, Cohen SP, Williams KA, Rowlingson AG, Wu CL. The analgesic effects of perioperative gabapentin on postoperative pain: a meta-analysis. *Reg Anesth Pain Med.* 2006;31:237–247.

145. Ho KY, Habib HS. Gabapentin and postoperative pain – a systematic review of randomized controlled trials. *Pain.* 2006;126:91–101.

146. Reuben SS, Buvanendran A, Kroin JS, Raghunathan K. Evaluation of the analgesic efficacy of administering celecoxib, pregabalin and their combination for spinal fusion surgery. *Anesth Analg.* 2006;103:1271–1277.

147. Menigaux C, Adam F, Guignard B, Sessler DI, Chauvin M. Preoperative gabapentin decreases anxiety and improves early functional recovery from knee surgery. *Anesth Analg.* 2005;100:1394–1399.

148. Kehlet H, Werner M, Perkins F. Balanced analgesia: what is it and what are its advantages in postoperative pain? *Drugs.* 1999;58:793–797.

149. Jin F, Chung F. Multimodal analgesia for postoperative pain control. *J Clin Anesth.* 2001;13:524–539.

150. Joshi GP. Multimodal analgesia techniques and postoperative rehabilitation. *Anesthesiol Clin North Am.* 2005;23:185–202.

151. Apfelbaum JL, Gan TJ, Zhao S, Hanna DB, Chen C. Reliability and validity of the preoperative opioid-related symptom distress scale. *Anesth Analg.* 2004;99:699–709.

152. Zhao SZ, Chung F, Hanna DB, Raymundo AL, Cheung RY, Chen C. Dose-response relationship between opioid use and adverse events after ambulatory surgery. *J Pain Symptom Manage.* 2004;28:35–46.

153. Gan TJ, Joshi GP, Zhao SZ, Hanna DB, Cheung RY, Chen C. Presurgical intravenous parecoxib sodium and follow-up oral valdecoxib for pain management after laparoscopic cholecystectomy surgery reduces opioid requirements and opioid-related adverse effects. *Acta Anaesthesiol Scand.* 2004;48:1194–1207.

154. Reuben SS, Raghunathan K, Cheung R. Dose-response relationship between opioid use and adverse events after spinal fusion surgery. *Anesthesiology.* 2006;105:A1646. [Abstract]

155. Wilmore DW, Kehlet H. Management of patients in fast track surgery. *BMJ.* 2001;322:473–476.

13

Oral and Parenteral Opioid Analgesics for Acute Pain Management

Raymond S. Sinatra

Opioids represent a class of analgesics that provide powerful dose-dependent pain relief for patients suffering moderate to severe pain. The class includes a large number of compounds with variable pharmacokinetics and pharmacodynamics, no hepatorenal toxic effects, and no ceiling effect for achievable pain relief. Opioids also offer dosing versatility and are marketed for oral, nasal, parenteral, transmucosal, transdermal, and neuraxial administration.

When defining this class of analgesics the term *opioid* is more precise than the overly broad definition *narcotic*, which includes other central-acting compounds such as cannabis, cocaine, and barbiturates.[1–3] Opioid analgesics include natural derivatives of opium, such as morphine; substituted semisynthetics, such as oxycodone; complex synthetics, including meperidine, fentanyl, and methadone; and endogenous ligands, such as enkephalin (Figure 13.1).[1,2]

Opioid use predates recorded history; however, earliest references describing opium extracts for pain control were associated with Egyptian and Sumerian cultures dating back to 3000 BC.[1–3] The active component of opium is morphine, named after Morpheus, the god of dreams. Morphine was isolated in the 1850s.[1,2] The use of morphine and intravenous syringes during the U.S. civil war (1860s) greatly improved pain management; however, misuse and overuse led to excessive rates of dependency and addiction.[1–4] Over 150 years later, misuse remains a problem, as the search for the opioid "holy grail," or compounds offering effective analgesia with reduced risk of abuse and serious adverse events, has been unsuccessful.

Historically, the use of opioids for pain management has oscillated from broad indiscriminate use a century ago to severe restrictions that left too many patients without adequate analgesia.[1–3] Fears of opioid addiction were responsible for the establishment of the U.S. Narcotic Control Acts of the early 1900s that limited opioid distribution and use.[1,2] Since the late 1980s, regulatory easements and greater medical acceptance have dramatically increased opioid dosing for patients suffering moderate to severe pain.[5,6] The Agency for Health Care Policy and Research and American Society of Anesthesiology have established pain treatment guidelines, and the Joint Commission on Accreditation of Health Care Organizations has included pain treatment in its evaluation of hospitals and health care providers.[6–9] Nevertheless, because of highly publicized cases of diversion and abuse, the pendulum has started to swing back toward increasing restriction, as evidenced by high-profile court cases and Food and Drug Administration/Drug Enforcement Administration statements discouraging high-dose opioid prescriptions.[10]

Despite the drawbacks of respiratory depression, other annoying adverse effects, and risk of misuse, parenteral and oral opioids remain the foundation of surgical and chronic pain management and essential therapy for managing moderately severe to severe pain. The benefits and drawbacks of opioid analgesics are outlined in Table 13.1.

OPIOID PHARMACOLOGY

Opioid Receptors

Opioids interact with specific transmembrane G-protein coupled binding sites termed *opiate* or *opioid receptors*. These receptors are located primarily in spinal dorsal horn, central gray, medial thalamus, amygdala, limbic cortex, and other regions of the central nervous system (CNS) that process affective and suffering aspects of pain perception.[1–4,11,12] Conversely, opioid receptors are not concentrated in the somatosensory cortex or other regions responsible for pain localization.[1–4,11] Opioid receptors serve as binding sites for endogenous ligands, including endorphins and the enkephalins, which naturally modulate pain transmission and perception.[1,3,11,12] Naturally occurring opiates and synthetic opioids have structural/chemical similarities that enable them to bind and activate opioid receptors resulting in powerful, dose-dependent analgesia.[1,2,10] As analgesics, opioids are highly selective in that they reduce or eliminate the suffering aspects of pain while preserving noxious localization.[10,11] With appropriate dosing, patients can precisely identify the site of tissue injury yet are less troubled by it.[1,12,13] Analgesic selectivity is also related to fact that opioids block noxious sensation without affecting other

Table 13.1: Oral and Intravenous Opioid Analgesics

Benefits

1. Rapid onset of analgesia for moderate, severe, and very severe pain
2. Highly effective analgesia: (no analgesic dose ceiling)
3. Selective analgesia: reductions in pain suffering, minimal effects on pain localization
4. No effects on key organs: cardiac, renal, hepatic, and hemostatic safety
5. Multiple agents and routes of administration are available
6. Relatively inexpensive (morphine, oxycodone)

Drawbacks

1. Annoying side effects: Nausea, pruritus, sedation, constipation
2. Clinically significant effects: ileus, bowel obstruction, severe vomiting, confusion, dysphoria
3. Life threatening effects: Airway obstruction, respiratory depression, respiratory arrest
4. Social effects: Dose escalation, physical dependence, diversion and abuse, addiction
5. May be expensive (sustained release opioids, oral buccal preparations

forms of sensory perception, such as light touch, pressure, and temperature.[1,2,11,12]

Three principal opioid receptor subtypes, designated as μ, κ, and δ, have been isolated and characterized. A fourth subtype, termed σ, is no longer characterized as a selective opioid receptor.[1,2] A newer receptor classification system uses the labels OPR$_1$, OPR$_2$, and OPR$_3$, which correspond to μ, κ, and δ receptors, respectively.[1,3,11,12] μ receptors (OPR$_1$) mediate supraspinal analgesia, as well as respiratory depression, nausea and vomiting, miosis, and bowel hypomotility. μ receptors also mediate euphoria and physical and psychological dependence and are responsible for increased release of prolactin and growth hormone.[1,2,12] Primary μ agonists include β-endorphin and morphine.

κ receptors (OPR$_2$) are believed to mediate spinal analgesia, visceral analgesia, and sedation but have a minimal effect on respiration.[1,3] Peripheral κ receptors have been identified in kidney, gastrointestinal tract, skin, muscle, and connective tissues. Receptors localized in kidney are associated with antidiuresis and clinically significant oliguria.[1,2] The primary endogenous ligand for κ receptors is dynorphin[1,3,12,14]; however, κ agonists are being developed that can activate peripheral receptors yet cannot penetrate the blood-brain barrier (BBB). These ligands may offer highly selective peripheral κ-mediated analgesia without central effects such as excessive sedation, euphoria, and respiratory depression.

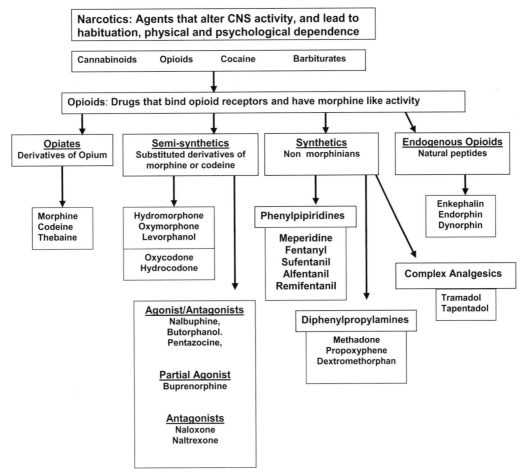

Figure 13.1: An overview of opioid compounds, including naturally occurring, semisynthetic, synthetic, and endogenous compounds.

Table 13.2: Opioid Receptor Subtypes and Binding of Selected Agonists[a]

Opioid	μ	κ	δ	σ	NMDA	α
Morphine	++	+	+	+	−	−
Hydromorphone	++	+	+	−	−	−
Oxymorphone	++	−	+	−	−	−
Oxycodone	++	+	+	−	−	−
Fentanyl	+++	−	−	−	−	−
Sufentanil	+++	−	−	−	−	−
Butorphanol	−	++	+	+	−	−
Buprenorphine	+	+	+	−	−	−
Methadone	++	?	+	−	+	+
Tramadol	+	−	−	−	-	+

[a] Based on information presented in Reisine and Pasternak (1997),[1] Gutstein and Akil (2002),[2] Pasero et al (1999),[3] Way et al (2004).[14]

δ receptors (OPR$_3$) are not as well characterized but appear to facilitate μ-receptor activity and enhance spinal and supraspinal analgesia. The primary ligand for δ receptors is enkephalin.[1,12] An additional, poorly characterized, receptor subtype, designated the σ$_1$ receptor, is activated by pentazocine. σ$_1$ receptors are no longer considered true opioid receptors because ligand binding is not antagonized by naloxone and other opioid antagonists. σ$_1$ receptors are believed to mediate opioid-related dysphoria, hallucinations, and confusion. Opioid receptor subtypes and sites of opioid activity are presented in Table 13.2.

Of all subtypes, the μ receptor has been most studied.[1,2,12,14] μ receptors are located at pre- and postsynaptic contacts between nociceptive cells and function to limit release of noxious transmitters and reduce neuronal excitation. The μ-receptor complex is activated following precise stereospecific attachment of agonist chemical groups, including a negatively charged hydroxyl group, the phenolic ring, and tertiary nitrogen to complimentary regions on the extramembrane binding site (Figure 13.2).[1,2,12,14] Receptor activation is followed by secondary activation of intracellular G proteins and an associated effector protein complex. Effector proteins inhibit adenylate cyclase and influence the activity of phosphokinases and other second messengers. These alterations decrease cyclic adenosine monophosphate (cAMP), limit potassium and calcium ion flux, and hyperpolarize nociceptive cells (see Chapter 1, *Pain Pathways and Acute Pain Processing*).[1,14]

Pharmacokinetics

Physiochemical and structural differences between opioid agonists can influence affinity and binding kinetics at μ receptors, as well as their ability to activate G proteins and other transducer molecules.[1,3,12,14] Receptor binding affinity influences agonist association/disassociation kinetics as well as pharmacological onset and duration of activity. The intrinsic efficacy of a given opioid agonist is related to its ability to activate coupled G proteins.[1,3,12,14] In general, potent opioids, such as fentanyl and sufentanil, have greater intrinsic efficacy at μ receptors than naturally occurring opiates such as morphine and codeine.[1,3] In clinical settings,' pharmacokinetic variables, such as lipid solubility, degree of ionization, and volume of distribution, play

Table 13.3: Pharmacological and Physiological Factors That Influence Onset, Duration, and Effectiveness of Opioid Analgesics

Pharmacological Correlates of Opioid Activity

Potency	High Lipid solubility
Onset	Low degree of ionization, High CNS penetration, High receptor affinity
Duration	High water solubility (CSF trapping), High receptor binding kinetics, Low hepatic/renal clearance, Active metabolites, Large volume of distribution
Safety	Mu receptor specificity, Lack of active of toxic metabolites
Efficacy	Multiple receptor specificity, high receptor affinity, high intrinsic efficacy

key roles in determining agonist potency, onset of effect, and analgesic duration (Table 13.3).[1,2,12,14] Analgesic onset is determined by the ability of an agonist to enter the CNS compartment and distribute into gray matter, where receptors are primarily localized. Drugs that are highly lipophilic and un-ionized easily enter the CNS and have a very rapid onset of effect. In contrast, hydrophilic, highly ionized opioids, such as morphine, have difficulty penetrating the BBB and have a delayed onset.[1,3] Opioid analgesic potency, or the amount of drug required to achieve an analgesic effect, is closely related to the octanol:water

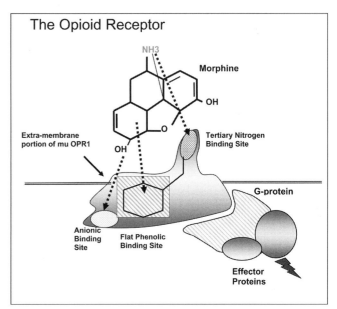

Figure 13.2: A schematic diagram of the extramembranous portion of the μ-opioid receptor and its interaction with morphine and associated effector proteins. Morphine and other opioid agonists attach to specific portions of the receptor, including an anion site, a flattened surface site that accepts the phenolic group, and a tertiary nitrogen attachment site. Attachment at the tertiary nitrogen binding site appears to be important for receptor activation and subsequent activation of the G protein. G proteins in turn activate other effector proteins within the complex that influence second messengers and neuronal ion flux. Opioid antagonists bind with high affinity to portions of the receptor; however, a bulky methyl or allyl group added to the tertiary nitrogen prevents receptor activation.

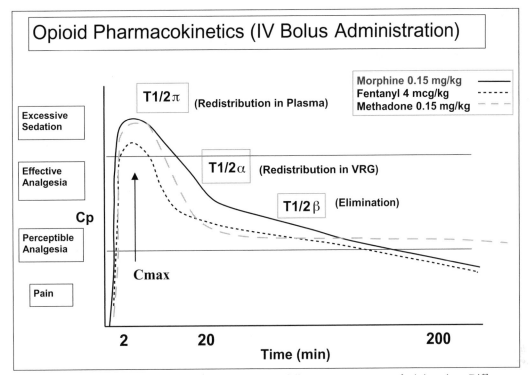

Figure 13.3: Plasma kinetics of selected opioid agonists following intravenous administration. Differences between perceptible and effective analgesia are dependent on plasma concentration (C_p). Following bolus administration, plasma levels at $T_{1/2\pi}$ represent drug redistribution thoughout the plasma compartment, $T_{1/2}$ α represents plasma concentration following redistribution into the vessel rich group, and $T_{1/2}$ β reflects plasma concentrations following hepatic elimination of free drug. Morphine and fentanyl have different lipid solubilities; however, their volume of distribution, $T_{1/2}$ α, and $T_{1/2}$ β redistribution kinetics are similar. Onset of analgesia with lipophillic opioids is related to time to maximum plasma concentration, T_{max}. Morphine's delay in onset reflects its difficulty in penetrating the BBB, not time to achieve T_{max}. Methadone has a more prolonged duration of effect as related to its very large volume of redistribution and delayed $T_{1/2}$ elimination kinetics.

coefficient (lipophilicity vs hydrophilicity) and intrinsic efficacy of the agonist.[1,2,12,14] As a rule, highly lipophilic opioids have significantly greater potency than less lipophilic or hydrophilic agents.[1,3,14]

Analgesic duration is related to several factors, including receptor dissociation kinetics, redistribution, elimination kinetics, and volume of distribution. Lipophilic opioids, including fentanyl and sufentanil, have dose-related durations of activity. With low doses duration is dependent on rapid $T_{1/2}$ α redistribution kinetics and is limited (Figure 13.3). With higher doses, duration correlates with $T_{1/2}$ β metabolism/elimination kinetics, which are dependent on enterohepatic reuptake, hepatic blood flow and extraction, and protein binding. Because $T_{1/2}$ β kinetics are time and enzyme dependent, administration of higher doses can markedly extend analgesic duration.[1,3,14] Morphine and methadone have unique attributes that also affect analgesic duration. Morphine's hydrophilic properties slow BBB egress and favor its sequestration in the cerebral spinal fluid (CSF). These factors prolong its duration despite declines in plasma morphine concentration. The formation of active metabolites (morphine-6-glucoronide) also tends to increase its duration of effect.[1,3,14] Methadone's large volume of distribution leads to a progressive prolongation in analgesic duration with repeated doses. After achievement of steady state, drug sequestered in peripheral compartments is taken up by the vasculature and maintains minimal effective plasma concentrations.

Opioid Tolerance and Hyperalgesia

Continued patient exposure to opioid analgesics leads to tolerance development and clinical manifestations such as physical dependence. Tolerance is defined as the progressive increases in dose required to maintain a desired pharmacological effect and is characterized by a shift to the right in the classic dose-response curve.[1,3] This physiological adaptation is observed in patients prescribed opioids for pain management, as well as those abusing this class of drug. Tolerance develops rapidly to the euphoric, sedative, and respiratory depressive effects of opioids, more slowly to their analgesic effects, and rarely to their inhibition of bowel function and constipatory effects.[1–3] Tolerance development has been related to upregulation of metabolic enzymes, enhanced drug elimination, downregulation of receptors, and receptor endocytotic efficacy. Endocytosis of μ-opioid receptors counteracts receptor desensitization and opioid tolerance by inducing fast reactivation and recycling. Opioid agonists have differing abilities to initiate endocytosis and regulate surface receptor concentrations.[15] Development of tolerance is delayed with opioids having high endocytotic efficacy; however, these compounds are associated with a more rapid onset of physical dependence.[15]

Intracellular changes associated with tolerance development include μ-receptor phosphorylation, G protein decoupling, activation of cAMP response element-binding protein, and compensatory upregulation of the cAMP pathway.[1,16] Receptor endocytosis also plays a role in cAMP pathway upregulation. Cyclic AMP upregulation counteracts opioid analgesic effects, increases neuronal excitation, and plays a role in physical dependence and withdrawal.[16] Physical dependence is a normal and commonly observed phenomenon in opioid-tolerant patients. On abrupt discontinuation of opioids, the cAMP pathway is further upregulated and parasympathetic tone is markedly increased.[16] Patients experience unpleasant, but rarely life threatening, withdrawal symptoms termed *the abstinence syndrome*, which includes sweating, shaking, cramping, and diarrhea.

Psychological dependence includes drug-seeking behavior and drug administration for purposes other than pain control. Addiction is a term describing an extreme form of psychological dependence where patients demonstrate impaired control, craving, compulsive use, and continued use despite harm. Although opioid addiction is driven primarily by psychological maladaptations, such behavior is also reinforced by physical dependence and fears of withdrawal.[1-3,14] Unlike physical dependence, opioid addiction is rarely observed in patients suffering moderate to severe acute pain.

A second clinical alteration observed in patients treated with opioids is termed *opioid-induced hyperalgesia* (OIH).[17] This phenomenon is characterized by paradoxical increases in pain intensity (*hyperesthesia*), the development of new pain complaints, and alterations in pain characteristics (*allodynia*) in response to continued administration or increased dosing of opioid analgesics.

Opioid-induced hyperalgesia is most often observed in tolerant patients but has also been observed in naive individuals exposed to rapid-acting/short-duration opioids, including remifentanil and alfentanil. Mechanisms responsible for opioid-induced analgesia are not completely understood; however, glutamate-induced activation of *N*-methyl-D-aspartic acid (NMDA) receptors and upregulation of cholecystokinin (CCK) and dynorphin that have antianalgesic excitatory effects have been proposed.[17] Excitatory effects of opioid metabolites (eg, morphine-3-glucoronide, hydromorphone-3-glucoronide) may also play a role in the development and progression of OIH. Early recognition of this clinical entity is the key to reestablishing effective pain control. Treatment of OIH includes discontinuation or dose reduction of the offending opioid/metabolite; opioid rotation, including administration of methadone; and administration of NMDA receptor antagonists.

GENETIC POLYMORPHISMS THAT INFLUENCE OPIOID ACTIVITY

Historically, leaders in pharmacology have believed that there were more similarities than differences between opioid analgesics used in clinical practice.[1,3,14] The marked interindividual variations in opioid dose response, agonist efficacy, side-effect profile, and rate of tolerance development underscores the inaccuracy of this statement. In recent years, opioid receptor pharmacogenomic research has uncovered significant μ-receptor polymorphisms with over two dozen different genetic variants detected.[18-21] Differences in μ-opioid receptor gene (*OPRM1*) expression do not effect ligand binding kinetics at the extracellular membranous portion of the receptor but appear to influence subsequent activation of associated proteins and second messengers.[1,18,19]

In the first "bench-to-bedside" evaluation of μ-opioid receptor polymorphism, *OPRM1* genotypes of patients undergoing

Table 13.4: A Variety of Genetic, Pharmacologic, and Pathophysiologic Factors Influence Patient Response to Opioid Analgesics[a]

Patient Variability in Opioid Response

1. Genetic polymorphisms
   a. OPRM1 encoding mu-opioid receptor
   b. Enzymes responsible for opioid metabolism (CYP450)
   c. Genes modifying receptor activation (transporter P-glycoprotein COMT)
2. Receptor endocytotic efficacy
3. Incomplete cross-tolerance
4. Extremes in patient age
5. Exposure to drugs that compete for metabolic enzymes
6. Exposure to drugs that increase CNS depression
7. Patient comorbidity (hepatic failure, CNS lesions, renal failure)

[a] Modified from Mogil JS (1999),[19] Pan (2005).[20]

total knee arthroscopy were analyzed preoperatively.[22] Seventy-four patients (62%) were homozygous for the A118 variant, 33 patients (27%) were heterozygous A118 and G118, and 13 patients (11%) were homozygous for the G118 variant. The authors found that patients homozygous G118 self-administered significantly more morphine during the first 48 hours following surgery (homozygous AA [25 mg], heterozygous AG [26 mg], homozygous GG [40 mg]).[22] This genetic variability was also observed in cancer pain management, with homozygous GG patients requiring an average morphine dose that was 93% higher than that needed by homozygous AA patients.[23]

Genetic variability of the catechol-*O*-methyl transferase (COMT) gene also influences morphine dose requirements. Patients homozygous for the Val:Val genetic variant required 63% more drug than Met:Met variants. Heterozygous Val: Met variants required 23% more. When the two genes are taken into account the AA Met/Met genotype required the least amount of morphine to maintain equivalent analgesic.[24] The transporter P-glycoprotein (ABCB1) system influences opioid clearance from cerebrospinal fluid. In a recent article, Park and coworkers[25] reported that genetic polymorphism in this enzyme system significantly influenced respiratory rate in patients exposed to 2.5 μcg/kg of fentanyl. Genetic variations of this enzyme system affect the clearance of morphine, methadone, and fentanyl, but not meperidine.[26]

The above-mentioned receptor polymorphisms and genetic variations in enzymes involved in metabolism and clearance, contribute to the wide range of patient responses to opioid analgesics.[1,2,27] If the clinician has been unable to achieve adequate pain control with acceptable adverse effects, an alternative opioid medication should be considered. At the present time, opioid rotation is the only method available to determine which patient will respond best to a particular drug.[28-30] Factors influencing patient responses to opioid-based analgesia are presented in Table 13.4.

Opioid Classification

According to their binding affinities and intrinsic activity at receptor subtypes, opioids are classified as either agonists, partial agonists, mixed agonist-antagonists, and complete

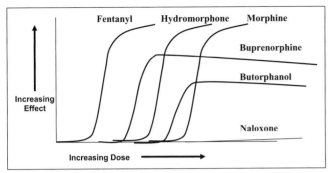

Figure 13.4: Dose-response curves of commonly employed agonists, partial agonists, mixed agonist-antagonists, and antagonists. Agonists all achieve maximum effect; however, dose requirements are dependent on potency. Mixed agonist-antagonists and partial agonists may have higher potency than agonists at low doses; however, analgesic efficacy is limited and maximum effect is not achieved. Antagonists have high affinity and can competitively displace agonists; however, they have no efficacy.

antagonists.[1–3] Opioid agonists include compounds such as morphine or fentanyl that bind receptors with moderate to high affinity, activate G proteins, and are capable of producing a maximal response following receptor activation. Partial agonists such as buprenorphine bind μ receptors with higher affinity than morphine, but activate the receptor and associated G proteins incompletely. The analgesic efficacy curve of partial agonists is bell shaped such that low doses provide increasing levels of analgesia to a point after which additional doses either do not increase pain relief or slightly diminish it.[1,2,14]

Agonist-antagonist-type opioids include butorphanol and nalbuphine. These compounds bind μ and κ receptors subtypes, but differ in activation efficacy. Generally they behave as agonists at κ receptors and antagonists at μ. At low doses, the analgesic properties of mixed agonist-antagonists are comparable to that of weak agonists, such as propoxyphene and codeine; however, at higher doses no additional analgesia is achieved.[1–3,14,22] This phenomenon, termed *the analgesic ceiling effect*, restricts their use to patients with mild to moderate pain.

Antagonists such as naloxone and naltrexone bind to all receptor subtypes with high affinity but do not activate the receptor and G proteins. Antagonists competitively block the activity of agonists by preventing or displacing their binding to the receptor. Although antagonists provide no direct analgesic effects, when administered in low dose they may alter receptor conformation and increase the intrinsic efficacy of opioid agonists.[1,2,14] In this regard, a low-dose continuous infusion of naloxone (0.25 mcg/kg/h) reduced concomitant patient-controlled analgesia (PCA) morphine dose requirements while maintaining equivalent analgesia in patients recovering from hysterectomy.[31] Dose-response curves for opioid agonists and mixed agonists are presented in Figure 13.4.

COMMONLY ADMINISTERED OPIOIDS

Morphine

Morphine remains the standard of comparison of all opioid analgesics and the most widely employed worldwide for acute and chronic pain management.[1–3,14,30,32] Morphine is a nonspecific agonist that binds to μ-, κ-, and δ-receptor subtypes. Clinically, it has moderate analgesic potency, a slow onset to peak effect, and an intermediate duration of activity.[1–2,30] Morphine's delayed onset of analgesia has been related to the fact that it is extremely hydrophilic and has difficulty penetrating the BBB.[1,2,14] Morphine has a variety of uses, including intravenous (IV) sedation, postoperative analgesia, posttrauma pain management, and chronic pain.[2,3,24,30–33]

Morphine is associated with clinically significant dose-dependent adverse effects.[1,2,23] These include annoying side effects, such as nausea, vomiting, and pruritus, and serious, occasionally life-threatening side effects such as excessive sedation and respiratory depression. Oral and IV doses of morphine release histamine, which may precipitate hypotension and bronchospasm.[1,2,23] Morphine also increases smooth muscle tone, and may induce or exacerbate biliary, tubular, and ureteral colic. Like other opioid agonists, morphine's effect on respiratory drive will increase Pa_{CO2} and may raise intracranial pressure.

Morphine undergoes enterohepatic recirculation and is predominately metabolized in the liver via glucoronidation (uridine diphosphate-glucuronosyl transferase).[34] Only 20%–30% of an oral dose of morphine is absorbed from the gastrointestinal tract. The principal hepatic metabolite morphine-6-glucoronide is renally excreted. This metabolite has significant analgesic and respiratory depressant activity and can accumulate and cause adverse events in patients with moderate to severe renal failure.[2,3,33,34] Morphine is available as an oral liquid, oral tablets, controlled release (CR) tablets (MS contin' Kadian[TM], Avinza[TM]), and parenteral injectable.[1,2,30,33]

Oxycodone

Oxycodone is a semisynthetic μ-receptor agonist that is widely prescribed for postoperative pain management.[1–3,23,35] There is some evidence to suggest that oxycodone is primarily a κ agonist.[36] Oxycodone has high oral bioavailability because of rapid gastrointestinal absorption and limited enterohepatic metabolism.[1,2,36] In clinical practice, oxycodone does not release significant amounts of histamine and may cause less sedation than equivalent doses of morphine.[1,23] Oxycodone, like codeine and hydrocodone, is primarily metabolized through the P450 microsomal cytokine P3A4 (CYP3A4) and/or CYP2D6 pathways.[1,2] The use of concomitant medications interacting with these pathways may affect the plasma levels of oxycodone, resulting in reduced analgesia or adverse events. Although most metabolites are inactive, up to 12% of oxycodone is 3-O-demethylated and converted to oxymorphone, a highly active compound.[1,2,37] Oxycodone is a versatile compound, available as an oral tablet, elixer (oxyIR), In Europe, an injectable form of oxycodone is available. Compounds containing oxycodone provide greater analgesic effects than oxycodone alone and include those containing acetaminophen (paracetamol), such as percocet and lortab, or ibuprofen (Combunox[TM]).[38] Controlled-release preparations of oxycodone (CR oxycodone, Oxycontin[TM]) are available and offer prolonged and uniform analgesia, avoiding troughs of effect observed with immediate release (IR) oxycodone. Controlled-release oxycodone has a unique composition, containing an outer rapid-acting component and slow-release inner matrix that provides up to 12 hours of pain relief.[39]

Hydrocodone

Hydrocodone is a μ-selective opioid agonist that is commonly prescribed for inpatient and outpatient acute pain management.

This semisynthetic derivative of codeine provides greater potency and analgesic efficacy, as well as improved tolerability, over that of the parent compound.[1,2,30] Although hydrocodone's oral analgesic potency is equivalent to that of oxycodone, many clinicians in the United States consider it to be a weaker drug with lower abuse potential. Hydrocodone tablets up to 15 mg and total 150 mg/d are less controlled (schedule III) than other semisynthetic opioids and generally do not require triplicate scripts. This lower level of regulation together with hydrocodone's reliability in relieving moderate pain explains why it is so widely prescribed.[1,4,7] Hydrocodone undergoes hepatic O-demethylation by CYP2D6 into the more active opioid, hydromorphone, which is eventually glucoronidated and renally excreted.[1,2,37] Patients who are extensive CYP2D6-hydrocodone metabolizers report greater analgesic benefits and fewer "bad opioid effects" than poor metabolizers.[37]

Hydromorphone

Hydromorphone is a semisynthetic, μ-selective opioid agonist developed in the 1920s and used for treatment of moderate to severe pain. Except for a ketone substitution at the 6 position of the phenanthrene ring, hydromorphone's chemical structure and molecular weight are similar to those of morphine.[1-3] Hydromorphone is less hydrophilic than morphine, and its ability to penetrate the BBB is greater. It has an analgesic potency 5–6 times greater than that of morphine, and its onset of effect is more rapid.[40,41]

Hydromorphone is associated with less histamine release than morphine and is less likely to precipitate hypotension and bronchoconstriction. In the United States, hydromorphone is often substituted for morphine in postsurgical settings. It is particularly useful in patients with severe pain unresponsive to morphine, individuals with high-grade opioid tolerance, and patients suffering adverse events with morphine.[3,33,40,41]

Hydromorphone provides useful IV sedation, postoperative analgesia, and epidural analgesia.[3,40,41] Its side-effect profile is similar to that of other opioids and includes dose-dependent nausea, sedation, and respiratory depression. Hydromorphone appears to have a lower incidence of pruritus and excessive sedation than morphine.[33,41,42]

Hydromorphone's elimination half-life is about 2.5 hours and the parent compound is primarily metabolized in liver by N-demethylation and glucuronidation.[2,3,43,44] Free drug as well as hydromorphone-3-glucuronide are excreted in urine. Drug accumulation and exaggerated effects can be expected in settings of hepatic and renal failure; however, its principal metabolite, hydromorphone-3-glucoronide, is inactive as an opioid. For this reason hydromorphone may be cautiously administered to patients with renal failure, with an increased are under the curve.[44] Hydromorphone is available as oral tablets, oral elixer, and parenteral injectable (Dilaudid). In some counties a controlled release preparation is also available.

Fentanyl

Fentanyl is a synthetic phenylpiperidine class, μ-specific opioid agonist related to meperidine.[1,2] It is highly potent (35–60X morphine) and has a rapid onset and variable dose-dependent duration of effect. Fentanyl's onset is related to its lipophilicity and its ability to rapidly penetrate the BBB and bind opioid receptors in CNS.[1-3] Fentanyl is associated with minimal effects on cardiac output or blood pressure. Because of its hemodynamic stability, it is safer than morphine for patients clinically significant cardiac and cerebral disease.[2,3,33,45] Fentanyl's side-effect profile is lower than that observed with morphine; however, dose-dependent nausea, sedation, and pruritus are commonly observed. Major adverse effects include rapid and profound respiratory depression and chest wall rigidity. Fentanyl is available as an injectable analgesic, transdermal patch, and transmucosal formulations such as the oral lozenge (Actiq™ oralet) and rapidly disintegrating tablet (Fentora™).[1,2]

Oxymorphone

Oxymorphone is a semisynthetic μ-selective opioid agonist related to thebane. Its parenteral potency is high, equivalent to 10 that times of morphine.[1,2,46] As a result of poor gastrointestinal absorption and high enterohepatic metabolism, its oral potency is reduced to one-tenth that of IV oxymorphone, and 3 times that of oral morphine. Like morphine, oxymorphone is primarily metabolized by hepatic glucoronidation.[1-3,46] Available data indicate that oral oxymorphone neither inhibits nor induces CYP450 metabolic pathways nor is it significantly metabolized by CYP450 enzymes.[1,2,4] These properties may offer clinical advantages over oxycodone and codeine for patients requiring nonanalgesic medications metabolized by this pathway.[4,33,46,47] Oxymorphone is available as an oral tablet and parenteral analgesic (Opana IR™, opana injectable). It is also available as a sustained release analgesic that provides a reliable 12-hour duration of effect (Opana ER™).[47] Sustained release oxymorphone is not recommended for surgical pain unless it is expected to be very severe and of prolonged duration.[47]

Methadone

Methadone is a synthetic phenylpropylamide-type opioid agonist with approximately 1.5–2 times the potency of morphine. Following chronic morphine exposure, the relative potency of oral morphine to methadone changes. With low doses, the relative potency is 3 to 1 (<100 mg/d of morphine) but increases to 12:1 with doses of morphine greater than 300mg /d.[1,2] Following oral administration, methadone is well absorbed, having a bioavailability that approaches 80%.[1,2] It also has a large volume of distribution and a very prolonged but variable (12 to 120 hours) plasma elimination half-life.[1,2,3,33]

Methadone dosing is complicated and over- and underdosage is common. Despite its prolonged elimination half-life, methadone's redistribution half-life and duration of effect are more limited. Initial doses provide up to 6 hours of analgesia; however, as the drug accumulates in the tissues, analgesic duration and risk of overdosing may increase substantially.[4,33,48] For this reason, it should only be employed by pain specialists or experienced caregivers. Some clinicians recommend initial once daily or three times daily administration for several days until effective plasma concentrations are achieved.[3,4,13,33] Thereafter, dosing is twice daily. In addition to its activity at opioid receptors, methadone appears to provide additional analgesic effects via interactions with NMDA and α-adrenergic receptors. Methadone has similar dose-dependent side effects as other opioids, particularly sedation, confusion, nausea, and vomiting, but it does not release significant amounts of histamine. Methadone blocks potassium channels expressed in myocardial cells. Therapeutic plasma levels are associated with time-related prolongation of the QTc interval and may initiate or exacerbate torsades de pointes and Wolff-Parkinson-White-type arrhythmias.[1–3,33] To minimize QTc interval prolongation, it is recommended that intravenous doses of methadone be given as a slow infusion rather than as a bolus.[49] A screening electrocardiogram may be necessary to evaluate the QTc interval when methadone doses exceed 60 mg/d.

Parenteral doses of methadone may be effective for patients with opioid tolerance and others suffering severe acute pain who are poorly responsive or unresponsive to morphine and hydromorphone.[4,33] Methadone may be employed as an adjuvant or as primary therapy. Adjuvant doses of 0.1–0.15 mg/kg provide rapid analgesic effects that may dramatically improve the pain relief provided by primary opioids. In acute pain settings, methadone doses of 0.25–0.3 mg/kg employed as monotherapy provide prolonged and highly effective analgesia for up to 24 hours, with many patients not requiring IV PCA opioids.[51,52] Following lower abdominal surgery, patients administered parenteral methadone (20 mg) intraoperatively followed by "as needed" (PRN) doses on the postanesthesia care unit reported less pain and need for supplemental opioids than others treated with similar doses of morphine.[51] In a very large 3954-inpatient series, methadone was effective for patients suffering prolonged and very painful postsurgical and medical-related acute pain.[53] Methadone is also advocated for patients suffering nerve injuries and neuropathic pain, as well as individuals who are highly opioid dependent or opioid hyperalgesic.[1,4,33,54,55] Plasma concentrations following an IV bolus dose of methadone as compared with morphine and fentanyl are presented in Figure 13.4.

Methadone is metabolized by the hepatic microsomal enzyme system undergoing N-demethylation or deamination into inactive compounds. Methadone is available as an injectable (Dolophine[TM]), oral elixir, or 20- to 40-mg oral tablet.

Meperidine

Meperidine is a weak phenylpiperidine-type opioid agonist with oral and parenteral potencies equivalent to one-tenth that of morphine.[1,2,3,27] Its analgesic onset is slightly more rapid than morphine; however, its duration of effect is only two-thirds as long. Meperidine was initially developed as an anticholinergic and provides a smooth muscle relaxing effect.[1,2,13,50] For this reason, it was initially advocated for controlling visceral pain and associated spasms. Meperidine is less commonly used in the United States as its renally cleared metabolite, normeperidine, is associated with anxiety, tremors, myoclonus, and seizures.[1,2,27,50] It should never be considered for chronic pain management.[4,33] Doses exceeding 1 gm/d or administration in patients with renal failure may result in neurotoxicity secondary to rising plasma concentrations of normeperidine. Meperidine elevates serotonin levels and can precipitate a serotonergic crisis when combined with other drugs that elevate serotonin such as monoamine oxidases.[50] Meperidine is available as an injectable or immediate release tablet (demerol).

Codeine

Codeine is a naturally occurring opiate-derived analgesic that is one-third to one-fourth as potent as morphine.[1–3] Codeine is used primarily in patients recovering from dental and ear-nose-and-throat (ENT) surgery. It offers no clinical advantages over semisynthetic ketone-substituted derivatives such as hydrocodone and oxycodone. Its analgesic efficacy is inferior to that of oxycodone, whereas its side-effect profile, particularly nausea and vomiting, is higher.[1–3,33,27] Codeine is a prodrug that must be metabolized to morphine by CYP2D6 to achieve analgesic effect.[1,2,13,27] This enzyme is very polymorphic, with most patients being rapid or intermediate metabolizers.[1,2,27] Approximately 20% of individuals are poor codeine metabolizers who are at have a high incidence of analgesic failure. Other patients may be extensive metabolizers who have an increased risk of excessive sedation and respiratory depression. Codeine is primarily administered as an oral tablet compounded with acetaminophen (Tylenol #3).

Butorphanol

Butorphanol is a synthetic mixed agonist-antagonist-type opioid. Low doses ranging from 2 to 4 mg are twice as potent as similar doses of morphine; however, higher doses are progressively less effective and are associated with increased sedation and dysphoria.[1,2,13,27] In the United States, butorphanol is used as a substitute for meperidine in patients complaining of moderate pain. Butorphanol and other mixed agonist-antagonists appear to be more effective in female patients and are primarily prescribed for visceral pain and headache.[51] It is used to control pain associated with ureteral and gall stones and is also employed for labor and delivery analgesia. Butorphanol is available as an injectable (Stadol[TM]) or nasal spray (Nasal Stadol[TM]).[1] Other mixed agonist-antagonists, such as nalbuphine and pentazocine, offer no clinical advantages over butorphanol, are rarely used, and are not discussed.

Tramadol

Tramadol is a weak μ-receptor opioid agonist with equivalent potency to codeine. Tramadol also has α-adrenergic analgesic effects that complement opioid-mediated effects.[1,2,13,33,52] It is not recommended for severe acute pain, but, is used for mild to moderate discomfort following minor surgery. In acute pain settings, doses of tramadol should not exceed 300 mg/d, and it should not be prescribed to patients taking monoamine oxidase inhibitors as it may induce psychotic behavior.[1–3,44] Tramadol is metabolized by CYP2D6 into an active metabolite that is 5 times as powerful as the parent compound. This O-demethylated metabolite has 200 times greater μ-receptor affinity, 2–4 times greater potency, and a longer half-life.[1,2,27,33,53,54] Like codeine, approximately 20% of individuals have CYP2D6 enzyme polymorphisms that result in poor metabolism. These patients cannot form the active metabolite, and are at increased risk for analgesic failure.[1,2,53,54] In the United States, tramadol is available only as an oral immediate release and controlled release preperations (Ultram[TM]).

Sufentanil

Sufentanil is a synthetic μ-specific opioid agonist related to fentanyl with extremely high potency, 500 to 700 times greater than that of morphine.[1,2,27] Sufentanil has high lipid solubility and opioid receptor affinity. It has an extremely rapid onset, powerful analgesic effect, and variable dose-dependent duration of effect. Sufentanil is associated with the least cardiac depression and has minimal to mild effects on blood pressure. For this reason it may offer a safer alternative to morphine for patients with cardiac and cerebral disease. This powerful opioid should be reserved for painful procedures/dressing changes or IV sedation and pain control in ventilator-dependent patients.

Buprenorphine

Buprenorphine is a partial agonist-type opioid that has been widely used as an intravenous analgesic in the EU. It exerts its analgesic effect via high affinity binding to μ receptors and very slow dissociation.[1,2,13,54] Nearly 100% of available μ-opioid receptors may be occupied following administration of 16 mg of sublingual buprenorphine.[1,54] As a result of buprenorphine's high receptor affinity and occupation rate, greater than normal doses of agonists or antagonists are required to displace it from opioid receptors.

A sublingual formulation of buprenorphine is commonly used as maintenance therapy for opioid-dependent patients. Patients presenting for surgery should continue taking this formulation during the perioperative period in addition to pain control provided by either neuraxial or regional techniques and nonopioid analgesics. Alternatively, patients treated with buprenorphine can be converted to 30–40 mg of methadone per day 1 week prior to surgery to prevent withdrawal and to avoid antagonism of standard opioid analgesics.[54]

Buprenorphine is supplied as a parenteral analgesic that can be administered subcutaneously IV and intramuscularly (IM). Buprenorphine is not available as an oral analgesic, as it is very poorly absorbed from the gastrointestinal tract, but a sublingual tablet is available. Analgesic doses for a variety of opioid agonists is presented in Table 13.4.

PARENTERAL OPIOID THERAPY

Because oral analgesics generally have low bioavailability and delayed onset and are poorly tolerated during the immediate postoperative period, parenterally (IV) administered opioids are commonly prescribed for pain management.[55] There are several situations where parenteral opioids are employed: (1) They are useful for patients advancing from IV PCA or epidural opioid based analgesia, who have moderate to severe discomfort, but have yet to tolerate oral diets. Parenteral dosing is of particular importance in patients who are nauseous or vomiting and therefore who might not absorb oral agents. (2) Several subsets of patients, including the elderly, the cognitively impaired, and overly dependent individuals, are poor candidates for IV PCA and may achieve better pain control with intravenous/intramuscular opioids administered by the clock or PRN. In these individuals, parenteral opioid requirements during early postoperative intervals may be used to provide a conversion guide for oral analgesic dosing that follows.[55–57] (3) Patients treated with continuous neural blockade or epidural analgesia may require occasional PRN doses of parenteral opioids for breakthrough pain control. The amount of opioid required during the first 24 hours of recovery may be so low as not to justify initiating IV PCA. Thereafter, patients may be advanced to oral opioids if required for breakthrough pain. Exceptions to this rule are opioid-dependent patients with significant tolerance development who, in addition to epidural or peripheral neural blockade for surgical pain, may require both IV PCA or parenteral opioid infusions for baseline pain management. (4) Patients recovering from ambulatory procedures generally require intravenous boluses of fentanyl, morphine, or

hydromorphone until stabilized and advanced to oral opioids. (5) High-risk patients and others who recover in the surgical intensive care unit (ICU) often require hemodynamic stabilization and postoperative ventilation and may not be candidates for IV or epidural PCA. These individuals may be treated with intravenous infusions of fentanyl, sufentanil, or hydromorphone that provide surgical analgesia, sedation, and improved tolerability of endotracheal intubation.[56,57]

Morphine remains the standard parenteral opioid analgesic for control of acute pain following surgical and traumatic injuries.[1,2,27,33] Ten milligrams of parenteral morphine is generally recommended as a starting dose for acute pain management in patients with a body weight over 50 kg.[1–3] More recent guidelines suggest that the initial bolus dose should be smaller (3–5 mg) and repeated in rapid succession until the patient is more comfortable.[3] Onset of analgesia with IV morphine is noted within 5–15 minutes, whereas duration ranges from 1 to 3 hours, depending on dose administered. We often employ small doses of IV morphine (2–5 mg every 1–2 hours) for breakthrough pain in patients treated with continuous regional blockade and epidural analgesia.[56] Parenteral boluses of morphine may also be administered to patients who were initially treated with IV PCA morphine or epidural analgesia yet remain nil per os (NPO).

Hydromorphone, oxymorphone, and, to a lesser extent, meperidine offer therapeutic alternatives for patients experiencing inadequate pain control with morphine or intolerant of its adverse effects. Meperidine's parenteral potency is one-tenth that of morphine with a duration of effect that is only two-thirds as long, thus doses of 100 to 120 mg may be required every 3 hours.[1,2,27,33] As mentioned previously, anecdotal reports suggest that meperidine is most effective in controlling visceral cramping and colicky pain. In this regard, we occasionally administer doses ranging from 75 to 150 mg to patients recovering from open cholycystectomy, ovarian and tubular procedures, and bladder surgery.[56] Despite its smooth muscle relaxation effects, meperidine is reported to be no more efficacious in treating biliary tract spasm than comparable doses of other μ opioids.[1–3] Nevertheless, we have found that, in some patients, low doses of meperidine (50–100 mg) are more effective than morphine in controlling visceral discomfort associated with acute pancreatitis and cholelithiasis.[56]

Intravenous hydromorphone has a more rapid onset of analgesia, a lower incidence of adverse effects, and a slightly shorter duration of effect than morphine.[1–3,13,57] Following IV administration, analgesic onset is noted in 2–5 minutes and peak effect in 10–15 minutes and duration averages 3.5 hours.[13,57] Parenteral doses of hydromorphone are a better choice than morphine for patients with very severe pain and offer a logical transitional analgesic for patients treated with IV PCA hydromorphone.[56] Because of the high concentration of marketed solutions (2–4 mg/mL), hydromorphone may also be administered subcutaneously with minimal discomfort to patients.

Oxymorphone has been available since the early 1960s and is currently marketed as a 1-mg vial for acute pain management. Oxymorphone's onset to peak effect is more rapid than that of morphine and its overall analgesic efficacy is superior.[46,58,59] Intravenous oxymorphone may be effectively employed in the postanesthesia care unit (PACU) for patients experiencing very severe pain. Rather than spending considerable time titrating repetitive doses of morphine to patients with high-grade opioid tolerance and others recovering from extremely painful procedures, 1–2 mg of IV oxymorphone can be administered to rapidly establish a powerful level of analgesia.[46] Onset is noted with 5 minutes, and, unlike fentanyl, the duration of effect may be prolonged for several hours.[57] For this reason it has been nicknamed the "fire extinguisher" by our PACU nurses.[56]

Parenteral doses of methadone are also advocated for patients with opioid tolerance and others suffering severe acute pain that is poorly responsive or unresponsive to morphine and hydromorphone. Methadone may be employed as an adjuvant or as primary therapy. Adjuvant doses of 0.1 mg/kg or less provide rapid analgesic effects that can augment the pain relief provided by primary opioids. In acute pain settings, methadone doses of 0.25–0.3 mg/kg employed as monotherapy provide prolonged and highly effective analgesia for up to 12 hours, with patients requiring little to no supplementation with IV PCA opioids.[60,61] Following lower abdominal surgery, patients treated with parenteral methadone (20 mg) intraoperatively followed by PRN doses in PACU reported less pain and need for supplemental opioids than others treated with similar doses of morphine.[60] Methadone was highly effective (85% achieving satisfactory pain relief) for patients suffering prolonged and very painful postsurgical and medical-related acute pain.[62] Methadone is also advocated for patients suffering nerve injuries and neuropathic pain, as well as individuals who are highly opioid dependent or opioid hyperalgesic.[62–64] Theoretical plasma concentrations following an IV bolus dose of methadone as compared with morphine and fentanyl is presented are Figure 13.4.

Fentanyl is best employed in patients with marked hemodynamic instability or well-documented allergies to naturally occurring or semisynthetic morphinians.[1–3,33,65] It is employed in two primary settings: (1) Doses of 50–200 μcg are commonly administered to patients recovering from ambulatory surgery and provide analgesia of rapid onset but short duration. Similar doses offer effective pain relief for patients requiring closed reductions and dressing changes.[56] (2) Intravenous infusions of fentanyl (0.5–5 μcg/kg/h) may be used to provide sedation and pain control for ventilated patients in the surgical ICU. In this setting, IV fentanyl infusions (1–2 μcg/kg/h) are often employed as a substitute for IV PCA in sedated, hemodynamically unstable, and ventilator-dependent patients.[56] Infusion rates are increased or diminished in response to inadequate pain control or to minimize adverse events. In addition, bolus doses of fentanyl (25–50 mcg), hydromorphone (0.5–1 mg), or methadone (5 mg) may be administered for breakthrough pain. The quality of analgesia provided by IV fentanyl infusions is excellent and equivalent to comparable doses administered epidurally, but with less pruritus.[65]

Fentanyl has recently been formulated as a patient-controlled transdermal system (Ionsys PCTS) that employs a low-intensity current to electrophorese the drug onto the skin, where it diffuses into the local circulation (see Chapter 20, *Novel Analgesic Drug Delivery Systems for Acute Pain Management*).

Buprenorphine is employed as a parenteral analgesic in the EU.[1,2,54,66,67] In an evaluation of PCA buprenorphine and morphine, both drugs provided adequate postoperative analgesia with no differences in visual analog pain scores, adverse events, and hospitalization period. Intravenous bolus doses of buprenorphine range from 5 to 15 mcg/kg.[67,68] Buprenorphine can also be administered intramuscularly. With this route analgesic onset is noted at 15 minutes, peak effect occurs at 1 hour, and the duration of action is 6 hours. Buprenorphine is also an effective analgesic when given subcutaneously and is particularly useful in patients with poor intravenous access.

The analgesic effectiveness of parenteral opioids may be potentiated with small doses of anticholinergic/antihistaminics, such as phenergan and vistaril; however, increased levels of sedation should be expected.[1,2,3,13,33] Other complications associated with parenteral opioids include respiratory depression, nausea and vomiting, pruritus, and postoperative bowel dysfunction.

ORAL ANALGESIC DOSING

Moderate to severe pain can persist for several days to weeks following major surgery. During the immediate postoperative period, anesthetic and surgical alterations in gastrointestinal function and perfusion markedly reduce the reliability and effectiveness of oral analgesics.[1–3,4,69] Once patients are able to tolerate a liquid diet they should be advanced to oral opioids, which should be continued during the convalescent and rehabilitative periods following surgery. Oral administration offers a safe, convenient, noninvasive, and cost-effective method of controlling acute pain that should always be considered in patients who continue to experience moderate to severe pain.[4,69]

Oral opioids, including morphine, meperidine, hydrocodone, and oxycodone, and compounded preparations containing acetaminophen, aspirin, and ibuprofen provide effective relief for patients complaining of moderate to severe pain. Orally administered morphine and meperidine are poorly absorbed and undergo significant enterohepatic metabolism. When compared to parenteral dosing, onset is delayed, duration is less predictable, and dose requirements are increased. In this regard, equianalgesic oral morphine and meperidine doses are 2–3 times higher than parenteral requirements.[1–3,13,33] McCormack and colleagues[69] evaluated the efficacy and tolerability of oral versus IM morphine in patients recovering from total hip arthroplasty. Patients in the oral and IM group received a 20-mg loading dose followed by 10 mg every 4 hours in blinded fashion. Although the incidence of adverse events was similar in both groups, patients treated with oral morphine reported lower pain intensity scores and required significantly less breakthrough medication during the first 48 hours.[69] Because oral morphine is inexpensive and effective, the authors suggested that it be considered an analgesic option for patients able to tolerate a liquid diet. In our experience, morphine oral elixir (20–40 mg) every 3–4 hours is generally more effective and better tolerated during the immediate postoperative period than similar doses of morphine tablets

Oxycodone and hydrocodone are more reliably absorbed than morphine, undergo limited first-pass glucoronidation, and have active metabolites that are more potent than their parent compounds.[1–3,27,70] Although parenteral forms of oxycodone are available in the EU,[70] only oral forms of administration have been approved for use in the United States.[1,2] Following oral administration, both oxycodone and hydrocodone have a rapid and predicable onset at 35 minutes, a peak effect at 60 minutes, and a duration of 3.5–4 hours.[1,2,3] Oral compounds containing oxycodone or hydrocodone with acetaminophen offer more effective analgesia than either opioid administered alone.[1,2] These preparations are well tolerated by patients recently advanced to oral diets and generally provide a smooth analgesic transition from IV PCA. They are also among the most widely prescribed analgesics for pain following hospital discharge. Nevertheless, the potential hepatotoxicity associated with acetaminophen-containing compounds places restrictions on the number of tablets that can be taken as well as total opioid dose. As a result, opioid dose can be subtherapeutic in selected patients.

Oral forms of oxycodone and hydrocodone compounded with ibuprofen have recently been formulated. The oxycodone compound (Combunox™) contains oxycodone (5 mg) and ibuprofen (400 mg) and is approved for short-term (7 days or less) management of acute and postoperative pain.[33,71] In a controlled evaluation of women recovering from abdominal surgery, compounded oxycodone plus ibuprofen provided superior pain relief, decreased the need for rescue opioids, and reduced the incidence of nausea and vomiting when compared to either oxycodone or ibuprofen alone. Oxycodone plus ibuprofen also had a more rapid onset of analgesia (22 min), and more prolonged duration of effect (7 hours) than either of its constituents.[71] The authors concluded that reductions nausea may be the result of opioid sparing, that is, a reduced need for rescue oxycodone, as well as ibuprofen's ability to block prostaglandin E_2 synthesis in the brainstem emesis center.

An oral compound containing hydrocodone (7.5 mg) plus ibuprofen (200 mg) is also available for short-term acute pain management and provides superior analgesia than hydrocodone alone. In a randomized controlled trial, this preparation was compared to an oxycodone (10 mg) plus acetaminophen (325 mg) compound and placebo for pain control following gynecologic surgery.[72] Patients treated with hydrocodone/ibuprofen experienced analgesia equivalent to those treated with higher doses of oxycodone and superior to individuals treated with placebo. One possible drawback of this preparation is that a 200-mg dose of ibuprofen may be inadequate to control the inflammatory aspects of acute surgical pain. A second potential drawback of this compound, as well as the previously mentioned oxycodone/ibuprofen preparation, is its nonselective nonsteroidal anti-inflammatory drugs (NSAID) component, which can increase risks of postsurgical bleeding and renal failure in susceptable patients.[73]

Oral immediate-release oxymorphone (Opana™) has recently been approved and is indicated for the relief of moderate to severe acute pain where the use of an opioid is appropriate.[4,47] Immediate-release oxymorphone was clinically evaluated in over 550 patients experiencing moderate to severe acute pain following abdominal and orthopedic surgeries.[74,75] In these trials, oxymorphone provided effective pain relief and was generally well tolerated. Absorption was rapid following oral administration with median time to peak concentration (T_{max}) of 0.5 hours. Its elimination half-life of 7 to 9 hours makes it well suited for dosing every 6 hours.[47,74] In a clinical trial of 300 patients recovering from orthopedic surgery, doses of immediate-release oxymorphone (10 and 20 mg) provided superior pain control and a more prolonged duration of effect than oxycodone (7.5 mg) or placebo.[75]

Sustained-release opioid preparations, including morphine (MS-contin), oxycodone (Oxycontin™), and oxymorphone (Opana ER™), offer several advantages, including less frequent administration intervals, avoidance of peak and trough plasma levels, and greater analgesic uniformity (Figure 13.5). These preparations provide 8–12 hours of pain relief and are best suited for patients suffering severe and prolonged postoperative pain.[47,76,77] Although not specifically approved for this indication, CR oxycodone has been prescribed for patients with

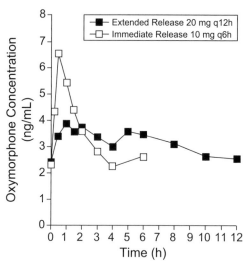

Figure 13.5: Plasma concentrations of oral IR oxymorphone and ER oxymorphone. The IR preparation was associated with a rapid onset to peak plasma concentration, T_{max}. The ER preparation avoided a high maximum concentration (C_{max}) and resulted in a more uniform plasma level for an extended duration of time. (McIlwain H, Ahdieh H. Safety, tolerability, and effectiveness of oxymorphone extended release for moderate to severe osteoarthritis pain: a one-year study. *Am J Ther.* 2005;12:106–112.)

severe pain during rehabilitation and for patients with significant opioid tolerance. In a randomized, open-label, multiple-dose study, patients treated with CR oxycodone administered every 12 hours following outpatient anterior cruciate ligament surgery benefited from more effective analgesia with fewer adverse effects than others receiving IR oxycodone prescribed either as fixed doses or PRN.[78] In a postoperative dose conversion study, Ginsberg and colleagues[79] evaluated the analgesic equivalency of CR oxycodone in patients discontinuing IV PCA. They found that the initial dose of CR oxycodone needed to maintain effective pain control was only 1.3–1.5 times higher than the prior day's dose of morphine (Table 13.5). We have found that the relationship is closer to 1:1, that is, if on the previous day the patient required 40 mg of IV morphine, the initial dose of CR oxycodone is 40 mg/d or 20 mg twice a day.[56]

An additional opioid preparation that may be considered for patients who cannot tolerate oral analgesics but continue to experience brief episodes of severe pain is fentanyl oralet (Actiq™). Fentanyl oralet releases between 100 and 400 μcg of fentanyl within 15 minutes with high bioavailability. Although not approved for acute pain management, this preparation can provide effective acute pain control when given 20–30 minutes prior to short painful procedures, such as closed reduction, dressing changes, and chest tube placement.[56]

Less potent opioid analgesics, such as tramadol and codeine, may be prescribed to patients recovering from dental and ENT surgeries and medical procedures associated with mild to moderate pain. A newer compounded form of tramadol (Ultracet™) provides greater effectiveness than tramadol. Ultracet is an oral, multimodal analgesic containing tramadol plus acetaminophen, approved for the short-term management of acute pain. In clinical trials tramadol (37.5 mg) plus acetaminophen (325 mg) compound was found as effective as hydrocodone (10 mg) and acetaminophen (650 mg), and superior to placebo

Table 13.5: Initial CR Oxycodone Dose and Current Pain Intensity at Baseline and 6 Hours after Initial CR Oxycodone Dose[a,b]

Surgery Type	n	IV Morphine in Prior 24 Hours (mg)	Initial CR Oxycodone Dose (mg Every 12 Hours)	Current Pain Intensity		P Value[c]
				Baseline	6 h Postdose	
Abdominal	44	$51 \pm .4$	27 ± 2	4.3 ± 0.4	2.9 ± 0.4	.0014
Orthopedic	42	$59 + 6$	34 ± 3	4.2 ± 0.4	3.5 ± 0.4	.1096
Gynecologic	29	39 ± 4	26 ± 3	3.9 ± 0.5	3.3 ± 0.4	.1444
All	116	51 ± 3	$29 \pm$	4.1 ± 0.2	3.3 ± 0.2	.0003

[a] Results are presented as mean $\pm$ SE.

[b] For those patients with both baseline and hour 6 pain intensity assessments only. Patients assessed pain intensity using an 11-point numerical scale of 0 = no pain to 10 = worst possible pain.

[c] Paired t test of change from baseline to hour 6. Modified from Ginsberg B et al (2003).[79]

in reducing pain following molar extraction surgery.[80] Tramadol/acetaminophen was better tolerated, having a lower incidence of nausea (19% vs 36%) and vomiting (12% vs 30%). When combined with an NSAID this compound offers significant multimodal benefits including μ-opioid, α-adrenergic, and acetaminophen-mediated analgesia as well as anti-inflammatory effects. These potentially additive analgesic effects may obviate the need to administer more potent opioids.

When initiating oral opioid therapy, the clinician should select a dosage and frequency based on the intensity of postsurgical pain, patient age, the presence of comorbid medical conditions, any concomitant therapy, and chronic opioid exposure.[3,13,27,33] Dosing and frequency recommendations should also be consistent with the manufacturer's prescribing information.

One may categorize parenteral opioids as first-tier agonists, such as hydrocodone, which are generally effective for opioid-naive patients with moderate to severe pain; more potent second-tier agonists, such as morphine and hydromorphone, for severe pain; and third-tier agonists, like oxymorphone, methadone, and fentanyl, for poorly controlled severe to very severe pain and for highly tolerant individuals.

The clinician must have a firm understanding of opioid dose equivalency and how to calculate parenteral to oral dose conversions. Equianalgesia refers to differences in opioid dose requirements necessary to provide equal levels of analgesia.[33,81] Equianalgesic dosing tables have been developed to aid with dosing conversions; however, they offer only approximate guidelines. Values provided in these tables are primarily based on single-dose evaluations and do not compensate for drug accumulation or active metabolites.[1,33,81] In postoperative settings, when converting from parenteral opioid such as hydromorphone to a different oral opioid, such as oxycodone, the clinician must compensate for differences in potency prior to calculating parenteral to oral dose equivalency. As a general rule, it is prudent to administer an initial IV to oral conversion dose somewhat 25%–33% lower than the calculated dose.[33,56] This more conservative approach offers greater patient safety by compensating for progressive reductions in postsurgical pain intensity and opioid requirements, as well as potentially greater analgesia efficacy gained by switching opioids (opioid rotation). An opioid potency and equianalgesic dosing table used by the Yale Pain Management Service[56] is presented in Table 13.6.

Short-acting oral opioids agents, such as IR morphine, IR hydrocodone, IR hydromorphone, IR oxycodone, and IR oxymorphone, may be favored initially because they are easy to titrate.[27,33] These agents are best employed in opioid-naive patients recovering from uncomplicated procedures that require relatively limited durations of treatment. Following extensive surgery with severe discomfort and prolonged and painful convalescence, sustained-release opioids may be considered. Short-acting opioids are characterized by a rapid rise and fall in serum opioid levels, whereas serum levels of sustained-release opioids increase slowly to therapeutic levels, remain there for an extended period, and then decline slowly (Figure 13.5).[76] With extensive and painful surgeries, we advance patients from epidural analgesia to CR oxycodone or CR morphine (10–15 mg twice a day) as well as IR oxycodone for breakthrough pain.[56] Such therapy is maintained for 3–7 days and is more likely to be effective than PRN doses of IR oxycodone or morphine alone. We also employ CR opioids to facilitate weaning opioid-dependent patients off of IV PCA.[56] Most opioid-dependent patients are treated with PCA for surgical pain plus a basal opioid infusion that controls their baseline chronic pain. Prior to weaning we initiate oral CR opioids in doses equivalent to the basal infusion. The basal infusion is discontinued and the patient is allowed to use PCA for an additional 8–24 hours. After this interval, PCA is discontinued and equivalent doses of IR oxycodone, hydrocodone, or morphine are substituted and administered PRN. Generally we are conservative when switching from IV to oral dosing and actually prescribe only one-half to two-thirds the equianalgesic dose.[47] For example, if after starting CR opioids, the patient has self-administered an additional 40 mg of morphine over 24 hours the equivalent dose of oral morphine required to replace PCA needs would be 120 mg over 24 hours (based on a 3:1 oral to IV dosing ratio). To assure patient safety, consider dosing only 60–90 mg morphine. If pain relief is inadequate, additional morphine may be provided as needed.

OPIOID-RELATED ADVERSE EVENTS

In settings of acute pain, most opioid-related adverse events are transient and tend to resolve with ongoing treatment.[2,3,73,74] Common adverse events associated with parenteral and orally administered opioids and their active metabolites include nausea, vomiting, sedation, pruritus, and constipation. In sensitive

Table 13.6: Equianalgesic Dosing Table

Dosing Guidelines for Oral and Parenteral Opioids

Opioid	Route	Potency	Dose (mg)	Onset	Duration	Metabolism	Comments
Morphine	PO	0.3	30 (15–45)	45 min	4–5 h	Glucoronidation	Poor oral effect
Morphine	IV	1.0	10 (5–15)	10 min	3.5–4 h	Glucoronidation	Histamine release
Meperidine	PO	0.02	200 (1–300)	45 min	3.5 h	N-demethylation	Toxic Metabolite
Meperidine	IV	0.1	100 (75–125)	10 min	3 h	N-demethylation	For visceral pain
Hydrocodone	PO	0.6	15 (7.5–15)	35 min	4–6 h	CYP450	Similar to oxycodone
Oxycodone	PO	0.8	10 (5–15)	30 min	4–6 h	CYP450	Good oral analgesic
Codeine	PO	0.2	50 (30–70)	45 min	3.5 h	CYP450	High side effect profile
Methadone	PO	1.0	10 (7.5–15)	10–20 min	6–8 h	Demethylation	Prolonged elimination
Methadone	IV	1.5	7.5 (5–10)	5–10 min	6–8 h	Demethylation	Difficult to titrate
Hydromorphone	PO	1.5	15 (7.5–15)	35 min	3.5–4 h	Glucoronidation	Well tolerated
Hydromorphone	IV	5.0	2 (1–3)	10–15 min	3.5–4 h	Glucoronidation	Useful for severe pain
Oxymorphone	PO	1.0	10 (5–15)	30 min	5–6 h	Glucoronidation	Useful for severe pain
Oxymorphone	IV	10	1 (0.5–2)	5–10 min	4 h	Demethylation	Useful for severe pain
Fentanyl	PO	40	0.2–0.4 mcg	5–10 min	60 min	Demethylation	Rapid onset
Fentanyl	IV	70	0.1–150 mcg	3–5 min	30 min	Demethylation	Very rapid onset
Tramadol	PO	0.1	100 (1–125)	40 min	4–6 h	O-demethylation	For mild-moderate pain

Note: Values listed represent approximations based on single dose calculations. According to this conversion scheme, IV morphine is assigned a potency of 1, whereas oral morphine is considered 0.3, because of its poor bioavailability and higher dose requirement. Methadone values represent single dose effects, accumulation of drug and duration of action will increase with continued dosing. To calculate oral to oral dose conversions, determine the prior 24-hour opioid dose (both scheduled and rescue doses) and then dose the new opioid according to the PO equianalgesic dose and potency listed above. Use the following proportion: potency of current opioid over 24 hour dose of current opioid vs potency of the new opioid over 24 hr dose of the new opioid (X). Solve for X by cross multiplying. Divide the 24-hour dose and administer as increments according to the duration of action of the new drug. For patient safety, we recommend using $\frac{1}{4}$ to $\frac{1}{3}$ less drug than the amount calculated. To calculate approximate IV to oral equianalgesic dose, use the table and multiply the potency of the currently used IV opioid by the prior 24-hour dose in milligrams and then divide this value by the potency of the PO opioid the patient will be converted to. This value is administered in divided doses based on the duration of the oral opioid. To provide greater patient safety divide this calculated dose by $\frac{1}{3}$ to $\frac{1}{2}$ and gauge its effectiveness. Subsequent dosing may be increased or decreased as necessary. Adapted from Reisine and Pasternak (1997),[1] Gutstein and Akil (2002),[2] Pasero et al (1999),[3] Fine and Portenoy (2004),[33] Mahler and Forrest (1975),[40] Palangio et al (2000),[72] Gordon et al (1999).[81]

individuals, the incidence and severity of these adverse events (AEs) may be so annoying and distressing that patients self-limit or discontinue opioid dosing and suffer poor pain control. Patients recovering from abdominal and gynecological surgery are generally at risk for opioid-induced bowel dysfunction and ileus, mandating that such therapy be supplemented with stool softeners, bulk laxatives, and occasional enemas. Most opioid-related AEs are dose dependent, which is why it is important to initiate therapy with the lowest effective dose and to utilize a multimodal analgesic approach. Some opioid-related AEs are often treated symptomatically, for example, by prescribing an antiemetic for nausea or a laxative for constipation.[82] Other side effects, such as sedation and pruritus, are typically addressed by decreasing the opioid dose rather than by treating the symptom.[82,83] In addition to dose reductions, other strategies that can be employed to minimize opioid-related AEs include changing the route of administration, switching to a different opioid or providing specialized pharmacologic therapy. Opioid-induced nausea and vomiting is perhaps the most troubling AE observed with oral and parenteral dosing.[82,83] We recommend aggressive treatment in highly symptomatic individuals, including opioid rotation and treatment with parenteral or rapidly disintegrating lingual ondansetron in doses of 4–8 mg.[27,33,84]

FUTURE DIRECTIONS WITH ORAL AND PARENTERAL OPIOIDS FOR ACUTE PAIN

In the near future improved and more selective opioid analgesics may be developed that better suit individual patient needs.[85]

1   Translation of research describing opioid receptor polymorphisms and genetic variations in metabolic enzymes[18–22] may spur the clinical development of novel agonists that provide optimal pain control with lowest side effect for patients with differing genetic profiles.

2   Rapidly disintegrating and readily absorbed lingual and buccal preparations avoid gastric absorption and first-pass hepatic and offer advantages of convenience and rapid analgesic onset. Although originally developed for breakthrough chronic pain, these routes of delivery may become available for acute pain management. Nasal and pulmonary delivered opioid preparations offer similar advantages as well as convenience and may displace the need for IV dosing and possibly IV PCA in patients who remain NPO.[86] It is not known whether these preparations will be associated with nasal irritation, epistaxis, or bronchospasm. The use of a morphine metabolite, morphine-6-glucoronide (M6G), may become

available as an alternative to morphine.[87] In a recent clinical trial in patients recovering from knee replacement surgery, doses of M6G provided significant morphine PCA-sparing effects with high tolerability and safety.[75]

3 Improved formulations may provide analgesic potentiation and opioid-sparing effects by compounding mixtures of opioids with NSAIDS, α_2 reuptake inhibitors (tapentadol), and α_2-δ antagonists. Peripherally acting κ-receptor agonists have been proposed that could provide effective relief of visceral pain (Ob-GYN, GU-renal colic), with low risk of μ-mediated respiratory depression.

4 Opioids formulated in crush-resistant, water-insoluble tablets may provide a lower risk for diversion, adulteration, and abuse (eg, snorting, injecting). Tablets containing mixtures of an agonist plus an antagonist, which are released if the tablet is adulterated are also being studied.

CONCLUSION

Parenteral and oral opioids remain the foundation for optimal acute pain management. Although more technologically sophisticated and invasive modalities, such as neuraxial and PCA-administered opioids, may provide superior analgesic efficacy the majority of patients experiencing acute pain are treated with oral or parenteral opioids.

Existing parenteral and oral analgesics offer effective pain relief; however, no agonist provides the optimal combination of high efficacy and low side effect profile for all patients. The application of new knowledge in receptor polymorphisms, novel delivery systems for existing opioids, and future development of new compounds will provide the pain specialist, surgeon, and primary care physician with powerful new tools for controlling moderate to severe pain.

REFERENCES

1. Reisine T, Pasternak G. Opioid analgesics and antagonists. In Goodman LS, Gilman A, eds. *The Pharmacologic Basis of Therapeutics.* 9th ed. New York, NY: Macmillan; 1997.

2. Gutstein HB, Akil H. Opioid analgesics. In: Hardman JG, Limbird LE, Gilman AG, eds. *Goodman & Gilman's The Pharmacological Basis of Therapeutics.* 10th ed. New York, NY: McGraw-Hill; 2002:569–619.

3. Pasero C, Portenoy RK, McCaffery M. Opioid analgesics. In: McCaffery M, Pasero C, eds. *Pain Clinical Manual.* St. Louis, MO: Mosby Inc, 1999:161–299.

4. Sinatra RS. Opioid analgesics in primary care: challenges and new advances in the management of noncancer pain. *Journal of the American Board of Family Medicine.* 2006;19(2):165–177.

5. Meldrum ML. A capsule history of pain management. *JAMA.* 2003;290:2470–2475.

6. Gilson AM, Joranson DE. Controlled substances and pain management: changes in knowledge and attitudes of state medical regulators. *J Pain Symptom Manage.* 2001;21:227–237.

7. Gilson AM, Joranson DE. U.S. policies relevant to the prescribing of opioid analgesics for the treatment of pain in in patients with addictive disease. *Clin J Pain.* 2002;18:S91–S98.

8. American Society of Anesthesiologists. A report by the American Society of Anesthesiologists Task Force on Pain Management, Chronic Pain Section. *Anesthesiology.* 1997;86:995–1004.

9. Joint Commission on Accreditation of Healthcare Organizations. JCAHO Standards for Pain Management [referenced from the Comprehensive Accreditation Manual for Hospitals, Update 3, 1999 (effective January 1, 2001)]. Available at: //www.texmed. org/has/prs/pop/jps.asp. Accessed August 5, 2003.

10. Kweder SL. USFDA Statement before Subcommittee on criminal justice, drug abuse, and human resources. Available at: //www. fda.gov/ola/2006/rxdrug abuse. 0726. Accessed July 26, 2006.

11. Sinatra RS, Bigham M: The anatomy and pathophysiology of acute pain. In: Grass JA, ed. *Problems in Anesthesiology.* Vol. 10. Philadelphia, PA: Lippincott-Raven; 1997:8–22.

12. Bonica JJ. Biochemistry and modulation of nociception and pain. In: Bonica, JJ, ed. *The Management of Pain.* 2nd ed. Philadelphia, PA: Lea & Febiger; 1990:94–121.

13. Beecher H. Pain in men wounded in battle. *Ann Surg.* 1946;123:96–105.

14. Way WL, Fields HL, Schumaker MA. Chapter 31- Opioid Analgesics. In: Katsung BG, ed. *Basic & Clinical Pharmacology.* 9th ed. New York, NY: Lange Medical Books/McGraw-Hill; 2004.

15. Zastrow M, Svingos A, Haberstock H, et al. Regulatory endocytosis of opioid receptors: cellular mechanisms and proposed role in physiological adaptation to opiate drugs. *Curr Opin Neurobiol.* 2003;13:348–353.

16. Nestler EJ, Aghajanian GK. Molecular and cellular basis of addiction. *Science.* 1997;278:58–63.

17. Angst MS, Clark JD. Opioid-induced hyperalgesia: a qualitative systematic review. *Anesthesiology.* 2006;104(3):570–587.

18. Galer BS, Coyle N, Pasternak GW, Portenoy RK. Individual variability in the response to different opioids: report of five cases. *Pain.* 1992;49:87–91.

19. Mogil JS. The genetic mediation of individual differences in sensitivity to pain and its inhibition. *Proc Natl Acad Sci USA.* 1999;96:7744–7751.

20. Pan YX, Xu J, Bolan E, Moskowitz HS, Pasternak GW. Identification of four novel exon 5 splice variants of the mouse mu opioid receptor gene. *Mol Pharmacol.* 2005;68:866–875.

21. Uhl GR, Sora I, Wang Z. The mu opiate receptor as a candidate gene for pain: polymorphisms, variations in expression, nociception, and opiate responses. *Proc Natl Acad Sci USA.* 1999;96:7752–7755.

22. Chou WY, Yang LC, Lu HF, Ko JY, Wang CH, Lin SH, Lee TH, Concejero A, Hsu CJ. Association of μ-opioid receptor gene polymorphism (A118G) with variations in morphine consumption for analgesia after total knee arthroplasty *Acta Anaesth Scand.* 2006;50:787–792.

23. Reyes Gibby CC, Shete S, et al. Exploring joint effects of genes and the clinical efficacy of morphine for cancer pain; OPRM1 and COMT gene. *Pain.* 2007;130:25–30.

24. Klepstad P, Dale O, Skorpen F, et al. Genetic variability and clinical efficacy of morphine. *Acta Anaesthesiol Scand.* 2005;49:902–908.

25. Park HJ, Shinn HK, Lee HS et al. Genetic polymorphism in the ABCB1 gene and the effects of fentanyl in Koreans. *Clin Pharm Therapeut.* 2007;81:539–546.

26. Hamabe W, Maeda T, Fukazawa Y, et al. Polymorphism in the ABCB1 transporter. *Pharmacol Biochem Behav.* 2006;85:629–636.

27. Ross JR, et al. *Pharmacogenetics J.* 2005;5:324–336. *Goodman & Gilman's Pharmacology.* 11th ed. McGraw-Hill. 2006.

28. Mercadante S. Opioid rotation for cancer pain: rationale and clinical aspects. *Cancer.* 1999;86:1856–1866.

29. Evans DA, Mahgoub A, Sloan TP, Idle JR, Smith RL. A family and population study of the genetic polymorphism of debrisoquine

oxidation in a white British population. *J Med Genet*. 1980;17:102–105.

30. Portenoy RK. Opioid therapy for chronic nonmalignant pain: a review of the critical issues. *J Pain Sympt Manag*. 1996;11:203–217.

31. Gan TJ, Ginsberg B, Glass PSA, et al. Opioid sparing effects of a low-dose infusion of naloxone in patient administered morphine sulphate. *Anesthesiology*. 1997;87(5):1075–1081.

32. Mahowald ML, Singh JA, Majeski P. Opioid use by patients in an orthopedics spine clinic. *Arthritis Rheum*. 2005;52:312–321.

33. Fine PG, Portenoy RK. *A Clinical Guide to Opioid Analgesia*. New York, NY: McGraw-Hill; 2004.

34. Yeh SY, Gorodetzky CW, Krebs HA. Isolation and identification of morphine-3 and 6-glucuronides, morphine 3,6 diglucuronide, morphine 3 ethereal sulfate, normorphine and normorphine 6-glucuronide as morphine metabolites in humans. *J Pharm Sci*. 1977;66:1288–1293.

35. Marco CA, Plewa MC, Buderer N, Black C, Roberts A. Comparison of oxycodone and hydrocodone for the treatment of acute pain associated with fractures: a double-blind, randomized, controlled trial. *Acad Emerg Med*. 2005;12:282–288.

36. Ross FB, Smith MT. The intrinsic antinociceptive effects of oxycodone appear to be kappa-opioid receptor mediated. *Pain*. 1997;73:151–157.

37. Otton SV, Schadel M, Cheung SW, Kaplan HL: CYP2D6 phenotype determines the metabolic conversion of hydrocodone to hydromorphone. *J Clin Therapeut*. 1993;54:463–472.

38. Combunox [package insert]. St Louis, MO: Forest Pharmaceuticals Inc.; 2004.

39. Stambaugh JE, Reder RF, Stambaugh MD, Stambaugh H, Davis M. Double-blind, randomized comparison of the analgesic and pharmacokinetic profiles of controlled- and immediate-release oral oxycodone in cancer pain patients. *J Clin Pharmacol*. 2001;41:500–506.

40. Mahler DL, Forrest WH. Relative analgesic potencies of morphine and hydromorphone in postoperative pain. *Anesthesiology*. 1975;42:602–607.

41. Inturrisi C, Portenoy R, Stillman M, et al. Hydromorphone bioavailability and pharmacokinetic-pharmacodynamic relationships. *Clin Pharm Ther*. 1988;43:162–169.

42. Keeri-Szanto M. Anesthesia time/dose curves IX: the use of hydromorphone in surgical anesthesia and post operative pain relief in comparison to morphine. *Can Anesth Soc J*. 1976;23:587–595.

43. Ritschel WA. Absolute bioavailability of hydromorphone after oral and rectal administration in humans. *J Clin Pharmacol*. 1987;27:647–653.

44. Babul N. Darke AC, Hagen N. Hydromorphone metabolite accumulation in renal failure. *J Pain Symptom Manage*. 1995;10(3):184–186.

45. Peng PW, Sandler AN. Fentanyl for postoperative analgesia: a review. *Anesthesiology*. 1999;90:576–599.

46. Sinatra RS, Harrison DM, Hyde N. Oxymorphone revisited. In: Katz R, ed. *Essays in Anesthesiology*. Vol. 8. 1988:208–215.

47. Opana ER(R) [package insert]. Chadds Ford, PA: Endo Pharmaceuticals Inc;). 2005.

48. Anderson A, Saiers JH, Abram S, Schlicht C. Accuracy in equianalgesic: dosing conversion dilemmas. *J Pain Symptom Manage*. 2001;21:397–406.

49. Wadam EF, Bigelow GE. Johnson RE, Nuzzo PA, Haigney MC. Qt interval effects of methadone, levomethadyl, and buprenorphine in a randomized trial. *Arch Intern Med*. 2007;167:2469–2475.

50. Latta K, Ginsberg B, Barken K. Meperidine: a critical review. *Am J Therapeut*. 2002;9:53–68.

51. Gear RW, Miaskowski C, Gordon NC, Paul SM, Heller PH, Levine JD. Kappa-opioids produce significantly greater analgesia in women than in men. *Nat Med*. 1996;2:1248–1250.

52. Sinatra RS, Sramcik J. Tramadol: its use in pain management. In: Hines RL, ed. *Anesthesiology Clinics of North America*. Vol. 2. Philadelphia, PA: Saunders, 1998;53–69.

53. Dayer P, Desmules J, Collart L. Pharmacology of tramadol. *Drugs*. 1997;53(Suppl 2):18–24.

54. Alford DP, Compton P, Samet JH. Acute pain management for patients receiving methadone or burenorphine therapy. *Arch Int Med*. 2006;144:127–134.

55. Sinatra RS, Torres J, Bustos AM. Pain management after major orthopaedic surgery: current strategies and new concepts. *J Am Acad Orthop Surg*. 2002;10:117–129.

56. Sinatra RS. Treatment guidelines and unpublished observations. Yale University Pain Management Service 2007.

57. Coda BA, Tanaka A, Jacobson RC: Hydromorphone analgesia after intravenous bolus administration. *Pain*. 1997;71:41–48.

58. Sinatra RS, Harrison DM. A comparison of oxymorphone and fentanyl as narcotic supplements in general anesthesia. *J Clin Anesth*. 1989;1:253–258.

59. Sinatra RS, Lodge K, Sibert K, et al. A comparison of morphine, meperidine, and oxymorphone as utilized in patient-controlled analgesia following cesarean delivery. *Anesthesiology*. 1989;70:585–590.

60. Richlin DM, Reuben SS. Postoperative pain control with methadone following abdominal surgery. *J Clin Anesthes*. 1991;3:112–116.

61. Chui PT Gin T. A double blind randomised trial comparing postoperative analgesia after perioperative loading doses of methadone or morphine. *Anesthesia Intensive Care* 1992;20:46–51.

62. Shir Y, Rosen G, Zeiden A, Davidson M. Methadone is safe for treating hospitalized patients. *Can J Anesthes*. 2001;48:1109–1113.

63. Rowbotham MC, Twilling L, Davies PS, Reisner L, Taylor K, Mohr D. Oral opioid therapy for chronic peripheral and central neuropathic pain. *N Engl J Med*. 2003;348:1223–1232.

64. Mitra S, Sinatra RS: Perioperative management of acute pain in the opioid-dependent patient. *Anesthesiology*. 2004;101:212–227.

65. Guinard JP Maurocordatos P Carpenter RL: A randomized comparison of intravenous versus lumbar and thoracic epidural infusions of fentanyl after Thoracotomy. *Anesthesiology*. 1992;77:1108–1115.

66. Abrahamsson J, Niemand D, Olsson AK, Tornebrandt K. Buprenorphine (Temgesic) as a perioperative analgesic: a multicenter sudy. *Anaesthesist*. 1983;32(2):75–79.

67. Ho ST, Wang JJ, Liu HS, Tzeng JI, Liaw WJ. The analgesic effect of PCA buprenorphine in Taiwan's gynecologic patients. *Acta Anaesthesiol Sin*. 1997;35(4):195–199.

68. Bullingham RE, McQuay HJ, Dwyer D, Allen MC, Moore RA. Sublingual buprenorphine used postoperatively: clinical observations and preliminary pharmacokinetic analysis. *Br J Clin Pharmacol*. 1981;12(2):117–122.

69. McCormack JP, Warnier CB, Levine M, Glick N. A comparison of oral dosed morphine sulfate and on demand IM morphine in the treatment of postoperative pain. *Can J Anesthes*. 1993;40:819–824.

70. Silvasti M, Rosenberg P, Seppala T, Svartling N, Pitkanen M. Comparison of analgesic efficacy of oxycodone and morphine in postoperative intravenous patient-controlled analgesia. *Acta Anaesthesiol Scand*. 1998;42:576–580.

71. Singla N, Pong A, Newman K. Combination oxycodone 5mg/ibuprofen 400mg for the treatment of pain after abdominal surgery in women. *Clin Therapeut*. 2005;27:45–57.

72. Palangio M, Wideman GL, Keffer M, Landau CJ. Combination hydrocodone and ibuprofen versus oxycodone and acetaminophen in the treatment of postoperative obstetric or gynecologic pain. *Clin Therapeut.* 2000;22:600–612.

73. Marret E, Kurdi O, Zufferey P, Bonnet F. Effects of nonsteroidal antiinflammatory drugs on patient-controlled analgesia morphine side effects: meta-analysis of randomized controlled trials. *Anesthesiology.* 2005;102:1249–1260.

74. Aqua K, Gimbel JS, Singla N, Ma T, Ahdieh H. Efficacy and tolerability of oxymorphone IR, for acute postoperative pain after abdominal surgery. *Clin Therapeut.* 2007;29:1000–1012.

75. Gimbel J, Ahdieh H. The efficacy and safety of oral immediate-release oxymorphone for postsurgical pain. *Anesth Analg.* 2004;99:1472–1477.

76. McCarberg BH, Barkin RL. Long-acting opioids for chronic pain: pharmacotherapeutic opportunities to enhance compliance, quality of life, and analgesia. *Am J Ther.* 2001;8:181–186.

77. Gabrail NY, Dvergsten C, Ahdieh H. Establishing the dosage equivalency of oxymorphone extended release and oxycodone controlled release in patients with cancer pain: a randomized controlled study. *Curr Med Res Opin.* 2004;20:911–918.

78. Reuben SS, Connelly NR, Maciolek H. Postoperative analgesia with controlled release oxycodone for outpatient anterior cruciate ligament surgery. *Anesth Analg.* 1999;48:1286–1291.

79. Ginsberg B, Sinatra RS, Adler LJ, et al. Conversion to oral controlled-release oxycodone from intravenous opioid analgesic in the postoperative setting. *Pain Med.* 2003;4(1):31–38.

80. Fricke JR, Karim R, Jordan D, Rosenthal N: A double-blind single-dose comparison of the analgesic efficacy of tramadol/acetaminophen combination tablets, hydrocodone/acetaminophen combination tablets and placebo after oral surgery. *Clin Ther.* 2002;24:953–968.

81. Gordon D, Stevenson K, Griffie J, et al. Opioid equianalgesic calculations. *J Palliat Med.* 1999;2:209–221.

82. Cherny N, Ripamonti C, Pereira J, et al. Strategies to manage the adverse effects of oral morphine: an evidence-based report. *J Clin Oncol.* 2001;19:2542–2554.

83. Wheeler M, Oderda GM, Asburn MA, Lipman AG. Adverse events associated with postoperative opioid analgesia: a systematic review. *J Pain.* 2002;3:159–180.

84. Zofran [package insert]. Research Triangle Park, NC: GlaxoSmithKline; 2004.

85. National Institutes of Health. *The NIH Guide: New Directions in Pain Research I.* Washington, DC: U.S. Government Printing Office; 1998.

86. Mather LE, Woodhouse A, Ward ME, Farr SJ. Pulmonary administration of aerosolised fentanyl: pharmacokinetic analysis. *Br J Anaesth.* 1998;46:37–43.

87. Romberg R, van Dorp E, Hollander J et al. A randomized double-blind placebo-controlled pilot study of morphine-6-glucoronide for postoperative pain relief after knee replacement surgery. *Clin J Pain.* 2007;23:197–203.

14

Intravenous Patient-Controlled Analgesia

Pamela E. Macintyre and Julia Coldrey

The concept of intravenous (IV) patient-controlled analgesia (PCA) as a technique that allows patients to self-administer intravenous opioids as required dates back to the mid-1960s, when it was shown that small IV doses of opioids could provide more effective pain relief than conventional intramuscular (IM) opioid regimens.[1] A little later, an "on-demand" system of analgesic administration was used as a measure of assessing a patient's pain,[2] as "pain can be described in terms of analgesic demand."[3] In this study, IV doses of the opioid were given by a nurse-observer at the patient's request.[2] It was noted that analgesic demands varied considerably within and between patients.

To more easily allow a patient access to repeated small IV doses of opioid (that is, without the need for a nurse to be readily available), an electronic device was developed that delivered 1 mL of the opioid solution after the patient pressed a demand button.[3] The opioids used in this study were morphine and meperidine (pethidine), and both were given in doses that would be considered small by today's standards (morphine 0.2 or 0.5 mg/mL and meperidine 2.0 or 5.0 mg/mL). However, PCA appeared to be a very effective way to treat postoperative pain.

Other early systems included the Demand Dropmaster and the Demanalg and the first commercially available PCA pump, the Cardiff Palliator.[4] This latter pump was developed for use on the labor wards. Although it preceded the microprocessor era, it was able to deliver drugs at a variety of rates and with adjustable parameters that were very similar to those of modern-day machines.[5] This device was used in various studies to show that pain relief and side effects were similar for morphine, meperidine, and nalbuphine.[4]

Another device, the on-demand analgesia computer (ODAC), incorporated monitoring of the patient's respiratory rate and limited the dose if a decrease in rate was detected.[6] The ODAC system, an early microprocessor-operated device, allowed the use of more complex PCA regimens.[7] It was also used to compare opioids such as alfentanil, fentanyl, and meperidine and to show that patients preferred PCA compared with previous experiences with conventional postoperative analgesia techniques.[4] Other devices developed in the early phases of PCA use in a clinical setting included the Prominject, Harvard PCA, and Abbott PCA machines.[7]

Over the years, further improvements were made to the design of PCA devices. These have resulted in increases in security and data output capacity, introduction of error reduction programs, and a choice of mains or battery power. In addition, a variety of disposable delivery systems are now available.

Discussion of the basic principles and features of the various PCA systems available, both programmable and disposable, is included in Chapter 21 (*Nonselective Nonsteroidal Anti-Inflammatory Drugs, COX-2 Inhibitors, and Acetaminophen in Acute Perioperative Pain*). The major advantage of programmable pumps is their flexibility of use, as adjustments can easily be made to parameters such as the size of the bolus dose and rate of delivery of both the bolus dose and a background infusion (if used). In addition, access to the syringe (or other drug reservoir) and the microprocessor program is possible only using a key or access code.

Disposable devices, however, have the advantages of being portable and simple to use, eliminating programming errors, and they may not require IV access (eg, some enable nasal and transdermal methods of drug delivery).[8] However, they do not allow as much flexibility in use and possible security issues may arise as the drug reservoirs for these devices are more readily accessible.[8] In addition, cost per patient may be high.

Although many studies were performed using PCA in the earlier years, the use of the technique in clinical practice did not become widespread until after the introduction of Acute Pain Services, first proposed and developed by Ready in the 1980s.[9] PCA has now become an accepted part of everyday safe and effective pain relief in the acute pain setting and, as such, the number of studies investigating it as a technique have declined significantly over recent years.

The overall effectiveness of any analgesic technique depends on both the degree of pain relief that can be achieved and the incidence of side effects or complications (ie, safety). Therefore, this chapter will cover the following:

- Analgesic efficacy of IV PCA, including comparison with other methods of pain relief and other routes use for PCA, and the various analgesic agents used

- Other patient outcomes, including satisfaction and effects on postoperative morbidity
- The preparation required before PCA is used in a clinical setting, including education of patients and staff, the provision of appropriate procedure protocols and orders, and the need to understand the influence of variations in the PCA "prescription" as well as how some patient factors (eg, psychological characteristics and concurrent comorbidities)
- Potential complications of IV PCA and the drugs used

The various types of equipment that can be used and the associated economic issues are also important; these are discussed in Chapters 21 (*Nonselective Nonsteroidal Anti-Inflammatory Drugs, COX-2 Inhibitors, and Acetaminophen in Acute Perioperative Pain*) and 43 (*Quality Improvement Approaches in Acute Pain Management*), respectively

ANALGESIC EFFICACY OF IV PCA

Comparisons with Other Analgesic Techniques

Conventional Opioid Analgesia

Dolin and Cashman[10] reviewed data obtained from many different kinds of published studies (cohort and case-controlled studies, audit reports and randomized-controlled trials) and concluded that IV PCA provided better pain relief than intermittent IM opioid analgesia. The incidence of moderate-severe pain and severe pain was 67.2% and 29.1%, respectively, for IM analgesia, whereas 35.8% of patients with IV PCA reported moderate-severe pain and 10.4% reported severe pain.[10] These authors also reviewed the incidence of side effects with these techniques – see later.

Three metaanalyses confirm these results. In two of them,[11,12] the magnitude of the difference in analgesia was small (5.9[11] and 8.0[12] on a pain scale of 0–100). In the third,[13] no difference in pain scores was found: analgesia with PCA was better only if all pain outcomes (pain relief, pain intensity, and need for rescue analgesia) were considered.

However, it is possible, especially in settings where there are high nurse to patient ratios and where it might be easier to provide analgesia truly on-demand (ie, follow the "PCA principle"[14]), that conventional forms of opioid administration may be as effective as IV PCA. A recent meta-analysis comparing the use of PCA versus nurse-administered analgesia following cardiac surgery[15] found no difference in analgesia at 24 hours, but significantly better pain relief with PCA at 48 hours. Similar results have been found in an emergency department setting, where IV PCA was as effective as nurse-administered IV bolus doses of opioid,[16] IM opioid analgesia after hysterectomy[17] and intermittent IV opioid administration after cardiac surgery.[18]

The ongoing popularity of PCA may seem at odds with the underwhelming results of Ballantyne et al,[11] Walder et al,[13] and Hudcova et al.[12] It is possible, under study conditions when greater attention is paid to the technique by investigators and staff alike, that conventional opioid analgesia may be effective. It is also possible, that the way in which PCA was used did not adequately allow for interpatient variations (eg, fixed program parameters) and significantly limited the flexibility, and thus efficacy, of the technique.[19]

Although opioid consumption may be higher with IV PCA compared with conventional opioid analgesia,[12,15] there appears to be no difference in the incidence of opioid-related side effects,[11,12,15] so that total opioid dose may be relatively unimportant.

Epidural Analgesia

Two recent meta-analyses have concluded that IV PCA is less effective than continuous epidural and patient-controlled epidural analgesia.[20,21] The exception to this is the use of a hydophilic opioid alone for epidural analgesia, when pain relief is no better than with IV PCA.[21] For more information on epidural and patient-controlled epidural analgesia, see Chapter 17 (*Regional Anesthesia*).

Comparisons with PCA Using Other Systemic Routes of Administration

Other routes that have been used with PCA include the subcutaneous (SC),[22,23] oral,[24] intranasal,[25,29] and transdermal[30] routes.

Subcutaneous PCA

Data on the effectiveness of SC PCA compared with IV PCA are inconsistent. Both significantly better[22,31] and comparable[23,32,33] pain relief has been reported, as well as the same[22,23,33,31] and a higher incidence[32] of nausea and vomiting. Compared with IV PCA, SC PCA may[22,23,32] or may not[33] result in higher opioid use.

Intranasal PCA

Metered-dose patient-controlled intranasal analgesia (PCINA) devices are available that allow the intranasal administration of a fixed dose of opioid. The opioid most commonly studied for use in PCINA is fentanyl. Toussaint et al[25] compared PCINA fentanyl (bolus dose = 25 µg) with IV PCA fentanyl (bolus dose = 17.5 µg), both with lockout intervals of 6 minutes, and found no difference in pain relief. The bioavailability of fentanyl via the intranasal route is 0.7,[27,28] therefore a PCINA bolus dose of 25 µg is equivalent to an IV PCA bolus dose of 17.5 µg.

Similar results have been noted by Paech et al[34] using a formulation that allows the delivery of larger bolus doses of fentanyl in a smaller volume (300 µg/mL fentanyl; 54 µg/180 µL dose). It has been suggested that the maximum volume given into each nostril should not exceed 150 µL.[27] Early PCINA devices delivered spray doses of a reasonable dose but large volume (eg, 25 µg fentanyl/0.5 mL[29,35]) or smaller volume, but with smaller doses than commonly used with IV PCA (eg, 9 µg fentanyl/180 µL[36]). The formulation developed by Paech et al[34] with a higher concentration of fentanyl allows delivery of a larger dose in a volume close to the suggested 150 µL limit. Patient satisfaction has also been assessed and was greater with PCINA fentanyl than nurse-administered analgesia after orthopedic surgery.[29]

Other drugs that have been administered by PCINA include diamorphine[28] and meperidine (pethidine).[37] Intranasal diamorphine was not as effective as IV diamorphine,[28] but PCINA meperidine was more effective than SC pethidine injections.[37]

Transdermal PCA

An iontophoretic transdermal PCA fentanyl system (Ionsys) is now available – see Chapter 22 (*Perioperative Ketamine for Better Postoperative Pain Outcome*) for more details. It uses a low-intensity electric current to drive the drug from the reservoir through the skin and into the systemic circulation.[38]

The Ionsys PCA system, which delivers a 40-μg-bolus dose over 10 minutes, has been shown to be more effective than placebo for pain relief after major surgery, when withdrawal from the study because of inadequate analgesia was the end point,[30,39] and as effective as IV PCA morphine (1-mg bolus dose), when patient satisfaction with the technique was the primary end point.[40]

In a study of pain relief after total hip arthroplasty, Hartrick et al[41] reported that pain relief and the incidence of side effects were similar with IV PCA (1 mg morphine, 5-minute lockout) and iontophoretic fentanyl PCA.

Comparison of the Different Opioids Used with IV PCA

On a population basis, little if any difference has been shown in the efficacy or incidence of side effects of the different opioids used with IV PCA,[42] although the results of individual studies are inconsistent.

For example, in comparisons of meperidine with morphine, various authors have noted less effective pain relief on movement with meperidine,[43,44–46] with no difference in nausea and vomiting[43,45–46] but less sedation[44] and pruritus.[44,47] This result, combined with the high incidence of adverse drug reactions,[48,49] including normeperidine (norpethidine) toxicity and serotonergic syndrome,[50–52] suggests that meperidine should not be used routinely for IV PCA.[42,50] Similarly, there appears to be no difference between morphine and fentanyl in terms of pain relief[47,53] or the incidence of side effects),[47,53] with the exception of pruritus, which is higher with morphine.[47]

Other comparisons with morphine include hydromorphone (no difference in pain relief or side effects),[54] tramadol (similar pain relief with an increase in nausea and vomiting[55] or no difference in side effects[56]), oxycodone (no difference in pain relief or side effects),[57] a morphine-alfentanil combination (again, no difference in analgesia or side effects),[58] and piritramide (equally effective, with similar side effects).[59]

Differences in cognitive function may be seen when different opioids are used in elderly patients. Herrick et al[60] reported that use of IV PCA fentanyl in elderly patients resulted in less depression of postoperative cognitive function and less confusion compared with IV PCA morphine. A retrospective audit of 1544 patients over the age of 65 years given morphine or fentanyl IV PCA after surgery reported that the incidence of postoperative confusion increased with age but that it was less likely to occur in patients prescribed fentanyl.[61] Overall, the incidence of confusion was 3.85% with fentanyl and 15.6% with morphine, but the differences were more marked the older the patient. In patients aged 65–75 years, the incidences of confusion with fentanyl and morphine were 2.6% and 10%, respectively; in patients aged 75–85 years these had increased to 3.8% and 20.5%, and in the oldest patients (85–95 years) the risk of confusion with fentanyl had increased to 8%, whereas 43% of patients receiving morphine became confused.[61]

Ng et al[62] reported no difference in postoperative cognitive function with tramadol and fentanyl. However, this might not have been a fair comparison, because the bolus doses used were not equianalgesic (tramadol 20 mg, fentanyl 10 μg) – not surprisingly, patients given tramadol had better pain relief with movement on the first day after surgery.

More recently, remifentanil has been used with IV PCA.[63,64] It has been found to provide at least equivalent analgesia compared with morphine[63,64] and fentanyl PCA[64] and may be associated with less nausea and vomiting.[63,64] It has potential advantages as an analgesic because of its very rapid onset/offset of action and lack of accumulation with repeated dosing. Concerns about respiratory depression with remifentanil (because of its potency) are not supported by the current literature.[63–65]

Even though on a population basis there are minimal differences between the different opioids, individual patients may gain benefit from one opioid over another. In a three-way crossover double-blinded randomized controlled trial comparing morphine, fentanyl, and pethidine, Woodhouse et al[47] showed that, whereas overall analgesia was equivalent for all three drugs, subjectively some patients found that they were better able to tolerate one or more of the opioids better than the other(s).

Individual patient responses to the PCA opioid may also be influenced by pharmacogenetic differences. Increased PCA morphine requirements in the postoperative period have been associated with polymorphism of the μ-opioid receptor at the 118 nucleotide position, encoding for a GG homozygote,[66,67] and other polymorphisms at genes encoding for morphine metabolism and transport across the blood-brain barrier have also been found to have an influence on the clinical efficacy of morphine.[68] Patients who have absent activity of the CYP2D6 enzyme have a poorer response to tramadol compared with those with normal enzyme activity.[69]

Efficacy of Other Drugs Added to PCA Opioid Regimens

Over the years, many drugs have been added to opioids in PCA in an attempt to either reduce side effects, improve analgesia, or both. Most of the literature relates to addition of ketamine and naloxone, but there is also some evidence for addition of other drugs (see Table 14.1).

Ketamine

The use of low-dose (ie, subanesthetic doses) ketamine run as a separate infusion in addition to PCA morphine or added to the PCA morphine solution, reduced morphine requirements in the first 24 hours after surgery as well as the incidence of postoperative nausea and vomiting.[70] No comment could be made regarding the best dose regimen, because of considerable variation in the doses of ketamine used in the included trials.

Of the four studies included in this metaanalysis that involved the addition of ketamine to the PCA morphine solution,[71–74] two showed a significant opioid-sparing effect,[72,74] and three noted lower pain scores.[71,72,74] The amount of ketamine added to PCA morphine varied from 0.75 mg to 2 mg per IV PCA bolus dose; side-effect profiles were similar.

Other authors have found that the incidence of pruritis may be reduced by the addition of ketamine,[73] and that there might be an increased incidence of dysphoria,[71] vivid dreams, and poor performance in cognitive testing.[75] However, the clinical significance of these results are questionable as there was a low rate of termination of the treatment because of these side effects.

Table 14.1: Efficacy of Analgesic Drugs Added to IV PCA Morphine

Drug	Comments	Reference
Ketamine	Morphine-sparing and improved pain relief	Burstal et al (2001), Javery et al (1996), Unlugenc et al (2003)[71,72,74]
Naloxone	Effect depends in dose used – see text	Cepeda et al. (2002, 2004)[76,77]
Tramadol	Morphine-sparing, but not better pain relief	Stiller et al (2007)[164]
Clonidine	Significantly less nausea and vomiting without an increase in sedation	Jeffs et al (2002)[165]
	Lower pain scores up to 12 hour	
	Higher patient satisfaction	
Magnesium	Morphine-sparing and better pain relief	Unlugenc et al (2003)[74]
Ketorolac	Opioid-sparing but no difference in pain relief or adverse effects	Chen et al (2005)[166]
	Earlier time to first bowel movement and first ambulation	
Lidocaine	No difference in pain relief, opioid use or nausea and vomiting	Cepeda et al (1996), Chia et al (1998)[167,168]
	Higher sedation scores in lidocaine group	

Naloxone

As naloxone may inhibit the excitatory opioid receptors that are involved in the development of hyperalgesia, and may possibly reduce the incidence of opioid-related side effects, it has also been added to PCA morphine (1 mg/mL) in varying doses. "Ultra-low" doses of naloxone (0.6 μg added to 1 mg PCA morphine) led to a lower incidence of nausea (not vomiting) and pruritus, with no change in pain relief or morphine use,[76] but a 10-fold increase in dose (6 μg added to 1 mg PCA morphine) resulted in increased pain and higher morphine requirements.[77] Sartain et al,[78] using a solution of 60 mg morphine and 800 μg naloxone in 30 mL (bolus dose = 1 mL) compared with morphine alone (1-mg bolus dose) were unable to show any difference in either pain relief or adverse effects.

PATIENT OUTCOMES

Patient Satisfaction

The evaluation of satisfaction appears to be complex as satisfaction scores may be more likely to indicate satisfaction with overall treatment or a reluctance to criticize treatment rather than reflect satisfaction with pain relief only.[79,80] Preoperative expectations for analgesia also appear to have an effect on postoperative satisfaction.[81] However, in the three metaanalyses by Walder et al,[13] Ballantyne et al,[11] and Hudcova et al,[12] patient satisfaction was significantly higher with IV PCA compared with conventional methods of opioid administration. High satisfaction may be correlated with lower pain ratings,[82,83] although some patients will report high levels of satisfaction and high pain scores[79,84,85] There is an additional, but definite, preference for PCA by nurses. They may feel that it reduces their workload[86] and helps to make the patient responsible for their own analgesia.[80]

Postoperative Morbidity

While epidural analgesia is the pain-relieving technique most likely to lead to lower postoperative morbidity (see Chapter 17, *Regional Anesthesia*), use of IV PCA may decrease the risk of postoperative pulmonary complications compared with conventional methods of opioid administration.[13,87] However, use of PCA has not been shown to reduce average length of stay in hospital.[11–13,15,17,86] Comparisons of patient outcomes between IV-PCA and other analgesic techniques are discussed in the relevant chapters of this book.

REQUIREMENTS FOR THE SAFE AND EFFECTIVE USE OF PCA

Before PCA can be used safely and effectively in a clinical setting, there are a number of issues that need to be considered. These include the following:

- education of patients and all medical and nursing staff involved with the use of PCA
- the provision of appropriate procedure protocols and orders
- a good understanding the influence of variations in the IV PCA "prescription," including programmable variables and how these can be adjusted to better suit individual patients
- a good understanding of how some patient factors may influence the success or otherwise of IV PCA

Education

One of the reasons for suboptimal management of acute pain is inadequate education of medical, nursing, and allied health staff and students, patients, and their families.[88] Inadequate knowledge, misconceptions, and the persistence of some of the myths that surround pain management continue to result in barriers that prevent optimal analgesia in many patients, even in those prescribed conventional forms of analgesia. If better pain relief is to be obtained, better education of all groups is needed. This is especially true if more sophisticated methods of pain relief (such as patient-controlled and epidural analgesia) are to be managed safely and effectively.

Patient Education

To enable patients to use PCA effectively, they should be given instructions about the technique before use. Information should be given to each patient and tailored to the needs of that patient.

Information can be presented in a number of ways: verbally, in a booklet, or on a video. It has been shown that providing patients with written information[89,90] or information on CD[91] significantly improves their knowledge and understanding of PCA compared with verbal instruction alone. It is known that most patients remember only a small part of any information presented at one time. Therefore, it will need to be repeated a number of times, including during treatment.

Patients should be made aware of a number of general factors important to their pain relief, including the following:

- treatment goals and benefits
- options available for the treatment of acute pain and possible side effects and complications
- how they will be monitored
- the need to communicate inadequate analgesia or side effects
- specialized education about IV PCA, including how to use the machine, safety aspects (eg. programming of the lockout interval, requirement for patient *only* to press button)

An example of an information sheet given to patients is in the Appendix.

Current literature regarding the benefits or otherwise of patient education gives conflicting results. Although use of a multimedia CD educational package may lead to improved pain relief,[91] better analgesia may not follow use of written[89,90,92] or standardized verbal information.[90,93] Similarly, structured preoperative patient education may[94] or may not[89–91,93] reduce the amount of IV PCA opioid consumed.

Lack of patient education was believed to be associated with fears held by patients about the risk of addiction (22% of patients) and overdose (30%) in a study where 43% of patients received no preoperative education and 24% received no instruction at any time during the study.[79] In later work by the same group,[89,90] it was found that, although the patients receiving written information were better informed about PCA, there was no difference in postoperative anxiety levels or fears of addiction and overdose. Preoperative anxiety levels, however, may be less in patients who receive preoperative education.[92]

Staff Education

Education of all staff involved in the use of PCA is also important if the technique is to be used safely and effectively. Education of junior medical staff needs to cover all aspects of the management of acute pain. In particular, they must be aware of the detrimental effects that unrelieved pain can have on patient well-being and outcome after trauma and surgery. Although they would not usually be directly responsible for more advanced, newer methods of pain relief, they must have a sound working knowledge of them and be aware of possible complications and drug interactions.[88]

Ward nurses are directly involved in the management of all forms of pain relief and play a key role in ensuring that analgesia, whether simple or sophisticated, is safely and effectively managed. Education and accreditation programs are therefore essential.

Many institutions require a nurse to complete an accreditation program before they can assume responsibility for a patient whose pain is being managed using IV PCA. Such programs often consist of verbal and written information (eg, lectures or workshops and booklets), written assessment (eg, multiple-choice questionnaires), and a practical assessment (eg, demonstration of ability to program IV PCA machines).[88]

The level of knowledge that nursing staff have about IV PCA may influence its effectiveness. Introduction of an APS nurse, whose role included staff and patient education, led to a 50% reduction in moderate to severe pain with PCA, a marked improvement in patient satisfaction, and significantly fewer side effects.[85] Similarly, when PCA was supervised by an APS compared with the primary service a year earlier, patients used significantly more opioids, the incidence of side effects was almost halved, and PCA bolus doses were altered more often to suit the individual patient.[95]

Standard Orders and Nursing Procedure Protocols

Standard Orders

To maximize both efficacy and safety, consideration should be given to standardizing a number of aspects of pain relief using IV PCA. As well as education of nursing and medical staff and patients, this would ideally include standardization of the following[88]:

- the drugs used – analgesic and nonanalgesic (eg, for the treatment of nausea and vomiting)
- drug doses and drug concentrations
- nondrug treatment (eg, supplemental oxygen)
- monitoring requirements (regular assessments of adequacy of analgesia and adverse effects)
- the response to inadequate analgesia
- the recognition and treatment of side effects

Many institutions incorporate all of these elements on specific preprinted orders (see example in the Appendix in Chapter 16, *Neuraxial Analgesia with Hydromorphone, Morphine, and Fentanyl: Dosing and Safety Guidelines*).

As with all guidelines, the aim is to try and improve the quality of clinical decision-making and reduce unnecessary variations in clinical practice – not to dictate practice. Standardized orders allow appropriate alterations to be made so maximum analgesia can be obtained with minimum possible side effects. For example, such orders may allow nursing staff to increase the bolus dose if pain scores are high, and to recognize and then treat common or serious side effects. Staff should also be required to reduce the bolus dose if there is increasing and excessive sedation.[88]

Nursing Procedure Protocols

Nursing procedure protocols should also be standardized. Key elements include the following[88]:

- statement of the institution policy toward accreditation for nursing staff responsible for PCA and who is responsible for PCA orders
- guides to the location of keys for the PCA machines and mechanisms for checking and discarding PCA opioids
- guidelines for the suitability of patients for PCA and instructions for patient education
- monitoring and documentation requirements as well as how to manage side effects and complications related to IV PCA
- detailed instruction on setting up and programming the PCA pump and the management of equipment faults and alarms
- the requirement for one-way antireflux and antisiphon valves

- instructions for the checking of the PCA settings against the prescription and the amount of drug delivered against the amount remaining in the syringe
- who to call if assistance or advice is required

Monitoring Requirements

In addition to regular assessments of the effectiveness of pain relief (usually using pain scores), patients should be monitored for the inset of any side effects related to the IV PCA opioid. Most importantly, impending respiratory depression must be picked at an early stage so that opioid doses can be reduced.

Traditionally, in patients receiving opioids, respiratory rate has been monitored and used as an indicator of respiratory depression. However, a decrease in respiratory rate has been found to be a late and unreliable sign of respiratory depression: conversely, a normal respiratory rate may coexist with marked rises in blood carbon dioxide levels[88] – see discussion under *Complications of PCA* later in this chapter.

Regular monitoring of oxygen saturation levels is also recommended. However, oxygen saturation readings may be unreliable indicators of an underlying problem if the patient is receiving supplemental oxygen, as is standard with for many patients receiving parenteral opioids.[88]

The PCA "Prescription"

The flexibility of use for electronic PCA pumps results from the variations that are possible in the parameters programmed into the device as part of the PCA "prescription." If both the efficacy and safety of PCA is to be maximized, a good understanding of the role of these variable parameters and the rationale for choosing a particular setting is important.

Loading Dose

Prior to commencing PCA, it is important for the patient to be adequately "loaded" – that is, they should be given enough opioid to be comfortable before they begin to take control of their own pain relief. Most if not all current electronic PCA machines have a "loading dose" facility that allows automatic administration of the dose before PCA proper starts. However, a set dose is unlikely to be effective for all patients because of enormous interpatient differences. It is preferable to titrate the loading for each patient prior to starting PCA.[88]

Bolus Dose

The size of the bolus dose (the amount of analgesic drug the patient receives after a successful demand) can influence the effectiveness or otherwise of PCA. A dose that is too small may mean that the patient is unable to achieve good pain relief; a dose that is too big may lead to excessive side effects and reduced safety.

The "optimal" PCA bolus dose is one that provides reliable, effective analgesia without producing excessive or dangerous side effects. However, evidence regarding the appropriate size of this dose is very limited.

Owen et al[96] studied patients randomly prescribed 0.5, 1, or 2 mg morphine. Patients prescribed 2-mg PCA bolus doses had a higher incidence of respiratory depression and most patients who self-administered 0.5 mg doses were unable to achieve good

pain relief. The authors concluded that a "dose of 1 mg was the best increment under the conditions of this study."

Another group[97] randomized patients to receive bolus doses of 1, 1.5, and 2 mg morphine and adjusted the lockout interval for these patient groups to 6, 9, and 12 minutes, respectively. This was so that the maximum amount of morphine each group could receive in 1 hour was 10 mg. They found no difference in pain relief or side effects between the groups but noted that patients receiving the 1-mg bolus dose recorded a higher number of demands within the lockout period and adjustments to the dose were required more often.[97]

In another attempt to determine an optimal morphine PCA dose, patients were allowed to choose among 0.5-, 1-, or 1.5-mg bolus doses of morphine using a specially designed handpiece.[98] Compared with a standard PCA machine, there were no differences noted in analgesia, total morphine doses, patient satisfaction, quality of sleep, or nausea and vomiting.

Different doses of fentanyl have also been investigated. Camu et al[99] compared the effectiveness and incidence of side effects of three different demand doses (20, 40, and 60 μg) delivered over 10 minutes. They concluded that 40 μg was the optimal dose as the frequency of adverse respiratory events was highest in the 60-μg group and the 20-μg group made more missed attempts.[97] Patient global assessment of "very good" or "excellent" and the absence of severe side effects was dose dependent and highest in the 60-μg group. However, delivery of an IV bolus dose over 10 minutes is not common clinical practice (the dose would usually be delivered over about 30 seconds). This may have limited the ability of the 20-μg dose to provide good analgesia and would be reflected in higher unsuccessful demand rate that was seen.

Another study looked at four different demand doses of fentanyl (10, 20, 30, and 40 μg) used for the management of pain during burn-dressing changes, pain relief was significantly better with the 30- and 40-μg doses; no patient became sedated or experiences nausea and vomiting.[100]

In clinical practice, relatively standard IV bolus doses such as morphine (1 mg), fentanyl (10–20 μg), tramadol (10 mg), and hydromorphone (0.2 mg) are commonly prescribed. However, it has been shown that postoperative PCA opioid requirements decrease markedly as patient age increases.[101–103] The reasons for this decrease have not yet been fully elucidated, but it is probably due more to changes in pharmacodynamic factors related to aging than age-related changes in pharmacokinetics.[104] It may therefore be reasonable to use a lower bolus dose in the older patient (eg, half the "standard" bolus dose in patients older than 70 years).[88]

If the prescribed dose is not "optimal" and as long it is not too small, the patient will be able to compensate to some degree by changing their demand rate.[96] However, they will only compensate to a certain degree. In the study by Owen et al,[96] patients who complained of pain made an average of only 4 demands per hour, even though they could have pressed the PCA button more frequently. It is possible that patients will not continue to activate the demand button if they do not feel they are getting good pain relief from a given bolus dose. This means that the size of the bolus dose will need to be increased or decreased according to subsequent reports of pain or the onset of any side effects. By making appropriate alterations to the bolus dose, PCA can be tailored to suit the individual patient.

It may be best to aim, in most patients, for a bolus dose size that requires the patient to administer, on average, no more that

2–3 bolus doses per hour. If analgesia is inadequate, and if they are averaging more than 2–3 doses each hour, it may be better to increase the size of the bolus dose rather than to encourage the patient to increase their rate of demand.[88] It follows that decreasing the lockout interval is unlikely to be of much benefit. Equally important is the need to reduce the size of the bolus dose should the patient become excessively sedated.[88] As Etches[105] observed, PCA is neither a "one size fits all" or a "set and forget" form of pain relief, and appropriate alterations need to be made if maximum effectiveness and safety with PCA are to be obtained.

BOLUS DOSES IN OPIOID-TOLERANT PATIENTS

In patients who are opioid tolerant, there is no one "optimal" size for the bolus dose. It is known that these patients have markedly higher PCA opioid requirements in the postoperative period compared with opioid-naive patients, as well as higher pain scores,[106] However, there is little good evidence on which to base the choice of bolus dose used and judging what dose to give can be difficult.

In an elegant study using pharmacokinetic simulation, Davis et al[107] calculated the size of the postoperative PCA fentanyl bolus doses according to preoperative requirements of fentanyl. The patients were given high-dose fentanyl infusions before surgery at a dose that led to a respiratory rate of less than 5 breaths per minute. From this, the effect site concentration required to reduce the respiratory rate to this level was used to calculate the postoperative effect site concentration for analgesia and the amount of fentanyl that would be needed. Half of this amount was then given as a background infusion and half as divided bolus doses; the doses were adjusted postoperatively so that patients required around 2–3 doses per hour.

Another method is to use a simple conversion so that the equivalent of the patient's usual opioid is given as the background infusion (if they cannot take it as normal) as the same figure is used as the starting bolus dose.[88] For example, if a patient is taking 150 mg of a controlled-release morphine preparation orally, this is equivalent to about 50 mg of parenteral morphine or approximately 2 mg/h. So a background infusion of 2 mg/h could be ordered (unless the patient can take his or her usual oral morphine dose) and a bolus dose of 2 mg of morphine prescribed.

Duration of Dose Delivery

Some PCA machines enable changes to be made in the rate at which the bolus dose is delivered. This can be useful if PCA bolus doses are given via the subcutaneous route when delivery of the dose can be painful if given too quickly.[88]

To investigate whether a slower rate of delivery might result in less nausea and vomiting, Woodhouse and Mather[108] compared the effects of different rates of delivery in patients after hysterectomy. Patients were allocated to receive either 1 mg morphine (in 1 mL) over 5 minutes using a 1-min lockout period or the same amount of morphine over 40 seconds with a 5-minute lockout interval. They reported no difference in pain relief or morphine use, but delivery over 5 minutes led to a significantly higher number of emetic episodes. Of interest, the overall incidence was surprisingly high with 90% of patients with the 40-second delivery and 100% patients with a 5-minute delivery reporting nausea. The only antiemetic used was metoclopramide, which is known to be much less ineffective than some other antiemetics in the postoperative setting – see later.

Lockout Interval

In clinical practice, lockout intervals (the time following the end of the delivery of one dose until the patient is able to successfully obtain another dose) of 5–10 minutes are commonly prescribed for IV PCA, regardless of the opioid used. This is despite the fact that the full effect of the opioid used most commonly in IV PCA (morphine) may not be seen for 15 minutes or more.[109] If the lockout interval is there to help prevent the patient demanding an excessive dose of opioid, it should be an indication of the time necessary for the patient to feel the effect of one bolus dose before another can be delivered. Therefore, this would vary according to the drug used and the time to peak effect of that drug. However, there are no studies showing that changing the lockout interval affects the efficacy of IV PCA. Ginsberg et al[109] investigated the differences between lockout intervals of 7 and 11 minutes for morphine and 5 and 8 minutes for fentanyl and reported no differences in analgesia, anxiety, or side effects.

In some centers, the practice is to decrease the lockout interval in response to patient reports of inadequate analgesia. However, as noted earlier, Owen et al[96] found that patients who complained of pain still made an average of only 4 demands per hour, even though they could have pressed the PCA button more frequently. Therefore, reductions in lockout interval, especially if intervals of 5 or 6 minutes are used, are probably going to be less effective than an increase in the size of the bolus dose.

Background Infusion

Conventional wisdom has it that the use of background (continuous) infusions with PCA in addition to patient demand reduces the safety of the technique. Indeed, most studies investigating the effect of background infusions have concluded that this practice results in higher opioid consumption[110,111,112] and an increased risk of respiratory depression.[111,113] Use of a night-only background infusion was also shown to increase the risk of programming errors as well as increase the incidence of hypoxia.[111] Introduced in the hope that it would improve pain relief, particularly at night, by reducing the frequency of demands required to maintain an analgesic plasma concentration, background infusions in general neither improve the effectiveness of analgesia[112] nor sleep[111] and do not reduce the number of demands made.[111]

A recent study of patients after cardiac surgery found that the addition of a background infusion did improve analgesia, as well as increase opioid consumption.[114] However, the parameters used – a lockout interval of 15 minutes and a bolus dose of just 0.015 mg/kg (ie, about 1 mg in an average 70 kg patient) – are not those commonly used with PCA and might have limited the effectiveness of IV PCA using patient demand mode only.

For the reasons noted above, the routine use of background infusions in adults is usually not recommended. However, their relative safety may be improved if a patient's opioid requirements are already known. For example, it may be suitable in patients who are opioid-tolerant, when it can be used to replace the patient's normal maintenance opioids, and may also be appropriate in patients requiring high doses of PCA opioid who are waking in pain at night[115] (anecdotal reports suggest that this is effective in many patients). To minimize risk, it is suggested that the background infusion comprise no more than 50% of the patient's total 24-hour hour requirement.[115]

Dose Limit

Interpatient opioid requirements vary enormously and there is no reliable method of determining how much opioid a patient will require for analgesia, far less how much will result in dangerous side effects. Although it is possible, in most pumps, to program a dose limit (commonly hourly or 4-hourly) that caps the total amount of drug that can be administered within a given time. Limits are sometimes placed on the dose that can be delivered over a set interval in an attempt to improve the safety of PCA. However, there is no good evidence to show that its use has resulted in a decrease in side effects related to PCA.[115]

Influence of Patients Factors

Psychological Factors

Patients using IV PCA are able to balance the degree of pain relief achieved against the severity of any side effects that may occur. That is, PCA affords patients a significant measure of control over both these aspects of their care – analgesia and analgesic-related adverse effects.

Some studies have shown a significant relationship between perceived control and higher satisfaction with lower pain ratings,[79,82] whereas others have failed to show any benefit.[116] In fact, the opposite may be true in some circumstances. Taylor et al[116] reported that some patients found the element of control disturbing, as it meant that they were also responsible for the production of unpleasant side effects.

PCA may have an important impact on the nurse-patient relationship. For example, patients may appreciate not having to call or bother the nurses. This may include that they preferred to be alone, that they felt the nurses were too busy, or that delays in getting nurse-administered pain relief were often too long.[117] These authors have also questioned whether the patient is really in control or is heavily influenced by medical and nursing staff, for whom PCA has certain advantages.

It is possible that different psychological factors, such as anxiety and depression, may influence the patient's satisfaction with IV PCA and the effectiveness of the technique, although results are inconclusive.[83,118] A recent study looked the correlation between a number of psychological factors and postoperative pain reports as well as analgesic consumption.[119] Emotional support and religious-based coping showed a positive correlation with postoperative morphine consumption; preoperative self-distraction coping correlated positively with pain while in the hospital; and preoperative distress, religious-based coping, behavioral disengagement, and emotional support positively predicted pain levels 4 weeks after surgery.[119]

Patient anxiety may also influence the efficacy of IV PCA. It has been shown that high anxiety levels are significantly related to higher pain scores and analgesic requirements in patients using PCA[84,118,120,121] and that anxiety may be associated with more frequent unsuccessful demands (ie, demands during the lockout period).[83,120]

Patient Comorbidities

It is not uncommon for studies looking at acute pain techniques and drugs to exclude certain groups of patients. However, it is often in these groups of patients that additional considerations are required if they are to obtain safe and effective pain relief using IV PCA. Examples of such groups include pediatric, elderly, and opioid-tolerant patients (acute pain management of these patient groups is covered in detail in other chapters of this book), and those with obstructive sleep apnea (OSA) or renal impairment.

PATIENTS WITH OBSTRUCTIVE SLEEP APNEA SYNDROME

It is commonly believed that patients with obstructive sleep apnea are at increased risk of respiratory depression when given opioids.[122] Concerns about the potential risks associated with administration of opioids in patients with OSA have led to suggestions that nonopioid or opioid-sparing acute pain management techniques should be used where possible.[123,124] However, good evidence comparing effects of various analgesic techniques in these patients is lacking.[125]

Case reports have led to conclusions that patients with OSA are at increased risk of respiratory depression when using IV PCA.[126–129] However, it is worth reading these reports in detail, as it would appear that there was an overreliance on the use of respiratory rate as an indicator of respiratory depression; the onset of respiratory depression was missed as vital signs were reported to be normal. The significance of increasing sedation (noted with these patients) as the better clinical indicator of early respiratory depression (see earlier) was not recognized.

As discussed later, it is wise to monitor patient sedation levels in all patients receiving opioids, including those prescribed IV PCA, and the PCA bolus dose should be reduced in any patient who becomes excessively sedated – preferably at a stage where they are still easy to rouse but have difficult staying awake rather than once they become unconscious.[88] This is especially important as many patients with undiagnosed OSA will be given opioids. The prevalence of OSA in the adult population is surprisingly high: it is said that up to 20% of adults have at least mild OSA, 7% have moderate to severe OSA, and that up to 75% of patients who could benefit from treatment remain undiagnosed.[130] Therefore, the chance of unknowingly giving opioids to a patient with OSA is significant.

Morbid obesity is significantly associated with OSA.[130] The use of PCA (without a background infusion) in these patients has been investigated and reported to be a safe and reasonably effective method of providing analgesia,[131–133] although the number of patients in these studies was small.

PATIENTS WITH RENAL IMPAIRMENT

Most opioids used on acute pain management are metabolized in the liver and their metabolites, as well as varying proportions of unchanged drug, are excreted by the kidney.

Patients with renal impairment may have reduced excretion of morphine-6-glucuronide (M6G) and morphine-3-glucuronide (M3G). M6G is an opioid agonist at least as potent as morphine, but its effects can be insidious as it crosses the blood-brain barrier very slowly.[134] Respiratory depression has been reported following IV PCA morphine in patients with renal impairment,[135] and the onset of this may be significantly delayed.[136] The 3-glucuronide (main) metabolites of morphine (M3G) and hydromorphone (H3G) are thought have neuroexcitatory effects and may also accumulate in patients with renal disease.[134] Accumulation of normeperidine (norpethidine) in patients with renal impairment has led to normeperidine (norpethidine) neurotoxicity.[137] As fentanyl has no active metabolites, it is suitable for use in patients with renal impairment[42] and

Table 14.2: Examples of Operator-Related Complications

Programming errors	Leading to patient death:
	Incorrect concentration[141,169,170]
	Leading to over-sedation and respiratory depression:
	Incorrect bolus dose size[171,172]
	Incorrect background infusions[173]
	Programming of background infusions when none were prescribed[140,173]
Wrong cassette	Cassette with wrong concentration of drug placed into PCA machine, leading to death; patient had been noted to be unrousable and snoring, but nothing was done as the nurse "considered the vital signs to be normal" (respiratory rate was 20 breaths per minute)[141]
Wrong drug	Syringe of bupivacaine and fentanyl intended for an epidural infusion in another patient placed in PCA pump – patient noticed to be "twitchy."[174]
Inappropriate patient selection or selection of opioid	Use of morphine in patients with renal failure leading to respiratory arrest[135]
	Use of meperidine in patients with renal impairment leading to normeperidine toxicity.[137]
	Use of a background infusion in a patients with obstructive sleep apnea[127]
Inappropriate prescription of concurrent medications	Inappropriate prescriptions of supplementary opioids (by other routes) or sedatives, including benzodiazepines and antihistamines (often involving inadequate knowledge about the risks of PCA and/or prescribing by more than one team) leading to oversedation and respiratory depression[126,140,175,176,177]

is probably the preferred opioid for use with IV PCA in these patients.[115]

An alternative opioid for use with IV PCA in these patients may be oxycodone, which is available for parenteral administration in many countries. The metabolites of oxycodone have very little clinical analgesic activity.[138] The major metabolite is noroxycodone, but this only has very weak analgesic activity and really plays no part on the pain-relieving effects of oxycodone; oxymorphone, on the other hand, is a potent opioid agonist, but it is produced in such small amounts that it has very little analgesic effect overall.[138]

COMPLICATIONS OF PCA

In general, complications relating to the use of PCA can be divided into four categories as follows:

- operator-related errors
- patient-related errors
- problems due to the equipment used
- side effects of the PCA opioid

Two large studies have looked at the type[139] and incidence[140] of operator-related and patient-related complications. The most common of the 5377 PCA-related errors examined by the United States Pharmacopeia (USP) were improper dose/quantity (38.9%), unauthorized drug (18.4%), omission error (17.6%), and prescribing error (9.2%); other errors included wrong administration technique, wrong drug preparation, wrong patient, and wrong route.[139] In the prospective survey of 3785 patients using IV PCA published by Ashburn et al,[140] 14 critical events were reported. These were 8 programming errors (all associated with the setting of a continuous infusion); 3 occasions when family members activated the PCA machine; 1 case of patient tampering; and 3 errors of clinical judgment. Other, more specific, examples of operator-related and patient-related errors as well as examples of problems involving the equipment used are given in the following sections.

Operator Errors

Operator errors include the following:

- those related to programming
- wrong drug
- inappropriate patient selection or selection of inappropriate opioid for a particular patient
- inappropriate prescription of concurrent medications

Although the mortality resulting from PCA programming errors is thought to be low (1 in 33 000 to 1 in 338 000),[141] around 30% of all PCA errors are believed to result from incorrect programming of PCA pumps.[142] This is twice as likely to result in injury or death than errors involving general-purpose infusion pumps and lead to more harm than errors from other types of medication administration.[142] These reports have led to suggestions that drug concentrations should be standardized within institutions.[142]

Examples of programming and other operator-related errors are given in Table 14.2. Changes that have been introduced in response to such problems include dose error reduction systems that use internal software to check the doses programmed against preset limits and then alert the programmer to inappropriate dose or continuous infusion settings.[142] Preset "standard" dosing protocols also can be used.[142]

Another innovation has been the introduction of integrated bar code readers that can identify the drug and drug concentration being used and, in some cases, automatically select the appropriate dosing protocol.[142]

Patient-Related Errors

Patient-related errors (see Table 14.3) include the following:

- failure to understand the technique adequately
- initiation of a demand by someone other that the patients ("PCA by proxy")
- tampering of the PCA machine by the patient

Table 14.3: Examples of Patient-Related Complications

Failure to understand PCA	Confusion between the nurse call and PCA demand button has been reported[175,178]
PCA by proxy	Unauthorized activation of the demand button by nurses[153,179] or family or visitors[113,140,153,180–182] leading to respiratory depression
Tampering	Could lead to administration of excessive opioid dose[146]

Most patients manage PCA well after just some initial education, but others may need reminding about its method of use. In addition, patients may have problems with some PCA demand buttons as some are small and not easy for elderly or disabled patients to use. In these patients, it may be possible to used a foot-activated[143] or breath-activated device (eg, attaching plastic tubing to the machine in place of the handset and asking the patients to blow into the tube[144,145]), allowing activation by the patient blowing into the tube.

As access to the syringe (or other drug reservoir) and the microprocessor program in electronic PCA pumps should only be possible using a key or access code, successful tampering would usually leave obvious signs of damage to the pump casing. However, this may not always be the case. Access to the syringe in a locked pump without a key has been reported.[146]

Problems Related to Equipment

Problems related to PCA equipment include the following:

■ spontaneous delivery of opioid
■ incorrect use of, or failure to use, antireflux and/or anti-syphon valves
■ incorrect placement of, or damage to, syringe/cartridge

In general, modern PCA pumps have a high degree of reliability. However, problems continue to be reported, as well as problems related to the disposable items required for each patient (see Table 14.4).

The routine inclusion of one-way antireflux valves and anti-siphon valves as integral parts of the infusion system has been recommended,[147] the former because retrograde flow of opioid along the intravenous line is a potential hazard and the latter because if the syringe or cassette is not correctly placed into the syringe carriage, there is a risk that the contents of the syringe may empty by gravity (siphon) into the patient.

Complications Related to the PCA Opioid

Recent meta-analyses have shown that the risk of side effects from opioids administered by PCA is similar to the risks related to traditional methods of systemic opioid administration (IV, IM, or SC).[12,13]

Wheeler et al[148] reviewed randomized-controlled trials reporting postoperative opioid-related adverse effects. When PCA was compared with IV/IM opioids combined, the respective incidences were respiratory depression (1.8% and 2.4%), gastrointestinal (mainly nausea and vomiting; 37.1% and 28.2%), and pruritus (14.7% and 17.5%), respectively.[148]

Table 14.4: Examples of Equipment-Related Complications

Spontaneous delivery of drug	Runaway pumps (machine unexpectedly changes the program and delivers an unprescribed dose of drug) when main electricity leads become loose or disconnected[176,183]
	Spontaneous triggering[184]
	Triggering as a result of an electrical short circuit (frayed wire in the demand apparatus)[185]
Use in unusual environment	Inability to reprogam PCA machine in hyperbaric chamber[186]
Incorrect use of, or failure to use, antireflux valves	Failure to incorporate an antireflux valve leading to respiratory depression[187]
	Wrongly connected Y-piece leading to respiratory depression[181]
Uncontrolled siphoning of syringe contents	Uncontrolled siphoning of syringe contents has been reported in association with:
	A syringe plunger not engaged in its carriage[188]
	A damaged drive mechanism failing to retain the syringe plunger[189]
	Improper cassette attachment[190]
	Cracked glass PCA syringes[191,192]

A later review of published cohort studies by Cashman and Dolin, case-controlled studies, and audit reports, as well as randomized-controlled trials, found reasonably similar incidences associated with the use of PCA: respiratory depression (1.2% to 11.5%; using hypoventilation and oxygen desaturation, respectively, as indicators), nausea (32%), vomiting (20.7%), and pruritus (13.8%).[149,150] The incidences reported for IM opioid analgesia were respiratory depression (0.8% to 37%; again using hypoventilation and oxygen desaturation, respectively, as indicators), nausea (17%), vomiting (21.9%), and pruritus (3.4%).[149,150]

Respiratory Depression

The true incidence of respiratory depression associated with PCA is very difficult to determine because of the variety of definitions used in published studies, including respiratory rate, hypercarbia, low oxygen saturation, and use of naloxone. Most commonly, when authors report on the incidence of respiratory depression, they use a decrease in respiratory rate as the indicator. However, there is still considerable debate as to the best way to monitor for opioid-induced respiratory depression in patients receiving opioids via IV PCA or other routes of administration.

A workshop convened by the Anesthesia Patient Safety Foundation (APSF) to discuss this issue in response to concerns about the safety if IV PCA recommended "the use of continuous monitoring of oxygenation (generally pulse oximetry) and ventilation in nonventilated patients."[122] This was despite recognizing the limitations of currently available monitors and despite the low sensitivity of continuous pulse oximetry in patients given supplemental oxygen (common in many countries).[122]

Another example of the low sensitivity of continuous pulse oximetry can be seen when the article referenced earlier by Cashman and Dolin,[149] which reports a much higher incidence of oxygen desaturation associated with IM analgesia (37% of patients) compared with PCA (11.5% of patients), is examined in conjunction with a later article by the same authors that reports on effectiveness of PCA and IM opioid analgesia. The much higher number of patients reporting moderate-to-severe or severe pain with IM opioid analgesia[10] would suggest that lower opioid doses were used in these patients, so it is highly unlikely that they also had a higher incidence of respiratory depression than patients using PCA. Unfortunately, monitoring of a patient's level of sedation, with an appropriate response to increasing sedation, was not among the recommendations from the APSF workshop.

A decrease in respiratory rate, often used as an indicator of decreasing ventilation, may be a late and unreliable sign of respiratory depression. Vila et al[151] described their results before and after the hospital-wide introduction of pain management standards. Only 3 of 29 patients reported to have respiratory depression exhibited a fall in respiratory rate, compared with 27 of the 29 who experienced a decrease in conscious state[151] Thus, the best early clinical indicator of respiratory depression is increasing sedation, which can be monitored using a simple sedation score.[88,151] Monitoring for opioid-related respiratory depression is covered in more detail in Chapter 28 (*Acute Pain Management in the Community Hospital Setting*).

The incidence of respiratory depression associated with the use of IV PCA is probably somewhere in the range of 0.1% to 1%.[122] As noted above, Cashman and Dolin[149] reported an incidence of PCA-related respiratory depression of 1.2% to 11.5% (depending on definition used). However, the incidence of sedation, reported by the same authors in a later article looking at other opioid-related side effects, was found to be just over 5%.[150] A more recent audit of 700 patients who received PCA for postoperative pain relief, reported that 13 patients (1.86%) developed respiratory depression; all had respiratory rates of <10 breaths per minute and 11 also had sedation scores of 2 (defined as "asleep but easily roused").[152]

A number of risk factors for respiratory depression have been identified. These include the use of concurrent (background) infusions, concurrent administration of sedatives or additional opioids, use in the elderly patient, nurse- or physician-controlled analgesia, inappropriate use of PCA by patients, and if the patient becomes hypovolemic.[105,113,140,153,154]

It may be possible to reduce the risk of respiratory depression. It has been shown that concurrent administration of NSAIDs significantly reduces PCA opioid requirements and the incidence of excessive sedation as well as opioid-related nausea and vomiting.[155]

Nausea and Vomiting

Although recent meta-analyses reported no difference in the incidence of nausea and vomiting with PCA compared with conventional methods of opioid delivery,[12,13] the review by Dolin and Cashman[150] referred to earlier, looking at published cohort studies, case-controlled studies, and audit reports, as well as randomized-controlled trials, reported that the incidence of nausea was higher with PCA (32%) than following IM opioid analgesia (17%) but there was no difference in the incidence of vomiting.[150]

It is possible that some of these differences may be related to opioid dose as the risk of nausea and vomiting is known to increase with increasing dose.[155,156] Concurrent administration NSAIDs leads to a reduction in PCA opioid requirements and a decrease in the incidence of nausea and vomiting.[155] However, a similar decrease is not seen when acetaminophen is added to the PCA opioid regimen, even though it too is opioid sparing.[157]

MANAGEMENT OF NAUSEA AND VOMITING ASSOCIATED WITH PCA OPIOID ADMINISTRATION

A detailed discussion of opioid-related nausea and vomiting and its management is outside the scope of this chapter (details are contained in Chapter 27 (*The Acute Pain Management Service: Organization and Implementation Issues*). However, there are some studies where antiemetics have been added to the PCA opioid (usually morphine) solution, and the benefits or otherwise of this strategy (some results conflict) are summarized in Table 14.5.

The antiemetic that has most commonly been studied as an additive to the PCA opioid solution is droperidol. Although it is effective in the prevention of both nausea and vomiting when administered in this way,[158,159] it may be more effective for nausea.[160] Adverse effects of droperidol are more likely when higher doses are administered.[158,160]

The practice of adding antiemetics to PCA remains controversial, as the risk of side effects may increase with increased use of PCA. In addition, although addition of antiemetics to the PCA opioid solution may provide effective prophylaxis against nausea and vomiting, separate administration of droperidol[161] and 5-HT$_3$ antagonists[162] can be just as effective.

Pruritus

The incidence of pruritus, thought to be a result of a μ-receptor-mediated mechanism rather than histamine release,[163] is significantly higher in patients given PCA compared with those receiving systemic opioids by other routes.[12] Dolin and Cashman[150] found that the incidence of pruritus was higher with PCA (13.8%) compared with IM/SC opioids (3.1%).

MANAGEMENT OF PRURITUS ASSOCIATED WITH PCA OPIOID ADMINISTRATION

A detailed discussion of opioid-related pruritus and its management is outside the scope of this chapter (details are contained in Chapter 27). However, there are some studies where antiemetics have been added to the PCA opioid solution. Both naloxone and droperidol have been shown to be effective in the prevention of opioid-induced pruritus.[163] The same is true when larger doses of droperidol (15 and 50 μg but not 5 μg added to 1 mg morphine) are added to PCA morphine solutions,[160] but not when 0.8 mg naloxone was added to 60 mg morphine.[78]

Normeperidine Toxicity

Reports of normeperidine (norpethidine) toxicity in patients using PCA meperidine started to appear in the early 1990s.[52] It has been suggested that no more than 600 mg meperidine should be given each day, for no more than a few days to reduce the risk of normeperidine toxicity, and that the drug should be avoided in patients with renal impairment.[51,88,42] In addition, because meperidine offers no benefit in terms of analgesic effect or incidence of adverse effects compared with other

Table 14.5: Effects of Different Antiemetics Added to PCA Morphine

Antiemetic	Effect	Reference
Droperidol	Decreased incidence nausea and vomiting	Tramer and Walder (1999)[158]
	NNT for nausea = 2.7; NNT for vomiting = 3.1	
	No dose response for antiemetic effects	
	Minor adverse effects more likely if >4 mg/d	
	Decreased incidence nausea and vomiting	Lo et al (2005)[159]
	Dose-response noted when added to 1 mg morphine: 5 μg no effect; 15 μg effective for nausea only; 50 μg effective for both nausea and vomiting	Culebras et al (2003)[160]
	NNT for nausea = 3.7; NNT for vomiting = 8.31	
	Increased risk of sedation with higher dose (50 μg)	
Ondansetron	Effective for prophylaxis of both nausea and vomiting	Cherian and Smith (2001)[162]
	Antivomiting but no antinausea effects	Tramer and Walder (1999)[158]
Promethazine	Reduced the incidence of nausea and vomiting	Silverman et al (1992)[193]
Diphenhydramine	Reduced the incidence of nausea and vomiting without increasing side effects such as sedation and dry mouth	Lin et al (2005)[194]
Cyclizine	Comparable incidences of severe nausea and vomiting compared with droperidol (50 μg) added to 1 mg PCA morphine	Laffey and Boylan (2002)[195]
Propofol	No benefit	Bree et al (1998)[196]
Nalmefene	Reduced the incidence of nausea and vomiting but did not reduce analgesia	Joshi et al (1999)[197]
Naloxone	No decrease in the incidence of nausea and vomiting (0.8 mg naloxone added to 60 mg morphine)	Sartain et al (2003)[78]

opioids used in PCA, it has been recommended that its use be discouraged.[42,50]

CONCLUSIONS

The technique of IV PCA has grown rapidly, from its initial development in the 1970s and increasing clinical use in the 1980s and 1990s, to one that is now a "standard" method of safe and effective acute pain management in the clinical setting. Although other forms of PCA are now available and increasing in popularity, the inherent flexibility of IV PCA as a method of administering systemic opioids means it will probably maintain a key role in the management of acute pain for some years to come.

APPENDIX: PATIENT GUIDE TO PATIENT-CONTROLLED ANALGESIA, ACUTE PAIN SERVICE, ROYAL ADELAIDE HOSPITAL (REPRODUCED WITH PERMISSION OF THE ROYAL ADELAIDE HOSPITAL)

Patient-controlled analgesia (or PCA for short) means that you have control over your own pain relief. A machine called a PCA pump can be used to give you a small dose of a strong pain-relieving drug such as morphine or fentanyl. Usually this machine will be attached to the drip (intravenous line or IV) in your arm. If you are uncomfortable, you press a button and the machine will pump a small dose of the drug into your drip. You can do this whenever you are uncomfortable – you do not need to tell the nurse first. The amount of pain medicine delivered by the machine each time you press the button, as well as other

settings on the machine, will be ordered by the anaesthetist from the APS. The PCA machine will be programmed by your nurse according to these orders.

How Often Can I Press the Button?

You can press the PCA button whenever you feel uncomfortable. However, once the button has been pushed and the PCA machine has delivered the dose, built-in timers in the machine will "lockout" further pushes for 5 minutes. This means that if you push the button within this time, the PCA machine will not deliver another dose. This is so that you have time to feel the effect of one dose of pain relieving drug before getting another dose. Remember, the aim is to make you comfortable – it is not always possible to be completely pain free.

Who is Allowed to Press the PCA Button?

The patient is the ONLY person allowed to press the button. Do not allow ANY hospital staff, relatives or friends to do so.

Will the Pain-Relieving Drug Work Immediately?

No. These drugs need to get to the brain and spinal cord so it may take 5 minutes or longer to get the full effect. If you are about to do something that you know will hurt, like coughing or moving, press the PCA button about 5 minutes *before* doing it.

What If the Pain Medicine Doesn't Work?

If you are pressing the PCA button quite frequently and are still uncomfortable, tell your nurse. They will firstly check that the IV is running properly. As long as you are not having problems staying awake, your nurse may increase the amount of pain medicine you get when you press the button. If necessary, your nurse will contact the APS.

Can I Overdose?

PCA is probably one of the safest ways of giving strong pain-relieving medicines. The dose that you get with each press of the button is very small. If you were getting just a little too much you would feel sleepy. This means that you would not press the button again. Your nurse would also notice this and would reduce the amount of drug delivered with each push of the button and, if necessary, treat the sleepiness.

How Long Will I Use PCA For?

When your doctors on the ward allow you to drink it means that your IV may soon be removed. PCA will usually stop at this time. You will be ordered other pain-relieving medicines should you need them.

More Information

While you have PCA, you will be seen at least once a day by an anaesthetist and nurse from the *Acute Pain Service* (APS) in addition to the doctors and nurses on your ward. The APS is part of the Department of Anaesthesia at the Royal Adelaide Hospital. Anaesthetists are the doctors who look after you during your anaesthetic, but they also specialise in pain relief. The APS also has an anaesthetist on-call 24 hours a day to help with pain control.

There is more information about the general management of acute pain in the information sheet about anaesthesia. Please read this as well as the information in this pamphlet.

REFERENCES

1. Roe BB. Are postoperative narcotics necessary? *Arch Surg.* 1963;87:912–915.
2. Sechzer PH. Objective measurement of pain. *Anesthesiology.* 1968;29:209–210.
3. Sechzer PH. Studies in pain with the analgesic-demand system. *Anesth Analg.* 1971;50:1–10.
4. White PF. Use of patient-controlled analgesia for management of acute pain. *JAMA.* 1988;259:243–247.
5. Evans JM, Rosen M, MacCarthy J, Hogg MI. Apparatus for patient-controlled administration of intravenous narcotics during labour. *Lancet.* 1976;1:17–18.
6. Hull CJ, Sibbald A. Control of postoperative pain by interactive demand analgesia. *Br J Anaesth.* 1981;53:385–391.
7. Harmer M, Rosen M, Vickers MD. eds. *Patient-Controlled Analgesia: Proceedings of the First International Workshop on Patient-Controlled Analgesia.* Oxford, UK: Blackwell; 1985.
8. Skryabina EA, Dunn TS. Disposable infusion pumps. *Am J Health Syst Pharm.* 2006;63:1260–1268.
9. Ready LB, Oden R, Chadwick HS, et al. Development of an anesthesiology-based postoperative pain management service. *Anesthesiology.* 1988;68:100–106.
10. Dolin SJ, Cashman JN, Bland JM. Effectiveness of acute postoperative pain management. I. Evidence from published data. *Br J Anaesth.* 2002;89:409–423.
11. Ballantyne JC, Carr DB, Chalmers TC, et al. Postoperative patient-controlled analgesia: meta-analyses of initial randomized control trials. *J Clin Anesth.* 1993;5:182–193.
12. Hudcova J, McNicol E, Quah C, et al. Patient controlled intravenous opioid analgesia versus conventional opioid analgesia for postoperative pain control: a quantitative systematic review. *Acute Pain.* 2005;7:115–132.
13. Walder B, Schafer M, Henzi I, Tramer MR. Efficacy and safety of patient-controlled opioid analgesia for acute postoperative pain:

a quantitative systematic review. *Acta Anaesthesiol Scand.* 2001; 45:795–804.
14. Lehmann KA. Recent developments in patient-controlled analgesia. *J Pain Sympt Manage.* 2005;29:S72–S89.
15. Bainbridge D, Martin JE, Cheng DC. Patient-controlled versus nurse-controlled analgesia after cardiac surgery: a meta-analysis. *Can J Anaesth.* 2006;53:492–499.
16. Evans E, Turley N, Robinson N, Clancy M. Randomised controlled trial of patient controlled analgesia compared with nurse delivered analgesia in an emergency department. *Emerg Med J.* 2005;22:25–29.
17. Choiniere M, Rittenhouse BE, Perreault S, et al. Efficacy and costs of patient-controlled analgesia versus regularly administered intramuscular opioid therapy. *Anesthesiology.* 1998;89:1377–1388.
18. Tsang J, Brush B. Patient-controlled analgesia in postoperative cardiac surgery. *Anaesth Intensive Care.* 1999;27:464–470.
19. Macintyre PE. Intravenous patient-controlled analgesia: one size does not fit all. *Anesthesiol Clin North Am.* 2005;23:109–123.
20. Werawatganon T, Charuluxanun S. Patient controlled intravenous opioid analgesia versus continuous epidural analgesia for pain after intra-abdominal surgery. *Cochrane Database Syst Rev.* 2005;CD004088.
21. Wu CL, Cohen SR, Richman JM, et al. Efficacy of postoperative patient-controlled and continuous infusion epidural analgesia versus intravenous patient-controlled analgesia with opioids: a meta-analysis. *Anesthesiology.* 2005;103:1079–1088.
22. Dawson L, Brockbank K, Carr EC, Barrett RF. Improving patients' postoperative sleep: a randomized control study comparing subcutaneous with intravenous patient-controlled analgesia. *J Adv Nurs.* 1999;30:875–881.
23. Urquhart ML, Klapp K, White PF. Patient-controlled analgesia: a comparison of intravenous versus subcutaneous hydromorphone. *Anesthesiology.* 1988;69:428–432.
24. Striebel HW, Scheitza W, Philippi W, et al. Quantifying oral analgesic consumption using a novel method and comparison with patient-controlled intravenous analgesic consumption. *Anesth Analg.* 1998;86:1051–1053.
25. Toussaint S, Maidl J, Schwagmeier R, Striebel HW. Patient-controlled intranasal analgesia: effective alternative to intravenous PCA for postoperative pain relief. *Can J Anaesth.* 2000;47:299–302.
26. Hallett A, O'Higgins F, Francis V, Cook TM. Patient-controlled intranasal diamorphine for postoperative pain: an acceptability study. *Anaesthesia.* 2000;55:532–539.
27. Dale O, Hjortkjaer R, Kharasch ED. Nasal administration of opioids for pain management in adults. *Acta Anaesthesiol Scand.* 2002;46:759–770.
28. Ward M, Minto G, Alexander-Williams JM. A comparison of patient-controlled analgesia administered by the intravenous or intranasal route during the early postoperative period. *Anaesthesia.* 2002;57:48–52.
29. Striebel HW, Olmann T, Spies C, Brummer G. Patient-controlled intranasal analgesia (PCINA) for the management of postoperative pain: a pilot study. *J Clin Anesth.* 1996;8:4–8.
30. Chelly JE, Grass J, Houseman TW, et al. The safety and efficacy of a fentanyl patient-controlled transdermal system for acute postoperative analgesia: a multicenter, placebo-controlled trial. *Anesth Analg.* 2004;98:427–433, table of contents.
31. Keita H, Geachan N, Dahmani S, et al. Comparison between patient-controlled analgesia and subcutaneous morphine in elderly patients after total hip replacement. *Br J Anaesth.* 2003;90:53–57.
32. White PF. Subcutaneous-PCA: an alternative to IV-PCA for postoperative pain management. *Clin J Pain.* 1990;6:297–300.
33. Munro AJ, Long GT, Sleigh JW. Nurse-administered subcutaneous morphine is a satisfactory alternative to intravenous

patient-controlled analgesia morphine after cardiac surgery. *Anesth Analg.* 1998;87:11–15.

34. Paech MJ, Lim CB, Banks SL, et al. A new formulation of nasal fentanyl spray for postoperative analgesia: a pilot study. *Anaesthesia.* 2003;58:740–744.

35. Striebel HW, Pommerening J, Rieger A. Intranasal fentanyl titration for postoperative pain management in an unselected population. *Anaesthesia.* 1993;48:753–757.

36. O'Neil G, Paech M, Wood F. Preliminary clinical use of a patient-controlled intranasal analgesia (PCINA) device. *Anaesth Intensive Care.* 1997;25:408–412.

37. Striebel HW, Bonillo B, Schwagmeier R, et al. Self-administered intranasal meperidine for postoperative pain management. *Can J Anaesth.* 1995;42:287–291.

38. Banga AK. Iontophoretic topical and transdermal drug delivery. *Drug Deliv Rep.* 2005;Autumn/Winter:51–53.

39. Viscusi ER, Reynolds L, Tait S, et al. An iontophoretic fentanyl patient-activated analgesic delivery system for postoperative pain: a double-blind, placebo-controlled trial. *Anesth Analg.* 2006;102:188–194.

40. Viscusi ER, Reynolds L, Chung F, et al. Patient-controlled transdermal fentanyl hydrochloride vs intravenous morphine pump for postoperative pain: a randomized controlled trial. *JAMA.* 2004;291:1333–1341.

41. Hartrick CT, Bourne MH, Gargiulo K, et al. Fentanyl iontophoretic transdermal system for acute-pain management after orthopedic surgery: a comparative study with morphine intravenous patient-controlled analgesia. *Reg Anesth Pain Med.* 2006;31:546–554.

42. Australian and New Zealand College of Anaesthetists. *Acute Pain Management: Scientific Evidence.* 2nd ed. Melbourne: Australian and New Zealand College of Anaesthetists; 2005.

43. Plummer JL, Owen H, Ilsley AH, Inglis S. Morphine patient-controlled analgesia is superior to meperidine patient-controlled analgesia for postoperative pain. *Anesth Analg.* 1997;84:794–799.

44. Sinatra RS, Lodge K, Sibert K, et al. A comparison of morphine, meperidine, and oxymorphone as utilized in patient-controlled analgesia following cesarean delivery. *Anesthesiology.* 1989; 70:585–590.

45. Bahar M, Rosen M, Vickers MD. Self-administered nalbuphine, morphine and pethidine. Comparison, by intravenous route, following cholecystectomy. *Anaesthesia.* 1985;40:529–532.

46. Stanley G, Appadu B, Mead M, Rowbotham DJ. Dose requirements, efficacy and side effects of morphine and pethidine delivered by patient-controlled analgesia after gynaecological surgery. *Br J Anaesth.* 1996;76:484–486.

47. Woodhouse A, Hobbes AF, Mather LE, Gibson M. A comparison of morphine, pethidine and fentanyl in the postsurgical patient-controlled analgesia environment. *Pain.* 1996;64:115–121.

48. Seifert CF, Kennedy S. Meperidine is alive and well in the new millennium: evaluation of meperidine usage patterns and frequency of adverse drug reactions. *Pharmacotherapy.* 2004;24:776–783.

49. Silverman ME, Shih RD, Allegra J. Morphine induces less nausea than meperidine when administered parenterally. *J Emerg Med.* 2004;27:241–243.

50. Latta KS, Ginsberg B, Barkin RL. Meperidine: a critical review. *Am J Ther.* 2002;9:53–68.

51. Simopoulos TT, Smith HS, Peeters-Asdourian C, Stevens DS. Use of meperidine in patient-controlled analgesia and the development of a normeperidine toxic reaction. *Arch Surg.* 2002;137:84–88.

52. Stone PA, Macintyre PE, Jarvis DA. Norpethidine toxicity and patient controlled analgesia. *Br J Anaesth.* 1993;71:738–740.

53. Howell PR, Gambling DR, Pavy T, et al. Patient-controlled analgesia following caesarean section under general anaesthesia: a com-

parison of fentanyl with morphine. *Can J Anaesth.* 1995;42:41–45.

54. Rapp SE, Egan KJ, Ross BK, et al. A multidimensional comparison of morphine and hydromorphone patient-controlled analgesia. *Anesth Analg.* 1996;82:1043–1048.

55. Pang WW, Mok MS, Lin CH, et al. Comparison of patient-controlled analgesia (PCA) with tramadol or morphine. *Can J Anaesth.* 1999;46:1030–1035.

56. Erolcay H, Yuceyar L. Intravenous patient-controlled analgesia after thoracotomy: a comparison of morphine with tramadol. *Eur J Anaesthesiol.* 2003;20:141–146.

57. Silvasti M, Rosenberg P, Seppala T, et al. Comparison of analgesic efficacy of oxycodone and morphine in postoperative intravenous patient-controlled analgesia. *Acta Anaesthesiol Scand.* 1998;42:576–580.

58. Ngan Kee WD, Khaw KS, Wong EL. Randomised double-blind comparison of morphine vs. a morphine-alfentanil combination for patient-controlled analgesia. *Anaesthesia.* 1999;54:629–633.

59. Dopfmer UR, Schenk MR, Kuscic S, et al. A randomized controlled double-blind trial comparing piritramide and morphine for analgesia after hysterectomy. *Eur J Anaesthesiol.* 2001;18:389–393.

60. Herrick IA, Ganapathy S, Komar W, et al. Postoperative cognitive impairment in the elderly. Choice of patient-controlled analgesia opioid. *Anaesthesia.* 1996;51:356–360.

61. Narayareswamy M, Smith J, Sprlaja A. Choice of opiate and incidence of confusion in elderly posstoperative patients. Paper presented at: the Australian and New Zealand College of Anaesthetists Annual Scientific Meeting: 2006: Adelaide, South Australia.

62. Ng KF, Yuen TS, Ng VM. A comparison of postoperative cognitive function and pain relief with fentanyl or tramadol patient-controlled analgesia. *J Clin Anesth.* 2006;18:205–210.

63. Kucukemre F, Kunt N, Kaygusuz K, et al. Remifentanil compared with morphine for postoperative patient-controlled analgesia after major abdominal surgery: a randomized controlled trial. *Eur J Anaesthesiol.* 2005;22:378–385.

64. Gurbet A, Goren S, Sahin S, et al. Comparison of analgesic effects of morphine, fentanyl, and remifentanil with intravenous patient-controlled analgesia after cardiac surgery. *J Cardiothorac Vasc Anesth.* 2004;18:755–758.

65. Krishnan K, Elliot SC, Berridge JC, Mallick A. Remifentanil patient-controlled analgesia following cardiac surgery. *Acta Anaesthesiol Scand.* 2005;49:876–879.

66. Chou WY, Yang LC, Lu HF, et al. Association of mu-opioid receptor gene polymorphism (A118G) with variations in morphine consumption for analgesia after total knee arthroplasty. *Acta Anaesthesiol Scand.* 2006;50:787–792.

67. Chou WY, Wang CH, Liu PH, et al. Human opioid receptor A118G polymorphism affects intravenous patient-controlled analgesia morphine consumption after total abdominal hysterectomy. *Anesthesiology.* 2006;105:334–337.

68. Klepstad P, Dale O, Skorpen F, et al. Genetic variability and clinical efficacy of morphine. *Acta Anaesthesiol Scand.* 2005;49:902–908.

69. Stamer UM, Lehnen K, Hothker F, et al. Impact of CYP2D6 genotype on postoperative tramadol analgesia. *Pain.* 2003;105:231–238.

70. Bell RF, Dahl JB, Moore RA, Kalso E. Perioperative ketamine for acute postoperative pain. *Cochrane Database Syst Rev.* 2006;CD004603.

71. Burstal R, Danjoux G, Hayes C, Lantry G. PCA ketamine and morphine after abdominal hysterectomy. *Anaesth Intensive Care.* 2001;29:246–251.

72. Javery KB, Ussery TW, Steger HG, Colclough GW. Comparison of morphine and morphine with ketamine for postoperative analgesia. *Can J Anaesth.* 1996;43:212–215.

73. Murdoch CJ, Crooks BA, Miller CD. Effect of the addition of ketamine to morphine in patient-controlled analgesia. *Anaesthesia.* 2002;57:484–488.

74. Unlugenc H, Ozalevli M, Guler T, Isik G. Postoperative pain management with intravenous patient-controlled morphine: comparison of the effect of adding magnesium or ketamine. *Eur J Anaesthesiol.* 2003;20:416–421.

75. Reeves M, Lindholm DE, Myles PS, et al. Adding ketamine to morphine for patient-controlled analgesia after major abdominal surgery: a double-blinded, randomized controlled trial. *Anesth Analg.* 2001;93:116–120.

76. Cepeda MS, Alvarez H, Morales O, Carr DB. Addition of ultralow dose naloxone to postoperative morphine PCA: unchanged analgesia and opioid requirement but decreased incidence of opioid side effects. *Pain.* 2004;107:41–46.

77. Cepeda MS, Africano JM, Manrique AM, et al. The combination of low dose of naloxone and morphine in PCA does not decrease opioid requirements in the postoperative period. *Pain.* 2002;96:73–79.

78. Sartain JB, Barry JJ, Richardson CA, Branagan HC. Effect of combining naloxone and morphine for intravenous patient-controlled analgesia. *Anesthesiology.* 2003;99:148–151.

79. Chumbley GM, Hall GM, Salmon P. Patient-controlled analgesia: an assessment by 200 patients. *Anaesthesia.* 1998;53:216–221.

80. Salmon P, Hall GM. PCA: patient-controlled analgesia or politically correct analgesia? *Br J Anaesth.* 2001;87:815–818.

81. Lebovits AH, Zenetos P, O'Neill DK, et al. Satisfaction with epidural and intravenous patient-controlled analgesia. *Pain Med.* 2001;2:280–286.

82. Pellino TA, Ward SE. Perceived control mediates the relationship between pain severity and patient satisfaction. *J Pain Sympt Manag.* 1998;15:110–116.

83. Jamison RN, Taft K, O'Hara JP, Ferrante FM. Psychosocial and pharmacologic predictors of satisfaction with intravenous patient-controlled analgesia. *Anesth Analg.* 1993;77:121–125.

84. Perry F, Parker RK, White PF, Clifford PA. Role of psychological factors in postoperative pain control and recovery with patient-controlled analgesia. *Clin J Pain.* 1994;10:57–63; discussion 82–85.

85. Coleman SA, Booker-Milburn J. Audit of postoperative pain control. Influence of a dedicated acute pain nurse. *Anaesthesia.* 1996;51:1093–1096.

86. Colwell CW, Jr., Morris BA. Patient-controlled analgesia compared with intramuscular injection of analgesics for the management of pain after an orthopaedic procedure. *J Bone Joint Surg Am.* 1995;77:726–733.

87. Gust R, Pecher S, Gust A, et al. Effect of patient-controlled analgesia on pulmonary complications after coronary artery bypass grafting. *Crit Care Med.* 1999;27:2218–2223.

88. Macintyre PE, Schug SA. *Acute Pain Management: A Practical Guide.* 3rd ed. London: Elsevier; 2007.

89. Chumbley GM, Hall GM, Salmon P. Patient-controlled analgesia: what information does the patient want? *J Adv Nurs.* 2002;39:459–471.

90. Chumbley GM, Ward L, Hall GM, Salmon P. Pre-operative information and patient-controlled analgesia: much ado about nothing. *Anaesthesia.* 2004;59:354–358.

91. Chen HH, Yeh ML, Yang HJ. Testing the impact of a multimedia video CD of patient-controlled analgesia on pain knowledge and pain relief in patients receiving surgery. *Int J Med Inform.* 2005;74:437–445.

92. McDonald S, Hetrick S, Green S. Pre-operative education for hip or knee replacement. *Cochrane Database Syst Rev.* 2004; CD003526.

93. Griffin MJ, Brennan L, McShane AJ. Preoperative education and outcome of patient controlled analgesia. *Can J Anaesth.* 1998;45:943–948.

94. Lam KK, Chan MT, Chen PP, Kee WD. Structured preoperative patient education for patient-controlled analgesia. *J Clin Anesth.* 2001;13:465–469.

95. Stacey BR, Rudy TE, Nelhaus D. Management of patient-controlled analgesia: a comparison of primary surgeons and a dedicated pain service. *Anesth Analg.* 1997;85:130–134.

96. Owen H, Plummer JL, Armstrong I, et al. Variables of patient-controlled analgesia. 1. Bolus size. *Anaesthesia.* 1989;44:7–10.

97. Badner NH, Doyle JA, Smith MH, Herrick IA. Effect of varying intravenous patient-controlled analgesia dose and lockout interval while maintaining a constant hourly maximum dose. *J Clin Anesth.* 1996;8:382–385.

98. Love DR, Owen H, Ilsley AH, et al. A comparison of variable-dose patient-controlled analgesia with fixed-dose patient-controlled analgesia. *Anesth Analg.* 1996;83:1060–1064.

99. Camu F, Van Aken H, Bovill JG. Postoperative analgesic effects of three demand-dose sizes of fentanyl administered by patient-controlled analgesia. *Anesth Analg.* 1998;87:890–895.

100. Prakash S, Fatima T, Pawar M. Patient-controlled analgesia with fentanyl for burn dressing changes. *Anesth Analg.* 2004;99:552–555, table of contents.

101. Macintyre PE, Jarvis DA. Age is the best predictor of postoperative morphine requirements. *Pain.* 1996;64:357–364.

102. Woodhouse A, Mather LE. The influence of age upon opioid analgesic use in the patient-controlled analgesia (PCA) environment. *Anaesthesia.* 1997;52:949–955.

103. Gagliese L, Jackson M, Ritvo P, et al. Age is not an impediment to effective use of patient-controlled analgesia by surgical patients. *Anesthesiology.* 2000;93:601–610.

104. Macintyre PE, Upton R, Ludbrook GL. Acute pain management in the elderly patient. In: Macintyre PE, Walker SM, Rowbotham DJ, eds. *Clinical Pain Management: Acute Pain.* London: Arnold; 2003.

105. Etches RC. Patient-controlled analgesia. *Surg Clin North Am.* 1999;79:297–312.

106. Rapp SE, Ready LB, Nessly ML. Acute pain management in patients with prior opioid consumption: a case-controlled retrospective review. *Pain.* 1995;61:195–201.

107. Davis JJ, Swenson JD, Hall RH, et al. Preoperative "fentanyl challenge" as a tool to estimate postoperative opioid dosing in chronic opioid-consuming patients. *Anesth Analg.* 2005;101:389–395, table of contents.

108. Woodhouse A, Mather LE. The effect of duration of dose delivery with patient-controlled analgesia on the incidence of nausea and vomiting after hysterectomy. *Br J Clin Pharmacol.* 1998;45:57–62.

109. Ginsberg B, Gil KM, Muir M, et al. The influence of lockout intervals and drug selection on patient-controlled analgesia following gynecological surgery. *Pain.* 1995;62:95–100.

110. Owen H, Szekely SM, Plummer JL, et al. Variables of patient-controlled analgesia. 2. Concurrent infusion. *Anaesthesia.* 1989; 44:11–13.

111. Parker RK, Holtmann B, White PF. Effects of a nighttime opioid infusion with PCA therapy on patient comfort and analgesic requirements after abdominal hysterectomy. *Anesthesiology.* 1992;76:362–367.

112. Dal D, Kanbak M, Caglar M, Aypar U. A background infusion of morphine does not enhance postoperative analgesia after cardiac surgery. *Can J Anaesth.* 2003;50:476–479.

113. Sidebotham D, Dijkhuizen MR, Schug SA. The safety and utilization of patient-controlled analgesia. *J Pain Symptom Manage.* 1997;14:202–209.

114. Guler T, Unlugenc H, Gundogan Z, et al. A background infusion of morphine enhances patient-controlled analgesia after cardiac surgery. *Can J Anaesth.* 2004;51:718–722.

115. Macintyre PE. Safety and efficacy of patient-controlled analgesia. *Br J Anaesth.* 2001;87:36–46.

116. Taylor NM, Hall GM, Salmon P. Patients' experiences of patient-controlled analgesia. *Anaesthesia.* 1996;51:525–528.

117. Taylor N, Hall GM, Salmon P. Is patient-controlled analgesia controlled by the patient? *Soc Sci Med.* 1996;43:1137–1143.

118. Thomas V, Heath M, Rose D, Flory P. Psychological characteristics and the effectiveness of patient-controlled analgesia. *Br J Anaesth.* 1995;74:271–276.

119. Cohen L, Fouladi RT, Katz J. Preoperative coping strategies and distress predict postoperative pain and morphine consumption in women undergoing abdominal gynecologic surgery. *J Psychosom Res.* 2005;58:201–209.

120. Gil KM, Ginsberg B, Muir M, et al. Patient-controlled analgesia in postoperative pain: the relation of psychological factors to pain and analgesic use. *Clin J Pain.* 1990;6:137–142.

121. Ozalp G, Sarioglu R, Tuncel G, et al. Preoperative emotional states in patients with breast cancer and postoperative pain. *Acta Anaesthesiol Scand.* 2003;47:26–29.

122. Weinger MB. Dangers of postoperative opioids. *APSF Newslett.* 2006–2007;61:67.

123. Benumof JL. Obesity, sleep apnea, the airway and anesthesia. *Curr Opin Anaesthesiol.* 2004;17:21–30.

124. Loadsman JA, Hillman DR. Anaesthesia and sleep apnoea. *Br J Anaesth.* 2001;86:254–266.

125. Gross JB, Bachenberg KL, Benumof JL, et al. Practice guidelines for the perioperative management of patients with obstructive sleep apnea: a report by the American Society of Anesthesiologists Task Force on Perioperative Management of patients with obstructive sleep apnea. *Anesthesiology.* 2006;104:1081–1093.

126. Etches RC. Respiratory depression associated with patient-controlled analgesia: a review of eight cases. *Can J Anaesth.* 1994;41:125–132.

127. VanDercar DH, Martinez AP, De Lisser EA. Sleep apnea syndromes: a potential contraindication for patient-controlled analgesia. *Anesthesiology.* 1991;74:623–624.

128. Parikh SN, Stuchin SA, Maca C, et al. Sleep apnea syndrome in patients undergoing total joint arthroplasty. *J Arthroplasty.* 2002;17: 635–42.

129. Lofsky A. Sleep apnea and narcotic postoperative pain medication: morbidity and mortality risk. *Anesthes Patient Saf Found Newslett.* 2002;17:24.

130. Young T, Skatrud J, Peppard PE. Risk factors for obstructive sleep apnea in adults. *JAMA.* 2004;291:2013–2016.

131. Choi YK, Brolin RE, Wagner BK, et al. Efficacy and safety of patient-controlled analgesia for morbidly obese patients following gastric bypass surgery. *Obes Surg.* 2000;10:154–159.

132. Kyzer S, Ramadan E, Gersch M, Chaimoff C. Patient-controlled analgesia following vertical gastroplasty: a comparison with intramuscular narcotics. *Obes Surg.* 1995;5:18–21.

133. Charghi R, Backman S, Christou N, et al. Patient controlled i.v. analgesia is an acceptable pain management strategy in morbidly obese patients undergoing gastric bypass surgery. A retrospective comparison with epidural analgesia. *Can J Anaesth.* 2003;50:672–678.

134. Lotsch J. Opioid metabolites. *J Pain Symptom Manage.* 2005;29: S10–S24.

135. Richtsmeier AJ, Jr., Barnes SD, Barkin RL. Ventilatory arrest with morphine patient-controlled analgesia in a child with renal failure. *Am J Ther.* 1997;4:255–257.

136. Angst MS, Buhrer M, Lotsch J. Insidious intoxication after morphine treatment in renal failure: delayed onset of morphine-6-glucuronide action. *Anesthesiology.* 2000;92:1473–1476.

137. Geller RJ. Meperidine in patient-controlled analgesia: a near-fatal mishap. *Anesth Analg.* 1993;76:655–657.

138. Kalso E. Oxycodone. *J Pain Symptom Manage.* 2005;29:S47–S56.

139. Patient-controlled analgesia pumps USP Quality Review [cited November 2006]. US Pharmacopeia Web site. http://www.usp.org/patientSafety/newsletters/qualityReview/qr812004-09-01.html.

140. Ashburn MA, Love G, Pace NL. Respiratory-related critical events with intravenous patient-controlled analgesia. *Clin J Pain.* 1994;10:52–56.

141. Vicente KJ, Kada-Bekhaled K, Hillel G, et al. Programming errors contribute to death from patient-controlled analgesia: case report and estimate of probability. *Can J Anaesth.* 2003;50:328–332.

142. ECRI. Patient-controlled analgesic infusion pumps. *Health Devices.* 2006;35:5–35.

143. Dawson P, Ashworth M. A footplate for conventional PCA demand buttons. *Anaesth Intensive Care.* 1990;18:585–586.

144. Southall L, Macintyre PE, Semple TG. PCA demand buttons. *Anaesth Intensive Care.* 1990;18:268.

145. Jastrzab G, Khor KE. Use of breath-activated Patient Controlled Analgesia for acute pain management in a patient with quadriplegia. *Spinal Cord.* 1999;37:221–223.

146. Peady C. Unauthorised access to the contents of a Graseby 3300 PCA pump. *Anaesthesia.* 2007;62:98–99; discussion 9.

147. Kluger MT, Owen H. Antireflux valves in patient-controlled analgesia. *Anaesthesia.* 1990;45:1057–1061.

148. Wheeler M, Oderda GM, Ashburn MA, Lipman AG. Adverse events associated with postoperative opioid analgesia: a systematic review. *J Pain.* 2002;3:159–180.

149. Cashman JN, Dolin SJ. Respiratory and haemodynamic effects of acute postoperative pain management: evidence from published data. *Br J Anaesth.* 2004;93:212–223.

150. Dolin SJ, Cashman JN. Tolerability of acute postoperative pain management: nausea, vomiting, sedation, pruritis, and urinary retention. Evidence from published data. *Br J Anaesth.* 2005;95:584–591.

151. Vila H, Jr., Smith RA, Augustyniak MJ, et al. The efficacy and safety of pain management before and after implementation of hospital-wide pain management standards: is patient safety compromised by treatment based solely on numerical pain ratings? *Anesth Analg.* 2005;101:474–480, table of contents.

152. Shapiro A, Zohar E, Zaslansky R, et al. The frequency and timing of respiratory depression in 1524 postoperative patients treated with systemic or neuraxial morphine. *J Clin Anesth.* 2005;17:537–542.

153. Fleming BM, Coombs DW. A survey of complications documented in a quality-control analysis of patient-controlled analgesia in the postoperative patient. *J Pain Symptom Manage.* 1992;7:463–469.

154. Looi-Lyons LC, Chung FF, Chan VW, McQuestion M. Respiratory depression: an adverse outcome during patient controlled analgesia therapy. *J Clin Anesth.* 1996;8:151–156.

155. Marret E, Kurdi O, Zufferey P, Bonnet F. Effects of nonsteroidal antiinflammatory drugs on patient-controlled analgesia morphine side effects: meta-analysis of randomized controlled trials. *Anesthesiology.* 2005;102:1249–1260.

156. Roberts GW, Bekker TB, Carlsen HH, et al. Postoperative nausea and vomiting are strongly influenced by postoperative opioid use in a dose-related manner. *Anesth Analg.* 2005;101:1343–1348.

157. Remy C, Marret E, Bonnet F. Effects of acetaminophen on morphine side-effects and consumption after major surgery: meta-analysis of randomized controlled trials. *Br J Anaesth.* 2005;94:505–513.

158. Tramer MR, Walder B. Efficacy and adverse effects of prophylactic antiemetics during patient-controlled analgesia therapy: a quantitative systematic review. *Anesth Analg.* 1999;88:1354–1361.

159. Lo Y, Chia YY, Liu K, Ko NH. Morphine sparing with droperidol in patient-controlled analgesia. *J Clin Anesth.* 2005;17:271–275.

160. Culebras X, Corpataux JB, Gaggero G, Tramer MR. The antiemetic efficacy of droperidol added to morphine patient-controlled analgesia: a randomized, controlled, multicenter dose-finding study. *Anesth Analg.* 2003;97:816–821.

161. Gan TJ, Alexander R, Fennelly M, Rubin AP. Comparison of different methods of administering droperidol in patient-controlled analgesia in the prevention of postoperative nausea and vomiting. *Anesth Analg.* 1995;80:81–85.

162. Cherian VT, Smith I. Prophylactic ondansetron does not improve patient satisfaction in women using PCA after Caesarean section. *Br J Anaesth.* 2001;87:502–504.

163. Kjellberg F, Tramer MR. Pharmacological control of opioid-induced pruritus: a quantitative systematic review of randomized trials. *Eur J Anaesthesiol.* 2001;18:346–357.

164. Stiller CO, Lundblad H, Weidenhielm L, et al. The addition of tramadol to morphine via patient-controlled analgesia does not lead to better post-operative pain relief after total knee arthroplasty. *Acta Anaesthesiol Scand.* 2007;51:322–330.

165. Jeffs SA, Hall JE, Morris S. Comparison of morphine alone with morphine plus clonidine for postoperative patient-controlled analgesia. *Br J Anaesth.* 2002;89:424–427.

166. Chen JY, Wu GJ, Mok MS, et al. Effect of adding ketorolac to intravenous morphine patient-controlled analgesia on bowel function in colorectal surgery patients–a prospective, randomized, double-blind study. *Acta Anaesthesiol Scand.* 2005;49:546–551.

167. Cepeda MS, Delgado M, Ponce M, et al. Equivalent outcomes during postoperative patient-controlled intravenous analgesia with lidocaine plus morphine versus morphine alone. *Anesth Analg.* 1996;83:102–106.

168. Chia YY, Tan PH, Wang KY, Liu K. Lignocaine plus morphine in bolus patient-controlled intravenous analgesia lacks post-operative morphine-sparing effect. *Eur J Anaesthesiol.* 1998;15:664–668.

169. ECRI. Abbott PCA Plus II patient-controlled analgesic pumps prone to misprogramming resulting in narcotic overinfusions. *Health Devices.* 1997;26:389–391.

170. ECRI. Medication safety: PCA pump programming errors continue to cause fatal overinfusions. *Health Devices.* 2002;31:342–346.

171. White PF. Mishaps with patient-controlled analgesia. *Anesthesiology.* 1987;66:81–83.

172. White PF, Parker RK. Is the risk of using a "basal" infusion with patient-controlled analgesia therapy justified? *Anesthesiology.* 1992;76:489.

173. Heath ML. Safety of patient controlled analgesia. *Anaesthesia.* 1995;50:573.

174. Wright DG. 'That chap on the PCAS is a bit twitchy today'. *Anaesthesia.* 1993;48:354.

175. Tsui SL, Irwin MG, Wong CM, et al. An audit of the safety of an acute pain service. *Anaesthesia.* 1997;52:1042–1047.

176. Notcutt WG, Morgan RJ. Introducing patient-controlled analgesia for postoperative pain control into a district general hospital. *Anaesthesia.* 1990;45:401–406.

177. Lotsch J, Skarke C, Tegeder I, Geisslinger G. Drug interactions with patient-controlled analgesia. *Clin Pharmacokinet.* 2002;41:31–57.

178. Farmer M, Harper NJ. Unexpected problems with patient controlled analgesia. *BMJ.* 1992;304:574.

179. Wheatley RG, Madej TH, Jackson IJ, Hunter D. The first year's experience of an acute pain service. *Br J Anaesth.* 1991;67:353–359.

180. Chisakuta AM. Nurse-call button on a patient-controlled analgesia pump? *Anaesthesia.* 1993;48:90.

181. Lam FY. Patient-controlled analgesia by proxy. *Br J Anaesth.* 1993;70:113.

182. Wakerlin G, Larson CP, Jr. Spouse-controlled analgesia. *Anesth Analg.* 1990;70:119.

183. Notcutt WG, Knowles P, Kaldas R. Overdose of opioid from patient-controlled analgesia pumps. *Br J Anaesth.* 1992;69:95–97.

184. Christie L, Cranfield KA. A dangerous fault with a PCA pump. *Anaesthesia.* 1998;53:827.

185. Doyle DJ, Vicente KJ. Electrical short circuit as a possible cause of death in patients on PCA machines: report on an opiate overdose and a possible preventive remedy. *Anesthesiology.* 2001;94:940.

186. Sanchez-Guijo JJ, Benavente MA, Crespo A. Failure of a patient-controlled analgesia pump in a hyperbaric environment. *Anesthesiology.* 1999;91:1540–1542.

187. Paterson JG. Intravenous obstruction and PCA machines. *Can J Anaesth.* 1998;45:284.

188. Grover ER, Heath ML. Patient-controlled analgesia. A serious incident. *Anaesthesia.* 1992;47:402–404.

189. Kwan A. Overdose of morphine during PCA. *Anaesthesia.* 1995;50:919.

190. ECRI. Improper cassette attachment allows gravity free-flow from SIMS-Deltec CADD-series pumps. *Health Devices.* 1995;24:84–86.

191. Thomas DW, Owen H. Patient-controlled analgesia–the need for caution. A case report and review of adverse incidents. *Anaesthesia.* 1988;43:770–772.

192. ECRI. Overinfusion caused by gravity free-flow from a damaged prefilled glass syringe. *Health Devices.* 1996;25:476–477.

193. Silverman DG, Freilich J, Sevarino FB, et al. Influence of promethazine on symptom-therapy scores for nausea during patient-controlled analgesia with morphine. *Anesth Analg.* 1992;74:735–738.

194. Lin TF, Yeh YC, Yen YH, et al. Antiemetic and analgesic-sparing effects of diphenhydramine added to morphine intravenous patient-controlled analgesia. *Br J Anaesth.* 2005;94:835–839.

195. Laffey JG, Boylan JF. Cyclizine and droperidol have comparable efficacy and side effects during patient-controlled analgesia. *Ir J Med Sci.* 2002;171:141–144.

196. Bree SE, West MJ, Taylor PA, Kestin IG. Combining propofol with morphine in patient-controlled analgesia to prevent postoperative nausea and vomiting. *Br J Anaesth.* 1998;80:152–154.

197. Joshi GP, Duffy L, Chehade J, et al. Effects of prophylactic nalmefene on the incidence of morphine-related side effects in patients receiving intravenous patient-controlled analgesia. *Anesthesiology.* 1999;90:1007–1111.

15

Clinical Applications of Epidural Analgesia

Daniel B. Maalouf and Spencer S. Liu

The use of epidural analgesia has shifted from a purely obstetrical practice to managing pain in patients undergoing multiple types of surgery, including thoracic, gastrointestinal, urologic, gynecologic, orthopedic, and vascular procedures. Epidural analgesia is the second most common form of pain management used in the United States after systemic opioids. More importantly, epidural analgesia has been shown to provide superior postoperative analgesia both at rest and with activity compared with systemic opioid administration. Epidural infusion provides more consistent pain relief resulting in a lower overall consumption of opioid and decreased related side effects.[1] Patients mobilize faster, are less sedated, and have improved respiratory functions compared to those receiving systemic analgesia only.[2] Optimal clinical application of local anesthetics, opioids, and other medications into the epidural space overcomes some of the potential disadvantages of this technique, including the increased nursing care, peaks and valleys in pain control, and increased cost. Epidural analgesia can be administered as a continuous infusion, demand only, or both. The advent of patient-controlled infusion pumps has allowed for more flexibility in infusion settings and resulted in an overall decrease in medication use and related side effects. This chapter discusses the application of epidural analgesia in the management of postoperative pain in patients undergoing thoracic, abdominal, urologic, gynecologic, orthopedic, and vascular surgery.

FACTORS AFFECTING EFFICACY OF EPIDURAL ANALGESIA

Epidural Catheter Location

The location of the epidural catheter placement affects the efficacy of epidural analgesia and influences patient outcomes.[3] Epidural catheters inserted in a location congruent to the incisional dermatome provide equal or superior analgesia compared to catheters placed at dermatomal levels away from the surgical site. This results in improved postoperative outcome and reduced incidence of side effects.[4-7] Thoracic epidural catheters placed for patients undergoing upper abdominal surgery and thoracic surgery provide a segmental blockade of the thoracic

dermatomes corresponding to the incision site. As a result, lesser volumes of the local anesthetic will be required, possibly improving the side-effect profile, including hypotension, urinary retention, and lower extremity weakness.[8-10] Discrepancy between epidural catheter insertion level and incision site may lead to an increased rate of side effects secondary to an increased infusion rate and increased volumes of local anesthetics used. This may prompt a reduction in the amount of medication administered in the epidural space and subsequently an interruption of analgesia. Inadequate pain relief can lead to early termination of epidural analgesia or mask the potential beneficial effects from epidural analgesia.[11-13]

Epidural Analgesics

Choice of Analgesic Agents

The choice of analgesic agents administered in the epidural space play a significant role in the achievement of optimal analgesia. The most common agents used are opioids and local anesthetics. These agents can be administered alone or in combination with other agents or adjuvants. Other agents used include clonidine (α_2-receptor agonist)[14-16] neostigmine (acetylcholinesterase inhibitor), adenosine (nucleotide by-product of ATP), isoproterenol (β_1- and β_2-receptor agonist)[17] verapamil (calcium channel blocker),[18] buprenorphine (partial mu receptor agonist), ketamine (*N*-methyl-D-aspartate [NMDA] receptor antagonist),[19,20] midazolam, and epinephrine.

Opioids

Opioid receptors are present in the dorsal horn of the spinal cord. Opioids have both presynaptic and postsynaptic effects in the dorsal horn and affect the modulation of nociceptive input but do not cause motor or sympathetic blockade.[21] Drugs placed in the epidural space will diffuse along a concentration gradient and into the surrounding tissues. The diffusion rate is determined by the Fick principle, which states that:

$$Q/t = KA[(C1 - C2)/D],$$

where Q/t = rate of diffusion, K = diffusion constant, A = surface area available for exchange, $C1$ = concentration of free drug in epidural space, C2 = concentration of free drug in blood or cerebrospinal fluid (CSF), and D = thickness of the diffusion barrier. The diffusion constant (K) of the drug depends on the physicochemical characteristics of the drug such as lipid solubility, degree of ionization, and molecular size. Consequently, hydrophobic opioids, such as fentanyl and sufentanil, diffuse preferentially into epidural fat as opposed to CSF. Alternatively, hydrophilic opioids in the epidural space, such as morphine, diffuse preferentially into the CSF and have greater bioavailability for spinal opioid receptors compared with their hydrophobic counterparts. The rate of diffusion, however, depends also on the nature and thickness of the diffusion barrier. The spinal meninges include the dura mater, the arachnoid mater, and the pia mater.

The dura mater is composed primarily of collagen and elastin fibers arranged longitudinally and circumferentially.[22] It is largely acellular, except for a layer of cells with a rich capillary network that forms the border between the dura and the arachnoid mater.[23] This capillary network acts to clear some of the opioid dose as it diffuses from the epidural space. Hydrophobic opioids may be cleared to a greater extent than are hydrophilic opioids because the former are much more permeable across capillary endothelial cell membranes. Further evidence of the importance of drug clearance taking place at the dura capillary network comes from animal studies demonstrating that epidural epinephrine reduces dura mater blood flow[24] in parallel with epinephrine's ability to reduce clearance of epidurally administered drugs.[25]

The arachnoid mater is composed of overlapping layers of epithelial cells with tight junctions, occluding junctions, and connective tissue fibers.[26] The arachnoid mater accounts for more than 90% of the resistance to drug diffusion.[27] There is a biphasic relationship between the rate of permeability of the drug and the rate of diffusion across the arachnoid mater. Drugs crossing the arachnoid must repeatedly partition into lipid bilayers of the arachnoid mater cells, diffuse across the lipid bilayer, and then partition into the aqueous extra or intracellular space. Hydrophobic opioids cross the lipid bilayer easily and their diffusion is halted in the aqueous layer. Similarly, hydrophilic drugs have the opposite problem, which slows their diffusion.[25]

The pia mater is adherent to the spinal cord and is composed of cells similar to those of the arachnoid mater. However, it is only one cell thick and does not contain occlusive intracellular junctions. The pia mater presents very little resistance to diffusion.

Cerebrospinal Fluid

Drugs move in the CSF by two mechanisms: simple diffusion and bulk flow. Pulsatile flow of blood into the CNS transiently increases the volume of the brain and to a lesser extent the spinal cord. The pulsating brain acts like a plunger forcing CSF down the dorsal surface of the spinal cord and up the ventral surface. The CSF flow carries with it any suspended drug molecules.[28] The principle cause of drug spread in the CSF is, therefore, the movement of the CSF itself. Opioid molecules are spread almost at the same rate, corresponding to the CSF flow and regardless of their hydrophilic or hydrophobic properties. The clearance rate is the determining factor in the clinical manifestation associated with rostral spread of opioid molecules in the CSF. Rapidly cleared drugs are in low concentration to cause significant supraspinal side effects (eg, sedation, respiratory depression) by rostral spread in the CSF.[29] However, hydrophobic opioids do cause supraspinal side effects, because they are rapidly

cleared into plasma and redistributed to the brainstem via the blood stream.

Opioids in the CSF must diffuse into the spinal cord to reach targeted opioid receptors. Herz and Teschemacher[30] administered radiolabeled morphine, dihydromorphine, and fentanyl into the CSF of the lateral ventricle of rabbits. At approximately 7 minutes, all 3 opioid molecules had penetrated to a 700-μm depth. However, as time progressed, fentanyl never penetrated any deeper into the brain and was completely cleared by 120 minutes. However, morphine and hydromorphone continued to move deeper and reached a depth of 3000 μm at 5 hours. More importantly, fentanyl demonstrated a pronounced preference for fiber structures (white matter), whereas hydrophilic opioids preferentially diffused into gray matter. White matter consists of approximately 80% lipids secondary to myelination of the axons. Gray matter lacks myelin and is relatively hydrophilic. As a result, hydrophobic opioids demonstrate a large volume of distribution and partition into white matter. Hydrophilic opioids remain in the extracellular fluid or diffuse into the gray matter and hence are bioavailable for a longer duration.[31]

All opioids administered into the epidural space produce analgesia, some of them for no other reason than that they diffuse into the capillaries and are redistributed to brainstem opioid receptors. As a result, analgesia obtained after an epidural dose of opioids is not proof, in and of itself, that the opioid has selective spinal site of action. To justify epidural administration of a drug, given the potential risks and increased expense of epidural dosing, one must prove that epidural opioids produce superior analgesia compared to equivalent doses administered intravenously (IV), intramuscularly, subcutaneously or transdermally, and result in fewer side effects, or both.

Epidural Morphine

Morphine is a hydrophilic opioid that has an analgesic effect that is primarily spinal.[3] It is usually administered as a single dose into the epidural space; however, continuous epidural infusion of morphine has been described in the treatment of post-thoracic surgery pain.[32] It has a slower onset but a longer duration of action and a higher incidence of side effects compared to hydrophobic opioids.[33] This may be due in part to a greater cephalad spread in the CSF.[34] As a result, hydrophilic opioids do not produce a segmental block when administered epidurally. They are transported rostrally in the CSF and bind receptors that may be some distance from the site of administration. Sedation and respiratory depression are seen when opioid molecules reach the brain stem.

Epidural morphine displays marked spinal selectivity as evidenced by dose sparing when compared to systemic administration. In a randomized clinical trial in women who had undergone cesarean section, epidural morphine was shown to provide better postoperative analgesia at a lower dose compared to intravenous and intramuscular morphine.[35] Women in the epidural group used one quarter the amount of morphine compared to the intravenous group, and they reported significantly better analgesia than women in both the intravenous and intramuscular groups. In patients undergoing more painful total joint replacement surgery, the relative potency of epidural morphine compared to self titrated IV PCA was 10:1.[36]

Epidural Hydromorphone

Hydromorphone is a hydrophilic μ₁ selective opioid agonist. Its structure and molecular weight are similar to that of morphine. Previous studies demonstrate modest spinally selective analgesia with a potency ratio of approximately 2:1 between epidural:systemic administration.[37]

Doses of 1–2 mg, epidurally, have been shown to relieve visceral and somatic pain after thoracic, abdominal, or pelvic surgery.[38] Continuous epidural infusion of hydromorphone has been used with decreased incidence of rostral spread of the opioid when compared to that encountered with bolus administration.

Epidural patient controlled analgesia using hydromorphone offers a greater advantage over intermittent boluses or continuous infusion mode. This setting reduces patients' opioid requirements while minimizing side effects and increasing patient satisfaction.[39,40] The incidence of pruritis is higher when hydromorphone is administered epidurally compared to the intravenous route. Clinical application of epidural hydromorphone is described in Chapter 16 (*Neuraxial Analgesia with Hydromorphone, Morphine, and Fentanyl: Dosing and Safety Guidelines*).

Epidural Fentanyl

The evidence for a spinal rather than a systemic action of fentanyl is conflicting. One body of evidence suggests that (1) fentanyl has an equivalent potency when given epidurally and intravenously, (2) that doses of fentanyl given epidurally and intravenously have equal blood levels and analgesic effects, and (3) that fentanyl does not provide a segmental analgesia when given epidurally. This suggests that when given epidurally, fentanyl is absorbed systemically and is redistributed via the bloodstream to supraspinal centers.

The second body of evidence suggests that fentanyl has a spinal site of action because (1) there is an increased potency of the molecule when given epidurally compared to intravenous administration, (2) there is a segmental analgesic effect when fentanyl is given epidurally, and (3) that there is a lack of correlation between the analgesic effect and the plasma concentration of fentanyl when given epidurally. Newer research suggests that this discrepancy may be related to the mode of administration of fentanyl into the epidural space. Although bolus administration provides a larger concentration gradient for the fentanyl molecules and enhances their diffusion into the CSF where they will act on the spinal opioid receptors, an infusion of fentanyl molecules does not achieve the same concentration gradient and the fentanyl molecules diffuse into the blood stream instead and act on supraspinal sites.[41]

Epidural Sufentanil

Sufentanil is significantly more hydrophobic than fentanyl. The analgesic effect of sufentanil is mediated by systemic uptake from the epidural space and redistribution to the brainstem opioid receptors.[42] A spinal site of action for sufentanil has not been demonstrated and, as a result, epidural administration of sufentanil is probably unwarranted.

Epidural Alfentanil

Alfentanil was not proven to have a spinal site of action. Studies suggest that alfentanil in the epidural space diffuses into blood vessels and is transported to the brainstem, where it exercises its effects. Because of its high lipid solubility, it is rapidly redistributed into tissues after initial administration and is cleared very rapidly into the plasma.[43]

Epidural Liposomal Morphine

Recently approved by the Food and Drug Administration for epidural analgesia, morphine encapsulated within liposomes provides extended release of morphine molecules and, subsequently, prolonged analgesia. It is administered as a single injection and has been shown to provide analgesia up to 48 hours postoperatively, following hip arthroplasty and cesarean section.[44] The advantages of such a formulation include a constant analgesia that is not affected by interruption of the epidural infusion. The analgesic gaps are fewer in number and are managed more easily with rescue medications. The need for epidural infusion pumps and catheters, maintenance, and cost is eliminated. The incidence of hypotension was less than that in the epidural local anesthetic group. Anticoagulation therapy can be initiated postoperatively without the associated risks of indwelling epidural catheters. The adverse events associated with using epidural liposomal morphine for postoperative analgesia include decreased oxygen saturation, hypotension, urinary retention, vomiting, nausea, constipation, pruritis, pyrexia, headache, and dizziness. Patients should be monitored postoperatively for respiratory depression for at least 24 hours because 90% of respiratory depression episodes occurred within the first 24 hours. The elderly and debilitated patients are at increased risk. Another major disadvantage associated with the administration of a long-acting medication is the prolonged manifestation of the side effects if they occur. Patients may have to endure side effects such as nausea or pruritis, which occur at significant rates, for 24 to 48 hours or longer. The need for monitoring for respiratory depression, and the potential for a prolonged manifestation of the side effects, should be taken into account when using liposomal morphine for postoperative analgesia.

Epidural Local Anesthetics

Local anesthetics bind to the sodium channels in nerve fibers, inhibit sodium conductance, and reduce action potential depolarization and subsequent nerve stimulus propagation. In the epidural space, local anesthetics penetrate axonal membranes of the nerve roots as they emerge from the spinal cord. As a result, epidural analgesia is segmental in nature and is affected by the location of the epidural catheter. It is also affected by the volume and dose of medication given. The larger the volume administered into the epidural space, the greater the spread, both cephalad and caudad. Increasing the dose of epidural medication will increase the concentration of the local anesthetic and result in a denser block that may include autonomic, sensory, and motor fibers. The effect of local anesthetics on nerve fibers is selective only for size and not type of nerve. Thinner nerve fibers are affected by lower concentrations of local anesthetics and both autonomic and somatic nerves are affected equally. Autonomic and pain fibers, C fibers, are the thinnest and are blocked first. As the concentration of local anesthetics increases, preganglionic sympathetic fibers, B fibers, are blocked, followed by touch, pressure sensation, and motor fibers, A fibers.[45] As a result, epidural local anesthetics block afferent and efferent signals to and from the spinal cord and consequently suppress the surgical stress response and may reduce perioperative morbidity and mortality.[46] Systemic absorption of local anesthetics from the epidural space may facilitate the return of gastrointestinal motility,[47] diminish inflammation, and decrease blood viscosity.[48]

Local anesthetics are not widely used as the sole agent in postoperative epidural analgesia because of the associated motor block and hypotension. To achieve effective analgesia using local anesthetics alone, patients will require higher concentrations of the drugs that will result in hypotension and motor block.

Table 15.1: Recommended Location for Epidural Catheter Placement for Surgical Procedures

Vertebral Level for Catheter	Location of Incision	Example of Surgery
T4–8	Thoracic	Thoracotomy
T6–8	Upper abdominal	Esophagectomy
T8–12	Mid-lower abdominal	Colectomy
L1–4	Lower extremity	Total knee replacement

Adapted from Etches et al (1997)[53] and Schug et al (1996).[52]

Infusion of bupivacaine (37.5–50 mg/h) via a thoracic epidural in postoperative thoracic surgery patients resulted in 80% hypotension and 30% inadequate analgesia.[49] Similar results were found when bupivacaine (24–45 mg/h) or ropivacaine (10–30 mg/h) were infused after upper and lower abdominal surgery.[50–52]

Nevertheless, epidural infusion of local anesthetics alone may be warranted in situations in which the side effects of opioids are troublesome to the patient.[3] Side effects from local anesthetics may be minimized by correct matching of epidural catheter site with location of incision (see Table 15.1).

The most commonly used local anesthetics in epidural analgesic preparations are bupivacaine, ropivacaine, and levobupivacaine. At low doses, these agents show a preferential sensory with minimal motor blockade.[54–56] The newer more expensive ropivacaine and levobupivacaine may be less cardiotoxic; however, this advantage may not be clinically important because of the relatively low doses of local anesthetics used for postoperative analgesia.

Local Anesthetics, Opioid Combination

Epidural analgesia is usually achieved using a combination of local anesthetics and opioid with or without an adjunct. Compared with epidural local anesthetics or opioids alone, a local anesthetic-opioid epidural provides superior postoperative analgesia.[57] Epidural local anesthetics decrease the incidence of postoperative gastrointestinal paralysis, PONV and pain after abdominal surgery compared to opioid-based analgesic regimens.[21,57,58] Clinical observations suggest that the combination of local anesthetics and opioids limit the regression of the sensory block seen with local anesthetics alone.[59] Whether the analgesic effects of local anesthetic-opioid combinations are synergistic or additive is not clear, but experimental studies imply a synergistic effect.[3] In addition to the superior analgesia provided by epidural local anesthetic-opioid combinations, a decreased dose requirement of each of the drugs used is also observed. The decrease in dose requirement leads to a decreased rate of side effects when compared to epidural local anesthetics and/or opioids alone. Side effects include hypotension and urinary retention when local anesthetics are used or pruritis, nausea, and vomiting in case of opioid use.

Many epidural combinations of opioids and local anesthetics have been used in clinical practice with clinically significant improvement in analgesia compared to intravenous opioid analgesia or epidural plain local anesthetic or opioid infusion. Table 15.2 shows randomized clinical trials comparing local anesthetics and opioid combination to plain local anesthetics or opioids. Epidural infusions containing dilute bupivacaine plus hydromorphone have been shown to provide effective analgesia and a favorable safety profile for parturients of varying parity and stages of labor and may prove effective in providing postoperative analgesia for surgical patients.[72]

Delivery Modes of Epidural Analgesia

Epidural analgesia can be achieved via different modes of delivery, including continuous infusion, demand only, or both. Patient-controlled epidural analgesia with a background infusion (PCEA) is the setting of choice. PCEA individualizes postoperative analgesic requirements, resulting in many advantages such as increased patients' satisfaction, superior analgesia, decreased amount of drug used, and decreased drug side effects.[3] Typical epidural analgesia solutions and PCEA settings are provided in Table 15.3.

Choice of Adjuvants

A number of agents have been used as adjuvants to improve the efficacy and/or safety of epidural analgesia. These include epinephrine, clonidine, ketamine, neostigmine, adenosine, isoproterenol, verapamil, buprenorphine, and midazolam. The most commonly used adjuvants are epinephrine and clonidine, however. Clinical studies comparing local anesthetic-opioid combinations with or without epinephrine and clonidine have shown that patients experienced better pain relief when the adjuvants are used (see Table 15.4).

The site and mode of action of adjuvants must be taken into account. Epinephrine is a vasoconstrictor that was associated with decreased resolution of the sensory block in patients and therefore markedly improving analgesia. However, the use of clonidine as an adjuvant in the epidural space was associated with improved analgesia and hypotension. The mechanism of action of clonidine may be through its diffusion and spread in the blood, and it may not have an advantage when administered epidurally compared to the intravenous route.

RISKS OF EPIDURAL ANALGESIA

The use of epidural analgesia is associated with potential complications or adverse effects, some of which are side effects of the medications being used, whereas others are related to the placement, migration, or removal of epidural catheters. Adverse effects from epidural medication include hypotension, motor blockade, respiratory depression, nausea, pruritis, and urinary retention.

Complications Related to the Placement, Migration, or Removal of the Catheter

Permanent neurological damage has been reported as a result of epidural catheter placement; its incidence ranges from 0.005% to 0.006%.[77,78] Auroy et al,[79] in a prospective study in France involving 30,413 epidurals inserted over a 5-month period, revealed an incidence of severe complications of 0.04%. The latter included 3 cardiac arrests, 4 convulsions, and 6 neurological injuries.[79]

Table 15.2: Randomized Clinical Trials Comparing the Effect of Epidural Local Anesthetic-Opioid Combinations with Epidural Opioids or Local Anesthetics Alone on Dynamic Pain Relief

Reference	Epidural Regimen	Type of Surgery/ Site of Epidural	Control	Dynamic Pain Relief Compared with Control
Scott et al (1989)[60]	Morphine 500 μg/h, 0.5% bupivacaine 25 mg/h	Upper abdominal/thoracic	0.5% bupivacaine 25 mg/h	Combination more effective
Dahl et al (1992)[61]	Morphine 200 μg/h, 0.25% bupivacaine 10 mg/h	Major abdominal/thoracic	Morphine 200 μg/h	Combination more effective
Crews et al (1999)[62]	Morphine 200 μg/h, 0.25% levobupivacaine 10 mg/h	Major abdominal/thoracic	Morphine 200 μg/h	Combination more effective for the first 8 hours
Lowson et al (1994)[63]	Diamorphine 250–600 μg/h, 0.167% bupivacaine 5–12 mg/h	Upper abdominal/thoracic	Diamorphine 250–600 μg/h	Combination more effective
Etches et al (1996)[64]	Pethidine 1 mg/mL, 0.1% bupivacaine	Thoracic/thoracic	Pethidine	NS difference
Paech et al (1994)[65]	Fentanyl 40 μg/h, 0.1% bupivacaine 4 mg/h	Major abdominal/thoracic	Fentanyl 40 μg/h	Combination more effective for the first 24 hours
Torda et al (1995)[66]	Fentanyl 50 μg + bupivacaine 12.5 or 25-mg bolus doses	Major abdominal/thoracic	Fentanyl 50 μg	NS difference
Mahon et al (1999)[67]	Fentanyl 50–100 μg/h, 0.1%–0.2% bupivacaine 5–20 mg/h	Thoracic/thoracic	Fentanyl 50–100 μg/h	NS difference after the first 2 hours
Kopacz et al (1999)[58]	Fentanyl 4 μg/mL, levobupivacaine 0.125%, PCEA 4 mL/h + 2 mL/10 min bolus	Arthroplasty/lumbar	Fentanyl 4 μg/mL or levobupivacaine 0.125% PCEA	Combination more effective
Scott et al (1999)[68]	Fentanyl 1–4 μg/mL, 0.2% ropivacaine PCEA 8 mL/h + 4 mL/30 min bolus	Major abdominal/thoracic	Ropivacaine 0.2%	Combination more effective
Mourisse et al (1992)[69]	Sufentanil 0.8 μg/mL, 0.125% bupivacaine 6–12 mg/h	Thoracic/thoracic	Sufentanil 0.8 μg/mL	Combination more effective
Wieblack et al (1997)[70]	Sufentanil 1 μg/mL, 0.17% bupivacaine PCEA 5 mL/h + 2 mL/20 min bolus	Thoracic, abdominal	0.17% bupivacaine	Combination more effective
Kampe et al (1999)[71]	Sufentanil 5–9 μg/h, 0.1% ropivacaine 5–9 mg/h	Orthopedic/lumbar	0.1% ropivacaine	Combination more effective

Table 15.3: Typical Solutions and Settings for Patient-Controlled Epidural Analgesia for Nonobstetric Use

Solution	Demand Bolus (mL)	Lockout (min)	Background Infusion (mL/h)
0.05% bupivacaine[a] + fentanyl 4 mcg/mL	2	10	4–6
0.2% ropivacaine + fentanyl 5 mcg/mL	2	20	5
0.05% ropivacaine + fentanyl 4 mcg/mL	2	10	4–6
0.06% bupivacaine + hydromorphone 10 mcg/mL	4	10	4

[a] Levobupivacaine may also be used in identical concentrations to bupivacaine.[9,73–75]

Transient neuropathy with eventual full recovery occurs more frequently, but is still relatively uncommon. Its incidence has been reported to range from 0.012% to 0.023%.[21]

Dural Puncture

The reported incidence of dural puncture is 0.32%–1.23% of epidural placement and can result in the development of a postdural puncture headache. In rare circumstances, a subdural hematoma can develop that may manifest in neurological deficit. There is a risk of pneumocephalus after a dural puncture if air is used in the loss of resistance technique. Using saline may help reduce the incidence and complications of pneumocephalus or venous air embolism that may encountered when using air in the loss of resistance technique.

Epidural Hematoma

Epidural hematomas occur as a result of epidural vessel puncture. The incidence of punctured vessels secondary to epidural

Table 15.4: Randomized Clinical Trials Comparing the Effect of Epidural Local Anesthetic-Opioid Combinations and Adjuvants on Dynamic Pain Relief

Reference	Epidural Regimen	Type of Surgery/ Site of Epidural	Adjuvant	Dynamic Pain Relief
Niemi et al (1998)[76]	Fentanyl 20 μg/h + 0.1% bupivacaine 10 mg/h	Thoracic/major abdominal and thoracic	Epinephrine 2 μg/mL	Better in the epinephrine group
Mogensen et al (1992)[14]	Morphine 100 μg/h + bupivacaine 5 mg/h	Thoracic/lower abdominal	Clonidine 18.75 μg/h	Better pain relief, but more hypotension
Paech et al (1997)[15]	Fentanyl 10 μg/h + 0.125% bupivacaine 7.5 mg/h + PCEA fentanyl	Thoracic/lower abdominal	Clonidine 2, 3, or 4 μg/mL at 5 mL/h	Better pain relief with clonidine 20 μg/h, but more hypotension

catheter placement occurs during 3%–12% of attempts.[80] Fortunately, subsequent development of epidural hematoma causing neurological damage is rare. For epidural blocks, the reported incidence is 1:150 000. The number of epidural hematomas has increased since the introduction of low-molecular-weight heparin in clinical practice in the United States. The incidence of epidural hematoma increased to as high as 1:6600 for epidural anesthetics.[3] Potential risk factors for the development of epidural hematoma after an epidural catheter insertion include haemostatic abnormality and/or anticoagulation and procedure difficulty. The timing of insertion or removal of epidural catheters in relation to the administration of anticoagulation may also increase the risk. The American Society of Regional Anesthesia and Pain Medicine have published consensus statements on neuraxial blockade and anticoagulation; one can refer to the Web site (www.asra.com) for the most updated guidelines.

Infection

The development of epidural abscess is a rare complication after epidural anesthesia or analgesia. There are many risk factors that are believed to increase the likelihood of epidural abscess formation. These include immunocompromised, septic, or bacteremic patients or patients with complicating disease states (malignancy, diabetes, multiple trauma, and chronic obstructive pulmonary disease), infection at the needle entry site, and prolonged catheterization time.

Patients with epidural abscesses usually present with back pain, erythema, leukocytosis, and progressive neurological deficit, from few days to several weeks after their epidural. Early diagnosis and treatment, which include the administration of antibiotics and possibly surgical decompression, is of essence to avoid permanent neurological deficits.

Catheter Migration/Dislodgement or Knotting

Epidural catheters can migrate intravenously or subdurally after insertion. The incidence of intrathecal migration has been reported as 0.15%–0.18%, with a similar rate of 0.18% for intravenous migration.[21] Unintentional delivery of local anesthetics into the bloodstream can result in toxicity with neurological and/or cardiac manifestation. In addition, intrathecal injection of an epidural dose of local anesthetics can result in a high block that may require invasive interventions and support. It is recommended that catheters be tested before the administration of an epidural bolus with a small dose of epinephrine containing

local anesthetic to rule out intravascular or intrathecal migration of the catheter. Dislodgement of epidural catheters typically occurs in 5.7% of the time. This can result in analgesic gap and pain if not detected early. Catheters that are threaded deep into the epidural space are at risk for knotting; one can avoid such complication by introducing the catheter only a few centimeters (4–6 cm) into the epidural space.

Hypotension

Hypotension results from the sympathetic blockade seen with epidural local anesthetic administration. The degree of hypotension depends on the level of the block, the dose of local anesthetic, and the volume status of the patient. High epidural blocks that reach the T1 to T5 levels block the cardiac accelerator fibers and may lead to bradycardia and hypotension. Unopposed parasympathetically mediated bronchoconstriction may lead to bronchospasm during epidural analgesia.[81] Lower concentrations of local anesthetics and PCEA infusion modes are used to minimize the decrease in blood pressure.

Motor Blockade

Unilateral or bilateral motor blockade or weakness has been reported in patients receiving epidural infusions, even with low doses of local anesthetics. Patients are, therefore, at an increased risk of fall and are not able to participate in physical therapy. The use of PCEA leads to decreased requirements in local anesthetic and may decrease the risk of motor block. Unilateral blocks may be avoided by using a multipore epidural catheter and limiting catheter insertion to 4–6 cm into the epidural space. The use of ropivacaine may produce less motor blockade compared to an equianalgesic dose of bupivacaine, especially when used in low concentration (0.1%) in combination with an opioid.

Respiratory Depression

Epidural opioids can lead to respiratory depression in some patients especially those over 70 years of age. The incidence of respiratory depression is higher when hydrophilic opioids, such as morphine, are used. The latter has a tendency to remain in the CSF, spread rostrally to brainstem respiratory centers and cause delayed respiratory depression. Hydrophobic opioids are less likely to cause a delayed respiratory depression; however, when given in an infusion, the cumulative dose can result in a decreased respiratory drive in some patients.

Table 15.5: Effective and Safe Management of Epidural Analgesia

Patient	Informed consent; careful selection based on a risk/benefit analysis and absence of contraindications
Regimen	Sterile technique; standard, pharmacy prepared or commercially produced low dose local anesthetics-opioid infusion Standard infusion pump (preferably different from intravenous PCA pumps) with PCEA capacity. Standard order sheets with check boxes. Identifiable administration sets without injection ports. Bacterial filter Transparent dressing
Staff	Training program/protocols/acute pain handbook with particular attention to: Recognition and management of complications including hypotension, respiratory depression, inadequate analgesia and motor blockade. Concurrent thrombophylaxis and anticoagulation therapy. Access to members of the acute pain team around the clock
Monitoring	Regular monitoring of dynamic pain scores, cardiorespiratory parameters, sedation scores, dermatomal level, and motor blockade. Daily inspection of the epidural site. Twice daily review by the APS
Audit	Audit and feedback to anesthesiologists, surgeons and nurses. Critical incident reporting[21]

ACUTE PAIN SERVICE

Providing effective and safe postoperative analgesia is a challenging task that involves many steps. Establishing an Acute Pain Service to handle this task is therefore essential. Epidural analgesia is a part of the multimodal approach that needs to be followed in achieving a successful APS practice. The practitioner must consider a few factors to provide a safe and effective management of postoperative epidural analgesia (see Table 15.5).

REFERENCES

1. Block BM, Liu SS, Rowlingson AJ, Cowan AR, Cowan JA, Wu CL. Efficacy of postoperative epidural analgesia: a metanalysis. *JAMA.* 2003;290:2455–2463.
2. Liu SS, Carpenter RL, Mackey DC, et al. Effects of perioperative analgesic technique on rate of recovery after colon surgery. *Anesthesiology.* 1995d;83:757–765.
3. Richman JM, Wu CL. (2005). Epidural analgesia for postoperative pain. *Anesthesiol Clin North Am.* 2005;23:125–140.
4. Rodgers A, Walker N, Schug S, et al. Reduction of postoperative mortality and morbidity with epidural or spinal anaesthesia: results from overview of randomized trials. *BMJ.* 2000;321:1493.
5. Wu CL, Fleischer LA. (2000a). Outcomes research in regional anesthesia and analgesia. *Anesth Analg.* 2000a;91:1232–1342.
6. Brodner G, Mertes N, Buerkle H, Marcus MA, Van Aken H. Acute pain management: analysis, implications and consequences after prospective experience with 6349 surgical patients. *Eur J Anaesthsiol.* 2000;17:566–675.
7. Liu SS, Bernards CM. Exploring the epidural trail. *Reg Anesth Pain Med.* 2002;27:122–124.
8. Chisakuta AM, George KA, Hawthorne CT. Postoperative epidural infusion of a mixture of bupivacaine 0.2% with fentanyl for upper abdominal surgery: a comparison of thoracic and lumbar routes. *Anaesthesia.* 1995;50:72–75.
9. Liu SS, Allen HW, Olsson GL. Patient controlled epidural analgesia with bupivacaine and fentanyl on hospital wards: prospective experience with 1,030 surgical patients. *Anesthesiology.* 1998;88:688–695.
10. Magnusdottir H, Kirno K, Ricksten SE, Elam M. High thoracic epidural anesthesia does not inhibit sympathetic nerve activity in the lower extremities. *Anesthesiology.* 1999;91:1299–1304.
11. Broekema AA, Gielen MJ, Hennis PJ. Postoperative analgesia with continuous epidural sufentanil and bupivacaine: a prospective study in 614 patients. *Anesth Analg.* 1996;82:754–759.
12. Kahn L, Baxter FJ, Dauphin A, et al. A comparison of thoracic and lumbar epidural techniques for post-thoracoabdominal esophagectomy analgesia. *Can J Anaesth.* 1999;46:415–422.
13. Ready LB. Acute pain: lessons learned from 25,000 patients. *Reg Anesth Pain Med.* 1999;24:499–505.
14. Mogensen T, Eliasen K, Ejlersen E, Vegger P, Nielsen IK, Kehlet H. Epidural clonidine enhances postoperative analgesia from a combined low-dose epidural bupivacaine and morphine regimen. *Anesth Analg.* 1992;75:607–610.
15. Paech MJ, Pavy TJ, Orlikowski CE, Lim W, Evans SF. Postoperative epidural infusion: a randomized, double-blind, dose-finding trial of clonidine in combination with bupivacaine and fentanyl. *Anesth Analg.* 1997;84:1323–1328.
16. Chia YY, Liu K, Liu YC, Chang HC. Adding ketamine in a multi-modal patient-controlled epidural regimen reduces postoperative pain and analgesic consumption. *Anesth Analg.* 1998;86:1245–1249.
17. Marcus MA, Vertommen JD, Van Aken H, Gogarten W, Buerkle H. The effects of adding isoproterenol to 0.125 % bupivacaine on the quality of epidural analgesia in laboring parturients. *Anesth Analg.* 1998;86:749–752.
18. Choe H, Kim JS, Ko SH, Kim DC, Han YJ, Song HS. Epidural verapamil reduces analgesic consumption after lower abdominal surgery. *Anesth Analg.* 1998;86:786–790.
19. Yaksh TL. Epidural ketamine: a useful, mechanistically novel adjuvant for epidural morphine? *Reg Anesth.* 1996;21:508–513.
20. Wu CT, Yeh CC, Yu JC, et al. Pre-incisional epidural ketamine, morphine and bupivacaine combined with epidural and general anaesthesia provides pre-emptive analgesia for upper abdominal surgery. *Acta Anaesthesiol Scand.* 2000;44:63–68.
21. Wheatley RG, Schug SA, Watson D. Safety and efficacy of postoperative epidural analgesia. *Br J Anaesth.* 2001;87:47–61.
22. Fink BR, Walker S. Orientation of fibers in human dorsal lumbar dura mater in relation to lumbar puncture. *Anesth Analg.* 1989;69:768.
23. Kerber CW, Newton TH. The macro and microvasculature of the dura mater. *Neuroradiology.* 1973;6:175–179.
24. Kozody R, Palahniuk RJ, Wade JG, Cumming MO, Pucci WR. The effect of subarachnoid epinephrine and phenylephrine on spinal cord blood flow. *Can Anaesth Soc J.* 1984;31:503–508.
25. Bernards CM. Understanding the physiology and pharmacology of epidural and intrathecal opioids. *Best Pract Res Clin Anaesthesiol.* 2002;16:489–505.
26. Vandenabeele F, Creemers J, Lambrichts I. Ultrastructure of the human spinal arachnoid mater and dura mater. *J Anat.* 1996;189:417–430.
27. Bernards CM, Hill HF. Morphine and alfentanil permeability through the spinal dura, arachnoid and pia mater of dogs and monkeys. *Anesthesiology.* 1990;73:1214–1219.
28. DiChiro GD, Hammock MK, Bleyer WA. Spinal descent of cerebrospinal fluid in man. *Neurology.* 1976;26:1–8.

29. Nordberg G, Hedner T, Mellstrand T, Dahlström B. Pharmacokinetic aspects of intrathecal morphine analgesia. *Anesthesiology.* 1984;60:448–454.

30. Herz A, Teschemacher H. Activities and sites of antinociceptive action of morphine-like analgesics and kinetics of distribution following intravenous, intracerebral and intraventricular application. In: Simmonds A, ed. Advances in Drug Research. London: Academic Press;1971:79–117.

31. Ummenhofer WC, Arends RH, Shen DD, Bernards CM. Comparative spinal distribution and clearance kinetics of intrathecally administered morphine, fentanyl, alfentanil, and sufentanil. *Anesthesiology.* 2000;92:739–753.

32. El-Baz NMI, Faber LP, Jensik RJ. Continuous epidural infusion of morphine for treatment of pain after thoracic surgery: a new technique. *Anesth Analg.* 1984;63:757–764.

33. Reisine T, Pasternak G. Opioid analgesics and antagonists. In: LS Goodman LS, Gilman A, eds. *The Pharmacologic Basis of Therapeutics.* 9th ed. New York, NY: Macmillan; 1997:494–534.

34. Grass JA. Epidural analgesia. In: Grass JA, ed. Problems in Anesthesia. Vol. 10, ed. Philadelphia, PA: Lippincott-Raven; 1998:445.

35. Kilbride MJ, Senagore AJ, Mazier WP, Ferguson C, Ufkes T. Epidural analgesia. *Surg Gynecol Obstet.* 1992;174:137–140.

36. Weller R, Rosenblum M, Conard P, Gross JB. Comparison of epidural and patient-controlled intravenous morphine following joint replacement surgery. *Can J Anaesth.* 1991;38:582–586.

37. Liu S, Carpenter RL, Mulroy MF, et al. Intravenous versus epidural administration of hydromorphone: effects on analgesia and recovery after radical retropubic prostatectomy. *Anesthesiology.* 1995b;82:682–688.

38. Halpern SH, Arellano R, Preston R, et al. Epidural morphine versus hydromorphone in post-caesarean section patients. *Can J Anaesth.* 1996;43:595–598.

39. Harrison DM, Sinatra R, Morgese L. Epidural narcotic and patient controlled analgesia for post-cesarean section pain relief. *Anesthesiology.* 1988;68:454–457.

40. White PW. Use of patient-controlled analgesia for management of acute pain. *JAMA.* 1998;259:243–247.

41. Ginosar Y, Riley ET, Angst MS. The site of action of epidural fentanyl in humans: the difference between infusion and bolus administration. *Anesth Analg.* 2003;97:1428–1438.

42. Miguel R, Barlow I, Morrell M, Scharf J, Sanusi D, Fu E. A prospective, randomized, double-blind comparison of epidural and intravenous sufentanil infusions. *Anesthesiology.* 1994;81:346–352.

43. Coda BA, Brown MC, Schaffer RL, Donaldson G, Shen DD. A pharmacokinetic approach to resolving spinal and systemic contributions to epidural alfentanil analgesia and side-effects. *Pain.* 1995;62:329–337.

44. Viscusi E. Emerging techniques in the management of acute pain: epidural analgesia. *Anesth Analg.* 2005;101:S23–S29.

45. Fotiadis RJ, Bavdie S, Weston MD, Allen-Mersh TG. Epidural analgesia in gastrointestinal surgery. *Br J Surg.* 2004;91:828–841.

46. Liu S, Carpenter RL, Neal JM. Epidural anesthesia and analgesia: their role in postoperative outcome. *Anesthesiology.* 1995c;82:1474–1506.

47. Kaba A, Laurent SR, Detroz BJ, et al. Intravenous Lidocaine infusion facilitates acute rehabilitation after laparoscopic colectomy. *Anesthesiology.* 2007;106:11–18.

48. Hollmann MW, Wieczorek KS, Smart M, Durieux ME. Epidural anesthesia prevents hypercoagulation in patients undergoing major orthopedic surgery. *Reg Anesth Pain Med.* 2001;26:215–222.

49. Conacher ID, Paes ML, Jacobseon L, Phillips PD, Heaviside DW. Epidural analgesia following thoracic surgery: a review of two year's experience. *Anaesthesia.* 1983;38:546–551.

50. Ross RA, Clarke JE, Armitage EN. Postoperative pain prevention by continuous epidural infusion: a study of the clinical effects and the plasma concentrations obtained. *Anaesthesia.* 1980;35;663–668.

51. Mitchell RW, Scott DB, Holmquist E, Lamont M. Continuous extradural infusion of 0.125% bupivacaine for pain relief after lower abdominal surgery. *Br J Anaesth.* 1988;60:851–853.

52. Schug SA, Scott DA, Payne J, Mooney PH, Hagglof B. Postoperative analgesia by continuous extradural infusion of ropivacaine after upper abdominal surgery. *Br J Anaesth.* 1996;76:487–491.

53. Etches RC, Writer WD, Ansley D, et al. Continuous epidural ropivacaine 0.2% for analgesia after lower abdominalsurgery. *Anesth Analg.* 1997;84:784–790.

54. Stevens RA, Bray JG, Artuso JD, Kao TC, Spitzer L. Differential epidural block. *Reg Anesth.* 1992;17:22–25.

55. White JL, Stevens RA, Beardsley D, Teague PJ, Kao TC. Differential epidural block: does the choice of local anesthetic matter? *Reg Anesth.* 1994;19:335–338.

56. Zaric D, Nydahl PA, Philipson L, Samuelsson L, Heierson A, Axelsson K. The effect of continuous lumbar epidural infusion of ropivacaine (0.1%, 0.2% and 0.3%) and 0.25% bupivacaine on sensory and motor block in volunteers: a double-blind study. *Reg Anesth.* 1996;21:14–25.

57. Jorgensen H, Wetterslev J, Moiniche S, Dahl JB. Epidural local anaesthetics versus opioid-based analgesic regimens on postoperative gastrointestinal paralysis, PONV and pain after abdominal surgery. *Cochrane Database Syst Rev.* 2000;CD001893.

58. Kopacz DJ, Sharrock NE, Allen HW. A comparison of levobupivacaine 0.125%, fentanyl 4microg/ml, or their combination for patient-controlled epidural analgesia after major orthopedic surgery. *Anesth Analg.* 1999;89:1497–1503.

59. Hjortso NC, Lund C, Mogensen T, Bigler D, Kehlet H. Epidural morphine improves pain relief and maintains sensory analgesia during continuous epidural bupivacaine after abdominal surgery. *Anesth Analg.* 1989;65:1033–1036.

60. Scott NB, Mogensen T, Bigler D, Lund C, Kehlet H. Continuous thoracic extradural 0.5% bupivacaine with or without morphine: effect on quality of blockade, lung function and the surgical stress response. *Br J Anaesth.* 1989;62:253–257.

61. Dahl JB, Rosenberg J, Hansen BL, Hjortso NC, Kehlet H. Differential analgesic effects of low-dose epidural morphine and morphine-bupivacaine at rest and during mobilization after major abdominal surgery. *Anesth Analg.* 1992;74:362–365.

62. Crews JC, Hord AH, Denson DD, Schatzman C. A comparison of the analgesic efficacy of 0.25% levobupivacaine combined with 0.005% morphine, 0.25% levobupivacaine alone, or 0.005% morphine alone for the management of postoperative pain in patients undergoing major abdominal surgery. *Anesth Analg.* 1999;89:1504–1509.

63. Lowson SM, Alexander JI, Black AMS, Bambridge AD. Epidural diamorphine infusions with and without 0.167% bupivacaine for postoperative analgesia. *Eur J Anaesthesiol.* 1994;11:345–352.

64. Etches RC, Gammer TL, Cornish R. Patient-controlled epidural analgesia after thoracotomy: a comparison of meperidine with and without bupivacaine. *Anesth Analg.* 1996;83:81–86.

65. Paech MJ, Westmore MD. Postoperative epidural fentanyl infusion-is the addition of 0.1% bupivacaine of benefit? *Anaesth Intensive Care.* 1994;22:9–14.

66. Torda TA, Hann P, Mills G, De Leon G, Penman D. Comparison of extradural fentanyl, bupivacaine and two fentanyl-bupivacaine mixtures for pain relief after abdominal surgery. *Br J Anaesth.* 1995;74:35–40.

67. Mahon SV, Berry PD, Jackson M, Russell GN, Pennefather SH. Thoracic epidural infusions for post-thoracotomy pain: a

comparison of fentanyl-bupivacaine mixtures vs. fentanyl alone. *Anaesthesia.* 1999;54:641–646.

68. Scott DA, Blake D, Buckland M, et al. A comparison of epidural ropivacaine infusion alone and in combination with 1, 2, and 4 µg/ml fentanyl for seventy-two hours of postoperative analgesia after major abdominal surgery. *Anesth Analg.* 1999;88:857–864.

69. Mourisse J, Hasenbos MA, Gielen MJ, Moll JE, Cromheecke GJ. Epidural bupivacaine, sufentanil or the combination for post-thoracotomy pain. *Acta Anaesthesiol Scand.* 1992:36:70–74.

70. Wieblack A, Brodner G, Van Aken H. The effects of adding sufentanil to bupivacaine postoperative patient-controlled epidural analgesia. *Anesth Analg.* 1997;85:124–129.

71. Kampe S, Weigand C, Kaufmann J, Klimek M, Konig DP, Lynch J. Postoperative analgesia with no motor block by continuous epidural infusion of ropivacaine 0.1% and sufentanil after total hip replacement. *Anesth Analg.* 1999;89:395–398.

72. Sinatra RS, Eige S, Chung JH, et al. Continuous epidural infusion of 0.05% bupivacaine plus hydromorphone for labor analgesia: an observational assessment in 1830 parturients. *Anesth Analg.* 2002;94:1310–1311.

73. Liu S, Angel JM, Owens, BD, Carpenter RL, Isabel L. Effects of epidural bupivacaine after thoracotomy. *Reg Anesth.* 1995a;20:303–310.

74. Liu SS, Moore JM, Luo AM, Trautman WJ, Carpenter RL. Comparison of three solutions of ropivacaine/fentanyl for patient controlled epidural analgesia. *Anesthesiology.* 1999;90:727–733.

75. Steinberg RB, Liu SS, Wu CL, et al. Comparison of ropivacaine/fentanyl PCEA vs IV PCA for perioperative analgesia and recovery after open colon surgery. *J Clin Anesth.* 2002;14:571–577.

76. Niemi G, Breivik H. Adrenaline markedly improves thoracic epidural analgesia produced by a low-dose infusion of bupivacaine, fentanyl and adrenaline after major surgery. A randomized, double-blind, cross-over study with and without adrenaline. *Acta Anaesthesiol Scand.* 1998;42:897–909.

77. Aromaa U, Lahdensuu M, Cozanitis DA. Severe complications associated with epidural and spinal anaesthesias in Finland 1987–1993: a study based on patient insurance claims. *Acta Anaesthesiol Scand.* 1997;41:445–452.

78. Kane RE. Neurologic deficit following epidural or spinal anesthesia. *Anesth Analg.* 1981;60:150–161.

79. Auroy Y, Narchi P, Messiah A, Litt L, Rouvier B, Samii K. Serious complications related to regional anesthesia; results of a prospective survey in France. *Anesthesiology.* 1997;87:479–486.

80. Schwander D, Bachmann F. Heparin and spinal or epidural anesthesia: decision analysis. *Ann Fr Anesth Reanim.* 1991;10:284–296.

81. Wang CY, Ong GS. Severe bronchospasm during epidural anaesthesia. *Anaesthesia.* 1993;48:514–515.

16

Neuraxial Analgesia with Hydromorphone, Morphine, and Fentanyl: Dosing and Safety Guidelines

Susan Dabu-Bondoc, Samantha A. Franco, and Raymond S. Sinatra

Neuraxial analgesia defines the administration of opioids alone, or in combination, with local anesthetics and, occasionally, clonidine into the spinal or epidural space. This form of analgesic delivery provides powerful and highly efficient anesthetic augmentation and pain relief in a variety of clinical settings (Table 16.1). Following epidural and spinal injection, a small fraction of opioid molecules leaves the cerebrospinal fluid (CSF) and binds to receptors in dorsal horn. Activation of these receptors effectively suppresses afferent noxious transmission at the first synapse with cells in the CNS (Figure 16.1). Epidural and intrathecally administered opioids provide greater analgesic potency than similar doses administered parenterally. In general, hydrophilic opioids such as morphine and hydromorphone are associated with gains in potency and duration of effect that are greater than those of highly lipophilic opioids. A second advantage noted with neuraxial opioids is the "selectivity" of analgesic effect that is maintained in the absence of sensory-motor or sympathetic blockade.[1,2] Please refer to Chapter 8 (*Pharmacokinetics of Epidural Opioids*) for a detailed overview of neuraxial opioid pharmacology. The following chapter provides practical dosing, delivery, and adverse event treatment guidelines for several postoperative neuraxial analgesic techniques. Although commonly administered opioids such as morphine and fentanyl are discussed, major emphasis is placed on hydromorphone, which is widely employed by our pain management service. Dosing guidelines reflect findings and recommendations from recent publications; however, unpublished anecdotal information gained from years of experience and data taken from classic, well-controlled clinical trials are also included.

SINGLE BOLUSES OF INTRATHECAL OR EPIDURAL OPIOIDS

Morphine (Astramorph™, Duramorph™) was first to receive Food and Drug Administration (FDA) approval for epidural and intrathecal use and remains the most widely investigated and extensively used spinal opioid. A single intrathecal bolus (0.2–1.0 mg) or multiple boluses of epidural morphine (2–10 mg)

may be used for pain control following thoracic, abdominal, and lower extremity orthopedic surgery.[2] Doses are usually administered via spinal needles or via epidural catheters inserted at thoracic or lumbar interspaces.

Intrathecal Bolus Dosing

Intrathecal morphine is commonly administered in conjunction with local anesthetic-based spinal anesthesia. The technique is highly efficient and effective for inpatients expected to have moderate to severe postsurgical pain that does not warrant placement of an epidural catheter. Intrathecal morphine has a 30-minute onset of analgesia and provides 12–24 hours of effective pain relief as well as significant intravenous (IV) or oral opioidsparing effects. At Yale-New Haven Hospital single doses of intrathecal morphine are routinely administered to patients undergoing total hip replacement surgery, vaginal hysterectomy, and less invasive rectal and urethral surgery to improve postsurgical analgesia and as a means to reduce IV patient-controlled analgesia (PCA) morphine requirements. The technique is of particular use in elderly patients and others who are intolerant of high-dose IV opioids and who have difficulty using PCA. In agreement with earlier findings from Kemper and Treiber[1] and Negre et al,[3] we have found that small to moderate doses of intrathecal/epidural morphine provide a 60%–75% reduction (opioid-sparing effect) in IV PCA requirements during the first 24 hours and 50% total dose reduction in patients recovering from hysterectomy, cesarean section, and major orthopedic surgery.[4] This combination of intrathecal morphine plus low-dose IV PCA may be employed as a substitute for continuous epidural analgesia in patients who are scheduled to receive postoperative anticoagulation. Alternatively, we have used intrathecal morphine plus a continuous femoral nerve block as an effective alternative for pain control following total knee arthroplasty for patients in which continuous epidural infusions are technically difficult or contraindicated. Intrathecal morphine dose is formulated according to several factors, including patient age, site and extent of surgery, and patient history of opioid dependency. In general doses of 0.2–0.4 mg are administered for lower

Table 16.1: Advantages and Disadvantages of Neuraxial Opioids

Advantages

1. Decreases MAC, shortens time to extubation
2. Faster onset of anesthesia/analgesia when combined with local anesthetic (LA)
3. Allows lower LA dose with faster recovery
4. Improves intraoperative spinal anesthesia
5. Selective postoperative analgesia (prolonged analgesia without motor block)
6. High analgesic efficacy (dose requirements reduced, analgesic effect superior to IV and IV PCA opioids)

Disadvantages

1. Sedation (less of a problem with lipophilic opioids)
2. Delayed respiratory depression (morphine)
3. Frequent pruritus (morphine, fentanyl)
4. Urinary retention
5. PONV (most severe with morphine)
6. Greater invasiveness and expense than parenteral opioids

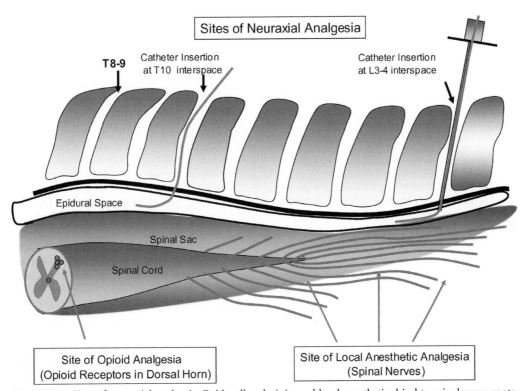

Figure 16.1: Sites of neuraxial analgesia. Epidurally administered local anesthetics bind to spinal nerve roots, dorsal root ganglion, and superficial layers of the spinal cord and block axonal conduction. Ultradilute solutions of bupivacaine and ropivacaine can provide differential blockade that specifically impedes noxious transmission in C and A-δ fibers. Epidural catheters placed at traditional vertebral interspaces (L2–L3 or L3–L4) permit local anesthetic solutions to accumulate at their primary sites of activity. Epidurally administered opioids bind and activate opioid receptors located in the dorsal horn (dots). Receptors that modulate pain from lower extremity and abdominal dermatomes are primarily localized in the lumbar-thoracic enlargement of the spinal cord between vertebral segments T8 and T10. Mixtures of local anesthetics and opioids provide additive multimodal analgesic effects with reductions in overall dose requirements. Hydrophilic agonists, such as morphine, provide nonsegmental analgesic effects as they can ascend in the CSF to bind and activate spinal opioid receptors. Highly lipophilic opioids, such as fentanyl, have difficulty ascending to these receptors as they are either trapped in epidural fat or are rapidly absorbed by the vasculature. Fentanyl molecules taken up from the epidural space are recirculated to the brain providing significant supraspinal analgesia. Hydromorphone's ability to spread rostrally is intermediate between morphine and fentanyl; however, infusions administered via L1–L2 catheters can ascend and activate receptors within the thoracolumbar enlargement. To overcome fentanyl's highly segmental properties, high infusion rates of dilute solution may employed to "push" enough molecules to the thoracolumbar region. It is recommended, however, that catheters be placed at higher vertebral segments (T10 or higher) to facilitate opioid receptor binding and improve analgesic efficacy.

Table 16.2: Recommended Doses of Intrathecal Morphine and Epidural Bolus Dose Morphine for Postoperative Analgesia (mg)

Surgical Procedure	Intrathecal Dose	Epidural Bolus Dose
Vaginal hysterectomy, cesarean section	0.15–0.2	2–3
Hip and knee surgery	0.2–0.5	2–5
Lower abdominal surgery	0.2–0.4	3–5
Upper abdominal surgery	0.4–0.6	5–7
Nephrectomy	0.4–0.6	5–7
Cholecystectomy	0.4–0.6	5
Abdominal aortic aneurysm	0.4–0.6	5–8
Whipple procedure	0.5–0.6	5–8
Retroperitoneal lymph node dissection	0.5–0.6	6–8
Thoracotomy	0.6–1.0	6–10

Note: Doses should be adjusted lower or higher depending on patient age, comorbidities, opioid tolerance, and so on.

abdominal and extremity surgery, whereas doses up to 0.8 mg may be required for larger upper abdominal procedures and thoracotomy (Table 16.2). In our experience, doses of intrathecal morphine should be reduced 25% or more in elderly and debilitated patients, whereas an increased dose is usually required in vigorous patients and is always required in those tolerant to opioid analgesics.[5]

Coadministration of injectable clonidine (Duraclon™) may further improve the neuraxial analgesic effects of intrathecal morphine. In patients recovering from total knee replacement surgery, intrathecal clonidine (25 or 75 μg) combined with intrathecal morphine (250 μg) decreased 24-hour IV morphine consumption and reduced pain intensity scores with movement when compared with morphine alone.[6] Patients receiving intrathecal morphine/clonidine combination may benefit from improved postoperative mobility that facilitates early rehabilitation and decreases the risk of deep vein thrombosis. One caution that should be considered when employing neuraxial clonidine is that the absorbed drug can slow the heart rate and drop blood pressure in high-risk patients. This is particularly true with epidural dosing in which higher doses of clonidine are required (refer later). Duraclon is approved for neuraxial administration but is expensive, and unless the pharmacy can divide the vial into separate patient doses, the majority of the contents will need to be discarded.

There have been very few clinical evaluations of intrathecal hydromorphone for postoperative analgesia.[7,8] The limited available data suggest that intrathecal hydromorphone (50–100 μg) produces analgesia and side effects similar to 100–200 μg of intrathecal morphine however, its duration of action may not be as prolonged.[7–9] In a double-blind study by Drakeford et al,[8] 60 patients scheduled for elective total hip or knee arthroplasty with tetracaine spinal anesthesia were randomly assigned to 1 of 3 treatment groups: group I received local anesthetic alone, group II received morphine (duramorph; 0.5mg), and group III received hydromorphone (0.002 mg/kg body wt). During the first 24 hours after the operation, the patients in groups II and III reported significantly less pain than those in group I. There were no significant differences between morphine and

hydromorphone with respect to the quality and duration of analgesia and incidence of adverse effects. Based on this and other studies demonstrating nonsuperiority, substitution of intrathecal hydromorphone for FDA-approved morphine preparations cannot be justified, except perhaps for patients with severe documented reactions to morphine.

Finally, intrathecal bolus doses of fentanyl (12.5–25 μg) provide less than 2 hours of analgesic effect and are not recommended for postoperative analgesia, except perhaps following same-day surgery. Intrathecal fentanyl can be coadministered with bupivacaine for augmentation of intraoperative spinal anesthesia.

Epidural Bolus Dosing

The analgesic superiority of single-dose epidural morphine over pain relief provided by parenteral opioids has been demonstrated in a variety of postsurgical settings.[2,10–12] In general, analgesic onset is appreciated after 30–60 minutes and its duration ranges from 12 to 24 hours, depending on the dose administered. Although single and intermittent doses of morphine provide effective analgesia that does not require sophisticated delivery systems, CSF morphine concentrations rise abruptly following each epidural bolus and may be associated with a high incidence of annoying and occasionally serious adverse effects. This is particularly true in elderly patients, for whom doses may need to be carefully adjusted. Ready and coworkers[13] studied age as a predictor of epidural morphine bolus dose requirements and found strong correlation among increasing patient age, increasing side effects, and effective epidural dose (milligrams of morphine per 24 hours).

We employ single-dose epidural morphine in settings where continuous epidural infusions are contraindicated (for example, patients who require postoperative anticoagulation). Single doses of epidural morphine are adjusted for patient age as well as the site and extent of surgery. In general, lower doses, 2–4 mg, are administered for lower abdominal surgeries, whereas doses are increased to 5–7 mg for upper abdominal procedures and up to 8–10 mg for thoracotomy (Table 16.1). Doses are reduced 25% or more in elderly patients and increased by 50%-100% in patients who will remain ventilated overnight and individuals who are highly opioid tolerant.

Epidural morphine-based analgesia may be augmented by the addition of clonidine. Thoracic epidural morphine (0.05 mg/kg), when combined with clonidine (3 μg/kg) in patients for radical gastrectomy[14] and 4 μg/kg in patients undergoing pancreatectomy,[15] provided postoperative analgesia superior to that of morphine alone. Analgesic onset was significantly faster, more powerful (requiring fewer rescue doses of parenteral morphine), and longer lasting. Likewise, following abdominal surgery, an epidural clonidine-fentanyl mixture doubled the duration of postsurgical analgesia compared to epidural fentanyl alone, although patients were troubled by increased drowsiness and hypotension.[16]

Hydromorphone (dilaudid), is a semisynthetic, μ-selective opioid agonist developed in the late 1920s and used for control of moderate to severe pain. Hydromorphone is associated with dose-dependent reductions in respiratory rate and minute ventilation; however, it is less sedating than morphine[17,18] and less likely to release histamine.[17,19] Because of its low side-effect profile, relatively rapid onset, and its availability as a preservative free solution, hydromorphone has been advocated and employed as a

Table 16.3: Bolus Dose Neuraxial Analgesia: Indications and Dosing Guidelines[5,9,44,77]

Opioid	Single Bolus Intrathecal	Single Bolus Epidural	Intermittent Bolus Epidural
Morphine	(0.2–1 mg) Postop analgesia	(2–10 mg) Postop/post trauma analgesia	(2–6 mg every 12 hours) Postop/post trauma analgesia
Meperidine	(10 mg) Postcesarean delivery analgesia	(40–80 mg) Same day surgery analgesia	Not recommended
Hydromorphone	(50–150 μg) Short stay surgery analgesia	(1 mg) Short stay surgery analgesia	(1–1.5 mg every 6 hours)
Fentanyl	(12.5–25 μg) Supplementation of Spinal anesthesia	(50–100 μg) Same day surgery and postcesarean analgesia	(50–75 μg every 2 hours) Not recommended

Note: Doses should be adjusted lower or higher depending on patient age, comorbidities, opioid tolerance, and so on.

neuraxial analgesic. Although not formally approved for neuraxial administration, hydromorphone was one of the first opioids tested in this setting, and its safety and analgesic efficacy have been evaluated in a number of clinical trials.[20–24]

Chestnut and colleagues[21] evaluated single-dose epidural hydromorphone (1 mg in 10 mL saline) for pain control following cesarean delivery. Patients assigned to the hydromorphone group benefited from superior pain control with 92% reporting good or excellent pain relief versus 56% in the control group. Time to first request for supplemental analgesia was extended (13 vs 3.1 hours), and 24-hour requirement for IV hydromorphone was reduced (4.7 vs 10.2 mg). In our experience, single-dose hydromorphone (1 mg) has a relatively short analgesic duration of 6–7 hours, and it is rarely employed for inpatient pain management. It may be considered for short-stay (less than 24 hours) settings, where patients are transitioned to oral analgesics within 5–12 hours following surgery. Epidural doses ranging from 0.5 to 1.0 mg (or one-fifth the recommended dose for morphine) may be co administered with epidural lidocaine (2%) for intaoperative anesthesia and for relief of postoperative pain following arthroscopic and less invasive pelvic/perineal surgery.[20–24] Guidelines for bolusing intrathecal and epidural opioids are outlined in Table 16.3.

CONTINUOUS EPIDURAL ANALGESIA

Continuous infusions of epidural opioids, opioids plus dilute local anesthetics, or concentrated local anesthetics alone provide more prolonged and uniform analgesia than single doses of epidural morphine.[25] Continuous infusions permit analgesia to be more precisely titrated to the level of pain stimulus and rapidly terminated if problems should occur. The technique avoids the high peak CSF concentrations that follow intermittent epidural boluses and reduces the risk of rostral CSF spread and delayed respiratory depression.[25,26] Other benefits include decreased time spent administering agents and assessing effect and a reduced risk of contamination and medication errors than intermittent dosing techniques. Continuous infusion techniques also provide greater therapeutic versatility because rapid-acting, short-duration opioids and dilute local anesthetic solutions may be coadministered.

Local Anesthetic Infusions

Epidural infusion of local anesthetics or central neural blockade offers reliable, segmental analgesia for patients recovering from orthopedic surgery or trauma. The technique is useful for patients with chronic obstructive pulmonary disease (COPD) and others who are exquisitely sensitive to opioids. However, such therapy is associated with sensory/motor and sympathetic blockade. In this regard, hypotension, motor weakness, and impaired micturition occur more frequently with epidural infusions of local anesthetics than with opioids. To maintain a balance between effective pain relief and unacceptable side effects, the epidural catheter tip should be placed at spinal interspaces immediately adjacent to the injury (ie, T12-L1 for hip surgery and T5, 6–7 for thoracotomy). Analgesia is maintained with solutions of 0.125%–0.25% bupivacaine or 0.2% ropivacaine, continuously infused at rates of 6–8 mL/h. Central neural blockade may be improved by adding clonidine to the local anesthetic solution; however, additive hypotensive effects should be anticipated. Analgesia may also be supplemented with IV ketorolac (7.5–15 mg every 6 hours) or Celecoxib™ (200 mg twice a day) unless contraindicated.

Fentanyl Infusions

Epidural fentanyl is commonly administered as continuous infusion because its rapid onset and short duration facilitates analgesic titration.[27] In earlier clinical trials, patients receiving continuous fentanyl infusions following upper abdominal surgery or cesarean section reported superior pain relief with less annoying side effects than individuals treated with parenteral opioids.[27–31] However, epidural dose requirements are high (30–60 μg/h), leading some investigators to question fentanyl's neuraxial specificity. In contrast to morphine, fentanyl has difficulty spreading to more rostral dermatomes as a significant portion of drug is either taken up by the vasculature or is trapped in epidural fat. Despite its more "segmental" analgesic effect, lumbar epidural infusions of fentanyl are used to control pelvic or lower extremity orthopedic pain involving lumbar/sacral dermatomes. Following these procedures, epidural fentanyl in concentrations of 2–5 μg/mL is usually infused at rates of 6–12 mL/h.

To achieve more effective analgesia, dilute concentrations of bupivacaine (0.0625%–0.1%) or ropivacaine (0.1%–0.2%) should be added to the fentanyl infusion unless contraindicated. Studies employing mixtures of fentanyl plus bupivacaine reported effective analgesia with much lower fentanyl dose requirements (20 μg/h or less).[32] Sjostrom et al[32] compared two concentrations of epidural bupivacaine and low-dose fentanyl for postoperative analgesia in 100 patients scheduled for colorectal surgery. Patients were randomized to receive infusions of either bupivacaine (0.12%) with fentanyl (2 μg/mL) or bupivacaine (0.24%) with fentanyl (4 μg/mL). Infusion rates were adjusted to insure postoperative patient comfort during the next 48 hours. The two groups required equal drug amounts of bupivacaine (10.8–11 mg/h) and fentanyl (18–18.4 μg/h), had low pain scores (VAS 3 or less), and experienced comparable and relatively few adverse effects.

A preoperative epidural bolus dose of fentanyl (100 μg) may be administered to increase the analgesic effectiveness of subsequent fentanyl plus bupivacaine infusions.[33] In a study of 40 patients undergoing subtotal gastrectomy, two groups were randomized to receive epidural fentanyl (100 μg) or saline prior to incision, followed by continuous epidural infusion of bupivacaine (0.2%) and fentanyl (30 μg/mL) at a rate of 0.7 mL/hr for 72 hours. Although the total analgesic rescue doses were comparative in both groups, the group that received preoperative fentanyl reported lower median pain scores up to 72 hours postoperatively.[33]

Finally, it should be appreciated that lumbar infusions of fentanyl plus bupivacaine are less effective in blunting pain from upper abdominal and thoracic incisions. In these settings, administration via catheters placed at higher interspaces (T8-T5) adjacent to the site of surgery is highly recommended. If thoracic catheters are difficult to place, lumbar infusion with large volumes of solution (10–14 mL/h) may promote rostral spread and better control pain at thoracic dermatomes; however, side effects may be increased.[34]

Morphine Infusions

Epidural infusions of morphine and hydromorphone also provide prolonged postsurgical analgesia for patients recovering from upper abdominal and thoracic procedures. Lumbar infusions of morphine provide nonsegmental analgesic effects that can control pain originating at higher spinal segments. Infusions of morphine are highly effective alone and may not require local anesthetic supplementation. This ability offers clinical advantages in settings such as hypovolemia, where coadministration of local anesthetics may be contraindicated. Addition of dilute local anesthetic (bupivacaine [0.0625%–0.1%] or ropivacaine [0.1%]) will, nevertheless, provide additive analgesic benefits, including reductions in infusion rate and morphine concentration.[35] Dahl and colleagues[36] reported that dilute concentrations of bupivacaine potentiated epidural morphine based analgesia in patients recovering from upper abdominal surgery. Pain intensity scores were similar at rest; however, assessments made during mobilization and cough were significantly reduced.

The continuous epidural morphine technique requires an intraoperative loading dose of 2–5 mg of epidural morphine with local anesthetic (bupivacaine [0.25%] or ropivacaine [0.2%]), as tolerated by the patient. Because morphine has a delayed onset to peak effect, we recommend that the loading dose be administered prior to surgical incision. The continuous infusion is initiated in the operating room near the end of surgery or in the postanesthesia care unit (PACU). Recommended infusion concentrations are 40–60 μg/mL alone or in combination with local anesthetic. In our experience, 40 μg/mL is associated with fewer and less severe adverse events, particularly pruritus and nausea; however, the 60 μg solution provides more reliable analgesic effects. Recommended rates of infusion range from 4 to 10 mL per hour depending on patient age, comorbidities, and the site and extent of surgery.

Combined Spinal Morphine Plus Epidural Infusion

Combined spinal plus epidural anesthesia/analgesia (CSE or CSEA) is another useful method by which an epidural catheter and spinal block are simultaneously placed to combine the rapid-onset, dense block of spinal anesthesia with the intra- and postoperative versatility of an epidural catheter. CSEA has been used for a wide variety of nonobstetric surgery in adults, including orthopedic, urologic, vascular, gynecologic, and general surgical procedures, and a variety of opioids and local anesthetics have been advocated.[37–41] The technique requires placement of either a standard or specialized 17-gauge needle into epidural space and then advancing a 24- to 25-gauge spinal needle through the epidural needle into the subarachnoid space. Subsequently, spinal local anesthetic, either bupivacaine (0.75%) or tetracaine (1%), is injected intrathecally. The spinal needle is then removed, and an epidural catheter is inserted in standard fashion. The catheter may then be used to prolong intraoperative anesthesia or to provide postoperative epidural analgesia. Recently, the technique has undergone several modifications designed to increase its safety and efficacy. A modification of the conventional CSE is the sequential CSE technique, in which spinal anesthesia is induced with local anesthetic and morphine (Astramorph™ or Duramorph™) to initiate anesthetic conditions that may then be extended with epidural top-ups of local anesthetic. A low-dose infusion of epidural fentanyl may be initiated following surgery for postoperative analgesia.[37] Preoperative administration of low-dose intrathecal bupivacaine plus morphine (0.2–0.4 mg) followed by a postoperative epidural infusion of fentanyl without local anesthetic may be particularly useful in high-risk patients in whom maintenance of stable hemodynamics is imperative. Teoh et al[42] demonstrated the advantages of an ultra-low-dose CSE (bupivacaine [3.75 mg], fentanyl [25 μg], morphine [100 μg] spinal plus additional epidural boluses of 1.5% lidocaine) versus a standard CSE (bupivacaine [9 mg] spinal) followed by boluses of 1.5% lidocaine intraoperatively and a postoperative epidural infusion of fentanyl plus dilute bupivacaine for surgical anesthesia and postoperative analgesia during uncomplicated cesarean deliveries. Intraoperatively, the low-dose spinal bupivacaine group had less motor block, more rapid sensory regression and motor recovery, less intraoperative hypotension, and equivalent postoperative analgesia. At Yale-New Haven Hospital, depending on the surgical procedure, patient's age, weight, and medical comorbidities, we administer intrathecal morphine (0.2–0.5 mg) plus bupivacaine (8–12 mg) preoperatively while simultaneously securing an epidural catheter for additional anesthesia. Postoperatively a dilute low rate (4–8 mL/h) epidural infusion of fentanyl plus bupivacaine or hydromorphone plus bupivacaine is initiated as required to maintain effective postoperative pain control.

Hydromorphone Infusions

Continuous epidural infusions of hydromorphone have been advocated for patients recovering from a variety of surgical procedures.[25,43] Chaplan and coworkers[25,44] compared a 3:1 dose ratio of morphine:hydromorphone for continuous epidural infusions. Patients in the hydromorphone group received between 0.15 and 0.2 mg/h, and experienced effective pain relief and less sedation and pruritus than patients receiving

Table 16.4: Advantages of Patient-Controlled Epidural Analgesia

Versus intravenous PCA

1. Superior pain relief

2. Reduced drug requirement

3. Reduction in drug related side effects

4. Shortened hospital stay?

Versus continuous epidural opioid infusion

1. Patient self-adjustment

2. Reduced hourly infusion requirement

3. Accommodation for changes in pain intensity (ie, ambulation)

4. Reduced anxiety, increased patient control

---

continuous infusions of morphine. Being moderately water soluble, vascular uptake of epidural hydromorphone is lower than that of fentanyl, although its ability to remain in CSF and spread rostrally is greater.[45] This property provides important clinical advantages: (1) like morphine, doses administered via high lumbar and low thoracic catheters can control pain at higher dermatomal segments and (2) epidural administration is associated with 3 times greater potency than similar amounts given IV. The safety and side-effect profile of epidural hydromorphone is superior to morphine as equianalgesic doses are associated with less pruritus and excess sedation.[25,44] For dosing and delivery guidelines, please refer to the section Epidural Hydromophone: How to Make It Work.

PATIENT-CONTROLLED EPIDURAL ANALGESIA

Patient-controlled epidural analgesia (PCEA) was developed in response to findings that epidural opioids provided superior pain relief, whereas IV PCA offers greater autonomy, higher patient satisfaction, and fewer troublesome side effects.[10,46] It seems reasonable to expect that epidural opioids could be combined with a self-administration dosing regimen, thereby providing the control and titratability of PCA as well as the greater effectiveness and potency gain associated with spinal analgesia.[10] The advantages of PCEA are outlined in Table 16.4.

Morphine PCEA

Most of the early work describing the concept of PCEA was performed at the University of Kentucky, where the technique was evaluated in over 4000 patients recovering from a variety of surgical procedures.[47,48] According to their protocol, patients were "loaded" with 2–3 mg of epidural morphine. Thereafter, a basal infusion (0.4 mg/h) was started, and patients were allowed to self-administer 0.2 mg morphine every 10–15 minutes with a maximal dose of 1.2 mg/h. In our experience, morphine's latency to peak effect and risk of delayed onset respiratory depression were undesirable characteristics for PCEA. In many centers, hydromorphone and fentanyl, which offer greater titratability and fewer adverse events, have become the agents of choice for PCEA.[44]

Fentanyl PCEA

Patients self-administering epidural fentanyl benefit from equivalent pain relief while requiring less drug than individuals treated with continuous fentanyl infusions.[49–52] The safety and effectiveness of bupivacaine-fentanyl PCEA (0.1% bupivacaine and 5 µg/mL fentanyl mixture) as compared with continuous epidural infusion (0.1 mL/kg/h) of same mixture was evaluated in 49 patients recovering from total knee arthroplasty.[52] Postoperative bupivacaine and fentanyl total dose requirement was significantly reduced in the PCEA group ($P < .001$) compared to the continuous epidural infusion group. Pain scores at rest and at leg raising, amount of rescue analgesics, and incidence of side effects were, nevertheless, similar in both groups. Because opioid related adverse effects are dose dependent, the reduction in fentanyl dosage observed with PCEA may offer clinical advantages that improve patient safety.

Liu et al[53] studied 1020 patients recovering from a wide variety of surgical procedures who utilized PCEA for pain control. They found that solutions containing bupivacaine (0.05%) plus fentanyl (4 µg/mL) administered at rate a of 2 mL every 10–15 minutes was safe, reliable, and effective. PCEA fentanyl has also been found to be safe and effective in elderly patients. Ishiyama et al[54] examined 40 elderly (>65 years old) and 40 young (20–64 years old) patients recovering from major abdominal procedures and treated with PCEA (ropivacaine [0.05%] plus fentanyl [4 µg/mL]). They found that both young and elderly self-administered similar amounts of PCEA fentanyl at rest. Elderly patients self-administered less medication during coughing and reported superior analgesia. The incidence of adverse effects (pruritus, nausea, respiratory depression, hypotension) were similar in both patient groups.

Buvanendran and coworkers[55] reported that pain relief, provided by PCEA fentanyl plus bupivacaine for patients recovering from total knee replacement, could be improved by administration of an oral cyclooxygenase 2 (COX-2) inhibitor, Rofecoxib™. They observed significant reductions in pain intensity scores, total infusate administered, and adverse effects, whereas patient functionality and rehabilitation were improved. Because Rofecoxib™ has been withdrawn, the COX-2 inhibitor Celecoxib™ (400-mg loading dose, followed by 200 mg twice a day) may be employed to achieve similar multimodal analgesic benefits.

We employ a PCEA fentanyl regimen that includes a basal infusion plus PCA bolus doses as required. This form of administration works well in elderly patients, who often forget to push the PCA delivery button and fall behind with their pain control. Most patients remain comfortable at rest with a 4- to 8-mL/h basal infusion of bupivacaine (0.05%) plus fentanyl (4 µg/mL). PCEA bolus doses of 2 mL every 6–8 minutes may then be administered to control breakthrough pain following cough, incentive spirometry, or ambulation. Because of fentanyl's segmental analgesic effects, thoracic epidural administration is recommended for pain control following upper abdominal and thoracic incisions. With thoracic infusions, the basal infusion may be further reduced to 2–6 mL/h.

Hydromorphone PCEA

Hydromorphone has also been advocated for epidural PCA. Parker and White[56] noted that patients self-administering epidural hydromorphone following cesarean section required 4-fold

Table 16.5: Dosing Guidelines for Epidural Opioid Infusions and PCEA[a]

Opioid	Site of Administration	Continuous Infusion Technique	Patient-Controlled Technique	Adjunctive Therapy[b]
Morphine	Lumbar catheters for incisions below T8, thoracic catheters for upper abdominal and thoracic surgery	2–4 mg bolus followed by infusion (40 μg/mL) at 6–12 mL/h for lumbar catheters; 4–8 mL/h for thoracic catheters	2–4 mg bolus followed by infusion (40 μg/mL) at 6–8 mL/h for lumbar catheters; 2–6 mL/h for thoracic. PCEA bolus dose 1–2 mL ever 15 min	Ketorolac (IV 7.5–15 mg every 6 hours), Celecoxib™ (200 mg twice a day); add epidural bupivacaine (0.05–0.1%) or less. Consider epidural clonidine?
Hydromorphone	Lumbar catheters for incisions below T10, thoracic catheters for upper abdominal and thoracic surgery	0.5- to 1.5-mg bolus followed by infusion (10–20 μg/mL) at 8–14 mL/h, for lumbar catheters; 4–8 mL/h for thoracic catheters	0.5- to 1.5-mg bolus followed by infusion (10–20 μg/mL) at 6–10 mL/h, lumbar catheters; 4–6 mL/h for thoracic PCEA bolus dose 1–3 mL every 6–8 minutes	Ketorolac (IV 7.5–15 mg every 6 hours), Celecoxib™ (200 mg twice a day); add epidural bupivacaine (0.05%) or less. Consider epidural clonidine?
Fentanyl	Lumbar catheters for incisions below T12, thoracic catheters for almost everything else	50–100 μg bolus followed by infusion (2–4 μg/mL) at 8–14 mL/hr for lumbar catheters; 4–8 mL/h, for thoracic catheters	50–100 μg bolus followed by infusion (2–4 μg/mL) at 6–10 mL/h, lumbar catheters 4–6 mL/h for thoracic PCEA bolus dose 1–3 mL every 6 min	Ketorolac (IV 7.5–15 mg every 6 hours), Celecoxib™ (200 mg twice a day); add epidural bupivacaine (0.1%) or less. Consider epidural clonidine?

[a] Dependent on age, physical status, height, extent of surgical dissection, degree of opioid tolerance, and so on.

[b] Unless contraindicated.

less drug to achieve effective analgesia than patients receiving IV PCA hydromorphone. Similarly, Liu and coworkers[57] found that patients self-administrating epidural hydromorphone (150 μg every 10–15 minutes) following radical prostatectomy required 50% less medication over the 72-hour study interval than patients treated with IV PCA. These findings of increased epidural versus intravenous potency suggested that hydromorphone had a primary spinal analgesic effect. Hydromorphone PCEA dosing guidelines are further discussed under *Epidural Hydromorphone: How to Make It Work.* Epidural dose requirements for single bolus techniques, continuous epidural infusion, and patient-controlled epidural infusion are presented in Table 16.5.

ADVERSE EFFECTS ASSOCIATED WITH SPINAL OPIOIDS

Epidural and intrathecally administered opioids are associated with a number of troublesome and occasionally serious adverse effects, including pruritus, nausea, urinary retention, somnolence, and respiratory depression.[2,58,59] These adverse events are most commonly observed with bolus doses of epidural and intrathecal morphine. Treatment protocols have been developed that can decrease the incidence and severity of side effects and improve patient safety while maintaining effective analgesia. The presence of side effects should be assessed frequently and treated quickly to minimize morbidity and patient dissatisfaction.

Respiratory Depression

Although rare in comparison with other side effects, respiratory depression is the most feared complication associated with epidural and intrathecally administered opioids.[2,20,59] Respiratory depression observed with intermittent doses of epidural/intrathecal morphine is gradual and insidious, occurring

Table 16.6: Factors That Increase the Risk of Spinal Opioid-Induced Respiratory Depression

Drug-related factors
  The use of morphine
  Excessive dose
  Large volume of injectate
  Excessive dose frequency
  Concomitant administration of parenteral opioids
Patient-related factors
  Age greater than 60 years
  Debilitated individuals
  Coexisting respiratory disease
  Raised intrathoracic pressure
  Trendelenberg position

8–12 hours following administration. This delayed onset of depressive symptoms has been related to rostral flow of CSF and delivery of morphine molecules to the brainstem respiratory centers.[2,59] Risk factors underlying delayed respiratory depression include excessive dose, extremes of age, pulmonary disease, morbid obesity, and concomitant administration of parenteral opioids (Table 16.6). In our experience, increasing nausea and vomiting and somnolence generally precede respiratory depression, and such patients should be closely monitored. Respiratory rates less than 10 per minute or evidence of diminished tidal volume should be treated promptly with naloxone (40–80 μg IV) followed by a naloxone infusion (300–400 μg/L of crystalloid every 8 hours). Naloxone infusions may provide prophylaxis of the worst aspects of opioid-induced respiratory depression in high-risk and elderly patients (>70 years).[60]

Pruritus

Generalized pruritus is often observed with morphine and to a lesser extent with hydromorphone and fentanyl. Occasionally, the intensity of itching is so annoying that it interferes with sleep.[2,58,61] Why pruritus occurs is poorly understood but its occurrence does not reflect an acute or excessive release of histamine, because peak effects are noted 3–6 hours following administration. Furthermore, pruritus is commonly observed with fentanyl, an opioid not associated with histamine release. Pruritus associated with epidural morphine is treated according to its severity. Mild facial pruritus may be relieved with cold compresses, whereas moderate generalized itching may respond to one or more doses of diphenhydramine (12.5–25 mg). Patients with moderate to severe pruritus are treated with IV boluses of naloxone (0.04 to 0.08 mg), which generally improves patient comfort without reversing spinal opioid analgesia.[62] One may conveniently maintain a continuous IV infusion by adding one or two ampules of naloxone (0.4 to 0.8 mg) to each liter of the patient's maintenance intravenous fluid. An infusion rate of 125 mL/h will deliver 50 to 100 μg/h of naloxone. Borgeat and colleagues[63] noted that subhypnotic doses (10 mg) of IV propofol could also be used to relieve spinal morphine-induced pruritus.

Nausea and Vomiting

Although nausea and vomiting is commonly observed in patients recovering from surgery, the incidence of symptoms is increased in patients treated with epidural and intrathecal opioids.[20,44,58] Nausea may result from either rostral spread of the drug in spinal fluid to the brainstem or vascular uptake and delivery to the vomiting center and chemoreceptor trigger zone.[58] In general, patients treated with intermittent boluses of morphine experience the highest incidence of nausea and vomiting, whereas patients receiving continuous hydromorphone infusions are less often affected.[44,45] The first step in reducing nausea and vomiting symptoms in patients not complaining of pain is to reduce the epidural opioid infusion rate. A variety of antiemetic agents may be administered to patients who remain symptomatic. Ondansetron is a highly effective antiemetic that has become our first-line treatment for opioid-induced nausea. Doses ranging from 4–8 mg may reduce the incidence and severity of symptoms.[64–66] Low doses of droperidol (0.625–1.25 mg) and metoclopramide (10 mg) administered either as prophylaxis or every 4–6 hours have also proven to be effective. The use of a transdermal scopolamine patch has also been reported to reduce the incidence of nausea and vomiting associated with epidural morphine, particularly during the first 10 hours following administration.[67] In the presence of intractable nausea, the infusion may be discontinued or switched to an epidural clonidine infusion. Intravenous boluses of naloxone followed by continuous infusion of 0.5–1 μg/kg/h should also be considered.

Urinary Retention

Spinal opioid-induced urinary retention is a commonly observed complication in general and orthopedic surgical patients. Urinary retention has been related to inhibition of sacral parasympathetic outflow that results in relaxation of the bladder detrusor muscle and an inability to relax the sphincter.[68] This adverse effect is less commonly observed with thoracic administration and may be relieved with intravenous naloxone; however, dose requirements are significant (0.8 mg), and reversal of analgesia may occur.[68]

EPIDURAL HYDROMORPHONE: HOW TO MAKE IT WORK

History and Evolution

At Yale-New Haven Hospital, the majority of patients recovering from extensive surgical procedures and major trauma are treated with continuous epidural infusions or epidural PCA. Since the late 1990s, hydromorphone has displaced both morphine and fentanyl and has become the epidural opioid of choice for patients recovering from thoracotomy, nephrectomy, upper abdominal surgery, and total knee replacement.

Modifications of dosing guidelines have improved the effectiveness and efficiency of hydromorphone infusions.[44,69] Early evaluations employed highly concentrated infusate solutions administered at relatively low rates per hour. The finding that epidural hydromorphone is associated with less rostral spread and more segmental analgesic effects than morphine led us to test whether its rate of delivery should conform to guidelines developed for more lipophilic opioids.[44,69] In a series of pilot trials, hydromorphone infusate concentration was gradually decreased from 50 to 30 μg/mL and eventually to 10 μg/mL, and hourly infusion rates increased from 2–5 mL/h to 10 to 12 mL/h.[44,69] The resulting "low-concentration/high-volume" technique resulted in a dosing regimen that reduced overall dose while extending dermatomal spread of analgesia. Benefits were most noticeable in settings where lumbar catheters were placed to control pain following upper abdominal and thoracic surgery. In these situations increasing the infusion rate from 3–5 mL/h of a 75-μg/mL solution to 10–15 mL/h of a 10–20 μg/mL solution reduced pain intensity and improved pulmonary function, but did not result in excessive sedation or respiratory depression. In agreement with previous reports,[70–72] we observed that the addition of ultradilute concentrations of bupivacaine (0.05%-0.03%) further improved the quality postsurgical analgesia, particularly effort dependent or dynamic pain, without increasing the incidence of orthostatic hypotension or interfering with safe, assisted ambulation.

Since 1995, nearly 13,000 patients recovering from major operative procedures and traumatic injuries at Yale-New Haven Hospital have been treated with epidural PCA or epidural infusions of hydromorphone (10–20 μg/mL) alone or in combination with dilute bupivacaine (0.625%–0.03%). In an evaluation of 2900 consecutive patients managed by our pain service,[73] the following information was obtained. The majority of patients were elderly (52% were age 65 years or greater) and/or had significant medical illness (56% American Society of Anesthesiologists [ASA] status III or IV). Twenty-nine percent of patients experienced none to mild pain (VAS 0–2 cm), 48% reported moderate discomfort (VAS 3–5), 15% reported moderate to severe discomfort (VAS 6–7), whereas 8% complained of poor pain control (VAS 8 or greater). Patients with inadequate analgesia were noted to have either improperly placed or dislodged epidural catheters or chronic pain/opioid dependence. The most common side effects included pruritus requiring treatment (12% incidence), nausea and vomiting (16%), and excessive sedation (6%). Life-threatening adverse events including airway obstruction and severe respiratory depression were extremely rare.

Seven patients experienced severe respiratory depression/code blue. Two elderly, emphysematous patients and one obese individual with chronic sleep apnea received inappropriately high loading doses of hydromorphone (1.2 mg or greater). All were resuscitated and none suffered long-term complications.[73]

Dosing Guidelines

Three protocols have been developed for continuous infusion and epidural PCA.

1 Patients undergoing lower extremity orthopedic and vascular procedures with epidural anesthesia or combined spinal plus epidural anesthesia plus conscious sedation receive an intraoperative epidural loading dose of 0.5–1.5 mg hydromorphone with appropriate doses of 0.5%-0.75% bupivacaine or ropivacaine to achieve surgical anesthesia. Alternatively, 0.25–0.3 mg of intrathecal morphine may be given with the spinal anesthetic portion of a CSE technique. In either case, supplemental boluses of local anesthetic may be administered as required during the procedure. On near completion of the procedure or following arrival in the PACU, a basal infusion of hydromorphone (10 μg–20 μg/mL) is initiated at a rate of 8–12 mL/h. The size of the loading dose and continuous infusion rate are influenced by patient age, extent of surgery, and location of the catheter. In this regard loading dose and infusion rates are reduced by one-third to one-half in patients greater than 70 years or when administered via thoracic catheters. When the patient becomes alert and oriented, Epi-PCA boluses (3–4 mL of solution) with a 6- to 8-minute lockout are added to supplement the continuous infusion.

2 Patients undergoing orthopedic, abdominal, and thoracic surgeries with general anesthesia plus epidural anesthesia/analgesia receive an intraoperative epidural loading dose of 0.5–1.5 mg hydromorphone, with 6–12 mL 0.25%–0.5% bupivacaine or 0.2%-0.75% ropivacaine depending on patient age and comorbidities. Ideally, the loading dose should be administered prior to surgical incision and, when possible, prior to induction of general anesthesia. Anesthesia should consist of a propofol induction and sevoflurane or desflurane maintenance. Doses of fentanyl may be administered during induction but sparingly during the procedure as required. To avoid confusion regarding the quality of epidural analgesia (and potential additive respiratory depression), long-acting opioids such as morphine and hydromorphone are restricted intraoperatively. Supplemental boluses of local anesthetic are administered as required during the case. In extremely prolonged surgeries, an additional bolus of hydromorphone (25%–50% of loading dose) is given 6 hours into the procedure. On arrival in the PACU, a basal infusion of hydromorphone (10–20 μg/mL) is initiated at a rate of 6–12 mL/h. When the patient becomes alert and oriented, Epi-PCA boluses (3–4 mL of solution) with a 6- to 8-minute lockout are added to supplement the continuous infusion.

3 An alternative approach, termed *epidural infusion-light general anesthesia*, is ideally suited for elderly-debilitated patients and for prolonged operative procedures. Patients receive a hydromorphone loading dose of reduced size (0.25–0.75 mg) with 3–5 mL 0.25% bupivacaine or 0.2% ropivacaine followed by an intraoperative infusion of dilute hydromorphone-0.03% bupivacaine. The infusion is set at a rate of 6–12 mL/h that is maintained during the course of a light sevoflurane- or desflurane-based general anesthetic. The combination epidural infusion-light general technique provides significant reduction in volatile anesthetic requirements, improves perioperative hemodynamic stability, and offers effective postsurgical analgesia. Epi-PCA dosing is added in the PACU, when the patient is alert and cooperative.

To further improve the overall quality of analgesia, supplemental doses of IV morphine (2–4 mg, every 2–4 hours) and ketorolac (7.5–15 mg ever 6 hours, unless contraindicated) and Celecoxib[TM] (200 mg twice a day), may be prescribed during the course of continuous epidural therapy.[55,72] The concept of employing nonopioid analgesics to augment hydromorphone based epidural analgesia was tested by Singh and coworkers.[72] They reported that the addition of IV ketorolac and dilute bupivacaine to Epi-PCA with hydromorphone significantly reduced pain scores during movement and improved peak expiratory flow rate on postoperative days 1 and 2.

Epidural-PCA is maintained for 2–4 days, depending upon the procedure and potential benefit to the patient. Most patients make a smooth transition to oral opioids such as oxycodone or oxycodone-acetaminophen compounds; however, some who remain nil per os (NPO) may require several days of low dose IV PCA therapy.[74] One exception to this rule is the opioid-dependent patient or the vigorous patient recovering from extensive and highly painful surgery. These patients are given a sustained-release morphine or oxycodone tablet at the time the continuous infusion is discontinued. We then continue epidural PCA boluses over the next several hours and gauge the analgesic effect of the sustained release preparation. If the level of relief is acceptable, the epidural catheter is removed and the patient is provided with immediate release opioid tablets for breakthrough pain.

We are increasingly asked to manage epidural hydromorphone infusions in opioid-dependent patients. Managing these patients can be difficult, even with a perfectly functioning epidural, as they not only demonstrate exaggerated acute pain related to their surgery, but are also troubled by chronic pain and physical dependence. In these individuals, we often increase the loading dose of epidural hydromorphone and intrathecal morphine by 50%–100% and the infusion concentration of hydromorphone by 100% or more to compensate for opioid tolerance and downregulation of spinal opioid receptors. Neuraxial analgesia may be further improved by the addition of epidural clonidine and more concentrated solutions of local anesthetic, unless contraindicated. Judicious use of IV ketamine infusions, methadone, and ketorolac or Celecoxib[TM] may be administered as adjuvants to further improve pain relief. In addition to the epidural infusion, the patient should always receive their baseline opioids either orally or parenterally to provide superspinal analgesic potentiation as well as avoiding opioid withdrawal.[73] (Refer to Chapter 34: *Acute Pain Management in Patients with Opioid Dependence and Substance Abuse*.) Occasionally, we will offer highly dependent patients who remain NPO IV PCA boluses of morphine or hydromorphone in addition to their continuous epidural infusion of hydromorphone plus local anesthetic. Many opioid-tolerant patients are poly-drug dependent and will require higher than usual doses of anxiolytics to control the emotional and affective components of pain perception.

Patients presenting with a history of ethanol abuse may also provide difficulties in management. These individuals often appear anxious, highly irritable, and dissatisfied with epidural pain therapy despite the fact that they are experiencing highly effective analgesia. In this setting anxiolytic therapy and ethanol withdrawal prophylaxis may dramatically improve patient cooperation and satisfaction.

Drug Preparation and Analgesic Assessment.

Epidural solutions are prepared by the department of pharmacy services. Solutions containing 10 μg/mL are prepared by adding 5 mg (0.5 mL) preservative free hydromorphone (taken from a multidose vial of dilaudid-HP 10 μg/mL) to a polyethylene bag containing 500 mL normal saline. Calculated volumes of 0.75% bupivacaine (generally without epinephrine) are added to achieve infusate concentrations of 0.0625%–0.031%. Infusion bags are prepared in batches and refrigerated at 40°F. Solutions prepared in this manner remain sterile and retain stability for prolonged periods.[75,76] A Hospira Gemstar pump with a 500-mL locking chamber (Hospira Inc., Lake Forest, IL) or similar device, which can be programmed to provide a continuous infusion and patient bolus delivery, is used to administer the epidural solutions.

The safety of epidural opioid analgesia depends on clear and specific postoperative orders, and frequent patient monitoring. Epidural dosing and rate of infusion must be individualized with regard to patient status and extent of surgery. Patients receiving continuous epidural analgesia are formally rounded on twice daily and additional visits by a member of the pain service as required. The adequacy of pain relief, level of sedation, and degree of sensory motor block are assessed and documented in the patients chart. Side effects including pruritus, nausea/vomiting, and urinary retention are treated by the floor nursing staff PRN as per specific orders (refer to the *Appendix*). We agree with recommendations that an acute pain service or knowledgeable 24-hour in-house personnel be immediately available to back up the nursing staff in settings of overdose or inadequate analgesia.[77,78]

Inadequate analgesia may be the result of catheter-related problems, undermedication, and patient related variability (anatomy, disease, medication history). The caregiver must first rule out catheter dislodgment by assessing the site and testing its function with dilute local anesthetic (5–10 mL 1% lidocaine or 0.125% bupivacaine). Following a negative test, the catheter may be repositioned or replaced. With functional catheters, an epidural bolus of 8–12 mL (80–120 μg) hydromorphone followed by an increase in epidural infusion rate generally improves patient comfort within 10–15 minutes. In patients with previously unrecognized chronic opioid dependence, effective interventions include switching to a more concentrated infusion of hydromorphone (20–40 μg/mL) and local anesthetic.[73]

Patient Monitoring and Safety with Hydromorphone

What is the most appropriate method of respiratory monitoring for patients treated with epidural/intrathecal opioids? This question is difficult, and no one solution appears applicable to every institution. The decision how best to monitor patients must be left to the judgment of the acute pain service in conjunction with the nursing staff. Pulse oximeters and apnea monitors have been employed to detect opioid-induced respiratory depression;

however, these devices share drawbacks of patient inconvenience, frequent and annoying false alarms, and an inability to detect hypercarbia. Vigilant nursing observation and documentation of inadequate respiratory effort, slow respiratory rate, or unusual somnolence represent the best form of monitoring.[77,78] The speed with which epidural hydromorphone-induced respiratory depression develops is not sudden but slowly progressive and is generally preceded by nausea/vomiting and increased sedation.[44,73] With appropriate staff education, and pain service backup, epidural hydromorphone may be administered to most patients recovering on the surgical ward.

Elderly individuals and patients with major organ dysfunction are at higher risk for opioid-induced respiratory depression, and may require intensive care unit (ICU) recovery.[44,61] Oxygen saturation, level of sedation, and respiratory rate should be monitored continuously in these patients, and arterial P_{CO_2} closely followed. Excessive doses of benzodiazepines and benadryl, compazine and vistaril are restricted in elderly patients in order to avoid excessive sedation, confusion, and airway obstruction. Patients with optimal levels of spinal opioid analgesia will almost always maintain an elevated P_{CO_2} (40–44 mm Hg).[44,73] Progressive increases in sedation and P_{CO_2} are corrected either by reducing the infusion rate or by initiating a low-dose intravenous infusion of naloxone (40–50 μg/h).

Precautions and Contraindications

Contraindications to continuous epidural hydromorphone infusions and other neuraxial techniques include patient refusal, spinal fracture, infection or tumor at the insertion site, septicemia, coagulopathy, and treatment with low-molecular-weight heparinoids. At Yale-New Haven Hospital epidural placement requires assessment of coagulation status and the absence vertebral fractures, instability, and neural deficit. In patients recovering from traumatic injuries, cervical spine imaging and clearance is highly desired, but difficult to perform, during the acute and early phases of recovery. We will not place catheters in patients with consumptive or drug-induced coagulopathy unless the underlying cause is corrected.

In the United States, significant concern has been raised regarding the safety of neuraxial analgesia in patients receiving anticoagulant-based prophylaxis of deep venous thrombosis (DVT). In December 1997, the FDA issued an advisory letter about the potential risk of epidural hematoma in patients receiving regional (spinal or epidural) anesthesia and low-molecular-weight heparin (LMWH). The American Society of Regional Anesthesia (ASRA) issued guidelines with respect to the safe use of anticoagulants in patients undergoing neuraxial anesthesia/analgesia (Table 16.7). The use of LMWH with spinal and epidural analgesic dosing is safe as long as published guidelines and recommendations from experienced clinical authorities are observed in all cases.

NOVEL OPIOIDS FOR NEURAXIAL ANALGESIA: BUPRENORPHINE

Buprenorphine is a partial μ agonist with a high receptor affinity and high lipid solubility. In addition, Molke et al[79] and Murphy et al[80] have shown that these factors may reduce rostral spread following epidural administration and associated side effects such as respiratory depression and nausea.

Table 16.7: Recommendations from the American Society of Regional Anesthesia Regarding the Use of LMWH and Neuraxial Anesthesia

1. Monitoring of platelets count

2. Use of antiplatelet medications, oral anticoagulant, and dextran must be avoided, because when combined with LMWH the risk of spinal hematoma is increased.

3. Presence of blood during epidural needle and catheter placement mandates that initiation of LMWH should be delayed for 24 hours postoperatively.

4. Patients on LMWH preoperatively and a single dose spinal anesthesia is going to be used, needle placement should occur at least 10 to 12 hours after the last dose of LMWH.

5. Low-molecular-weight heparin should not be started for at least 2 hours after the epidural catheter has been removed.

6. The use of LMWH in the presence of indwelling catheter is not recommended. If epidural analgesia is expected to continue longer than 24 hours, consider delaying the use of LMWH and start prophylaxis with heparin or coumadin.

7. Statistically, a certain number of patients will experience an epidural hematoma without anticoagulant therapy; the risk of epidural hematoma is estimated to be less than 1 in 200 000 cases for spinal anesthesia and less than 1 in 150,000 cases for epidural anesthesia

Buprenorphine is not presently approved for use in the United States; however, a number of studies performed in the EU suggest that it is safe and effective. Epidural buprenorphine has an analgesic potency greater than or equal to that provided by epidural morphine, with potentially greater safety. Miwa et al[81] found that buprenorphine in a dose of 4 or 8 $\mu g/kg^{-1}$ provides postoperative analgesia as effective as epidural morphine in doses of 80 $\mu g/h$. A buprenorphine dose of 15 $\mu g/h$ appears to be optimal for post operative pain relief after lower abdominal surgery. In a study by Giebler et al,[82] only one patient of 4000 who received epidural buprenorphine suffered clinically significant respiratory depression. Buprenorphine has also been used epidurally in the management of pain associated with multiple rib fractures.[83–85] In the study by Govindarajan et al,[83] nausea, vomiting, and pruritis were the only complications. There was no hypotension, urinary retention, or respiratory depression. Mehta et al[86] compared the effectiveness of buprenorphine in lumbar (LEA) versus thoracic (TEA) epidurals for postoperative analgesia in high-risk patients recovering from coronary artery bypass graft (CABG) surgery. Patients received epidural buprenorphine (0.15 mg) with a top-up dose of buprenorphine (0.15 mg) if the VAS score was 3 or more at 1-hour assessment. In addition, intramuscular ketorolac (30 mg) was given for breakthrough pain treatment. The results of the study showed that both the TEA and LEA groups experienced similar VAS pain scores from 1 to 24 hours postoperatively. Side-effect profiles and total ketorolac dose were also similar. In essence, the quality of analgesia with either lumbar or thoracic epidural catheters is excellent for patients recovering from CABG surgery. The mode and site of analgesic action of epidural buprenorphine was studied in human gastrectomy patients by Inagaki et al.[87] Their study found that epidural buprenorphine produces segmental spinal analgesia; however; a significant portion of the dose is rapidly absorbed into the systemic circulation, resulting in supraspinal analgesic effects equivalent to intravenous doses.

CONCLUSION

In the years that have followed publication of our first pain textbook[88] application of neuraxial opioid analgesia has changed dramatically. These techniques have been refined to the point that they offer improved safety while providing highly efficient opioid dosing and superior reductions in pain intensity. When initiated preincisionally and maintained for several days, continuous epidural infusions and epidural-PCA have the potential to significantly reduce or prevent pain perception. The technique is associated with analgesic gaps, particularly related to catheter malpositioning, dislodgement, and infusion device malfunction. The effectiveness of neuraxial analgesia provided by low infusate concentrations of morphine and hydromorphone is critically dependent on an optimally placed catheter, whereas more lipophilic opioids may continue to provide adequate supraspinal analgesia if the catheter is dislodged from the epidural space.

Despite well-documented advantages, the role of neuraxial analgesia for acute pain management has declined since the the late 1990s and its future is uncertain. Reasons responsible for this decline are varied; however, the move toward less invasive and laparoscopic procedures, the increased use of low-molecular-weight heparinoids, the increasing availability, and the potentially greater safety of peripheral neural blockade have had a significant negative impact. In addition, the release of prolonged duration epidural morphine (DepoDur) has displaced the need for indwelling catheters and continuous epidural infusions. Refer to Chapter 20, *Novel Analgesic Delivery Systems*. At our institution and many others, the risk to benefit ratio of continuous epidural infusions can no longer be justified for less painful procedures such as caesarean section and hysterectomy in relatively healthy patients. In these settings, we continue to employ single-dose intrathecal morphine for postoperative pain. Continuous epidural infusions of opioid plus local anesthetic remains the "state of the art" pain management technique, and therapy of choice for high-risk patients and those recovering from invasive and extremely painful surgeries. Infusions of hydromorphone and dilute local anesthetic have been embraced at our institution and many others because of the spinal potency gain, analgesic efficacy and patient safety such therapy provides. It remains unclear whether epidural administration of novel analgesics such as buprenophine offer measurable clinical advantages that would encourage future use.

APPENDIX

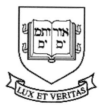

Yale Pain Management Service Epidural PCA Orders and Patient Management Guidelines

1 Patients admitted to the Yale Pain Service must have a CCSS (or other electronic order set) generated surgical or medical

"request for consultation" form inserted into the medical record.

2   Standardization of orders and documentation follow-up is essential for delivery of safe and effective pain control. *Orders* are pre-written on the CCSS system under Dept Orders, pain management adults. Screens which follow provide standardized orders for IV PCA, continuous regional blockade, continuous epidural and PCEA, and single dose epidural. Orders for medication, adjunctive agents, and monitoring must be activated for each patient admitted to the Service.

3   Pain service orders are discontinued when the patient is referred back to the primary care team. The pain service will recommend analgesics and doses for continued in-patient management and for patient discharge, however, the primary caregiver is responsible for all prescriptions.

4   In addition to catheters placed for postoperative analgesia, the trauma team may request a "stat" epidural for pain control and to improve pulmonary function. These after hours requests are rarely a true emergency and can often be postphoned until the morning team arrives. Epidural insertion should always be delayed in settings of ill defined fever, impaired coagulation, r/o cervical injury, and inability to obtain informed consent.

Patient Management: Epidural Patient-Controlled Analgesia, (EPI-PCA)

Epidural patient-controlled analgesia involves placement of an epidural catheter, administration of an analgesic loading dose (opioids, local anesthetic, or both), and initiation of patient-activated epidural boluses in combination with a continuous epidural infusion. Thoracic epidurals improve analgesic specificity for upper abdominal and thoracic procedures (improve pain relief and reduce dose requirement). Ideally, the catheter tip should be placed at epidural segments immediately adjacent to the injury/surgical site (i.e. T5–7 for thoracotomy incision, L3–4 for lower extremity procedures).

Patients receiving Epi-PCA are "loaded" with 2–5 mg of epidural morphine or 0.5–1.5 mg hydromorphone +/ − variable doses of local anesthetic in the operating room. The size of the loading dose is influenced by patient age, extent of surgery, and location of the catheter. In extremely prolonged surgeries, an additional bolus of hydromorphone (25–50% of loading dose) may be given 6 hours into the procedure. Thereafter, an epidural infusion is started either in the OR or upon arrival in the PACU. The infusate is contained in 500-ml bags and is administered by a dedicated infusion pump. Five hundred ml epidural solution bags are prepared by the department of pharmacy services and refrigerated at 40 degrees F. to maintain sterility and stability. Infusate bags contain either hydromorphone 10–20 μg/ml or hydromorphone 10–20 μg/ml plus bupivacaine 0.15–0.031%. The plain hydromorphone solution is recommended for all patients who are hypovolemic or at risk for hypovolemia, and for Gyn oncology patients (surgeons request). After patients are awake and alert they are given the PCA button and allowed to self-administer hydromorphone every 6–8 minutes as needed.

Duration of therapy: Functional epidural catheters are maintained for 24–48 hours in patients recovering from pelvic and lower extremity procedures, 48 hours following thoracotomy, and 48–72 hours following upper abdominal surgeries. Epidural catheters and site of insertion are inspected daily on morning rounds. Exceptional situations requiring early discontinuation of therapy include the following: 1. inadequate pain control, 2. intractable side effects, 3. initiation of low molecular wt heparin, 4. 12-hours after initiation of Coumadin, 5. Sustained high fever/sepsis. Clinically significant hypovolemia/hypotension does not necessarily mandate discontinuation of therapy, however local anesthetic should be removed from the epidural infusate. Bupivacaine should also be discontinued in setting where the patient complains of excessive sensory motor blockade. Discontinuance of therapy requires that the pain resident/nurse carefully remove the catheter and document this process in the medical record. The resident is instructed never to pull a "stuck" catheter as this increases risks of neural injury or a piece breaking and remaining at the site. With attending assistance the stuck catheter can often be removed by flexing and extending the patients back and carefully pulling on the catheter.

When the epidural infusion is discontinued, the resident must return the pump, electrical cord, and the PCEA button to the shelf in the Anesthesiology workroom. These pumps are expected to be replaced in the condition that they were found (i.e.: placed on the shelf with the electrical cord + PCEA button carefully stored in the locked solution containment box).

Inadequate Pain Control: Inadequate analgesia may be the result of catheter related problems, undermedication (lack of, or a suboptimal hydromorphone loading dose), and patient related variability (anatomy, disease, high grade opioid dependence). If patients complain of severe discomfort (VAS 7 or greater) the resident/attending team must first rule out catheter dislodgment by assessing the site and testing its function with dilute local anesthetic (5–10 ml 1% lidocaine). Following a negative test (lack of sensory block to temperature or pinprick) the catheter is promptly repositioned or replaced. With evidence of catheter functionality, an 8–12 ml (80–120 μg) hydromorphone bolus dose followed by an increase in epidural infusion rate generally improves patient comfort within 10–15 minutes. In patients presenting with chronic opioid dependence, effective interventions include switching to a more concentrated infusion of hydromorphone (20–40 μg/ml), increasing the rate of epidural infusion, supplementation with chronic pain medications, or co-administration of parenteral opioids (IV boluses of morphine or IV-PCA).

Treatment of Respiratory Depression and Other Adverse Effects

Epidural infusions of hydromorphone are associated with less sedation, nausea, and pruritus than morphine however, these side effects may occur in 10–20% of patients. Delayed respiratory depression is also less likely, however, close attention to dose must be made in high risk settings (patients greater than 70 years, history of severe COPD, history of sleep apnea, and morbid obesity). These patient are best recovered in the ICU or floors that can provide continuous oxygen saturation monitoring. Clinically significant respiratory depression is highly unlikely in opioid tolerant patients. As a general rule, adverse effects/events are dose dependent, therefore, in patients experiencing effective pain control your first and often best option to reduce their incidence or severity is to reduce the epidural infusion rate by 33% to 50%. Reductions in epidural bolus dose may also be considered. Prophylactic treatment should also be considered including: initiation of a IV-naloxone infusion to minimize sedation/respiratory depression in high risk patient populations); Intraoperative and post-surgical "by the clock" doses of ondansetron in patients at high risk for nausea and vomiting.

Hourly monitoring of respiratory rate and level of sedation are utilized to detect respiratory compromise. Oxygen saturation and respiratory rate should be monitored continuously in these patients, and arterial Pco$_2$ closely followed. Excessive doses of benzodiazepines and benadryl are restricted in elderly patients in order to avoid sedation, confusion, and airway obstruction. Patients with optimal levels of spinal opioid analgesia will almost always maintain an elevated Pco$_2$ (40–44 mmHg). Further increases in sedation and Pco$_2$ are corrected either by reducing the hydromorphone infusion rate or by initiating a low dose intravenous infusion of naloxone. The addition of naloxone (1 amp, 400 µg) to the patient's IV bag running at a rate of 100–125 ml/hr will reverse sedative and mild respiratory depressive effects of neuraxially administered opioids, while not antagonizing analgesia. Patients experiencing more profound depression, should receive naloxone boluses 100–200 µg titrated to effect, followed by an infusion. In the most severe cases (1 per 1,000 patients) patients will require airway management and ventilatory support to correct the CNS depressive effects of hypercarbia/respiratory acidosis. If severe respiratory depression/arrest should occur, please have the resident draw a plasma sample for toxicity screen and secure the epidural-PCA pump (do not remove the infusate bag or unplug the device, as important history will be lost).

Nausea following visceral surgery may be controlled with metoclopramide (10 mg) while droperidol (0.125 mg) is recommended following non-abdominal surgery. Not all episodes of N&V are related to neuroaxial opioids, the resident should always rule out (and correct) surgical related factors such as hypotension, hypovolemia, raised ICP, blocked NG tube etc. Severe opioid mediated nausea must be treated aggressively. Ondansetron (2–4 mg) should be administered promptly to patients complaining of nausea unresponsive to treatment with first line agents.

Moderate to severe pruritus is a common and often quite annoying adverse effect observed with neuraxially administered opioids. Avoid administering Benadryl, as the itching generally does not respond to antihistaminics, and its CNS depressive effects may result in profound sedation. Naloxone infusions (20–50 µg/hr) are recommended and effectively control cases of mild to moderate pruritus. Severe pruritus often requires 1–2 boluses of naloxone (100 µg), followed by a higher concentration infusion (up to 100 µg/hr). Boluses of propofol 10 mg/hr are effective and may be employed for patients recovering in the ICU. In unresponsive cases, consider switching to epidural fentanyl (5 µg/ml plus bupivacaine 0.031%, at rates of infusion employed with hydromorphone) or discontinuing therapy and converting to IV-PCA. The former is recommended during the first 24 hrs, particularly for high-risk patients recovering from painful procedures.

Yale Pain Management Service Epidural Patient Controlled Analgesia (EPCA) Order Set

1 Patient has an epidural catheter for postoperative pain control and will be managed by the Anesthesiology Pain management service Beeper 128-3154
2 Catheter is placed at ___ interspace.

3 Please check the insertion site per shift. Notify the pain service if any of the following is observed (Leaking of infusate, redness, bleeding, pain at insertion site)
4 Epidural Analgesic Solution:
   Hydromorphone ___ µg/ml plus bupivacaine ___ %
   Hydromorphone ___ µg/ml plus ropivacaine ___ %
   Hydromorphone ___ µg/ml
   Fentanyl ___ µg/ml plus bupivacaine ___ %
5 Epidural Continuous Infusion rate ___ ml/hr
6 Epidural Bolus dose ___ ml, per ___ min
7 Four hour dose limit ___ ml
8 Adjunctive analgesia: Ketorolac ___ mg, (IV), q ___ hrs
   Celecoxib ___ mg, (PO), q ___ hrs
9 Treatment of Adverse Events:
   ___ (Pruritus) Naloxone infusion (400 µg/liter, infuse at ___ ml/hr
   ___ (Nausea) Ondansetron ___ mg, ___ hrs
   ___ (Nausea) Droperidol ___ mg, ___ hrs
   ___ (Respiratory Depression) Naloxone ___ µg
10 Notify The Anesthesiology pain service if the patient has a respiratory rate of 10 or less, oxygen saturation 90% or less. Is troubled by pain intensity greater than 5, or is troubled by nausea, vomiting and pruritus unresponsive to standard therapy.

REFERENCES

1. Kemper PM, Treiber H. Neuraxial morphine plus PCA-a new method in post-cesarean analgesia. *Analg Anesth.* 1990;70:S198.
2. Cousins MJ, Cherry DA, Gourlay GK. Acute and chronic pain: Use of spinal opioids. In: Cousins MJ, Bridenbaugh PO, ed. *Neural Blockade in Clinical Anesthesia and Management of Pain.* 2nd ed. Philadelphia, PA: JB Lippincott; 1988:993–996.
3. Negre I, Gueneron JP, Jamali SJ, et al. Preoperative analgesia with epidural morphine. *Anesth Analg.* 1994;79:298–302.
4. Sinatra RS. Unpublished observations, Yale University Acute Pain and Obstetrical Anesthesiology Services; 2007.
5. Sinatra RS, Dabu-Bondoc S. Unpublished data, Yale University Acute Pain and Obstetrical Anesthesiology Services; 2007.
6. Sites BD, Beach M, Biggs R, et al. Intrathecal clonidine added to a bupivacaine-morphine spinal anesthetic improves postoperative analgesia for a total knee arthroplasty. *Anesth Analg.* 2003;96(4):1083.
7. Abram SE, Mampilly GA, Milosavljevic D. Assessment of the potency and intrinsic activity of systemic versus intrathecal opioids in rats. *Anesthesiology.* 1997;87:127–134.
8. Drakeford MK, Pettine KA, Brookshire L, Ebert F. Spinal narcotics for postoperative analgesia in total joint arthroplasty: a prospective study. *J Bone Joint Surg Am.* 1991;73:424–428.
9. Rathmell JP, Lair TR, Nauman B. The role of intrathecal drugs in the treatment of acute pain. *Anesth Analg.* 2005;101(suppl 5):30–43.
10. Harrison DM, Sinatra R, Morgese L. Epidural narcotic and patient controlled analgesia for post-cesarean section pain relief. *Anesthesiology.* 1988;68:454–457.
11. Loper KA, Ready LB. Epidural morphine after anterior cruciate ligament repair: a comparison with PCA morphine. *Anesth Analg.* 1989;68:350–352.
12. Shulman M, Sandler An, Bradley JW, et al. Post-thoracotomy pain and pulmonary function following epidural and systemic morphine. *Anesthesiology.* 1984;61:569–575.

13. Ready LB, Chadwick HS, Ross B. Age predicts effective epidural morphine dose after abdominal hysterectomy. *Anesth Analg.* 1987;66:1215–1218.

14. Anzai Y, Nishikawa T. Thoracic epidural clonidine and morphine for postoperative pain relief. *Can.J.Anaesth.* 1995;42(4):292–297.

15. Rockemann MG, Seeling W, Brinkmann A, et al. Analgesic and hemodynamic effects of epidural clonidine, clonidine/morphine, and morphine after pancreatic surgery – a double-blind study. *Anesth Analg.* 1995;80(5):869–874.

16. Rostaing S, Bonnet F, Levron JC, Vodinh J, Pluskwa F, Saada M. Effect of epidural clonidine on analgesia and pharmacokinetics of epidural fentanyl in postoperative patients. *Anesthesiology.* 1991;75(3):420–425.

17. Reisine T, Pasternak G. Opioid analgesics and antagonists. In: Goodman LS and Gilman A, ed. *The Pharmacologic Basis of Therapeutics.* 9th ed. New York: Macmillan; 1997.

18. Rapp SE, Ross BK, Wild LM, et al. A multidimensional comparison of morphine and hydromorphone patient-controlled analgesia. *Anesth Analg.* 1996;82(5):1043–1048.

19. Coda BA, Tanaka A, Jacobson RC. Hydromorphone analgesia after intravenous bolus administration. *Pain.* 1997;71:41–48.

20. Bromage PR, Camporesi E, Chestnut D. Epidural narcotics for postoperative analgesia. *Anesth Analg.* 1980;59:473–480.

21. Chestnut DH, Choi WW, Isbell TJ. Epidural hydromorphone for postcesarean analgesia. *Obstet Gynecol.* 1986;68(1):65–69.

22. Henderson SK, Matthew EB, Cohen H, et al. Epidural hydromorphone: A double blind comparison with intramuscular hydromorphone for postcesarean section analgesia. *Anesthesiology.* 1987;66:825–830.

23. Halpern SH, Arellano R, Preston R, et al. Epidural morphine versus hydromorphone in post-caesarean section patients. *Can J Anaesth.* 1996;43(6):595–598.

24. Dougherty TB, Baysinger CL, Heneberger JC, Gooding DJ. Epidural hydromorphone with and without epinephrine for post-operative analgesia after cesarean delivery. *Anesth Analg.* 1989;68:318–322.

25. Chaplan SR, Duncan SR, Brodsky JB, Brose WG. Morphine and hydromorphone epidural analgesia: a prospective, randomized comparison. *Anesthesiology.* 1992;77:1090–1094.

26. El-Baz NM, Faber LP, Jensik RJ. Continuous epidural infusion of morphine for treatment of pain after thoracic surgery: a new technique. *Anesth Analg.* 1984;63(8):757–764.

27. Bailey PW, Smith BE. Continued epidural infusion of fentanyl for postoperative analgesia. *Anesthesia.* 1980;35:1002–1006.

28. Welchew EA, Thornton JA. Continuous thoracic epidural fentanyl. *Anaesthesia.* 1982;37:309–316.

29. Salomaki TE, Laitinen JO, Vainionpaa V, Nuutinen LS. 0.1% bupivacaine does not reduce the requirement for epidural fentanyl infusion after major abdominal surgery. *Reg Anesth.* 1995;20(5):435–443.

30. Berti M, Fanelli G, Casati A, Lugani D, Aldegheri G, Torri G. Comparison between epidural infusion of fentanyl/bupivacaine and morphine/bupivacaine after orthopaedic surgery. *Can J Anaesth.* 1998;45(6):545–550.

31. Silvasti M, Pitkanen M. Continuous epidural analgesia with bupivacaine-fentanyl versus patient-controlled analgesia with i.v. morphine for postoperative pain relief after knee ligament surgery. *Acta Anaesthesiol Scand.* 2000;44(1):37–42.

32. Sjostrom S, Blass J. Postoperative analgesia with epidural bupivacaine and low-dose fentanyl–a comparison of two concentrations. *Acta Anaesthesiol Scand.* 1998;42(7):776–782.

33. Doi K, Yamanaka M, Shono A, Fukuda N, Saito Y. Preoperative epidural fentanyl reduces postoperative pain after upper abdominal surgery. *J Anesth.* 2007;21(3):439–441.

34. Birnbach DJ, Arcurio T, Johnson MD, et al. Effect of diluent volume on analgesia produced by epidural fentanyl. *Anesth Analg.* 1988;60:13–14.

35. Hjortso NC, Lund C, Mogensen T, et al. Epidural morphine improves pain relief and maintains sensory analgesia during continuous epidural bupivacaine after abdominal surgery. *Anesth Analg.* 1986;65:1033–1036.

36. Dahl JB, Rosenberg J, Hansen BL, et al. Differential analgesic effects of low-dose epidural morphine and morphine-bupivacaine at rest and during mobilization after major abdominal surgery. *Anesth Analg.* 1992;74:362–365.

37. Rawal N, Holmstrom B, Crowhurst JA, Van Zundert A. The combined spinal-epidural technique. *Anesthesiol Clin N Am.* 2000;18:267–295.

38. Rawal N, Schollin J, Wesström G. Epidural versus combined spinal epidural block for caesarean section. *Acta Anaesthesiol Scand* 1988;32:61–66.

39. Holmstrom B, Laugaland K, Rawal N, Hallberg S. Combined spinal epidural block versus spinal and epidural block for orthopaedic surgery. *Can J Anaesth.* 1993;40(7):601–606.

40. Cazeneuve JF, Berlemont D, Pouilly A. Value of combined spinal and epidural anesthesia in the management of peroperative analgesia in prosthetic surgery of the lower limb: prospective study of 68 cases. *Rev Chir Orthop Reparatrice Appar Mot.* 1996;82(8):705–708.

41. Stamenkovic D, Geric V, Slavkovic Z, Raskovic J, Djordjevic M. Combined spinal-epidural analgesia vs. Intermittent bolus epidural analgesia for pain relief after major abdominal surgery: a prospective, randomized, double-blind clinical trial. *Int J Clin Pract.* 2007.

42. Teoh WH, Thomas E, Tan HM. Ultra-low dose combined spinal-epidural anesthesia with intrathecal bupivacaine 3.75 mg for cesarean delivery: a randomized controlled trial. *Int J Obstet Anesth.* 2006;15(4):273–278.

43. Brodsky JB, Chaplan SR, Brose WG, Mark JBD. Continuous epidural hydromorphone for postthoracotomy pain relief. *Ann Thorac Surg.* 1990;50:888–893.

44. Sinatra RS, Levin S, Ocampo CA. Neuroaxial hydromorphone for control of postsurgical, obstetric, and chronic pain. *Semin Anesth Periop Med Pain.* 2000;19:108–131.

45. Brose WG, Tanelian DL, Brodsky JB, et al. CSF and blood pharmacokinetics of hydromorphone and morphine following lumbar epidural administration. *Pain.* 1991;45:11–15.

46. White P. Use of patient-controlled analgesia for management of acute pain. *JAMA.* 1998;259:243–247.

47. Wamsley PNH. Patient-controlled epidural analgesia. In: Sinatra RS, Hord AH, Ginsberg B, Preble LM, ed. *Acute Pain Mechanisms and Management.* St Louis: Mosby; 1992.

48. Wamsley PNH, McDonnell FJ, Colclough GW, et al. A comparison of epidural and intravenous PCA after gynecological surgery. *Anesthesiology.* 1990;73:A1268.

49. Grant R, Dolman J, Harper J, et al. Patient controlled lumbar epidural fentanyl compared with patient controlled intravenous fentanyl for post-thoracotomy pain. *Can J Anaesth.* 1992;39:214–219.

50. Hodgson PS, Liu SS. A comparison of ropivacaine with fentanyl to bupivacaine with fentanyl for postoperative patient-controlled epidural analgesia. *Anesth Analg.* 2001;92(4):1024–1028.

51. Kostamovaara PA, Laurila JJ, Alahuhta S, Salomaki TE. Ropivacaine 1 mg x ml(-1) does not decrease the need for epidural

fentanyl after hip replacement surgery. *Acta Anaesthesiol Scand.* 2001;45(4):489–494.

52. Silvasti M, Pitkanen M. Patient-controlled epidural analgesia versus continuous epidural analgesia after total knee arthroplasty. *Acta Anaesthesiol Scand.* 2001;45(4):471–476.

53. Liu SS, Allen HW, Olsson GL. Patient-controlled epidural analgesia with bupivacaine and fentanyl on hospital wards: prospective experience with 1,030 surgical patients. *Anesthesiology.* 1998;88(3):688–695.

54. Ishiyama T, Iijima T, Sugawara T, et al. The use of patient-controlled epidural fentanyl in elderly patients. *Anaesthesia.* 2007;62(12):1246–1250.

55. Buvanendran A, Kroin JS, Tuman KJ, et al. Effects of perioperative administration of a Cox-2 inhibitor on pain management and return to functionality after knee replacement surgery. *JAMA.* 2003; 290:2411–2418.

56. Parker RK, White PF. Epidural patient-controlled analgesia: an alternative to intravenous patient-controlled analgesia for pain relief after cesarean delivery. *Anesth Analg.* 1992;75:245–251.

57. Liu S, Carpenter RL, Mulroy MF, et al. Intravenous versus epidural administration of hydromorphone. *Anesthesiology.* 1995;82:682–688.

58. Bromage PR, Camporesi EM, Durant PAC, et al. Non-respiratory side effects of epidural morphine. *Anesth Analg.* 1982;61:490–495.

59. Kafer ER, Brown J, Scott D, et al. Biphasic depression of ventilatory responses to CO2 following epidural morphine. *Anesthesiology.* 1983;58:418–427.

60. Johnson A. Influence of intrathecal morphine and naloxone intervention on postoperative ventilatory regulation in elderly patients. *Acta Anaesthesiol Scand.* 1992;36:436–444.

61. Rawal N, Schott U, Dahlstrom B, et al. Influence of naloxone infusion on analgesia and respiratory depression following epidural morphine. *Anesthesiology.* 1986;64(2):194–201.

62. Rawal N. Nonnociceptive effects of intraspinal opioids and their clinical applications. *Int Anesthesiol Clin.* 1986;24(2):75–91.

63. Borgeat A, Saiah M, Wildersmith O, et al. Subhypnotic doses of propofol relieves pruritus induced by epidural and intrathecal morphine. *Anesthesiology.* 1992;76:510–512.

64. Tramer MR, Reynolds DJ, Moore RA, McQuay HJ. Efficacy, dose-response, and safety of ondansetron in prevention of postoperative nausea and vomiting: a quantitative systematic review of randomized placebo-controlled trials. *Anesthesiology.* 1997;87(6):1277–1289.

65. Millo J, Siddons M, Innes R, Laurie PS. Randomised double-blind comparison of ondansetron and droperidol to prevent postoperative nausea and vomiting associated with patient-controlled analgesia. *Anaesthesia.* 2001;56(1):60–65.

66. Yazigi A, Chalhoub V, Madi-Jebara S, Haddad F, Hayek G. Prophylactic ondansetron is effective in the treatment of nausea and vomiting but not on pruritus after cesarean delivery with intrathecal sufentanil-morphine. *J Clin Anesth.* 2002;14(3):183–186.

67. Kotelko DM, Rottman RL, Wright WC, et al. Transdermal scopolamine decreases nausea and vomiting following cesarean section in patients receiving epidural morphine. *Anesthesiology.* 1989;71:675–679.

68. Rawal N, Mollefors K, Axelsson K, et al. An experimental study of urodynamic effects of epidural morphine and naloxone reversal. *Anesth Analg.* 1984;62:641–647.

69. Sinatra RS, Eige S, Chung JH, et al. Continuous epidural infusion of 0.05% bupivacaine plus hydromorphone for labor analgesia:

an observational assessment in 1830 parturients. *Anesth Analg.* 2002;94(5):1310–1311, table of contents.

70. Liu S, Angel JM, Owens BD, Carpenter RL, Isabel L. Effects of epidural bupivacaine after thoracotomy. *Reg Anesth.* 1995;20(4):303–310.

71. Parker RK, Sawaki Y, White PF. Epidural patient-controlled analgesia: influence of bupivacaine and hydromorphone basal infusion on pain control after cesarean delivery. *Anesth Analg.* 1992;75(5):740–746.

72. Singh H, Bossard RF, White PF. Epidural PCA: effect of ketorolac vs. bupivacaine coadministration during patient-controlled hydromorphone epidural analgesia after thoracotomy. *Anesth Analg.* 1997;84:564–569.

73. Ayoub C, Sinatra RS. Postoperative analgesia: epidural and spinal techniques. In: Chestnut DH, ed. *Obstetric Anesthesia: Principles and Practice.* Vol. III. St Louis: Mosby; 2004.

74. Brown D, O'Neill O, Beck A. Post-operative pain management: transition from epidural to oral analgesia. *Nurs Stand.* 2007;21(21):35–40.

75. Sevarino FB, Welchek-Pizarro C, Sinatra RS. Sterility of epidural solutions recommendations for cost-effective use. *Reg Anesth Pain Med.* 2000;25(4):368–371.

76. Christen C. Johnson CE, Walters JJR. Stability of bupivacaine hydrochloride and hydromorphone hydrochloride during simulated epidural coadministration. *Health Syst Pharm.* 1996;53(2):170–173.

77. Ready LB, Loper KA, Nessly M, Wild L. Postoperative morphine is safe on surgical wards. *Anesthesiology.* 1991;75:452–456.

78. Ready LB, Oden R, Chadwick HS, et al. Development of an anesthesiology-based postoperative pain management service. *Anesthesiology.* 1988;68:100–106.

79. Molke JF, Jensen NH, Holk IK, Revenborg N. Prolonged and biphasic respiratory depression following epidural buprenorphine. *Anaesthesia.* 1987;42:470–475.

80. Murphy DF MM. Pain relief after epidural buprenorphine after spinal fusion: a comparison with intramuscular morphine. *Acta Anaesthesiol Scand.* 1984;28:144–146.

81. Miwa Y, Yonemura E, Fukushima K. Epidural administered buprenorphine in the perioperative period. *Can J Anaesth.* 1996;43(9):907–913.

82. Giebler RM, Scherer RU, Peters J. Incidence of neurologic complications related to thoracic epidural catheterization. *Anesthesiology.* 1997;86(1):55–63.

83. Govindarajan R, Bakalova T, Michael R, Abadir AR. Epidural buprenorphine in management of pain in multiple rib fractures. *Acta Anaesthesiol Scand.* 2002;46(6):660–665.

84. Daghfous M, Nafaa N, Abderrahim N, et al. Analgesia in thoracic injuries: a comparative study of 2 techniques of loco-regional analgesia. *Tunis Med.* 1998;76(2):1047–1051.

85. Kariya N, Oda Y, Yukioka H, Fujimori M. Effective treatment of a man with head injury and multiple rib fractures with epidural analgesia. *Masui.* 1996;45(2):223–226.

86. Mehta Y, Juneja R, Madhok H, Trehan N. Lumbar versus thoracic epidural buprenorphine for postoperative analgesia following coronary artery bypass graft surgery. *Acta Anaesthesiol Scand.* 1999;43(4):388–393.

87. Inagaki Y, Mashimo T, Yoshiya I. Mode and site of analgesic action of epidural buprenorphine in humans. *Anesth Analg.* 1996;83(3):530–536.

88. Sinatra RS, Hord AH, Ginsberg B, Preble LM. *Acute Pain Mechanisms and Management.* St Louis: Mosby; 1992.

17

Regional Anesthesia

James Benonis, Jennifer Fortney, David Hardman, and
Gavin Martin

Surgery of the upper and lower limbs presents anesthesiologists with an alternative to general anesthesia, that being regional anesthesia. Even if we do not utilize a regional technique for anesthesia we certainly can do so for postoperative analgesia. For years neuroaxial techniques were used as the sole regional anesthetic of choice for the lower limb. The advent of low-molecular-weight heparins (eg, enoxaparin, fondaparinux) and the potential risk for the development of epidural hematomas has severely limited their use and led to a much higher use of peripheral nerve blocks in everyday practice. Since the mid-2000s, great improvements have been made in the equipment used to perform peripheral nerve blocks, including stimulating peripheral nerve catheters and the use of ultrasound to identify nerves.[1]

In addition, recent literature has shown a growing body of evidence supporting the benefit of regional anesthesia versus general anesthesia with respect to mortality, morbidity, postoperative analgesia, and functional recovery. In a metaanalysis study, Rodgers et al[2] showed a reduction in mortality of 33%. They also showed a significant decrease in the incidence of myocardial ischemic events, respiratory depression, rate of deep vein thrombosis (DVT) formation, and blood loss. Adequate pain management following surgery using a multimodal technique, including the use of cycloxygenase-2 inhibitors (COX-2 inhibitors), pregabalin or gabapentin, and peripheral nerve blocks, plays an important role in the management of acute postoperative pain and possibly the prevention of subsequent chronic pain syndromes.[3,4] The development of chronic pain syndromes following surgery may be correlated to the severity of acute pain in the postoperative period.

In this chapter, we will describe the commonly used peripheral nerve blocks that can be performed for some of the more common upper and lower limb surgery. This chapter will include new developments in this fast growing area of regional anesthesia and describe how we perform these blocks in our every day practice.

MULTIMODAL ANALGESIA

Pain management has made great strides with regards to post-operative pain management but many patients fail to receive this basic requirement.[5] Classically, physician often bases their perioperative pain management plan on the use of a single agent, usually an opioid. The evidence is clear that a multimodal approach to pain management is beneficial to our patient.[6,7] The benefits are derived from the fact that using multiple agents blocks the pain pathways at different sites and that the effects of these agents are not only additive but often synergistic. This allows the use of lower doses of analgesics and thus reduces the dose-dependent side effects of the agents used. At our institution, we commonly use celecoxib (400 mg) on the day of surgery followed postoperatively (200 mg twice daily), unless its use is contraindicated because of a sulfur allergy or cardiovascular and renal comorbidities. All COX-2 inhibitors were tainted with the rofecoxib scandal, which showed increased incidence in myocardial events leading to death in long-term high-dose studies.[8,9] Celecoxib is the only remaining COX-2 on the market. Studies looking at the effect of all nonsteroidal anti-inflammatory drugs (NSAIDs) have shown this drug to be no worse than other NSAIDS such as ibuprofen with regard to myocardial events.[10] However, this drug should be used with caution in any patient with significant cardiovascular risk factors or renal insufficiency. The role of COX-2 inhibitors with regard to the inhibition of bone healing following fractures or orthopedic surgery is inconclusive, with a few animal and human studies showing a deleterious effect.[11] What appears to be the current feeling with regard to this issue is that short-term use of COX-2 inhibitors may reduce the rate of bone healing, but the rate of bone growth returns to normal very shortly after stopping the COX-2 inhibitors.[12] Gabapentin, a commonly used antiepileptic, has been found to also have analgesic properties following acute as well as chronic pain and is commonly used in the perioperative setting in doses ranging between 400 and 1200 mg daily.[13–15] The limiting factor for gabapentin use is that its absorption from the gastrointestinal tract involves an active transport system and this process is saturable limiting absorption of higher doses. Pregabalin has properties similar to gabapentin with both drugs blocking the α_2-δ subunits of the calcium channel. However, within clinically useful doses pregabalin has linear kinetics: the more administered, the higher the plasma concentration. A study looking at opioid usage after spinal fusion surgery showed that pregabalin had a synergistic effect when combined with celecoxib in reducing opioid requirements by about 60%.[16] We commonly prescribe 150 mg pregabalin on the day of surgery, followed by 75 mg twice daily for 3 days postoperatively. This dose is adjusted depending on the age of the patient and renal function. The main adverse effects are oversedation and dizziness, with both side effects having a higher incidence in the elderly.

In addition to the combination of an NSAID and anticonvulsant, we often perform a peripheral nerve block and if possible use an indwelling nerve catheter that remains in place for 2–3 days postoperatively to extend the beneficial effect of the nerve block. Single-shot nerve blocks tend to wear off late at night and because the patients at this stage may have no opioids within their system this leads to a period of severe pain, normally when the physicians are not present in the hospital. The presence of peripheral nerve block catheters and a continuous infusion of local anesthetics avoid this problem.

ANTICOAGULATION AND THE MANAGEMENT OF PERIPHERAL NERVE CATHETERS

Deep vein thrombosis (DVT) poses a serious threat to patients undergoing orthopedic procedures. A multitude of anticoagulant techniques are used, often dictated by the preference of the orthopedic surgeon, with no uniform evidence-based criteria to optimize DVT prophylaxis. There are no definitive studies attesting to whether coumadin is superior to low-molecular-weight heparin (LMWH) or vice versa.[17–19] In the study by Freedman et al,[17] the risk of proximal DVT was lowest with coumadin (6.3%) when compared to LMWH (7.7%), but there was no difference in the incidence of PEs and mortality. Miric et al[18] found that LMWH was better than coumadin in preventing DVTs in total hip replacements: 4% versus 12%, respectively. What is clear is that the use of unfractionated heparin does not offer enough DVT prophylaxis to patients undergoing joint replacement procedures and that, when LMWH is compared to coumadin, there is increased incidence of minor and major wound blood loss.[17,20]

The latest recommendations from The Seventh American College of Chest Physicians Consensus Conference advise that only coumadin, fondaparinux, and LMWH are adequate forms of DVT prophylaxis when used alone for hip or knee replacement surgery.[21] Pharmacological agents should always be combined with mechanical prophylaxis, which should begin intraoperatively, if possible. Mechanical prophylaxis, however, should be used alone only when there is a significant risk of bleeding. The use of newer anticoagulants, in particular LMWH, has resulted in anesthesiologists having to modify their anesthetic plan. Vandermeulen demonstrated a significant increase in the incidence of epidural hematomas when epidural anesthesia/analgesia is used in conjunction with LMWH.[22] This resulted in the Food and Drug Administration adding a black box warning to limit the use of LMWH in patients with an epidural.[23] Guidelines have been developed by the American Society of Regional Anesthesia (ASRA) for the use of regional techniques in the presence of a variety of anticoagulants.[24] These guidelines are for neuraxial techniques but have been extrapolated for the use of peripheral nerve blocks. It is important to remember that these are guidelines and that when deciding on performing a regional peripheral nerve block in the presence of a potential coagulation issues the clinician needs to balance the risk of regional technique versus the risk imposed by a general anesthetic. Based on the guidelines, a peripheral nerve block should not be performed on a patient with suspected coagulation problems. A peripheral nerve block should not be performed within 12 hours of the last dose of LMWH if a standard prophylactic dose (LMWH 40 mg) is used. With higher doses such as 1 mg/kg a period greater than 24 hours should have passed prior to nerve block placement. Nerve catheters if placed can be used in the presence of LMWH but should be removed 2 hours prior to next dose of LMWH. The ASRA guidelines for patients receiving platelet inhibitors suggest that clopidogrel should be stopped for 7 days prior to a major nerve block, whereas ticlopeidine would delay the placement for 10 days. Other NSAIDs and aspirin can be safely used in the presence of nerve blocks.

LOGISTICS AND EQUIPMENT NEEDED FOR THE PERFORMANCE OF REGIONAL ANESTHESIA

To perform these peripheral nerve blocks with a high degree of efficiency and safety, it is important to have the right equipment. A preoperative block area with full monitoring and resuscitation equipment is needed, as this will allow the placement of blocks prior to the start of surgery. Complications some of them being life-threatening may follow the initiation of regional techniques, thus mandating the availability of the resuscitative equipment. Recent data suggest 20% intralipid may be of benefit during resuscitation of a cardiovascular events following the inadvertent intravascular injection of higher doses, suggesting that it should be readily available.[25,26] The presence of a block resident in preoperative area can help with maintaining turnover and at the same time can lead to improved training of the residents.[27]

The following list represents the equipment and drugs required to perform peripheral nerve blocks:

- insulated stimulating needles (1, 2, 4, and 6 inches long)
- stimulating and nonstimulating peripheral nerve block catheters
- infusion pumps
- ultrasound machines with software specifically for regional anesthesia
- sterile sheaths for ultrasound probes
- peripheral nerve block stimulators
- long-acting local anesthetics
  ropivacaine (0.5% or 0.75%)
  bupivacaine (0.5%)
  for postoperative analgesia
    ropivacaine (0.1% or 0.2%)
    bupivacaine (0.125% or 0.25%)
- short-acting local anesthetics
  mepivacaine (1.5%)
  lidocaine (2%)

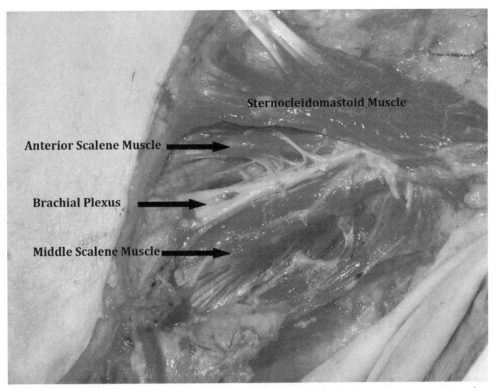

Figure 17.1: Anatomical dissection demonstrating the brachial plexus within the interscalene groove. See color plates.

for post operative analgesia only:
  mepivacaine (0.75%)
  lidocaine (1%)
  Epinephrine to make 1/400 000 solution
- sterristrips, benzoin tincture and tagederm for securing of nerve block catheters
- marker pens for landmarks
- resuscitative drugs
  - midazolam for sedation and management of seizures
  - intralipid: may be of benefit for the management of local anesthesia arrhythmias.
  - thiopentone for management of resistant seizures
- resuscitative equipment
  - oxygen
  - ambubag
  - endotracheal tube and laryngoscope

Follow-up of patients with peripheral nerve block catheters is essential for the monitoring of both efficacy and safety. The acute pain service (APS) or an anesthesiologist readily undertakes this function. The APS make important decisions about adjustment of infusion rates, the addition of adjuvants for pain management, and the timing of peripheral nerve block catheter removal with special reference to the administration of anticoagulants.

PERIPHERAL NERVE BLOCKS OF THE UPPER LIMB

The innervations of the upper limb are derived almost completely from the brachial plexus. Complete blockade of the upper limb unlike the lower limb can thus be achieved by means of a single injection.[28,29] The site of injection into the brachial plexus depends on the location of the surgery. These blocks can be performed either for anesthesia or analgesia or both. Single injection can be made or continuous nerve blocks can be performed using continuous nerve catheters. Paraesthesia, nerve stimulation, or ultrasound techniques[30,31] can be employed in the performance of these blocks.

Anatomy of the Brachial Plexus

The brachial plexus is derived from the 5 anterior rami of the spinal nerves C5–T1, sometimes receiving contributions from C4 and T2.[32–35] These roots emerge from the spinal column by exiting through intervertebral foramen and pass between the muscle bellies of anterior and middle scalene. The anterior scalene muscle originates from the anterior tubercles of the transverse processes of C3–C6 and inserts on the scalene tubercle of the upper surface of the first rib. The anterior scalene muscle separates the subclavian vein anteriorly from the subclavian artery. The middle scalene muscle originates from the posterior tubercles of the transverse processes of C2–C7 and inserts on the upper surface of the first rib behind the subclavian groove, over which the subclavian artery passes. This groove between these two muscle bellies constitutes the interscalene groove and is the landmark that is traditionally sought when performing an interscalene nerve block (Figure 17.1). These roots merge to form three trunks that lie on top of each other: superior (C5–C6), middle (C7), and inferior (C8–T1). Each trunk just above the clavicle then splits to form six divisions: anterior division of the superior, middle, and inferior trunks and the posterior division

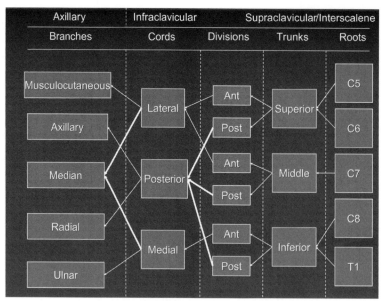

Figure 17.2: Simplified diagram of brachial plexus.

of the superior, middle, and inferior trunks. These six divisions will regroup distal to the first rib to become the three cords. Just above the clavicle, the brachial plexus comes to lie in close approximation to the subclavian artery. The brachial plexus is normally situated posterior lateral to the subclavian artery. The cords are named according to their position in respect to the axillary artery. The posterior cord is formed from the three posterior divisions of the trunks (C5–T1). The lateral cord is the anterior divisions from the upper and middle trunks (C5–C7), and the medial cord is simply a continuation of the lower trunk (C8–T1). The big picture overview of the anatomy of the brachial plexus is as follows (Figure 17.2): 5 roots of the brachial plexus (C5–T1) converge into 3 trunks (superior, middle, inferior), which then diverge into 6 divisions (3 anterior, 3 posterior), which then converge into 3 cords (lateral, posterior, medial), which finally diverge into 5 terminal nerves. In summary, the pattern of divergence and convergence is 5 > 3 < 6 > 3 < 5, terminating with the following 5 terminal nerve branches:

- axillary nerve and radial nerve: terminal nerve branches of the posterior cord
- musculocutaneous nerve: terminal nerve branch of the lateral cord
- ulnar nerve: terminal nerve branch of the medial cord
- median nerve: terminal nerve branch of the medial and lateral cord

The phrenic nerve (C3–C5) runs on the ventral surface of the anterior scalene muscle. Winnie and colleagues[36] popularized the concept that a fascial sheath envelops the nerves of the brachial plexus. The sheath arises from the prevertebral fascia originating from the cervical transverse process and terminates in the axilla. The presence of a sheath according to Winnie et al[36] would allow the plexus to be completely blocked with a single injection. The literature, however, shows that multiple injections into the plexus may result in a higher success rate, quicker onset of block and a lower volume of local anesthetic.

INTERSCALENE BLOCKADE

Halsted first performed an interscalene brachial plexus nerve block in 1884, after blocking the nerve roots in the neck with a cocaine solution. Halsted performed this block by direct injection into the plexus after surgical exposure of the plexus. July Etienne in 1925 described the first percutaneous technique of blocking the brachial plexus at the interscalene level. It was not until 1970, when Alon Winnie and colleagues[36] described the percutaneous technique of palpating for the interscalene groove between the anterior and middle scalene muscles, that this technique gained popularity.

When blocking the brachial plexus using the interscalene approach, the cervical plexus is also blocked, making it an ideal block for shoulder surgery. The use of interscalene nerve blocks alone or in combination with general anesthesia for anesthesia and analgesia offers patients a significant advantage in terms of pain scores, time to ambulation, time to discharge, and need for unexpected admission compared with general anesthesia.[37] Shoulder replacements are on the increase with the development of newer prostheses and the aging population. Pain management following shoulder replacement surgery can be problematic as this is a procedure associated with severe postoperative pain and many patients are already receiving chronic opioid management. A variety of techniques can be used for postoperative pain, including interscalene nerve block, intra-articular infusions of local anesthetics, and suprascapular nerve blocks. Suprascapular nerve blocks have been shown to be superior compared with patient-controlled intravenous analgesia.[38] Potential benefits of a suprascapular nerve block compared with an interscalene nerve block are ease of performance, lower volumes of local anesthetics needed, and fewer complications such as phrenic nerve paralysis and intrathecal injection. The major drawback compared with interscalene nerve block is the requirement for suprascapular nerve block to be combined with general anesthesia, thus necessitating the need for airway manipulation and the deleterious physiological changes associated with general anesthesia. Intra-articular infusions have become a popular method of providing postoperative pain management but some studies have shown intra-articular infusion of local anesthetic to have minimal benefit compared with placebo. A systematic review of intra-articular local anesthetic after arthroscopic knee surgery has shown a mean difference in VAS score of 11 mm (7 to 14 mm) in favor of the intra-articular group.[39] Singelyn et al[40] in a prospective randomized trial, compared intra-articular analgesia, suprascapular nerve block, and interscalene brachial plexus nerve block in patients undergoing arthroscopic shoulder surgery. No significant difference in pain scores was observed between the intra-articular group and the control group, who received general anesthesia alone. The suprascapular group and interscalene group, when compared to the control group and intra-articular group, had significantly lower pain scores at rest at 4 and 24 hours and on movement at 24 hours. Patients receiving an interscalene nerve block had the highest satisfaction scores. The satisfaction scores at 24 hours were 82 + 17, 80 + 19, 87 + 12, and 73 + 16 for the suprascapular, intra-articular, interscalene, and control groups, respectively. Only the interscalene group showed a significant reduction in total morphine requirements during the 24-hour follow-up period.

The interscalene block is performed as the nerve roots coalesce into the superior, middle, and inferior trunk as they pass between the anterior and middle scalene muscles. The interscalene groove is the most important landmark in the identification of the brachial plexus when using the classical nerve stimulation technique. One can imagine that the trunks lie on top of each other in the coronal plane with the inferior trunk (C8–T1) lying deepest, thus making it extremely difficult to block the inferior trunk. The inferior trunk gives rise to the ulnar nerve that will innervate major portions of the hand limiting the usefulness of the interscalene technique for anesthesia of the hand.

Indications

The interscalene block is ideally suited for anesthesia of the shoulder area as the axillary nerve one of the earliest branches of the brachial plexus is blocked by the interscalene approach but not when performing more distal brachial plexus blocks, such as a supraclavicular block. The axillary nerve innervates the deltoid area of the shoulder. The interscalene nerve block also results in blockade of the superficial cervical plexus that is essential for shoulder surgery. Blockade of the interscalene brachial plexus will also result in blockade of the cervical sympathetic chain with a resultant Horner's syndrome. More importantly an interscalene nerve block will also result in phrenic nerve involvement with resultant diaphragmatic paralysis and possible reduction in respiratory reserve. This may be of extreme importance in a patient with chronic obstructive airway disease and already decreased respiratory reserve. A study by Urmey et al[41] showed 100% blockade of the diaphragm following an interscalene block using 34–52 mL of local anesthetic. A subsequent study showed minimal diaphragmatic involvement but still good analgesia with 10 mL bupivacaine (0.25%).[42] The consequence of diaphragmatic paralysis in a patient with severe chronic obstructive pulmonary disease is questionable as in most of these patients there is very little diaphragmatic movement and inspiration and expiration is largely dependant on the accessory muscles. Diaphragmatic paralysis may be significant in morbidly obese patients as abdominal contents may push into the chest. This may be relieved by elevating the head of the bed.

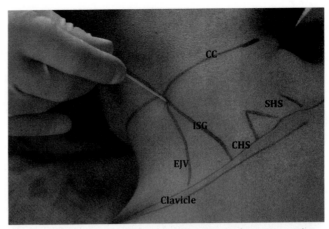

Figure 17.3: Needle position performing interscalene nerve stimulation technique. Abbreviations: CC = line from cricoid cartridge corresponding to C6 level; ISG = interscalene groove; EJV = external jugular vein; SHS = sternal head of sternocleidomastoid muscle; CHS = clavicular head of sternocleidomastoid muscle.

Block Techniques

The interscalene blocks can be placed using classic landmarks, nerve stimulation techniques, or ultrasound.

Nerve Stimulation Technique

1 When performing the interscalene block using a nerve stimulator technique, it is important to first identify the cricoid cartilage of the trachea. This corresponds to approximately C6 (Figure 17.3).
2 From this point the fingers are moved backward in an attempt to locate the interscalene groove at the level of C6 (Figure 17.3).
3 A 1-inch (25 mm) stimulating needle is inserted into the interscalene groove at this point perpendicular to the skin with a slight caudal direction (Figure 17.3). The caudal direction of the needle reduces the potential for the needle passing through the intervertebral foramen and into the subarachnoid space with a resultant total spinal anesthetic.[43,44]
4 The plexus is normally located approximately 1–2 cm beneath the skin.
5 Stimulation of the phrenic nerve with resultant diaphragm contraction requires redirection of the needle in a more posterior direction. As explained, the phrenic nerve crosses over the anterior scalene muscle and thus lies anterior to the plexus.
6 Likewise, stimulation of the trapezius or serratus anterior muscle, because of stimulation of the accessory or thoracodorsal nerves, respectively, requires movement of the needle in an anterior direction.
7 A response at between 0.3 and 0.5 mA is required to ensure a high rate of success.[45] An adequate response consists of contraction of the muscles of the forearm, biceps, or symmetrical contraction of the deltoid muscle.[46]
8 Once the desired contraction is achieved 30 mL of local anesthetic (ropivacaine [0.5%] or mepivacaine [1.5%]) is injected. One milliliter of local anesthetics should result in abolition of the nerve stimulation. If this does not occur, the

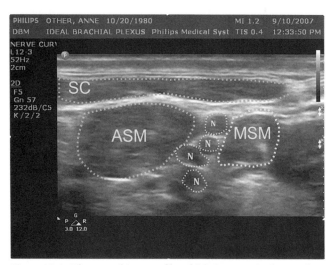

Figure 17.4: Ultrasound image of brachial plexus at the interscalene level. Abbreviations: SCM = sternocleidomastoid muscle; ASM = anterior scalene muscle; MSM = middle scalene muscle; N = nerve.

injection of local anesthetics should be stopped as the needle may be intravascular or intrathecal.

9 The local anesthetic is injected in 5-mL aliquots followed by aspiration for blood. The local anesthetic should have epinephrine added to the solution that acts as an intravascular marker (0.075 mL of 1/1000 epinephrine mixed with 30 mL local anesthetic to make a solution of 1/400 000). The addition of epinephrine may also reduce the absorption of the local anesthetic, thus reducing the potential for central nervous system and cardiovascular toxicity, and may lengthen the block duration.

10 An interscalene catheter is a suitable option if analgesia is required for a prolonged period. Two options are available: a stimulating or nonstimulating catheter. A stimulating catheter is preferable as it increases the chance of successful postoperative analgesia.[47] No local anesthetic should be injected into the plexus prior to correct placement of the catheter. The space into which the catheter is to be passed can be dilated with 5% dextrose water, but this is not essential. After location of the brachial plexus the stimulating catheter is inserted into the plexus. If the stimulation is lost the catheter is withdrawn back into the needle and the stimulation is reacquired. Simply turning the needle through 90° is all that is often needed to restore stimulation. It is important not to move the needle while the catheter tip is distal to the needle as this may damage the catheter. Once the catheter is in the correct position a 1-mL injection of local anesthetic through the catheter should abolish the stimulation. This is followed by the injection of the remaining 30 mL of local anesthetic.

Ultrasound-Guided Technique

The interscalene block is ideally suited for the use of ultrasound. An ultrasound machine with a high frequency (10–14 MHz) linear array probe is required to identify the brachial plexus that is fairly superficial, normally at a depth of approximately 1–2 cm from the skin. The higher the frequency of the probe, the greater the resolution of the picture but with limited penetration.

The plexus shows up as a hypoechoiec region lying between the anterior and middle scalene muscles (Figure 17.4).

1 The ultrasound probe is held so that the ultrasound beams cut across the brachial plexus at 90° (Figure 17.5). When using the probe, it is important to remember that this is a dynamic process and the probe must be moved up and down to allow tracking of the nerves and also to achieve the best picture.

2 There are two schools of thought regarding the relationship of the needle relative to the ultrasound, the so-called in-plain and out-plain views. We favor the in-plain approach, as the needle can be visualized along its entire length. In the in-plain approach, the needle is directed along the long axis of the ultrasound probe (Figure 17.5).

3 The needle is advanced until it lies between the superior and middle trunk of the plexus.

4 Approximately 15–20 mL of local anesthetic (ropivacaine [0.5%] or mepivacaine [1.5%]) is injected watching for the distribution of the local anesthetic around the trunks of the plexus. The use of ultrasound allows a smaller volume of local anesthetic to be used when performing nerve blocks.[48] Casati et al[48] showed a 42% reduction in the minimum effective volume of ropivacaine (0.5%) required to block the femoral nerve as compared to the nerve stimulation guidance.

5 The local anesthetic is injected in 5-mL aliquots, followed by aspiration for blood. All local anesthetic has epinephrine added to make a solution of 1/400 000 (0.075 mL of 1/1000 epinephrine mixed with 30 mL local anesthetic makes a 1/400 000 solution), which acts as an intravascular marker.

6 If the distribution is inadequate the needle can be repositioned and the injection continued. This is a major advantage over the conventional nerve stimulation technique that does not allow for visualization of local anesthetic distribution or repositioning of the needle.

7 The peripheral nerve catheter is then threaded into the interscalene space by a second person, all the time watching with the ultrasound where the catheter passes in relationship to the nerve trunks.

8 Final confirmation of the catheter placement is confirmed by injection through the catheter of a couple of milliliters of local anesthetic and again confirming proximity to brachial plexus with the ultrasound.

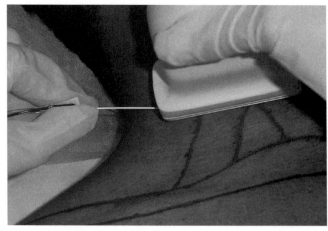

Figure 17.5: Ultrasound and needle position performing an interscalene nerve block.

9   For this block, we routinely use a nonstimulating catheter but a stimulating catheter can also be used. If a stimulating catheter is to be used, no local anesthetic can be injected prior to assuring correct placement of the stimulating catheter. In a study looking at the placement of 144 interscalene catheters using ultrasound a success rate of 98% was achieved with a single apical pneumothorax being reported (0.7%).[49]

For postoperative pain management a ropivacaine solution (0.1%–0.2 %) is routinely infused as part of a multimodal technique, including NSAIDS and or anticonvulsants. Studies have shown a patient-controlled regional analgesia technique (PCREA) to be superior to a constant infusion of local anesthetic with respect to amount of local anesthetic infused and thus potentially toxic side effects.[50,51] Commonly, the infusion pump is set to deliver a background infusion of 5 mL/h, with the patient having the ability to administer a further 5 mL of local anesthetic every 30 minutes. This would allow a maximum of 20 mL of ropivacaine per hour (20–40 mg ropivacaine [0.1%–0.2%]). The catheter will be removed when indicated, often on day 2 postsurgery. The multimodal technique is continued and supplemented with oral opioids if necessary. The removal of the catheter should be timed to coincide with the lowest risk of perioperative anticoagulants.

Complications of Interscalene Nerve Blocks

A number of complications are associated with an interscalene block. Some of these complications are more common and in fact can be viewed as side effects that occur because of the anatomical relationship of the brachial plexus to other important structures. Diaphragm paralysis due to phrenic nerve involvement occurs in almost 100% of cases and may result in a feeling of shortness of breath and in patients with respiratory insufficiency may result in respiratory failure. Horner's syndrome resulting from blockade of the sympathetic chain occurs in approximately 70%–90% of patients and will result in mydriasis, dropping of the ipsilateral eyelid, and anhydrous. Blockade of the recurrent laryngeal nerve on the left side will result in hoarseness (2%–6%). More serious complications consist of intrathecal injection and a total spinal, pneumothorax, and vertebral artery puncture and arterial injection of local anesthetics, with possible resultant seizures.

Pearls

■   The external jugular vein offers an important landmark for the position of the interscalene groove.
■   A slight caudal direction of the needle will help prevent the stimulating needle passing through the intervertebral foramen, thus reducing the potential for a total spinal.
■   Stimulation of the diaphragm reflects stimulation of the phrenic nerve and requires repositioning of the stimulating needle in a posterior direction.
■   Likewise. stimulation of the trapezius or serratus anterior muscle due to stimulation of the accessory or thoracodorsal nerves, respectively, requires movement of the needle in anterior direction.
■   Symmetrical contraction of the deltoid muscle caused by stimulation of the axillary nerve will result in adequate anesthesia for shoulder surgery

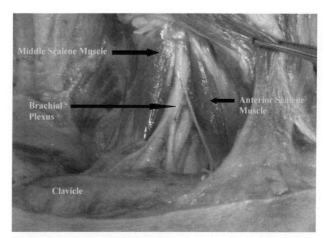

Figure 17.6: Anatomical dissection of the brachial plexus in the supraclavicular region. See color plates.

SUPRACLAVICULAR NERVE BLOCK

Kulenkampff first described this block in 1910. In this original description, the needle was inserted in a downward medial direction toward the dome of the lung, leading to a high incidence of pneumothorax. More recent descriptions, such as the Winnie and Collin's[52] perivascular subclavian approach, have led to a much better safety profile. In fact, in a study of 1001 supraclavicular blocks no clinical pneumothorax were detected.[53] Brown et al[54] introduced the "plumb-bob" technique in 1993 to simplify the approach. In this technique, the needle is introduced above the clavicle, just lateral to the sternocleidomastoid muscle, and advanced perpendicularly to the plexus in an anteroposterior direction. There is, however, still a small potential for pneumothorax. We commonly use the perivascular supraclavicular block in our practice to anesthetize any part of the arm distal to the midhumerus. The supraclavicular block has a fast onset that is accompanied by a very dense block. A supraclavicular block anesthetizes the divisions of the brachial plexus as they pass over the first rib under the clavicle (Figure 17.6). The divisions are tightly grouped together just posterolateral to the subclavian artery and medial to the middle scalene muscle. The anterior scalene muscle separates the subclavian artery from the subclavian vein that lies anterior to the artery. Blockade of the axillary nerve at this level is not possible, thus making this block less useful for surgery involving the shoulder area. Blockade of the brachial plexus at this level as with the interscalene approach may result in diaphragmatic paralysis with resultant respiratory distress in certain patients with restricted respiratory lung functions. This effect was shown not to occur as frequently as with an interscalene nerve block and did not result in respiratory difficulties in healthy subjects.[55]

Block Techniques

Nerve Stimulation Technique

When performing the perivascular subclavian approach with a nerve stimulator the following steps are followed:

1   The interscalene grove is identified at the C6 level (see interscalene approach) and then traced downward toward the supraclavicular region.

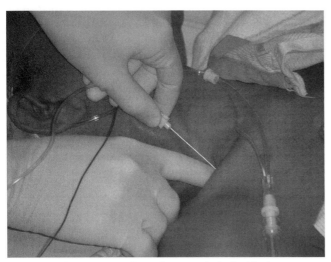

Figure 17.7: Perivascular supraclavicular block.

2   The point of entry for the needle should be into the inter-scalene groove just posterolateral to the subclavian impulse, if palpable (Figure 17.7).

3   The needle should be directed into the interscalene groove in the direction of the ipsilateral arm while ensuring that the needle is held parallel to the bed (Figure 17.7). It is important to ensure that the needle direction is never in a medial direction to reduce the possibility of a pneumothorax.

4   If no response is found the needle should be moved in an anterior posterior direction and may also be moved laterally to search for the plexus. Movement of the needle in a medial direction may result in a pneumothorax.

5   The end response that is favored to achieve a high success rate is contraction of the muscles of the hand again at a current strength between 0.3 and 0.5 mA.

6   A 1-mL injection of local anesthetic should, like all nerve blocks, result in abolition of the muscular contraction.

7   Approximately 30–35 mL of local anesthetic is then injected as done for the interscalene nerve block.

Ultrasound-Guided Technique

Ultrasound can be used to perform the supraclavicular nerve block. The brachial plexus is easily visible at this level.[56]

1   Again, a linear array ultrasound probe with a high frequency (10–14 MHz) is preferred. The probe is held in the supra-clavicular fossa as shown in Figure 17.8.

2   The ultrasound beam transects the plexus at right angles. Identification of the subclavian artery lying just above the first rib is used as important landmark as the plexus lies either lateral or posteriolateral to the pulsating artery.

3   The plexus will show up as hypoechoiec round structures, normally tightly grouped together, with the appearance of a bunch of grapes (Figure 17.9).

4   A 4-inch (100-mm) stimulating needle is inserted in the long access of the probe and is directed so as to lie within the plexus.

5   By bringing in the needle from the posterior edge of the ultrasound probe one can enter the plexus without needing to pass through the subclavian artery. Placing the patient

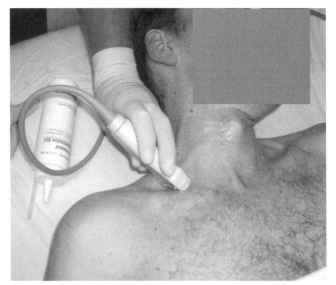

Figure 17.8: Ultrasound probe position for supraclavicular nerve block.

in a slight lateral position allows for easier insertion of the stimulating needle posterior to the ultrasound probe (Figure 17.10).

6   It is important when moving the needle to ensure that the needle is always visualized to prevent inadvertent puncture of the lung. The pleura of the lung are in close proximity to the plexus (1–2 cm) (Figure 17.9).

7   Ten to 20 mL of local anesthetic is then injected; look for distribution of the local anesthetic. Correct injection of local anesthetic often results in a donut appearance around the plexus as visualized on ultrasound.

8   Catheters can be inserted just as described in the interscalene approach using either a stimulating or nonstimulating catheter. A peripheral nerve stimulator technique can be combined with the ultrasound technique when performing this block as in any other ultrasound nerve block. However, the technique of combining stimulator technique with ultrasound has not been shown to increase efficacy of performing an ultrasound supraclavicular block.[57]

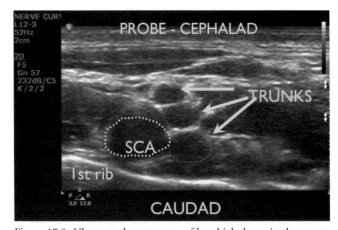

Figure 17.9: Ultrasound appearance of brachial plexus in the supra-clavicular region. SCA = subclavian artery.

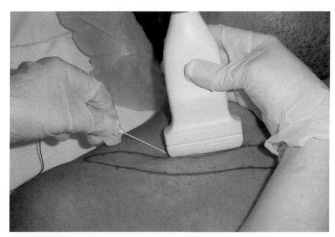

Figure 17.10: Needle position for the performance of a supraclavicular nerve block.

A recent study by Williams et al[58] showed that the ultrasound technique was superior to nerve stimulator technique with regard to quality of block, success, and time to perform the block. Surgical anesthesia without supplementation was achieved in 85% of patients in the ultrasound group and 78% of patients in the nerve stimulator group ($P = .28$). No patient in the ultrasound group and 8% of patients in nerve stimulator group required general anesthesia ($P = .12$). The quality of ulnar block was significantly inferior to the quality of block in other nerve territories in the nerve stimulator group but not in the ultrasound group. The block was performed in an average of 9.8 minutes in the nerve stimulator group and 5.0 minutes in the ultrasound group ($P = .0001$).[58]

Complications of Supraclavicular Nerve Block

The major complications associated with this approach are pneumothorax and subclavian artery puncture. The potential for the development of a pneumothorax has resulted in this block not being routinely performed by anesthesiologists. However, as shown with the subclavian perivascular approach the potential for this complication should be minimal and the use of ultrasound should further reduce these complications.

INFRACLAVICULAR BRACHIAL PLEXUS BLOCKS

The infraclavicular block provides good anesthesia for surgery involving the distal humerus, elbow, forearm, and hand. It is not useful for surgery involving the shoulder or proximal humerus. Not having to abduct the arm or perform separate blocks for the musculocutaneous and intercostobrachial/medial brachial cutaneous nerves is an advantage of the infraclavicular block when compared to axillary block. By virtue of the anatomy of the infraclavicular approach provides excellent conditions for fixation of continuous catheters.

The axillary approach provides anesthesia for surgery of the forearm and hand. It is not effective for surgery involving the elbow or upper arm. The superficial location of the axillary artery allows easier compression in case of puncture than the infraclavicular approach.

Anatomy of Brachial Plexus below Clavicle

As the brachial plexus crosses beneath the pectoralis minor, the nerve divisions rejoin to become three cords. These cords are named by their relationship to the axillary artery: posterior, lateral, and medial. The lateral cord is the most superficial, whereas the medial cord is the deepest and is below the axillary artery. The cords are classically described as being at 3, 6, and 9 o'clock in relation to the axillary artery, but significant anatomic variability exists.

The axillary and radial nerves come from the posterior cord. The axillary nerve supplies the deltoid muscle and upper shoulder, whereas the radial nerve innervates the extensor muscles of the wrist and hand, thumb abductor muscles, and sensory innervation to most of the back of the hand. Additionally, the radial nerve supplies the triceps and brachioradialis muscle. Stimulation of the radial nerve results in extension of the wrist and fingers and abduction of the thumb. The triceps muscle extends the elbow joint, whereas the brachioradialis muscle (classified as an extensor) actually flexes the elbow. This can lead to confusion as to whether the radial (posterior cord) or median nerve (lateral or medial cord) is actually being stimulated. However, if wrist and hand extensors are activated as well, one can be assured of a radial, and therefore posterior cord stimulation.

From the medial cord, the ulnar nerve and the medial half of the median nerve arise. The ulnar nerve supplies sensation to the medial half of the fourth digit and the entire fifth digit, the ulnar aspect of the palm, and the ulnar aspect of the posterior hand. It also provides innervation to the adductor pollicis and all interosseus muscles, which results in contraction of the fourth and fifth digits and adduction of the thumb when stimulated. The median nerve fibers from the medial cord innervate the flexors in the first three and a half fingers, adduction of the thumb, and provide sensation in the palm.

The musculocutaneous nerve, which is responsible for contraction of the biceps muscle and sensation in the lateral forearm, arises from the lateral cord. The lateral portion of the median nerve also arises from the lateral cord and innervates the flexor and pronator muscles of the forearm, along with the thenar muscle of the thumb. It also contributes to the finger flexors and to sensation from the thumb to the lateral half of the fourth finger.

As the plexus crosses into the apex of the axilla, the cords form the axillary, musculocutaneous, radial, ulnar, and median nerves. The last three follow the course of the axillary artery. The axillary nerve leaves the plexus at the coracoid process and heads in a very lateral and dorsal direction. It is not affected by the axillary approach to brachial plexus blockade. The musculocutaneous nerve also leaves the plexus at the level of the coracoid process and runs laterally into the coracobrachialis muscle. From there, it travels downward, ventral to the humerus, between the biceps and brachialis, which it innervates. The lateral sensory cutaneous nerve is the termination of the musculocutaneous nerve and provides sensory innervation to the lateral aspect of the forearm. Looking at a cross section of the arm at the axilla, the median and musculocutaneous nerves lie superior to the artery, whereas the radial and ulnar nerves lie inferior to the artery. The median and ulnar nerves are more superficial, whereas the radial and musculocutaneous nerves lie deeper. There is anatomic variability in the location of the nerves, however, which may make localization with nerve stimulation difficult at this level.

INFRACLAVICULAR BLOCK

Bazy first described brachial plexus blockade below the clavicle in 1914. Multiple refinements on his technique were proposed over the years, but this approach fell out of favor until Raj reintroduced the technique in 1973. However, it was not until the 1990s, when an increased interest in regional anesthesia techniques arose, that the infraclavicular approach to the brachial plexus gained stature. As many practitioners had difficulty reproducing Raj's success with the technique, Kilka, Whiffler, Klaastad and others suggested further modifications.

Block Techniques

Nerve Stimulator Technique

Multiple approaches have been described for this technique. This discussion will be limited to the modified Raj, vertical infraclavicular, and coracoid approaches, which are the most popular.

Bony landmarks common to most approaches are the jugular notch, the clavicle, and the acromioclavicular joint and coracoid process. For the modified Raj approach, a line is drawn from the jugular notch to the acromioclavicular joint. From the midpoint of that line, a perpendicular line is drawn 2.5–3 cm caudal. The needle is inserted at this point and angled at 45°–60° toward the axillary artery in the axilla. This approach requires a 4-inch needle.

The coracoid approach utilizes a point 2 cm lateral and 2 cm inferior to the tip of the coracoid process. A four-inch needle is inserted perpendicular to all planes.

The vertical infraclavicular block, like the Raj technique, marks the midpoint of a line between the jugular notch and the acromioclavicular joint. However, with this approach, a needle is inserted just below the clavicle at an angle of 90°. A 2-inch (50-mm) needle is utilized.

1   The patient should be lying supine, with the arm to be blocked lying by the patient's side, and a grounding electrode placed. The practitioner will be standing by the arm to be blocked.
2   An injection site is marked, 2 cm lateral and two centimeters distal from the tip of the coracoid process. After sterile prepping and draping, the skin should be anesthetized with a small amount of local anesthetic, using a 25-gauge sterile needle.
3   With the 4-inch stimulator needle connected to the nerve stimulator and the current set to 1.0 mA, the needle tip is inserted at an angle of 90° to all planes. Care must be taken to avoid directing the needle in a medial direction to avoid puncturing the pleura.
4   The cords will be contacted at an average depth of 4–5 cm from the skin. If the plexus is not located immediately, the needle may be sequentially redirected in a cephalad or caudal direction by 10°. If the plexus is still not located, landmarks should be reassessed.
5   When a response has been obtained, the current should be decreased slowly and needle position fine-tuned to achieve stimulation with a current less than 0.5 mA.
6   If needle aspiration is negative for blood, slowly inject local anesthetic of choice with frequent repeated aspirations. The infraclavicular block is a large volume block, and 30–40 mL of local anesthetic will be required for successful neural blockade.

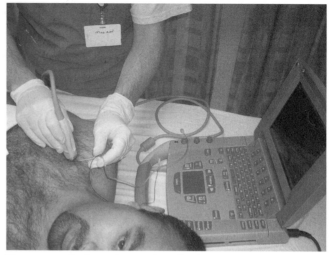

Figure 17.11: Probe position and needle entry point for infraclavicular block.

Ultrasound-Guided Technique

In the infraclavicular area, the brachial plexus can best be visualized with a linear probe in the 4- to 7-MHz range, with the probe in a parasaggital plane just medial to the coracoid process (Figure 17.11). The axillary artery and vein will be seen below the pectoralis major and minor muscles. The cords will appear as hyperechoic, with the lateral cord cephalad to the artery and the posterior cord posterior to the artery. The medial cord is typically between the artery and vein but may be difficult to visualize (Figure 17.12).

1   With area sterilely prepped and draped, sterile ultrasound gel is placed over the insertion site. The probe, as noted above, is placed in a parasaggital position medial to the coracoid process.
2   When the plexus has been visualized, a 4-inch stimulator needle is inserted from a cephalad direction, along the plane of the probe. The lateral cord will be the first part of the plexus contacted, and 10–15 mL of local anesthetic should be injected. Redirecting the needle to a steeper angle, the needle may be passed posterior to the artery, where the posterior cord is located. When contacted, an additional 10–15 mL of local anesthetic should be injected.
3   The needle should be withdrawn again, and redirected in a shallower angle, to pass the needle between the artery and vein. When this is achieved, an additional 10–15 mL of local anesthetic should be injected.
4   When done correctly, the artery and cords should appear to be surrounded by a "donut" shaped lucent ring.
5   It is not necessary to use a peripheral nerve stimulator for this technique, but as with the axillary block, it may be useful when anatomy is difficult.

Complications of Infraclavicular Nerve Block

Vascular puncture is the most frequent complication with this block, with rates as high as 50% depending on technique utilized. However, in patients with normal coagulation, both venous and arterial punctures have been reported with no major complications. Pneumothorax is a relatively rare complication, even with blind techniques. There have been no reports of pneumothorax

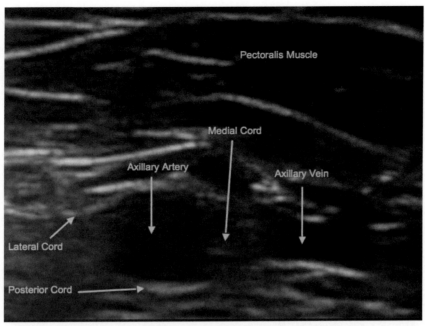

Figure 17.12: Ultrasound image of the infraclavicular brachial plexus.

with the ultrasound-guided approach, providing another reason for practitioners to add this technique to their repertoire. Muscle pain and hematoma formation are not uncommon, but have not been noted to be persistent problems Nerve damage has been a rare complication.

Pearls

- Compared to the axillary approach, the infraclavicular approach provides greater coverage. There is no need for separate injections to block the musculocutaneous or intercostobrachial nerves.
- Anatomic variability exists and the position of the cords may vary along the course of the axillary artery.
- Errors that increase the risk of pneumothorax include the following: too medial insertion of the needle, too medial angle of the needle, and depth of insertion exceeding 6 cm.
- No reported pneumothorax has occurred when ultrasound guidance has been used for this block.
- Single versus multiple injections are controversial with nerve stimulator techniques. However, with ultrasound guidance, injections can be individualized to optimize the spread of local anesthetic.

AXILLARY BRACHIAL PLEXUS BLOCKADE

Hall described the surgical technique of axillary blockade in 1884, followed by Hirschel's description of the percutaneous technique in 1911. In 1958, Burnham[59] recommended the technique of filling the axillary sheath with local anesthetic to simplify block placement. However, several investigators found problems with lack of proximal spread of the local anesthetic, despite multiple techniques claiming to promote such spread. Anatomic studies to explain the cause of incomplete block were not conclusive. In 2002, Klaastad et al[60] investigated the spread of local anesthetic through an axillary catheter using magnetic

resonance imaging (MRI) scanning. They found that, in most patients, the spread of local anesthetic was uneven and thus the sensory blockade was not adequate. Those findings made it clear why other investigators, notably Koscielniak-Nielson et al[61,62] and Sia and coworkers,[63,64] had discovered that multiple-nerve stimulation was superior (in both block success and speed of onset) to the single- and double-nerve stimulation methods used earlier. A Cochrane review by Handoll and coworkers in 2006 validated these conclusions.[65] With the advent of ultrasound technology for nerve blocks, needle placement can be more precise and should thus reduce the difficulty and increase the success rate for axillary blockade.

Anatomy of the Brachial Plexus at the Axillary Level

It is important to remember that the axillary approach to the brachial plexus blocks all of the terminal nerve branches of the brachial plexus, with the exception of the axillary nerve. This is in contrast to the progressively more proximal approaches to the brachial plexus, such as the infraclavicular approach, which blocks the cords of the brachial plexus, followed by the supraclavicular approach and interscalene approaches, which respectively block the trunks and the roots of the plexus. The terminal nerves of the brachial plexus are as follows: axillary and radial nerve, which is a terminal nerve branche of the posterior cord. The musculocutaneous nerve is a terminal nerve branch of the lateral cord. The ulnar nerve is the terminal nerve branch of the medial cord. Last, the median nerve is the terminal nerve branch of the medial and lateral cord. The median nerve is located lateral (or superior) to the axillary arterial pulse, the radial nerve is posterior to the axillary artery, and the ulnar nerve is located medial (or inferior) to the axillary artery (Figure 17.13). Although these three nerves are located fairly closely to one another in the axillary sheath, the musculocutaneous nerve is a lone ranger and lies the most posterior (deepest to the skin) and lateral of all the terminal nerves, coursing through the belly of the coracobrachialis muscle as it passes from the medial aspect of the arm

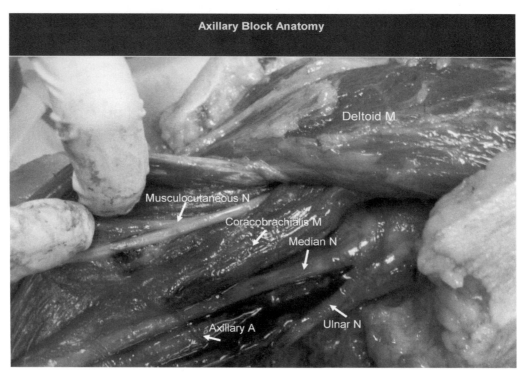

Figure 17.13: Axillary block anatomy. See color plates.

to the lateral aspect of the elbow, running in the fascial planes separating the biceps muscle from the brachialis muscle, anterior to the humerus (Figure 17.13).

These nerves take care of all of the sensory and motor innervation of the upper limb, with the exception of the axillary nerve (sensation over the deltoid "cap" of the shoulder and motor abduction of the shoulder) and the intercostobrachial nerve. The intercostobrachial nerve is a sensory nerve only and innervates the skin of the medial axilla and medial upper arm. Remember, the intercostobrachial nerve is not part of the brachial plexus per se, and is merely a spinal sensory nerve, with variable nerve root origins that may include T1 and T2.

An understanding of the dynamic anatomy of these structures is essential to have a three-dimensional picture in your mind's eye as these structures progress from the proximal axilla to the elbow and forearm. Once you understand where the nerves and vessels are going, you then have the ability to supplement an incomplete axillary block at multiple downstream sites. In fact, one of the unheralded advantages of using portable ultrasound for peripheral nerve blockade is that it allows you visualize the changing location of these nerves as you scan along the length of the arm, and seeing these images on a regular basis reinforces your anatomical understanding of three-dimensional anatomy.

For instance, when visualizing the array of nerves around the axillary artery, one can easily identify the radial nerve by scanning distally along the arm from the axilla to the elbow. The radial nerve is the first nerve to diverge from the neurovascular bundle, and it does so in the proximal third of the arm, as it is the only nerve to pass behind (posterior) the humerus and then run in the radial groove and leave in the fascial plane sandwich between the lateral and medial head of the triceps. Ultimately, the radial nerve emerges on the lateral side of the distal arm and forearm between the brachialis and brachioradialis muscle.

In contrast, the median and ulnar nerve stay in close proximity to the brachial artery until the distal third of the arm, at which point the ulnar nerve dives into the medial intermuscular septum and emerges in the posterior compartment of the arm and then runs immediately lateral to the medial epicondyle. The median nerve continues to run alongside the brachial artery as it course from the axilla to the cubital fossa. Unlike the ulnar nerve, the median nerve remains in the anterior compartment of the arm, eventually running in the sandwich fascial layer between the short head of the biceps and the brachialis muscle. As the median nerve approaches the cubital fossa, it crosses from the lateral side of the brachial artery to the medial side of the brachial artery.

Indications

The axillary approach to the brachial plexus should be considered to be one of the primary regional techniques that provide complete surgical anesthesia (and/or postoperative analgesia) for all procedures on the fingers, hand, wrist, forearm, and distal third of arm, including the elbow.[66] This approach may also be used to supplement an incomplete or failed proximal approach to the brachial plexus, involving infraclavicular or supraclavicular approaches, while maintaining careful attention to total local anesthetic exposure to prevent neurotoxic or cardiotoxic events.

The axillary approach will not provide adequate anesthesia and analgesia for open and closed procedures involving the shoulder, as the axillary nerve primarily innervates this area. This nerve branches early from the posterior cord and is not accessible to blockade from the distal axilla.

Block Techniques

There are currently four different methods used to perform the axillary block, including paraesthesia approach, transarterial

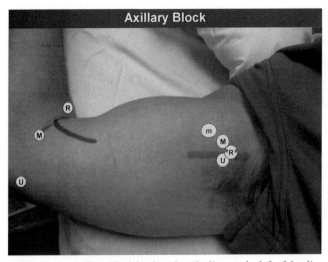

Figure 17.14: Axillary block landmarks. The line on the left of the diagram indicates the brachial artery pulse. The circles indicate the positions of the terminal nerve branches of the branchial plexus. Abbreviations: M = median nerve, R = radial nerve; U = ulnar nerve; m = musculocutaneous nerve. The mark in the elbow flexor crease represents the brachial arterial pulse, whereas the black line indicates the medial border of the biceps tendon.

approach, neurostimulation approach, and ultrasound-guided approach (with or without simultaneous neurostimulation).[67–70] Each of these methods have their own advocates and associated equipment costs, along with varying levels of training requirements to gain proficiency.

The paraesthesia method is probably the most difficult to learn and requires the greatest level of anatomical knowledge and training. It is also probably the least well accepted from a patient satisfaction standpoint, due to the minimal amount of sedation that is normally used. However, the transarterial approach is probably the easiest to learn and requires minimal knowledge of anatomy. The neurostimulation method is probably the most commonly used method today; because most of today's practicing anesthesiologists were trained using this technique.[71] In contrast to the eliciting-eliciting methods of axillary blockade, neurostimulation techniques provide clear objective end points and allow for a greater level of sedation, if necessary,to keep patients comfortable throughout the procedure. An understanding of the motor innervation of the musculocutaneous, median, radial, and ulnar nerves are necessary to be successful. And finally, ultrasound-guided methods are the latest advance in technology, with the benefit of being able to directly visualize the nerves and see the spread of local anesthetic around the nerve bundles. However, ultrasound use requires a slightly different kind of anatomical knowledge than that required for neurostimulation. A major disadvantage of using ultrasound, as compared to all other methods, is an increase of several orders of magnitude in equipment-related costs.

Nerve Stimulator Technique

One should palpate the axillary artery as high in the axilla as possible and draw a horizontal line with a marking pen overlying the skin along the long axis of the artery. If you cannot feel the pulse, it is frequently located just lateral (or superior) to the axillary hair line. The artery is located inferior to the coracobrachialis muscle and superior to the triceps (Figure 17.14). The median and musculocutaneous nerves lie superior to the artery,

whereas the radial and ulnar nerves are inferior to it. The median nerve is generally more superficial than the musculocutaneous, whereas the ulnar nerve is typically more superficial than the radial nerve. The radial nerve location can be quite variable, occasionally being found posterior to the artery.

1   The arm to be blocked should be placed in 90° abduction, with the forearm flexed comfortably. For a nerve stimulator technique, a ground electrode is placed on the patient proximal to the area being blocked. The positive electrode is then connected to the nerve stimulator.

2   Axillary block using neurostimulation techniques enjoys a 95% success rate but only when multi-injection techniques are used that isolated and stimulate at least 3 nerve branches.

3   After sterile prepping and draping of the axilla, the arterial pulse is palpated as high in the axilla as possible. A local anesthetic skin weal is placed over the needle insertion site using the 25-gauge needle. The nerve stimulator should be set between 0.5 and 1 mA at 2 Hz. The block needle, a 22- or 24-gauge, short-bevel, 50-mm-long, insulated stimulating needle is inserted in a direction almost perpendicular to the axillary artery figure. The needle will then be directed above the artery to stimulate the median nerve (Figure 17.15). As the needle penetrates the superficial brachial fascia, a characteristic "pop" can often be felt. Stimulation of the median nerve may elicit pronation of the forearm, flexion at the wrist, flexion of the thumb, and/or flexion of the fingers. If stimulation is maintained with a current <0.5 mA, 5–10 mL of local anesthetic solution is injected slowly while aspirating periodically to reduce the risk of intravascular injection.

4   The needle is then withdrawn to the subcutaneous tissue and redirected below the artery, above the triceps muscle. When the fascia is penetrated, the needle is advanced until any of the following are seen: supination of forearm, extension of wrist, and/or extension of fingers and thumb (radial nerve). Again, when stimulation is present with current <0.5 mA, an additional 5–10 mL of local anesthetic solution is injected, with periodic aspiration of the needle.

5   Remove the needle from the skin and insert it just medial to the axillary pulse and remember that the ulnar nerve is as

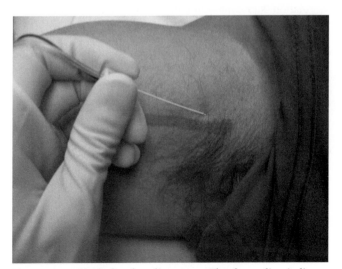

Figure 17.15: Blockade of median nerve. The drawn line indicates Brachial Artery Pulse.

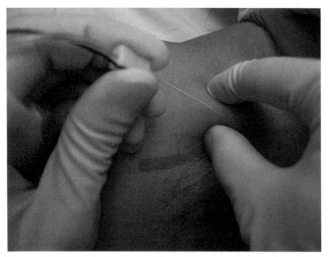

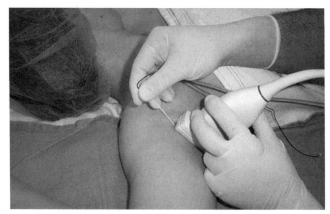

Figure 17.17: Ultrasound and Needle Position for Axillary Brachial Plexus.

Figure 17.16: Blockade of musculocutaneous nerve. The drawn line indicates the brachial artery pulse. The coracobrachialis muscle is being pinched by the thumb nd index fingers of the right hand.

superficial as the median nerve. Successful stimulation of the ulnar nerve will cause any of the following motor responses: abduction or adduction of the fingers (fingers spreading apart and then coming back together), ulnar deviation of the wrist, flexion of the fourth and fifth digits and adduction of the thumb. Note, it can be easy to mistakenly confuse the flexion of the fourth and fifth digits and thumb adduction with median nerve stimulation. Often, the ulnar nerve will be encountered prior to reaching the radial nerve, with thumb adduction and flexion of the last two fingers. If this occurs, 5–10 mL of local anesthetic is injected before increasing needle penetration to locate the radial nerve.

6 Pinch the coracobrachialis muscle in the bicipital groove, just lateral (or superior) to the axillary pulse line (Figure 17.16). After depositing a 1–2 mL skin wheal, advance your stimulating needle at a 90° angle to the skin until stimulation of the musculocutaneous nerve occurs resulting in elbow flexion or the periosteum of the humerus is encountered. Do not be misled by direct local stimulation of the short head of the biceps resulting from direct intramuscular stimulation. An additional 5–10 mL of local anesthetic is injected when stimulation is present with current noted above. If you do not stimulate the nerve on the first needle pass, then withdraw the needle to just below the skin surface and redirect the needle more laterally initially. In the event that you still fail to obtain stimulation, then withdraw the needle back to the surface, and this time advance in a more medial direction.

7 For intercostobrachial nerve block, remove the needle from previous entry site and then infiltrate approximately 5–10 mL of local anesthetic solution subcutaneously in the axilla over the arterial pulse, injecting in a medial to lateral direction. Although not always necessary for procedures on the upper extremity, this should be done whenever an upper arm tourniquet is used to minimize tourniquet discomfort.

Ultrasound-Guided Technique

In addition to the equipment noted above, use a portable ultrasound machine, a 10- to 15-MHz linear ultrasound probe, ultrasound gel, and either a sterile sheath for the probe or a sterile, transparent surgical dressing to cover the surface of the probe.[72,73]

Ultrasound-guided axillary blocks free the operator from the constraints of traditional surface landmarks and afford the regional anesthesiologist the freedom to block the nerves wherever they are best visualized. In addition, unlike any other method of neural block, the ability to visualize the spread of local anesthetic around the nerve in real time gives the operator multiple opportunities to readjust the needle position to obtain optimum spread of local anesthetic around the nerve bundle. The visual effect is that of a doughnut ring of local anesthetic, surrounding the interior "hole" or nerve bundle.

Just like the nerve stimulation technique, this block is also performed as a multi-injection technique and as follows[74,75]:

1 Arm position and sterile prep and drape are identical to the nerve stimulator technique. The probe is positioned as high in the axilla as possible, perpendicular to the long axis of the arm (Figure 17.17). This will allow a transverse view of the neurovascular bundle.

2 The axillary artery is easily identified by its pulsations (Figure 17.18). The axillary vein is nonpulsatile and may be

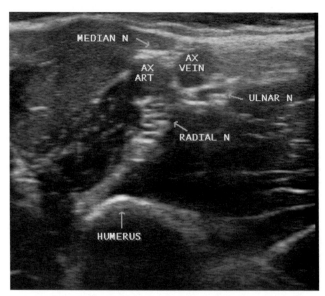

Figure 17.18: Ultrasound image of brachial plexus in axilla. Abbreviations: AX ART = axillary artery; AX VEIN = axillary vein.

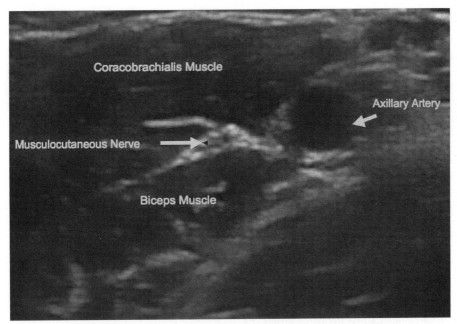

Figure 17.19: Ultrasound image of musculocutaneous nerve in axilla.

easily compressed. The nerves are typically hypoechoic, with some hyperechoic areas internally. They may sometimes not appear as discrete entities, but as areas with irregular borders, whose echo densities differ from surrounding tissues. If in doubt, the nerve may be traced distally. As the nerves leave the axilla, they separate and may be more distinct. This is especially true of the radial nerve. Observing that the radial nerve is the first nerve to move away from the brachial artery in the midhumeral region, whereas the ulnar nerve is the last nerve to move away in the distal arm, can serve to identify individual nerves.

3   The musculocutaneous nerve leaves the neurovascular bundle more proximally in the axilla and can be identified as a hyperechoic structure located between the coracobrachialis and biceps muscles (Figure 17.19). It runs a short distance between the muscles before penetrating the body of the coracobrachialis muscle.

4   Once the nerves have been identified, a skin wheal is placed at either the lateral or medial edge of the transducer long axis, and the 22-gauge, short-bevel needle is inserted in the plane (IP) of the long axis of the transducer (Figure 17.17). After the needle tip is visualized, the needle shaft is slowly advanced toward the nerve bundle, taking care to keep the entire shaft visible in the plane of the ultrasound beam. Alternatively, an insulated stimulating needle may be used to help identify the terminal nerve by observing the unique motor twitch elicited as the needle tip approaches the nerve bundle.

5   As the needle tip approaches within 1 mm of the nerve bundle boundary, a test dose of 1 mL of local anesthetic is injected, and the spread of the local anesthetic solution is noted. If perineural spread is observed, and resistance to injection is low, then approximately 5–10 mL of local anesthetic solution is injected surrounding each nerve.

6   It is also possible to perform this block using a needle approach out-of-plane (OOP) to the transducer, with the needle tip being inserted in the skin adjacent to the

midpoint of the transducer length, with a much shorter pathway to the nerve bundle.

7   Block the intercostobrachial nerve as previously described with a subcutaneous infiltration of local anesthetic. This nerve is not well visualized with ultrasound.

Paraesthesia and Transarterial Technique[62,76,77]

A 22-gauge or smaller short-bevel needle, 50 mm in length, is normally used for this technique. Advance the needle using anatomical knowledge of nerve locations to obtain paraesthesia in desired nerve distribution, or transfix axillary artery, and after careful negative aspiration, deposit local anesthesia posterior to artery and then withdraw the needle until it is located just anterior to artery. After repeat negative aspiration, deposit additional local anesthetic. Total volume of local anesthetic should not exceed 40 mL of bupivacaine (0.5%) or 20 mL of ropivacaine (0.75%).

Complications of Axillary Brachial Plexus Block

Vascular puncture is not uncommon, especially when ultrasound is not utilized. Intravascular injection of local anesthetic can produce symptoms ranging from lightheadedness to seizure and cardiac arrest. Frequent aspiration during injection is necessary to avoid this complication. However, if venous puncture has occurred, negative pressure from the syringe during aspiration may collapse the wall of the vein against the needle lumen, preventing blood from entering the needle. For this reason, even with negative aspiration of blood, the local anesthetic should be injected slowly, with close observation for any signs of early anesthetic toxicity.

Toxicity may also occur from LA absorption into the axillary vasculature. As opposed to the immediate symptoms seen with intravascular injection, absorption toxicity may not become apparent for 5–30 minutes after injection. Symptoms are similar to those of intravascular injection and can be treated with oxygen, benzodiazepines, and airway support if necessary.

Hematoma formation may occur after vascular puncture, especially arterial puncture. Steady pressure should be applied to the site for at least 5 minutes after needle removal to reduce the chances of hematoma formation.

Peripheral nerve injury can be secondary to direct needle injury, intraneural injection, and tourniquet pressure, positioning difficulties, or direct surgical injury. Surgical injuries are typically distal to the block site and can be differentiated from needle trauma on that basis. Needle trauma or intraneural injection produces deficits in the distribution of the affected nerve, whereas ischemic injuries from tourniquet use tend to be more diffuse. The majorities of injuries are neuropraxia and resolve within several weeks.

Pearls

- Some practitioners prefer to start with a higher stimulator current, causing stimulation at a greater distance from the nerve, and then decrease the current to fine tune needle placement. Others prefer to start with low current (0.5 mA). This may make nerve location more difficult initially but will decrease patient discomfort when the nerve enters the axillary sheath.

- Local anesthetic should not be injected if stimulation occurs with current <0.2 mA, as the needle may be intraneural. Withdraw needle slightly until stimulation requires a current of 0.3–0.5 mA.

- When using an ultrasound-guided technique, it is not necessary to use a nerve stimulator. However, nerve stimulation may be a useful adjunct to verify correct needle placement when anatomy is difficult or the practitioner is less experienced in ultrasound techniques.

- The axillary approach to brachial plexus will not block T1, T2, which innervate the underside of the upper arm near the axilla. Pneumatic tourniquets are commonly used for hand and arm surgery to allow for bloodless conditions in areas where visibility may be obscured by even a minimal amount of bleeding. As these tourniquets may produce significant pressure pain, an intercostobrachial (T2) and medial brachial cutaneous (C8, T1) blocks are typically performed along with the axillary block. These blocks may be accomplished by subcutaneous infiltration of local anesthetic in the axilla in a plane perpendicular to the long axis of the arm.

- When the needle tip is observed under ultrasound to be in contact with the peripheral nerve, approximately 25% of the time there will be no apparent motor twitch response when the nerve stimulator is turned on.

ELBOW BLOCKS

The elbow block is suitable for any procedure on the forearm, wrist, hand, and fingers, as long as an upper arm tourniquet is not required.[78] Surgery on the hand and wrist can be performed with this block, as long as the surgeon is willing to use a forearm tourniquet. At the same time, there are many procedures on the hand, wrist, and forearm that do not require tourniquet use.

The major advantage to this block is the fact that it allows for greater mobility of the arm postoperatively and that a smaller total volume of local anesthetic can be used, therefore, further reducing the potential for local anesthetic toxicity. However, the major disadvantage is that this block is shorter acting when compared to an axillary block, and greater patient cooperation is required during the procedure because the patient is able to flex the forearm.

Perhaps the best reason to understand how to perform this approach is that it can be easily used to supplement an incomplete axillary block. Once you have determined which terminal nerve branch needs to be supplemented, then you can isolate the nerve at the elbow and inject a small volume of local anesthetic solution to achieve complete surgical anesthesia of the forearm and distal structures.

It may be useful to think of the elbow block as the "ankle block" of the elbow, because, just like the ankle block, there are five separate nerve injections that need to be made. In addition to blocking the median, radial, and ulnar nerves, to achieve complete surgical analgesia of the forearm, the lateral antebrachial cutaneous nerve (terminal extension of the musculocutaneous nerve) and the medial antebrachial cutaneous nerves must be blocked. Surgery involving the hand and fingers, but distal to the wrist, does not require blockade of these last two nerves, unless a forearm tourniquet is going to be utilized during the procedure.

Anatomy

Locate the cubital fossa at the level of the humeral intercondylar line (Figures 17.20 and 17.21). The radial nerve is located lateral to the bicipital aponeurosis and is a deep structure, emerging between the biceps and brachialis muscle and then diving under the brachioradialis muscle. The lateral antebrachial cutaneous nerve (terminal branch of the musculocutaneous nerve) emerges epifascially between the brachialis and biceps muscles and lies subcutaneously on the lateral aspect of the cubital fossa. Moving medially, the pulse of the brachial artery is palpated just medial to the biceps aponeurosis, and the median nerve is located immediately medial to the brachial artery. As the nerve continues its passage into the forearm, it passes distally while diving under the muscle belly of the pronator teres. The medial antebrachial cutaneous nerve (a branch of the medial cord) runs in the subcutaneous tissue of the medial aspect of the cubital fossa. The ulnar nerve is the only nerve that is located in the posterior compartment of the elbow and runs relatively superficially in the groove between the olecranon and medial epicondyle of the humerus. Frequently, the nerve can be palpated and rolled in the groove. As the ulnar nerve passes into the forearm, it moves into the anterior compartment on the medial surface and then runs in conjunction with the ulnar artery at the midpoint of the forearm.

Block Techniques

Nerve Stimulator Technique

This block can be performed using landmarks only (blind technique) or with the aid of neurostimulation or ultrasound. The motor responses to stimulation of the median, radial, and ulnar nerves have been previously referenced in this document. After the landmarks are drawn, and sterile prep of the cubital fossa is accomplished, a 22- or 24-gauge, short-bevel insulated needle is advanced 1–2 cm below the skin surface at a 90° angle to the skin while searching for a paraesthesia or the appropriate motor stimulation. After a threshold current stimulation of <0.5 mA is obtained, and negative

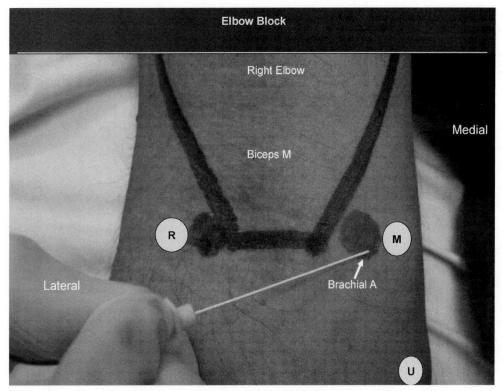

Figure 17.20: Elbow block. The circles demonstrate the position of the radial, median, and ulnar nerves.

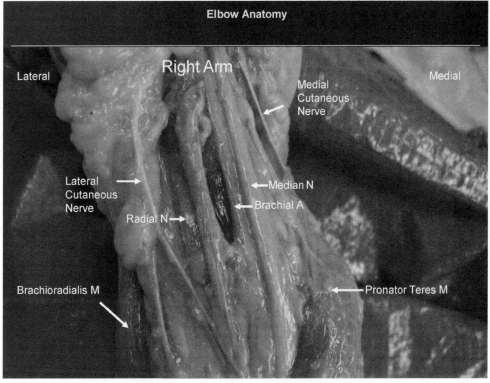

Figure 17.21: Elbow block anatomy. See color plates.

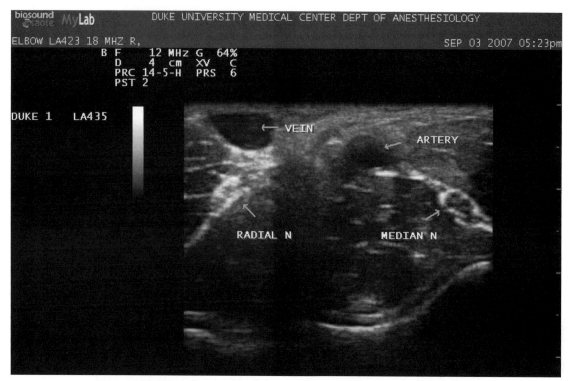

Figure 17.22: Elbow flexor crease ultrasound anatomy of radial and median nerves.

aspiration occurs, then approximately 5–7 mL of a local anesthetic solution is deposited near the median, radial, and ulnar nerves.

Ultrasound-Guided Technique

Under ultrasound, the medial and radial nerves assume the shape of a bitapered oval, with the radial nerve seen arcing away from the cubital vein, whereas the median nerve arcs away from the brachial artery. The radial and median nerves appear hyperechoic under ultrasound (Figure 17.22). Just as during an axillary block, the needle may be advanced in the long-axis plane of the transducer, or out-of-plane, depending on user preference, and the needle may be readjusted to obtain optimal spread of local anesthetic solution around the nerve.

You should be cautious when attempting to block the ulnar nerve at the elbow because of the potential for spearing the nerve with a needle in the olecranon groove – I recommend instead that you inject distal or proximal to the groove, using either stimulation or ultrasound. The ulnar nerve is easily visualized under ultrasound and appears as a hyperechoic, honeycombed structure (Figures 17.23 and 17.24). Another approach is to identify the ulnar nerve, approximately 5 cm distal to the elbow flexor crease in the forearm (Figure 17.24). Once the nerve passes distal to the olecranon groove, it moves from the posterior surface of the arm to the anterior surface of the forearm, thereby moving in a medial to lateral direction. The ulnar nerve is easily identified at this point, because it is relatively superficial, and local anesthetic can be deposited around the nerve without danger of nerve entrapment in a closed space.

Finally, the lateral and medial antebrachial cutaneous nerves are superficial nerves and can be blocked with a subcutaneous infiltration of 5–7 mL of local anesthetic solution across the lateral and medial aspect of the cubital fossa, injecting laterally and then medially to the biceps tendon aponeurosis.

Complications of an Elbow Block

There is a potential for intraneuronal injections, especially when attempting to perform an ulnar nerve block in the olecranon groove. There is also a potential for pressure-related ischemic damage to the nerve if a large volume of local anesthetic is injected into a closed space. The other major problem that can occur is hematoma formation secondary to brachial artery puncture, especially when performing this block in patients who are anticoagulated. This can be easily prevented and treated with direct manual pressure and compression. Finally, the risk of local anesthetic toxicity is extremely low, because of the small volume of local anesthetic that is injected close to the veins and arteries of the cubital fossa.

WRIST BLOCK

The wrist block can be considered a primary block for procedures involving multiple digits or for procedures involving the dorsal and palmar aspects of the hand whenever a tourniquet is not required for surgery.[79–81] This block can be used in lieu of an axillary or elbow block to allow greater postoperative mobility of the upper extremity. Most importantly, a thorough understanding of the wrist block will let you use your anatomical knowledge to supplement an incomplete axillary or elbow block for procedures involving the hand and fingers. Patient selection and cooperation is essential to successfully use this technique in your practice, because motor function of the arm and forearm

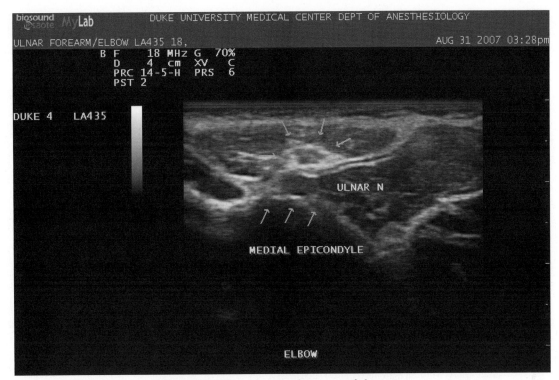

Figure 17.23: Elbow ultrasound anatomy of ulnar nerve.

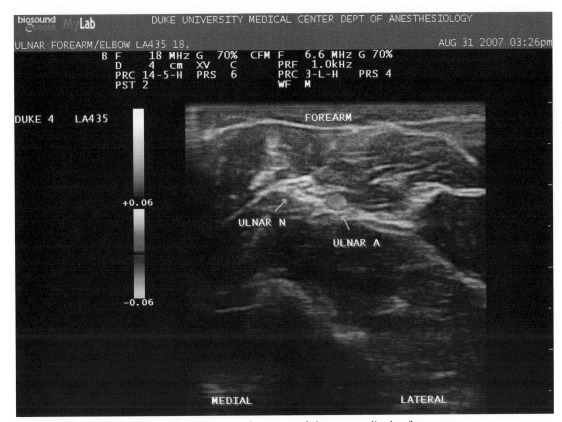

Figure 17.24: Elbow ultrasound anatomy of ulnar nerve, distal to flexor crease.

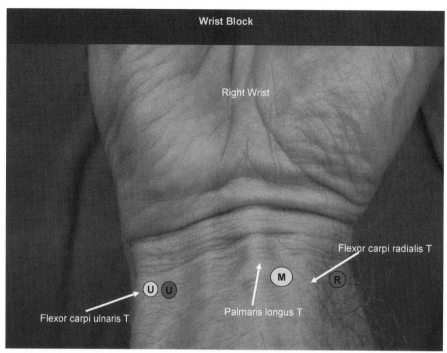

Figure 17.25: Wrist block surface anatomy. Abbreviations: U in yellow = ulnar nerve; U in red = ulnar artery; M = median nerve; R = radial artery.

are preserved, allowing the uncooperative patient to move the arm at will. You can consider a supplemental block of the musculocutaneous nerve at the axillary level, with 5–7 mL of a short acting local anesthetic, which will render the forearm and hand immobile.

Anatomy

Unlike the elbow block, there are only three nerves to block in the wrist block: the ulnar, median, and superficial radial nerves (Figures 17.25 and 17.26). The superficial radial nerve is a sensory nerve only and lies subcutaneously on the lateral side of the wrist, crossing the anatomical snuffbox (extensor pollicus tendons) and then continuing along the posterior surface of the wrist. Motor function of the thumb is supplied by the posterior interosseus nerve, which is a branch of the interosseus nerve, which is itself a branch of the deep radial nerve. It cannot be blocked at the wrist, so if motor paralysis of the thumb and motor paralysis of wrist extension is required, then the radial nerve must be blocked at the elbow or axilla

The median nerve is located between the tendons of the flexor carpi radialis and the palmaris longus and lies deep to the tendons, with the tendons being encased by the flexor retinaculum connective tissue. If you ask a patient to flex their wrist slightly and then oppose their thumb to their little finger, the palmaris longus tendon is the most prominent surface tendon. The flexor carpi radialis tendon is located immediately lateral and toward the base of the thumb. Note that the median nerve also gives off a palmar cutaneous branch, so the nerve should be blocked at least 5 cm proximal to the wrist flexor crease prior to the takeoff of the palmar cutaneous branch.

That leaves us with the ulnar nerve, which is on the medial side of the wrist, and located between the flexor carpi ulnaris

tendon and the ulnar arterial pulse. The flexor carpi ulnaris is the most medial of all the tendons in the wrist and can be easily palpated by asking the patient to flex and extend at the wrist. Just like the median nerve, the ulnar nerve is located under the roof of the flexor retinaculum connective tissue. And also like the median nerve, the ulnar nerve gives off a dorsal cutaneous branch that supplies the back of the hand. This nerve branch can be blocked with a subcutaneous infiltration of 5 mL of local anesthetic solution, injected 5 cm proximal to the wrist crease, and extending from the ulnar aspect of the forearm to the dorsal aspect of the wrist.

Block Techniques

A wrist block can be performed via a landmark-guided blind technique (Figure 17.25) (most popular) or with the aid of a nerve stimulator or ultrasound.

Blind

1 Superficial radial nerve: 5–10 mL of local anesthetic injected subcutaneously with a 25-gauge needle from the lateral aspect of the wrist, extending over the anatomical snuffbox and dorsal aspect of wrist (Figure 17.27).
2 Median nerve: 3–5 mL of local anesthetic of local anesthetic injected between the tendons of palmaris longus and flexor carpi radialis, 5 cm proximal to wrist flexor crease (Figure 17.25). Insert a 22- to 24-gauge short-bevel needle at a 90° angle to the skin, pop through the flexor retinaculum, and advance 1–2 cm until a paraesthesia elicited or the periosteum of the radius is encountered. Withdraw slightly and inject. If resistance to injection is encountered, then continue to withdraw the needle until resistance decreases.

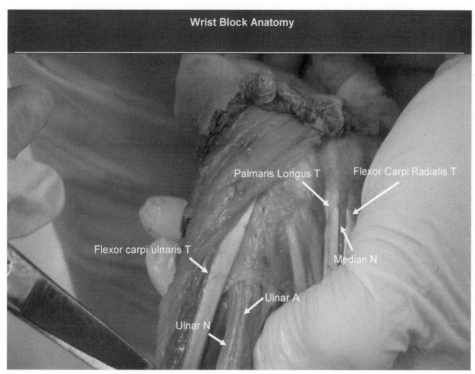

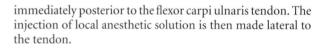

Figure 17.26: Wrist block anatomy. See color plates.

3 Ulnar nerve: 3–5 mL of local anesthetic solution injected between the flexor carpi ulnaris tendon and ulnar artery, approximately 5 cm proximal to the wrist flexor crease (Figure 17.28). Insert a 22- to 24-gauge short-bevel needle at a 90° angle to the skin, pop through the flexor retinaculum, and advance until a paraesthesia is elicited or the periosteum of the ulna is encountered. Aspirate to avoid injection into ulnar artery and then inject local anesthetic solution. Again, if resistance is initially encountered, withdraw the needle until resistance to injection decreases. An alternative approach to the needle entry direction is to position the needle on the medial aspect of the wrist, pointed at a 90° angle to the long axis of the forearm, with the needle entry point immediately posterior to the flexor carpi ulnaris tendon. The injection of local anesthetic solution is then made lateral to the tendon.

Peripheral Nerve Stimulation

1 Can be utilized to localize the median and ulnar nerves but not the superficial radial nerve, which is a purely sensory nerve.

2 Sometimes it is difficult to obtain a motor response from the median nerve, and in this case, a paraesthesia or a blind injection is acceptable. Make sure that you are injecting lateral to the palmaris longus tendon and not medial to the tendon, as sometimes the palmaris longus tendon is confused with the flexor carpi radialis tendon.

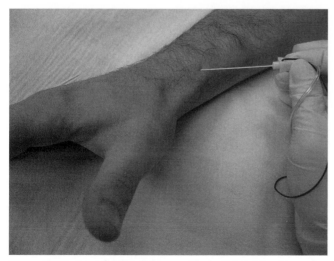

Figure 17.27: Superficial radial nerve block. Inject lateral to pulse, superficially, and extend to soral aspect of wrist.

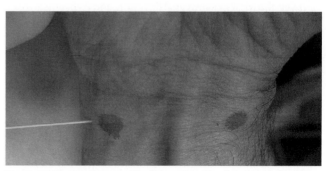

Figure 17.28: Ulnar nerve block at wrist. The left dot in the lower part of the figure represents the ulnar arterial pulse; the dot in the lower right part of the figure represents the radial arterial pulse. The prominent tendon in the center of the figure is the palmaria longus tendon, with the median nerve located immediately lateral to the tendon.

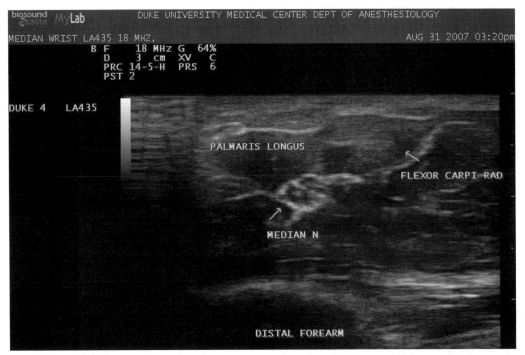

Figure 17.29: Ultrasound image of median nerve and flexor tendons at wrist flexor crease.

Ultrasound-Guided Technique

1 The median and ulnar nerves are well visualized as hyperechoic honeycombed structures (especially the median), and ultrasound is useful to separate the median nerve from the surrounding tendons and to avoid direct neural injection (Figure 17.29).

2 The ulnar artery is a useful landmark to help identify the ulnar nerve, because the ulnar nerve lies immediately medial to the artery (Figure 17.30).

3 The superficial radial nerve is not well visualized on ultrasound.

4 It is easy to confuse nerves and tendons at the wrist under ultrasound, as they both have a similar appearance. However, as you move the probe away from the wrist in a distal to proximal direction, it is easy to separate the nerves from the tendons. The median nerve tends to run more deeply from the surface than the tendons, whereas the ulnar nerve continues to run adjacent to the ulnar artery, moving away from the wrist in a proximal direction, and is therefore easily distinguished from the flexor carpi ulnaris tendon.

Complications of a Wrist Block

Excessively large volumes of local anesthetic solutions in tight fascial compartments of the wrist can lead to a compartment syndrome, resulting in ischemic damage to the median and ulnar nerves and potentially leading to a permanent residual neuropathy. Take care to limit the total injection volumes for these nerves.

PERIPHERAL NERVE BLOCKS OF THE LOWER LIMB

The innervation of the lower extremity is derived from both the lumbar and the sacral plexus. As discussed above, the anatomy of the peripheral nervous system of the upper extremity is conveniently contained entirely within the brachial plexus, allowing for single peripheral nerve blocks that can provide anesthesia or analgesia to the entire extremity. The neural anatomy of the lower extremity is not as conveniently organized for the regional anesthesiologist, requiring at least two peripheral nerve blocks to provide complete anesthesia or analgesia to the entire lower extremity. Both single injection nerve blocks as well as continuous peripheral nerve catheters may be utilized to provide analgesia or anesthesia or both. The sites of injection along the course of the nerves of the lumbosacral plexus are determined by the operative site and will result in varying distributions of sensory and motor blockade.

Anatomy of the Lumbosacral Plexus

The ventral rami of L1-L4 emerge from the vertebral foramen and course anterior to the transverse processes of the lumbar vertebral bodies and into the psoas major muscle, where they collectively form the lumbar plexus. The terminal branches that emerge from the body of the psoas muscle and their respective contributions from the lumbar plexus are as follows: (1) iliohypogastric (L1), (2) ilioinguinal (L1), (3) genitofemoral (L1, L2), (4) lateral femoral cutaneous nerve of the thigh (L2, L3), (5) obturator nerve (L2, L3, L4), and (6) femoral nerve (L2, L3, L4) (Figure 18.30). The saphenous nerve is a terminal sensory branch of the femoral nerve. The nerve branches of the lumbar plexus provide motor innervation to the lower abdomen, hip flexors, thigh adductors, and quadriceps muscles and sensation to the lower abdomen, groin, lateral and anteromedial thigh, and the medial aspect of the lower leg and foot.

The sacral plexus is formed by the ventral rami of the L4–S3 nerve roots. These roots begin to merge on the anterior surface of the lateral sacrum and come together to form the sciatic nerve on the anterior surface of the piriformis muscle. The sciatic nerve is the main terminal branch of the sacral plexus and it is

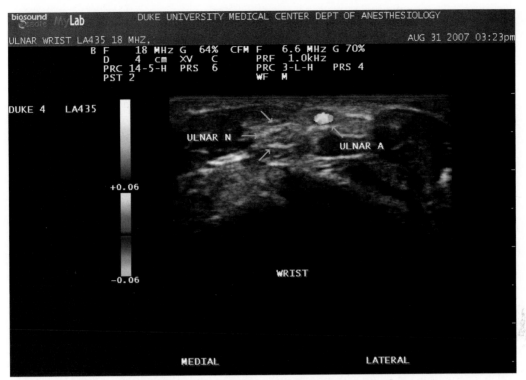

Figure 17.30: Ultrasound image of ulnar nerve and artery at wrist flexor crease.

the largest nerve in the human body, approximately the size of the thumb at its origin. Shortly after its formation, the sciatic nerve exits the pelvis through the sciatic foramen, gives rise to the posterior cutaneous nerve of the thigh, descends between the greater trochanter of the femur and ischial tuberosity, and finally divides at a variable distance, from 0 to 11.5 cm above the popliteal crease, as shown in a cadaver study, to form the tibial nerve and common peroneal nerves.[82] The sciatic nerve also gives off various articular and muscular branches along its course.

BLOCKS OF THE LUMBAR PLEXUS

Psoas Compartment Blockade (Posterior Approach to the Lumbar Plexus)

Winnie et al[83] first described the posterior approach to the lumbar plexus in 1974. Winnie reported that blockade of both the lumbar and sacral plexuses could be achieved with his approach. Chayen et al, and Parkinson et al reported various modifications of this technique.[84,85] Chayen et al modified Winnie et al's approach and named their approach the *psoas compartment block* and, contrary to Winnie et al's reports, determined that it would be necessary to perform a separate sciatic nerve block in addition to a lumbar plexus block to achieve complete anesthesia or analgesia of the leg.[85] Winnie had previously reported the anterior approach to the lumbar plexus, also known as the femoral "3-in-1" approach, and claimed that a large volume of local anesthetic placed within a femoral nerve sheath would spread proximally to the lumbar plexus, achieving blockade of the obturator and lateral femoral cutaneous nerves in addition to the femoral nerve.[86] Parkinson et al[85] reported that reliable blockade of the obturator and lateral femoral cutaneous nerves could not be obtained with the "3-in-1" technique. They modified the two approaches of Winnie and Chayen with the

addition of nerve stimulation and reported no difference in efficacy between the two approaches. Further cadaver investigation showed no such femoral nerve "sheath" that would be capable of allowing proximal spread of local anesthetic to the lumbar plexus from an inguinal perivascular approach.[87]

Thus, the psoas compartment block is the only technique that provides consistent blockade of the femoral, lateral femoral cutaneous, and obturator nerves, resulting in complete anesthesia or analgesia to the region of the lower extremity innervated by the lumbar plexus. Blockade of the ilioinguinal, iliohypogastric, and genitofemoral nerves, the more proximal branches of the lumber plexus, is more variable with this technique. When the psoas compartment block is used in conjunction with a sciatic nerve block anesthesia and analgesia of the entire leg is achieved.[85] The clinical applications of the psoas compartment block include surgery on the hip, anterior thigh, and knee. Because of its significant clinical utility, the posterior lumbar plexus block is gaining popularity and is heavily used in some practices, particularly for procedures involving the hip or knee.

When compared to general anesthesia for knee arthroscopy in an outpatient setting, a lumbar plexus block with mepivacaine resulted in more frequent PACU bypass, lower pain VAS scores postoperatively, and decreased requirements for analgesics prior to same-day discharge.[88] Even greater benefit is observed when lumbar plexus blockade is used for more invasive procedures. In patients undergoing arthroscopic repair of the anterior cruciate ligament (ACL), Matheny et al[89] showed an 89% reduction in opioid requirements and a resultant decrease in opioid side effects in patients who received continuous lumbar plexus catheters when compared to a group of patients who received intravenous patient-controlled analgesia (IV PCA).

A number of studies have examined the benefit of lumbar plexus blockade for total knee arthroplasty (TKA). Patients

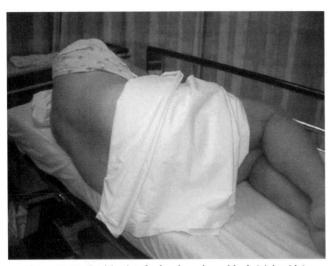

Figure 17.31: Positioning for lumbar plexus block (right side).

report an easier and more comfortable recovery with continuous lumbar plexus block compared to their own previous experience with general anesthesia and IV PCA.[90] Campbell at al compared continuous lumbar plexus infusions to epidural infusion and showed no significant differences in opioid consumption, range of motion, or pain scores at rest or with movement; however, patients with epidural catheters had a 3-fold increase in incidence of bladder catheterization. Raimer et al[91] compared continuous lumbar plexus and sciatic catheters to both epidurals and IV PCA. The groups with continuous peripheral nerve catheters and epidurals had superior analgesia with respect to pain levels, opioid requirements, and patient satisfaction. Patients who received lumbar plexus and sciatic catheters had fewer side effects than patients in the epidural and IV PCA groups. Watson et al[92] evaluated the benefit of a continuous lumbar plexus catheter over a single injection. Compared with single-shot blocks, patients who received continuous lumbar plexus catheters had decreased opioid requirements and earlier mobilization after TKA. In addition to improved patient satisfaction, superior analgesia, decreased side effects, and earlier mobilization, a recent study has shown that the addition of a continuous lumbar plexus catheter to a spinal anesthetic resulted in decreased leukocyte count and plasma levels of C-reactive protein showing that continuous peripheral catheters for postoperative analgesia may contribute to the attenuation of the systemic inflammatory response.[93] Lumbar plexus blockade has also proven to be beneficial for both total hip arthroplasty (THA) and hip fracture.[94–97] Several studies have shown that psoas compartment block results in lower pain VAS scores and decreased opioid use after THA in the postoperative period.[95,98] In addition to decreased pain scores and opioid use, Stevens et al reported that a lumbar plexus block resulted in decreased blood loss associated with THA.[96] Although studies of single-injection lumbar plexus blocks have shown improved analgesia over IV PCA from 6 to 24 hours postoperatively, prolonged analgesia may be obtained with a continuous lumbar plexus catheter.[97,99–101] Capdevila et al[100] showed a reduction in VAS scores for greater than 48 hours postoperatively. When compared to epidural analgesia for THA, a continuous lumbar plexus catheter was equally effective in providing analgesia, reducing opioid use and increasing patient satisfaction. A continuous lumbar plexus catheter was superior to an epidural in regards to side effects, with a reduc-

tion of more than 80% in the incidence of orthostatic hypotension, PONV, and urinary retention. In addition, patients with lumbar plexus catheters ambulated earlier than patients with epidurals.[101] In an anesthesia protocol that emphasized continuous lumbar plexus nerve catheters for both THA and TKA, Hebl et al demonstrated decreased side effects, decreased postoperative cognitive dysfunction, earlier postoperative ambulation, and earlier hospital discharge in patients who received a continuous peripheral lumbar plexus catheter compared to controls.[97]

Although it is clear that a lumbar plexus block can be beneficial to patients undergoing surgery of the hip or knee, overall benefits and their duration will likely be dependant on whether a lumbar plexus single injection or continuous catheter technique is utilized. The addition of a sciatic nerve block may also play a role in the efficacy of this technique.

Techniques

Peripheral Nerve Stimulation

To block the lumbar plexus from a posterior approach, the patient is positioned with the operative side up in the lateral decubitus position with a slight forward rotation. The hips and knees are flexed and the leg on the side to be blocked should be easily visible so that twitches of the quadriceps and the resulting patellar tendon snap can be easily observed (Figure 17.31).

The landmarks for this technique include the spinous processes, iliac crest, and posterior-superior iliac spine. The exact needle entry point varies somewhat, depending on the author, but all have yielded similar results and similar complication rates. The technique below describes Winnie's approach.

1 The spinous processes of the lumbar vertebrae are palpated. A line connecting the spinous processes is drawn, representing midline.
2 The iliac crest is palpated and a perpendicular line is drawn from the iliac crest to the midline. This is the intercristal line, which is at the approximate level of the L4 spinous process (Figure 17.32).
3 The posterior-superior iliac spine (PSIS) is palpated and marked (Figure 17.32).
4 A paramedian line is drawn from the PSIS parallel to midline and intersecting the intercristal line at 90° (Figure 17.32).

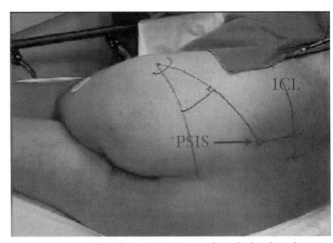

Figure 17.32: Winnie's posterior approach to the lumbar plexus.

5 The needle insertion site described by Winnie and colleagues is at the intersection of the intercristal line and the paramedian line from the PSIS (Figure 17.32). The needle bevel is oriented caudally and laterally, directed along the course of the plexus and away from the epidural and subarachnoid spaces.

6 Prepare the area with an antiseptic solution and anesthetize the insertion site with a subcutaneous infiltration of local anesthetic.

7 The nerve stimulator is set to deliver 1.0–1.5 mA and a 4-inch (100 mm) stimulating needle is inserted perpendicular to all planes (taking into account the forward tilt of the patient).

8 This should place the needle tip between the transverse processes of L4 and L5. The plexus should be sought at an approximate depth of 7–9 cm. The depth of the plexus is correlated to body-mass index and tends to be deeper in men than women.[100]

9 If no twitch is obtained and there is no contact with bone, the needle should be withdrawn and redirected 10°–15° medially.

10 If the transverse process is contacted, the needle should be withdrawn toward skin and redirected 10°–15° caudally. The plexus should be sought at a depth no more than 2 cm past the transverse process.

11 If no twitch is obtained, the needle should be withdrawn and redirected cephalad, above the transverse process.

12 Motor response of the quadriceps and associated snap of the patellar tendon at a current of 0.3–0.5 mA is the objective endpoint.

13 Once the desired contraction is achieved and after negative aspiration, 30 mL of local anesthetic (ropivacaine [0.5%] or mepivacaine [1.5%]) is injected. One milliliter of local anesthetic should result in abolition of the muscle twitch. If this does not occur the injection of local anesthetic should be stopped as the needle may be intravascular or within a dural sleeve.

14 The local anesthetic is injected in 5-mL aliquots followed by aspiration for blood. Epinephrine (1:400 000) is routinely added to the solution to serve as an intravascular marker. The addition of epinephrine may also reduce the absorption of the local anesthetic, thus reducing the potential for central nervous system and cardiovascular toxicity, and may lengthen the block duration with shorter acting local anesthetics.

15 There are obvious benefits from the prolonged analgesia that can be provided with a continuous lumbar plexus catheter, including decreased opioid consumption, decreased nausea and vomiting, decreased pruritus, earlier ambulation, improved patient satisfaction, and accelerated recovery after surgery.[97,102,103]

Stimulating or nonstimulating catheters may be placed via a stimulating Tuohy needle. If a stimulating catheter is used the space may be dilated with dextrose (D5W) prior to catheter placement. The catheter is advanced 4–8 cm past the tip of the needle.

Ultrasound Guidance

The limits of current portable ultrasound technology often make visualization of nerves of the lumbar plexus difficult or impossible, except in the thinnest of patients or in pediatric patients.[104] The location of the plexus just anterior to the bony transverse processes, which do not permit the transmission of ultrasound waves, is a major limiting factor in the utility of ultrasound for this technique. The depth of the nerves, particularly in obese patients, is another limitation. As a result, real-time ultrasound-guided psoas compartment blocks are often not practical and not widely used. By scanning with a low-frequency probe, however, one can often visualize important surrounding structures, including the vertebral bodies, spinous processes, transverse processes, and kidney. These structures can provide a guide for proper needle insertion site and expected depth to the transverse process and lumbar plexus.[105–107]

Complications

The lack of mainstream enthusiasm for the psoas compartment block is likely from the fact that it is a deep block that is technically more challenging than many of the other peripheral nerve blocks. This is a technique that should be employed only after appropriate training and many anesthesiologists have had little or no exposure to this technique during their training. Grant et al[108] showed that even in institutions that use this technique on a regular basis, there was much greater variability among those with less experience in the ability to identify the appropriate landmarks.

Because of the deep needle placement into the body of the psoas muscle there is risk for vascular puncture and hematoma. There have been case reports of large retroperitoneal hematomas with this block. This, along with the larger volumes of local anesthetic that are generally used, increases the potential for systemic toxicity. The close relation of the roots of the lumbar plexus to the epidural space and the extension of dural sleeves out along the nerve roots carries the risk of epidural or subarachnoid spread of local anesthetic. Spread of local anesthetic to the epidural space may occur in as many as 15% of patients and results in bilateral lower extremity sympathectomy and resultant hypotension. These risks necessitate careful selection of the local anesthetic to be administered as well as the dose to be given.

Pearls

- Ensure the spine is properly aligned and not overrotated.
- Appropriate sedation is necessary as this procedure can be uncomfortable because of multiple factors, including needle contact with periosteum, needle passage through muscles, and nerve stimulation. This is best started after patient positioning and prior to marking the anatomical landmarks, as sedation may then be sufficiently titrated.
- Always use bony landmarks rather than skin folds, which can be misleading, particularly in obese patients.
- It is best to palpate the iliac crest with the palpating hand on the pelvis and the fingertips pressing down on the crest.
- If one has difficulty palpating PSIS, it is often helpful to palpate the edge of the pelvis from the iliac crest posteriorly and caudally to the point of the PSIS.
- The paramedian line from the PSIS is approximately 6–7 cm from midline in the average patient.
- Remember to account for the forward tilt of the patient when directing the needle.
- The landmarks of Winnie often result in an entry point that is too lateral. This can be overcome with medial angulation of the needle; however, this may carry a higher incidence of epidural spread of local anesthetic. Capdevila et al have

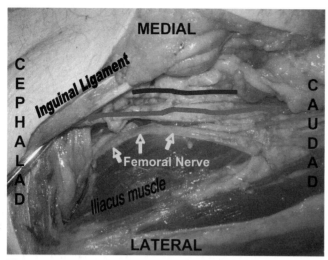

Figure 17.33: Femoral nerve lying on top of iliacus muscle as it passes under the inguinal ligament. Key: blue line = femoral vein; red line = femoral artery. See color plates.

suggested a modified approach based on anatomical studies. Rather than using the intersection of the paramedian line and the intercristal line, their modified insertion point is the junction of the medial two-thirds and lateral one-third of the intercristal line between midline and Winnie's insertion site. In the average patient the paramedian line is approximately 6 cm from midline. Two-thirds of that distance, or 4 cm from midline in the average patient, would be the insertion site for the modified approach described by Capdevila. Many clinicians therefore simply mark the midline and the intercristal line with an insertion site 4 cm from midline on the intercristal line. It is important to note that there is potential for error in outlying patients when using predetermined distances rather than patient-specific landmarks.[100]

- If local twitch of the paraspinous muscles is obtained, the needle tip is too shallow and should be advanced further.
- If hamstring twitches are obtained the needle is in contact with the sacral plexus. The needle should be withdrawn and angled more lateral or more cephalad.
- Presence of muscle stimulation after injection of local anesthetic likely represents intravascular injection or misplacement of the needle tip within a dural sleeve. The injection should be stopped and the needle repositioned.
- Avoid fast injection of local anesthetic and injection under high pressure, which have been associated with nerve injury.

FEMORAL NERVE BLOCKADE

Winnie et al described the 3-in-1 block as an inguinal paravascular approach to the lumbar plexus in 1973, 1 year before describing the posterior approach to the lumbar plexus. A number of studies have since called into question the reality of the 3-in-1 block, showing inconsistent results in the ability to obtain blockade of the obturator and lateral femoral cutaneous nerves in addition to the femoral nerve[85,87,109–112] In 1997 Marhoffer et al[113] first described how the use of ultrasound may improve on well-established techniques for femoral nerve blockade.

A femoral nerve block provides anesthesia and analgesia to the anterior thigh, femur, knee, and medial lower leg and foot.

Anesthesia of the entire leg from the level of the middle of the thigh can be achieved when combined with a sciatic nerve block. Despite the inability to consistently obtain blockade of all three of the nerves as with the posterior approach to the lumbar plexus, the femoral nerve block is a relatively basic technique with a high success rate, low incidence of complications, and broad clinical utility for both surgical anesthesia and postoperative analgesia. As such, it is no surprise that it is the most common lower extremity nerve block performed.[114]

The femoral nerve originates from the ventral rami of the L2–L4 nerve roots and is the largest terminal branch of the lumbar plexus. The femoral nerve lies flat on the iliacus muscle as it exits the pelvis under the inguinal ligament (Figure 17.33). At the level of the inguinal crease the orientation of the neurovascular structures can be remembered by the acronym "NAVEL." The orientation, from lateral to medial, is femoral nerve, artery, vein, empty space, lymphatics. The femoral nerve lies deep to two fascial planes, the fascia lata and the fascia iliaca. The nerve is located approximately 1–2 cm or, perhaps more accurately, 1 patient thumb width[115] lateral to the artery and is separated from the artery medially by the ligamentum iliopectineus. A triangle is formed by the ligamentum iliopectineus medially, the fascia lata superficially, and the iliacus muscle deep to the nerve. The femoral nerve is located within this triangular boundary, which is an important concept for ultrasound guided femoral nerve blocks.

Several studies looked at the potential benefits of femoral nerve block for knee arthroscopy. Patel et al[116] compared femoral nerve block to general anesthesia and showed a high patient acceptance, decreased need for analgesics in the postanesthesia care unit (PACU), and decreased hospital length of stay.

Other studies did not show a great advantage offered by femoral nerve block for knee arthroscopy, likely because of the minimally invasive nature and relatively low pain scores associated with the procedure.[117–121]

When used for a more invasive procedure, such as ACL repair, a femoral nerve block has been associated with improved analgesia for up to 23 hours postoperatively, decreased opioid use, and facilitated hospital discharge.[122–125] Similar results have been obtained with catheter based techniques.[126] There are, however, other reports in the literature of femoral nerve block for ACL repair that have failed to show similar benefits[127,128] It has been postulated that this may be in part because of the fact that a sciatic nerve block is needed in addition to a femoral nerve block to provide posterior coverage[129,130] Williams et al[131] compared a regional technique with a femoral and sciatic nerve block to general anesthesia for ACL repair in an ambulatory surgical center setting. In addition to the reduced pain and opioid requirements that other studies have shown, they found increased PACU bypass and same-day discharge with a regional technique. In their center, where they perform 250 ACL repairs in 1 year, they estimated an annual cost savings of $98 613.

Perhaps the procedure for which the femoral nerve block is most widely used and has the most clinical utility is the TKA. Ng et al demonstrated the analgesic benefits of even a single-shot femoral nerve block.[132] Studies have shown that, compared to IV PCA, a continuous femoral nerve block may result in lower pain scores, reduced opioid requirements, decreased incidence of side effects, earlier hospital discharge, improved rehabilitation, and increased joint range of motion.[133–136] When compared to neuraxial techniques, a continuous femoral nerve catheter has shown to provide similar analgesia with fewer side effects.[134,135,137,138] As with continuous femoral nerve catheters for ACL repair, there are studies that have failed to show benefits of a continuous peripheral nerve catheter for TKA.[139] Again, it has been speculated that this lack of benefit may be due to pain in a sciatic nerve or perhaps even obturator or lateral femoral cutaneous nerve distribution.

Excellent results have been obtained when combining a femoral nerve block with a sciatic nerve block for TKA. Cook et al reported that the addition of a single shot sciatic nerve block to a femoral nerve block resulted in improved analgesia and decreased opioid requirements.[140] By adding a sciatic nerve catheter in addition to a femoral nerve catheter investigators have demonstrated prolonged analgesia and lower pain scores.[141,142] When compared to epidural analgesia, a combined sciatic nerve block resulted in decreased opioid consumption, decreased incidence of PONV, and earlier hospital discharge.[143] A combined femoral-sciatic block has also resulted in lower pain scores and reduced opioid consumption compared to a spinal anesthetic with intravenous opioids for postoperative analgesia.[144,145] The good safety profile and relative ease of performance of the femoral nerve block make it an excellent and popular choice for analgesia after surgery on the femur and knee. With the increasing number of patients undergoing knee surgery and the intense pain associated with these surgeries the utilization of the femoral nerve block is likely only to increase in the years to come.

Techniques

Blockade of the femoral nerve can be accomplished via landmarks, paraesthesia, nerve stimulation, and ultrasound guidance, either alone or in combination. There are several studies showing evidence for the clinical superiority of ultrasound guidance over other techniques. Marhofer et al found that ultrasound guidance improves sensory block, hastens onset time, and reduces the amount of local anesthetic necessary for femoral nerve blocks.[113,146] Casati et al[48] reported a 42% reduction in the minimum amount of ropivacaine (0.5%) to achieve femoral nerve blockade with ultrasound guidance compared to a peripheral nerve stimulation technique.

Nerve Stimulator Technique

1 Position the patient in the supine position with the legs extended.
2 Identify the femoral crease.
3 Palpate and mark the location of the femoral artery in the femoral crease.
4 Mark a needle insertion site 1–2 cm, or one patient thumbbreadth,[115] lateral to the femoral artery in the femoral crease.
5 Prepare the area with an antiseptic solution and anesthetize the insertion site with a subcutaneous infiltration of local anesthetic.
6 The nerve stimulator is set to deliver 1.0 to 1.5 mA.
7 With one hand palpating the artery, insert a 2-inch (50-mm) needle in the sagital plane with a slight cephalad angulation.
8 Twitch of the quadriceps muscle resulting in cephalad movement of the patella (patellar snap) at a current of 0.2 to 0.5 mA is the goal motor response.
9 Once the desired contraction is achieved and after negative aspiration, 20 mL of local anesthetic (ropivacaine [0.5%] or Mepivacaine [1.5%]) is injected. One milliliter of local anesthetic should result in abolition of the muscle twitch. If

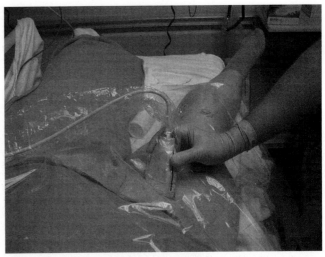

Figure 17.34: Probe positioning for ultrasound guided femoral nerve block.

this does not occur the injection of local anesthetic should be stopped as the needle tip may be intravascular.
10 The local anesthetic is injected in 5-mL aliquots followed by aspiration for blood. Epinephrine (1:400 000) is routinely added to the solution to serve as an intravascular marker. The addition of epinephrine may also reduce the absorption of the local anesthetic, thus reducing the potential for central nervous system and cardiovascular toxicity, and may lengthen the block duration with shorter acting local anesthetics.
11 One may place a continuous femoral nerve catheter, which have resulted in improved and prolonged analgesia, decreased opioid requirements, reduced incidence of side effects, decreased hospital stay, and improved postoperative rehabilitation and joint mobilization.[133–136]

Ultrasound-Guided Technique

The femoral nerve has a much more superficial location, allowing for real-time ultrasound-guided nerve blockade.[113,146–149]

1 Position the patient supine with the ultrasound machine positioned opposite the side to be blocked (Figure 17.34).
2 Place a high-frequency linear probe on the operative leg in an axial plane at the level of the inguinal crease (Figure 17.34).
3 Locate the femoral vein and artery, with the artery lateral to the vein. Color Doppler and occlusion of the vein by pressure applied with the probe can help to identify the femoral vessels.
4 Scan proximally and distally on the leg to identify the split of the femoral artery into the common femoral artery, profunda femoral artery, and lateral circumflex femoral artery (Figure 17.35). Once the arterial division is identified, scan proximally to find a view of the artery and vein cephalad to the arterial division.
5 The femoral nerve lies approximately 1–2 cm lateral to the artery. The nerve lies on top of the iliacus muscle and deep to the fascia lata and fascia iliaca (Figures 17.33 and 17.36). It is contained within a triangular-shaped fascial sheath formed by the ligamentum iliopectineus that separates the artery medially, the fascia lata superficially, and the iliacus muscle

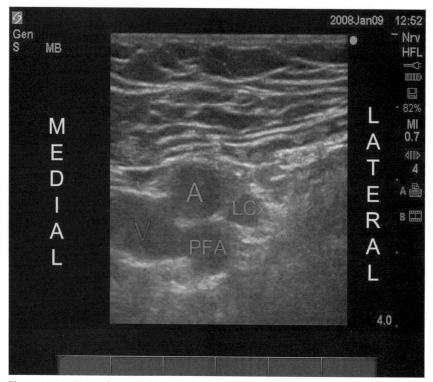

Figure 17.35: Femoral vessels distal to arterial divisions, at the level of a classic, landmark based approach. Abbreviations: V = femoral vein; A = femoral artery; PFA = profunda femoral artery; LCx = lateral circumflex femoral artery.

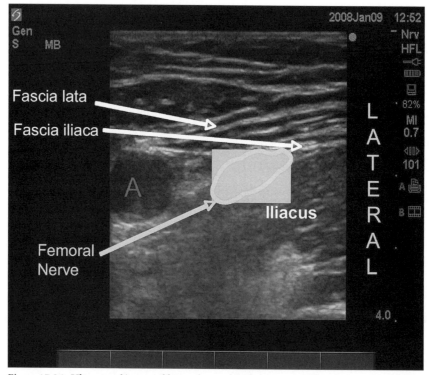

Figure 17.36: Ultrasound image of femoral nerve block anatomy. Abbreviation: A = femoral artery.

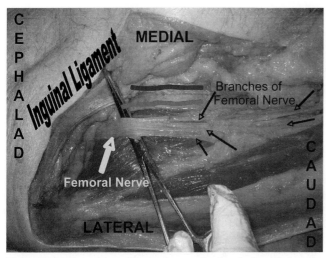

Figure 17.37: Branching of femoral nerve distal to the inguinal crease. Key: blue line = femoral vein; red line = femoral artery. See color plates.

deep to the nerve. The nerve lies directly on the iliacus muscle at the level of the inguinal crease and appears as a hyperechoic density (Figure 17.36). The fasica iliaca lies on top of both the iliacus muscle and the femoral nerve. Occasionally, the nerve itself can be difficult to visualize prior to the injection of local anesthetic, at which point it becomes more clearly delineated.

6 The femoral nerve branches as it courses distally down the leg from the level of the inguinal ligament (Figure 17.37). The motor branch of the femoral nerve, which, when stimulated, produces the classic quadriceps contraction and cephalad movement of the patella, or "patellar snap," is usually located laterally within the nerve and laterally within the fascial triangle.

7 Prepare the area with an antiseptic solution and anesthetize the insertion site with a subcutaneous infiltration of local anesthetic.

8 A 2-inch (50-mm) block needle can be inserted in line with the ultrasound beam, as with the upper extremity blocks (Figure 17.34) or, alternatively, the needle may be inserted perpendicular to the probe. Although in-line needle orientation allows for visualization of the needle tip at all times, a perpendicular orientation may allow for technically easier block placement, especially when performing a continuous catheter technique. The needle should be repositioned under ultrasound guidance as necessary to ensure local anesthetic spread within the triangular sheath surrounding the nerve. It is important to visualize spread of local anesthetic deep to the fascia iliaca.

Complications

As with all peripheral nerve blocks, complications such as local anesthetic toxicity and nerve injury have been associated with the femoral nerve block; however, the superficial location of the femoral nerve in the inguinal crease, the compressibility of the nearby vessels, and its distance from the spinal cord and vital organs make it a relatively safe peripheral nerve block with few complications. One of the most common concerns with a continuous femoral nerve block is the possibility of infection. In a large,

multicenter, prospective analysis of 1 416 continuous catheters at various sites, including but not limited to femoral catheters, Capdevila et al found colonization of 28.7% of the catheters overall. The median duration of catheters was 56 hours. Rate of actual local inflammatory signs was only 3%. There were no serious infectious complications other than one case of a psoas abscess in a diabetic patient. Risk factors for local inflammation and infection included stay in an intensive care unit postoperatively, catheter duration greater than 48 hours, male sex, and lack of antibiotic prophylaxis. From this analysis and from central line data, it may be prudent to limit the duration of a femoral catheter to 48 hours, with close monitoring of catheters left in longer than 48 hours.[150] As with other lower extremity nerve blocks there is a risk of falling postoperatively due to a weak or insensate limb.[151] Vascular puncture and hematoma are another set of possible complications.[152] The compressibility of the femoral vessels, however, makes this complication less of an issue compared to the posterior approach to the lumbar plexus.

Pearls

- Use the mnemonic NAVEL to remember the orientation of the neurovascular structures from lateral to medial.
- In obese patients it is important to optimize patient positioning and exposure of the inguinal crease. Placing a "bump" of sheets or pillows under the hips may help to bring the artery more superficial for landmark techniques. For ultrasound or landmark techniques, the pannus can be retracted superiorly and out of the field and held in place with several large pieces of two inch silk tape attached to the contralateral bed rail.
- For stimulation techniques, some operators prefer to stand facing the patient's feet, resting the hand on the ASIS. This allows the person performing the block to stabilize his or her hand without interference from the contracting quadriceps muscles. It also allows easy visualization of the quadriceps contractions.
- The goal twitch for stimulator techniques is quadriceps contraction resulting in cephalad movement of the patella, or "patellar snap," at a current less than 0.5 mA. Have an assistant place a hand on the patellar tendon below the patella to ensure proper twitch response.
- Often times contraction of the sartorius muscle may be elicited (Figure 17.38). This results in a contraction of the straplike muscle from the ASIS laterally, across the thigh, to the medial aspect of the knee. This can be misleading, as it can mean one of three things:
  1 The needle tip is too superficial and eliciting stimulation of the anterior branch of the femoral nerve, which innervates the sartorius. The needle should be advanced deeper.
  2 The needle tip is in the sartorius muscle itself at a level proximal to where the sartorius crosses the femoral nerve, causing direct muscle stimulation. The needle should be withdrawn and directed medially.
  3 The needle tip is in the sartorius muscle at a level distal to where the sartorius crosses the femoral nerve, causing direct muscle stimulation. The needle should be withdrawn and directed laterally.
- When using a stimulation technique, keep the fingertips of the palpating hand on the femoral artery.

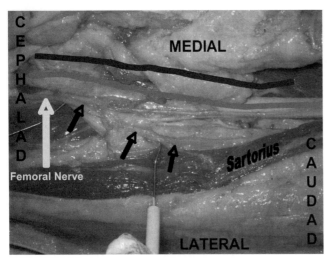

Figure 17.38: Relation of sartorious muscle to femoral nerve. Key: black arrows = anterior branch of femoral nerve to sartorius muscle; top line = femoral vein; bottom line = femoral artery.

- If blood is aspirated the needle tip has likely punctured the femoral vein or artery or one of the arterial branches. The needle should be withdrawn and reinserted 1 cm laterally.
- When using an ultrasound-guided technique, ensure the spread of local anesthesia below the fascia iliaca.

BLOCKS OF THE SACRAL PLEXUS

Sciatic Nerve Block

The sciatic nerve is the main nerve of the sacral plexus, formed from the L4–S3 nerve roots. It gives off the posterior cutaneous nerve of the thigh shortly after exiting the sciatic foramen and then branches into the tibial and peroneal nerves in the popliteal fossa. The sciatic nerve can be blocked at a number of locations by a wide variety of approaches, both proximally and distally. Some of the most commonly employed and most clinically useful techniques for blocking the sciatic nerve are the classic sciatic (Labat) approach and ultrasound-guided infragluteal sciatic nerve block proximally and the popliteal and ultrasound-guided popliteal sciatic nerve blocks distally.

Classic Sciatic (Labat)

NERVE STIMULATOR TECHNIQUE

1 Position the patient with the operative side up in the lateral decubitus position, tilted slightly forward, with the operative leg flexed slightly more than the dependant leg and the operative foot resting on the dependant leg. This is also known as the Sim's position.
2 Palpate and mark the greater trochanter of the femur (Figure 17.39).
3 Palpate and mark the PSIS. Draw a line connecting the PSIS and the greater trochanter (Figure 17.40).
4 Palpate and mark the sacral hiatus. Draw a line connecting the sacral hiatus and the greater trochanter (Figure 17.40).
5 From the midpoint of the line connecting the greater trochanter and PSIS drawn in step 3, draw a perpendicular line in the caudad direction. Where this line intersects the line from the sacral hiatus to the greater trochanter is

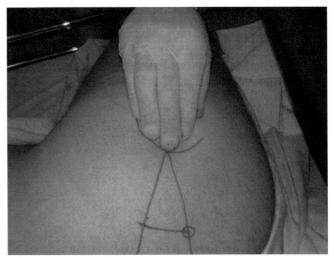

Figure 17.39: Palpation of the apex of the greater trochanter of femur.

marked as the needle insertion site. This should be approximately 4–6 cm along the perpendicular bisecting line (Figure 17.40).
6 Prepare the area with an antiseptic solution and anesthetize the insertion site with a subcutaneous infiltration of local anesthetic.
7 Set the nerve stimulator to deliver 1.0 to 1.5 mA.
8 Insert a 4-inch (100-mm) needle perpendicular to all planes.
9 The expected depth of the sciatic nerve is 6 to 8 cm.
10 As the needle is advanced, local contraction of the gluteus and piriformis muscles are observed prior to reaching the sciatic nerve.
11 Stimulation of the sciatic nerve may result in twitches in the hamstring, calf, foot, or toes. Stimulation of the tibial component of the sciatic nerve resulting in plantarflexion of the toes at a current of 0.2 to 0.5 mA will yield the best results.

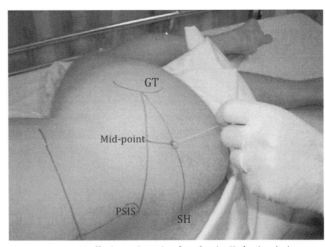

Figure 17.40: Needle insertion site for classic (Labat) sciatic nerve block. A line is dropped perpendicularly from the midpoint of the line joining the posterior-superior iliac spine and the greater trochanter. Four to five centimeters along this line is the point of needle insertion. The line joining the sacral hiatus and greater trochanter transects this point. Abbreviations: PSIS = posterior-superior iliac spine; GT = greater trochanter; SH = sacral hiatus.

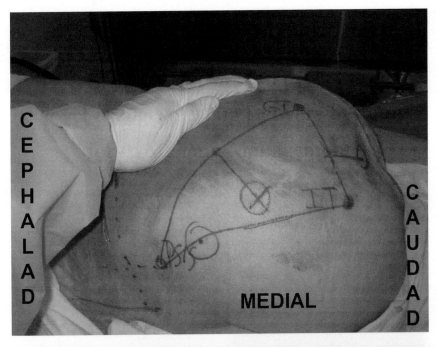

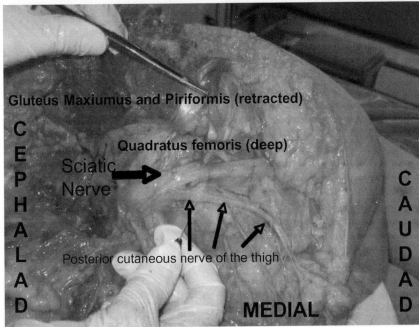

Figure 17.41: Sciatic nerve cadaver anatomy. (Above) Landmarks showing approximate insertion sites for parasacral (Maseur), classic (Labat), and Raj sciatic nerve blocks. (Below) Dissection reveals proximal takeoff of the posterior cutaneous nerve of the thigh.

12 Once the desired contraction is achieved and after negative aspiration, 20 mL of local anesthetic (ropivacaine [0.5%] or mepivacaine [1.5%]) is injected. One milliliter of local anesthetic should result in abolition of the muscle twitch. If this does not occur the injection of local anesthetic should be stopped as the needle tip may be intravascular.

13 The local anesthetic is injected in 5-mL aliquots followed by aspiration for blood. Epinephrine (1:400 000) may be added to the solution to serve as an intravascular marker. The addition of epinephrine may also reduce the absorption of the local anesthetic, thus reducing the potential for central nervous system and cardiovascular toxicity, and may lengthen the block duration with shorter acting local anesthetics. Some argue the avoidance of epinephrine for sciatic nerve blockade as the epinephrine may compromise the blood supply to the nerve, increasing the risk of nerve damage.

14 A continuous sciatic nerve catheter may be placed for prolonged analgesia

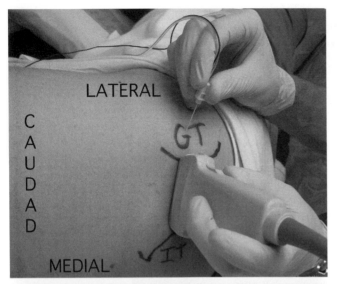

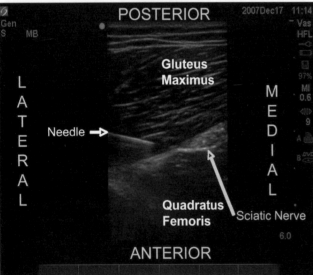

Figure 17.42: Probe positioning, needle insertion site, and ultrasound appearance of an ultrasound-guided subgluteal sciatic nerve block.

PEARLS

■ Mark the inner boundaries of the bony landmarks so that the line connecting them is as short as possible.

■ Local contraction of the gluteus and piriformis muscles is a good sign the needle is being advanced in the correct direction. If contraction of these muscles is not present the needle entry point or direction may need adjusting.

■ If contraction of the hamstrings is elicited the needle tip is likely too medial and should be withdrawn and redirected 5° more laterally along the perpendicular bisecting line.

■ If eversion of the foot or dorsiflexion of the foot and toes is obtained the needle tip is likely too lateral. The needle should be withdrawn and redirected 5° more medially along the perpendicular bisecting line.

■ If blood is aspirated the needle tip may have punctured the inferior gluteal artery and should be withdrawn and directed laterally.

Infragluteal Sciatic
ULTRASOUND-GUIDED TECHNIQUE

1 Position the patient in the Sim's position as described above.
2 Palpate and mark the greater trochanter of the femur and the ischial tuberosity (Figure 17.42).
3 Place a low frequency ultrasound probe transversely between the greater trochanter and ischial tuberosity and scan in an axial plane.
4 Identify the greater trochanter as the hyperechoic semicircle located laterally.
5 Identify the ischial tuberosity as the hyperechoic semicircle located medially.
6 Identify the fibers of the gluteus maximus muscles running between the greater trochanter and ischial tuberosity (Figure 17.42).
7 The sciatic nerve lies between the two bony structures and between the anterior border of the gluteus maximus superficially and the posterior border of the quadratus femoris deep. It appears as a hyperechoic oval-shaped density (Figure 17.42).
8 Prepare the area with an antiseptic solution and anesthetize the insertion site with a subcutaneous infiltration of local anesthetic.
9 Use a 4- to 6-inch (100- to 150-mm) needle depending on patient size and depth of the nerve. The block needle should be inserted in line with the ultrasound beam. A lateral approach will be easier ergonomically and has the benefit of decreasing the likelihood of puncturing the inferior gluteal artery.
10 A nerve stimulator may be used to provide confirmation that the needle is within close proximity of the sciatic nerve.
11 Once the position of the needle tip is satisfactory, aspirate to ensure the needle is not intravascular and then inject 20 mL of local anesthetic (ropivacaine [0.5%] or mepivacaine [1.5%]) in incremental doses. One milliliter of local anesthetic should result in abolition of the muscle twitch if using a nerve stimulator. The needle should be repositioned under ultrasound guidance as necessary to ensure circumferential spread of local anesthetic around the sciatic nerve.[153,154]

PEARLS

■ If the sciatic nerve is not immediately visible, first identify the bony landmarks as reference points. The sciatic nerve lies between these two landmarks.

■ Tilting and rocking the probe may make the nerve more visible. This is an ultrasound property known as anisotropy.

■ To help confirm that a potential target is the sciatic nerve attempt to trace it with the ultrasound probe along its course down the leg into the popliteal fossa.

■ Insert the needle a few centimeters lateral from the edge of the probe to allow for a more-shallow needle-probe angle and better needle visualization.

Popliteal Sciatic
TECHNIQUES
NERVE STIMULATOR TECHNIQUE

1 The patient is positioned prone. The foot on the operative side should be hanging off the bed or the leg elevated on a pillow so the foot is free to move in response to neurostimulation.

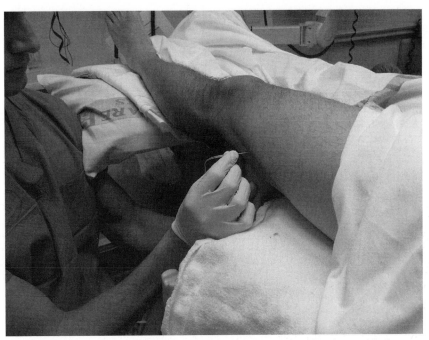

Figure 17.43: Supine positioning for ultrasound-guided popliteal nerve block.

2 Mark the popliteal fossa crease.

3 Mark a line along the tendon of the biceps femoris laterally.

4 Mark a line along the tendon of the semimembranosus and semitendinosus medially.

5 The needle insertion site is marked at the midpoint between the tendons of the biceps femoris and the semimembranosus and semitendinosus at a point 7-cm cephalad from the popliteal crease.

6 Prepare the area with an antiseptic solution and anesthetize the insertion site with a subcutaneous infiltration of local anesthetic.

7 Set the nerve stimulator to deliver 1.0 to 1.5 mA.

8 Insert a 2-inch (50-mm) needle perpendicular to all planes.

9 The expected depth of the sciatic nerve is 3 to 5 cm.

10 Stimulation of the sciatic nerve in the popliteal fossa may result in twitches in the calf, foot, or toes. Stimulation of the tibial component of the sciatic nerve resulting in plantarflexion of the toes at a current of 0.2 to 0.5 mA will yield the highest success rate.

11 Once the desired contraction is achieved and after negative aspiration, 30–40 mL of local anesthetic (ropivacaine [0.5%] or mepivacaine [1.5%]) is injected. One milliliter of local anesthetic should result in abolition of the muscle twitch. If this does not occur the injection of local anesthetic should be stopped as the needle tip may be intravascular.

12 The local anesthetic is injected in 5-mL aliquots followed by aspiration for blood. Epinephrine (1:400 000) may be added to the solution to serve as an intravascular marker. The addition of epinephrine may also reduce the absorption of the local anesthetic, thus reducing the potential for central nervous system and cardiovascular toxicity, and may lengthen the block duration with shorter acting local anesthetics. Some argue the avoidance of epinephrine for sciatic nerve blockade as the epinephrine may compromise the blood supply to the nerve, increasing the risk of nerve damage.

13 A continuous sciatic nerve catheter may be placed for prolonged analgesia.

PEARLS

■ Elevate the leg on a pillow to allow free movement of the foot as well as to aid in the identification of the popliteal crease and tendons.

■ Local twitches of the hamstring muscles are a sign that the needle insertion site is too medial when semitendinosus or semimembranosus contractions are observed or too lateral when biceps femorus contractions are observed.

■ If stimulation of the peroneal branch of the sciatic nerve is obtained the needle should be withdrawn and redirected slightly medially. If stimulation of the tibial component is not achieved with very small changes in needle position this may be a sign that the needle entry point is below the division of the sciatic nerve. One may attempt to stimulate and block the branches separately or change the needle insertion site a few centimeters more proximally up the leg.

■ Aspiration of blood likely indicated puncture of the popliteal artery or vein and is an indication that the needle insertion is too deep and/or medial.

■ It may be impossible to elicit muscle twitches at a current of less than 0.5 mA in patients with diabetes, peripheral vascular disease, or peripheral neuropathy. In this subset of patients it is advisable to change to a higher current (2–3 mA) and accept a higher current as an end point if initial attempts do not produce a motor response.

ULTRASOUND-GUIDED TECHNIQUE

1 The patient may be positioned prone, lateral, or supine (Figures 17.43, 17.44, and 17.45). If the patient is positioned supine, the operative leg may be elevated on a support stand.

2 Place a linear, high-frequency ultrasound probe transversely in the popliteal crease. Scan in the axial plane.

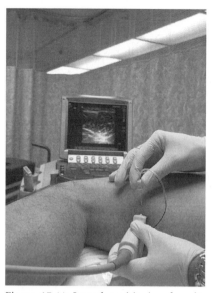
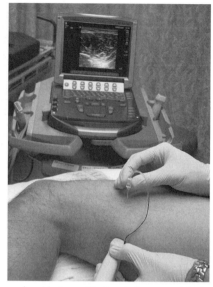

Figure 17.44: Lateral positioning for ultrasound-guided popliteal sciatic nerve block. (Left) Needle entry adjacent to probe. (Right) Lateral needle entry.

3 Attempt to locate the popliteal artery, which appears as a pulsatile, anechoic circle. The vein often lies posterior lateral (superficial) to the artery. Color flow Doppler and occluding pressure applied with the probe can be used for confirmation (Figure 17.46).

4 Posterior lateral to the artery and vein identify the tibial nerve, which often appears as a hyperechoic circle with hypoechoic honeycombing. The common peroneal nerve is located lateral to the tibial nerve (Figures 17.46 and 17.47).

5 By tracing these nerves proximally up the leg, the branch point of the sciatic nerve into the tibial and peroneal nerves can be located (Figure 17.47).

6 If the tibial and peroneal nerves are unable to be located in the popliteal fossa one can look for the sciatic nerve more proximally in the thigh, positioned at the apex of the intermuscular groove between the biceps femoris and semimembranosis and semitendonosis.

7 Prepare the area with an antiseptic solution and anesthetize the insertion site with a subcutaneous infiltration of local anesthetic.

8 A 4-inch (100-mm) needle is introduced from the lateral aspect of the thigh, in plane with the ultrasound beam. Alternatively, an out-of-plane needle approach may be used by directing the needle tangential to the ultrasound beam in a cephalad direction. Some practitioners prefer this approach when placing a continuous catheter.

9 A nerve stimulator may be used to provide confirmation that the needle is within close proximity of the sciatic nerve.

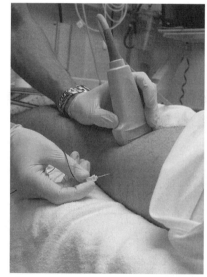
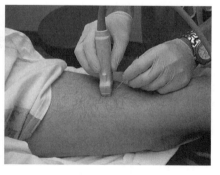

Figure 17.45: Prone positioning for ultrasound-guided popliteal sciatic nerve block. (Left) In-plane needle orientation. (Right) Out-of-plane needle orientation.

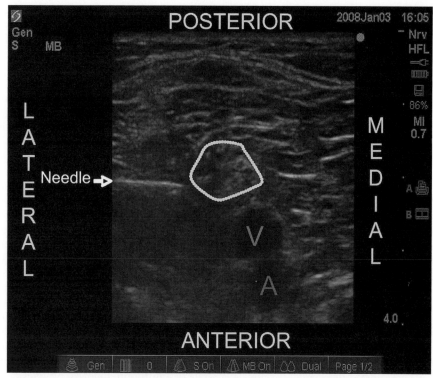

Figure 17.46: Ultrasound-guided lateral popliteal sciatic nerve block Abbreviations: V = vein; A = artery. Key: dotted yellow line = sciatic nerve proximal to division in popliteal fossa.

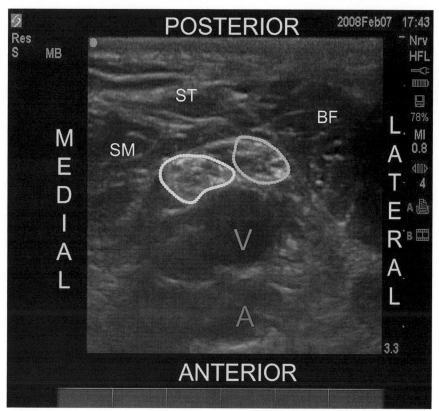

Figure 17.47: Division of sciatic nerve in popliteal fossa. Abbreviations: V = vein; A = artery; BF = biceps femoris; ST = semitendinosus; SM = semimembranosus. Key: left dotted line = tibial nerve; right dotted line = peroneal nerve.

10 Once the position of the needle tip is satisfactory, aspirate to ensure the needle is not intravascular and then inject 30 mL of local anesthetic (ropivacaine [0.5%] or mepivacaine [1.5%]) in incremental doses. One milliliter of local anesthetic should result in abolition of the muscle twitch if using a nerve stimulator. The needle should be repositioned under ultrasound guidance as necessary to ensure circumferential spread of local anesthetic around the sciatic nerve.[155–158]

PEARLS

- Squeezing the calf muscle while using color flow Doppler may help to visualize the popliteal vein.
- The division of the sciatic nerve is variable. Identifying the division of the nerve into the tibial and peroneal branches helps confirm the sciatic nerve.
- Changing the angle of incidence of the ultrasound probe may help to make the nerve more hyperechoic and therefore more visible under ultrasound.
- The nerve may be blocked anywhere along its course. Blocking the nerve more proximally requires less volume of local anesthetic and results in faster onset of nerve blockade.
- For more distal blocks, injecting local anesthetic at the point of the division of the nerve may maximize nerve surface area to local anesthetic and may hasten the onset of the block.

COMPLICATIONS

Many of the complications of other nerve blocks hold true for the sciatic nerve block. These include infection, vascular puncture, hematoma, local anesthetic toxicity, and nerve injury. One should keep in mind that the inferior gluteal artery runs along the medial side of the sciatic nerve at proximal injection sites and the popliteal artery and vein are in close proximity at the popliteal level. Perhaps more specific to the sciatic nerve block is the risk for postoperative fall resulting from foot drop and the associated gait disturbance.[151] Patients should be carefully evaluated and given specific instructions prior to receiving a sciatic nerve block to help avoid postoperative falls.

COMPLICATIONS OF PERIPHERAL NERVE BLOCKS

There are many complications that can occur when performing peripheral nerve blocks.[159,160] Insuring adequate training can reduce the occurrence of many of these complications. What is adequate training is in itself a difficult question to answer. How best to teach regional techniques and how many of each block is required to obtain an adequate level has been looked at in many studies. How to apply this in a residency program is extremely difficult to ascertain.

Complications have been listed under each block but we will focus on two important complications, namely local anesthetic toxicity and nerve injury.

Toxicity

Local Anesthetic Toxicity

The mechanism of action of most local anesthetics is via blockade of voltage-gated sodium channels of the peripheral neurons. Unfortunately, local anesthetic has the potential to block other important cellular structures, thus resulting in a variety of complications with central nervous system and cardiovascular toxicity being the two most important complications. Documented sites of toxic action include sodium,[161] potassium,[162] and calcium ion channels and the β-adrenergic and lysophosphatidate signaling pathways. Systemic toxic reactions to local anesthetics are manifested by a progressive spectrum of neurological symptoms as blood levels rise. The two most common causes for these complications are either direct intravascular injection of local anesthetic or an excessive total dose of local anesthetic. Direct intravascular injection of local anesthetic will result in these complications irrespective of the total dose injected. For example, a few milliliters of local anesthetic injected into the intervertebral artery when performing an interscalene block can result in seizures. Intravascular injection will normally result in the development of complications soon after injection and are more commonly associated with regional techniques in the neck. The seizures associated with this type of injection tend to be short lived as only small quantities of local anesthetic have been injected. In the case of an excessive local anesthetic dose the process first requires absorption of the local anesthetic from the subcutaneous tissue into the blood stream so the presentation may occur 20–30 minutes later. The concentration of local anesthetic in the bloodstream may remain elevated for a much longer period, resulting in prolonged convulsions. Classically, intercostal nerve blocks have the highest rate of absorption, followed by epidural blocks, brachial plexus blocks, and subcutaneous injection. When running continuous infusion of local anesthetic postoperatively it is important to be aware of the potential of toxicity if large doses of local anesthetics are being infused. The safe infusion rates of local anesthetic are not clearly defined.[163] It has been suggested that 400 and 800 mg of bupivacaine and ropivacaine, respectively, over a 24-hour period can be safely infused. Following a number of important steps when administrating any local anesthetic can reduce the potentials for these complications, with the restriction of the total dose being essential. The other important steps consist of using epinephrine (5–15 μg) in the local anesthetic, aspiration prior to injection, and slow incremental injections in 5-mL aliquots. The 5-mL aliquots should be injected over a period of 10 seconds followed by a delay of 40 seconds prior to continuing the local anesthetic injection. This will leave enough time for the effect of the epinephrine to occur. Further important steps that can be taken to reduce the potential for local anesthetic toxicity include the use of benzodiazepines for sedation that may increase the seizure threshold and the prevention of oversedation with the resultant hypercarbia that may lower seizure threshold. It is very important to be able to recognize an intravascular injection as soon as possible to reduce the dose of local anesthetic injected as well as to start resuscitative measures as soon as possible. Intravascular injection of local anesthetics with an epinephrine marker will result in the following potential changes: increase in heart rate and blood pressure and T wave changes on the electrocardiogram (EKG). In fact, especially in the elderly or patients on β-blockers, the EKG changes are the most reliable markers of intravascular injection. In most patients, a positive response to 15 μg of epinephrine is defined as an increase in heart rate by >15 bpm, increase in systolic blood pressure >15mmHg, or a 25% decrease in lead II T-wave amplitudes.

The risk of systemic toxicity following peripheral nerve blocks has been studied, and is now relatively uncommon. The major reason for the decrease in toxicity is probably related to the changes in practice introduced since Albright highlighted this issue in 1981. Auroy looked at complications of regional anesthesia in France. A total of 56 major complications in 158 083 regional anesthesia procedures were reported.[160] Most were related to neuroaxial techniques and only 1 death was related to a peripheral nerve block that was reported as a posterior lumbar plexus block. Auroy's rate was 7.5 systemic toxic reactions per 10 000 peripheral nerve blocks. Borgeat and Ekatodramis[164] found a frequency of 20 per 10 000 in brachial plexus blocks.

Central Nervous System Toxicity

Local anesthetics block the neurons of the central nervous system. Borgeat et al reported a frequency of central nervous system toxicity of 0.2% during interscalene nerve block.[164] The symptoms of central local anesthetic toxicity occur at a lower local anesthetic plasma concentration than the cardiovascular side effects thus can be a warning sign of impeding cardiovascular collapse. Symptoms and signs of central nervous toxicity will include tinnitus, perioral numbness, lightheadedness, dizziness, agitation, excitability, muscle twitching, and seizures. Treatment consists of stopping further injection of local anesthetic, ABC of resuscitation. The seizures can be terminated by the use of midazolam or even thiopentone if refractory. Propofol may be of some benefit in the management of the seizures produced by local anesthetic toxicity. It is important to observe for cardiovascular side effects such as ventricular arrhythmias in any patient with central nervous system excitation as this may be a prelude to cardiovascular collapse.

Cardiovascular Toxicity

In the cardiovascular system, local anesthetics block sodium channels and thus decrease the rate of nerve conduction in the Purkinje fibers and myocardium, as well as cause direct myocardial depression. Arrhythmias after local anesthetic overdose include conduction delays, from bundle branch block to complete heart block, sinus arrest or asystole. Ventricular ectopic beats can occur that may progress to ventricular tachycardia, torsades de pointes, and ventricular fibrillation. There have been multiple case reports of cardiac arrest and arrhythmias following bupivacaine injection. Many have been associated with difficult and prolonged resuscitation. This whole dilemma, highlighted by Albright in 1979,[165] followed multiple reports of women dying during delivery from cardiac arrest following the use of bupivacaine (0.75%). The cardiotoxicity of the aminoamides was shown to result from the R-enatiomer. The L-enatiomer has been shown to be less cardiotoxic and this led to the development of newer aminoamides, such as ropivacaine and L-bupivacaine, both pure L-enatiomers. Ropivacaine appears in clinical practice to be a safer alternative than bupivacaine when using large doses of local anesthetic to perform peripheral nerve blocks. There is some concern that the potency of ropivacaine is less than bupivacaine, so much so that higher doses of ropivacaine would be needed to obtain a comparable block to bupivacaine thus negating its safety.

Management of Local Anesthetic Toxicity

The management of local systemic toxicity is largely based on animal experiments and case reports. As in any cardiovascular resuscitation the ACLS guidelines should be followed, but it is important to realize that many of the drugs used in the ACLS may be deleterious in the setting of local anesthetic toxicity. Epinephrine can exacerbate arrhythmias associated with local anesthetic overdose.[166] Vasopressin has been added to the ACLS guidelines as an alternative to epinephrine and it may be useful if a vasopressor is required in resuscitation of local anesthetic toxicity.[167] Amiodarone is a primary drug in the ACLS management of arrhythmias. Amiodarone inhibits ion channels that are implicated in local anesthesia toxicity thus theoretically may be deleterious in local anesthetic toxicity management. However in an animal model, survival after bupivacaine-induced arrhythmias was higher with amiodarone than with placebo, but not statistically significant.[168] Lidocaine has been shown to be both beneficial and deleterious in the presence of bupivacaine-induced toxicity again giving further credence to use of amiodarone. Agents that should definitely be avoided include calcium channel blockers and phenytoin.

The use of 20% intralipid may be a new treatment of choice for local anesthetic toxicity.[25] Case reports of successful resuscitation in bupivacaine-induced cardiac arrests and animal studies have shown great promise in this area.[169] Two mechanisms of actions have been postulated with regard to the mode of action of intralipid in the management of local anesthetic toxicity. The intralipid may provide a lipid sink, into which bupivacaine is absorbed drawing the local anesthetic out of the myocardial cells. A second mechanism is the fact that it has been shown that bupivacaine inhibits the transport of fatty acids into the cardiac mitochondria. High fatty acid plasma concentrations may thus reverse such as inhibition. The current protocol for local anesthetic-induced cardiac toxicity that is unresponsive to standard therapy recommends an initial bolus of intralipid (20%) at 1.5 mL/kg over a minute, followed by an infusion at a rate of 0.25 mL/kg/min. The bolus can be repeated every 3 to 5 minutes up to a dose of 3 mL/kg. The infusion should be continued once circulation is restored. The infusion rate can be increased up to 0.5 mL/kg/min if hypotension persists. A total of dose of 8 mL/kg is recommended (http://www.lipidrescue.org).

Peripheral Nerve Injuries

It is believed that regional anesthesia is more prone to result in nerve damage than general anesthesia. However, looking at the closed claim reports of the American Society of Anesthesiologists database in 1980 and 1990 it was found that 60% of nerve injuries were related to general anesthesia.[170] The complications related to peripheral nerve blocks are rare, making it difficult to estimate the incidence of complications. The overall incidence of long-term nerve injury ranges between <0.02% and 0.4%.[171] Auroy in this study reported 4 neural lesions among 21 278 single-shot nerve blocks.[160] In a prospective study over a 1-year period, 1422 patients having a peripheral nerve block were followed for efficacy and complications. The overall incidence of postoperative neurological deficit in this study was 0,21%.[150]

Damage to the nerve may result from an ischemic injury, direct trauma, or neurotoxicity. Ischemia may be from generalized hypotension, as has been seen with some spinal cord lesions, but this is not a problem per se with regional anesthesia as this can occur in the presence of general anesthesia alone. Ischemia resulting directly from peripheral nerve blocks may be secondary because of external compression (hematoma) or internal compression (intraneural injection) causing a decrease in arterial perfusion of the nerve. Direct trauma to the nerve by the needle can result in neurological complications. The shape of the bevel and the presence of paraesthesia are two factors that may contribute to the incidence of nerve damage. It is felt that the elicitation of paraesthesia with the needle during the performance of the nerve block or during injection increases the incidence of persistent neurological complications. Whether the use of a nerve stimulator to find the nerve decreases the incidence of complications is unclear. It seems prudent to perform these peripheral nerve blocks on patients not under general anesthesia as this will allow the patient to report any paraesthesia during nerve replacement. The use of ultrasound to perform peripheral nerve blocks may change this thinking, but at this stage the evidence is not available. Short-beveled needles are also thought to reduce the incidence of complications. The type of local anesthetic, concentration, and duration of exposure may also cause neurological complications, as has been implicated with lidocaine (5%). The addition of epinephrine to local anesthetics in some animal models has shown to produce perfusion injuries to nerves but this has not been seen with the concentration (epinephrine [1/200 000–1/400 000]) of epinephrine commonly used in the performance of regional anesthesia.

The presentation of the nerve injury may occur soon after surgery up to 30 days after the procedure. The normal presentation is paraesthesia or dysathesia, with motor impairment being very uncommon. A full neurological examination is required to document the deficit. Further evaluation may consist of imaging techniques such as an MRI to exclude conditions such as hematomas that may be compressing the nerves. Neurophysiologic testing such as nerve conduction studies and electromyography may be useful to define the presence and extent of nerve injury as well as monitor the progress of the lesion. NSAIDs and drugs such as gabapentin or pregabalin may also be beneficial in the management of the symptoms related to the nerve damage.

REFERENCES

1. Marhofer P, Chan VW, Marhofer P, Chan VWS. Ultrasound-guided regional anesthesia: current concepts and future trends. *Anesth Analg.* 2007;104:1265–1269.
2. Rodgers A, Walker N, Schug S, et al. Reduction of postoperative mortality and morbidity with epidural or spinal anaesthesia: results from overview of randomised trials. *BMJ.* 2000;321:1493.
3. Reuben SS, Buvanendran A. Preventing the development of chronic pain after orthopaedic surgery with preventive multimodal analgesic techniques. *J Bone Joint Surg,* 2007;89:1343–1358.
4. Kehlet H, Jensen TS, Woolf CJ, Persistent postsurgical pain: risk factors and prevention. *Lancet.* 2006;367:1618–1625.
5. Apfelbaum JL, Chen C, Mehta SS, Gan TJ. Postoperative pain experience: results from a national survey suggest postoperative pain continues to be undermanaged. *Anesth Analg.* 2003;97:534–540.
6. Kehlet H, Dahl JB. Anaesthesia, surgery, and challenges in postoperative recovery. *Lancet.* 2003;362:1921–1928.
7. Kehlet H, Wilmore DW. Multimodal strategies to improve surgical outcome. *Am J Surg.* 2002;183:630–641.
8. Bresalier RS, Friedewald VE, Jr., Rakel RE, Roberts WC, Williams GW. The editor's roundtable: cyclooxygenase-2 inhibitors and cardiovascular risk. *Am J Cardiol.* 2005;96:1589–1604.
9. Bresalier RS, Sandler RS, Quan H, et al. Adenomatous polyp rrevention on Vioxx trial I: cardiovascular events associated with rofecoxib in a colorectal adenoma chemoprevention trial. *N Engl J Med.* 2005;352:1092–1102.
10. McGettigan P, Henry D. Cardiovascular risk and inhibition of cyclooxygenase: a systematic review of the observational studies of selective and nonselective inhibitors of cyclooxygenase 2. *JAMA.* 2006;296:1633–1644.
11. Meunier A, Aspenberg P. Parecoxib impairs early metaphyseal bone healing in rats. *Arch Orthopaed Trauma Surg.* 2006;126:433–436.
12. Reuben SS, Ekman EF. The effect of cyclooxygenase-2 inhibition on analgesia and spinal fusion. *J Bone Joint Surg.* 2005;87: 536–542.
13. Kong VK, Irwin MG: Gabapentin: a multimodal perioperative drug? *Br J Anaesth.* 2007;99:775–786.
14. Tiippana EM, Hamunen K, Kontinen VK, Kalso E: Do surgical patients benefit from perioperative gabapentin/pregabalin? A systematic review of efficacy and safety. *Anesth Analg.* 2007;104:1545–1556.
15. Seib RK, Paul JE. Preoperative gabapentin for postoperative analgesia: a meta-analysis. *Can J Anaesth.* 2006;53:461–469.
16. Reuben SS, Buvanendran A, Kroin JS, Raghunathan K. The analgesic efficacy of celecoxib, pregabalin, and their combination for spinal fusion surgery. *Anesth Analg.* 2006;103:1271–1277.
17. Freedman KB, Brookenthal KR, Fitzgerald RH, Jr, Williams S, Lonner JH. A meta-analysis of thromboembolic prophylaxis following elective total hip arthroplasty. *J Bone Joint Surg Am.* 2000;82-A:929–938.
18. Miric A, Lombardi P, Sculco TP. Deep vein thrombosis prophylaxis: a comprehensive approach for total hip and total knee arthroplasty patient populations. Am J Orthoped 2000;29:269–274.
19. Fitzgerald RH, Jr, Spiro TE, Trowbridge AA, et al. Prevention of venous thromboembolic disease following primary total knee arthroplasty. A randomized, multicenter, open-label, parallel-group comparison of enoxaparin and warfarin. *J Bone Joint Surg Am.* 2001;83-A:900–906.
20. Stern SH, Wixson RL, O'Connor D. Evaluation of the safety and efficacy of enoxaparin and warfarin for prevention of deep vein thrombosis after total knee arthroplasty. *J Arthroplasty.* 2000;15:153–158.
21. Hirsh J, Raschke R. Heparin and low-molecular-weight heparin: the Seventh ACCP Conference on Antithrombotic and Thrombolytic Therapy. *Chest.* 2004;126:188S–203S.
22. Vandermeulen E. Guidelines on anticoagulants and the use of LR anesthesia. *Acta Anaesthesiol Belg.* 2001;52:425–429.
23. Dolenska S. Neuroaxial blocks and LMWH thromboprophylaxis. *Hospital Med.* 1998;59:940–943.
24. Horlocker TT, Wedel DJ, Benzon H, et al. Regional anesthesia in the anticoagulated patient: defining the risks (the second ASRA Consensus Conference on Neuraxial Anesthesia and Anticoagulation). *Reg Anesth Pain Med.* 2003;28:172–197.
25. Weinberg G. Lipid infusion resuscitation for local anesthetic toxicity: proof of clinical efficacy. *Anesthesiology.* 2006;105:7–8.
26. Weinberg G. Lipid rescue resuscitation from local anaesthetic cardiac toxicity. *Toxicol Rev.* 2006;25:139–145.
27. Martin G, Lineberger CK, MacLeod DB, El-Moalem HE, Breslin DS, Hardman D, D'Ercole F. A new teaching model for resident training in regional anesthesia. *Anesth Analg.* 2002;95:1423–1427.
28. De Andres J, Sala-Blanch X. Peripheral nerve stimulation in the practice of brachial plexus anesthesia: a review. *Reg Anesth Pain Med.* 2001;26:478–483.
29. Neal JM, Hebl JR, Gerancher JC, et al. Brachial plexus anesthesia: essentials of our current understanding. *Reg Anesth Pain Med.* 2002;27:402–428.
30. Gray A. Ultrasound-guided regional anesthesia: current state of the art. *Anesthesiology.* 2006;104:368–373. [review]
31. Hadzic A. *Textbook of Regional Anesthesia and Acute Pain Management.* 1st ed. New York, NY: McGraw-Hill Medical; 2007.

32. Agur A, Dalley A. *Grant's Atlas of Anatomy*. 11th ed. New York, NY: Lippincott Williams & Wilkins; 2004.

33. Clemente C. *Anatomy: A Regional Atlas of the Human Body*. 5th ed. New York, NY: Lippincott Williams & Wilkins; 2006.

34. Meier G, Buettner J. *Peripheral Regional Anesthesia: An Atlas of Anatomy and Techniques*. Stuttgart: Thieme Medical Publishers; 2007.

35. Partridge B, Katz J, Benirschke K. Functional anatomy of the brachial plexus sheath: implications for anesthesia. *Anesthesiology*. 1987;66:743–747.

36. Winnie AP, Ramamurthy S, Durrani Z, Radonjic R. Interscalene cervical plexus block: a single-injection technic. *Anesth Analg*. 1975;54:370–375.

37. Bishop JY, Sprague M, Gelber J, Krol M, Rosenblatt MA, Gladstone J, Flatow EL. Interscalene regional anesthesia for shoulder surgery. *J Bone Joint Surg*. 2005;87:974–979.

38. Ritchie ED, Tong D, Chung F, Norris AM, Miniaci A, Vairavanathan SD. Suprascapular nerve block for postoperative pain relief in arthroscopic shoulder surgery: a new modality? *Anesth Analg*. 1997;84:1306–1312. [see comment]

39. Moiniche S, Mikkelsen S, Wetterslev J, Dahl JB. A systematic review of intra-articular local anesthesia for postoperative pain relief after arthroscopic knee surgery. *Reg Anesth Pain Med* 1999;24:430–437.

40. Singelyn FJ, Lhotel L, Fabre B. Pain relief after arthroscopic shoulder surgery: a comparison of intraarticular analgesia, suprascapular nerve block, and interscalene brachial plexus block. *Anesth Analg*. 2004;99:589–592.

41. Urmey WF, Talts KH, Sharrock NE. One hundred percent incidence of hemidiaphragmatic paresis associated with interscalene brachial plexus anesthesia as diagnosed by ultrasonography. *Anesth Analg*. 1991;72:498–503.

42. al-Kaisy AA, Chan VW, Perlas A. Respiratory effects of low-dose bupivacaine interscalene block. *Br J Anaesth*. 1999;82:217–220.

43. Ward ME. The interscalene approach to the brachial plexus. *Anaesthesia*. 1974;29:147–157.

44. Mulroy MF. Regional anesthetic techniques. *Int Anesthesiol Clin*. 1994;32:81–98.

45. Bashein G, Haschke RH, Ready LB. Electrical nerve location: numerical and electrophoretic comparison of insulated vs insulated needles. *Anesth Analg*. 1984;63:919–924.

46. Silverstein WB, Saiyed MU, Brown AR. Interscalene block with a nerve stimulator: a deltoid motor response is a satisfactory endpoint for successful block. *Reg Anesth Pain Med*. 2000;25:356–359. [see comment]

47. Birnbaum J, Kip M, Spies CD, et al. The effect of stimulating versus nonstimulating catheters for continuous interscalene plexus blocks in short-term pain management. *J Clin Anesth*. 2007;19:434–439.

48. Casati A, Baciarello M, Di Cianni S, et al. Effects of ultrasound guidance on the minimum effective anaesthetic volume required to block the femoral nerve. *Br J Anaesth*. 2007;98:823–827.

49. Bryan NA, Swenson JD, Greis PE, Burks RT. Indwelling interscalene catheter use in an outpatient setting for shoulder surgery: technique, efficacy, and complications. *J Shoulder Elbow Surg*. 2007;16:388–395.

50. Eledjam JJ, Cuvillon P, Capdevila X, et al. French study g: Postoperative analgesia by femoral nerve block with ropivacaine 0.2% after major knee surgery: continuous versus patient-controlled techniques. *Reg Anesth Pain Med*. 2002;27:604–611.

51. Singelyn FJ, Vanderelst PE, Gouverneur JM. Extended femoral nerve sheath block after total hip arthroplasty: continuous versus patient-controlled techniques. *Anesth Analg*. 2001;92:455–459. [see comment]

52. Winnie AP, Collins VJ. The subclavian perivascular technique of brachial plexus anesthesia. *Anesthesiology*. 1964;25:353–363.

53. Franco CD, Vieira ZE. 1,001 subclavian perivascular brachial plexus blocks: success with a nerve stimulator. *Reg Anesth Pain Med*. 2000;25:41–46.

54. Brown DL, Cahill DR, Bridenbaugh LD. Supraclavicular nerve block: anatomic analysis of a method to prevent pneumothorax. *Anesth Analg*. 1993;76:530–534.

55. Neal JM, Moore JM, Kopacz DJ, Liu SS, Kramer DJ, Plorde JJ. Quantitative analysis of respiratory, motor, and sensory function after supraclavicular block. *Anesth Analg*. 1998;86:1239–1244.

56. Chan VW, Perlas A, Rawson R, Odukoya O. Ultrasound-guided supraclavicular brachial plexus block. *Anesth Analg*. 2003;97:1514–1517.

57. Beach ML, Sites BD, Gallagher JD. Use of a nerve stimulator does not improve the efficacy of ultrasound-guided supraclavicular nerve blocks. *J Clin Anesth*. 2006;18:580–584.

58. Williams SR, Chouinard P, Arcand G, Harris P, Ruel M, Boudreault D, Girard F. Ultrasound guidance speeds execution and improves the quality of supraclavicular block. *Anesth Analg*. 2003;97:1518–1523.

59. Burnham PJ. Regional block of the great nerves of the upper arm. *Anesthesiology*. 1958;19:281–284.

60. Klaastad O, Smedby O, Thompson GE, et al. Distribution of local anesthetic in axillary brachial plexus block: a clinical and magnetic resonance imaging study. *Anesthesiology*. 2002;96:1315–1324.

61. Koscielniak-Nelson Z, Hesselbjerg L, Fejlberg V. Comparison of transarterial and multiple nerve stimulation techniques for an initial axillary block by 45 ml of mepivcaine 1% with adrenaline. *Acta Anaesthesiol Scand*. 1998;42:570–575.

62. Koscielniak-Nielsen Z, Stens-Pedersen H, Lippert K. Readiness for surgery after axillary block: single or multiple injection techniques. *Eur J Anaesthesiol*. 1997;14:164–171.

63. Sia S, Lepri A, Ponzecchi P. Axillary brachial plexus block using peripheral nerve stimulator: a comparison between double and triple injection techniques. *Reg Anesth Pain Med*. 2001;26:499–503.

64. Sia S, Lepri A, Campolo M, et al. A comparison between axillary and midhumeral approaches. *Anesth Analg*. 2002;95:1075–1079.

65. Handoll H, Koscielniak-Nelson Z. Single, double, or multiple injection techniques for axillary brachial plexus block for hand, wrist, or forearm surgery. *Cochrane Database Syst Rev*. 2006; Jan 25(1):CD003842.

66. Schwemmer U, Markus C, Greim C, Brederlau J, Roewer N. Ultrasound-guided anaesthesia of the axillary brachial plexus: efficacy of multiple injection approach. *Ultraschall Med*. 2005;26:114–119.

67. Baranowski A, Pither C. A comparison of three methods of axillary brachial plexus anaesthesia. Anaesthesia 1990;45:362–365.

68. Goldberg M, Greff C, Larijani G, Norris M. A comparison of three methods of axillary approach to the brachial plexus blockade for upper extremity surgery. Anesthesiology 1987;66:814–816.

69. Winnie AP, Radonjic R, Akkineni SR, et al. Factors influencing distribution of local anesthetic injected into the brachial plexus sheath. *Anesth Analg*. 1979;58:225–234.

70. Winnie AP. *Plexus Anesthesia: Perivascular Techniques of Brachial Plexus Block*. Philadelphia, PA: W.B. Saunders; 1990.

71. Tuominen M, Pitkanen M, Nummien M, Rosenberg P. Quality of axillary brachial plexus block: comparison of success rate using perivascular and nerve stimulator techniques. *Anaesthesia*. 1987;42:20–22.

72. Retzl G, Kapral S, Greher M, et al. Ultrasonographic findings of the axillary part of the brachial plexus. *Anesthes Analg*. 2001;92:1271–1275.

73. Sites B, Beach M, Spence B, et al. Ultrasound guidance improves the success rate of perivascular axillary plexus block. *Acta Anaesthesiol Scand.* 2006;50:678–684.

74. Casati A, Danelli G, Baciarello M, et al. A prospective, randomized comparison between ultrasound and nerve stimulation guidance for multiple injection axillary brachial plexus block. *Anesthesiology.* 2007;106:922–926.

75. Lavoie J, Martin R, Tetrault JP, et al. Axillary plexus block using a peripheral nerve stimulator: single or multiple injections. *Can J Anaesth.* 1992;39:583–586.

76. Koscielniak-Nelson Z, Nielsen P, Nielsen S, Gardi T, Hermann C. Comparison of transarterial and multiple nerve stimulation techniques for axillary block using a high dose of mepivacaine with adrenaline. *Acta Anaesthesiol Scand.* 1999;43:398–404.

77. Vester-Andersen T, Broby-Johansen U, Bro-Rasmussen F. Perivascular axillary block VI: the distribution of gelatine solutions injected into the axillary neurovascular sheath of cadavers. *Acta Anaesthesiol Scand.* 1986;30:18–22.

78. Dilger J, Wells R. The use of peripheral nerve blocks at the elbow for carpal tunnel release. *J Clin Anesth.* 2005;17:621–623.

79. Delaunay L, Chelly J. Blocks at the wrist provide effective anesthesia for carpal tunnel release. *Can J Anaesth.* 2001;48:656–660.

80. Gebhard RE, Al-Samsam T, Greger J, et al. Distal nerve blocks at the wrist for outpatient carpal tunnel surgery offer intraoperative cardiovascular stability and reduce discharge time. *Anesth Analg.* 2002;95:351–355.

81. Macaire P, Choquet O, Jochum D, Travers V, Capdevila X. Nerve blocks at the wrist for carpal tunnel release revisited: the use of sensory nerve and motor nerve stimulation techniques. *Reg Anesth Pain Med.* 2005;30:536–540.

82. Vloka JD, Hadzic A, April E, Thys DM. The division of the sciatic nerve in the popliteal fossa: anatomical implications for popliteal nerve blockade. *Anesth Analg.* 2001;92:215–217.

83. Winnie AP, Ramamurthy S., Durrani Z, Radonjic R. Plexus blocks for lower extremity surgery. *Anesthesiol Rev.* 1974;1:1–621.

84. Chayen D, Nathan H, Chayen M. The psoas compartment block. *Anesthesiology.* 1976;45:95–99.

85. Parkinson SK, Mueller JB, Little WL, Bailey SL. Extent of blockade with various approaches to the lumbar plexus. *Anesth Analg.* 1989;68:243–248. [see comment]

86. Winnie AP, Ramamurthy S, Durrani Z. The inguinal paravascular technic of lumbar plexus anesthesia: the "3-in-1 block." *Anesth Analg.* 1973;52:989–996.

87. Ritter JW. Femoral nerve "sheath" for inguinal paravascular lumbar plexus block is not found in human cadavers. *J Clin Anesth.* 1995;7:470–473.

88. Jankowski CJ, Hebl JR, Stuart MJ, et al. A comparison of psoas compartment block and spinal and general anesthesia for outpatient knee arthroscopy. *Anesth Analg.* 97:1003–1009.

89. Matheny JM, Hanks GA, Rung GW, Blanda JB, Kalenak A. A comparison of patient-controlled analgesia and continuous lumbar plexus block after anterior cruciate ligament reconstruction. *Arthroscopy.* 1993;9:87–90.

90. Luber MJ, Greengrass R, Vail TP. Patient satisfaction and effectiveness of lumbar plexus and sciatic nerve block for total knee arthroplasty. *J Arthroplasty.* 2001;16:17–21.

91. Raimer C, Priem K, Wiese AA, et al. Continuous psoas and sciatic block after knee arthroplasty: good effects compared to epidural analgesia or i.v. opioid analgesia: a prospective study of 63 patients. *Acta Orthopaed.* 2007;78:193–200.

92. Watson MW, Mitra D, McLintock TC, Grant SA: Continuous versus single-injection lumbar plexus blocks: comparison of the effects on morphine use and early recovery after total knee arthroplasty. *Reg Anesth Pain Med.* 2005;30:541–547.

93. Bagry H, Asenjo JF, Bracco D, Carli, F. Effect of a continous peripheral nerve block on the inflammatory response in knee arthroplasty. *Reg Anesth Pain Med.* 2008;33:17–23.

94. de Visme V, Picart F, Le Jouan R, Legrand A, Savry C, Morin V. Combined lumbar and sacral plexus block compared with plain bupivacaine spinal anesthesia for hip fractures in the elderly. *Reg Anesth Pain Med.* 2000;25:158–162.

95. Biboulet P, Morau D, Aubas P, Bringuier-Branchereau S, Capdevila X. Postoperative analgesia after total-hip arthroplasty: comparison of intravenous patient-controlled analgesia with morphine and single injection of femoral nerve or psoas compartment block. A prospective, randomized, double-blind study. *Reg Anesth Pain Med.* 2004;29:102–109.

96. Stevens RD, Van Gessel E, Flory N, Fournier R, Gamulin Z. Lumbar plexus block reduces pain and blood loss associated with total hip arthroplasty. *Anesthesiology.* 2000;93:115–121.

97. Hebl JR, Kopp SL, Ali MH, et al. A comprehensive anesthesia protocol that emphasizes peripheral nerve blockade for total knee and total hip arthroplasty. J Bone Joint Surg. 2005;87(suppl 2):63–70.

98. Hevia-Sanchez V, Bermejo-Alvarez MA, Hevia-Mendez A, Fervienza P, Franch M, Diaz ML. Bloqueo posterior del plexo lumbar para analgesia postoperatoria de artroplastias de cadera. *Rev. Esp lAnestesiol Reanim.* 2002;49:507–511.

99. Buckenmaier CC, 3rd, Xenos JS, Nilsen SM. Lumbar plexus block with perineural catheter and sciatic nerve block for total hip arthroplasty. *J Arthroplasty.* 2002;17:499–502.

100. Capdevila X, Macaire P, Dadure C, et al. Continuous psoas compartment block for postoperative analgesia after total hip arthroplasty: new landmarks, technical guidelines, and clinical evaluation. *Anesth Analg.* 94:1606–1613. [see comment]

101. Turker G, Uckunkaya N, Yavascaoglu B, Yilmazlar A, Ozcelik S. Comparison of the catheter-technique psoas compartment block and the epidural block for analgesia in partial hip replacement surgery. *Acta Anaesthesiol Scand.* 2003;47:30–36.

102. Chelly JE, Casati A, Al-Samsam T, Coupe K, Criswell A, Tucker J. Continuous lumbar plexus block for acute postoperative pain management after open reduction and internal fixation of acetabular fractures. *J Orthopaed Trauma.* 2003;17:362–367.

103. Chudinov A, Berkenstadt H, Salai M, Cahana A, Perel A: Continuous psoas compartment block for anesthesia and perioperative analgesia in patients with hip fractures. *Reg Anesth Pain Med.* 1999;24:563–568.

104. Kirchmair L, Enna B, Mitterschiffthaler G, et al. Lumbar plexus in children: a sonographic study and its relevance to pediatric regional anesthesia. *Anesthesiology.* 2004;101:445–450.

105. Grau T, Leipold RW, Horter J, Martin E, Motsch J. Colour Doppler imaging of the interspinous and epidural space. *Eur J Anaesthesiol.* 2001;18:706–712.

106. Greher M, Kirchmair L, Enna B, et al. Ultrasound-guided lumbar facet nerve block: accuracy of a new technique confirmed by computed tomography. *Anesthesiology.* 2004;101:1195–1200.

107. Greher M, Scharbert G, Kamolz LP, et al. Ultrasound-guided lumbar facet nerve block: a sonoanatomic study of a new methodologic approach. *Anesthesiology.* 2004;100:1242–1248.

108. Grant SA, Breslin DS, MacLeod DB, et al. Variability in determination of point of needle insertion in peripheral nerve blocks: a comparison of experienced and inexperienced anaesthetists. *Anaesthesia.* 2003;58:688–692.

109. Lang SA, Yip RW, Chang PC, Gerard MA. The femoral 3-in-1 block revisited. *J Clin Anesth.* 1993;5:292–296.

110. Marhofer P, Nasel C, Sitzwohl C, Kapral S. Magnetic resonance imaging of the distribution of local anesthetic during the three-in-one block. *Anesth Analg.* 2000;90:119–124. [see comment]

111. Cauhepe C, Oliver M, Colombani R, Railhac N. Le bloc "trois-en-un": mythe ou realite? *Ann Francaises Anesth Reanim.* 1989;8:376–378.

112. Seeberger MD, Urwyler A. Paravascular lumbar plexus block: block extension after femoral nerve stimulation and injection of 20 vs. 40 ml mepivacaine 10 mg/ml. *Acta Anaesthesiol Scand.* 1995;39:769–773.

113. Marhofer P, Schrogendorfer K, Koinig H, Kapral S, Weinstabl C, Mayer N. Ultrasonographic guidance improves sensory block and onset time of three-in-one blocks. *Anesth Analg.* 1997;85:854–857. [see comment]

114. Klein SM, Pietrobon R, Nielsen KC, Warner DS, Greengrass RA, Steele SM. Peripheral nerve blockade with long-acting local anesthetics: a survey of the Society for Ambulatory Anesthesia. *Anesth Analg.* 94:71–76.

115. Schulz-Stubner S, Henszel A, Hata JS. A new rule for femoral nerve blocks. *Reg Anesth Pain Med.* 2005;30:473–477.

116. Patel NJ, Flashburg MH, Paskin S, Grossman R. A regional anesthetic technique compared to general anesthesia for outpatient knee arthroscopy. *Anesth Analg.* 1986;65:185–187.

117. Goranson BD, Lang S, Cassidy JD, Dust WN, McKerrell J. A comparison of three regional anaesthesia techniques for outpatient knee arthroscopy. *Can J Anaesth.* 1997;44:371–376.

118. De Andres J, Bellver J, Barrera L, Febre E, Bolinches R. A comparative study of analgesia after knee surgery with intraarticular bupivacaine, intraarticular morphine, and lumbar plexus block. *Anesth Analg.* 1993;77:727–730.

119. Casati A, Cappelleri G, Berti M, Fanelli G, Di Benedetto P, Torri G. Randomized comparison of remifentanil-propofol with a sciatic-femoral nerve block for out-patient knee arthroscopy. *Eur J Anaesthesiol.* 2002;19:109–114.

120. Cappelleri G, Casati A, Fanelli G, et al. Unilateral spinal anesthesia or combined sciatic-femoral nerve block for day-case knee arthroscopy: a prospective, randomized comparison. *Minerva Anestesiol.* 2000;66:131–136; discussion 137.

121. Casati A, Cappelleri G, Fanelli G, et al. Regional anaesthesia for outpatient knee arthroscopy: a randomized clinical comparison of two different anaesthetic techniques. *Acta Anaesthesiol Scand.* 2000;44:543–547.

122. Mulroy MF, Larkin KL, Batra MS, Hodgson PS, Owens BD. Femoral nerve block with 0.25% or 0.5% bupivacaine improves postoperative analgesia following outpatient arthroscopic anterior cruciate ligament repair. *Reg Anesth Pain Med.* 2001;26:24–29.

123. Edkin BS, McCarty EC, Spindler KP, Flanagan JF. Analgesia with femoral nerve block for anterior cruciate ligament reconstruction. *Clin Orthopaed Relat Res.* 1999:289–295.

124. Peng P, Claxton A, Chung F, Chan V, Miniaci A, Krishnathas A: Femoral nerve block and ketorolac in patients undergoing anterior cruciate ligament reconstruction. *Can J Anaesth.* 1999;46:919–924.

125. Williams BA, Kentor ML, Vogt MT, et al. Femoral-sciatic nerve blocks for complex outpatient knee surgery are associated with less postoperative pain before same-day discharge: a review of 1,200 consecutive cases from the period 1996–1999. *Anesthesiology.* 2003;98:1206–1213.

126. Lynch J, Trojan S, Arhelger S, Krings-Ernst I. Intermittent femoral nerve blockade for anterior cruciate ligament repair. Use of a catheter technique in 208 patients. *Acta Anaesthesiol Belg.* 1991;42:207–212.

127. Schwarz SK, Franciosi LG, Ries CR, et al. Addition of femoral 3-in-1 blockade to intra-articular ropivacaine 0.2% does not reduce analgesic requirements following arthroscopic knee surgery. *Can J Anaesth.* 1999;46:741–747.

128. Frost S, Grossfeld S, Kirkley A, Litchfield B, Fowler P, Amendola A. The efficacy of femoral nerve block in pain reduction for outpatient hamstring anterior cruciate ligament reconstruction: a double-blind, prospective, randomized trial. *Arthroscopy.* 2000;16:243–248.

129. Mansour NY, Bennetts FE. An observational study of combined continuous lumbar plexus and single-shot sciatic nerve blocks for post-knee surgery analgesia. *Reg Anesth.* 1996;21:287–291.

130. Nakamura SJ, Conte-Hernandez A, Galloway MT. The efficacy of regional anesthesia for outpatient anterior cruciate ligament reconstruction. *Arthroscopy.* 1997;13:699–703.

131. Williams BA, Kentor ML, Vogt MT, et al. Economics of nerve block pain management after anterior cruciate ligament reconstruction: potential hospital cost savings via associated postanesthesia care unit bypass and same-day discharge. *Anesthesiology.* 2004;100:697–706.

132. Ng HP, Cheong KF, Lim A, Lim J, Puhaindran ME. Intraoperative single-shot "3-in-1" femoral nerve block with ropivacaine 0.25%, ropivacaine 0.5% or bupivacaine 0.25% provides comparable 48-hr analgesia after unilateral total knee replacement. *Can J Anaesth.* 2001;48:1102–1108.

133. Edwards ND, Wright EM. Continuous low-dose 3-in-1 nerve blockade for postoperative pain relief after total knee replacement. *Anesth Analg.* 1992;75:265–267.

134. Singelyn FJ, Deyaert M, Joris D, Pendeville E, Gouverneur JM. Effects of intravenous patient-controlled analgesia with morphine, continuous epidural analgesia, and continuous three-in-one block on postoperative pain and knee rehabilitation after unilateral total knee arthroplasty. *Anesth Analg.* 1998;87:88–92.

135. Capdevila X, Barthelet Y, Biboulet P, Ryckwaert Y, Rubenovitch J, d'Athis F. Effects of perioperative analgesic technique on the surgical outcome and duration of rehabilitation after major knee surgery. *Anesthesiology.* 1999;91:8–15.

136. Serpell MG, Millar FA, Thomson MF. Comparison of lumbar plexus block versus conventional opioid analgesia after total knee replacement. *Anaesthesia.* 1991;46:275–277.

137. Tarkkila P, Tuominen M, Huhtala J, Lindgren L. Comparison of intrathecal morphine and continuous femoral 3-in-1 block for pain after major knee surgery under spinal anaesthesia. *Eur J Anaesthesiol.* 1998;15:6–9.

138. Schultz P, Anker-Moller E, Dahl JB, Christensen EF, Spangsberg N, Fauno P. Postoperative pain treatment after open knee surgery: continuous lumbar plexus block with bupivacaine versus epidural morphine. *Reg Anesth.* 1991;16:34–37.

139. Hirst GC, Lang SA, Dust WN, Cassidy JD, Yip RW. Femoral nerve block: single injection versus continuous infusion for total knee arthroplasty. *Reg Anesth.* 1996;21:292–297.

140. Cook P, Stevens J, Gaudron C. Comparing the effects of femoral nerve block versus femoral and sciatic nerve block on pain and opiate consumption after total knee arthroplasty. *J Arthroplasty.* 2003;18:583–586.

141. Weber A, Fournier R, Van Gessel E, Gamulin Z. Sciatic nerve block and the improvement of femoral nerve block analgesia after total knee replacement. *Eur J Anaesthesiol.* 2002;19:834–836.

142. Ben-David B, Schmalenberger K, Chelly JE. Analgesia after total knee arthroplasty: is continuous sciatic blockade needed in addition to continuous femoral blockade? *Anesth Analg.* 98:747–749.

143. Chelly JE, Greger J, Gebhard R, et al. Continuous femoral blocks improve recovery and outcome of patients undergoing total knee arthroplasty. *J Arthroplasty.* 2001;16:436–445.

144. McNamee DA, Convery PN, Milligan KR. Total knee replacement: a comparison of ropivacaine and bupivacaine in combined

femoral and sciatic block. *Acta Anaesthesiol Scand.* 2001;45:477–481.

145. Allen JG, Denny NM, Oakman N. Postoperative analgesia following total knee arthroplasty: a study comparing spinal anesthesia and combined sciatic femoral 3-in-1 block. *Reg Anesth Pain Med.* 1998;23:142–146.

146. Marhofer P, Schrogendorfer K, Wallner T, Koinig H, Mayer N, Kapral S. Ultrasonographic guidance reduces the amount of local anesthetic for 3-in-1 blocks. *Reg Anesth Pain Med.* 1998;23:584–588.

147. Gruber H, Peer S, Kovacs P, Marth R, Bodner G. The ultrasonographic appearance of the femoral nerve and cases of iatrogenic impairment. *J Ultrasound Med.* 2003;22:163–172.

148. Soong J, Schafhalter-Zoppoth I, Gray AT. The importance of transducer angle to ultrasound visibility of the femoral nerve. *Reg Anesth Pain Med.* 2005;30:505.

149. Sutin KM, Schneider C, Sandhu NS, Capan LM. Deep venous thrombosis revealed during ultrasound-guided femoral nerve block. *Br J Anaesth.* 2005;94:247–248.

150. Capdevila X, Pirat P, Bringuier S, et al. French Study Group on Continuous Peripheral Nerve B: continuous peripheral nerve blocks in hospital wards after orthopedic surgery: a multicenter prospective analysis of the quality of postoperative analgesia and complications in 1,416 patients. *Anesthesiology.* 2005;103:1035–1045.

151. Muraskin SI, Conrad B, Zheng N, Morey TE, Enneking FK. Falls associated with lower-extremity-nerve blocks: a pilot investigation of mechanisms. *Reg Anesth Pain Med.* 2007;32:67–72.

152. Wiegel M, Gottschaldt U, Hennebach R, Hirschberg T, Reske A. Complications and adverse effects associated with continuous peripheral nerve blocks in orthopedic patients. *Anesth Analg.* 104:1578–1582.

153. Chan VW, Nova H, Abbas S, McCartney CJ, Perlas A, Xu DQ. Ultrasound examination and localization of the sciatic nerve: a volunteer study. *Anesthesiology.* 104:309–314.

154. van Geffen GJ, Gielen M. Ultrasound-guided subgluteal sciatic nerve blocks with stimulating catheters in children: a descriptive study. *Anesth Analg.* 103:328–333. [see comment]

155. McCartney CJ, Brauner I, Chan VW. Ultrasound guidance for a lateral approach to the sciatic nerve in the popliteal fossa. *Anaesthesia.* 2004;59:1023–1025.

156. Minville V, Zetlaoui PJ, Fessenmeyer C, Benhamou D. Ultrasound guidance for difficult lateral popliteal catheter insertion in a patient with peripheral vascular disease. *Reg Anesth Pain Med.* 2004;29:368–370.

157. Rivas Ferreira E, Sala-Blanch X, Bargallo X, Sadurni M, Puente A, De Andres J. Bloqueo popliteo posterior guiado por ecografia. *Rev Esp Anestesiol Reanim.* 2004;51:604–607.

158. Sinha AK, Joshi BP, Sharma A, Goel HC, Prasad J. Ultrasound-assisted conversion of toxic beta-asarone into nontoxic bioactive phenylpropanoid: isoacoramone, a metabolite of Piper marginatum and Acorus tararinowii. *Nat Prod Res.* 2004;18:219–223.

159. Auroy Y, Narchi P, Messiah A, et al. Serious complications related to regional anesthesia: results of a prospective survey in France. *Anesthesiology.* 1997;87:479–486.

160. Auroy Y, Benhamou D, Bargues L, et al. Major complications of regional anesthesia in France: the SOS Regional Anesthesia Hotline Service. *Anesthesiology.* 2002;97:1274–1280.

161. Valenzuela C, Snyders DJ, Bennett PB, Tamargo J, Hondeghem LM. Stereoselective block of cardiac sodium channels by bupivacaine in guinea pig ventricular myocytes. *Circulation.* 1995;92:3014–3024.

162. Valenzuela C, Delpon E, Tamkun MM, Tamargo J, Snyders DJ. Stereoselective block of a human cardiac potassium channel (Kv1.5) by bupivacaine enantiomers. *Biophys J.* 1995;69:418–427.

163. Rosenberg PH, Veering BT, Urmey WF. Maximum recommended doses of local anesthetics: a multifactorial concept. *Reg Anesth Pain Med.* 2004;29:564–575; discussion 524.

164. Borgeat A, Ekatodramis G. Nerve injury associated with regional anesthesia. *Curr Top Med Chem.* 2001;1:199–203.

165. Albright GA. Cardiac arrest following regional anesthesia with etidocaine or bupivacaine. *Anesthesiology.* 1979;51:285–287.

166. Heavner JE, Pitkanen MT, Shi B, Rosenberg PH. Resuscitation from bupivacaine-induced asystole in rats: comparison of different cardioactive drugs. *Anesth Analg.* 1995;80:1134–1139.

167. Krismer AC, Hogan QH, Wenzel V, et al. The efficacy of epinephrine or vasopressin for resuscitation during epidural anesthesia. *Anesth Analg.* 2001;93:734–742.

168. Haasio J, Pitkanen MT, Kytta J, Rosenberg PH. Treatment of bupivacaine-induced cardiac arrhythmias in hypoxic and hypercarbic pigs with amiodarone or bretylium. *Reg Anesth.* 1990;15:174–179.

169. Rosenblatt MA, Abel M, Fischer GW, Itzkovich CJ, Eisenkraft JB. Successful use of a 20% lipid emulsion to resuscitate a patient after a presumed bupivacaine-related cardiac arrest. *Anesthesiology.* 2006;105:217–218.

170. Lee LA, Posner KL, Domino KB, Caplan RA, Cheney FW. Injuries associated with regional anesthesia in the 1980s and 1990s: a closed claims analysis. *Anesthesiology.* 2004;101:143–152.

171. Urban MK, Urquhart B. Evaluation of brachial plexus anesthesia for upper extremity surgery. *Reg Anesth.* 1994;19:175–182.

18

Regional Anesthesia for Acute Pain Management in the Outpatient Setting

Holly Evans, Karen C. Nielsen,
Marcy S. Tucker, and Stephen M. Klein

Ambulatory surgery includes procedures following which, the patients are discharged from a health care facility within 23 hours. Advances in minimally invasive surgical technique have contributed to the frequency of outpatient procedures. Institutional fiscal pressures have further promoted a reduction in patient length of stay. Perioperative patient care has evolved to meet the needs of the outpatient.

Ambulatory anesthesia incorporates techniques that provide rapid emergence and return to preoperative function but that also provide effective postoperative analgesia with minimal side effects. Regional anesthesia and local anesthetic based techniques provide postoperative analgesia to the surgical site, minimize the requirement for opioid analgesia and reduce the risk of opioid-related side effects.[1,2] This chapter outlines the application of peripheral nerve blocks as well as the use of wound infiltration of local anesthetic for postoperative analgesia in outpatients.

PATIENT SELECTION FOR AMBULATORY REGIONAL ANESTHESIA AND ANALGESIA

A comprehensive preoperative assessment is performed for all patients scheduled for ambulatory surgery. Prior to planning ambulatory regional anesthesia for postoperative analgesia, both the surgical procedure and the patient are evaluated as to their suitability for this modality of pain control. The planned analgesic modality must provide comprehensive pain control for the anticipated surgical insult. For example, a superficial wound catheter may be insufficient for surgery that also involves extensive deep dissection of painful structures. Single injection peripheral nerve block or wound infiltration is considered for surgical procedures with mild to moderate postoperative pain (ie, knee arthroscopy), whereas continuous catheter techniques are applicable for procedures with significant postoperative pain (ie, shoulder rotator cuff repair).

It is imperative that appropriate patients be selected for ambulatory regional anesthesia (Table 18.1). Patients must demonstrate adequate comprehension and responsibility to ensure safe implementation of the technique. Patient education is designed to ensure acceptable analgesia and to prevent patient injury following hospital discharge. Patients must appreciate the implications of sensory and motor nerve block that results from the regional anesthetic technique. They must be able to properly care for their insensate extremity or body part by keeping it well padded and unrestricted. Patients must avoid use of the numb or weak extremity. For example, those with a numb lower extremity must avoid weight bearing on the affected leg because this may lead to falls. Patients must wear a protective sling or brace to safeguard the affected extremity. Patients must be informed about and understand the anticipated duration of action of the analgesic modality. They must be familiar with the indications for and dosing of oral analgesic adjuncts (eg, acetaminophen, cyclooxygenase 2 inhibitors, opioids) and they must understand the preemptive use of these medications in anticipation of the regression of the effects of the regional anesthesia technique.

Patients who receive an ambulatory perineural or wound infusion must be able to recognize the symptoms of local anesthetic toxicity. They must be able to stop the pump and seek medical care should toxicity symptoms occur. Patients must understand additional basic ambulatory pump function, including how to administer patient-controlled boluses. Patients must have a reliable caregiver with them at all times during the infusion. They must be comfortable with removal of the perineural or wound catheter at home; alternatively, they must agree to return to the hospital for removal. All of the above information should be provided in writing and reinforced verbally prior to hospital discharge.

All patients discharged home following a long-acting peripheral nerve block or with a continuous perineural or wound infusion of local anesthetic must receive adequate postoperative follow-up. All patients should be given contact information for their anesthesiologist in case they have questions, concerns, or an adverse reaction. All patients should receive telephone follow-up by the anesthesiology department until the sensorimotor block has fully resolved and the continuous infusion pump and catheter have been removed.

Table 18.1: Patient Inclusion Criteria for Ambulatory Perineural or Wound Infusions

Able to protect insensate extremity

Able to understand basic ambulatory pump function

Able to monitor for potential side effects

Able to participate in appropriate follow-up

Able to understand the use of analgesic adjuncts

Presence of reliable caregiver

Table 18.2: Onset Time, Duration of Effect and Maximum Recommended Dose of Local Anesthetics Used for Perineural or Wound Injection

	Onset (min)	Duration (hours)	Maximum Dose (mg/kg) of Epinephrine-Containing Solution
Chloroprocaine	10–20	1–2	14
Lidocaine	10–20	2–3	7
Mepivacaine	10–20	3–6	7
Bupivacaine	15–30	6–12	3
Ropivacaine	15–30	6–12	3.5

LOCAL ANESTHETICS AND EQUIPMENT FOR AMBULATORY REGIONAL ANESTHESIA AND ANALGESIA

Local anesthetic solutions and continuous infusion pumps used to provide postoperative analgesia must be tailored to the specific needs of outpatients. Table 18.2 summarizes the basic pharmacology of commonly used local anesthetics. Chloroprocaine, lidocaine, or mepivacaine is used when rapid onset and/or short duration of effect is required. These agents may be selected when minimal postoperative pain is anticipated. Alternatively, they may be used when resolution of the initial block is desired prior to starting a continuous infusion of local anesthetic. Ropivacaine or bupivacaine is selected for extended duration of action. Wound and perineural analgesia typically involves the injection of large doses of local anesthetic; consequently, ropivacaine's superior safely profile is advantageous. A single perineural injection of ropivacaine provides 12–24 hours of postoperative analgesia.[3] In addition to its duration of action and safety profile, the ability to provide selective sensory anesthesia with limited motor weakness[4] makes ropivacaine well suited for use in continuous wound or perineural infusion.

A number of adjuvants are added to local anesthetic either to increase safety or to enhance analgesic efficacy (Table 18.2). Epinephrine is commonly added to the local anesthetic as a 1:200 000 to 1:400 000 solution. It acts as a marker of intravascular injection by causing a rise in heart rate and blood pressure when inadvertently injected into an artery or vein. Epinephrine causes localized vasoconstriction; as a result, it can reduce the systemic absorption of local anesthetic and reduce the risk of toxicity. The addition of epinephrine to the local anesthetic solution may also enhance analgesia.[5] Epinephrine is avoided with local anesthetic infiltration of the fingers, toes, nose and penis because of the risk of distal ischemia. Clonidine is an α_2 agonist with analgesic properties. A perineural dose of 1–2 μg/kg enhances the quality and duration of analgesia provided by peripheral nerve blocks performed with short-acting local anesthetics.[6] Similar effects have not been conclusively demonstrated when clonidine is used in conjunction with long-acting local anesthetics.[7,8] Associated hypotension, bradycardia, and sedation potentially limit the use of clonidine in the ambulatory population. Many other local anesthetic adjuvants (Table 18.3) have been studied; however, results have been conflicting and use is not routine.[9–16]

A variety of continuous infusion pumps are available for ambulatory perineural or wound analgesia. A nondisposable or a disposable pump can be selected. Nondisposable pumps are typically electronic and have the capability to program a range of bolus, lockout, and continuous infusion settings. These pumps have greater initial costs but lower ongoing costs associated with them compared to disposable pumps. Patients must return nondisposable pumps to the medical center either in person or by mail. Some authors have reported great success and patient compliance in returning pumps when an envelope with prepaid postage is provided.[17] Disposable infusion pumps are available in elastomeric or electronic options. Elastomeric pumps rely on the tensile strength of the fluid reservoir to generate output of local anesthetic solution. Many elastomeric pumps currently available have the ability to vary the continuous infusion rate and the capacity to provide patient-controlled boluses. In a series of studies, Ilfeld et al present data on the infusion rate accuracy and reliability for specific pumps used for ambulatory local anesthetic infusion.[18–21]

PERIPHERAL NERVE BLOCKS FOR POSTOPERATIVE ANALGESIA IN OUTPATIENTS

Peripheral nerve blocks involve the injection of local anesthetic in close proximity to a nerve or nerve plexus. This modality achieves sensory, motor, and sympathetic block in the territory supplied by the nerve in question. Single-injection techniques are of finite duration, whereas continuous perineural catheters provide the potential for prolonged postoperative analgesia.

The advantages of peripheral nerve blocks are well documented. In a meta-analysis, Liu et al[1] compared regional anesthesia versus general anesthesia for ambulatory surgical procedures. They summarized 7 trials with 1003 patients and found that single injection peripheral nerve blocks enhanced analgesia and reduced side effects in the immediate postoperative period. Patients who received peripheral nerve blocks had lower visual analog pain scores (by 24 mm), reduced analgesic requirements (odds ratio [OR] 0.11), and decreased incidence of nausea (OR 0.17) compared to those patients who received general anesthesia. These advantages decreased the mean time spent in the postanesthesia care unit (PACU) by 24 minutes and even enabled a greater proportion of peripheral nerve block patients to bypass the PACU (OR 14) when compared to those who received general anesthesia. Overall, patient satisfaction was higher among the group who received peripheral nerve blocks (OR 4.7).

Table 18.3: Local Anesthetic Adjuvants

	Dose	Therapeutic Effect	Side Effects
Epinephrine	1:400 000 to 1:200 000	Reduces systemic absorption of local anesthetic Acts as marker of intravascular injection of local anesthetic Analgesic	Hypertension and tachycardia with intravascular injection
Clonidine	1–2 μg/kg	Analgesic	Hypotension Bradycardia Sedation

In another meta-analysis, Richman et al[2] evaluated continuous peripheral nerve blocks versus opioids for postoperative analgesia. They summarized 19 trials with 603 patients of which 51% involved the use of a continuous femoral nerve or lumbar plexus block, 35% evaluated a continuous interscalene brachial plexus block, and the remaining 13% involved catheters placed at other perineural locations. Although this meta-analysis involved many in-patient studies, the effects are still illustrative of the benefits of continuous peripheral nerve blocks. Results demonstrated superior analgesia from continuous peripheral nerve blocks as evidenced by lower visual analog pain scores for 72 hours after surgery ($P < .001$) and reduced morphine consumption in the first 48 hours (20.8 mg vs 54.1 mg; $P < .001$) compared to opioid analgesia alone. Furthermore, the continuous peripheral nerve block group had a lower incidence of nausea/vomiting, sedation, and pruritus (number needed to treat 4, 4, and 6, respectively). Motor block was the only adverse effect seen with greater frequency in the continuous peripheral nerve block group.

Although the benefits of peripheral nerve blocks are evident, careful consideration of potential adverse effects is warranted. Several large series provide information concerning the incidence of side effects related to these techniques. Klein et al[22] prospectively followed 1791 ambulatory patients who were discharged home following 2382 peripheral nerve blocks with long-acting local anesthetic. They included data on 733 interscalene, 193 supraclavicular, 193 axillary, 338 lumbar plexus, 263 femoral, and 662 sciatic nerve blocks. Short-term postoperative analgesia was excellent; however, many patients required opioid analgesia following nerve block regression. Immediate complications occurred in 11 patients and included oversedation (n = 4), preseizure excitation following an axillary block (n = 1), epidural spread from lumbar plexus block (n = 1), and other minor side effects (n = 5). During telephone follow-up, persistent numbness was identified in 10% of patients contacted at 24 hours and in 0.9% at 7 days and persistent weakness occurred in 7% at 24 hours and 0.7% at 7 days. Only 12 patients (0.5% of peripheral nerve blocks) had long-lasting postoperative neurological symptoms. Most of these cases were likely multifactorial in etiology with contributions from the patient's underlying disease and the surgical procedure. Most neurological symptoms recovered by 6 months. Finally, one fall occurred when a patient who was discharged with femoral and sciatic nerve blocks was exiting the car. No injury resulted.

Capdevila et al[23] prospectively studied 1416 inpatients who received continuous peripheral nerve block analgesia following orthopedic surgery and collected data on the neurologic and infectious risks of this technique. The most common side effect involved technical problems in 253 patients (17.9%). Issues consisted primarily of catheter kinking, blockage or displacement, leakage of fluid around the catheter entry site, and infusion pump malfunction. Neurologic side effects were also identified. Persistent postoperative numbness occurred in 42 patients (3%), prolonged motor block resulted in 31 patients (2.2%), and uncomfortable paresthesias or dysesthesias were experienced by 21 patients (1.5%). There were 3 abnormal electromyograms following femoral nerve blocks; 1 patient had complete resolution of symptoms in 36 hours, whereas the others required 8 to 10 weeks for full recovery. Risk factors for the development of neurologic side effects included postoperative intensive care admission (relative risk 9.8), age 18-39 years (relative risk 3.9), and the use of bupivacaine (relative risk 2.8). Bacterial colonization was demonstrated in 278 of the 969 catheter tips cultured (28.7%). Colonization usually occurred with a single organism, most commonly *Staphylococcus epidermidis*, gram-negative bacillus, or *Staphylococcus aureus*. Only one diabetic patient having knee arthroplasty required antibiotic treatment for a psoas muscle abscess and cellulitis that resulted from a femoral nerve catheter. Identified risk factors for the development of local inflammation or infection included postoperative intensive care admission (relative risk 5.07), catheter duration greater than 48 hours (relative risk 4.61), male sex (relative risk 2.1), and the absence of prophylactic antibiotics (relative risk 1.92). Other rare complications of continuous peripheral nerve blocks identified in this study included respiratory failure (n = 2) and swallowing difficulties (n = 2) after interscalene block, epidural spread with hemodynamic instability (n = 3) after psoas compartment block, and intravascular catheter migration without local anesthetic toxicity (n = 1).

Auroy et al[24] performed a nationwide survey of regional anesthesia practice in France. The incidence of neuropathy following peripheral nerve blocks was 12 in 43 946 (2.7:10 000) in the immediate postoperative period and 7 in 43 946 (1.6:10 000) at 6 months. Seizure from local anesthetic systemic absorption occurred in 6 patients (1.4:10 000); however, no arrhythmias were noted. There were 2 cases of respiratory failure and one case of fatal cardiac arrest that followed lumbar plexus block. All were presumed to be related to inadvertent intrathecal injection.

What follows is a description of the various peripheral nerve block techniques used for ambulatory anesthesia and analgesia. Nerve block performance technique is briefly summarized and followed with an evidence-based description of the benefits and potential drawbacks of each modality in its application to outpatient surgery. An in-depth description of each nerve block technique, including the use of ultrasound, is beyond the scope of this chapter and the reader is referred to other sources.[25,26]

Interscalene Brachial Plexus Block

The interscalene approach is the most proximal of the brachial plexus blocks and is summarized in Table 18.4. It targets the roots of the brachial plexus (C5 to T1). When using a nerve stimulator, a 25- to 50-mm nerve block needle is inserted in the interscalene groove at the level of C6 (the cricoid cartilage) and directed slightly posterior and caudad until a deltoid or biceps twitch is elicited. Ultrasound guidance enables needle positioning and injection of local anesthetic in close proximity to the C6 nerve root under direct vision.

Table 18.4: Interscalene Brachial Plexus Block

Anatomy	Block of the roots of the brachial plexus
Surgical applications	Shoulder
	Upper arm
Nerve block needle	25–50 mm
Local anesthetic volume	30–40 mL
Clinical effects: single injection block[31]	Reduces pain
	Facilitates bypass of phase 1 recovery
	Facilitates return to ambulation and oral intake
	Facilitates timely same day discharge
Clinical effects: continuous perineural infusion[32,34]	Reduces pain and opioid use
	Reduces nausea, sedation, and insomnia
	Improves cognitive function
	Improves sleep quality
Potential adverse effects[29,30]	Transient phrenic nerve block
	Transient cervical sympathetic ganglion block
	Transient recurrent laryngeal nerve block
	Transient neurologic deficit (2.84 per 100 patients)
	Vertebral artery injection ($<0.2\%$)
	Pneumothorax ($<0.2\%$).
	Subarachnoid or epidural block ($<0.2\%$)

This interscalene block produces excellent anesthesia in the C5–C8 dermatomes.[27] Consequently, this block is well suited for analgesia following shoulder and upper arm procedures. In contrast, the interscalene block may not provide complete anesthesia of the inferior nerve roots of the brachial plexus (ie, T1). As a result, this block is less reliable for distal upper extremity surgical procedures. Furthermore, the interscalene block does not provide anesthesia to the medial aspect of the upper arm because this area is innervated by the intercosto-brachial nerve. This nerve is derived from the T2 nerve root and is not part of the brachial plexus. Individual T1 and T2 paravertebral blocks are used to supplement an interscalene block when extensive shoulder surgery is performed (ie, shoulder arthroplasty).

Common side effects associated with the interscalene block include block of the phrenic nerve, cervical sympathetic ganglion, and recurrent laryngeal nerve. This can lead to dyspnea, Horner's syndrome (ptosis, miosis, anhydrosis), and hoarseness, respectively. Symptoms are usually mild and rarely prevent same-day discharge of healthy ambulatory patients. Nevertheless, patients with more serious underlying pulmonary disease can be significantly affected by the transient reduction in lung volumes by up to 40% that typically occurs in association with a phrenic nerve block.[28] Following review of the literature, Brull et al[29] suggest that the interscalene brachial plexus block specifically carries the greatest risk of transient neurological deficit with an incidence of 2.84 per 100 (95% confidence interval 1.33–5.98 per 100). Nevertheless, chronic brachial plexus injury and other serious complications, such as vertebral artery injection, pneu-

mothorax, subarachnoid, or epidural block, are rare ($<0.2\%$) when proper technique is used.[30]

Hadzic et al[31] studied patients having ambulatory open rotator cuff repair and compared interscalene block versus general anesthesia. Patients who received interscalene block anesthesia and analgesia had improved analgesia, fewer side effects, and more rapid postoperative recovery. Expedited recovery related to interscalene block was demonstrated by a greater proportion of patients bypassing phase 1 recovery (76% vs 16%; $P < .001$) and a more rapid return to ambulation (84 minutes vs 234 minutes; $P < .001$) and oral intake (64 minute vs 201 minute; $P = .005$). Furthermore, same-day discharge was achieved more expeditiously (123 minutes vs 286 minutes; $P < .001$) and by a greater proportion of patients (100% vs 84%; $P = .05$) who received interscalene block compared to general anesthesia. Nevertheless, by 24 hours postoperatively, the single injection interscalene block failed to confer any long-term analgesic or recovery benefit over opioid analgesia.

Continuous ambulatory interscalene block can further prolong these benefits.[32,33] Ilfeld et al[32] studied patients having open or arthroscopic rotator cuff repair, subacromial decompression, or acromioplasty. They placed an interscalene catheter in all patients, dosed it initially with mepivacaine, and then randomized patients to receive a perineural infusion of either ropivacaine or saline for 2 days postoperatively. Those who received the ropivacaine infusion had lower pain scores ($P < .05$) and reduced opioid consumption for 2 days. Furthermore, the incidence of side effects, including nausea, sedation and insomnia, were significantly lower over the first 2 days postoperatively in the ropivacaine group. Other investigators have also cited the benefit of interscalene block on postoperative cognitive function and quality of sleep.[34]

Further illustrating the advantages of regional anesthesia for ambulatory surgery, continuous interscalene blocks have also been used to facilitate same-day discharge following total shoulder arthroplasty. Ilfeld et al[35] described a series of 6 patients who took part in a pilot project. Five patients were discharged home directly from the PACU and one patient was admitted for one night due to significant perioperative blood loss. The perineural infusion of 0.2% ropivacaine was maintained for 4-6 days and provided adequate analgesia with minimal opioid requirements or side effects. Additional evidence suggests that continuous interscalene nerve block enhances early postoperative achievement of rehabilitation goals following total shoulder arthroplasty.[36]

Supraclavicular Brachial Plexus Block

The roots of the brachial plexus combine to form the superior, middle, and inferior trunks. The supraclavicular approach to the brachial plexus block targets the trunks of the brachial plexus (Table 18.5). When using a nerve stimulator technique, a 50-mm nerve block needle is placed in the distal interscalene groove about 1 cm cephalad to the clavicle and superolateral to the subclavian artery. The needle is advanced toward the ipsilateral axilla in a plane parallel to the bed and a distal upper extremity motor response is sought (ie, finger flexion or finger extension). Ultrasound guidance enhances appropriate needle positioning and local anesthetic deposition but can also be used to avoid puncture of the pleura or blood vessels.

The supraclavicular block can be used for plastic, orthopedic, and vascular procedures of the elbow, forearm, wrist, and

Table 18.5: Supraclavicular Brachial Plexus Block

Anatomy	Block of the trunks of the brachial plexus
Surgical applications	Elbow
	Forearm
	Wrist
	Hand
Nerve block needle	50 mm
Local anesthetic volume	30 mL
Benefits	Rapid onset
Potential adverse effects (<0.5%)[3]7	Pneumothorax
	Hematoma
	Intravascular injection of local anesthetic
	Transient nerve injury

Table 18.6: Infraclavicular Brachial Plexus Block

Anatomy	Block of the cords of the brachial plexus
Surgical applications	Elbow
	Forearm
	Wrist
	Hand
Nerve block needle	50–75 mm
Local anesthetic volume	30 mL
Benefits	Performed with head and arm in neutral position
Clinical effects: single injection block[39]	Reduces pain scores and opioid use
	Reduces nausea, vomiting, fatigue, and poor concentration
	Facilitates bypass of phase 1 recovery
	Facilitates postoperative ambulation and oral intake
	Facilitates timely hospital discharge
Clinical effects: continuous perineural infusion[40]	Reduces pain and opioid use
	Reduces nausea and sedation
	Improves sleep quality
Potential adverse effects	Pneumothorax
	Hematoma
	Intravascular injection of local anesthetic
	Transient nerve injury

hand. The supraclavicular block is performed where the brachial plexus is most compact; consequently, it produces reliable, rapid onset anesthesia and is particularly useful in a fast-paced ambulatory surgery center. This block alone may not be sufficient for shoulder surgery because the axillary nerve is inconsistently anesthetized. A separate intercostobrachial nerve block is added when anesthesia of the medial upper arm is required (ie, for tourniquet anesthesia). A subcutaneous injection of 5–10 mL of local anesthetic is deposited in a ring medial to the pulsation of the axillary artery at the level of the axilla.

Although few randomized trials investigate the effects of supraclavicular nerve blocks in outpatients, several large series provide support for their efficacy and safety.[22,37,38] Despite the frequently cited risk of pneumothorax, 2 groups[37,38] have shown a 0% incidence of pneumothorax following over 1000 supraclavicular blocks using the subclavian perivascular approach. Other complications are also rare and include hematoma (0.5%), intravascular injection of local anesthetic (0.3%), and transient nerve injury (0.1%).[37]

Infraclavicular Brachial Plexus Block

As the brachial plexus passes over the lateral aspect of the first rib, each trunk branches to form anterior and posterior divisions. The divisions subsequently rejoin to form the medial, lateral, and posterior cords. The infraclavicular approach involves injection of local anesthetic in close proximity to the cords of the brachial plexus as they surround the subclavian artery. This block is summarized in Table 18.6. When a nerve stimulator is used for the coracoid approach, a 50- to 75-mm nerve block needle is inserted 2 cm inferior and 2 cm medial to the coracoid process. The needle is advanced perpendicular to the skin until a distal upper extremity motor response is elicited (ie, finger flexion with medial cord stimulation or finger extension with posterior cord stimulation). Alternatively, an ultrasound-guided block enables needle and local anesthetic placement under direct vision.

The infraclavicular brachial plexus block is used for procedures of the elbow, forearm, wrist, and hand. The axillary nerve may be spared as this nerve exits the brachial plexus sheath proximal to the level of the infraclavicular block. In addition, supplemental block of the intercostobrachial nerve is required for anesthesia of the medial arm. The infraclavicular block pro-

vides several advantages over other distal brachial plexus blocks. It can be performed with both the patient's head and arm in a neutral position that can be beneficial for trauma patients. In addition, this approach provides a relatively clean and immobile site for continuous catheter placement and fixation. Complications of the infraclavicular block may include vascular puncture due to the close proximity of the subclavian artery as well as the rare risk of pneumothorax or nerve injury.

Hadzic et al[39] provided evidence for the benefit of infraclavicular block when they compared this technique to general anesthesia for patients having ambulatory hand and wrist surgery. The infraclavicular nerve block provided superior analgesia as demonstrated by lower VAS scores ($P < .001$) and a smaller proportion of patients requiring analgesia (0 vs 48%; $P < .001$) while in the hospital, when compared to the general anesthetic. The infraclavicular nerve block afforded additional recovery advantages, including a lower incidence of nausea/vomiting (8% vs 32%; $P < .001$), sore throat (4% vs 36%; $P < 0.001$), fatigue (32% vs 68%; $P < .001$), and inability to concentrate (8% vs 56%; $P < .001$). Furthermore, recovery occurred more expeditiously among nerve block patients as evidenced by more frequent phase 1 PACU bypass (76% vs 25%; $P < .001$) as well as by decreased time to oral intake, ambulation (82 minutes vs 145 minutes; $P < .001$), and hospital discharge (121 minutes vs 218 minutes; $P < .001$). Despite these advantages, there was no difference between groups in pain scores or analgesic requirements in the first 48 hours following hospital discharge. This may be related to the use of short-acting chloroprocaine for the infraclavicular

Table 18.7: Axillary Brachial Plexus Block

Anatomy	Block of the branches of the brachial plexus
Surgical applications	Elbow
	Forearm
	Wrist
	Hand
Nerve block needle	50 mm
Local anesthetic volume	40 mL
Benefits	Pulsatile landmark
	Vessels compressible if punctured
Clinical effects: single injection block[43]	Reduces pain and opioid use
	Reduces nausea and vomiting
	Facilitates bypass of phase 1 recovery
	Facilitates timely outpatient discharge
Potential adverse effects	Incomplete anesthesia due presence of septae
	Multiple injections required
	Mobile catheter site
	Risk of infection from perineural catheter

nerve block; however, it is most likely from the minimal pain experienced following such minor surgical procedures (ie, carpal tunnel release, ganglion cyst excision).

Ilfeld et al[40] demonstrated the advantage of continuous ambulatory infraclavicular block for moderately painful orthopedic surgery of the upper extremity. They placed an infraclavicular catheter, dosed it with a mepivacaine solution for surgical anesthesia, and randomized patients to receive a continuous infusion of 0.2% ropivacaine or saline for postoperative analgesia. The treatment group had lower pain scores for the 2-day duration of the infusion ($P < .05$) and decreased opioid consumption for 3 days ($P < .05$). Patients receiving the ropivacaine infusion had a lower incidene of nausea ($P = .028$) and sedation ($P = .037$) on the first postoperative day as well as improved sleep quality during the first 2 nights ($P < .002$) when compared to the placebo group.

The benefits of continuous ambulatory infraclavicular nerve block have been applied to further expand the scope of outpatient surgery. Ilfeld et al[41] published a case report describing ambulatory total elbow arthroplasty facilitated by a continuous perineural infusion of local anesthetic at home for 6 days. Analgesia was effective and no complications resulted.

Axillary Brachial Plexus Block

The cords of the brachial plexus combine to form the axillary, musculocutaneous, median, radial, and ulnar nerves. The axillary brachial plexus block involves injection of local anesthetic in close proximity to these terminal branches of the brachial plexus. Table 18.7 summarizes the key features of this peripheral nerve block.

With the arm abducted and the elbow flexed, a 50-mm nerve block needle is advanced superior, posterior, or inferior to the axillary artery to elicit median (finger flexion), radial (finger

extension), or ulnar (supination) nerve motor response, respectively. Multiple injections enhance block success and onset time because of the presence of fibrous septae within the brachial plexus sheath at this level.[42] The musculocutaneous nerve exits the brachial plexus sheath proximal to the level of this block; consequently, a supplementary musculocutaneous nerve is required for lateral forearm anesthesia. This is performed by injecting 5 mL of local anesthetic solution into the substance of the coracobrachialis muscle. A separate intercostobrachial nerve block is required for medial arm anesthesia. The axillary nerve is typically spared as it branches away from the brachial plexus promixal to the axilla. The axillary brachial plexus block with supplementation of the musculocutaneous and intercostobrachial nerves provides anesthesia of the elbow and the distal upper extremity; consequently, this block can be used for procedures of the elbow, forearm, wrist, and hand.

The advantages of the axillary block include a readily identifiable pulsatile landmark, ease of performance, and low incidence of serious side effects. The needle insertion site in the axilla is accessible and compressible. Compression of the nerve block site can reduce the severity of hematoma when accidental or intended vascular puncture occurs or when this block is performed in patients with mild systemic coagulopathy.

Disadvantages of this block include the need for multiple injections, the risk of toxicity because of the large dose of local anesthesic used, and the prolonged onset time. Dislodgement and the maintenance of sterility are concerns when continuous axillary catheters are employed.

McCartney et al[43] have investigated the effects of a single-injection axillary brachial plexus block for ambulatory hand surgery. They randomized patients to receive an axillary block with lidocaine versus general anesthesia. The axillary nerve block provided superior immediate postoperative analgesia and was associated with reduced pain scores, longer time to first analgesic (97.6 minutes vs 29.9 minutes; $P < .001$), and decreased opioid consumptions while in the hospital. In addition, fewer patients in the axillary block group experienced nausea or vomiting prior to hospital discharge (6% vs 24%; $P < .05$). Axillary nerve block anesthesia accelerated immediate postoperative recovery, allowing a greater proportion of patients to bypass the PACU (98% vs 54%; $P < .001$) and reducing the time to discharge (100.4 minutes vs 142.6 minutes; $P < .001$). Despite these early postoperative advantages, there was no difference between the two treatment groups in terms of pain, opioid consumption, or opioid-related side effects following hospital discharge. This is likely related to the use of lidocaine, a short-acting local anesthetic, for the single-injection nerve block. As previously discussed, a continuous catheter technique can be used to extend the duration of postoperative analgesia at home.[44]

Distal Upper Extremity Nerve Blocks

The terminal nerves of the brachial plexus can be individually blocked at any point along their course distal to the axilla. The advantage of this approach is the ability to provide site-specific anesthesia while sparing those nerves not involved in surgical site innervation. Moreover, individual nerve blocks may be valuable for supplementation of an incomplete brachial plexus block.

In the midhumeral brachial plexus block, the musculocutenaous, median, radial, and/or ulnar nerves are blocked midway

Table 18.8: Lumbar Plexus Block

Anatomy	Block of the L1 to L4 nerve roots
Surgical applications	Anterior knee and thigh
	Knee (in combination with sciatic nerve block)
Nerve block needle	100 mm
Local anesthetic volume	30 mL
Benefits	Produces more reliable anesthesia of the femoral, obturator and lateral femoral cutaneous nerves than femoral nerve block
Clinical effects: single injection block[45]	Reduces pain
	Reduces nausea, sore throat and difficulty concentrating
	Facilitates bypass of phase 1 recovery
	Facilitates oral intake
	Facilitates ambulatory discharge
Potential adverse effects	Hip flexor weakness
	Epidural anesthesia
	Nerve injury
	Bowel or kidney injury
	Retroperitoneal hematoma
	Total spinal anesthesia

between the axilla and the elbow. Similarly, a small volume of dilute local anesthetic can be used to block the median and/or radial nerves at the elbow. The ulnar nerve is located in the ulnar groove at the elbow and nerve block should rarely be performed here because of the high risk of nerve injury. The ulnar, median, and/or radial nerves can be blocked at the wrist for surgical procedures of the hand or fingers.

Intravenous Regional Anesthesia

Intravenous regional anesthesia, or Bier block, produces surgical anesthesia distal to the elbow. A double tourniquet is placed on the upper arm and the arm is exsanguinated using an Esmarch bandage. Lidocaine is injected into a vein in the exsanguinated arm. Anesthesia results from diffusion of lidocaine to nearby nerves. Advantages of this technique include its simplicity. Disadvantages include the potential for local anesthetic toxicity related to faulty tourniquet placement or inadvertent deflation, limited duration of surgical anesthesia because of tourniquet pain and limb ischemia, as well as a lack of postoperative analgesia.

Lumbar Plexus Block

The L1 to L4 nerve roots combine to form the lumbar plexus and its terminal branches – the femoral, lateral femoral cutaneous, and obturator nerves. The lumbar plexus block is summarized in Table 18.8. It involves injection of local anesthetic close to the proximal part of the lumbar plexus in a paravertebral location. A 100-mm needle is inserted at the intersection of the intercristal line and a paraspinal line through the posterior superior iliac

spine. The needle is advanced slightly medially and caudal to the transverse process of L4 until knee extension is elicited at 0.5 mA.

This nerve block produces anesthesia of the three terminal branches of the lumbar plexus. This results in sensory anesthesia of the anterolateromedial thigh and medial calf and motor block of the hip flexors, quadriceps, and thigh adductor muscles. When used alone, the lumbar plexus block is effective for procedures of the anterior thigh such as muscle biopsy. The lumbar plexus block is combined with a sciatic nerve block to provide complete knee anesthesia for procedures such as arthroscopy, ligament reconstruction, or arthroplasty.

Hip flexor weakness can result from a lumbar plexus block and may make early postoperative ambulation difficult for some outpatients. Even the use of a walker or crutches can be challenging in the presence of hip flexor weakness. An epidural block can result from inadvertent epidural spread of local anesthetic and this can significantly delay hospital discharge. Other serious complications occur in 1.3%,[24] and these may include local anesthetic toxicity, retroperitoneal hematoma, nerve injury, and renal damage. Although extremely rare, there has been a death reported following lumbar plexus block[24] and the etiology was felt to be unintentional subarachnoid local anesthetic injection.

Hadzic et al[45] compared a combined lumbar plexus-sciatic nerve block versus "fast-track" general anesthesia for patients having knee arthroscopy. Patients who received the lumbar plexus-sciatic nerve blocks reported lower visual analog pain scores ($P = .02$). The nerve block group also had a lower incidence of nausea ($P < .001$), sore throat (28% vs 60%; $P = .045$), and difficulty concentrating (25% vs 56%; $P = .04$) in the immediate postoperative period compared to the group who received general anesthesia. Peripheral nerve blocks were associated with a more rapid early postoperative recovery as documented by more frequent phase 1 PACU bypass (72% vs 24%; $P < .002$), a shorter time to oral intake (69 minutes vs 125 minutes; $P = .001$), and reduced time to hospital discharge (162 minutes vs 226 minutes $P = .009$). Nevertheless, there were no differences between the groups in terms of analgesia following hospital discharge. The use of the short-acting local anesthetic chloroprocaine may have prevented any long-term benefits from the peripheral nerve blocks; alternatively, patients having knee arthroscopy may experience minimal pain following hospital discharge regardless of anesthetic technique. Certainly, a careful analysis of the risk-benefit ratio should be considered when lumbar plexus-sciatic nerve block is considered for minimally invasive surgery such as knee arthroscopy.

Greater benefit from the lumbar plexus block is likely to result when a continuous perineural catheter is used for invasive surgery. Klein et al[46] have reported the successful use of an ambulatory lumbar plexus catheter for multiligament knee reconstruction. Ilfeld et al[47] further extended the application of this technique for ambulatory total hip arthroplasty.

Femoral Nerve Block

The femoral nerve block is summarized in Table 18.9. It involves injection of local anesthetic close to the femoral nerve below the inguinal ligament. When using a nerve stimulator, a 50-mm needle is inserted lateral to the pulsation of the femoral artery at the level of the inguinal crease and advanced cranially until

Table 18.9: Femoral Nerve Block

Anatomy	Block of the femoral nerve at the inguinal ligament
Surgical applications	Anterior knee and thigh
	Knee (in combination with sciatic nerve block)
Nerve block needle	50 mm
Local anesthetic volume	20 mL
Benefits	Pulsatile landmark
	Easily compressible in the event of vascular puncture
Clinical effects: single injection block[50,52]	Reduces incidence of unanticipated hospital admissions
	Cost savings
Potential adverse effects	Risk of instability and falls
	Mobile catheter site
	Risk of infection with prolonged perineural catheter

Table 18.10: Proximal Sciatic Nerve Block

Anatomy	Block of the sciatic nerve in the gluteal region
Surgical applications	Knee (in combination with lumbar plexus or femoral nerve block)
	Ankle (in combination with femoral or saphenous nerve block)
	Foot
Nerve block needle	100 mm
Local anesthetic volume	20 mL
Benefits	Analgesia
Clinical effects: single injection block[50]	Reduces opioid use
Potential adverse effects	Instability and falls

quadriceps contraction occurs at 0.5 mA. Ultrasound guidance enables needle insertion and injection of local anesthetic under direct vision.

A femoral nerve block produces sensory anesthesia of the anterior thigh, anterior knee, and medial calf as well as motor block of the quadriceps muscles. The lateral femoral cutaneous and obturator nerves are inconsistently blocked; consequently, the "3-in-1" block is infrequently achieved.[48] Most patients can ambulate with isolated unilateral quadriceps weakness and can achieve discharge criteria after a femoral nerve block. This technique is advantageous in its simplicity and in the ready compressibility of the site should vascular puncture occur. Catheter dislodgement and insertion site infection are potential drawbacks of continuous femoral nerve blocks; however, serious complications are rare (<0.03%).[24]

Although a single injection femoral nerve block can provide effective analgesia following knee arthroscopy, no advantage was found compared to an intra-articular injection of local anesthetic.[49] When more painful anterior cruciate ligament reconstruction is considered, a femoral nerve block can provide superior analgesia compared to opioid analgesia[50] and intra-articular local anesthetic.[51] In a retrospective review of 1200 patients, Williams et al[50] documented the benefit of peripheral nerve blocks for patients having knee surgery. A single-injection femoral nerve block (with or without additional sciatic nerve block) reduced the rate of unanticipated hospital admission for patients having "more invasive" knee surgery compared to those treated with opioid analgesia (P ≤ .002). Furthermore, the combined femoral-sciatic nerve block reduced the requirement for analgesics in the step-down recovery unit following "more invasive" surgery compared to femoral nerve block alone or opioid analgesia (7% vs 22%; P < .001). In addition to the enhanced quality of patient care, these benefits can also translate to cost savings for the health care institution.[52]

A femoral catheter and continuous infusion of local anesthetic can prolong postoperative analgesia. This technique has

been employed to facilitate ambulatory total knee arthroplasty[53] and has also been shown to reduce costs associated with hospital admission.[54]

Fascia Iliaca Block

The fascia iliaca block involves injection of local anesthetic below the fascia iliaca in attempt to produce spread of solution to the lumbar plexus. A 50-mm needle is inserted 0.5–1 cm inferior to the junction of the lateral third and medial two-thirds of the inguinal ligament. The needle is advanced perpendicular to the skin and loss of resistance can be felt twice as the needle passes through the fascia lata and the fascia iliaca. Advantages of the fascia iliaca block include the ease of performance. Applications and potential complications are as for the femoral nerve block.

Proximal Sciatic Nerve Block

The sciatic nerve is formed from the L4 to S3 nerve roots. Even at its most proximal point, the nerve is divided functionally and anatomically into three components: the posterior cutaneous nerve of the thigh and the common peroneal and the tibial nerves. A number of approaches to the proximal sciatic nerve block have been described (ie, classic, subgluteal, lateral, anterior) and a detailed description of each approach is available in standard textbooks of regional anesthesia.

The proximal sciatic nerve block is summarized in Table 18.10. It produces sensory anesthesia of the posterior thigh, posterior knee, anteroposterolateral calf, ankle, and foot. It results in motor block of the hamstrings, the muscles involved in ankle movement, as well as the toe flexors and extensors. Alone, this block has few applications; consequently, it is more commonly used with lumbar plexus/femoral nerve block for knee surgery as previously described.

A proximal sciatic nerve block supplemented with a femoral or saphenous nerve block can be used for procedures of the ankle (ie, ankle arthroscopy, fusion, or arthrodesis), foot (ie, fracture reduction, hallux valgus repair), or toes. The saphenous nerve is the terminal branch of the femoral nerve. It provides

Table 18.11: Distal Sciatic Nerve Block in the Popliteal Fossa

Anatomy	Block of the sciatic nerve in the popliteal fossa
Surgical applications	Ankle (in combination with femoral or saphenous nerve block)
	Foot
Nerve block needle	50–75 mm
Local anesthetic volume	40 mL
Benefits	Greater preservation of lower extremity motor strength than proximal sciatic block
Clinical effects: single injection block[56]	Reduces pain and opioid use
	Reduces length of hospital stay
Potential adverse effects	Rare

sensation to the medial calf and can be blocked by subcutaneous infiltration medial to the tibial tuberosity or by injection of local anesthetic deep to the sartorius muscle at the level of the proximal patella.

The proximal sciatic nerve block produces more extensive lower extremity weakness than block of the sciatic nerve in the popliteal fossa. Consequently, ambulation is more significantly affected following a proximal sciatic nerve block. Serious complications are rare (<0.05%).[24]

Distal Sciatic Nerve Block in the Popliteal Fossa

The common peroneal and tibial components of the sciatic nerve physically separate 5-10 cm cephalad to the popliteal fossa.[55] The popliteal sciatic nerve block is summarized in Table 18.11. It is achieved by injection of local anesthetic proximal to the separation of the common peroneal and tibial nerves. The patient is positioned prone and a 50- to 75-mm needle is inserted 7–10 cm proximal to the popliteal crease and 1 cm lateral to the midpoint of the fossa. When a nerve stimulator is used, the needle is advanced cephalad until toe flexion, extension, or foot inversion is elicited at 0.5 mA. Ultrasound guidance enables needle placement and local anesthetic injection under direct vision.

A popliteal fossa block produces sensory anesthesia in the distribution of both the common peroneal and tibial nerves. This correlates to the posterior knee, anteroposterolateral calf, ankle, and foot. A supplementary femoral or saphenous nerve block can be used to produce comprehensive anesthesia distal to the knee. Consequently, this technique is suitable for foot and ankle surgery. The popliteal sciatic nerve block provides motor block to the muscles involved in ankle movement as well as the toe flexors and extensors. The hamstring muscles are spared and so ambulation is usually minimally affected. Serious complications from the popliteal sciatic nerve block are rare.[24,56]

White et al[56] performed a popliteal fossa nerve block with bupivacaine for patients having foot or ankle surgery and subsequently randomized them to receive a continuous perineural infusion of either bupivacaine or saline. The patients in the treatment group reported lower pain scores for 2 days ($P < .05$) and required less opioid analgesia in the first 24 hours compared to patients in the placebo group (10.3 mg vs 34.7 mg;

$P < .05$). In addition, mean length of hospital stay was shorter in the group who received a bupivacaine infusion compared those who received saline (0.7 days vs 1.4 days; $P = .05$).

Ankle Block

The ankle block involves injection of local anesthetic close to the terminal nerves of the lower extremity at the ankle. The femoral nerve terminates as the saphenous nerve. The distal branches of the sciatic nerve include the superficial and deep peroneal nerves (from the common peroneal nerve), the tibial nerve, and the sural nerve (from both the tibial and common peroneal nerves). The saphenous nerve is blocked with a subcutaneous injection of 5 mL of local anesthetic solution anterior to the medial malleolus, close to the saphenous vein. The superficial peroneal nerve is blocked with a subcutaneous injection of 10 mL of local anesthetic solution in a ring around the anterior aspect of the ankle from the medial to the lateral malleolus. The deep peroneal nerve is blocked with an injection of 5 mL of local anesthetic solution lateral to the pulsation of the dorsalis pedis artery. The tibial nerve is blocked with infiltration of 5–10 mL of local anesthetic solution posterior to the pulsation of the tibial artery behind the medial malleolus. The sural nerve is blocked with infiltration of 5 mL of local anesthetic posterior to the lateral malleolus. All or selected nerves can be blocked according to the location of the surgical procedure. Epinephrine-containing local anesthetic is avoided because of the risk of distal ischemia.

Advantages of the ankle block include ease of performance and preservation of lower extremity motor function. Drawbacks include a lack of tourniquet anesthesia and the inability to prolong analgesia by catheter techniques. Serious complications are rare.

Paravertebral Nerve Block

The paravertebral nerve block is summarized in Table 18.12. This technique involves injection of local anesthetic in close proximity to a segmental spinal nerve as it courses through the paravertebral space. The paravertebral space is a wedge-shaped region on either side of the vertebral column bounded at each segmental level by the parietal pleura, vertebral body, and the superior costotransverse ligament that extends from the transverse process above to the rib below.

The patient can be positioned sitting, prone, or lateral decubitus with the side to be blocked uppermost. The levels to be blocked should be chosen according to the surgical procedure performed (Table 18.13), bearing in mind that the thoracic spinal nerves exit below their respective transverse processes that, in turn, are located at the same horizontal level as the spinous process of the vertebra above. A 10-cm, 22-gauge Tuohy needle is inserted 2.5 cm lateral to the cephalad border of the appropriate spinous process (ie,, needle inserted beside T5 spinous process to effect block of T6 spinal nerve). The needle is advanced caudad and 1 cm deep to the transverse process until a change in resistance is appreciated as the superior costotransverse ligament is pierced.

Paravertebral blocks have been compared to general anesthesia with opioid analgesia for breast surgery. The nerve blocks were associated with lower pain scores, reduced opioid consumption, decreased incidence of nausea and vomiting, shorter hospital stay, as well as improved arm motion.[57,58] Similar benefits

Table 18.12: Paravertebral Nerve Block

Anatomy	Block of the segmental spinal nerves in the paravertebral space
Surgical applications	Breast
	Hernia (inguinal, incisional, umbilical)
Nerve block needle	100-mm Tuohy
Local anesthetic volume	3–5 mL per segment
Benefits	Analgesia
Clinical effects: single injection block[57,58–61]	Reduces pain and opioid use
	Reduces nausea and vomiting
	Reduces hospital length of stay
	Improves ipsilateral arm mobility
Potential adverse effects[62,63]	Hematoma
	Epidural anesthesia
	Brachial plexus block
	Horner's syndrome
	Local anesthetic toxicity
	Pneumothorax
	Total spinal anesthesia
	Pulmonary hemorrhage
	Nerve injury

Table 18.13: Segmental Anesthesia Required for Various Surgical Procedures

Surgical Procedure	Levels Blocked
Mastectomy	T2–T6
Mastectomy with axillary dissection	T1–T6 with superficial cervical plexus block
Breast biopsy	Level of lesion with one level above and below
Inguinal hernia repair	T10–L2
Umbilical hernia repair	T9–T11 bilaterally
Incisional hernia repair	According to level of repair
Adjunct for shoulder surgery (subdeltoid incision)	T1–T2
Iliac crest bone harvesting	T11–L1

of local anesthetic toxicity is related to the large volumes of local anesthetic used to obtain an adequate block and to the significant systemic absorption that occurs in this highly vascular area.

Ilioinguinal and Iliohypogastric Nerve Block

These nerves are branches of the lumbar plexus and can be blocked in the anterior abdominal wall as they course between the external and internal oblique muscles. The iliohypogastric nerve supplies sensation to the suprapubic area; the ilioinguinal nerve innervates the superomedial thigh and a portion of the genitals. Ilioinguinal and iliohypogastric nerve block can be used for analgesia following inguinal hernia, orchidopexy, and hydrocele repairs and is advantageous in its simplicity. The patient is positioned supine, the skin disinfected, and local skin infiltration performed. A 50-mm needle is inserted 1–2 cm medial and 1–2 cm superior to the anterior superior iliac spine along a line drawn from it to the umbilicus. A loss of resistance can be appreciated as the needle pierces the external oblique muscle. Side effects include inadvertent femoral nerve block that may impair the mobility of an outpatient.

WOUND INFILTRATION FOR POSTOPERATIVE ANALGESIA IN OUTPATIENTS

Infiltration of local anesthetic at the surgical site can enhance postoperative analgesia following a variety of surgical procedures. Although this technique is simple and safe, even long-acting local anesthetics provide analgesia of limited duration.

Insertion of a wound catheter for continuous infusion of local anesthetic can prolong the duration of effect from this analgesic modality. At the conclusion of the surgical procedure, the surgeon places the wound catheter. This is easily and efficiently accomplished. Catheters can be placed in a number of sites – subcutaneous, subfascial, supraperiosteal, intra-articular, and intraperitoneal. Wound catheters can be attached to ambulatory local anesthetic infusion pumps, making this technique suitable for outpatient use. The cost of this technique varies according to the ambulatory pump used.

were observed in studies involving patients having inguinal[59,60] and umbilical[61] hernia repair.

In two large series, pneumothorax occurred in 0.3%–2.1%.[62,63] This complication can have obvious implications for outpatients. The risk of local anesthetic toxicity can be minimized by using a precalculated dose of local anesthetic based on the patient's weight and by adding epinephrine to the local anesthetic solution. Other potential adverse effects are extremely rare and include epidural or intrathecal injection with associated hypotension, total spinal anesthesia, or post dural puncture headache.[62,63]

Intercostal Nerve Block

The intercostal nerve block involves placement of local anesthetic in close proximity to the intercostal nerve. The intercostal nerve courses between the pleura and internal intercostal medial to the angle of the rib and between the internal and innermost intercostal lateral to the angle of the rib. The intercostal nerve block provides segmental anesthesia to the skin and intercostal muscles in a dermatomal distribution. The patient is placed prone and the segmental levels to be blocked are identified according to the surgical procedure. A 25-mm needle is inserted at the angle of the rib (5–9 cm from midline) along its inferior border. Blocking the nerve in this location, proximal to the take-off of its branches, ensures more complete anesthesia. The nerve block needle is inserted to contact rib, redirected caudally and advanced 3–5 mm deep to the rib. After negative aspiration for blood, 3–5 mL of local anesthetic is injected and the block is repeated at each of the desired levels.

Intercostal nerve block is indicated for analgesia following breast or chest wall procedures. Pneumothorax is rare (0.42%)[64] despite the close proximity of the lung and pleura. The risk

Rawal et al.[44] reported the use of this technique for outpatients following maxillofacial surgery and iliac crest bone harvesting. Prior to surgical closure, the surgeon placed a 22-gauge, multiorificed epidural catheter in the wound just above the periosteum and tunneled the catheter 4–5 cm subcutaneously to enhance fixation. They attached the catheters to disposable, elastomeric pumps containing 50 to 100 mL of 0.25%–0.5% bupivacaine and instructed patients on how to self-administer intermittent boluses every 60 minutes at home. The dosing regimen involved a bolus dose of 2.5 mL for maxillofacial procedures and 5–10 mL for other surgical wounds. Analgesia was effective for 90% of patients. Each bolus dose onset within 5 minutes and lasted 2–8 hours.

Since Rawal's description, other investigators have studied the efficacy of local anesthetic wound infusions for analgesia following a variety of surgical procedures. In a systematic review, Liu et al[65] summarized the results of 44 randomized trials with 2141 patients to determine the efficacy of continuous wound catheters. A subgroup analysis was also performed for cardiothoracic, general, gynecologic-urologic, and orthopedic surgical procedures. The investigators found that the wound catheters decreased visual analog pain scores at rest by a mean of 10 mm (95% CI 7- to 13-mm reduction; $P < .001$) and this remained significant for all subgroups. Wound catheters decreased visual analog pain scores with activity by a mean of 15 mm (95% CI 9- to 22-mm reduction; $P < .001$); however, in the subgroup analysis this effect was not significant for cardiothoracic or general surgical procedures. Wound catheters reduced the requirement for opioid rescue by a mean 41% (vs 66%; OR 0.15; $P < .001$) and decreased the daily morphine consumption by a mean of 11 mg (95% CI 7- to 14-mg reduction; $P < .001$). However, when subgroup analysis was performed, the reduction in daily opioid consumption among patients having orthopedic surgery was not significant. Among those with wound catheters, there was a greater proportion of patients who rated their analgesia as "excellent" (43% vs 13%; OR 7.7; $P = .007$); however, subgroup analysis found this only to be significant for those having orthopedic procedures. Wound catheters were associated with a reduction in the incidence of postoperative nausea and vomiting (24% vs 40%, OR 0.45; $P < .001$). Moreover, length of hospital stay was reduced by 1 day in the continuous wound catheter group (7 days vs 8 days; $P < .05$). There were no cases of local anesthetic toxicity. The incidence of pump failure was 1.1%. Furthermore, the incidence of wound infection was 0.7% among those patients receiving treatment and 1.2% among those in a control group.

The meta-analysis by Liu et al[65] primarily involved inpatients having significantly painful surgical procedures. Nevertheless, several studies have investigated the use of ambulatory continuous local anesthetic wound infusions. Four randomized, controlled trials explored the use of continuous subfascial wound catheters for analgesia following outpatient inguinal hernia repair.[66–69] Investigators compared an infusion of bupivacaine (0.5%) at 2 mL/h for 48 to 60 hours postoperatively versus a saline placebo infusion,[68,69] opioid analgesia without a subfascial catheter,[66] or both.[67] Three of the four studies[66–68] demonstrated lower visual analog pain scores with continuous local anesthetic wound infusion though the duration of analgesic benefit varied from 24 to 80 hours. Nevertheless, no reduction in opioid consumption was apparent. Sanchez et al[70] found similar results with a subcutaneous catheter that was dosed with 2 mL/h of either bupivacaine (0.25%) or saline.

A number of randomized, controlled trials have investigated the analgesic efficacy of continuous local anesthetic infusion via intra- and periarticular catheters placed following orthopedic surgical procedures. Seven trials evaluated the use of intra-articular catheters for operative shoulder arthroscopy.[71–77] These trials are difficult to compare because the local anesthetic solution and infusion regimen varied (ie, ropivacaine vs bupivacaine, 0.2% vs 0.5%, no additional adjuvants vs added morphine or epinephrine, continuous infusion only vs patient-controlled boluses, infusion duration 24 vs 72 hours). Nonetheless, continuous intra-articular local anesthetic infusion appears to reduce visual analog pain scores for several days (range 0-7 days) and to decrease opioid consumption following arthroscopic shoulder surgery (range 0-88% dose reduction). No effect on postoperative nausea and vomiting or patient satisfaction was apparent.

In contrast to the arthroscopic approach, open shoulder surgery can be associated with greater postoperative pain. Two randomized, controlled trials have investigated the use of continuous periarticular local anesthetic infusion as an analgesic modality following open shoulder surgery. Gottschalk et al.[78] infused 5 mL/h of study solution via a subcutaneous catheter. They found that patients who received 0.375% ropivacaine had reduced visual analog pain scores at rest and with activity for 48 hours ($P < .005$), decreased opioid consumption by 58% ($P < .05$), and less postoperative nausea and vomiting (19% vs 29%) compared to those who received saline. In contrast, Boss et al[79] placed a subacromial catheter and infused 6 mL/h of bupivacaine (0.25%) versus saline for 48 hours and found no difference in visual analog pain scores, opioid consumption, incidence of postoperative nausea and vomiting, or patient satisfaction. The analgesic efficacy of periarticular local anesthetic infusion for open shoulder surgery requires further elucidation.

Two randomized controlled trials have examined intra-articular local anesthetic infiltration as an analgesic modality following anterior cruciate ligament repair. Alford et al[80] combined a single injection femoral nerve block with an intra-articular catheter infusing 2 mL/h of bupivacaine (0.25%) versus saline. They found that the treatment group had lower visual analog pain scores for 4 days compared to the control group; however, there was no difference between groups in opioid consumption or postoperative nausea and vomiting. A study by Hoenecke et al[81] obtained similar results.

Several studies have compared periarticular versus perineural administration of local anesthetic for postoperative analgesia. Singelyn et al[82] randomized patients having arthroscopic acromioplasty to receive one of four analgesic modalities – a suprascapular nerve block, an intra-articular injection of local anesthetic, an interscalene brachial plexus nerve block, or intravenous patient controlled opioid analgesia. All local anesthetic techniques were single injections and no continuous catheters were used in this study. The interscalene block provided the best analgesia as measured by visual analog pain scores and morphine consumption. The intraarticular injection provided no advantage over opioid analgesia. In a study involving continuous catheter techniques, Dauri et al[83] randomized patients having arthroscopically assisted anterior cruciate ligament repair to receive one of three postoperative analgesic modalities – continuous epidural, continuous peripheral nerve block, or intra-articular catheter. All analgesic modalities involved an infusion of ropivacaine (0.2%) with sufentanil 0.2 μg/mL with a basal rate of 5 mL/h and with patient-controlled boluses of 5 mL every

2 hours. Peripheral nerve blocks included a continuous inguinal paravascular femoral 3-in-1 block and a single-injection sciatic nerve block. Each nerve block was dosed with ropivacaine (0.75%) initially. The visual analog pain scores were higher in the intra-articular catheter group compared to the epidural group at 24 hours (40 mm vs 17.5 mm; $P < .05$); however, there was no significant difference between the intra-articular and peripheral nerve block groups. The dose of supplemental opioid and nonopioid analgesia administered was greater in the intraarticular group compared to the other two groups (6 patient-controlled opioid boluses vs 2; $P < .001$ and 75 mg ketorolac vs 30 mg; $P < .005$). Urinary retention occurred more frequently in the epidural group; however, the incidence of side effects was otherwise no different between groups. Patient satisfaction was greater in the epidural group compared to the intraarticular group (3.1 ± 0.64 vs 2.3 ± 0.86; $P < .005$); however, no difference was observed between the intra-articular and peripheral nerve block groups.

Continuous ambulatory infusion of local anesthetic into the surgical wound offers a number of advantages in the management of postoperative pain for outpatients. Wound catheter placement is simple and efficient. Local anesthetic administered into the surgical wound provides acceptable analgesia. Some studies have shown that this technique can reduce opioid consumption and related side effects as well as enhance postoperative recovery and mobilization.[84] Finally, this technique is reasonably well tolerated and most patients feel comfortable caring for and removing their wound catheters and pumps at home.

Despite these advantages, wound catheters may be associated with several concerns. Adverse effects include fluid leakage from the insertion site,[85] catheter dislodgement, catheter entrapment,[85] and, in some cases, inadequate analgesia.[85] The catheter represents a foreign body and can be associated with wound infection. Infusion of local anesthetic into a wound may adversely affect wound healing or cause tissue necrosis. A report on home continuous wound infusions of local anesthetic from the United States Food and Drug Administration[86] summarizes 40 adverse event reports. In this series a surgical wound infection occurred in 15 patients, cellulitis developed in 13 patients, and tissue necrosis, an extremely rare surgical complication, resulted in 17 patients. In addition, Gomoll et al[87] demonstrated evidence of bupivacaine-induced chondrotoxicity following intra-articular infusion in a rabbit shoulder model. Certainly, the benefits of this technique need to be fully elucidated and weighed against the potential risks.

CONCLUSION

Peripheral nerve blocks provide excellent postoperative analgesia following ambulatory surgery and minimize the requirement for opioid analgesia. Single-injection blocks with long-acting local anesthetic provide up to 24 hours of pain relief. Analgesia is extended for several days using a continuous perineural infusion of local anesthetic. Adequate pain relief and the absence of opioid-related side effects, such as nausea, vomiting, and sedation, greatly enhance the quality of postoperative recovery. Furthermore, these benefits frequently result in a reduced length of hospital stay. Additional advantages of peripheral nerve block analgesia include enhanced postoperative rehabilitation and improved sleep.

Infiltration and infusion of local anesthetic directly into the surgical wound consists of another technique for postoperative analgesia in outpatients. The analgesic efficacy of this technique has been proven for a number of surgical procedures; however, the usefulness of this modality for other operations remains controversial.

Outpatient surgery is attractive to patients, health care providers, and hospital administration alike. Increasingly complex procedures, such as total joint arthroplasty, are being performed on an outpatient basis. Peripheral nerve blocks and local anesthetic wound infusions facilitate accelerated discharge and improve patients' quality of recovery at home.

REFERENCES

1. Liu SS, Strodtbeck WM, Richman JM, Wu CL. A comparison of regional versus general anesthesia for ambulatory anesthesia: a meta-analysis of randomized controlled trials. *Anesth Analg.* 2005;101:1634–1642.
2. Richman JM, Liu SS, Courpas G, et al. Does continuous peripheral nerve block provide superior pain control to opioids? A meta-analysis. *Anesth Analg.* 2006;102:248–257.
3. Casati A, Borghi B, Fanelli G, et al. A double-blinded, randomized comparison of either 0.5% levobupivacaine or 0.5% ropivacaine for sciatic nerve block. *Anesth Analg.* 2002;94(4):987–990.
4. Wang RD, Dangler LA, Greengrass RA. Update on ropivacaine. *Exp Opin Pharmacother.* 2001;2(12):2051–2063.
5. Niemi G, Breivik H. Epinephrine markedly improves thoracic epidural analgesia produced by a small-dose infusion of ropivacaine, fentanyl, and epinephrine after major thoracic or abdominal surgery: a randomized, double-blinded crossover study with and without epinephrine. *Anesth Analg.* 2002;94(6):1598–1605.
6. Bernard JM, Macaire P. Dose-range effects of clonidine added to lidocaine for brachial plexus block. *Anesthesiology.* 1997;87(2):277–284.
7. Erlacher W, Schuschnig C, Koinig H, et al. Clonidine as adjuvant for mepivacaine, ropivacaine and bupivacaine in axillary, perivascular brachial plexus block. *Can J Anaesth.* 2001;48(6):522–525.
8. El Saied AH, Steyn MP, Ansermino JM. Clonidine prolongs the effect of ropivacaine for axillary brachial plexus blockade. *Can J Anaesth.* 2000;47(10):962–967.
9. Lee IO, Kim WK, Kong MH, et al. No enhancement of sensory and motor blockade by ketamine added to ropivacaine interscalene brachial plexus blockade. *Acta Anaesthesiol Scand.* 2002;46(7):821–826.
10. Bone HG, Van Aken H, Booke M, Burkle H. Enhancement of axillary brachial plexus block anesthesia by coadministration of neostigmine. *Reg Anesth Pain Med.* 1999;24(5):405–410.
11. Bouaziz H, Paqueron X, Bur ML, Merle M, Laxenaire MC, Benhamou D. No enhancement of sensory and motor blockade by neostigmine added to mepivacaine axillary plexus block. *Anesthesiology.* 1999;91(1):78–83.
12. Flory N, Van-Gessel E, Donald F, Hoffmeyer P, Gamulin Z. Does the addition of morphine to brachial plexus block improve analgesia after shoulder surgery? *Br J Anaesth.* 1995;75(1):23–26.
13. Bourke DL, Furman WR. Improved postoperative analgesia with morphine added to axillary block solution. *J Clin Anesth.* 1993;5(2):114–117.

14. Viel EJ, Eledjam JJ, De La Coussaye JE, D'Athis F. Brachial plexus block with opioids for postoperative pain relief: comparison between buprenorphine and morphine. *Reg Anesth.* 1989;14(6):274–278.

15. Jarbo K, Batra YK, Panda NB. Brachial plexus block with midazolam and bupivacaine improves analgesia. *Can J Anaesth.* 2005;52(8):822–826.

16. Van Elstraete AC, Pastureau F, Lebrun T, Mehdaoui H. Neostigmine added to lidocaine axillary plexus block for postoperative analgesia. *Eur J Anaesthesiol.* 2001;18(4):257–260.

17. Ilfeld BM, Enneking FK. Continuous peripheral nerve blocks at home: a review. *Anesth Analg.* 2005;100:1822–1833.

18. Ilfeld BM, Morey TE, Enneking FK. Portable infusion pumps used for continuous regional analgesia: delivery rate accuracy and consistency. *Reg Anesth Pain Med.* 2003:424–432.

19. Ilfeld BM, Morey TE, Enneking FK. The delivery rate accuracy of portable infusion pumps used for continuous regional analgesia. *Anesth Analg.* 2002;95(5):1331–1336.

20. Ilfeld BM, Morey TE, Enneking FK. Delivery rate accuracy of portable, bolus-capable infusion pumps used for patient-controlled continuous regional analgesia. *Reg Anesth Pain Med.* 2003;28(1):17–23.

21. Ilfeld BM, Morey TE, Enneking FK. New portable infusion pumps: real advantages or just more of the same in a different package? *Reg Anesth Pain Med.* 2004:371–376.

22. Klein SM, Nielsen KC, Greengrass RA, Warner DS, Martin A, Steele SM. Ambulatory discharge after long-acting peripheral nerve blockade: 2382 blocks with ropivacaine. *Anesth Analg.* 2002;94(1):65–70.

23. Capdevila X, Pirat P, Bringuier S, et al. Continuous peripheral nerve blocks in hospital wards after orthopedic surgery: a multicenter prospective analysis of the quality of postoperative analgesia and complications in 1,416 patients. *Anesthesiology.* 2005;103(5):1035–1045.

24. Auroy Y, Benhamou D, Bargues L, et al. Major complications of regional anesthesia in France: the SOS Regional Anesthesia Hotline Service. *Anesthesiology.* 2002;97:1274–1280.

25. Hadzic A, ed. *Textbook of Regional Anesthesia and Acute Pain Management.* New York, NY: McGraw-Hill; 2007.

26. Evans H, Nielsen KC, Steele SM. Regional Anesthesia for Ambulatory Surgery. In: Twersky RS, Philip BK, eds. *Handbook of Ambulatory Anesthesia.* New York, NY: Springer-Verlag; 2007.

27. Lanz E, Theiss D, Jankovic D. The extent of blockade following various techniques of brachial plexus block. *Anesth Analg.* 1983;62(1):55–58.

28. Urmey WF, Gloeggler PJ. Pulmonary function changes during interscalene brachial plexus block: effects of decreasing local anesthetic injection volume. *Reg Anesth.* 1993;18(4):244–249.

29. Brull R, McCartney CJ, Chan VW, El-Beheiry H. Neurological complications after regional anesthesia: contemporary estimates of risk. *Anesth Analg.* 2007;104:965–974.

30. Borgeat A, Ekatodramis G, Kalberer F, Benz C. Acute and nonacute complications associated with interscalene block and shoulder surgery: a prospective study. *Anesthesiology.* 2001;95(4):875–880.

31. Hadzic A, Williams BA, Karaca PE, et al. For outpatient rotator cuff surgery, nerve block anesthesia provides superior same-day recovery over general anesthesia. *Anesthesiology.* 2005;102(5):1001–1007.

32. Ilfeld BM, Morey TE, Wright TW, Chidgey LK, Enneking FK. Continuous interscalene brachial plexus block for postoperative pain control at home: a randomized, double-blinded, placebo-controlled study. *Anesth Analg.* 2003;96(4):1089–1095.

33. Klein SM, Grant SA, Greengrass RA, et al. Interscalene brachial plexus block with a continuous catheter insertion system and a disposable infusion pump. *Anesth Analg.* 2000;91(6):1473–1478.

34. Nielsen KC, Greengrass RA, Pietrobon R, Klein SM, Steele SM. Continuous interscalene brachial plexus blockade provides good analgesia at home after major shoulder surgery-report of four cases. *Can J Anaesth.* 2003;50(1):57–61.

35. Ilfeld BM, Wright TW, Enneking FK, et al. Total shoulder arthroplasty as an outpatient procedure using ambulatory perineural local anesthetic infusion: a pilot feasibility study. *Anesth Analg.* 2005;101:1319–1322.

36. Ilfeld BM, Wright TW, Enneking FK, Morey TE. Joint range of motion after total shoulder arthroplasty with and without a continuous interscalene nerve block: a retrospective, case-control study. *Reg Anesth Pain Med.* 2005;30(5):429–433.

37. Franco CD, Vieira ZE. 1,001 subclavian perivascular brachial plexus blocks: success with a nerve stimulator. *Reg Anesth Pain Med.* 2000;25(1):41–46.

38. Vaghadia H, Chan V, Ganapathy S, Lui A, McKenna J, Zimmer K. A multicentre trial of ropivacaine 7.5 mg x ml(-1) vs bupivacaine 5 mg x ml(-1) for supra clavicular brachial plexus anesthesia. *Can J Anaesth.* 1999;46(10):946–951.

39. Hadzic A, Arliss J, Kerimoglu B, et al. A comparison of infraclavicular nerve block versus general anesthesia for hand and wrist day-case surgeries. *Anesthesiology.* 2004;101(1):127–132.

40. Ilfeld BM, Morey TE, Enneking FK. Continuous infraclavicular brachial plexus block for postoperative pain control at home: a randomized, double-blinded, placebo-controlled study. *Anesthesiology.* 2002;96(6):1297–1304.

41. Ilfeld BM, Wright TW, Enneking FK, Vandenborne K. Total elbow arthroplasty as an outpatient procedure using a continuous infraclavicular nerve block at home: a prospective case report. *Reg Anesth Pain Med.* 2006;31(2):172–176.

42. Partridge BL, Katz J, Benirschke K. Functional anatomy of the brachial plexus sheath: implications for anesthesia. *Anesthesiology.* 1987;66(6):743–747.

43. McCartney CJ, Brull R, Chan VW, et al. Early but no long-term benefit of regional compared with general anesthesia for ambulatory hand surgery. *Anesthesiology.* 2004;101(2):461–467.

44. Rawal N, Axelsson K, Hylander J, et al. Postoperative patient-controlled local anesthetic administration at home. *Anesth Analg.* 1998;86(1):86–89.

45. Hadzic A, Karaca PE, Hobeika P, et al. Peripheral nerve blocks result in superior recovery profile compared with general anesthesia in outpatient knee arthroscopy. *Anesth Analg.* 2005;100(4):976–981.

46. Klein SM, Greengrass RA, Grant SA, Higgins LD, Nielsen KC, Steele SM. Ambulatory surgery for multi-ligament knee reconstruction with continuous dual catheter peripheral nerve blockade. *Can J Anaesth.* 2001;48(4):375–378.

47. Ilfeld BM, Gearen PF, Enneking FK, et al. Total hip arthroplasty as an overnight-stay procedure using an ambulatory continuous psoas compartment nerve block: a prospective feasibility study. *Reg Anesth Pain Med.* 2006;31(2):113–118.

48. Parkinson SK, Mueller JB, Little WL, Bailey SL. Extent of blockade with various approaches to the lumbar plexus. *Anesth Analg.* 1989;68(3):243–248.

49. Goranson BD, Lang S, Cassidy JD, Dust WN, McKerrell J. A comparison of three regional anaesthesia techniques for outpatient knee arthroscopy. *Can J Anaesth.* 1997;44(4):371–376.

50. Williams BA, Kentor ML, Vogt MT, et al. Femoral-sciatic nerve blocks for complex outpatient knee surgery are associated with less postoperative pain before same-day discharge: a review of 1,200 consecutive cases from the period 1996–1999. *Anesthesiology.* 2003;98(5):1206–1213.

51. Mulroy MF, Larkin KL, Batra MS, Hodgson PS, Owens BD. Femoral nerve block with 0.25% or 0.5% bupivacaine improves postoperative analgesia following outpatient arthroscopic anterior cruciate ligament repair. *Reg Anesth Pain Med.* Jan-Feb 2001;26(1):24–29.

52. Williams BA, Kentor ML, Vogt MT, et al. Economics of nerve block pain management after anterior cruciate ligament reconstruction: potential hospital cost savings via associated postanesthesia care unit bypass and same-day discharge. *Anesthesiology.* 2004;100(3):697–706.

53. Ilfeld BM, Gearen PF, Enneking FK, et al. Total knee arthroplasty as an overnight-stay procedure using continuous femoral nerve blocks at home: a prospective feasibility study. *Anesth Analg.* Jan 2006;102:87–90.

54. Ilfeld BM, Mariano ER, Williams BA, Woodard JN, Macario A. Hospitalization costs of total knee arthroplasty with a continuous femoral nerve block provided only in the hospital versus on an ambulatory basis: a retrospective, case-control, cost-minimization analysis. *Reg Anesth Pain Med.* 2007;32(1):46–54.

55. Vloka JD, Hadzic A, April E, Thys DM. The division of the sciatic nerve in the popliteal fossa: anatomical implications for popliteal nerve blockade. *Anesth Analg.* 2001;92(1):215–217.

56. White PF, Issioui T, Skrivanek GD, Early JS, Wakefield C. The use of a continuous popliteal sciatic nerve block after surgery involving the foot and ankle: does it improve the quality of recovery? *Anesth Analg.* 2003;97(5):1303–1309.

57. Naja MZ, Ziade MF, Lonnqvist PA. Nerve-stimulator guided paravertebral blockade vs. general anaesthesia for breast surgery: a prospective randomized trial. *Eur J Anaesthesiol.* 2003;20(11):897–903.

58. Klein SM, Bergh A, Steele SM, Georgiade GS, Greengrass RA. Thoracic paravertebral block for breast surgery. *Anesth Analg.* 2000;90(6):1402–1405.

59. Klein SM, Pietrobon R, Nielsen KC, et al. Paravertebral somatic nerve block compared with peripheral nerve blocks for outpatient inguinal herniorrhaphy. *Reg Anesth Pain Med.* 2002;27(5):476–480.

60. Naja MZ, el Hassan MJ, Oweidat M, Zbibo R, Ziade MF, Lonnqvist PA. Paravertebral blockade vs general anesthesia or spinal anesthesia for inguinal hernia repair. *Middle East J Anesthesiol.* 2001;16(2):201–210.

61. Naja Z, Ziade MF, Lonnqvist PA. Bilateral paravertebral somatic nerve block for ventral hernia repair. *Eur J Anaesthesiol.* 2002;19(3):197–202.

62. Naja Z, Lonnqvist PA. Somatic paravertebral nerve blockade: incidence of failed block and complications. *Anaesthesia.* 2001;56(12):1184–1188.

63. Lonnqvist PA, MacKenzie J, Soni AK, Conacher ID. Paravertebral blockade. Failure rate and complications. *Anaesthesia.* 1995;50(9):813–815.

64. Moore DC, Bridenbaugh LD. Pneumothorax: its incidence following intercostal nerve block. *JAMA.* 1962;182:1005–1008.

65. Liu SS, Richman JM, Thirlby RC, Wu CL. Efficacy of continuous wound catheters delivering local anesthetic for postoperative analgesia: a quantitative and qualitative systematic review of randomized controlled trials. *J Am Coll Surg.* 2006:914–932.

66. Lau H, Patil NG, Lee F. Randomized clinical trial of postoperative subfascial infusion with bupivacaine following ambulatory

open mesh repair of inguinal hernia. *Digest Surg.* 2003;20(4):285–289.

67. Oakley MJ, Smith JS, Anderson JR, Fenton-Lee D. Randomized placebo-controlled trial of local anaesthetic infusion in day-case inguinal hernia repair. *Br J Surg.* 1998;85(6):797–799.

68. Schurr MJ, Gordon DB, Pellino TA, Scanlon TA. Continuous local anesthetic infusion for pain management after outpatient inguinal herniorrhaphy. *Surgery.* 2004;136:761–769.

69. LeBlanc KA, Bellanger D, Rhynes VK, Hausmann M. Evaluation of continuous infusion of 0.5% bupivacaine by elastomeric pump for postoperative pain management after open inguinal hernia repair. *J Am Coll Surg.* 2005;200(2):198–202.

70. Sanchez B, Waxman K, Tatevossian R, Gamberdella M, Read B. Local anesthetic infusion pumps improve postoperative pain after inguinal hernia repair: a randomized trial. *Am Surg.* 2004;70(11):1002–1006.

71. Axelsson K, Nordenson U, Johanzon E, et al. Patient-controlled regional analgesia (PCRA) with ropivacaine after arthroscopic subacromial decompression. *Acta Anaesthesiol Scand.* 2003;47(8):993–1000.

72. Barber FA, Herbert MA. The effectiveness of an anesthetic continuous-infusion device on postoperative pain control. *Arthroscopy.* 2002;18(1):76–81.

73. Harvey GP, Chelly JE, al Samsam T, Coupe K. Patient-controlled ropivacaine analgesia after arthroscopic subacromial decompression. *Arthroscopy.* 2004;20(5):451–455.

74. Klein SM, Nielsen KC, Martin A, et al. Interscalene brachial plexus block with continuous intraarticular infusion of ropivacaine. *Anesth Analg.* 2001;93:601–605.

75. Park JY, Lee GW, Kim Y, Yoo MJ. The efficacy of continuous intrabursal infusion with morphine and bupivacaine for postoperative analgesia after subacromial arthroscopy. *Reg Anesth Pain Med.* 2002;27:145–149.

76. Quick DC, Guanche CA. Evaluation of an anesthetic pump for postoperative care after shoulder surgery. *J Shoulder Elbow Surg.* 2003;12:618–621.

77. Savoie FH, Field LD, Jenkins RN, Mallon WJ, Phelps RA, 2nd. The pain control infusion pump for postoperative pain control in shoulder surgery. *Arthroscopy.* 2000;16(4):339–342.

78. Gottschalk A, Burmeister MA, Radtke P, et al. Continuous wound infiltration with ropivacaine reduces pain and analgesia requirement after shoulder surgery. *Anesth Analg.* 2003;97:1086–1091.

79. Boss AP, Maurer T, Seiler S, Aeschbach A, Hintermann B, Strebel S. Continuous subacromial bupivacaine infusion for postoperative analgesia after open acromioplasty and rotator cuff repair: preliminary results. *J Shoulder Elbow Surg.* 2004;13(6):630–634.

80. Alford JW, Fadale PD. Evaluation of postoperative bupivacaine infusion for pain management after anterior cruciate ligament reconstruction. *Arthroscopy.* 2003;19(8):855–861.

81. Hoenecke HRJ, Pulido PA, Morris BA, Fronek J. The efficacy of continuous bupivacaine infiltration following anterior cruciate ligament reconstruction. *Arthroscopy.* 2002;18:854–858.

82. Singelyn FJ, Lhotel L, Fabre B. Pain relief after arthroscopic shoulder surgery: a comparison of intraarticular analgesia, suprascapular nerve block, and interscalene brachial plexus block. *Anesth Analg.* 2004;99(2):589–592.

83. Dauri M, Polzoni M, Fabbi E, et al. Comparison of epidural, continuous femoral block and intraarticular analgesia after anterior cruciate ligament reconstruction. *Acta Anaesthesiol Scand.* 2003;47:20–25.

84. Kirchhoff R, Jensen PB, Nielsen NS, Boeckstyns ME. Repeated digital nerve block for pain control after tenolysis. *Scand J Plastic Reconstruct Surg Hand Surg.* 2000;34(3):257–258.

85. Klein SM, Steele SM, Nielsen KC, et al. The difficulties of ambulatory interscalene and intra-articular infusions for rotator cuff surgery: a preliminary report. *Can J Anaesth.* 2003;50(3):265–269.

86. Brown SL, Morrison AE. Local anesthetic infusion pump systems adverse events reported to the Food and Drug Administration. *Anesthesiology.* 2004;100(5):1305–1307.

87. Gomoll AH, Kang RW, Williams JM, Bach BR, Cole BJ. Chondrolysis after continuous intra-articular bupivacaine infusion: an experimental modal investigating chondrotoxicity in the rabbit shoulder. *Arthroscopy.* 2006;22(8):813–819.

19

Patient-Controlled Analgesia Devices and Analgesic Infusion Pumps

Benjamin Sherman, Ikay Enu, and
Raymond S. Sinatra

Patient-controlled analgesia (PCA) describes the conceptual framework for on-demand, intermittent administration of opioid and nonopioid analgesics under patient control.[1] The broader concept of PCA should neither be restricted to a single route or mode of administration, nor should PCA imply a mandatory need for a sophisticated or expensive infusion device. This chapter reviews the history, scientific validity, and available technology of three different forms of PCA, including intravenous PCA (IV PCA), neuraxial PCA, and ambulatory PCA, all of which offer the patient autonomy and control in the management of their pain.

INTRAVENOUS SYSTEMS

Opioid analgesics remain the mainstay for the treatment of moderate to severe postoperative pain. Traditionally, they are administered on an as-needed (PRN) basis via oral and intravenous routes and, less often, intramuscularly. To achieve optimal analgesic benefit, several pharmacokinetic principles must be appreciated. (1) Therapeutic plasma levels and adequate central nervous system (CNS) delivery must be achieved to assure sufficient occupancy and activation of opiate receptors. (2) Therapeutic concentrations for different opioid agonists exhibit wide interpatient variability. (3) For most opioids, the therapeutic window is relatively narrow; hence, underdosing and overdosing can easily occur. In light of these variables, and in the attempt to optimize analgesic benefits, the use of IV PCA offers a reliable and titratable administration option.[1]

Plasma and CNS concentrations are most uniform when opioids are administered by either continuous infusion or as multiple small doses. Prior to the introduction of IV PCA systems, analgesic dosing regimens were dependent on clinical care variables such as nursing assessment of pain severity, the speed of nursing response to the patient complaints, preparation of the syringe, and administration of the drug (Figure 19.1). Furthermore, the efficacy of IV-administered opioids is also dependent on individual patient characteristics such as degree of pain perception, absorption from the administration site, pharma-

cokinetics and pharmacodynamics, opioid receptor polymorphisms, and psychologic variables. A patient interactive dose delivery system is usually better able to accommodate for these variabilities. IV PCA allows patients to self titrate drugs in proportion to the degree of perceived pain intensity, as well as dosing adjustments in response to changes in the painful stimulus (Figure 19.2).[2]

Early History

In their landmark study published in the mid-1970s, Marks and Sachar[3] exposed the endemic practice of analgesic undermedication in a large proportion of hospitalized patients. They also showed that physicians and nurses were misinformed and lacked sophistication regarding safe and effective use of opioid analgesics. Thus began attempts to improve analgesic delivery by optimizing its mode of administration.

The concept of IV PCA was initially described by a clinical anesthesiologist, Phillip Sechzer,[4] in 1968. He theorized that the behavior of patients controlling their own analgesia could be structured in a fashion analogous to that of an animal terminating a painful stimulus by pressing a bar. He hypothesized that patients could respond to their pain by pressing an analgesic "activation button" until a personal threshold of relief was attained. The frequency of analgesic demands or button pushing provided an important measure of pain intensity while the cumulative dose administered correlated with the adequacy of pain relief. In designing an automatic drug administration pump, Sechzer believed that the following criteria were essential for safe and dependable function: (1) administration of sterile analgesic solutions of known concentration, (2) precise, consistent, and replicable delivery of a set dose, and (3) ease of standardization and calibration.[5] The first IV PCA device to meet these requirements was a modified Holter roller pump, which was evaluated in over 118 medical and surgical patients during a 2-year trial period. Despite its primitive nature, most patients utilizing these devices were able to safely and effectively control the intravenous administration of opioids and achieve effective pain relief. Nevertheless, the main

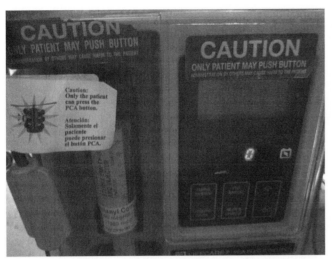

Figure 19.1: A method to reduce PCA by proxy. Labels are placed on the pump indicating that only the patient may activate the PCA device. The photograph shows labels used by the pain service at Duke University Medical Center. A new label provides instructions in Spanish in addition to the English language sticker (figure courtesy of Dr Brian Ginsberg).

application for IV PCA during the decade after its introduction was for the treatment of intractable chronic pain and for the evaluation of equianalgesic dosing in drug trials. More widespread application and use in postoperative settings awaited further development of prototypical PCA devices.

Prototypical IV PCA devices included the Cardiff Palliator (Graseby Medical LTD, UK), the On Demand Analgesia Computer or ODAC (Janssen Scientific Instruments, Belgium), and the Prominiject (Pharmacia AB, Sweden). The Cardiff Palliator was designed by investigators at the Welsh National School of Medicine. Although it was the first IV PCA device to be commercially marketed, its large size, non-tamper-proof dosage and interval settings, and notoriety for being difficult to use (patients

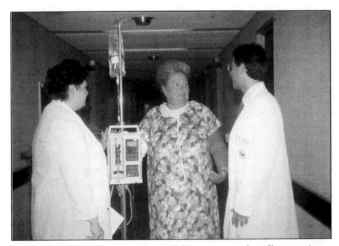

Figure 19.2: IV PCA is an analgesic delivery system that allows patients to self-titrate analgesics in response to the magnitude of their perceived pain stimulus. It accommodates for interindividual differences in analgesic pharmacokinetics and pharmacodynamics, as well as psychosocial responses to discomfort. Such therapy may facilitate ambulation because patients can administer additional doses of analgesics to compensate for an increasing intensity of incident pain.

were required to press the activation button twice within 1 second to successfully administer a demand dose) minimized widespread acceptance. The ODAC, a highly innovative device developed by Hull and coworkers, incorporated a pneumograph that prevented further drug delivery if respiratory depression was detected. It also incorporated a miniature audio system that provided prompts to remind the patient that additional analgesia was available and how to administer the drug. Unfortunately, this device shared many of the deficiencies seen with the Cardiff Palliator, as well as excessive false-positive detections of respiratory depression.[1]

The Prominiject PCA infusion pump was designed to provide demand doses as well as split incremental doses. The split dose consisted of an incremental bolus dose followed by a preset tail dose infused over a 10 minute interval. This large device incorporated a built-in printer and locked syringe chamber; however, drug volume was limited to what could be contained in a 25-mL syringe. Although commercially available, this device was soon superseded by smaller first-generation PCA pumps marketed by Abbott, Pharmacia, and Bard.[1]

Design Theory

The pharmacologic principles that form the basis for IV PCA were elucidated by Austin et al[6] in 1980, who described the concept of minimum effective analgesic concentration (MEAC). Following administration of opioid boluses, these authors measured plasma concentrations, assessed pain intensity scores, and developed concentration-therapeutic effect curves. The lowest opioid concentration at which pain was reliably relieved was termed the *minimum effective analgesic concentration*. Furthermore, they showed that whereas opioids consistently provide effective analgesia, therapeutic plasma concentrations varied considerably among individuals. This finding suggested that pharmacodynamic variability in opioid response accounts for a major proportion of interindividual differences in dose requirements.[6] Intravenous PCA technology allows individuals to self-direct and self-titrate opioid delivery to an acceptable level of relief, thereby achieving MEAC (Figure 19.3). More consistent plasma opioid concentrations are maintained, avoiding peaks and troughs that are characteristic of PRN intramuscular (IM)/IV injections.[7]

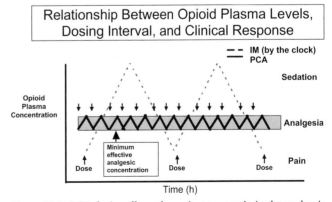

Figure 19.3: PCA dosing allows the patient to remain in the analgesic therapeutic window (shaded region) for a greater proportion of the dosing interval than by the clock IM dosing. (Modified from Ferrante FM et al. *Anesth Analg.* 1988;67:457–461.[11])

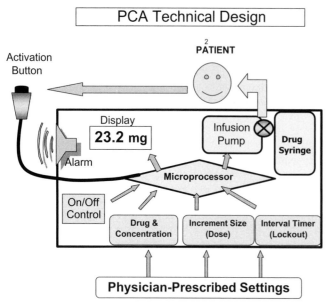

Figure 19.4: Technical schematic of a typical patient-controlled analgesia device. Microprocessors allow caregivers to program drug, dose, and lockout interval, whereas the patient determines dosing time and total dose administered. Incremental bolus doses are administered via a patient control button and cumulative dose is displayed on a small screen. The syringe or bag containing drug is placed in a locked, tamper-resistant portion of the device.

Basic Considerations

Since the early 1980s, a large number of IV PCA systems, incorporating many unique features and several modes of operation were developed and approved for use. The feature most modern systems have in common is a microprocessor that allows the patient to interact (within preset dose limits and lockout intervals) with an infusion pump connected to an intravenous line (Figure 19.4). The device is activated by pressing a remote activation button connected to the machine. Each button push is termed an *analgesic demand*. Successful pump activation results in the delivery of an "incremental" or "bolus" dose. The bolus dose may be delivered according to the drug concentration (milligrams per milliliter), volume of solution (milliliters), or both.[1,7,8] With appropriate patient education and opioid dose, the ratio of analgesic demands versus incremental doses delivered should approach 1.0.[1]

Whereas earlier IV PCA devices allowed for entry parameters of just milliliters or milligrams, many of the newer models also allow for entry of microgram units, thereby reducing the potential for programming errors when using fentanyl or sufentanil.[7] Most IV PCA pumps include audible beeps and visual cues with successful delivery of an incremental bolus, thus providing the patient important dosing reinforcement. A lockout interval is simultaneously engaged at the time the incremental dose is delivered thereby assuring that another dose cannot be administered within a preset time limit. This dose delay represents one of the key safeguards associated with IV PCA. It is designed to protect the patient from potential overdosage secondary to patient confusion or when proxy doses are given by overly concerned visitors. The lockout interval in effect limits the number of incremental boluses a patient can self-administer over a period of time. Increased sedation and sleep usually ensues before the patient is able to administer amounts great

enough to cause overdosage. Many devices store the number of attempts (demands) as well as the total number of incremental boluses delivered over the previous 12 and 24 hours of therapy. A second safety mechanism that helps minimize overdose is the maximum dose limit. This added safeguard is usually set as either a 1- or 4-hour cumulative milligram or microgram dosing limit.[1]

Initial loading dose, demand dose, background infusion rate, and lockout intervals are clinician programmed functions of most IV PCA systems. The patient controls the frequency at which the boluses are given. Choosing the size of the incremental bolus and the lockout interval depends mainly on the plasma kinetics and CNS penetration of the particular drug employed. The incremental bolus should be of adequate size to provide the patient with approximately 15 minutes to 1 hour of analgesia before additional doses are required, but not so large that excessive sedation is experienced.

Following IV administration, plasma opioid concentrations decline rapidly as the drug redistributes from the blood to the peripheral tissues. Thus, when IV PCA is initiated, a loading dose is generally required to achieve therapeutic plasma concentrations. Fentanyl and other highly lipid-soluble opioids have large volumes of distribution and require a high frequency of boluses to maintain therapeutic plasma concentrations during the first few hours after initiation. Longer duration nonlipophillic agents such as morphine and hydromorphone generally require fewer bolus doses per hour.[1]

The relationship between the size of demand doses and lockout intervals is also important in a PCA regimen.[8,9] A small demand dose (0.5 mg morphine or equivalent) programmed with a short 6-minute lockout may represent the safest and most appropriate dose in a variety of situations, including elderly and morbidly obese patients or others with pulmonary diseases. However, despite providing equivalent analgesia, use of smaller demand doses with short lockouts usually requires increased PCA attempts per hour for some patients and less overall satisfaction than regimens employing higher 1-mg doses of morphine and moderate lockouts (8–10 minutes).[9] Conversely, larger doses of morphine (1.5–2 mg) with prolonged lockout intervals (15 minutes) may result in patient dissatisfaction as such dosing is associated with increased side effects, excessive number of failed attempts, and patient mistrust.

Individual patient characteristics influence total dose delivered, bolus dose requirements, and overall effectiveness. Age, gender, and body weight are often assumed to be important factors influencing any pharmacologic therapy. With regard to IV PCA, studies have shown that age inversely affects opioid dosing and the is best predictor of IV PCA morphine requirements during the first 24 hours after surgery.[10] Gender and body weight, however, do not predict opioid requirements.[7,10] It has long been understood that patients who are tolerant to opioids, and those with a history of chronic pain, have increased PCA total dose requirements. These individuals must be supplied with their baseline opioid dose in addition to their postoperative analgesic requirements (please refer to Chapter 34: *Acute Pain Management in Patients with Opioid Dependency and Substance Abuse*) Although IV PCA can be used successfully in opioid-tolerant patients, the addition of regional analgesia and adjuvant therapies should always be considered. Other factors that may influence IV PCA dosing requirements include psychological factors, genetic variations in opioid receptor binding (μ-opioid receptor polymorphisms) and metabolism, and concomitant illnesses.[7] The individual's decision to press the PCA button remains essential to successful use of IV PCA. In this regard, cognitive disorders and psychological factors, such as fear and confusion, may override pharmacodynamic considerations so that patients may accept worse pain or be unable to attain maximum benefit from IV PCA.[11]

Clinical Management

In a recent systematic review on the safety and efficacy of PCA for acute postoperative pain, Walder et al[12] analyzed the data from 288 randomized controlled trials, comparing opioids administered by IV PCA with conventional opioid analgesia (intravenous, subcutaneous, and intramuscular) in postoperative patients. This review presented data suggesting that, IV PCA therapy provided superior postoperative pain control. Analgesic efficacy end points were in favor of PCA and the combined data indicated that the difference was statistically significant. Furthermore, this review presented evidence that patients prefer PCA for the autonomy it allows them (Figure 19.2). However, the amount of opioids consumed was no different with the two methods, and the incidence of opioid-related adverse reactions (ie, respiratory depression, hypoxia, nausea and vomiting, sedation, urinary retention) was similar with both therapies.[12]

Mu opioid receptor agonists are the mainstays of acute postoperative pain management and have been successfully administered via IV PCA (Table 19.1) They provide powerful, dose-dependent analgesic effects. However, annoying and, occasionally intolerable, side effects may result in a "clinical analgesic ceiling." This ceiling may limit further dosing and the achievement of adequate pain relief. The μ agonists are equally effective at equianalgesic doses (eg, 10 mg of morphine = 1 mg of oxymorphone, = 2 mg of hydromorphone = 100 mg of meperidine.) Similarly, there are only minor differences in side-effect profiles of pure μ-agonists, although individual patients may experience excessive nausea and vomiting or pruritis with one drug, but not another. With standard IV PCA doses, morphine, meperidine, and fentanyl have similar effects on GI motility and biliary pressure. Metabolites and routes of elimination differ markedly between μ agonists providing one rationale for choosing one opioid over another for IV PCA.[7]

Morphine, the most commonly used opioid for IV PCA in the United States, has an active metabolite, morphine-6-glucuronide, that also produces analgesia, sedation, and res-piratory depression. Whereas morphine is metabolized mainly by glucuronidation, its active metabolite relies predominantly on renal excretion for elimination. Prolonged and profound delayed onset of respiratory depression has been reported in patients with renal failure receiving IV morphine.[13,14]

Hydromorphone is metabolized primarily in the liver and excreted primarily as an inactive glucuronide metabolite. It is 5 to 6 times as potent as morphine, thus a demand dose of 0.2 mg is considered equianalgesic to 1 mg of morphine. Because of its increased potency, hydromorphone is well suited for opioid-tolerant patients, allowing for greater intervals between refilling of the drug reservoir.[15]

Fentanyl is considered 50–75 times as potent as morphine. However, it has a much shorter duration of action because of redistribution pharmacokinetics. It has been successfully used for PCA. For IV PCA, fentanyl demand doses of 25 to 30 μg are approximately equianalgesic to 1 mg of morphine. Fentanyl has a more rapid onset of analgesia than morphine because of its high lipid solubility and CNS penetration. For patients with renal failure, it is a suitable choice because it is metabolized by the liver only and does not rely on renal excretion for elimination.[7]

Meperidine has traditionally been the second most common μ-opioid agonist prescribed for IV PCA; however, because of its neurotoxic, renally cleared metabolite, normeperidine, its routine use for IV PCA has been limited. Although normeperidine has no analgesic properties, accumulation of normeperidine causes CNS excitation, resulting in a range of toxic reactions from anxiety and tremors, to grand mal seizures.[16] Meperidine is absolutely contraindicated for IV PCA in patients with renal dysfunction, seizure disorders, and in those taking monoamine oxidase inhibitors (MAOIs) because of the potential for a lethal drug interaction causing malignant hyperpyrexia syndrome. For these reasons, it is recommended that meperidine be used for short durations, in carefully monitored doses, and only in patients who have demonstrated intolerance to all other opioids.[16] A 10-mg demand dose of merperidine is equianalgesic to 1 mg of morphine.

Oxymorphone (numorphan, Opana injectable) has also been advocated for IV PCA.[17] In a randomized postsurgical evaluation, PCA boluses of oxymorphone (0.3 mg) provided highly effective pain control that was superior to morphine and meperidine in terms of time to achieve peak analgesic effect, incidence of excessive sedation, and maximum reduction in pain intensity scores. Patients treated with oxymorphone particularly with basal infusions of 0.3 mg/h were troubled by a higher incidence of nausea. Based on this information, it is recommended that PCA bolus doses should be reduced to 0.15–0.2 mg and basal infusions eliminated in opioid naive patients.

Sufentanil, alfentanil, and remifentanil also have been used for PCA with sufentanil having been the most studied. In contrast to the longer acting opioids, a small background infusion is essential to sustain analgesia with fentanyl, sufentanil, and alfentanil. When using sufentanil, an initial demand dose of 2–4 μg appears to be most appropriate.[18] Alfentanil is a weak pure opioid agonist, and it may be a poor choice for IV PCA therapy because it lacks an optimal dose and its duration of effect is very limited.[19] Remifentanil is probably appropriate for IV PCA use only in severe episodic pain conditions, such as labor pain, because of its ultrashort duration.[20]

In some countries, tramadol, a central-acting analgesic with opioid and nonopioid mechanisms, is widely employed for IV PCA. Tramadol binding affinity at μ-receptors is approximately

Table 19.1: Available Parenteral Opioids[a]

μ-Agonists	Agonist-Antagonists	Partial Agonists
Morphine	Butorphanol	Buprenorphine
Fentanyl	Nalbuphine	
Hydromorphone		
Oxymorphone		
Meperidine		
Sufentanil		
Alfentanil		

[a] Adapted from Grass, JA, *Anesth. Analg.* 2005;101(suppl 5): 44–61.[7]

600-fold less than that of morphine. A demand dose of 10 mg of tramadol is equianalgesic to 0.5–1 mg of morphine.[21] The M1 mono-*O*-desmethyl metabolite of tramadol has a greater affinity for opiate receptors and contributes to its analgesic effects. Tramadol also inhibits central uptake of norepinephrine and serotonin. Thus, its antinociceptive effect is mediated by multiple mechanisms, which interact synergistically to relieve pain.[22]

Pharmacologic strategies to reduce IV PCA-induced postop nausea and vomiting include treatment with antiemetics such as serotonin or dopamine antagonists (ie, ondansetron or droperidol, respectively) or corticosteroids, such as dexamethasone. Common treatments for IV PCA-related pruritis include the use of antihistamines such as diphenhydramine and hydroxyzine or the slow infusion of pure opioid antagonists, such as nalaxone. Individual patients differ in the degree of sedation in response to particular opioids. Patients with altered renal function experience sedation with the accumulation of active morphine metabolites. Opioid-sparing strategies, such as coadministration of around-the-clock nonsteroidal anti-inflammatory drugs (NSAIDS), and COX-2 inhibitors may reduce sedation.[7]

Postoperative confusion or delirium, particularly in elderly patients, is a relatively common phenomenon. Although PCA opioids may contribute to confusion, deficits in dosing and suboptimal analgesia may further increase confusion and agitation.[23] Many elderly and cognitively impaired patients forget how to self-administer opioids or lose track of the control button. These patients will require more frequent observation and reinstruction to optimize PCA (refer to Chapter 31, *Acute Pain Management for Elderly "High-Risk" and Cognitively Impaired Patients: Rationale for Regional Analgesia*).

Safety

A major complication of IV PCA therapy is respiratory depression often from overmedication or use of basal infusions. Patient risk factors for respiratory depression with IV PCA include advanced age, head injury, sleep apnea, obesity, respiratory failure, concurrent use of sedative medications, hypovolemia, and renal failure.[24]

Most incidents of overmedication involving IV PCA are typically associated with the entry of an incorrect programming parameter such as drug concentration, bolus dose size, or continuous or basal flow rates. An erroneously programmed drug concentration, for example, will cause the pump to deliver an excessive amount of drug, thus, causing an overdose.[25] The Institute for Safe Medication Practices (ISMP) have collected research on adverse outcomes including overdose and death in patients using IV PCA. They have found several common factors and caregiver errors that increase risk of overdose and have suggested corrective steps to minimize adverse outcomes (Table 19.2).

Adverse events may also occur in settings where prescription and pump programming are correct. The clinical effects of opioids may be difficult for caregivers to anticipate. Thus, a dose that is insufficient for one patient may oversedate another, depending on each individual's unique physiology, metabolic variability, and μ-receptor polymorphisms.[26] Also, overdosage may occur when family members or clinicians activate the delivery request button on the patient's behalf. This inappropriate method of dosing is termed *PCA by proxy* (Figure 19.5).[27]

Another way to reduce overmedication incidents is through the use of standardized protocols. IV PCA pumps are often programmed according to facility-wide protocols that allow for

Table 19.2: PCA Overdose Reports

1. The Institute for Safe Medical Practice (ISMP) database received 425 incidents involving narcotic infusion pumps during the years 1987–2003. These incidents were associated with 135 injuries, 23 deaths, and 127 potential deaths requiring pump deactivation and naloxone administration

2. Methods to reduce PCA and analgesic infusion pump injuries and death include the following:

   1. Adequate nurse training and refresher training

   2. "High-alert" medication labeling

   3. Two nurses must program pump

   4. "Concerned loved one" proxy-administration safeguards

   5. Programming safeguards (smart pumps)

Ref: U David. http://www.ismp-canada.org/download/OHA-20040614.pdf.

standardized drug concentrations and dosing regimens for typical patient characteristics. Using standardized protocols reduces medication errors by limiting the number of choices a physician needs to make when prescribing, and by reducing transcription and programming errors related to hard-to-read orders.[28] Table 19.3 provides an overview of factors responsible for overmedication.

All PCA systems must include protection against accidental purging because of the large amount of drugs that could potentially be infused into the patient. However, because modern IV PCA devices are designed to fail in a noninfusion mode

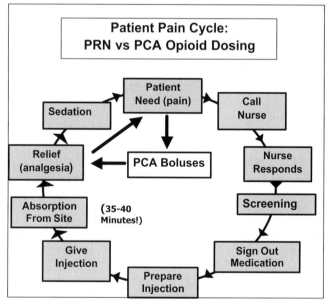

Figure 19.5: The pain cycle. Patients recovering from surgery or traumatic injury are often treated with IM or IV analgesics given on a PRN basis. This inefficient and labor-intensive method requires screening, preparation, and nurse administration that may be delayed 35–40 minutes on busy floors. Absorption variables further increase the onset of analgesic effects. Patients finally appreciate relief and some degree of sedation, only to experience increasing pain several hours later. This cycle repeats itself every 3–4 hours during the postoperative period. In theory, PCA dosing eliminates the pain cycle by allowing more frequent patient-directed analgesic dosing.

Table 19.3: Institute for Safe Medication Practices: Safety Issues with PCA: How Errors Occur

1. Improper patient selection

   Avoid patients with cognitive, physical, psychological dysfunction, or comorbid conditions (eg, obesity, asthma, sleep apnea)

2. Misprogramming errors (the most frequent reason for overdose)

   Most programming errors involve improper concentration or drug

3. Drug selection errors

   Prefilled syringes of different opioids and different concentrations are packaged in similar-looking boxes. Name similarities (eg, morphine, hydromorphone, oxymorphone) lead to mix-ups

4. Inadequate staff training

   Nurses may not always receive adequate training in pump programming, or they may not retain their proficiency once trained

5. Inadequate monitoring

   1. Level of consciousness and respiratory rate checked infrequently

   2. Pulse oximetry offers false security since saturation can be maintained with low respiratory rates, if nasal oxygen is provided

6. PCA by proxy

   Sedated patients will not press the button to deliver more opiate; however, family members and health care professionals may administer proxy doses, trying to keep patients comfortable (with increasing toxicity!)

7. Inadequate patient education

   1. Activation button may be confused as the nurse call button

   2. Alert, intelligent patients may misunderstand the directions for use, believing that they must press the button every 6 minutes

8. Prescription errors

   Mistakes in converting an oral opioid dose to the IV route (the most problematic opioids are oxymorphone and hydromorphone [oral IV conversion range of 3:1 to 5:1])

Ref: Safety Issues With Patient-Controlled Analgesia-Part I-How Errors Occur. [Institute for Safe Medication Practices Web site http://www.ismp.org/Newsletters/acutecare/articles/20030710.asp]

(preventing a pump runaway) and incorporate antisiphon and backflow valves, overdosage related to pump malfunction is less likely to occur. Although pumps are tested by the manufacturer before shipping, calibration and flow rate checks should be performed on delivery and every 6 months thereafter by the hospital's medical engineering staff, which is stated in the manufacturer's guidelines.[1]

A recent safety feature that has been integrated into some IV PCA pumps, is the ability for physiologic monitoring. Some pumps now include monitoring modules to identify patients with respiratory depression, a common hazard of IV PCA therapy. These modules provide continuous monitoring of patients via recorded physiologic values, including oxygen saturation (SPO_2) and end-tidal CO_2 ($ETCO_2$). They also include prompts and alarms to alert the clinician whenever physiologic values fall below specified limits. Many manufacturers continue to develop methods of detecting and preventing dose-related infusion errors and the programming of incorrect infusion settings.

Three types of "advanced error reduction features" used for IV PCA "smart pumps" include bar coding, dose error reduction systems, and computer-based pump-programming software.[29]

Integrated bar-code readers using preset pump programming allow clinicians to initiate therapy without manually entering the information into the pump. When a drug vial's bar code is scanned and inserted, pump settings such as drug name and concentration are entered automatically (Figure 19.6). Some systems can automatically populate the pump with patient-specific or drug vial-specific dosing protocols and dosing limits. The limitations of integrated bar-code readers, however, are that they cannot identify inappropriate continuous or bolus dose settings or provide dosing limits on subsequent reprogramming.[29]

Dose error reduction systems help guide manual programming by comparing programmed doses with preset limits stored in drug libraries downloaded to the pump. These systems alert clinicians to programmed doses that exceed these preset limits and can either require confirmation before beginning delivery or not allow delivery at all. Pumps with dose error reduction systems store the alert and event log information that results from clinical use of drug libraries. Thus, hospitals can retrieve these data for insight into their own medication practices to improve their drug libraries and clinical practices. A disadvantage of dose error reduction systems, however, is that they do not ensure that the right drug is selected from the library.[29]

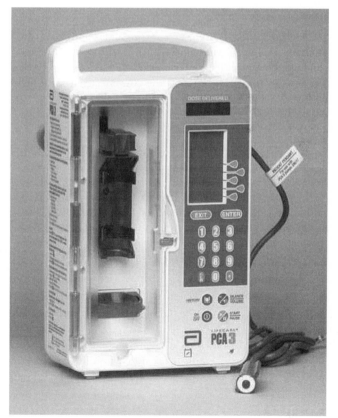

Figure 19.6: Third-generation Hospira PCA device. This device has been designed to help reduce medication errors, enhance utility, and increase efficiency. A built-in bar code reader automatically identifies drug name and concentration thereby minimizing programming errors. Stored speed protocols that include drug, standard concentration, and dose limits save time and improve compliance with standing orders (figure courtesy of Hospira, Inc, Chicago, IL).

Computer-based pump-programming applications are also capable of programming pumps automatically. This software allows a clinician to program an IV PCA pump by selecting and downloading preset dosing protocols from a computer to a pump via a wired connection. Once the clinician sends a protocol to a pump, the pump is populated with a drug name, starting dose, time-based dosing limit, and lockout intervals, thus eliminating entry errors that occur often during initial programming. In some cases, the pump receives protocol specific dosing limits (similar to those offered by dose error reduction systems) for subsequent reprogramming over the course of therapy. One advantage of computer-based pump programming software is the ability of pumps to offer the software without needing larger, more complex data storage, displays, and user menus. Another advantage of this system is that facilities can quickly revise dosing protocols by simply updating them using lap-top and hand-held computers. The implementation of computer-based pump programming requires a hard-wired connection between the pumps and a a hand held computer. This may not be possible in small facilities with limited budgets.[29]

All three error reduction technologies encourage facilities to standardize protocols based on a limited number of drugs, concentrations, and dosing limits. When implemented effectively, these advanced features can be powerful tools for reducing infusion errors caused by misprogramming.[29]

Cost-Effectiveness

An important consideration and possible downside of PCA therapy is its cost. Expenses involved in the provision of analgesia include direct cost of drugs, consumables, equipment, and labor. There is a lack of valid data on the cost-effectiveness of these devices.[30]

When analyzing the overall cost of treatment, one must consider both direct costs and indirect costs. Direct costs include the cost of equipment, drugs, and consumables, such as disposable tubing, batteries, and syringes. The indirect costs include the labor costs of pharmacy, nursing, and biomedical central supply personnel required to store, check, and maintain the PCA pumps. The pumps and syringes also have to be set up and the pump correctly programmed by trained personnel.[30] One also needs to consider the expense of treating the side effects of PCA opioid therapy, and also the indirect costs of morbidity and mortality, such as litigation costs.[7] With PCA technology, however, nursing time involved in the provision of analgesia is usually much less compared with conventional forms of pain relief (Figure 19.1). Therefore, in a busy ward, where the number of appropriately qualified nurses may be limited, the use of PCA in some patients may allow more time for nurses to attend to more pressing duties. Much more extensive cost analysis studies need to be done to accurately find the cost burden of PCA.

Systems

Since the advent of PCA, several delivery options have been approved by the Food and Drug Administration (FDA). They include incremental bolus on demand, incremental bolus on demand with a continuous (basal) infusion, continuous infusion, and incremental bolus with a tail dose (Figure 19.7).[1] The

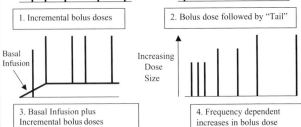

Figure 19.7: Forms of PCA delivery: (1) Standard incremental bolus dosing. Plasma levels fall rapidly following each dose. (2) Bolus dose followed by tail over the lock out interval maintains effective analgesic plasma levels for a more prolonged period. (3) Basal infusion plus incremental bolus doses also maintains plasma levels of analgesic by providing a subtherapuetic infusion. (4) Smart pumps to be developed will increase or decrease the size of the incremental bolus in proportion to the frequency of patient demands.

most popular and simplest mode of patient-controlled administration is incremental bolus dose on demand. This dosing option is completely dependent on patient control within preprogrammed dose and lockout interval constraints. One major drawback to this form of delivery is that patients may awaken in severe pain, because they cannot activate the system during periods of sleep.[83]

Bolus dose on demand plus a continuous infusion (also termed basal infusion) provides a background, subtherapeutic plasma level of opioid on which patient demands permit titration to an individualized MEAC (Figure 19.3). The addition of a continuous infusion offers the theoretical advantage of allowing sleep to occur without considerable reductions in opioid plasma levels. It also allows the bolus dose to be made smaller while increasing the interval between successive demands.[8]

A PCA pump set to a continuous mode alone allows the physician to fully control analgesic delivery. The simplest infusion regimen consists of a loading dose followed by a constant infusion. Infusion regimens ideally should be based on the drug's pharmacokinetics, so that a desired drug concentration is achieved and maintained.[1] This mode of administration should be reserved for patients who are incapable of self-dosing. Because continuous infusions reduce the inherent safety of PCA, patients should be even more closely monitored.

In addition to the device selected, other practical issues must be taken into account when considering PCA, including the availability of trained personnel, standardized policy and procedure guidelines, and adequate patient monitoring.[1] The advantages versus disadvantages of IV PCA are outlined in Table 19.4.

Analgesic Infusion Pump Technology

Infusion pumps can be divided into two major groups: positive displacement pumps or gravimetric controllers. With gravimetric devices, controllers regulate gravity induced flow of infusate. These pumps have minimal safeguards and are rarely used for

Table 19.4: Potential Advantages versus Disadvantages of IV PCA

Advantages

- Rapid onset of effect (5–10 min)
- Minimizes the interval between analgesic request and pain relief
- Breaks the pain cycle
- Accommodates for inter-individual differences in analgesic requirements
- Compensates for pharmacokinetic, pharmacodynamic, and genetic differences
- High degree of patient acceptance, control and satisfaction

Disadvantages

- It requires expensive infusion devices, syringes, and tubing
- It requires IV access, generally a dedicated line
- Overdosage may occur when relatives/nurses administer doses for the patient ("PCA by proxy" dosing)
- Overdosage may occur as a result of programming errors or use of basal infusions
- Elderly patients may not understand the concept of "self-administration"

opioid analgesics. Positive displacement pumps can be further divided into two broad categories based on their pumping mechanisms: peristaltic pumps and syringe pumps.

Peristaltic pumps deliver flow by an action similar to that of the human enteral tract. They occlude and release specialized tubing sets in a distally migrating periodic pattern that propels boluses of fluid at a rate that is controlled by the microprocessor, producing an intermittent flow pattern.

Syringe-driven pumps deliver flow by a turning lead screw mechanism that forces the plunger into the barrel of the syringe reservoir. Many of the larger PCA pumps employ rotating lead screws, which provide accurate delivery while preventing free flow when the syringe is being changed. Because drug delivery is limited to the volume of drug within the syringe (25 to 60 mL), the frequency of syringe changes may be excessive unless the drug is formulated in a concentrated solution.

Another distinction on pump technology is pump size and portability. PCA pumps are either designed to be larger pole mounted units or smaller ambulatory units. Pole-mounted units are usually large and cannot be carried by the patient. Advantages include that they usually have built-in rechargeable batteries (which offer lower cost than disposable batteries), are robust and more resistant to physical damage, and are less likely to be stolen or tampered with. These units normally run on 110-volt AC current from a wall source. Ambulatory pumps are smaller and lightweight and usually run on battery power. They have the advantage of being very portable, having a large capacity for drug solutions, and do not require large efforts to store and transport. The disadvantages are that they are more fragile and prone to theft and tampering. Ambulatory pumps are further discussed later in the chapter.

There have been many different models of PCA pumps developed since the late 1980s, each with strengths and weaknesses. With corporate mergers and acquisitions, the selection of commercially available pumps available in 2008 has decreased from the number marketed in the 1990s. Improvements in technology and increased clinical experience has helped companies to introduce safer and more reliable products. When considering purchase of PCA devices, it is extremely important to analyze which features are available and desirable for particular hospital settings.

The power supply is a critically important element of any PCA device. All nonambulatory pumps today have two power sources; power provided via a 110- or 220-V wall outlet and a battery backup system. Ideally, any pump should automatically transition to battery power without the loss of prescription information or patient use history. Ideally, PCA pumps should run for approximately 24 hours on battery power alone.

All PCA pumps must have accidental purging mechanisms to prevent unintentional overdose of medication to the patient. Pumps today are designed to fail in a noninfusion mode and incorporate antisiphon and backflow valves to minimize or prevent accidental overdose. The FDA collects and gathers reports on accidental injuries caused by medical products online, and it is called the Manufacturer and User Facility Device Experience Database (MAUDE; http://www.fda.gov/cdrh/maude.html). These reports are extremely helpful in identifying trends in problematic pumps. An example of MAUDE data can be seen in Table 19.5. All pumps require periodic scheduled maintenance by the biomedical engineer's office to ensure accurate dosing as well.

The cost of administration sets, drug reservoirs, prefilled syringes, and disposable batteries are another important consideration when evaluating a particular PCA device. Pumps that require specialized infusion tubing and drug reservoirs will, within a short amount of time, eclipse the purchase price of the device. If the device utilizes generic components, one must also consider the preparation costs of the medications and the cost of training personnel to ensure the quality and quantity of

Table 19.5: FDA Manufacturer and User Facility Device Experience Database (MAUDE) Analgesic Undermedication Findings[a]

Device-related events (n = 82)

   58 were battery, software, or display malfunctions

   10 were failed alarms

   8 were because of defective pendants

   6 were because of faulty syringe injectors

Operator errors (n = 6)

   3 resulted from improper analgesic loading

   2 occurred when the tube clamp was not removed

   1 resulted from programming error

[a] MAUDE data represent reports of adverse events involving medical devices. Between 2003 and 2004, there were 19 spontaneous user reports of adverse events involving PCA devices. Of 2009 patient reports, 89 (4.4%) specifically documented underdelivery of analgesia. Of the 89 reports, 31 cases in which duration without any analgesic was recorded; mean duration of undermedication was 26 hours.

Ref: *Manufacturer and User Facility Device Experience Database-Maude* [US Food and Drug Administration Center for Devices and Radiological Health Web site]. http://www.fda.gov/cdrh/maude.html.

Table 19.6: General Considerations for PCA Systems

Power supply
  Alternating current
  Rechargeable, alkaline or lithium battery
  Battery run time
Mode of administration
  Intravenous
  Epidural
  Ambulatory or nonambulatory patients
Modes of operation
  On-demand parameters
  Continuous-infusion parameters
  On-demand plus continuous infusion parameters
Delivery system
  Unit dimensions
  Standard tubing versus dedicated tubing provided by the manufacturer
  Standard syringes versus syringe/reservoir provided by the manufacturer
  Pharmacy preparation of drug versus purchase of prefilled syringes produced by the manufacturer
Programmability
  By concentration or volume, or both
  Maximum dose available
  Bolus or dose-size parameters
  Lockout time parameters
  Infusion-rate parameters
Safety features
  Security access codes
  Keyed access
  Tamperproof mechanisms
  Anti-siphon and backflow valves
  Physiologic monitoring capabilities
  Error reduction software
  Networking capabilities with data analysis

Table 19.7: Desirable IV PCA Features

Convenient to use with simple protocols for set up and change in dose prescriptions

Patient activator button must be sturdy yet simple to use

Versatile, must be easily adaptable for different types of administration modes

Ability to record and retrieve drug usage and patient demand history

Provide security against drug tampering

Portable for ambulatory patients; primary and backup batteries with prolonged duration of activity

Clear display of drug and dosages

Alarms for pump microprocessor malfunction, occlusion, and disconnect

Automatic priming of administration set

Prevention of free flow

Printer capabilities

Size and weight of the unit; smaller allow easier ambulation

Integrates with physiologic monitoring easily and accurately

the medications. General considerations and desired features of PCA devices are outlined in Tables 19.6 and 19.7.

Future IV-PCA Technology: Pharmacokinetic Drug Delivery Systems

The ideal system for PCA would be one that is noninvasive and provides continuous analgesia with minimal side effects. No cumbersome equipment would be needed, it would not limit patient mobility, and it would not require extensive labor for setup, maintenance, or storage. It would also have the ability to self titrate to avoid unwanted side effects.

Current PCA technology uses analgesic dosing based on empirical determinants, such as body weight or fixed intervals, and often leads to an unacceptably high incidence of over- and underdosing because of large interpatient variability in pharmacokinetics and pharmodynamics of opioid analgesics. Plasma opioid concentration is a dynamic variable that is dependent

on the ability of the drug to equilibrate with the multiple compartments in the body and gain access to the CNS.[31] Age, sex, lean body mass, hepatic and kidney function, and the method of drug delivery can all influence a drugs plasma concentration. The current success of IV PCA is, in large part, because of the fact that the patient judges the magnitude of pain or the adequacy of pain relief.[32] Thus, adequate plasma opioid concentration is deduced by patient feedback. This method of titration often leads the physician to drift outside of the therapeutic window and requires multiple adjustments to the dose and treating unwanted side effects.

Opioid analgesics exhibit multicompartment pharmacokinetics. That is, plasma concentrations decline exponentially after a bolus dose. To produce a stable plasma concentration of opioids, a sufficient amount of drug must be given to fill the central compartment (blood and rapidly equilibrating tissues) to a preselected concentration. Then, a constant-rate infusion must be initiated to compensate for drug loss by elimination and the redistribution of drugs from the central compartment to the deeper peripheral tissues. When the plasma opioid concentration is held constant in this manner, there will be a direct relationship between plasma drug concentration and the concentration of drugs at opioid receptors in the CNS. Hence, in theory, drug effect should be proportional to plasma concentration, thus insuring effective pain relief.[33]

One possibility for improvement of patient-controlled analgesia is the development of infusion-based systems that allow patients to adjust plasma opioid concentration around an initially effective target value to obtain better pain relief while minimizing side effects. Pain is not a static state but rather a dynamic one that increases and decreases with changes in patients activity. Appropriately designed variable-rate target-controlled infusions, which factor multiple compartment model pharmacokinetics, may minimize the disequilibrium of opioid concentrations between blood and CNS.[32]

In a randomized controlled trial involving bone marrow transplant patients requiring opioid analgesia for prolonged periods, Hill et al[32] compared pharmacokinetic-based IV PCA dosing (PKPCA) with conventional, bolus-dose morphine IV PCA. The main purpose of this study was to compare the effectiveness of PKPCA with conventional IV PCA morphine for oral mucositis pain control. Pharmacokinetically based IV PCA used a computer with the patient's individualized PK information and a bolus elimination transfer algorithm to control a patient's dose. The authors found that patients who self-administer morphine by PKPCA reported less pain throughout the study than compared to patients treated with conventional IV PCA. This increased margin of pain relief by PKPCA was accompanied by increased morphine consumption and a modest, time-limited increase in the intensity of some side effects, most notably sedation.[32]

The future of IV PCA technology is ideally headed toward a target plasma controlled system. The advancement in computer technologies allows for small devices to accomplish highly complex physiologic calculations quickly and also potentially take serum samples in real time. A pump can then maintain a plasma concentration and adjust the dose accordingly. Target-controlled infusion systems are available in Europe, but the technology is mostly being used perioperatively for anesthetic uses.[34]

Another area where PCA technology is advancing is in the mode of drug delivery. Currently, PCA must be administered invasively, either through an intravenous catheter or percutaneously into the epidural, intrathecal or soft tissue space. These modes of delivery can be limiting because of a patient's anticoagulation status or tend to decease patient mobility because of the attached pump apparatus. A new concept of drug delivery that is currently being tested is called iontophoresis, where charged molecules penetrate the skin in the presence of an electrical field. This technology has been applied to many different medications, including pain medications. Fentanyl works well for this application due to its small sized molecules, lipophilicity, potency, and lack of active metabolites.[35] A recent randomized controlled trial by Viscusi et al[35] showed that this method of drug administration was equivalent to that of standard morphine IV PCA in both pain relief and incidence of side effects (Figure 19.8; please refer to Chapter 20, *Novel Analgesic Delivery Systems for Acute Pain Management*).

Commercially Available IV-PCA Infusion Devices

IV PCA pumps introduced since the year 2000 that are still currently available for purchase include The Alaris System PCA module, Curlin Medical 400 CMS, Hospira Gemstar, Hospira Lifecare PCA 3, and Smiths Medical CADD-Prizm PCS II.

Alaris System PCA Module

The Alaris PCA model (introduced in December 2004; Alaris Medical Systems, Inc, subsidiary of Cardinal Health, Inc, San Diego, CA, USA) is a syringe-driven pump sold as a component of the pole-mounted Alaris system (Figure 19.9). This component can be bundled with $ETCO_2$ and SPO_2 monitoring. The system may be used solely for PCA or for use in combination with other general purpose infusions or monitoring modules. The Alaris PCA module comes equipped with Alaris's Guardrails software. This software provides a number of applications, including a dose error reduction system, as well as wireless pump connectivity that allows the pump to send event logs to and receive drug libraries from a central server. An integrated bar-code imaging module for clinician, patient, and drug-container identification was released in 2005. The activation button for PCA dosing is ergonomically contoured with a lighted push button.[29]

The Alaris system has a large, comprehensive display screen that is easy to use and interrogate, and it provides comprehensive history, including the total amount of drug delivered, doses requested, and doses delivered for the previous 24, 12, 8, 4, 2, or 1 hours. The pump's data logs can be downloaded to a computer using an application of the Guardrails software known as Continuous Quality Improvement (CQI). This software allows for the analysis of the dose error reduction system alarms and event logs to help hospitals better tailor the drug library to its clinical needs and improve clinical practice.[29]

General safety features of the Alaris PCA module include escalating alarm volume and clear text, with diagrams that state the alarm's cause and provide the user with instructions for appropriate follow-up. The Guardrails software includes a computer-based drug library editor for developing and maintaining facility-customized drug libraries and data mining. Guardrails also allows hospitals to customize drug-specific or therapy-specific drug entities. These entities include dosing limits (that may or may not be overridden) for continuous or bolus delivery settings, lockout limits, and clinical advisories for each drug. When coupled to physiologic monitoring modules, Guardrails software includes the ability to automatically interrupt PCA therapy if the patient's SPO_2 or breaths per minute fall below hospital specified limit. Audible and visual alerts signal any programming parameters that are outside the limits for the particular drug entity selected.[29]

Curlin Medical 4000 CMS

The Curlin Medical 4000™ clinical management system (CMS) (introduced in 2001; Curlin Medical LLC, Huntington Beach, CA, USA) is a multitherapy pump, configurable to PCA only, that can be used for hospital or home care applications (Figure 19.10). Accessories for the pump include a pole-mounting bracket and lockboxes.[29]

The 4000 CMS incorporates a PC-based CMS programming application. This application can send a standardized dosing protocol via a wired connection from a computer or hand-held PC to the pump. The CMS software allows for automatic pump programming in home care environments.[29] A key attribute of this device includes its ambulatory design, which allows fluid delivery from a wide variety of bags or syringes. Also, the pump provides displays in two font sizes: large and small. Large font screens alternate with two small-font screens that display all delivery information.[29]

Advanced error reduction features of the 4000 CMS include the PC-based pump-programming software. This program allows a hospital to develop drug-specific, therapy-specific, or patient-specific dosing protocols that are stored on a computer or PDA, and sent via a connecting cable to a pump. Pump settings, such as drug concentration, continuous and bolus delivery settings, lockout interval, and time based dosing limits, will automatically be programmed into the system. The pump also offers audible and visual alerts for any programming parameters that are outside the limits of the protocol.[29]

Hospira Gemstar

The Hospira Gemstar (introduced in March 2000; Hospira, Inc, Lake Forest, IL, USA) is a multitherapy ambulatory pump

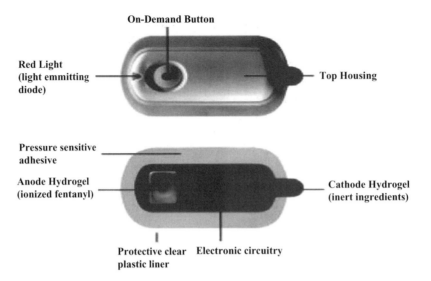

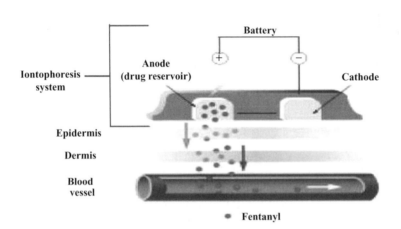

Figure 19.8: Fentanyl hydrochloride patient-controlled transdermal system (PCTS, Ionsys) is a self-contained, needle-free, credit-card-sized fentanyl-delivery system that is worn on the arm or chest. The system uses iontophoretic technology to actively deliver preprogrammed doses of fentanyl into the systemic circulation when the on-demand button is pressed. (Adapted from Koo, PJ 2005)

(configurable to PCA only) sold with optional pole-mounting brackets, an ambulatory carrying case, and multiple power sources (Figure 19.11). The Gemstar infusion system comes in 3 variations, each with a unique color. The blue pump has intravenous as well as epidural capabilities, whereas the yellow pump has capability for only IV pain management. The gray pump is not marketed for pain therapy, but is for other types of infusions such as parenteral nutritional and blood component therapies. The Gemstar is intended for hospital use or home care. An advantage of the Gemstar's ambulatory design is that it allows fluid delivery from a wide variety of bags, syringes, vials, and bottles. General safety features include an occlusion alarm that allows the user to select from among three pressure limits: low (7 psi), medium (14 psi), and high (30 psi). This may be useful in reducing nuisance alarms in high-pressure therapies, such as epidural administration, whereas providing a low-pressure setting for IV administration. Unfortunately, this pump does not include any advanced error reduction features such as bar coding.[29]

Hospira LifeCare PCA 3

The Hospira LifeCare PCA 3 (introduced in October 2002; Hospira, Inc, Lake Forest, IL, USA) is a large pole-mounted syringe driven infusion pump that delivers medications from 30-mL Hospira syringes (Figure 19.6). The pump has an integrated bar code reader to identify the drug name and concentration of labeled syringes as they are loaded into the pump. Its large comprehensive screen displays the drug name and concentration at all times as verified by the bar code scanner, as well as step-by-step prompts that are easy to follow. Furthermore, the display screen clearly indicates the cause of alarms and provides the user with instructions for appropriate follow-up. The device allows the user to retain pump settings if the drug vial has the same drug name and concentration as the previous drug vial, as indicated by the bar code.[29]

One of the advanced error reduction features of the Hospira LifeCare PCA 3 is the integrated bar code reader that identifies a syringe's drug name and concentration. By eliminating manual entry, this reader eliminates errors in entering

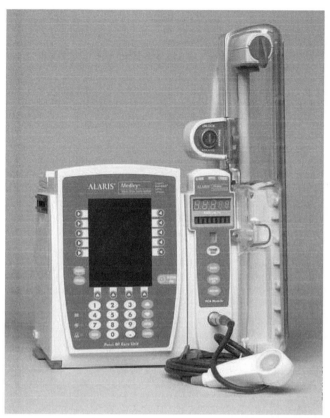

Figure 19.9: The Alaris System is the forefront of PCA safety technology. Its platform is capable of intergrating PCA, SPO$_2$, capnography (ETCO$_2$), and bar coding for all infusions, with wireless connectivity to transmit pertinent data to existing clinical information systems and electronic patient records. (Figure courtesy of Alaris Medical Systems, Inc, subsidiary of Cardinal Health, Inc, San Diego, CA.)

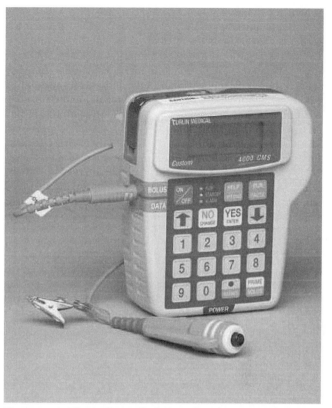

Figure 19.10: The Curlin Medical 4000 Clinical Management System (CMS) is a multitherapy pump that can be configurable to PCA only and is versatile for either home or hospital use. (Figure courtesy of Curlin Medical LLC, Huntington Beach, CA.)

drug concentration and in entering initial programming parameters.[29] A second error reduction feature of the Hospira LifeCare PCA 3 is its ability for automatic pump programming. This feature allows a facility to develop up to 10 delivery protocols specific to this pump. Each protocol contains information about specific drug vials and about pump settings such as delivery mode (PCA only, PCA plus continuous, or continuous only), continual and basal delivery settings, lockout time, and 1- or 4-hour dosing limits.[29]

In 2006, Hospira introduced the Hospira LifeCare PCA, an enhanced version of the LifeCare 3, but integrated with Hospira's MedNet dose error reduction system software. This software offers a computer-based drug library editor for developing facility specific drug libraries and has the ability to data mine alert and alarm logs for continuous quality improvement.[29]

Smiths Medical CADD-Prizm PCS II

The Smiths Medical CADD-Prizm PCS II™ (introduced in August 2004; Smith Medical MD, Inc, St Paul, MN, USA) is an ambulatory pump that can be used either for hospital or home care applications (Figure 19.12). Two variations are available, a purple pump that can be adapted for intravenous PCA and a yellow pump for epidural PCA (EPCA). Accessories for the pump include a pole-mounting bracket, medication cassette reservoirs (either 50 or 100 mL), lockboxes, administration sets that can be used with medication bags and syringes.[29] The device utilizes a report key that offers quick interrogation of doses requested

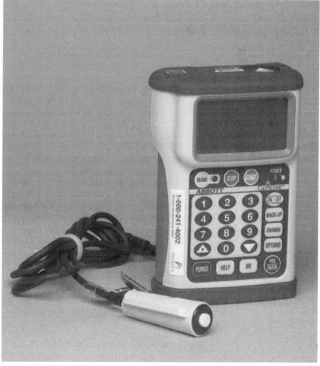

Figure 19.11: The GemStar Medication Management System is an ambulatory, small, lightweight, single-channel pump with advanced software for customized configuration and usage with multiple therapeutic modalities. (Figure courtesy of Hospira, Inc, Chicago, IL.)

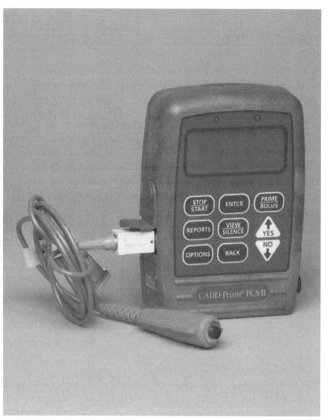

Figure 19.12: The CADD-Prizm PCS ambulatory infusion pump is a small ambulatory-style pump that can be used for either hospital or home care treatments. (Figure courtesy of Smith Medical MD, Inc, St Paul, MN.)

versus doses delivered, cumulative doses given, and a patient pain scale.[29]

The Prizm PCS II incorporates the Sentry PC-based pump-programming application, which can send (via a wired connection) standardized dosing protocols and dosing limits for subsequent computer-to-pump programming changes.[29] The CADD-Sentry programming software allows a hospital to develop drug-specific dosing protocols that are stored on a computer and sent via a connecting cable or modem to the pump. The protocols automatically program pump settings such as drug concentration, continuous and bolus delivery settings, lockout interval, time-based dosing limits, and fixed limits on continual and bolus delivery and lockout settings. This feature may limit errors because the pump will not allow the user to select programming parameters that are outside the set limits for a particular protocol. Thus, to set the pump outside these fixed limits, the user must have a code to access a protected "BioMed toolbox menu" that is unlikely for the user to have access to, or they can connect the pump to a computer and download another protocol that will allow this setting (Tables 19.8 and 19.9).[29]

NEURAXIAL AND PATIENT CONTROLLED ANALGESIA SYSTEMS

Background

Neuraxial drug administration describes a technique of delivering medication into the vicinity of the spinal cord. Two primary

methods of neuraxial drug administration include the *epidural* technique and the *subarachnoid* (intrathecal) technique. Subarachnoid analgesia is achieved by injecting a bolus dose of drug directly into the subarachnoid space. The drug is then dispersed in the cerebrospinal fluid (CSF), a medium that is in direct contact with neural structures of the spinal cord. Epidural analgesia describes the bolus injection or continous infusion of medications via an indwelling catheter positioned in the epidural space. Epidural dosing depends on diffusion of drug through the dura mater to produce an effect on spinal nerve roots or spinal cord.[36] The injection of local anesthetics into the epidural space was first described in the late 1800s, before the development of spinal anesthesia. However, practical application was not established until the 1930s. The technique was perfected in the 1970–1980s, when it was utilized for labor and delivery analgesia, which continues to be one of its major applications.[37] It was not until 1976, that the direct and powerful effects of opioids acting at spinal cord receptors led to the utilization of epidural dosing for acute pain management.[37] Currently, several classes of analgesics and methods of administration have been described. These include continuous epidural infusions and epidural patient controlled epidural analgesia (PCEA), both using combinations of opioids plus local anesthetics or local anesthetics or opioids alone.[37] In this section, we discuss patient-controlled and continuous epidural dosing and the systems available for providing such therapy.

Design Theory

The proposed theory for the effectiveness of PCEA, also termed epidural patient controlled analgesia (EPCA) for acute pain management, embodies many of the described assumptions underlying the efficacy and versatility of IV PCA. PCEA systems are also designed to take advantage of spinal cord pain processing as well as the unique pharmacokinetics of opioids and local anesthetics within the neuraxis. Most PCEA pumps share similar design and technology as pumps designed for IV PCA. In this regard, many of the devices designed for IV PCA can be used for PCEA and vice versa. The minimum requirements for a pump to possess the capability for PCEA include the ability to deliver sufficient driving pressure to overcome the resistance of a narrow gauge epidural catheter, the ability of the patient to initiate delivery of a bolus of medication, as well as a high rate infusion, a large lockable drug box, and safety features that minimize patient tampering.[38]

Basic Considerations

When compared to IV PCA, PCEA is the second most frequently used and second most studied method of analgesic self-administration. It is, by far, the most commonly used form of patient-controlled neuraxial analgesia.[7] PCEA optimizes analgesic efficacy by titrating delivery of epidural analgesics to provide individual dose requirements while minimizing adverse effects. PCEA demand doses are most commonly set at 2–4 mL using dilute concentrations of local anesthetics, with small amounts of an opioid. The optimal PCEA delivery variables (demand dose, lockout interval, and continuous background infusion) have not been clearly determined; however, continuous/basal infusion rates are essential and percentage of total dose is generally 3 times greater than that required with IV PCA. Infusion rates are usually set between 4 to 16 mL/h depending

Table 19.8: Specifications of Currently Marketed PCA Devices

Device	Maker	Specifications	Reservoir	Pump Mechanism	Dosing Modes	Flow Rates	Error Reduction Features
Alaris System PCA Module	Cardinal Health	4.5 (w) × 15.0 (h) × 7.5 (d) inches; weight = 5.5 lbs; power source: AC and backup rechargable battery	Up to a 60-mL syringe	Positive displacement	PCA	0.1 to 999 mL/h	Bar coding capacity; physiologic monitoring capacity ($ETCO_2$ and PulseOx), wireless networking capacity
Curlin Medical 4000 CMS	Curlin Medical	5.1 × 4.0 × 2.5 inches; weight 17.5 oz; power sources: 2 C alkaline batteries; AC and external rechargeable battery pack	1.0 to 9999 mL	Peristaltic pumping	Five-therapy ambulatory electronic infusion pump comprising continuous, PCA (IV, epidural, subcutaneous), TPN, intermittent, and variable modes.	0.1 mL to 400 mL/h	PC-based pump-programming software
Hospira GemStar	Hospira	5.5 (h) × 3.8 (w) × 2.0 (d) inches; weight 17 oz; power source: AC with backup rechargable alkaline batteries; 2 AA	1.0 to 9999 mL	Peristaltic pumping	Seven therapy pump (blue): TPN, pain management, intermittent, continuous, weight dosed, mL/h only, and variable time; six-therapy pump (gray): above minus pain management pump (yellow): only pain management (intravenous, epidural, subcutaneous, or arterial)	Blue and Gray: 0.1 to 1000; mL/h yellow: 0.1 to 25 mL/h	No advanced error reduction features
Hospira LifeCare PCA 3	Hospira	8 (w) × 13 (h) × 6 (d); weight approx. 10 lbs; power source: AC with battery backup	30-mL syringe	Positive displacement	PCA, continuous or PCA with continuous	Delivery rates variable depending on mode; PCA = 1 mL/35 s	Integrated bar code coupled to profiles, automatic pump programming; the LifeCare PCA has MedNet software
Smiths Medical Cadd-Prizm PCS II	Smiths Medical	Size 1.7 × 4.1 × 5.6 inches; weight 20 oz; power: 9-V battery with AC backup	1-9999 mL	Peristaltic pumping	PCA, continuous or PCA with continuous; suitable for intravenous, intra-arterial, epidural, intrathecal, subcutaneous, or intraperitoneal	40 to 125 mL/h	No advanced error reduction features

on the location of the surgery, the level of the catheter, and the age of the patient. For instance, lower rates of continuous infusions are used for thoracic level catheters and in elderly patients.[7]

Clinical Management

The clinical application of neuraxial analgesia was initially limited to bolus dose administration of pain medications through needles or catheters inserted in the epidural space. Later, it was broadened to continuous analgesic infusions via indwelling epidural catheters.[36] The optimal solution for epidural infusions

and PCEA is still a matter of much debate; however, combinations containing a long-acting local anesthetic and an opioid, such as fentanyl, morphine, or hydromorphone, are widely employed (refer to Chapters 15, *Clinical Application of Epidural Analgesia*, and 16, *Neuraxial Analgesia with Hydromorphone, Morphine, and Fentanyl*). Although opioids such as morphine and hydromorphone can be used effectively alone, they are commonly combined with dilute concentrations of long-acting local anesthetics such as bupivicaine (0.031%–0.125%), levobupivicaine (0.05%–0.125%), and ropivicaine (0.1%–0.2%).[7,38] Combination dosing improves the overall quality of analgesia, reduces

Table 19.9: Pros and Cons of Currently Marketed PCA Devices

Device	Summary	Pros	Cons
Alaris System PCA Module	Attributes for this pump include its ease of use, a comprehensive and configurable dose error reduction system, and its integration with physiologic monitoring	(1) Guardrails dose error reduction software offers dosing limits and gives analysis of logged alerts and alarms; (2) bar code function available; (3) ergonomic lighted dosing button	None worth mentioning
Curlin Medical 4000 CMS	This pump is easy to use with good flow accuracy and continuity; a good pump for outpatient clinics, home care applications, and hospitals that prefer small ambulatory style pumps	(1) CMS programming software; (2) ambulatory design that allows a wider range of bags and syringes for medication storage	(1) Increased workflow needed to use the automated pump programming feature; (2) dose review is not required after programming is set; (3) lockbox cannot stand upright, must be pole mounted
Hospira GemStar	Easy to use pump without many operational disadvantages; however, this pump does not have any advanced error reduction features	(1) Wide variety of containers for fluid delivery; (2) several operational options on power-up; (3) provides clear displays and straightforward prompts	(1) No advanced error reduction features; (2) "Check IV Set" alarm ambiguous; (3) lockbox can be difficult to assemble and load; (4) transformer is large and difficult to transport
Hospira LifeCare PCA 3 and LifeCare PCA	Easy to use pump with few disadvantages; this pump is an excellent choice for hospitals wishing to purchase prefilled syringes.	(1) Bar code reader to eliminate wrong drug or concentration errors; (2) profiles software offers limited standardized automatic programming associated with specific hospira prefilled syringes; (3) Large, straightforward, comprehensive display; (4) MedNet dose error reduction software (only available in LifeCare PCA)	(1) Accepts only Hospira syringes; (2) releases post occlusion bolus averaging 1.5 mL if specific protocol is not followed: (3) no advanced error software available in the LifeCare PCA 3
Smiths Medical Cadd-Prizm PCS II	Although a good choice for outpatient clinics and home use because of its compact and rugged design, it has a few disadvantages.	(1) CADD-Sentry pump programming software; (2) ambulatory design allows fluid delivery from a wide range of containers	(1) Large workflow needed to accommodate the software; (2) poor flow continuity when set at low flows (0.1mL/h); (3) does not continuously display dosing parameters; (4) manually entering new programming is time-consuming and confusing; (5) "check cassette" alarm is ambiguous; (6) pump's "automatic review" function after settings are entered can be cumbersome

Adapted from ECRI health devices Jan 2006.

the dose requirements of individual drugs, and minimizes local anesthetic exposure and related side effects.[37,39,40]

Neuraxially administered opioids exert their effects as a result of activation of opioid receptors in the spinal cord, as well as central effects following vascular absorption. The relative contribution of each of these mechanisms is dependent on dose, site of administration, and the physiochemical properties of the specific opioid administered.[37] Lipophilicity is a variable that greatly affects the properties of opioids. Lipophilic fentanyl has a more rapid onset and a shorter duration of epidural activity than hydrophilic opioids such as morphine. Lipophilic opioids are absorbed rapidly by neural (and fatty) tissues and, therefore, exhibit a narrower band of segmental analgesia. Extensive vascular absorption provides significant supraspinal contribution to their analgesic effects.[37]

Hydrophilic opioids such as morphine and hydromorphone penetrate neural tissue slower than lipophilic opioids, result-

ing in a delayed onset of analgesia. Hydrophilic opioids have a delayed elimination, allowing widespread CSF distribution. Thus, nonsegmental analgesia can be achieved at dermatomes distant from the catheter site.[37]

Respiratory depression is the most serious and potentially life-threatening adverse effect of neuraxial opioid administration. This side effect can occur as a consequence of systemic absorption or rostral spread of opioid to brainstem respiratory centers.[39] The elderly appear to display increased sensitivity to opioid-induced CNS depression, including sedation and respiratory depression.[41]

Systems

There are four parameters that must be set prior to initiating PCEA therapy. These include bolus size, lockout interval, continuous infusion rate, and maximum 4-hour dose for each 2- to

4-hour period. In general, epidural solutions are programmed as milliliters of solution rather than as milligrams of analgesic. The bolus dose is the volume of drug that a patient self-administers when they press the PCEA button. The volume, which is set by the caregiver, must be large enough to spread through the epidural space and be effective, yet small enough to be safe. For example, elderly patients generally require small volumes of drug (1–2 mL), whereas more vigorous individuals and those with large incisions may require larger volumes (4–5 mL). The lockout interval is a set amount of time usually ranging from 4 to 15 minutes before which a patient cannot self-administer another bolus dose. In general, the lockout interval should be chosen to match the time the dose becomes effective, that is, 5–6 minutes for rapid-acting opioids such as fentanyl and 10–15 minutes for slower agents such as morphine.[38]

The continuous background infusion is the volume of drug set per hour that the patient receives continuously without need for request. The necessity of the background infusion is that it reduces analgesic variability over time by providing a baseline level of pain control on which the patient self-administers additional analgesics in response to changes in clinical setting (ie, ambulation, physical therapy deep breathing). Ideally lipophilic opioids should be administered at spinal segments immediately adjacent to the site of surgery. High rates of infusion may be required when lipophilic opioids are administered via catheters placed at interspaces distant from the site of surgery. Lower rates of infusion are required for hydrophilic opioids that spread rostrally. A major drawback of continuous infusions alone is that patients cannot control analgesic delivery in response to an increasing pain stimulus (ie ambulation).[38]

Safety

Intravenous PCA and EPCA therapy share similar hazards and potential for programming errors and device/catheter malfunction. Epidural infusion devices are predisposed to preparation and administration errors, including incorrect drug or drug concentrations and rates of infusion. That may lead not only to overdose, but also to the risk of neurotoxicity. For example, bags prepared for IV infusion may be confused and substituted for epidural solutions with potentially serious complications.[42]

The ISMP is an organization that works on reducing medical errors in the health care setting. They collect data on medical errors and have identified how most injuries from PCA/PCEA technologies occur (see Table 19.3). They also have identified methods that may be employed for the prevention of PCEA medication and pump errors and they include (1) perform a failure mode and effects analysis (identify the possible failure mode causes and effects and assess the situation for each and determine an overall hazard score); (2) design a certification or privileging process that includes how to order PCA/PCEA, how to use the pump, and to review the signs and symptoms of opioid toxicity; (3) design standard order sets for the pumps; (4) establish patient selection criteria; (5) establish standard concentrations for medications and only stock those concentrations; (6) set maximum dose limits in the computer ordering system; and (7) require two clinicians to double check the correct patient, order, drug concentration, and pump settings.[30]

Other hazards specific to PCEA include the possibility of local infection or meningitis because epidural catheters can serve as an entry point for bacterial contamination. Strict aseptic technique and in-line filters may reduce the overall incidence of infection. Epidural hematoma, particularly in anticoagulated patients, remains as a rare, but potentially catastrophic, complication of indwelling epidural catheter. The American Society of Regional Anesthesia (ASRA) recommends that such therapy would contraindicate placement or necessitate removal of epidural catheters (please refer to ASRA guidelines).[30]

Commercially Available PCEA Infusion Devices

Hospira Gemstar

The Hospira Gemstar (introduced in March 2000; Hospira, Inc, Lake Forest, IL, USA) is a multitherapy ambulatory pump (configurable to PCA only) sold with optional pole-mounting brackets, an ambulatory carrying case, and multiple power sources (Figure 19.11). The Gemstar infusion system comes in three variations, each with a unique color. The blue pump offers epidural functions. An advantage of the GemStar's ambulatory design is that it allows fluid delivery from a wide variety bags, syringes, vials, and bottles. General safety features include an occlusion alarm that allows the user to select from among three pressure limits: low (7 psi), medium (14 psi), and high (30 psi). This may be useful in reducing nuisance alarms in high-pressure epidural administration. Other than the pressure alarm and locking code designed to prevent tampering, the device does not include advanced error reduction features.[29]

Smiths Medical CADD-Prizm PCS II

The Smiths Medical CADD-Prizm PCS II (introduced in August 2004; Smith Medical MD, Inc, St Paul, MN, USA) is an ambulatory pump that can be used for either hospital or home care applications (Figure 19.12). The pump comes with two variations, a purple pump, which can be adapted for intravenous PCA, or a yellow pump for EPCA. Accessories for the pump include a pole-mounting bracket, medication cassette reservoirs (either 50 or 100 mL), lockboxes, and administration sets that can be used with medication bags and syringes.[29] The report key offers quick access to reports such as doses requested versus doses delivered, cumulative doses given, and patient pain scale.[29]

Curlin Medical 4000 CMS

The Curlin Medical 4000 CMS (introduced in 2001; Curlin Medical LLC, Huntington Beach, CA, USA) is a multitherapy pump, configurable to PCA only, that can be used for hospital or home care applications (Figure 19.10). Accessories for the pump include a pole-mounting bracket and lockboxes.[29]

Perineural Ambulatory Analgesia Systems

Background

Perineural drug administration involves the infusion of drug over a single or several nerve roots or peripheral nerves that correspond to a particular dermatome or myotome. In the past decade, there has been an increasing interest in continuous peripheral nerve blocks. This technique involves the percutaneous insertion of a catheter directly adjacent to the peripheral nerves supplying the affected surgical site. Local anesthetic is then infused via the catheter providing potent, site-specific analgesia. Combining a perineural catheter with a portable infusion pump allows outpatients to experience the same level of analgesia previously afforded only to those remaining hospitalized.[43] This technique has been utilized to provide continuous analgesia in such varied anatomic locations as paravertebral, interscalene, intersternocleidomastoid, infraclavicular, axillary, psoas, femoral, sciatic, popliteal, and tibial nerve placements.

There are two main classes of pumps employed for continuous perineural analgesia. These include electronic and nonelectronic pumps. Electronic pumps used for perineural analgesia employ similar design, technology, and mechanisms as pumps used for PCA and PCEA. Thus, in this section, we focus on nonelectronic (mechanical) pumps that include elastomeric infusion pumps, spring-powered infusion pumps, and negative pressure (vacuum) infusion pumps.

Ganapathy et al[44] evaluated 7 patients who received popliteal-sciatic continuous regional anesthetic blocks, with an initial dose of 30 mL of ropivicaine (0.5%) via a perineural cathter placed prior to elective ankle and foot surgery. On discharge, the popliteal catheter was connected to an Eclipse elastomeric pump containing 50 mL of ropivicaine (3%). All patients evaluated reported that they were "very satisfied" with the technique and indicated that they would use the technique again. Two patients had mild nausea. Six required tylenol 3 for mild surgical pain. All patients, except 1, could remove the catheters by themselves. Two patients fell asleep after opening the bolus clamp resulting in delivery of the total content of the pump without any adverse effects. The authors concluded that patient selection is very important and a certain level of education is necessary for the patient to comprehend the use of such a device, removal of an indwelling catheter, and sterile precautions. Patients who live alone are not good candidates for this device.[44] This study underscores the potiential for the future expansion of ambulatory regional pain therapies.

Design Theory

Nonelectronic disposable infusion pumps have been in clinical use since the early 1980s. This technology has expanded in recent times, and they are currently employed in hospitals and home care settings to deliver therapies such as chemotherapy, antimicrobials, analgesia, and anesthesia, as well as for postoperative pain control and chronic pain management.

All nonelectronic disposable pumps use the same mechanical principles. Flow of medication is determined by the variables of pressure and resistance, very similar to Ohm's law. The pressure on the fluid is generated by a variety of mechanisms, including stretched elastomers, compressed springs, vacuum drives, or pressure supplied from a cartridge of pressurized gas. The pressure generated by disposable pumps on fluid is typically within the range of 250 to 600 mmHg, compared with a fluid reservoir pressure for electric pumps of 5 to 1200 mmHg.[45]

Resistance is due restriction within the flow path, and in ambulatory pumps, the restriction of flow is caused by sections of narrow-bore tubing. The smaller the diameter increases the resistance and decreases the device's flow rate. Other variables to consider are temerature and the pumps spacial reationship to the patient. Temperature will have an impact on the viscosity of the fluid, affect the pressure of the driving gas, and also potentially alter the diameter of the flow restrictors. Flow restrictors are usually made of materials whose dimensions change little with temperature in order to maintain accuracy. Typical materials used are glass and plastic. It is recommended to avoid exposing the ambulatory pumps to any extremes in temperature for this reason.

Spatial relationship to the patient must be considered because large elevations above the infusion site could increase flow rate.[45]

Disposable pumps can infuse at flow rates of 0.5–500 mL/h, with running times from 30 minutes to 12 days. Reservoir volume usually ranges from 60 to 500 mL.[45]

Systems

In elastaomeric pumps, the driving pressure on the fluid is generated by the force of a stretched elastomer. These pumps consist of an elastomeric membrane which contains the drug, and an outer protective shell. The membranes are made of various elastomers, both natural and synthetic (eg, isoprene, rubber, latex, and silicon), and can be made of a single or multiple layers. The type of elastomer and the geometry of the elatomeric balloon determine the pressure generated on the fluid when the balloon is stretched. Multiple-layer elastomeric membranes can generate higher pressures than the single-layer membranes.[45]

All elastomeric pumps share a common flow pattern, where the flow rate at the beginning of an infusion is higher than during most of the infusion, with a second increase close to the end of the delivery. These nonlinear flow-rate patterns are due to variations in the force exerted by the stretched elastomeric membrane. Although this variation in flow rate is considered to be clinically acceptable, it is useful for clinical users to be aware of this performance.[45]

Positive-pressure spring-powered pumps are powered by energy stored in a compressed spring. These pumps often contain reusable components and are made from durable materials such as Teflon, stainless steel, or polycarbonate.[45] The flow-rate patterns for simple-spring disposable pumps have typical characteristics, with the flow rate being significantly higher at the beginning of the infusion than at the end. These variations result from fluctuations of the pressure applied on the fluid by the compressed spring. The pressure decreases with the volume of drug remaining in the reservoir, such that the flow rate decreases steadily during the course of the delivery.[45]

Negative-pressure pumps or vacuum pumps exert a driving pressure via the pressure difference across two sides of the pump's low-pressure chamber wall. The vacuum chamber's pressure gradient is created by the user while filling the device. Expansion of the drug reservoir by the addition of fluid causes simultaneous expansion of the reduced pressure chamber, thus, creating a significant vacuum. During infusion delivery, pressure on the movable wall plunger is generated by the large pressure difference between its two sides, causing it to move and compress the fluid in the drug containing chamber. These devices have driving pressures around 600 mmHg, which is the highest pressure achievable for disposable pumps. Flow rate patterns for negative-pressure pumps are more constant than that of elastomeric or spring driven pumps, but this has not been shown to be clinically different.[45]

Basic Considerations

With today's current technologies of nerve stimulators and ultrasound guidance, single shot peripheral nerve blocks's have become quite common and orthopedic patients are the largest group who undergo peripheral nerve blocks (PNB). Peripheral neural blockade provides excellent postoperative analgesia and has been reported to decrease hospital stay, and reduce the rate of unanticipated hospital readmission (refer to Chapter 17, *Regional Anesthesia*). Despite the use of long-acting local anesthesia in peripheral nerve blocks (PNB), some patients still report wound pain during the first 24 to 48 hours postoperative hours, and an even greater number require opioid analgesics

7 days after surgery. Continuous infusions of local anesthetics via non-electronic patient controlled perineural analgesia has proved efficacious in this patient population in controlling postoperative pain.[46]

A number of studies have been published comparing the efficacy of nonelectronic perineural ambulatory pumps to traditional electronic patient-controlled systems. Ilfeld et al[47] compared the efficacy of an elastomeric pump with two electronic pumps for patient-controlled perineural analgesia patients recovering from orthopedic surgery. Intraoperative anesthesia was provided with 0.5% ropivicaine via indwelling catheters, and postoperative pain was managed with patient-controlled perineural analgesia. Patients were divided to receive either an elastomeric pump or a more traditional electronic pump for the administration of the perineural infusions. Patients were transferred to the surgical ward for the first postoperative night and then discharged the following day with the catheter in place. A home care nurse visited the patient twice daily to access VAS pain scores. This study demonstrated that disposable nonelectronic pumps are as effective as the electronic PCA pumps for postoperative pain relief, and are associated with fewer technical problems, and consequently, better satisfaction scores. These results also demonstrated the safety and convenience of disposable elastomeric pumps for patient recovery at home.

Continuous peripheral analgesia via elastomeric pumps has also been evaluated in children recovering from orthopedic surgery by Dadure et al[48] in 2003. Postoperatively, a continuous infusion of 0.2% ropivicaine was administered at 0.1mL/kg/h in 25 ASA I and II children (age range from 1 to 15 years) using disposable elastomeric pumps. A total of 11 popliteal, 9 femoral, and 5 axillary nerve blocks were performed. No block failures were noted. Thirteen disposable pumps with a flow of 2 mL/h, 9 with 5 mL/h, and 3 with 7 mL/hr were used over a 45.5-hour period. The median dose of ropivicaine administered was 10.1 mg/kg. The children experienced effective pain control. No local site reactions, evidence of local anesthetic toxicity, or neurological symptoms were observed. Advantages of nonelectronic elastomeric pumps in this study included minimal use of rescue analgesia, simplicity of use and function, and the freedom of movement these pumps provide children, making it easier for them to play.

Clinical Management and Safety

Outpatient perineural infusions may be used after mildly painful procedures to decrease opioid requirements and opioid-related side effects. However, because not all patients desire, or are capable of accepting, the extra responsibility that comes with managing the catheter and pump, appropriate patient selection is crucial for safe ambulatory local anesthetic infusion. As some degree of postoperative cognitive dysfunction is common after surgery, investigators often require patients to have a caretaker at least through the first postoperative night. Complications that could be managed routinely within the hospital may take longer to identify or be more difficult to manage in medically unsupervised patients at home. Investigators often exclude patients with known hepatic or renal insufficiency in an effort to avoid local anesthetic toxicity. For infusions that may affect the phrenic nerve and ipsilateral diaphragm function (ie, interscalene or cervical paravertebral catheters), patients with heart or lung disease are often excluded because continuous interscalene local anesthetic infusions have been shown to cause frequent ipsilateral

diaphragm paralysis. Furthermore, among the adopted criteria for discharging patients home is the ability to ambulate; therefore, discharge with lower extremity peripheral nerve blocks remains controversial.[43]

One major difference between inpatient and ambulatory infusions is the catheter site will not be observed daily by an experienced medical professional. Therefore, optimal sterile technique must be maintained when placing the catheter to avoid infection, and every effort must be made to optimally secure the catheter for outpatients.[43]

When selecting infusion pumps for perineural analgesia, several factors must be considered to determine the optimal device for a given clinical application. They include infusion rate accuracy, consistency, and reliability, as well as patient-controlled bolus capability and volume of local anesthetic required.

Poor flow accuracy of disposable pumps is a major disadvantage of these devices and makes them inappropriate for therapies that require extremely accurate drug delivery. Ilfeld et al[48] studied the flow rate accuracy and consistency of various ambulatory infusion pumps. Results showed that the elastomeric and spring-powered pumps infused at higher than expected rates initially. They found that raising the flow-regulator temperature a few degrees above room temperature increased infusion rates approximately 10% in one elastomeric pump (Infusor LV5), but less than 5% in the other (Accufuser Plus). Furthermore, other factors, like viscosity, atmospheric pressure, and back pressure, affect the accuracy of delivery of most nonelectronic pumps.[45] These differences in flow rate accuracy may have implications for patient care when applied to continuous perineural analgesia. Health care providers must be aware of pump infusion profiles to maximize patient safety and benefit.

Identification of clinical situations appropriate for disposable pump use is critical and should be considered a first step in selecting the optimal device. Such variables as acceptable infusion rate accuracy, patient-controlled bolus dose availability, desired infusion duration, infusion rate profile, and total drug volume of reservoir should be taken into account.[48]

Cost-Effectiveness

The typical price range for disposable infusion pumps is $30–$86. The price range for electric pumps is wide, but typically in the range of $1200–$3500. Although these initial costs favor disposable perineural pumps, the long-term cost savings is not as obvious, and there has been no concensus on which is a clearly better value.[48] In a few studies, the long-term use of low-price disposable devices was more costly than the one-time purchase of an electronic infusion pump. There are many factors that need to be taken into account when analyzing the cost of perineural therapies, such as the cost of the filling apparatus for disposable pumps, as well as the cost of using pharmacy facilities.[48]

Commercially Available Nonelectronic Perineural Infusion Devices

Elastomeric Pumps
ON-Q C-BLOC CONTINUOUS PERIPHERAL NERVE BLOCK SYSTEM
The ON-Q C-Bloc Post-Op Pain Relief System (I-Flow Corp., Lake Forest, CA, USA), manufactured by I-Flow, is a nonelectronic elastomeric infusion pump that maintains a continuous perineural infusion of local anesthetics for the management of postoperative pain (Figure 19.13). While maintaining continuous neural blockade, this ambulatory drug delivery system

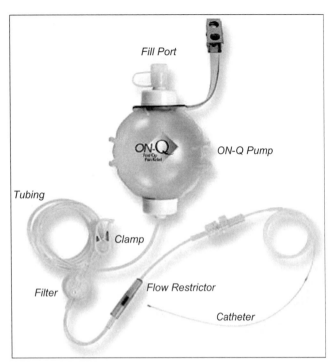

Figure 19.13: The On-Q Painbuster pump, a product of the I-Flow Corporation, is an example of a gas-pressurized elastomeric infusion device. (Figure courtesy of I-Flow Corporation, Lake Forest, CA.)

decreases the amount of oral and IV/IM opioids required by a patient and dose-dependent side effects. With the C-Bloc, dilute local anesthetic solutions are delivered via a catheter at a rate that does not impair motor function, but maintains pain control.

The pump consists of a multilayer membrane with a protective PVC cover. The strain of the elastomeric membrane provides a positive pressure of approximately 10 psi (500 mm Hg), and a capillary orifice controls the flow rate. The pump consists of three layers; an inner layer that is a synthetic thermoplastic elastomer that contains the drug and is nonlatex, a middle layer composed of natural rubber latex, and an outer protective layer made of PVC. This pump possesses a 1.2-μ particulate filter and a 0.02 air-eliminating filter.

A variety of sizes and flow rates are available, providing dosing flexibility. Depending on the model selected, the device may hold from 35 mL to 550 mL of local anesthetic with infusion duration ranging from 12 hours to 5 days.

Local anesthetics often used with the On-Q C-Bloc system include lidocaine (1%), bupivicaine (0.25%), and ropivicaine (0.2%). The system has an on-demand feature so the patient can deliver an additional dose of medication if there is break-through pain. The ON-Q C-Bloc System can also be used during a procedure for pain relief.

The ON-Q C-Bloc system with onDemand has an added feature that allows patients to give a 5 mL-bolus every hour in addition to the continuous 2–8-mL/h rate. The on demand has a 1-hour refill. This lockout mechanism prevents the patient from receiving a full bolus dose if the patient presses the bolus button before 1 hour. Medication doses should be calculated at the total average rate of 7–13 mL/h (2–8 mL basal + 5 mL bolus).

The major disadvantage of the ON-Q C-Bloc system is a flow rate/delivery accuracy of ±15% of the labeled infusion rate. As mentioned, this may be inappropriate for therapies that require extremely accurate local anesthetic drug delivery.

Another disadvantage of the ON-Q C-Bloc system is the effect of temperature on the accuracy of drug delivery. The ON-Q C-Bloc system is calibrated to the patient's body temperature, thus the flow restrictor must be in contact with the patient's skin. If the restrictor is away from the body, the medication will infuse at a slower than expected flow rate.[49]

Spring-Powered Pumps
PAIN CARE 3000, 3200, AND 4200

The Pain Care 3000, 3200, and 4200 series (BREG. Vista, CA) are spring-powered nonelectronic perineural ambulatory infusion pumps. The local anesthetic solution anesthetic is delivered through a latex-free radio-opaque, multiport infusion catheter.

The Pain Care 3000 pump can hold up to 100 mL of local anesthetic, whereas the 3200 and 4200 models have a capacity of up to 200 mL. Average local anesthetic delivery ranges from 2 mL/h (Pain Care 3000 and Pain Care 4200) to 4 mL/h (Pain Care 3200). The Pain Care 3000, 3200, and 4200 series of pumps combine a continuous infusion with the benefit of a patient-controlled 4-mL bolus that can be obtained by squeezing the pump. Average times for bolus refill of the Pain Care 3000 and 4200 pumps is 2 hours, and for the 3200 model, it is 1 hour. Complete local anesthetic infusion usually occurs in 2 days in the Pain Care 3000 and 3200 models (Figure 19.14) and 4 days in the 4200 model.

Like their elastomeric counterparts, the Pain Care pumps provide continuous perineural/surgical site infusion of local anesthetics. Local anesthetics used with these devices include lidocaine and/or bupivicaine. A flow indicator on the pump

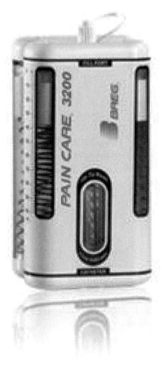

Figure 19.14: The Pain Care 3200 is a spring-driven device made by BREG, which is used for local wound site infusion of nonnarcotic anesthetic for the management of postoperative pain. (Figure courtesy of BREG, Inc, Vista, CA.)

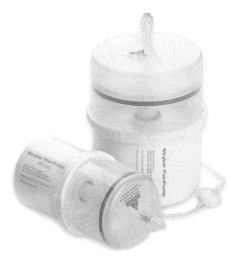

Figure 19.15: The Stryker Pain Pump 1, a vacuum-driven pain management device, is a portable, single-use, disposable pain management device that helps deliver a continuous, controlled infusion of local anesthetic to the surgical site. (Figure courtesy of Stryker Medical, Kalamazoo, MI.)

gives immediate feedback on flow, and graduation marks provide visibility of amount of medication delivered. Use of these pumps results in decreased need for oral, IM, or PCA narcotic medications, thus, they can be used effectively for outpatient surgery.

A disadvantage of spring-powered pumps is the propensity for variable flow rates. Flow rate accuracy with spring-powered pumps can also be affected by the temperature of the surrounding environment.[50]

Negative-Pressure Pumps

PAIN PUMP 1

The Stryker Pain Pump 1 (Stryker, Kalamazoo, MI) (Figure 19.15) is a vacuum-driven (negative-pressure) nonelectronic ambulatory infusion pump. It is a single-use pain management device that can deliver a continuous infusion of local anesthetic to the surgical site. The Pain Pump 1 is available in two sizes, one with a 120-mL container and the other with a volume capacity of 270 mL. Flow rates can be adjusted on these pumps from a minimum of 0.6 mL/h (for a 7-day infusion) to a maximum of 4 mL/h (for a 1-day infusion) for the 120-mL pump. With the 270-mL pump, flow rates may range from 2 mL/h (for a 5day infusion) to 8 mL/h infusion (for a 1.5-day infusion). Duration of infusion is set by the physician, and the patient is unable to adjust the flow rate. Visible volume scale allows one to confirm that medication is flowing through the pump and determine the amount of consumed medication and remaining time.

The latex-free system of the Pain Pump 1 includes a puncture-resistant canister design with a protective hard outer shell. With the Pain Pump 1, extended fenestrated catheters of varying lengths (0.5, 2.5, 5.0, and 10 inches) can be tunneled in either one or two sites and connected to the pump.[51]

CONCLUSION

Since its introduction to clinical pain management in the early 1980s, PCA and continuous analgesic infusion devices have provided safe and effective analgesia for millions of patients and have played a major role in reducing the incidence of analgesic undermedication in the postsurgical period.

Intravenous PCA is expensive and requires direct IV access and has been is associated with pump failures and misprogramming errors that lead to underdosage and overdosage. Smart pump technology, including the use of bar coding, built-in wireless pulse oximetry, and patient monitoring capabilities, have added an extra layer of patient safety. These safety improvements do not imply that caregivers should let down their vigilance by not double checking programming and maintaining close patient observation. Continuing improvements including disposable needlefree transdermal PCA may further reduce technology failures inherent with electronic devices. The same improvements are at hand with PCEA devices and perineural infusion pumps. These devices have become smaller and more user friendly, encouraging patient ambulation and possible continuation of therapy on discharge to home or rehabilitation facility. The trend toward inexpensive elastomeric analgesic infusions provides simplicity while maintaining safety, and will further encourage home-based continuation of regional analgesia.

REFERENCES

1. Sinatra RS. Acute Pain: Mechanisms & Management. St Louis, MO: Mosby; 1992.
2. Graves DA, Foster TS, Batenhorst RL, Bennett RL, Baumann TJ. Patient-controlled analgesia. Ann Intern Med. 1983;99(3):360–366.
3. Marks RM, Sachar EJ. Undertreatment of medical inpatients with narcotic analgesics. Ann Intern Med. 1973;78(2):173–181.
4. Sechzer PH. Objective measurement of pain. Anesthesiology. 1968;29:209–210.
5. Sechzer PH. Patient-controlled analgesia (PCA): a retrospective. Anesthesiology. 1990;72(4):735–736.
6. Austin KL, Stapleton JV, Mather LE. Relationship between blood meperidine concentrations and analgesic response: a preliminary report. Anesthesiology. 1980;53(6):460–466.
7. Grass JA. Patient-controlled analgesia. Anesth Analg. 2005;101 (suppl 5):44–61.
8. White PF. Clinical uses of intravenous anesthetic and analgesic infusions. Anesth Analg. 1989;68(2):161–171.
9. Owen H, Plummer JL, Armstrong I, Mather LE, Cousins MJ. Variables of patient-controlled analgesia. 1. Bolus size. Anaesthesia. 1989;44(1):7–10.
10. Burns JW, Hodsman NB, McLintock TT, Gillies GW, Kenny GN, McArdle CS. The influence of patient characteristics on the requirements for postoperative analgesia. A reassessment using patient-controlled analgesia. Anaesthesia. 1989;44(1):2–6.
11. Ferrante FM, Orav EJ, Rocco AG, Gallo J. A statistical model for pain in patient-controlled analgesia and conventional intramuscular opioid regimens. Anesth Analg. 1988;67(5):457–461.
12. Walder B, Schafer M, Henzi I, Tramer MR. Efficacy and safety of patient-controlled opioid analgesia for acute postoperative pain: a quantitative systematic review. Acta Anaesthesiol Scand. 2001;45(7):795–804.
13. Sear JW, Hand CW, Moore RA, McQuay HJ. Studies on morphine disposition: influence of renal failure on the kinetics of morphine and its metabolites. Br J Anaesth. 1989;62(1):28–32.
14. Osborne RJ, Joel SP, Slevin ML. Morphine intoxication in renal failure: the role of morphine-6-glucuronide. Br Med J 1986;292(6535):1548–1549.

15. Parab PV, Ritschel WA, Coyle DE, Gregg RV, Denson DD. Pharmacokinetics of hydromorphone after intravenous, peroral and rectal administration to human subjects. *Biopharm Drug Dispos.* 1988;9(2):187–199.

16. Simopoulos TT, Smith HS, Peeters-Asdourian C, Stevens DS. Use of meperidine in patient-controlled analgesia and the development of a normeperidine toxic reaction. *Arch Surg.* 2002;137(1):84–88.

17. Sinatra RS, Harrison DM. Oxymorphone in patient-controlled analgesia. *Clin Pharm.* 1989;8(8):541–544.

18. Lehmann KA, Gerhard A, Horrichs-Haermeyer G, Grond S, Zech D. Postoperative patient-controlled analgesia with sufentanil: analgesic efficacy and minimum effective concentrations. *Acta Anaesthesiol Scand.* 1991;35(3):221–226.

19. Owen H, Brose WG, Plummer JL, Mather LE. Variables of patient-controlled analgesia. 3: test of an infusion-demand system using alfentanil. *Anaesthesia.* 1990;45(6):452–455.

20. Balcioglu O, Akin S, Demir S, Aribogan A. Patient-controlled intravenous analgesia with remifentanil in nulliparous subjects in labor. *Exp Opin Pharmacother.* 2007;8(18):3089–3096.

21. Pang WW, Mok MS, Lin CH, Yang TF, Huang MH. Comparison of patient-controlled analgesia (PCA) with tramadol or morphine. *Can J Anaesth.* 1999;46(11):1030–1035.

22. Scott LJ, Perry CM. Tramadol: a review of its use in perioperative pain. *Drugs* 2000;60(1):139–176.

23. Lynch EP, Lazor MA, Gellis JE, Orav J, Goldman L, Marcantonio ER. The impact of postoperative pain on the development of postoperative delirium. *Anesth Analg.* 1998;86(4):781–785.

24. Macintyre PE. Safety and efficacy of patient-controlled analgesia. *Br J Anaesth.* 2001;87(1):36–46.

25. Medication safety: PCA pump programming errors continue to cause fatal overinfusions. *Health Devices* 2002;31(9):342–346.

26. Klepstad P, Rakvag TT, Kaasa S, et al. The 118 A > G polymorphism in the human u-opioid receptor gene may increase morphine requirements in patients with pain caused by malignant disease. *Acta Anaesthesiol Scand* 2004;48(10):1232–1239.

27. Wuhrman E, Cooney MF, Dunwoody CJ, Eksterowicz N, Merkel S, Oakes LL, American Society for Pain Management Nursing. Authorized and unauthorized ("PCA by Proxy") dosing of analgesic infusion pumps: position statement with clinical practice recommendations. *Pain Manag Nurs.* 2007;8(1):4–11.

28. Husch M, Sullivan C, Rooney D, et al. Insights from the sharp end of intravenous medication errors: implications for infusion pump technology. *Qual Saf Health Care.* 2005;14(2):80–86.

29. ECRI. Patient-controlled analgesic infusion pumps. *Health Devices* 2006;35(1):5–35.

30. Viscusi ER, Schechter LN. Patient-controlled analgesia: finding a balance between cost and comfort. *Am J Health Syst Pharm* 2006;63(8 suppl 1):3,13; quiz 15–16.

31. van den Nieuwenhuyzen MC, Engbers FH, Vuyk J, Burm AG. Target-controlled infusion systems: role in anaesthesia and analgesia. *Clin Pharmacokinet.* 2000;38(2):181–190.

32. Hill HF, Mackie AM, Coda BA, Iverson K, Chapman CR. Patient-controlled analgesic administration: a comparison of steady-state morphine infusions with bolus doses. *Cancer* 1991;67(4):873–882.

33. Mather LE, Owen H. The scientific basis of patient-controlled analgesia. *Anaesth Intensive Care.* 1988;16(4):427–436.

34. Van Poucke GE, Bravo LJ, Shafer SL. Target controlled infusions: targeting the effect site while limiting peak plasma concentration. *IEEE Trans Biomed Eng.* 2004;51(11):1869–1875.

35. Viscusi ER, Reynolds L, Chung F, Atkinson LE, Khanna S. Patient-controlled transdermal fentanyl hydrochloride vs intravenous morphine pump for postoperative pain: a randomized controlled trial. *JAMA.* 2004;291(11):1333–1341.

36. Franco A, Diz JC. The history of the epidural block. *Curr Anaesth Crit Care.* 2000;11(5):274.

37. Schug SA, Saunders D, Kurowski I, Paech MJ. Neuraxial drug administration: a review of treatment options for anaesthesia and analgesia. *CNS Drugs.* 2006;20(11):917–933.

38. van der Vyver M, Halpern S, Joseph G. Patient controlled epidural analgesia versus continuous infusion labour analgesia: a meta-analysis. *Br J Anaesth.* 2002;89:459–465.

39. de Leon-Casasola OA, Lema MJ. Postoperative epidural opioid analgesia: what are the choices? *Anesth Analg.* 1996;83(4):867–875.

40. George KA, Wright PMC, Chisakuta A. Continuous thoracic epidural fentanyl for post-thoracotomy pain relief: with or without bupivacaine?. *Anaesthesia.* 1991;46(9):732–736.

41. Tsui BC, Wagner A, Finucane B. Regional anaesthesia in the elderly: a clinical guide. *Drugs Aging.* 2004;21(14):895–910.

42. Orunta I, Cairns C, Greene R. Improving the safety of epidural analgesia. *Pharmaceut J.* 2005;275:228–231.

43. Ilfeld BM, Enneking FK. Continuous peripheral nerve blocks at home: a review. *Anesth Analg.* 2005;100(6):1822–1833.

44. Ganapathy S, Amendola A, Lichfield R, Fowler PJ, Ling E. Elastomeric pumps for ambulatory patient controlled regional analgesia. *Can J Anaesth.* 2000;47(9):897–902.

45. Skryabina EA, Dunn TS. Disposable infusion pumps. *Am J Health Syst Pharm.* 2006;63(13):1260–1268.

46. Capdevila X, Macaire P, Aknin P, Dadure C, Bernard N, Lopez S. Patient-controlled perineural analgesia after ambulatory orthopedic surgery: a comparison of electronic versus elastomeric pumps. *Anesth Analg.* 2003;96(2):414, 417, table of contents.

47. Ilfeld BM, Morey TE, Enneking FK. Portable infusion pumps used for continuous regional analgesia: delivery rate accuracy and consistency. *Reg Anesth Pain Med.* 2003;28(5):424–432.

48. Dadure C, Pirat P, Raux O, et al. Perioperative continuous peripheral nerve blocks with disposable infusion pumps in children: a prospective descriptive study. *Anesth Analg.* 2003;97(3):687–690.

49. On-Q PainBuster®- Post-op Pain Relief System (U.S.). Available at: http://www.iflo.com/prod_onq_classic.php. Accessed 12/3/2007, 2007.

50. Paincare 3000 – BREG. Available at: http://www.breg.com/products/pain_management/paincare_3000/default.html. Accessed 12/3/2007, 2007.

51. Post Operative Pain Pumps – PainPump 1: Stryker. Available at: http://www.stryker.com/myhsp/exercise/PainManagement/AnestheticInfusionDevices/PainPump1and1.5/index.htm. Accessed 12/3/2007, 2007.

20

Novel Analgesic Drug Delivery Systems
for Acute Pain Management

James W. Heitz and Eugene R. Viscusi

In spite of the attention focused on the treatment of acute pain in the previous decade, there is evidence that many hospitalized patients continue to experience inadequate pain relief. One might argue that limitations in resources or education are still a significant factor in the undertreatment of pain. However, this is at least also partially attributable to deficiencies in our tools used for analgesia as many of our currently available technologies fail to provide consistent analgesic benefit for many patients. Although most clinicians are acutely aware of dose-limiting side effects that accompany opioid analgesia, the inherent failure rate of intravenous patient-controlled analgesia (IV PCA) or continuous epidural analgesia is less well understood.

Moreover, the technology associated with the delivery of analgesia may introduce or increase the risk of complications. Epidural catheters increase the risks of spinal hematoma formation in the presence of anticoagulation. Intravenous catheters have been associated with infection. There are also growing concerns about medication errors and pump-programming errors related to pump technology resulting in patient harm. Although little work has been done examining the effect of patients' time tethered to equipment, it is easy to imagine that tubing, pumps, and catheters limit movement, physical therapy, and activities of daily living. Even less understood are the costs associated with maintaining cumbersome pump and infusion technologies for pain management.

New therapies for acute pain management may reduce analgesic gaps, complications associated with indwelling catheters, medication errors, and the burdens of health care providers while simultaneously liberating patients from awkward technologies. This chapter presents recently approved and emerging technologies for acute pain management. Most of the data are available from studies intended for the drug approval process. Hence, the studies may not represent "real-world" application of the products and leaves clinicians to interpret the information and incorporate it appropriately into clinical use.

ADVANCES IN TRANSDERMAL DRUG DELIVERY

The skin is the largest organ in the human body and its large surface area is easily accessible for medication administration. In addition to convenience, transdermal administration of medication confers distinct clinical advantages compared with other modalities. Unlike intravenous drug administration, transdermal drug delivery does not require the use of needles or functioning venous access. Unlike oral drug administration, transdermal drug delivery does not require the ability and willingness to swallow pills or liquids and avoids hepatic first-pass metabolism of the drug. Transdermal drug delivery also offers the possibility of sustained plasma concentrations of drugs, avoiding the peaks and troughs associated with parenteral or oral bolus dosing. These factors make the transdermal route a potentially desirable mode for drug delivery in the treatment of acute pain with a high degree of patient acceptability.

However, before entering the systemic circulation, a drug applied to the skin must traverse the epidermis and some portion of the dermis to reach the capillaries that exist near the dermis-epidermis junction. One of the many functions of intact skin is to provide a barrier to keep the external environment externalized. The primary barrier to drug absorption occurs at the most superficial layer of the epidermis, the stratum corneum. The stratum corneum is composed of dead keratinized epidermal cells interposed with lipids typically ranging in thickness from 10 to 20 μ, depending on the area of the body.[1] Transdermal drug delivery across the stratum corneum is believed to occur primarily through these lipid deposits that form the intracellular pathways.[2]

The stratum corneum is an effective barrier to the absorption of most drugs. Therefore, transdermal therapeutic systems (TTS) that rely on passive diffusion of drugs along a concentration gradient are limited to lipophilic compounds of relatively low molecular weight (<500 Da) that can achieve clinical effect at low plasma levels.[3] These restrictive criteria severely limit the number of drugs that can be used clinically by transdermal administration. Three drugs are currently approved for transdermal administration for the purpose of analgesia in the United States by the Food and Drug Administration (FDA), namely fentanyl (molecular weight 336.5 Da), lidocaine (molecular weight 234.3 Da), and diclofenac epolamine (molecular weight 411.3 Da), however, the transdermal formulation of the antihypertensive drug clonidine (molecular weight 230 Da) may be used in "off-label" fashion for its α_2-adrenergic agonist properties in the treatment of acute pain.

Fentanyl was the first analgesic to be commercially marketed for delivery by transdermal formulation. Many of the physical properties of fentanyl make it uniquely well suited to transdermal administration. It has a low molecular weight and high lipophility with an octanol:water partition coefficient of 717 and has a skin flux 1000 times greater than morphine.[4] The fentanyl patch TTS (Duragesic: Ortho-McNeil, Titusville, NJ) was approved by the FDA in 1990. The fentanyl patch has gained widespread acceptance for the treatment of pain by clinicians in the past 2 decades and annual sales of brand name and generic fentanyl patches now exceed $1.2 billion dollars in the United States. However, the pharmacokinetics of fentanyl patch TTS limit its clinical utility.

The patch is applied for a period of 72 hours delivering an average hourly dose of fentanyl equal to the strength labeling on the patch. After initial application of the patch, the process of passive diffusion of fentanyl is slow. Plasma levels are virtually undetectable in the first 2 hours,[5,6] and peak plasma levels may not be achieved for 12 to 48 hours.[7–10] Conversely, a subcutaneous deposit of fentanyl persists that may contain as much as approximately one-third of the total dose delivered,[11,12] and continues to allow for drug delivery after removal of the patch. Therefore, opioid-mediated depression of ventilation may be delayed after application of the fentanyl patch TTS, and may persist even after patch removal. Cutting or otherwise damaging the polyester film cover to the drug reservoir can cause the patch to release unregulated amounts of the active drug. In 2004, a manufacturing defect allowing for the excessive release of fentanyl led to the recall of some of the 75-µg/h patches. Apparent opioid overdose has also been reported when the fentanyl patch TTS was placed beneath a forced-air heating blanket.[13] Fentanyl patch TTS is indicated for treatment of moderate to severe pain in opioid-tolerant individuals. Because of the slow onset of analgesia and the sustained diffusion of opioid after removal, the fentanyl patch TTS is not indicated for the treatment of acute postoperative pain and a 4% incidence of opioid-mediated ventilatory depression has been reported in this setting.[14] For similar reasons, the fentanyl patch TTS is not suitable for the therapy of intermittent pain.

The lidocaine patch (5%) (Lidoderm: Endo Pharmaceuticals, Chadds Ford, PA) was approved by the FDA for treatment of postherpetic neuralgia in 1999. Although it utilizes passive transdermal diffusion along a concentration gradient similar to the fentanyl patch, there are important distinctions between the two. Unlike fentanyl, the clinical efficacy of lidocaine is achieved by its local effects on the peripheral nerves and not by its systemic absorption. Analgesia is produced without production of a complete sensory block. Technically, the efficacy of the lidocaine is derived from topical penetration of the drug; therefore, the lidocaine patch (5%) is not a true transdermal drug delivery system (which implies systemic absorption). Consequently, the lidocaine patch (5%) must be applied directly over the area of discomfort and can be used only if the skin there is intact. The

patch is 10×14 cm and contains 700 mg of lidocaine. The patch can be reduced to the desired size by cutting prior to removal of the polyethylene terephthalate film release liner without causing uncontrolled liberation of the active drug.

The manufacturer recommends use of no more than 3 patches at one time and to wear the patches for no more than 12 hours in any 24-hour period. Systemic absorption of lidocaine is negligible when used at recommended doses. The application of 3 patches (2100 mg lidocaine over 420 cm^2) results in peak plasma concentrations of 130 ng/mL, an order of magnitude less than plasma concentrations generally considered therapeutic in the treatment of cardiac dysrrhymias.[15] Local anesthetic toxicity is unlikely; the side-effect profile is mostly limited to local reactions such as skin irritation and rash. Caution should be exercised prescribing the lidocaine patch (5%) with the concurrent administration of oral Class I antiarrhythmics (especially mexilitene), because of the potential for synergistic toxicity. After 12 hours of application, 97% ± 2% of the active drug remains in the patch.[16] As the discarded patch still contains approximately 675 mg of lidocaine, there is the theoretical risk of systemic toxicity if patch were licked or chewed and discarded patches should be disposed of away from children or household pets.

The lidocaine patch (5%) has demonstrated efficacy in the treatment of postherpetic neuralgia (PHN).[14,17,18] Although the lidocaine patch (5%) currently only has FDA approval for treatment of PHN, clinically it has been used to treat a variety of etiologies of neuropathic pain. There are published reports of its use in focal neurological pain syndromes,[19] carpal tunnel syndrome,[20] complex regional pain syndrome type II,[21] chronic low back pain,[22] as well as a variety of other chronic pain syndromes, including peripheral ischemia,[23] postthoracotomy syndrome, postmastectomy pain,[23,24] meralgia paresthetica, complex regional pain syndrome type I, and neuromas at various body sites.[24] The efficacy of the lidocaine patch (5%) in the therapy of acute pain is less well established. The use of the lidocaine patch (5%) for the acute (less than 4 weeks) therapy of musculoskeletal injuries among professional football and basketball athletes has been reported.[25] One potential factor limiting its utility in the therapy of acute pain, is that the patch must be applied over intact skin and should not be placed over incisions, lacerations, or other disruptions of the skin. Because systemic absorption of lidocaine from the lidocaine patch (5%) is minimal, the use of the patch in doses and or durations in excess of manufacturer recommendations still may be safe. In healthy volunteers, application of the 4 patches for 18 hours per 24 hour cycle over a 3-day period resulted in peak plasma levels only nominally greater than those obtained by adhering to the recommended 3 patches for 12 hours per 24 hour cycle.[26] For therapy of subacute pain, application of as many as 4 patches for 24 hours each day for a duration as long as 8 weeks has been reported without evidence of systemic toxicity.[27,28] Extended therapy at recommended doses for as long as 7 years has also been reported in a geriatric population and appears to be safe.[29]

The diclofenac epolamine topical patch (1.3%) (Flector Patch; Alpharma Pharmaceuticals, LLC, Piscataway, NJ) is a novel transdermal nonsteroidal anti-inflammatory drug (NSAID) expected to be available in the United States in 2008. Although clinical experience with transdermal diclofenac is limited in the United States, this product has been marketed in other countries under various trade names for a few years. The diclofenac epolamine topical patch (1.3%) is also supplied as a 10 cm × 14 patch that should be applied directly to the skin over the most painful area twice daily. Each patch contains 180 mg of diclofenac epolamine (13 mg per gram of adhesive), a salt form of the NSAID diclofenac in an aqueous base.

Like other formulations of NSAIDS, the diclofenac epolamine topical patch (1.3%) has pharmacodymanic effects that include analgesia as well as anti-inflammatory and antipyretic activities. Peak plasma concentrations in the range of 0.7–6 ng/mL were reported 10–20 hours after application of a single patch; there is some accumulation of drug with repeated dosing and plasma levels between 32%–47% have been reported with twice daily application over a 5-day period.[30] The primary analgesic benefit is derived from local activity of the NSAID; therefore, the patch must be applied over the area of pain and can be used only on a surface area where the skin is intact. It is indicated for the treatment of minor sprains, muscle strains, and contusions. Side effects are mostly cutaneous reactions, including pruritus, dermatitis, and burning, but the usual precautions for using NSAIDS apply. All NSAIDS, including the diclofenac epolamine topical patch (1.3%), should be used with caution in patients with a history of asthma, congestive heart failure, renal disease, or gastrointestinal bleeding.

In contrast to the lidocaine patch (5%), the primary clinical indication of the diclofenac epolamine topical patch (1.3%) is the short-duration treatment therapy of acute musculoskeletal pain. In a double-blind, randomized, placebo-controlled study of 222 subjects with an assortment of minor sports-related sprains, strains, and contusions, 2-week therapy with diclofenac epolamine topical patch (1.3%) resulted in statistically significant less pain scores on treatment days 3, 7, and 14, but statistically insignificant differences in side effects than placebo.[31] A similar study of 120 athletes with blunt soft tissue injury demonstrated significant reduction in pain scores over a 6-day period with a side-effect profile indistinguishable from that of placebo.[32] The diclofenac epolamine topical patch (1.3%) performed equally well as a eutectic mixture of local anesthetics (EMLA) in decreasing the discomfort associated with peripheral venous cannulation and both performed better than placebo, among 450 American Society of Anesthesiologists Physical Status I and II patients having elective outpatient therapy.[33] As clinical experience grows with this agent, its indications for treatment of mild to moderate acute pain may expand accordingly.

ALTERNATIVES TO TRADITIONAL TRANSDERMAL THERAPEUTIC SYSTEMS

Although transdermal drug administration is advantageous from the perspective of both the patient and the clinician, technical challenges have limited the number of drugs that can be administered via a transdermal modality. The first transdermal patch was FDA approved in 1981, but less than a dozen drugs are currently available for delivery by transdermal patch. Because neither the lidocaine patch (5%) nor the diclofenac epolamine topical patch (1.3%) derive their effect from systemic absorption of the drug, the fentanyl patch TTS remains the only analgesic patch commercially marketed that achieves therapeutic plasma levels. Efforts to improve transdermal delivery of analgesics have focused on improving either patch design or drug penetration through the stratum corneum of the skin.

One modification of patch design has been developed by Cygnus Pharmaceuticals (USA) for delivery of fentanyl. The fentanyl transdermal delivery system (FTDS) replaces the fentanyl reservoir with a rate control membrane design of the fentanyl patch TTS with an unsealed multilaminate matrix system in which the fentanyl is embedded.[34] Elimination of the rate control membrane produces faster delivery of fentanyl with a significantly faster onset time of 4 to 6 hours.[35] However, fentanyl FTDS proved to be unacceptable in the treatment of acute postoperative pain. Pharmacokinetic studies of fentanyl FTDS demonstrated as much as a 20-fold variation in hourly fentanyl delivery, much greater than the variation seen with fentanyl patch TTS. Severe opioid-mediated depression of ventilation was reported in 2 of 14 postoperative patients when the 60 cm^2 (90–100 mcg/h) fentanyl FTDS patch was used for analgesia in the postanethesia care unit (PACU).[36] Several other trials demonstrated a high incidence of ventilatory depression with lesser strength fentanyl FTDS patch as well.[9]

There are a number of potential strategies for breaching the barrier properties of skin to allow for a greater variety of medications to be transdermally delivered to the patient. The addition of absorption enhancers, particularly terpene derivatives and phenols, may improve movement of some compounds across the stratum corneum. Absorption enhancers facilitate transdermal migration of drugs by disturbing the integrity of the stratum corneum by fluidization of the lipid channels and disruption of proteins but do so at clinical price of causing skin irritation. Also, the addition of compounds that cause dilation of the dermal microcirculation (eg, nitroglycerin) could improve systemic absorption the drug. Conversion of some drugs to prodrugs with better absorption properties that could later be converted to active drug by intrinsic enzymes may facilitate transdermal absorption. For example, valeryol naltrexone and hepnaltrexone have been demonstrated to have increased skin flux compared with naltrexone in animal models.[37] However, these approaches are attempts to improve passive transdermal diffusion across a concentration gradient as still limited in the types of molecules that can be delivered.

The use of energy to actively drive diffusion across the skin has demonstrated the capacity to deliver a wider variety of molecules, including macromolecules such as insulin. Phonophoresis uses ultrasound energy to promote the transdermal migration of certain compounds. However, thus far the best success has been achieved with absorption enhancement by electrical energy. Electrical energy could aid in transdermal drug migration by 1 of 2 mechanisms. Electroporation involves the use of electricity to temporarily increase the permeability of the lipid pores of the stratum corneum, allowing for the increased migration of hydrophilic compounds.[2] Electricity can also be utilized to directly affect the movement of charged particles across skin, a process known as iontophoresis. All of these techniques have demonstrated some success in the laboratory, but iontophoresis is the first enhancement to transdermal drug delivery to realize commercial and clinical success.

IONTOPHORESIS

Iontophoresis uses the energy of an electric field to drive charged particles through the skin.[38] The fundamental components of an iontophoretic system include a direct current energy source with a positive electrode (anode) and a negative electrode (cathode) and 2 reservoirs, one containing an active drug in ionic form and the second containing a salt. Similar charges repel each other; therefore, a charged molecule placed under the appropriately

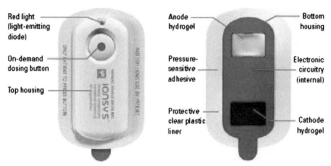

Figure 20.1: Fentanyl iontophoretic transdermal system: Front and back view.

charged electrode will repel the molecule. Cathodal and anodal iontophoresis have been developed, depending on the charge of the drug molecule.[39] Cathodal iontophoresis can deliver anions across the skin, whereas anodal iontophoresis delivers cations. Passive diffusion across a concentration gradient is a very minor component of transdermal drug delivery; drug delivery is primarily via electromigration of charged drug molecules as well as by electroosmosis of drug by current-driven water transport.[40] A wide variety of drugs have been delivered by iontophoresis. Two self-contained units are commercially marketed for iontophoretic delivery of the analgesics fentanyl and lidocaine.

FENTANYL IONTOPHORETIC TRANSDERMAL SYSTEM

The fentanyl iontophoretic transdermal system (fentanyl ITS) (Ionsys; Ortho-McNeil, Inc, Raitan, NJ) was approved by the FDA in 2006. Fentanyl ITS is a self-contained and disposable unit for the anodal iontophoretic delivery of fentanyl hydrochloride (molecular weight 372.9 DA, octanol:water partition coefficient is 860). Therefore, fentanyl ITS is capable of delivering measured doses of fentanyl on patient demand. The fentanyl ITS is preprogrammed to deliver 40 μg of fentanyl over 10 minutes after two sequential depressions of the recessed demand button within a 3-second interval. An audible tone signals that the device has been successfully activated and a dose of fentanyl HCL is being dispensed. An indicator light located above the demand button shows readiness to dispense medication. A solidly lit red light indicates the unit is dispensing medication, and a flashing red light indicates the unit ready to deliver a demand dose. The unit cannot be activated while a dose is being dispensed and the solid red light is on. The pattern of the flashing encodes the approximate number of doses already delivered.[41]

The fentanyl ITS is composed of an approximately credit card size 2-piece unit.[42] The battery (3 V) and the operational electronics, including the indicator light and the activation button, are contained in a white plastic housing top. Two hydrogel reservoirs, one anode containing the fentanyl HCL and one cathode containing inactive ions, and a polyisobutylene skin adhesive are contained in a bottom housing made of red plastic (Figures 20.1 and 20.2). The anodal hydrogel is positioned under the patient dose activation button. The unit is completely programmed and will remain operational for either 80 doses or 24 hours. At maximal usage, 80 doses can be achieved in 13 hours and 20 minutes. On the completion, if desired, the unit should be replaced with a fresh device. The red bottom housing of the

spent device still contains significant amounts of fentanyl HCL and should be separated from the top housing and disposed of properly.[41]

The quantity of fentanyl delivered by iontophoresis correlates directly with the magnitude of current utilized to deliver it.[43–45] Fentanyl ITS delivers each demand dose slowly over 10 minutes. A current of 170 μA has been demonstrated to iontophoretically delivery 40 μg of fentanyl HCL.[46] Therefore, the unit is programmed to deliver a 170-uA current with each successful, a dose extrapolated from the use of IV PCA (fentanyl) to provide analgesia with an acceptable safety profile.[47] The quantity of fentanyl HCL delivered by activation of the unit has been demonstrated to be independent of patient age, sex, or race, but dependent on the location of the device on the body.[48] Fentanyl ITS is designed to be applied to the upper arm or chest of the patient. Placement on the lower arm results in lower dose delivery; placement on other areas of the body remains unstudied. Hence, recommended locations for placement are the upper chest or upper outer arm. Sites should be rotated for each application. Bioavailability of the delivered dose increases with repeated use, rising from 41% of the first dose to nearly 100% after the 20th dose.[49] Key pharmacokinetic parameters are similar for 80 μg fentanyl delivered by fentanyl ITS (two doses) and 80 μg fentanyl delivered intravenously, including T_{max} (0.65 vs 0.58 h), $t_{1/2}$ (11.0 vs 12.6 h), and C_{max} (1.37 vs 1.82 ug/L).[46]

Fentanyl ITS is novel compared to other forms of transdermal fentanyl. In contrast to transdermal administration of fentanyl by patch, fentanyl ITS is indicated for the treatment of acute postoperative pain in the hospital setting. Unlike the fentanyl patch, fentanyl ITS is capable of delivering patient-controlled demand doses. Unlike fentanyl TTS, fentanyl ITS does not create significant deposits of fentanyl and serum levels begin to fall almost immediately after removal of the dispensing unit from the skin.

However, the most clinically relevant comparison is with IV PCA. In the postoperative period, fentanyl ITS is associated with significantly fewer analgesic gaps compared with IV PCA.[50] Moreover, the spectrum of system-related events associated with fentanyl ITS was smaller than those associated with IV PCA. Device failure occurs infrequently (26 in 641 patients) with a much smaller incidence of analgesic gaps arising from patient noncompliance associated with inability to understand the use of the device (3 of 641 patients), inability to locate the demand

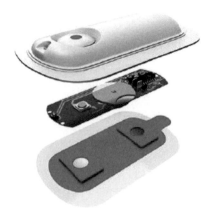

Figure 20.2: Fentanyl iontophoretic transdermal system: Electronic and drug components.

button (4 of 641 patients), or nonuse because of side effects (2 of 641 patients). Intravenous PCA was associated with a similar, but lower incidence of device failures (26 of 658 patients) or patient noncompliance because of inability to understand use of the device (2 of 658 patients) or locate the demand button (3 of 658 patients) but was also associated with analgesic gaps associated with a plethora of reasons related to IV access, including infiltration (17 of 658 patients), no IV access (8 of 658 patients), concurrent administration of incompatible medication or product via the IV (4 of 658 patients), leaking IV tubing (4 of 658 patients), air in line (1 of 658 patients), and phlebitis (1 of 658 patients). Analgesic gaps were also noted to occur during IV PCA from programming errors (5 of 658 patients) or deliberate patient or family tampering with the programming (3 of 658 patients) that did not occur with the preprogrammed fentanyl ITS system. Fentanyl ITS requires significantly less nursing time compared with IV PCA.[51] In many hospitals where nursing time is an increasingly scare commodity reductions in time spent on tasks related to postoperative analgesia might correlate with improvement in other nursing tasks. Patients rated fentanyl ITS easier to use and having less impact on movement than standard IV PCA. Nurses and physical therapists found caring for patients easier with fentanyl ITS compared to standard IV PCA.[52] Further studies are needed to fully evaluate the ease of care benefits of this less invasive and less cumbersome technology.

The efficacy and safety profile of fentanyl ITS has been demonstrated by several clinical trials. In a study of 189 patients after major abdominal, orthopedic, or thoracic surgery, fentanyl ITS was associated with lower pain scores and higher patient satisfaction than placebo among patients with access to "as needed" intravenous opioid rescue doses.[53] There was no significant ventilatory depression with either group. Limitations of the study included a potential bias from a 3 to 1 randomization scheme between the fentanyl ITS and placebo groups and a lack of control for initial pain score on entry into the study.[54] A larger second study with 484 enrolled patients compared fentanyl ITS to placebo in postoperative patients with pain scores by use of the visual analog scale of 5 or less at the time of enrollment.[55] Supplemental IV fentanyl was available to each group if requested. Fewer patients in the fentanyl ITS group dropped out of the study because of inadequate analgesia than in the placebo group. Pain intensity scores in the fentanyl ITS group were lower as well; patient global assessment and investigator global assessment scores were higher. Again, there were no episodes of significant ventilatory depression in either group. Comparison with IV PCA better emulates clinical practice. A number of clinical trials have demonstrated similar efficacy between fentanyl ITS and IV PCA morphine.[52,56,57] Pooled data from were analyzed for a combined 1941 patients randomized in these three trials to either fentanyl ITS or IV PCA morphine.[58] The patients were disproportionately female (>67%) and white (>81%) and were primarily status post total hip replacement or pelvic surgery. Mean last pain intensity scores in the first 24 hours were equivalent in the fentanyl ITS and IV PCA morphine groups, as were the percentages of patients who reported their patient global assessment to be "good" or "excellent." The incident of treatment-related hypoxia was similar between the fentanyl ITS and IV PCA morphine groups (3.6% vs 3.7%). Pruritus was more common among the IV PCA morphine group, whereas headache was more common among the fentanyl ITS group.

Pharmacoeconomic analysis is warranted to evaluate relative expense of fentanyl ITS compared with IV PCA. However,

fentanyl ITS compares favorably with IV PCA morphine for efficacy and safety of postoperative analgesia. It offers the added benefits of reduced nursing time and fewer analgesic gaps. Additional benefits remain to be determined, including potential benefits associated with improved patient mobility, physical therapy, and reduction in medication errors and pump programming errors.

LIDOCAINE IONTOPHORESIS

A self-contained unit for the iontophoretic delivery of lidocaine is also available. The Lidosite Topical System (Vyteris Inc., Fairlawn, NJ) received FDA approval in 2004. It is a 2-part device composed of a reusable Lidosite controller that contains a battery, a microprocessor, and an LCD display and a single-use, disposable 5-cm^2 Lidosite patch containing 100 mg of lidocaine and 1.05 mg of epinephrine. The Lidosite Topical System is FDA approved for topical anesthesia for venipuncture and IV catheter insertion and superficial dermatological procedures. Because a small quantity of epinephrine is also delivered iontophoretically with the lidocaine, application of the device over areas supplied by end arteries is contraindicated.[59] Clinical trials are being conducted to evaluate its efficacy in providing analgesia prior to certain types of painful injections.

EXTENDED RELEASE EPIDURAL MORPHINE

Neuraxial opioids are well established clinically in the treatment of acute postoperative pain. Epidural analgesia in all its pharmacological permutations has been demonstrated in large meta-analysis to provide pain control superior to IV PCA.[60,61] However, the duration of action of a single bolus of preservative-free morphine is less than 24 hours. This necessitates either rebolusing or continuous infusion via an epidural catheter. The failure rate of epidural infusions approaches 30% in the postoperative period.[62] This can contribute to analgesic gaps. Additionally, the presence of an indwelling epidural catheter may be a concern if there is a need for anticoagulation for prevention of deep vein thrombosis.

The development of a novel carrier, DepoFoam, allows for an increased duration of action of epidural morphine without the need for an indwelling epidural catheter (Figures 20.3 and 20.4). DepoFoam consists of microscopic multivesicular liposome particles that serve as a carrier for the active drug, which is encapsulated in aqueous pockets. Degradation of the liposomal structure allows for predictable release of drug. The lipids are biodegradable and absorbed by the body. DepoDur (EKR Therapeutics, Inc., Cedar Knolls, NJ) was approved by the FDA in 2004 and utilizes DepoFoam technology to create extended release epidural morphine (EREM) with a duration of action up to 48 hours without redosing.

The pharmacokinetics of EREM has been established in studies on rats[63] and dogs.[64] Peak morphine levels in the cerebrospinal fluid (CSF) are approximately one-third compared with standard epidural morphine are significantly delayed after administration. A 5-mg dose of standard epidural morphine injected into the epidural space of a dog reaches peak CSF concentrations in 5 minutes, whereas a 10-mg dose of EREM did not reach peak CSF concentration for 3 hours.[63] Peak serum concentrations are delayed as well and are about 1/15th those achieved

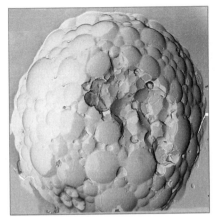

Figure 20.3: DepoFoam: electron micrograph of 20-μ-diameter particle.

with standard epidural morphine, perhaps in part attributable to reduced lymphatic and hematogenous uptake of the drug because of the relative large size of the multivesicular lysomal structure of the DepoFoam.

In an open-labeled study of 39 American Society of Anesthesiologists Physical Status (ASA PS) I-II patients undergoing total hip arthroplasty, a 5-mg dose of standard epidural morphine was compared with 10-, 15-, 20-, 25-, and 30-mg doses of EREM.[65] Patients were also provided with fentanyl by IV PCA. Time to first request for additional analgesia was 3 to 6 times longer in the EREM group and overall fentanyl consumption was less. Patient satisfaction was better in the EREM groups, despite the lower fentanyl usage. It should be noted that this was an early study and the 25- and 30-mg doses of EREM were not marketed by the manufacturer.

Four randomized, double-blinded controlled trials examined the use of EREM for postoperative analgesia. In a study of 200 patients undergoing total hip arthroplasty, doses of 15-, 20-, or 25-mg EREM were compared with placebo.[66] Patients were additionally randomized to spinal anesthesia or general anesthesia, but intraoperative opioid dosing was standardized at 250 μg. Mean time to first request was reduced across all doses compared with placebo (21.3 hours vs 3.1 hours) as was cumulative fentanyl use (510 ± 708 μg vs 2,901 ± 1803 μg). No additional analgesia was required by 25% of the EREM compared with just 2% of the placebo group. In a similar study of 162 randomized patients undergoing total knee athroplasty, 20- and 30-mg EREM doses were compared with placebo.[67] Additional

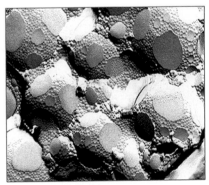

Figure 20.4: DepoFoam: detail of chambers filled with aqueous solution of drug.

analgesia was available in protocol employing IV bolus and IV PCA morphine, IV hydromorphone, and IV PCA placebo. Time to first request for analgesia was again significantly increased in the EREM groups (6.8–7.9 hours vs 3.3 hours), although the effect was not as profound as in the THA study. Total supplement opioid use was similarly decreased. The study with the greatest total number of patients performed so far was a study of 541 patients undergoing a variety of lower abdominal surgeries.[68] A variety of surgical procedures requiring subumbilical incisions were included, but laparoscopic procedures, appendectomy, transuretheral procedures, caesarian sections, and vascular procedures were excluded. Patients were randomized into 1 of 6 arms of postoperative epidural analgesia, either 5 mg of standard epidural morphine or 5-, 10-, 15-, 20-, or 25-mg EREM. IV PCA fentanyl was available to all patients. Unlike the two studies on orthopedic patients with placebo controls, time to first request for additional analgesia was not significantly different among any of the 6 arms. However, total fentanyl use was significantly reduced in patients receiving 10-mg EREM or more and visual analog pain scores were significantly reduced despite reduced opioid use. In a study of 73 women undergoing cesarian section under intrathecal bupivacaine (12–15 mg) and intrathecal fentanyl (10 μg), patients were randomized to postoperative epidural analgesia with 5 mg standard epidural morphine or 5-, 10-, or 15-mg EREM.[69] As with the previous study with an active treatment control, time to request for first analgesia was not significantly different among the 4 arms. However, total opioid use in the 48-hour postoperative period was reduced among patients receiving the 10- and 15-mg EREM doses.

These studies support the 48-hour extended duration of analgesia with reduced analgesic gaps requiring supplemental opioids. The cesarean section study provides a further dimension examining the effects of EREM on patient functionality. This study supports an outcome of improved patient function for patients who received EREM (10 mg) compared to other standard therapies.

The need for naloxone rescue for significant depression of ventilation was greater in the EREM groups than placebo controls in the 2 orthopedic surgery studies.[66,67] In the study on patients undergoing lower abdominal surgery comparing the 5 doses of EREM to 5 mg of epidural morphine, the need for naloxone rescue was significantly greater than control only in the 20- and 25-mg EREM groups and the latter dose was not marketed by the manufacturer.[68] There were 3 deaths among patients randomized to the EREM dose. One occurred before the study drug was administered, and 1 occurred because of a postoperative myocardial infarction believed to be unrelated to the study drug. However, there was 1 death that was felt to be possibly related to the EREM. This occurred in a patient who received the EREM and then had her surgery cancelled for other reasons. Aspiration and ventilatory embarrassment occurred 21 hours after administration of EREM. Although investigators felt this event was most likely not attributable to the study drug, a contributory component from EREM could not be excluded from the adverse event. Regardless, this event illustrates one of the possible drawbacks to EREM. Therapy cannot be discontinued once administered as it can be with a continuous infusion. Therefore, a patient could have the effects of epidural opioid therapy for an extended duration unopposed by the potentially protective stimulation from a surgical procedure. Other side effects seen during these studies included pruritus, urinary retention, and hypotension. It should also be noted that these studies excluded ASA PS IV patients as well as patients with a history of severe pulmonary disease, obstructive sleep apnea, or opioid-tolerance. Efficacy and safety in these patient groups has not been established.

EREM is a packaged as a 10-mg/mL suspension available in 10-, 15-, and 20-mg vials. It should be kept in refrigerated storage at a temperature of 2°C–8°C. Once drawn from the vial, it must be either used or discarded within 4 hours. Prior to withdraw, the vial should be gently inverted but not vigorously shaken to resuspend the liposomes that settle toward the bottom during storage. Current manufacturer dosing recommendations include up to 15 mg for major orthopedic procedures of the lower extremity, up to 10–15 mg for lower abdominal surgery, and up to 10 mg after clamping of the umbilical cord for cesarean section.[70] No other medications should be administered into the epidural space for 48 hours after administration of EREM, including local anesthetics. Because unintentional intrathecal administration of DepoDur could lead to profound depression of ventilation, a conventional "test" dose of local anesthetic with epinephrine is permissible prior to administration. In clinical practice, many clinicians administer EREM through the epidural needle rather than an epidural catheter, obviating the need for a test dose.

DepoFoam has the potential to increase the duration of action of other drugs. It is currently also used to slow the release of certain antiviral agents and chemotherapeutics.[71] An extended-release bupivacaine formulation using this drug delivery platform is also being developed.

When examining the preliminary studies for EREM, it is important to recognize that these were designed for the drug approval process. Many of the doses studied were significantly higher than doses used in clinical practice subsequent to approval. Further, most clinicians practice multimodal analgesia that reduces dose requirements and improves the side effects. Many clinicians are using doses between 7.5 and 10 mg routinely in this fashion. If additional analgesia is required, nonopioid oral agents should be used, followed by oral agents. Many patients will benefit from using oral supplemental analgesics, thus avoiding the addition of a PCA pump.

Patient selection is also important to using EREM successfully. Elderly patients and patients with sleep apnea or a history of airway obstruction may be more sensitive to opioids and will require special consideration. EREM has not been studied in opioid-tolerant patients, hence, there are no recommendations for dosing these patients.

CONCLUSION

New products offer new opportunities to patients and clinicians.[72] Smaller, less invasive technologies may improve patient mobility and reduce the hazards of infection and bleeding associated with indwelling systems. Preprogrammed systems may reduce medication errors and programming errors. Extended delivery systems may reduce analgesic gaps and the need for more cumbersome PCA and epidural pumps. However, further studies are required to support these concepts even though they may appear self-evident.

Ultimately, it lies in the hands of clinicians to capitalize on these potential benefits. A nurse who spends less time caring for pumps, catheters, and infusions may be able to focus more attention on the patient versus the technology. A patient less encumbered by tethering may be able to participate more fully in activities if they are offered. Judicious use of multimodal analgesia and oral analgesic supplement may reduce the need for PCA. Hence, clinicians will have to take active roles in utilizing new technologies for their fullest capacity.

REFERENCES

1. Proksch E, Jensen JM. Skin as an organ of protection. In: Wolff K, Goldsmith LA, Katz SI, Gilchrest BA, Paller AS, Leffell DJ, eds. Fitzpatrick's Dermatology in General Medicine. 7th ed. New York, NY: McGraw-Hill; 2008;383–395.
2. Prausnitz MR, Bose VG, Lagner R, Weaver JC. Electroporations of mammalian skin: a mechanism to enhance transdermal drug delivery. *Proc Natl Acad Sci USA.* 1993;90:10504–10508.
3. Scheindlin S. Transdermal drug delivery: past, present, future. *Mol Interven.* 2004;4:308–332.
4. Grond S, Radbruch L, Lehmann KA. Clinical pharmacokinetics of transdermal opioids: focus on transdermal fentanyl. *Clin Pharmacokinet.* 200:38–59.
5. Gourlay GK, Kowalski SR, Plummer JL, Cherry DA, Gaukroger P, Cousins MJ. The transdermal administration of fentanyl in the treatment of postoperative pain: pharmacokinetcs and pharmacodynamic effects. *Pain.* 1989;37:193–202.
6. Gourlay GK, Kowalski SR, Plummer JL, Cousins MJ, Armstrong PJ. The efficacy of transdermal fentanyl in the treatment of postoperative pain: a double-blind comparison of fentanyl and placebo systems. *Pain.* 1990;40:21–28.
7. Broome IJ, Wright BM, Bower S, Reilly CS. Postoperative analgesia with transdermal fentanyl following lower abdominal surgery. *Anaesthesia.* 1995;50:300–303.
8. Duthie DJ, Rowbotham DJ, Wyld R, Henderson PD, Nimmo WS. Plasma fentanyl concentrations during transdermal delivery of fentanyl to surgical patients. *Br J Anaesth.* 1988;60:614–618.
9. Grond S, Radbruch L, Lehmann KA. Clinical pharamacokinetics of transdermal opioids: focus on transdermal fentanyl. *Clin Pharmacokinet.* 200:38:59–89.
10. Holley FO, van Steennis C. Postoperative analgesia with fentanyl: pharmacokinetics and pharmacodynamics of constant-rate i.v. and transdermal delivery. *Br J Anaesth.* 1988;60:608–613.
11. Varvel JR, Shafer SL, Hwang SS, Coen PA, Stanski DR. Absorption characteristics of transdermally administered fentanyl. *Anesthesiology.* 1989;70:928–934.
12. Peng P, Sandler A. A review of the use of fentanyl in analgesia in management of acute pain in adults. *Anesthesiology.* 1999;90:576–599.
13. Frolich M, Giannotti A, Modell JH. Opioid overdose in a patient using a fentanyl patch during treatment with a warming blanket. *Anesth Analg.* 2001;93;647–648.
14. Food and Drug Administration. Fentanyl transdermal system approved for chronic pain. *JAMA.* 1990;264:1802.
15. Rowbotham MC, Davies PS, Verkempinck C, Galer BS. Lidocaine patch: double-blinded controlled study of a new treatment method for post-herpetic neuralgia. *Pain.* 1996;65:39–44.
16. Lidoderm (lidocaine patch 5%) [package insert]. Chadds Ford, PA: Endo Pharmaceuticals; 2006.
17. Galer, BS, Rowbotham MC, Perander J, Friedman E. Topical lidocaine patch 5% relieves postherpetic neuralgia more effectively than a vehicle topical patch: results of an enrichment enrollment study. *Pain.* 1999;80:533–538.
18. Katz HP, Gammaitoni AR, Davis MW, Dworkin RH and the Lidoderm Patch Study Group. Lidocaine patch 5% reduces pain intensity and interference with quality of life in patients with

postherpetic neuralgia: an effectiveness trial. *Pain Med.* 2002; 3:324–332.

19. Meier T, Wasner G, Faust M, et al. Efficacy of lidocaine patch 5% in the treatment of focal peripheral neuropathic pain syndromes: a randomized, double-blind, placebo-controlled study. *Pain.* 2003;106;151–158.

20. Nalamachu S, Crockett RS, Gammaitoni A, Gould AR, Errol M. A comparison of lidocaine patch 5% vs naproxen 500 mg twice weekly for the relief of pain associated with carpal tunnel syndrome: a 6-week, randomized, parallel-group study. *Medscape Gen Med.* 2006;8:33.

21. Karmarkar A, Lieberman I. Management of complex regional pain syndrome type II using lidoderm 5% patches. *Br J Anesth.* 2007;98:261–262.

22. Hines R, Keaney D, Moskowitz MH, Prakken S. Use of lidocaine patch 5% for chronic low back pain; a report of four cases. *Pain Med.* 2002;3:361–365.

23. Argyra E. 5% lidocaine patch in the treatment of neuropathic pain of diverse origin. [abstract]. Eur J Pall Care-Abstract book 9 Congress of the European Association for Palliative Care. 2003;80.

24. Devers A, Galer B. Topical lidocaine patch relieves a variety of neuropathic pain conditions: an open-label study. *Clin J Pain.* 200:16(3):205–208.

25. Benoist JL. Gammaitoni AR. The 5% lidocaine patch reduces pain intensity in professional athletes with sports injury pain without significant systemic effects or cognitive and performance impairment. *Arch Phys Med Rehab.* 2005;86.e34.

26. Gammaitori AR, Davis MW. Pharmacokinectics and tolerability of lidocaine patch 5% with extended dosing. *Ann Pharmacother.* 2002;236–240.

27. Barbano RL, Hermann DN, Galer BS, et al. Effectiveness of lidocaine patch 5% in diabetic neuropathy patients with or without allodynia (2003) Abstract presented at: the 7th International Conference on the Mechanisms and Treatment of Neuropathic Pain; September 18–20; San Francisco, CA.

28. J. Gimbel M, Hale R, Linn BS, Galer, E. Kurkimilis E, Gammaitor AR. Lidocaine patch 5% in patients with acute/subacute chronic low back pain: Impact on pain intensity, pain relief, and pain interference with QOL (2003) Abstract presented at: the 22nd Annual Meeting of the American Pain Society; March 20–23; Chicago, IL.

29. Galer BS. More than 7 years of consistent neuropathic pain relief in geriatric patients. *Arch Intern Med.* 2003;163:628.

30. Flector (diclofenac epolamine topical patch 1.3%), [package insert]. Sanbonmatsu, Kagawa, Japan: Teikoku Seiyaki Co, Ltd; 2007.

31. Galer BS, Rowbothman M, Perander J, Devers A, Friedman E. Topical diclofenac patch relieves minor sports injury pain: results of a multicenter controlled clinical trial. *J Pain Symptom Manage.* 2000;19:287–294.

32. Predel HG, Koll R, Pabst H, et al. Diclofenac patch for topical treatment of acute impact injuries: a randomised, double blinded, placebo controlled, mutlicenre study. *Br J Sports Med.* 2004;38:318–323.

33. Argarwal A, Gautam S, Gupta D, Singh U. Transdermal diclofenac patch vs eutectic mixture of local anesthetics for venous cannulation pain. *Can J Anesth.* 2007;54:196–200.

34. Reinhart DJ, Goldberg ME, Roth JV, et al. Transdermal fentanyl system plus im ketorolac for the treatment of postoperative pain. *Can J Anaesth.* 1997;44377–44384.

35. Miguel R, Kreitzer JM, Reinhart D, et al. Postoperative pain control with a new transermal fentanyl delivery system: a multicenter trial. *Anesthesiology.* 1995;83:470–477.

36. Fiset P, Cohane C, Browne S, et al. Biopharmaceutics of a new transdermal fenanyl device. *Anesthesiology.* 1995;83:459–469.

37. Hammell DC, Stolarczyk EI, Klausner M, et al. Bioconversion of Naltrexone and Its 3-O-Alkyl-Ester Prodrugs in a Human Skin Equivalent. *J Pharm Sci* 2005;94:828–836.

38. Viscusi ER, Witkowski TA. Iontophoresis: the process behind noninvasive drug delivery. *Reg Anesth Pain Med.* 2005;30:292–294.

39. Batheja P, Kaushik D, Hu L, Michniak-Kohn BB. Transdermal iontophoresis. *Drug Deliv.* 2007.

40. Curdy C, Kalia Y, Guy RH. Non-invasive assessment of the effects of iontophoresis on human skin in-vivo. *J Pharm Pharmacol.* 2001;52:769–777.

41. Ionsys (fentanyl iontophoretic transdermal system) [package insert]. Raritan NJ: Ortho-McNeil, Inc; August 2006.

42. Minkowitz HS. *Fentanyl Iontophoretic Transdermal System: A Review. Techniques in Regional Anesthesia and Pain Management.* 2007;11(1):3–8.

43. Gupta SK, Southam M, Santhyan G, Klausner M. Effect of current density on pharmacokinetics following continuous or intermittent input from a fentanyl electrotransport system. *J Pharm Sci.* 1998;87:976–981.

44. Gupta SK, Bernstein KJ, Noorduin H, van Peer A, Saythan G, Haak K. Fentanyl delivery from a electrotransport system. Delivery is a function of total current, not duration of current. *J Clin Pharmacol.* 1998;48:951–958.

45. Gupta SK, Sathyan G, Phipps B, Klausner M, Southam M. Reproducible fentanyl doses delivered intermittently at different time intervals from an electrotransport system. *J Pharm Sci.* 1999;88:835–841.

46. Sathyan G, Jaskowiak J, Evashenk M, Gupta S. Characterisation of the pharmacokinetics of fentanyl HCL patient-controlled transdermal system (PTCS): effect of current magnitude and multiple-day dosing, and comparison with IV fentanyl administration. *Clin Pharmacokinet.* 2005;44(suppl 1):7–15.

47. Camu F, Van Aken H, Bovill JG. Postoperative analgesic effects of three demand dose sizes of fentanyl administered via patent controlled analgesia. *Anesth Analg.* 1998;87:890–895.

48. Gupta SK, Hwang S, Southam M, Sathyan G. Effects of application site and subject-controlled demographics on the pharmacokinetics of fentanyl HCL patient-controlled transdermal system (PCTS). *Clin Pharmacokinet.* 2005;44:25–32.

49. Sathyan G, Zomorodi K, Gidwani S, Gupta SK. The effect of dosing frequency on the pharmacokinetics of a fentanyl HCL patient-controlled transdermal system (PCTS). *Clin Pharmacokinet.* 2005;44:17–24.

50. Panchal SJ, Damaraju CV, Nelson WW, Hewitt DJ, Schein JR. System-related events and analgesic gaps during postoperative pain management with the fentanyl iontophoretic transdermal system and morphine intravenous patient-controlled analgesia. *Anesth Analg.* 2007;105:1437–1441.

51. Evans C, Schein J, Nelson W, et al. Improving patient and nurse outcomes: a comparison of nurse tasks and time associated with two patient-controlled analgesia modalities using Delphi panels. *Pain Manage Nurs.* 2007;8:86–95.

52. Hartrick CT, Bourne MH, Gargiulo K, Damaraju CV, Vallow S, Hewitt DJ. Fentanyl iontophoretic transdermal system for acute-pain management after orthopedic surgery : a comparative study with morphine intravenous patient-controlled analgesia. *Reg Anesth Pain Med.* 2006;31(6):546–554.

53. Chelly JE, Grass J, Houseman TW, Minkowitz, Pue A. The safety and efficacy of a fentanyl patient-controlled transdermal system for acute postoperative analgesia: a multicenter, placebo-controlled trial. *Anesth Analg.* 2004;98:427–433.

54. Koo PJS. Postoperative pain management with a patient-controlled transdermal delivery system for fentanyl. *Am J Health-Syst Pharm.* 2005;62:1171–1176.

55. Viscusi ER, Reynolds L, Tait S, Melson T, Atkinson LE. Iontophoretic fentanyl patient-activated analgesic delivery system for post-operative pain: a double-blind, placebo-controlled trial. *Anesth Analg.* 2006;102:188–194.

56. Viscusi ER, Reynolds L, Chung F, Atkinson LE, Khanna S. Patient-controlled transdermal fentanyl hydrochloride vs intravenous morphine pump for postoperative pain: a randomized controlled trial. *JAMA.* 2004;291:1333–1341.

57. Minkowitz HS, Rathmell JP, Vallow S, Gargiulo K, Damaraju CV, Hewitt DJ. Efficacy and safety of the fentanyl iontophoretic transdermal (ITS) and intravenous patient-controlled analgesia (IV PCA) with morphine for pain management following abdominal or pelvic surgery. *Pain Med.* 2007;8(8):657–668.

58. Viscusi ER, Siccardi M, Damarju CV, Hewitt DJ, Kershaw P. The safety and efficacy of fentanyl iontophoretic transdermal system compared with morphine intravenous patient-controlled analgesia for post-operative pain management: an analysis of pooled data from three randomized, active-controlled clinical studies. *Anesth Analg.* 2007;105:1428–1436.

59. Lidosite Topical System [package insert. Fairlawn NJ: Vyteris Inc; 2004.

60. Block BM, Liu SS, Rowlingson AJ Cowan AR, Cowan JR, Wu CL. Efficacy of postoperative epidural analgesia: a meta-analysis. *JAMA.* 2003;290:2456–2463.

61. Wu CL, Cohen SR, Richman JM, et al. Efficacy of postoperative patient-controlled and continuous infusion epidural analgesia versus intravenous patient-controlled analgesia with opioids: a meta-analysis. *Anesthesiology.* 2005;103:1079–1088.

62. Ready LB. Acute pain: lessons learned from 25,000 patients. *Reg Anesth Pain Med.* 1999;24:499–505.

63. Kim T, Murdande S, Gruber A, Kim S. Sustained-release morphine for epidural analgesia in rats. *Anesthesiology.* 1996;85:331–338.

64. Yaksh TL, Provencher JC, Rathburn ML, Kohn FR. Pharmacokinetics and efficacy of epidurally delivered sustained-release encapsulated morphine in dogs. *Anesthesiology.* 1999;90:1402–1412.

65. Viscusi ER, Kopacz D, Hartrick CT, Martin G, Manvalien G. Single-dose extended-release epidural morphine for pain following hip arthroplasty. *Am J Therapeut.* 2006;13:423–431.

66. Viscusi ER, Martin G, Hartrick CT, Forty-eight hours of postoperative pain relief after total hip arthroplasty with a novel, extended-release epidural morphine formulation. *Anesthesiology.* 2005;102:1014–1022.

67. Hartrick CT, Martin G, Kantor G, Koncelik J, Manvelian G. Evaluation of a single-dose extended-release epidural morphine formulation for pain after knee athroplasty. *J Bone Joint Surg.* 2006;88A:271–281.

68. Gambling D, Hughes T, Martin G., Horton W, Manvelian G for the Single-Dose EREM Study Group. A comparison of DepoDur,™ a novel, single-dose extended-release epidural morphine, with a standard epidural morphine for pain relief after lower abdominal surgery. *Anesth Analg.* 2005;100:1065–1074.

69. Carvalho B, Riley E, Cohen SE, et al, for the DepoDur Study Group. Single-dose, sustained-release epidural morphine in the management of postoperative pain after elective cesarean section: results of a multicenter randomized controlled study. *Anesth Analg.* 2005;100:1150–1158.

70. [package insert]. San Diego CA: SkyePharma Inc; 2007.

71. Angst MS, Drover DR. Pharmacology of drugs formulated with Depofoam™: a sustained release drug delivery system for parenteral administration using mutlivesicular liposome technology. *Clin Pharmacokinet.* 2006;45:1153–1176.

72. Rathmell JP, Wu CL, Sinatra RS, et al. Acute post-surgical pain management: a critical appraisal of current practice, December 2–4, 2005. *Reg Anesth Pain Med.* 2006;31(4 suppl 1):1–42.

21

Nonselective Nonsteroidal Anti-Inflammatory Drugs, COX-2 Inhibitors, and Acetaminophen in Acute Perioperative Pain

Jonathan S. Jahr, Kofi N. Donkor, and
Raymond S. Sinatra

Notwithstanding the noteworthy advances that have been made in using analgesic drugs in managing acute pain, the effective treatment of acute postsurgical pain poses unique challenges for practitioners.[36,73,77,157,158] The increasing number and complexity of surgical procedures being performed on an outpatient basis, the need for patients undergoing day care procedures to have analgesic therapy that is effective with minimal adverse effects, is intrinsically safe, and can be easily managed, has contributed to the challenges practitioners are currently facing.[36,73,77,135,156,157]

Opioid-based analgesics have traditionally been the primary drugs used in managing severe postoperative pain, but their use has been associated with complications and adverse effects like respiratory depression, sedation, drowsiness, pruritus, skin rash, urinary retention, ileus, constipation, and postoperative nausea and vomiting (PONV).[36,73,77,135,157,158] These limitations ultimately restrict patients from early mobilization and discharge after surgical procedures. These issues are crucial to health care institutions, because the current standard of practice for postoperative pain management is currently focused on early mobilization and rapid discharge of patients after surgery.[35,36,73,77,135,157,158]

The combination of multiple modalities of analgesic therapies (see Figure 21.1[a]), otherwise called *balanced analgesia* or *multimodal analgesia*, has been proposed as the rational approach to pain management and many consider this concept as the most effective way in managing acute postoperative pain; this practice has evolved rapidly.[77] The rationale behind this concept has been that analgesic drugs, acting through different mechanisms, result in additive or synergistic analgesia. Multiple drugs such as opiates and regional blocking agents, which attenuate the pain-related signals in the central nervous system (CNS), nonselective nonsteroidal anti-inflammatory drugs (NSAIDs), selective cyclooxygenase 2 inhibitors (COX-2 inhibitors), which act mainly in the periphery and ultimately block the synthesis of prostaglandins PG, (the primary noxious mediator released

from damaged tissues and primarily involved in peripheral inflammation; see Figure 21.1[b]), acetaminophen (paracetamol, *N*-acetyl-*p*-aminophenol [APAP]), which may act to inhibit PG synthesis in the central nervous system (CNS) and, to a lesser extent, through a peripheral action by blocking pain-impulse generation, and adjuvant drugs like the *N*-methyl-D-aspartate (NMDA) receptor antagonists, when used in an evidence-based manner with the appropriate dose, route, and combination of therapy, may be administered to maximize perioperative analgesia while minimizing adverse effects (see Figure 21.2).[35,36,72,77,135] In fact, the World Health Organization's (WHO) pain relief ladder for cancer pain includes the use of nonopioid analgesics as first-line drugs, adding opioids for moderate and severe pain (see Figure 21.3).

Preemptive analgesia, a form of antinociceptive treatment that prevents the establishment of central sensitization caused by incisional and inflammatory injury has been evaluated with NSAIDs, COX-2 inhibitors and acetaminophen, either as a single agent, or in combination with other analgesics.[81] In an effort to evaluate the use of the nonopiate analgesics in perioperative pain therapy, this chapter evaluates the NSAIDs, COX-2 inhibitors, and acetaminophen and their use in preemptive analgesia and in combination with other analgesics in multimodal analgesic therapy.

The value of NSAIDs in minor, moderate, and severe postoperative pain has been well documented in clinical trials. Even though they represent the ideal alternative component in the multimodal approach to postoperative pain, their use as the sole analgesic in more severe pain states remains questionable because of their limited efficacy and their adverse effect profile.[35,36,135,150,157] The vast variations in the pharmacokinetics and pharmacodynamic properties of the different NSAIDs makes these groups of drugs vary considerably in many ways, including their degree of adverse effects. The perioperative inhibition of COX-1, the enzyme that is involved in generating cytoprotective prostanoids such as prostaglandins

Minor Surgery	Wound infiltration with local anesthethetic
	Peripheral nerve blockade with local anesthetic
	Oral or parenteral NSAIDs and/or APAP
	Oral or parenteral opioid with or without APAP for breakthrough pain

Intermediate Surgery	Wound infiltration with local anesthesia
	Peripheral nerve blockade with local anesthetic
	Intravenous PCA opioids
	Oral or parenteral NSAIDS and/or APAP
	Single injection intrathecal or epidural opioid

Major Surgery	Wound infiltration with local anesthesia
	Peripheral nerve blockade with local anesthetic
	Epidural local anesthetic and opioid
	Oral or injectable NSAIDs
	Systemic opioid (intravenous, intermittent, or PCA)

Figure 21.1(a). Recommended approach to analgesia in patients undergoing surgical procedures. Jin F et al. J Clin. Anesth 2001.[72]

and prostacyclin, has resulted in complications that include renal injuries, gastric ulcerations, and potential operative site bleeding complications. Nevertheless, as previously stated, current evidence supports the use of NSAIDs in perioperative pain management.[35,36,73,77,150,157,158]

The effort to minimize the gastrointestinal damage and the potential surgical site bleeding complications associated with the NSAIDs led to the increasing utilization of the COX-2 inhibitors as an adjuvant for managing perioperative pain. Current evidence suggests that the preoperative and postoperative administration of the COX-2 inhibitors results in significant opioid-sparing effects, reduced adverse effects, and improved quality of recovery and patient satisfaction with postoperative pain management.[35,36,57,73,77,98,135] However, there have been emerging controversies regarding the potential adverse cardiovascular risks associated with the use of the COX-2

Prostaglandins (PG)

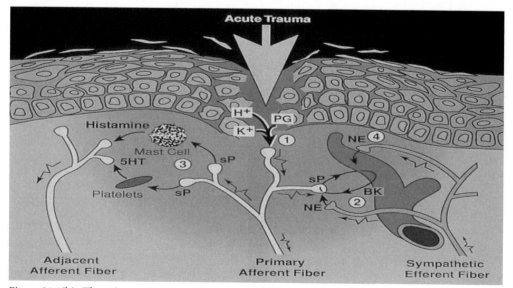

Figure 21.1(b). The primary noxious mediator released from damaged tissue is prostaglandin (PG). PG is responsible for nociceptor activation and sensitization and they play a major role in peripheral inflammation. NSAIDs and COX-inhibitors effectively block PG synthesis.

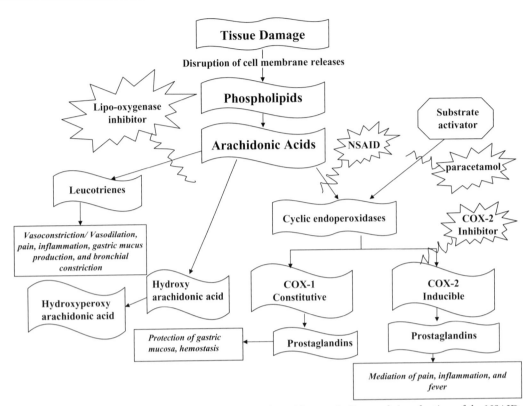

Figure 21.2. Tissue damage, the arachidonic acid cascade and its metabolites, and site of action of the NSAIDs and COX-2 inhibitors and possible site of action of paracetamol. Modified from Dahl et al[36] and Sinatra RS.[143]

inhibitors and whether these compounds truly overcome the perceived limitations associated with NSAIDs, following long-term use.[35,36,57,73,77,98,135,150]

Acetaminophen is a well-known analgesic drug that has been well documented in postoperative pain management. Acetaminophen has been described as a less potent analgesic when compared to that of NSAIDs, but it seems to have an additional analgesic efficacy when given in combination with NSAIDs. The intravenous preparation of paracetamol, and its prodrug, propacetamol, has been shown to be efficacious as a postoperative analgesic therapy. There are currently increasing concerns about renal toxicity when these drugs are used in combination with NSAIDs in vulnerable patients. The thera-

peutic window of acetaminophen has been found to be narrow, and even modest overdosing has resulted in serious liver damage.[36,73,77,135,157,158]

This chapter focuses on the clinical uses, dosing, opioid-sparing effects, safety, and efficacy of the nonopioid analgesics (NSAIDs, COX-2 inhibitors, and APAP) for the management of acute postoperative pain. Because of the broad nature of this topic, the diverse number of NSAIDs and COX-2 inhibitors, and the prodigious amount of literature available on these analgesics, it is challenging to review all available studies on the various NSAIDs, COX-2 inhibitors, and APAP. To ensure the highest quality of systematic reviews of the available literature, clinical trials were included based on the Bandolier method of evaluating clinical trials and the Oxford Pain Validity Scale (OPVS) (Table 21.1).[104] These techniques allow for the largest possible databases of patients to be evaluated, while avoiding actual meta-analyses. Based on the OPVS, scores that were greater than 13 were used in this chapter. Occasionally, studies with lower scores or single blinded studies were included if the particular analgesic in question is a commonly used analgesic and the study in question is the only study available for inclusion. Literature searches of perioperative analgesic clinical trials of these nonopioid analgesics were conducted in the Cochrane Central Register of Controlled trials in the Cochrane Library and the MEDLINE database (1966 to December of 2006). The database search strategy involved a Boolean search of [ketorolac or diclofenac or ibuprofen or indomethacin or naproxen nabumetone or ketoprofen or piroxicam or celecoxib or etoricoxib or lumiracoxib or flosulide or meloxicam or nimesulide or parecoxib or rofecoxib or valdecoxib or paracetamol or propacetamol] and [postoperative or surgery or surgical] and [randomized, double-blinded controlled trials or systemic reviews or metaanalysis].

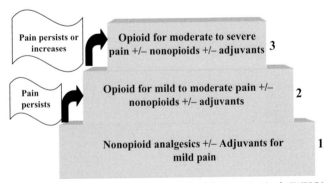

Figure 21.3. Modified from the World Health Organization's (WHO) pain relief ladder. If pain occurs, there should be prompt administration of drugs in the order as displayed. Begin with nonopioid analgesics (NSAIDs, COX-2 inhibitors, APAP) and then, as necessary, use mild opioids and then move to strong opoids if pain relief is still not achieved.

Table 21.1: Method Used in Evaluating Trials in This Chapter[a]

Item		Score
Blinding[b]	1. Trial was convincingly double blinded	6
	2. Trial was not convincingly double-blinded	3
Size of trial groups	1. The start group start size was ≥40	3
	2. Start group start size was between 30 and 39	2
	3. The start group start size was between 20 and 29	1
	4. The start group start size was between 10 and 19	0
Outcomes	1. The study included results from at least 1 pre hoc desirable outcome and used the outcome appropriately	2
	2. The study did not include results from any of the pre hoc desirable outcomes or the pre hoc desirable outcomes were not used appropriately	0
Demonstration of internal sensitivity	1. For all treatment groups, baseline levels were sufficient to be able to measure a change following the intervention or the trial demonstrated internal sensitivity	1
	2. Baseline levels were insufficient to measure a change following the intervention or baseline levels could not be assessed or the trial did not demonstrate internal sensitivity	0
Data analysis	1. The trial defined the relevant outcomes clearly, including where relevant, exactly what "improved," "successful treatment," etc, represented	1
	2. The study failed to describe outcomes clearly	0
	1. The study presented either mean data with standard deviations, dichotomous outcomes, median with range, or sufficient data to enable extraction of any of the above data	1
	2. The study presented none of the above data	0
	1. The trial used appropriate statistical test, with corrections for multiple tests where relevant	1
	2. The study used inappropriate statistical tests and/or multiple testing with no corrections or no statistics were carried out	0
	1. The dropout rate reported was either ≤10% or >10% and includes an intention-to-treat analysis in which dropouts were included appropriately	1
	2. The dropout rate was >10% and dropouts were not included in the analysis, or it is not possible to calculate dropout rate from data presented	0
	Total Score[c]	

[a] Adopted from the Oxford Pain Validity Scale (OPVS).[8,104]

[b] This chapter focused mostly on randomized, controlled double-blinded studies, all other studies were excluded unless otherwise stated.

[c] A minimum score of 13 was needed in the chosen clinical trials for it to be included.

Trials reported in abstract forms, single-blinded clinical trials, and case reports were rarely evaluated.

Systematic review articles and metaanalyses were also included in some sections to add perspective to results and conclusions, but they were not used to provide definitive statements. It is the authors' hope that in providing only best available research, our conclusions regarding these broad classes of nonopioid analgesics can be refined and distilled into significant recommendations.

USE OF THE NSAIDS IN THE MANAGEMENT OF SURGICAL PAIN

NSAIDs have long been used in the treatment of nonoperative pain syndromes because of their analgesic, anti-inflammatory, and antipyretic properties. Their mechanism of action is through the nonspecific inhibition of COX, which therefore blocks both the constitutive COX-1 isoform, responsible for gastric protection and platelet function, and the inducible proinflammatory isoform, COX-2 (see Figure 21.2).[151] Thus, the actions of the NSAIDs result in both the desired analgesic effects and

the unwanted adverse effects of the COX isoforms. With the development of parenteral NSAIDs (eg, ketorolac, diclofenac, ketoprofen, and others), the concerns regarding opioid-related adverse effects (eg, PONV, ileus, biliary spasm, urinary retention, respiratory depression), the evolution of the concept of multi-modal analgesia, and the many randomized, controlled trials that have proved the opioid-sparing effects following the use of the NSAIDs in surgical procedures, the use of these drugs have become increasingly frequent in the management of perioperative pain.[36,150,158] There are currently more than 20 different NSAIDs that have been developed (Table 21.2), and even though these NSAIDs represent diverse chemical entities and exert a wide range of chemical effects, they all generally achieve their hyperalgesic suppressing effects by reducing the concentration of PG peripherally and centrally. Analgesic efficacy is obtained at the level of tissue injury by inhibiting local mediators of pain and inflammation and preventing peripheral sensitization, as well as centrally by inhibiting COX in the spinal cord, thereby reducing neuronal input from peripheral inflammation during the postoperative period.[36,72,78,150,151]

Systematic reviews of published randomized controlled trials of NSAIDs like ketorolac, diclofenac, naproxen, piroxicam, and

Table 21.2: NSAIDs

Generic Name	Brand Name(s)[a]	Dosage Forms[b]	Suggested Doses in Acute Pain[c]	Common Adverse Effects[d]
Acetylsalicylic acid, aspirin, ASA	Ecotrin, Bayer, others	Oral capsule, delayed release: 81 mg Oral Tablet: 81 mg, 325 mg, 486 mg, 500 mg, 650 mg, 800 mg Oral tablet, chewable: 81 mg Oral tablet, enteric coated: 81 mg, 162 mg, 325 mg, 487.5 mg, 500 mg, 650 mg, 975 mg Oral tablet, extended release: 650 mg, 800 mg, 975 mg Rectal suppository: 1.2 g, 60 mg, 125 mg, 200 mg, 325 mg, 650 mg Oral gum: 227 mg	325 to 650 mg PO/PR every 4 h; MAX: 3.9 g/24 h	Indigestion, nausea and vomiting, gastrointestinal ulcers, bleeding, tinnitus, bronchospasm, angioedema, Reye's syndrome
Diclofenac sodium[e]	Voltaren, cataflam	Oral tablet, enteric coated: 25 mg, 50 mg, 75 mg Oral tablet, extended release: 75 mg, 100 mg	50–100 mg PO/IM/IV	Edema, pruritus, rash, abdominal pain, constipation, diarrhea, flatulence, indigestion, nausea, increased liver function test, dizziness, headache, tinnitus, burning sensation, congestive heart failure, hypertension, myocardial infarction, thrombotic tendency observations, gastrointestinal hemorrhage, gastrointestinal perforation, gastrointestinal ulcer
Etodolac	Lodine	Oral capsule: 200 mg, 300 mg Oral tablet: 400 mg, 500 mg Oral tablet, extended release: 400 mg, 500 mg, 600 mg	200 to 400 mg PO every 6 to 8 h as needed; MAX: 1200 mg/d	Edema, abdominal pain, diarrhea, flatulence, indigestion, nausea, dizziness, malaise, congestive heart failure, hypertension, myocardial infarction, thrombotic tendency observations, gastrointestinal hemorrhage, gastrointestinal perforation, inflammatory disorder of digestive tract, melena
Fenbufen	Afiancen, others	Oral tablet: 300 mg, 450 mg Oral capsule: 300 mg	600–1000 mg PO every day twice a day	Nausea, vomiting, abdominal discomfort, epigastralgia, hearburn, headache, dizziness, skin rash and/or pruritus, interstitial nephritis, toxic epidermal necrolysis, liver dysfunction, aplastic anemia
Fenoprofen	Nalfon	Oral capsule: 200 mg, 300 mg Oral tablet: 600 mg	200 mg PO every 4 to 6 h PRN	Edema, anemia, increased liver function test, hypertension, myocardial infarction, thrombotic tendency observations, scaling eczema, Stevens-Johnson syndrome, gastrointestinal perforation, inflammatory disorder of digestive tract, hepatitis, jaundice, liver failure, anaphylactoid reaction, cerebrovascular accident, acute renal failure, bronchospasm
Flurbiprofen[f]	Ansaid	Oral tablet: 50 mg, 100 mg	50 mg PO every 4–6 h PRN	Edema, rash, abdominal pain, constipation, diarrhea, flatulence, indigestion, nausea, vomiting, dizziness, headache, somnolence, tinnitus, nervousness, urinary symptoms, rhinitis, malaise, congestive heart failure, hypertension, myocardial infarction, thrombotic tendency observations, gastrointestinal perforation, gastrointestinal ulcer, inflammatory disorder of digestive tract, melena

Generic Name	Brand Name(s)[a]	Dosage Forms[b]	Suggested Doses in Acute Pain[c]	Common Adverse Effects[d]
Ibuprofen[g]	Motrin	Oral capsule: 200 mg Oral capsule, Liquid filled: 200 mg Oral suspension: 100 mg/ 5 mL, 50 mg/2.5 mL, 40 mg/mL, 50 mg/1.25 mL Oral tablet: 100 mg, 200 mg, 300 mg, 400 mg, 600 mg, 800 mg Oral tablet, chewable: 50 mg, 100 mg	300 to 800 mg PO three times a day	Body fluid retention, rash, abdominal pain, constipation, diarrhea, heartburn, indigestion, nausea, stomatitis, vomiting, increased liver function test, dizziness, headache, somnolence, tinnitus, congestive heart failure, hypertension, myocardial infarction, thrombotic tendency observations, gastrointestinal hemorrhage, gastrointestinal perforation, gastrointestinal ulcer, inflammatory disorder of digestive tract, melena
Indomethacin[g]	Indocin	Oral capsule: 25 mg, 50 mg Oral capsule, extended release: 75 mg Oral suspension: 25 mg/ 5 mL Rectal suppository: 50 mg	25–50 mg PO/PR/IM twice a day	Abdominal pain, anal irritation, constipation, diarrhea, indigestion, nausea, tenesmus, vomiting, dizziness, headache, somnolence, tinnitus, depression, fatigue, cardiac dysrhythmia, chest pain, congestive heart failure, edema, hypertension, myocardial infarction, gastrointestinal perforation, gastrointestinal ulcer, inflammatory disorder of digestive tract
Ketoprofen[h]	Orudis, others	Oral capsule: 25 mg, 50 mg, 75 mg Oral capsule, extended release: 100 mg, 150 mg, 200 mg Oral tablet: 12.5b mg	25 to 50 mg PO every 6–8 h as needed, MAX: 300 mg/d	Edema, rash, abdominal pain, constipation, diarrhea, flatulence, indigestion, nausea, dizziness, headache, insomnia, tinnitus, congestive heart failure, hypertension, myocardial infarction, thrombotic tendency observations, gastrointestinal hemorrhage, gastrointestinal perforation
Ketorolac Tromethamine	Toradol	Injection solution: 15 mg/mL, 30 mg/mL Intramuscular solution: 30 mg/mL Intravenous solution: 15 mg/mL, 30 mg/mL Oral tablet: 10 mg	15–30 mg PO/IM/IV	Edema, hypertension, injection site pain, pruritus, rash, sweating symptom, abdominal pain, constipation, diarrhea, flatulence, indigestion, nausea, stomatitis, vomiting, anemia, purpuric disorder, dizziness, headache, somnolence, myocardial infarction, palpitations, syncope, thrombotic tendency observations, gastrointestinal hemorrhage (rare), gastrointestinal perforation (rare), inflammatory disorder of digestive tract, melena (rare)
Meclofenamate	Meclomen	Oral capsule: 50 mg, 100 mg	50 mg PO every 4 to 6 h, MAX: 400 mg/d	Edema, increased liver function test, hypertension, myocardial infarction, thrombotic tendency observations, scaling eczema, Stevens-Johnson syndrome, gastrointestinal perforation, gastrointestinal ulcer, inflammatory disorder of digestive tract
Mefenamic Acid	Ponstel	Oral capsule: 250 mg	500 mg, followed by 250 mg PO every 6 h PRN, not longer than 1 week	Edema, increased liver function test, hypertension, myocardial infarction, thrombotic tendency observations, scaling eczema, Stevens-Johnson syndrome, gastrointestinal perforation, gastrointestinal ulcer, inflammatory disorder of digestive tract
Meloxicam	Mobic	Oral suspension: 7.5 mg/ 5 mL Oral tablet: 7.5 mg, 15 mg	7.5 mg PO qd; MAX: 15 mg	Edema, pruritus, rash, abdominal pain, diarrhea, flatulence, indigestion, nausea, anemia, increased liver function test, arthralgia, back pain, dizziness, headache,

(*continued*)

Table 21.2 (*continued*)

Generic Name	Brand Name(s)[a]	Dosage Forms[b]	Suggested Doses in Acute Pain[c]	Common Adverse Effects[d]
				insomnia, urinary tract infectious disease, pharyngitis, upper respiratory infection, angina, cardiac dysrhythmia, congestive heart failure, hypertension, myocardial infarction, thrombotic tendency observations, vasculitis, erythema multiforme, scaling eczema, Stevens-Johnson syndrome, toxic epidermal necrolysis, gastrointestinal hemorrhage, gastrointestinal perforation, gastrointestinal ulcer, inflammatory disorder of digestive tract, melena, pancreatitis
Nabumetone	Relafen	Oral tablet: 500 mg, 750 mg	1000–2000 mg PO every day	Edema, pruritus, rash, abdominal pain, constipation, diarrhea, flatulence, indigestion, nausea, occult blood in stools, dizziness, headache, insomnia, tinnitus, hypertension, myocardial infarction, erythema multiforme (rare), scaling eczema, Stevens-Johnson syndrome, toxic epidermal necrolysis, gastrointestinal hemorrhage, gastrointestinal perforation, inflammatory disorder of digestive tract, melena, anemia, thrombocytopenia, hepatitis, increased liver function test, jaundice
Naproxen	Naprosyn, Anaprox	Oral suspension: 25 mg/mL Oral tablet: 250 mg, 375 mg, 500 mg Oral tablet, enteric coated: 375 mg, 500 mg	May initiate at 500 mg; maintenance: 250 mg PO every 6–8 h as needed or 500 mg every 12 h as needed; MAX: initial dose 1250 mg/d, then 1000 mg/d	Edema, pruritus, rash, abdominal pain, heartburn, indigestion, nausea, stomatitis, anemia, dizziness, headache, lightheadedness, vertigo, tinnitus, dyspnea, congestive heart failure, myocardial infarction, pulmonary edema, vasculitis, scaling eczema, Stevens-Johnson syndrome, toxic epidermal necrolysis, gastrointestinal hemorrhage, gastrointestinal perforation, inflammatory disorder of digestive tract, pancreatitis, agranulocytosis
Nimesulide	Antiflogil, others	Oral drops: 50 mg/mL Satchet: 100 mg Oral suspension: 50 mg/5 mL Tablet: 100 mg	200 mg PO twice a day	Skin rash, pruritus, erythema, flushing, facial edema, diaphoresis, heartburn, epigastric pain, nausea, diarrhea, vomiting, purpuric skin lesion, sleep disorders, vertigo, hyperexcitability, drowsiness, headaches, gastrointestinal hemorrhage, acute hepatitis, irreversible liver failure, acute renal failure
Oxaprozin	Daypro	Oral tablet: 600 mg	1200 mg PO daily, MAX: 1800 mg/d	Rash, abdominal pain, constipation, diarrhea, indigestion, nausea, vomiting, tinnitus, dysuria, increased frequency of urination, edema, hypertension, myocardial infarction, palpitations, thrombotic tendency observations, cerebrovascular accident, gastrointestinal hemorrhage, gastrointestinal perforation, inflammatory disorder of digestive tract
Piroxicam	Feldene	Oral capsule: 10 mg, 20 mg	20 mg PO daily	Edema, pruritus, rash, abdominal pain, constipation, diarrhea, flatulence, heartburn, indigestion, nausea, vomiting, dizziness, headache, congestive heart failure, hypertension, myocardial infarction, tachyarrhythmia, thrombotic tendency observations

Generic Name	Brand Name(s)[a]	Dosage Forms[b]	Suggested Doses in Acute Pain[c]	Common Adverse Effects[d]
Sulindac	Clinoril	Oral tablet: 150 mg, 200 mg	200 mg PO twice a day for 7–14 days; MAX: 400 mg/d	Edema, pruritus, rash, abdominal pain, constipation, diarrhea, indigestion, nausea, dizziness, headache, tinnitus, nervousness, myocardial infarction, thrombotic tendency observations, vasculitis, erythema multiforme, scaling eczema, Stevens-Johnson syndrome, gastrointestinal hemorrhage, gastrointestinal perforation, inflammatory disorder of digestive tract, pancreatitis
Tenoxicam	Tenotec, others	Injection powder: 20 mg Oral tablet: 20 mg	20–40 mg PO/PR/IA/IV	Nausea, dyspepsia, epigastric pain, indigestion, diarrhea, vomiting, flatulence, dizziness, headache, vertigo, tiredness, depression, peptic ulcer, severe hematuria
Tolmetin	Tolectin	Oral capsule: 400 mg Oral tablet: 200 mg, 600 mg	200–600 mg PO three times a day, MAX 1800 mg	Edema, weight gain, weight loss, abdominal pain, diarrhea, flatulence, indigestion, nausea, vomiting, asthenia, dizziness, headache, congestive heart failure, hypertension, myocardial infarction, thrombotic tendency observations, cerebrovascular accident, acute renal failure, hematuria, proteinuria, bronchospasm

Abbreviations: PO = by mouth; PR = per rectum; MAX = maximum dose; IM = intramuscular; IV = intravenous; h = hours; PRN = as needed.

[a] Only a number of brand names are listed in this section.

[b] Dosage forms listed are based on information given in micromedex and/or used in clinical trials.

[c] Suggested doses in acute pain are those that have been suggested in micromedex, and/or used in clinical trials. Doses listed do not necessarily apply to all patients, recommended doses in clinical pratice should depend on a clinician's best judgement and should be patient specific.

[d] The table does not give a full list of all the adverse effects that have been reported, only some of the most common adverse events that have been reported in clinical trials are stated in this section.

[e] There is a diclofenac injectable that is currently not available on the market, but undergoing clinical trials.

[f] Flurbiprofen also has an injection form called flurbiprofen axetil, but it is currently not available in the market.

[g] Ibuprofen and indomethacin have parenteral forms available, but they are currently not indicated in pain management, they are currently used for the closure of patent ductus arteriosus in infants.

[h] Ketoprofen has an injectable form, but it is currently not available on the market, but has been studied in clinical trials.

indomethacin have evaluated their use in acute postoperative pain, and most of these reviews concluded positively regarding the effectiveness and safety of the NSAIDs in acute perioperative pain. One of these reviews was inconclusive about the effectiveness of indomethacin for acute postoperative pain.[11,47,95,96,148] Some systematic reviews have concluded that there are no significant differences in the analgesic efficacy between different NSAIDs, but they do have different levels of toxicities, especially at high or increased doses.[61,73] Some authors have therefore suggested that, because there is no documented evidence of superiority of any particular NSAID for use in surgical pain, the choice of NSAIDs should depend on the route of administration, toxicity, duration of analgesia, and cost.[73] There is also a quantitative systematic review of published randomized, controlled trials that concluded that the bioavailability of most NSAIDs are generally high after oral administration and low after rectal administration.[153] In a systematic review, with metaanalysis, that was performed to determine the analgesic efficacy and adverse effects of single doses of ketorolac through the oral and parenteral routes of administration, the authors concluded that the oral route of administration was

equivalent to that of the parenteral route, and, therefore, in patients who have no contraindication to NSAIDs and can swallow, the oral routes could be used instead of the parenteral route.[73,148]

The goal of this section of the chapter is to review the most important and current evidence available on the efficacy and opiate-sparing effects of some of the NSAIDs (including those that have not yet been approved for use by the U.S. Food and Drug Administration [FDA]). As stated previously, because of the many and diverse nature of NSAIDs, and the numerous clinical trials that have been performed in evaluating their efficacy in surgical pain, this chapter will not review all the available literature, but rather will present the most robust studies based on the type of surgery, the frequency of use or importance of the NSAID involved, and the study design used in evaluating the efficacy of the NSAID. The aim will be to provide the readers with accurate information on the use of the NSAIDs in surgical pain. Evidence supporting the preemptive, perioperative, and/or postoperative use of some of these NSAIDs will be evaluated and a summary of all the clinical trials that are cited in this section may be viewed in Tables 21.3 and 21.4.

Table 21.3: Preemptive Use of the NSAIDs: Summary of Clinical Trials

Ref	Dose and Route of NSAID (n)	Dose and Route of Comparators	Type of Surgery	Duration/Timing of Dose	Outcome Measures[a]	Analgesic Efficacy Results[b]
108	Before surgery and tourniquet placement: 30 mg IV **K** (23)	After surgery and tourniquet placement: 30 mg IV **K** (25)	Ankle fracture surgery	Preoperatively: before tourniquet inflation Postoperatively: 15 min after surgery and tourniquet placement	1. Visual analog scale pain scores 2. Morphine PCA consumption 3. Nausea and vomiting 4. Postoperative bleeding	Preemptive analgesic efficacy of **K** > postoperative use of **K** (short lived ~ 6 hours, no difference in opiate consumption) Preemptive nausea score < postoperative nausea score Postoperative bleeding was not reported for any subject
134	Before surgery: 30 mg IV **K** + intraarticular injection of 20 mL ropivacaine 0.25% and 2 mg morphine and epinephrine 1:200 000 + femoral nerve block with 20 mL ropivacaine 0.25% (20)	After surgery: 30 mg IV **K** + intraarticular injection of 20 ml ropivacaine 0.25% and 2 mg morphine and epinephrine 1:200 000 + femoral nerve block with 20 ml ropivacaine 0.25% (20)	Arthroscopic knee ligament repair	Preoperatively: 15 min before procedure Post-operatively: immediately after skin incision	1. Verbal pain rating scores 2. PCA morphine consumption	Preemptive analgesic efficacy of multimodal therapy > postoperative analgesic efficacy (no measurable long-term advantage for preemptive analgesia)
52	Before surgery: 60 mg IV **K** (20)	After surgery: 60 mg IV **K** (20) **P** (20)	Total hip replacement surgery	Preoperatively: immediately after arriving in the operating room Postoperatively: at the time of skin closure	1. Visual analog pain score 2. Adverse effects (sedation, respiratory depression, nausea, perioperative bleeding)	Preemptive analgesic efficacy of **K** > postoperative use of **K** (benefit was not sustained with time) > **P** No statistical difference in the number of transfusions in all groups
113	Before surgery: 30 mg IV **K** (32)	After surgery: 30 mg IV **Tr** (32)	Oral surgery	Preoperatively: just before procedure	1. Pain intensity hourly for 12 hours 2. Median time to rescue analgesia 3. Postoperative acetaminophen consumption 4. Patients global assessment	Analgesic efficacy of the preemptive use of **K** > preemptive use of **Tr**
114	Before surgery: 30 mg IV **K** (34)	After surgery: 30 mg IV **K** (34)	Oral surgery	Preoperatively: 30 min before procedure Postoperatively: immediately after surgery (crossover study)	1. Pain intensity scores over 12 hours 2. Time to rescue analgesic 3. Postoperative analgesic consumption Patient's global assessment	Analgesic efficacy of the preemptive use of **K** > postoperative use of **K**
88	Group **K**: 60 mg IV **K** + 20 mg IM **CPM** (20) Group **DM + K**: 60 mg IV **K** + 40 mg IM **DM** (20)	Group **DM**: (40 mg **DM** + 20 mg of CPM) IM + 2 ml NS IV (20) Control: 20 mg IM **CPM** + 2 ml IV NS (20)	Laparoscopic-assisted vaginal hysterectomy	Preoperatively: 30 min before skin incision	1. Visual analog scale pain scores 2. Time to PCA request for pain relief 3. Total opiate consumption	**DM + K** > **DM** or **K** > Control

Ref	Dose and Route of NSAID (n)	Dose and Route of Comparators	Type of Surgery	Duration/Timing of Dose	Outcome Measures[a]	Analgesic Efficacy Results[b]
100	0.5 mg/kg IM **k** + 0.6 mg/kg IM **Mep** (24)	P (**25**)	Ambulatory laparoscopic cholecystectomy	Preoperatively: 45 min before induction of anesthesia	1. Pain scores 2. Nausea 3. Postoperative recovery	Analgesic efficacy of the preemptive use of **K + Mep** > **P** Incidence of nausea in K < P
3	75 mg IV **D** (36)	60 mg IV **K** (31) P (**32**)	Major orthopedic surgery	Preoperatively: before induction of anesthesia	1. Visual analog scale 2. Verbal pain score 3. Sedation score 4. Frequency of opioid adverse effects 5. Morphine consumption	Analgesic efficacy of the preemptive use of **D** = preemptive use of **K** > **P**
56	50 mg PR **D** (24)	P (22)	Gynecological laparoscopy	Preoperatively: prior to induction of anesthesia	1. Visual analog scale pain score 2. Postoperative analgesic requirement 3. Adverse effects	Analgesic efficacy of the preemptive use of **D** > preemptive use of **P** No difference in incidence of adverse effects
119	50 mg PO **D** + ropivacaine (39) 50 mg PO **D** + saline	P + ropivacaine (36) P + saline (37)	Day-case knee arthroscopy	Preoperatively: 60 min before procedure	1. Visual analog scale pain score 2. Adverse effects	**D** + ropivacaine = **D** + saline > **P** + ropivacaine, **P** + saline
120	50 mg PO **D** (100)	10 mg PO **Dia** (100)	Day-case varicose vein repair	Preoperatively: 60 min before procedure	1. Visual analog scale pain score 2. Postoperative analgesic requirement	Analgesic efficacy of the preemptive use of **D** > preemptive use of **Dia**
30	550 mg PO **N** (26)	P (40)	Arthroscopic knee surgery	Preoperatively: 30–60 min before procedure	1. Visual analog scale pain score 2. Postoperative analgesic requirement 3. Length of day surgery stay	Analgesic efficacy of the preemptive use of **N** > **P** (both in the preoperative period and 24 hours after completion of surgery)
31	550 mg PO **N** (21)	P (23)	Outpatient laparoscopic tubal ligation	Preoperatively: less than 1 h before procedure	1. Visual analog scale pain score 2. Analgesic requirement 3. Adverse effects 4. Length of day surgery stay	Analgesic efficacy of the preemptive use of **N** > **P** (no increase in analgesic adverse effect)
111	2 h preoperatively: 20 mg PO **PIRO** (20) Immediately before induction: 20 mg PO **PIRO** (20)	1 h postoperatively: 20 mg PO **PIRO** (20)	Gynecological laparoscopic surgery	Preoperatively: 2 h before procedure Preoperatively: immediately before induction Postoperatively: 1 h after procedure	1. Visual analog scale pain score 2. Analgesia requirement	**PIRO** given 2 hours preoperatively > **PIRO** given immediately before induction or 1 hour postoperatively
62	Preoperatively: 40 mg SL **PIRO** (25)	Postoperatively: 40 mg SL **PIRO** (27)	Laparoscopic bilateral inguinal hernia repair	Preoperatively: 2 h before procedure Postoperatively: 10 min after procedure	1. Visual analog scale pain score 6 h after surgery 2. Consumption of **Tr**	**PIRO** given 2 hours preoperatively > **PIRO** given 10 min postoperatively

(continued)

Table 21.3 (*continued*)

Ref	Dose and Route of NSAID (n)	Dose and Route of Comparators	Type of Surgery	Duration/Timing of Dose	Outcome Measures[a]	Analgesic Efficacy Results[b]
69	40 mg PO **PIRO** (25)	**P** (24)	Oral surgery	Preoperatively: 2.5 h before procedure	1. Time at which analgesia was first received 2. Total amount of analgesics consumed in 24 h	**PIRO > P**
1	20 mg IV **T** (40)	**P** (40)	Laparoscopic cholecystectomy or groin hernia repair	Preoperatively: immediately before induction	1. Postoperative analgesic requirement 2. Perioperative adverse effects 3. Visual analog scale pain score 4. Hospitalization time	**T > P**
146	Group **T**: 40 mg IV **T** + 20 mg IM **CPM** (20) Group **DM** + **T**: 40 mg IV **T** + 40 mg IM **DM** (20)	Group **DM**: (40 mg **DM** + 20 mg of CPM) IM + 4 ml NS IV (20) Control: 20 mg IM **CPM** + 4 ml IV NS (20)	Laparoscopic cholecystectomy	Preoperatively: 30 min before skin incision	1. Visual analog scale pain score 2. Time to first request of **Mep** for pain relief 3. Total **Mep** consumption	**DM** + **T** > **DM** > **T** > Control
116	1600 mg PO **IBU** SR, then 1600 mg PO **IBU**, 24 h after the initial dose	P	Lower abdominal gynecological surgery	Preoperatively: 2–4 hours before procedure, then 24 h after the first dose	1. Pain scores 2. Occurrence of adverse events 3. Morphine consumption	**IBU > P** (no increase in adverse effects)
101	800 mg PO **IBU**	**60 mg IV K**	Elective laparoscopic hernia repair	Preoperatively: **IBU** given 1 h before procedure Preoperatively: **K** given at time of trocar insertion	1. Postoperative pain in 18 and 24 h	**IBU = K**
16	Preoperatively: 100 mg IV **Ket** Postoperatively: 100 mg IV Ket	**Preoperatively: 2 gm IV** Prop Postoperatively: 2 gm IV Prop	Laparoscopic cholecystectomy	Preoperatively: before induction Postoperatively: immediately after surgery	1. Visual analog scale pain score 2. Nalbuphine consumption	Preoperative **Ket** > Postoperative **Ket** Preoperative **Ket** > Preoperative **Prop** and postoperative **Prop**

Abbreviations: Ref = reference; n = number of patients in group; mg = milligrams; g = grams; IV = intravenous route; IM = intramuscular; PR = per rectum; PO = by mouth; SL = sublingual; **K** = ketorolac; PCA = patient-controlled analgesia; **P** = placebo; **Tr** = tramadol; **DM** = detromethorphan; **CPM** = chlorpheniramine; **Mep** = meperidine; **D** = diclofenac; **Dia** = diazepam; **N** = naproxen sodium; **Ket** = ketoprofen; **PIRO** = piroxicam; **T** = tenoxicam; NS = normal saline; **IBU** = ibuprofen; **Prop** = propacetamol.

[a] Outcome measures/endpoints presented in summary table might not be all the end points that were presented in the study.

[b] Analgesic efficacy results presented in table are a general summary of author(s)' conclusions.

Preincisional Use of NSAIDs for Surgical Pain

Given the mechanism of action and pharmacodynamic and pharmacokinetic properties of the NSAIDs, nociceptor modulation necessitates their administration in advance of the anticipated time for the patient to achieve the desired analgesic effect.[150] However, the use of the NSAIDs in preemptive analgesic therapy in surgical procedures has been debated extensively and is still controversial.[78,79,81,102,112] Because of the effects of the nonselective NSAIDs on platelet aggregation, some studies recommend that NSAIDs should not be used in the immediate pre- or perioperative period, because they may increase the risk of bleeding.[132,144] However, Slappendel et al,[146] studying patients undergoing total hip surgery and the use of the NSAID nabumetone, showed that the preoperative pain intensity that occurred after stopping NSAIDs is directly related to, and determines, the postoperative morphine dose that would

Table 21.4: Postoperative Use of NSAIDs: Summary of Clinical Trials

Ref	Dose and Route of NSAID (n)	Dose and Route of Comparator(s)	Type of Surgery	Duration/Timing of Dose	Outcome Measures[a]	Analgesic Efficacy Results[b]
35	20 mg PO **K** followed by 10 mg PO **K** 4–6 hours after the first dose (66)	10 mg/1000 mg PO **H/A** followed by 10 mg/1000 mg PO **H/A** 4–6 hours later (59)	Anterior cruciate ligament reconstruction	Postoperatively: 1st dose: at least 48 hours after surgery 2nd dose: 4–6 hours after 1st dose	1. Pain intensity 2. Pain score 3. Adverse events	**K** > **H/A** (no bleeding problems observed in either group)
36	10 mg PO **K** every 6 hours for up to 3 days (83)	7.5 mg/750 mg PO **H/A** every 6 hours for up to 3 days (82) **P**(87)	Ambulatory arthroscopic or laparoscopic tubal ligation	Postoperatively: after awakening with moderate to severe pain	1. Pain intensity 2. Pain score 3. Adverse effects	**K** = **H/A** > **P** (overall tolerability favored the **K** group)
37	120 mg IV **K** over 24 hours	**P**	Lower abdominal surgery	Postoperatively: Immediately after surgery	1. Cumulative morphine consumption 2. Pain score at rest 3. Occurrence of adverse events	**K** > **P** (there was no difference between treatments in the incidence of adverse respiratory effects, nausea, or vomiting)
38	30 mg IV **K** 30 mg IV K + 0.1 mg/kg morphine (503)	Morphine (500)	Different types of surgeries: Abdominal surgery, orthopedic surgery, craniofacial surgery, thoracic surgery, spinal surgery	Postoperatively: **K** or morphine started after surgery. If pain intensity is 5 or more (on a scale of 1–10) 30 minutes after analgesic administration, patients were given 2.5 mg of morphine every 10 minutes until pain intensity was 4 or less	1. Proportion of patients who reported a decrease in pain intensity 30 minutes after the initiation of analgesics 2. Opioid-related adverse effects	Morphine > **K** (adding **K** to morphine reduced opioid consumption and morphine related adverse effects)
39	30 mg IV **K** (loading dose) followed by 15 mg IV **K** every 6 hours (20) or 60 mg IV **K** (loading dose) followed by 30 mg IV **K** every 6 hours (21)	**P** (21)	Intraabdominal gynecologic surgery	Postoperatively: immediately at the end of surgery	1. Visual analog pain and satisfaction scores 2. Opioid consumption 3. Frequency and severity of adverse effects	**K** > **P**
40	1.5 mg/mL IV **K** + 5 mg/ml **Tr** (30)	10 mg/mL **Tr** (30)	Major abdominal surgery	Postoperatively: at the beginning of wound closure	1. Total analgesic consumption 2. Sedation score	**K** + **Tr** = **Tr** (sedation score was significantly lower in the **K** + **Tr**)
44	40 mg IV **Teno** (256)	**P** (258)	Abdominal or orthopedic surgery	Postoperatively: at the end of surgery and then 24 hours later	1. Analgesic efficacy 2. Incidence of adverse effects	**Teno** > **P** (**Teno** was associated with minimal adverse effects and high tolerability)
45	20 mg IV **Teno** (45)	**P** (48)	Cesarean section	Postoperatively: at the end of surgery	1. Wound pain 2. Uterine cramping pain 3. Opioid consumption	**Teno** > **P** (no additional effect on wound pain)

(continued)

Table 21.4 (*continued*)

Ref	Dose and Route of NSAID (n)	Dose and Route of Comparator(s)	Type of Surgery	Duration/Timing of Dose	Outcome Measures[a]	Analgesic Efficacy Results[b]
46	500 mg PO **NAP** + morphine (40)	P + morphine (40)	Cesarean section	Postoperatively: every 12 hours after surgery	1. Visual analog scale pain score (incision pain, uterine cramping, gas pain) 2. Analgesic use 3. Adverse effects	**NAP** > **P** (does not reduce the incidence of inadequate analgesia)
47	100 mg IV **Ket** (25) (all patients received morphine and propacetamol)	P (25)	Spinal fusion surgery	Postoperatively: every 8 hours after surgery	1. Visual analog scale pain score 2. Morphine consumption	**Ket** > **P**
48	100 mg IV **Ket** + 2 g IV **Prop** (32) 100 mg IV **Ket** (33)	2 g IV **Prop** (33)	Thyroidectomy	Postoperatively: 30 minutes before the end of surgery, then every 6 hours	1. Visual analog scale pain score 2. Tramadol consumption	**Ket** = **Ket** + **Prop** > **Prop**
49	100 mg PR **D** (40)	P (42)	Cesarean section	Postoperatively: every 12 hours after surgery	1. Visual analog scale pain score 2. Need for rescue analgesics 3. Adverse effects	**D** > **P** (the average level of postoperative pain was lower in the diclofenac group, but was not significant. No difference in adverse effects)
50	100 mg PR **D** + 1 g PR **Acet** (17) 100 mg PR **D** (17)	1 g PR **Acet** (20)	Cardiac surgery	Postoperatively, 2 hours after surgery: **D** – every 18 hours after surgery for 24 hours **Acet**- every 6 hours after surgery for 24 hours	1. Visual analog scale pain score 2. Morphine consumption 3. Sedation	**D** + **Acet** = **D** > **Acet**
51	100 mg PR **Ind** + morphine (44)	P + morphine (46)	Major abdominal surgery	Postoperatively: every 8 hours for 3 days	1. Postoperative subjective pain assessment 2. Analgesic requirement 3. Respiratory function	**Ind** + morphine > **P** + morphine
52	100 mg PR **Ind** + morphine (25)	P + morphine (25)	Total hip arthroplasty	Postoperatively: every 8 hours for 5 doses	1. Visual analog scale pain score 2. Morphine consumption	**Ind** + morphine > **P** + morphine

Abbreviations: Ref = reference; n = number of patients in group; mg = milligrams; g = grams; IV = intravenous route; IM = intramuscular; PR = per rectum; PO = by mouth; SL = sublingual; **K** = ketorolac; **Ket** = ketoprofen; PCA = patient-controlled analgesia; **P** = placebo; **Tr** = tramadol; **Teno** = tenoxicam; **D** = diclofenac; **H/A** = hydrocodone/acetaminophen; **NAP** = naproxen sodium; NS = normal saline; **Ind** = indomethacin; **Acet** = acetaminophen; **Prop** = propacetamol.

[a] Outcome measures/end points presented in summary table might not be all the end points that were presented in the study.

[b] Analgesic efficacy results presented are a general summary of author(s)' conclusions.

be needed for surgical pain (see Figure 21.4), which therefore means that a patient who does not have any contraindication to the use of NSAIDs would benefit by requiring less opiate postsurgically (and hence less prone to the opiate adverse effects) if NSAIDs are used preemptively during surgical procedures. The efficacy of some of the nonselective NSAIDs (eg, ketorolac, diclofenac, naproxen, piroxicam, tenoxicam, flurbiprofen, indomethacin, ketoprofen, fenbufen, and several others) in preemptive analgesic therapy have been evaluated in clinical trials and this section of the chapter evaluates these studies to provide information about the role of the NSAIDs in preemptive analgesic therapy.

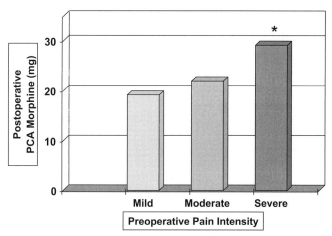

Figure 21.4. Pain intensity after stopping NSAIDs determines the postoperative morphine dose required for analgesia. Slappendel et al (1999).[146]

The preemptive use of ketorolac (alone and in combination with other analgesics) has been evaluated in orthopedic surgery, oral surgery, abdominal surgery, and vaginal hysterectomy. In a study that evaluated patients who were undergoing ankle fracture repair surgery, a 30-mg intravenous dose of ketorolac given once preemptively was shown to prevent an increase in pain from baseline rather than when given after the surgery. There was no difference in opiate consumption between the two groups, but the preemptive group had a lower nausea score.[108] In a study that evaluated the preemptive versus the postoperative effectiveness of a multimodal analgesic regimen that included a 30-mg intravenous (IV) dose of ketorolac, an intraarticular injection of 20 mL of ropivacaine (0.25%) with 2 mg of morphine and epinephrine, and a femoral nerve block of 20 mL ropivacaine (0.25%) in patients undergoing arthroscopic knee repair surgery, the preemptive use of the multimodal analgesic regimen resulted in lower pain scores and a lower opiate consumption in the initial stay in the postanesthesia care unit (PACU). There was, however, no measurable long-term advantage associated with preemptive multimodal drug administration, when compared to its postoperative use.[134] In another study that evaluated the preemptive use of a 60-mg IV dose of ketorolac, when compared to its postoperative use and placebo in patients undergoing total hip replacement surgery, the preemptive use of ketorolac had a greater analgesic effect in the immediate postoperative period than when it was administered after the surgical procedure. There was no statistical difference in the number of blood transfusions that occurred in the study groups.[52] In studies that evaluated patients undergoing oral surgery, the preemptive use of a 30-mg IV dose of ketorolac was shown to be more efficacious than when it is used postoperatively. It was also found to be more effective than the preemptive use of tramadol.[113,114] The preoperative cotreatment of ketorolac with dextromethorphan (an NMDA receptor antagonist) in patients undergoing laparoscopic-assisted vaginal hysterectomy was shown to be more efficacious than either dextromethorphan or ketorolac alone.[88] In patients undergoing ambulatory laparoscopic cholecystectomy, the preoperative cotreatment of ketorolac with meperidine was also shown to be more effective than placebo.[100] The preemptive use of diclofenac has also been assessed in several types of surgical procedures. In one study that evaluated the morphine-sparing effects of diclofenac sodium compared to ketorolac in patients undergoing

major orthopedic surgeries, the preoperative administration of a 75-mg IV dose of diclofenac or 60-mg IV dose of ketorolac significantly reduced morphine requirements and associated adverse effects after major orthopedic surgeries.[3] In patients undergoing gynecological laparoscopy, a 50-mg dose of diclofenac given rectally before induction of anesthesia was shown to result in better pain relief and less postoperative analgesic consumption, when compared to placebo.[56] In patients undergoing day case knee arthroscopy and varicose vein repair, a 50-mg oral dose of diclofenac given preemptively was shown to be very effective in reducing analgesic requirements postoperatively in these procedures.[119,120]

The use of naproxen sodium as a preemptive analgesic has been studied in arthroscopic knee surgery and patients undergoing outpatient laparoscopic tubal ligations. In both procedures, a single preoperative oral dose of 550 mg naproxen sodium was effective in reducing postoperative pain, postoperative analgesic requirement, without any increase in morbidity.[30,31]

Use of a 20-mg oral dose of piroxicam given 2 hours preoperatively in patients undergoing gynecological laparoscopic surgery reduced pain scores, time to first analgesia, and postoperative analgesic requirements compared to its administration prior to induction or 1 hour postoperatively.[111] In another study that evaluated patients undergoing laparoscopic bilateral inguinal hernia repair, a 40-mg sublingual dose of piroxicam given 2 hours before the procedure was shown to be more effective than when it was administered postoperatively.[62] In dental surgery, the use of a 40-mg oral dose of piroxicam, given 2.5 hours before surgery, was shown to be opioid sparing with a reduction in postoperative analgesic requirement when compared to placebo.[69]

In a study that proposed to investigate the postoperative pain relief effect of preoperative tenoxicam usage in patients undergoing laparoscopic cholecystectomy or inguinal hernia repair, a 20-mg intravenous dose of tenoxicam given immediately before induction was shown to be safe and effective for postoperative pain relief after surgery when compared to that of placebo.[1] However, another study evaluated the preemptive use of tenoxicam and dextromethorphan in patients undergoing laparoscopic cholecystectomy, and the results suggested that the pretreatment of tenoxicam alone did not provide significant preemptive analgesia in patients after the surgery. In that study, the use of tenoxicam in combination with dextromethorphan, and dextromethorphan alone, provided significant pain relief (see Figure 21.4).[146]

The preemptive use of sustained release ibuprofen as an adjunct to morphine PCA was evaluated in a study that involved patients scheduled for lower abdominal gynecological surgery. In this study, 1600 mg of ibuprofen was given preoperatively and then 24 hours after the first dose, and its postoperative analgesic effect monitored after the surgery. Patients who received ibuprofen reported significantly less pain when compared to placebo.[116] A study that compared the preemptive use of an oral dose of 800 mg ibuprofen with that of a 60-mg IV dose of ketorolac in patients scheduled for elective laparoscopic inguinal hernia repair showed that pain relief from ibuprofen given preemptively is not statistically different from that obtained with the preemptive use of ketorolac.[101]

In a study that evaluated the preemptive use of a 100-mg IV dose of ketoprofen in laparoscopic cholecystectomy as compared to its postoperative use, and the use of a 2-g dose of propacetamol (preemptively and postoperatively), the preemptive use of ketoprofen was shown to be opioid sparing and more effective in improving postoperative analgesia than all the other comparators.[16]

There are many other studies that have evaluated the preemptive use of the NSAIDs in various types of surgical procedures and different routes of administration and, in most of these, NSAIDs have proved to be efficacious and opioid sparing with little to no adverse effects when compared to placebo or their active comparators. There are other studies on the preemptive use of the NSAIDs that have not demonstrated a clear benefit to the adjunctive use of the NSAIDs.[19,38,151] It is also known that NSAIDs are capable of increasing bleeding time because of the effect they have on platelet aggregation, but in most of the studies that were evaluated, the risk of bleeding was not significantly different from placebos or their active comparators. However, the opioid-sparing effect of the NSAIDs and the analgesic effect of the NSAIDs were significant in most of these studies.[16,31,56,88,101,114,116] The current recommendation for the preemptive use of the NSAIDs is controversial and it is still not a universally accepted method of managing postoperative pain.

Postoperative Use of the NSAIDs

The post- and perioperative use of NSAIDs like ketorolac, diclofenac, indomethacin, piroxicam, tenoxicam, naproxen, and several others have been evaluated in several types of surgical procedures and in several dosage forms either as a single therapy compared with other analgesics or placebo or in a multimodal approach in combination with different kinds of analgesics to determine their efficacy, opiate-sparing effects, and safety.

In abdominal surgery, the postoperative use of a 120-mg dose of ketorolac, given as an IV infusion over 24 hours, as an adjunct to opiates, significantly reduced morphine requirements.[15] In patients who have undergone anterior cruciate ligament reconstruction, the use of oral ketorolac, given after a loading dose of parenteral ketorolac, was shown to have a better pain reduction with similar safety profile when compared to hydrocodone/acetaminophen.[10] In yet another study that evaluated the efficacy of oral ketorolac to that of hydrocodone/acetaminophen in patients who have undergone ambulatory arthroscopic or laparoscopic tubal ligation procedures, the investigators found no difference in the analgesic efficacy between ketorolac or hydrocodone/acetaminophen, but overall tolerability to the medications favored the ketorolac group.[159] A large trial, involving 1003 adult patients undergoing a diverse number of surgical procedures (eg, abdominal surgery, orthopedic surgery, craniofacial surgery, thoracic surgery, spinal surgery), showed that a combination of a 30-mg dose of intravenous ketorolac and 0.1 mg/kg morphine, when compared to either ketorolac or morphine alone, significantly reduced morphine requirements and opioid-related adverse effects in the immediate postoperative period.[21] In patients recovering from intraabdominal gynecologic surgery, the use of a 30-mg IV loading dose of ketorolac followed by a 60-mg dose every 6 hours or a 60-mg loading dose followed by a 30-mg dose every 6 hours were shown to be significantly effective, opioid-sparing, and safer than placebo.[141] The postoperative use of ketorolac in combination with tramadol in patients who underwent abdominal surgery was found to be as safe and effective with similar pain relief when compared to a higher dose of tramadol when used as a monotherapy in these patient population.[85]

The postoperative use of a 40-mg IV dose of tenoxicam in patients who have undergone abdominal or orthopedic surgery was shown to provide reliable analgesia, reduction in opioid consumption, and minimal adverse effects when compared to placebo.[155] In patients who have undergone cesarean section, the use of a 20-mg IV dose of tenoxicam was shown to be opioid sparing and able to potentiate opioid analgesic effects.[67] The postoperative use of a 500-mg oral dose of naproxen given every 12 hours was also shown to lead to improved analgesia in patients who have undergone cesarean delivery.[4]

In patients who underwent spinal fusion surgery and were already receiving morphine and propacetamol, the addition of a 100-mg IV dose of ketoprofen every 8 hours reduced morphine requirements and improved postoperative analgesic requirements.[7] Another study that was performed in patients who underwent thyroidectomy showed no improvement in analgesia in the concomitant use of ketoprofen with propacetamol compared to when propacetamol was administered alone.[53]

In patients undergoing cesarean section, the use of a rectal dose of 100 mg diclofenac given every 12 hours after surgery was shown to be opioid sparing with no significant adverse effects.[37] In cardiac surgery, the use of diclofenac alone or its combined use with rectal acetaminophen was shown to have significant opioid-sparing effects and improvement in pain relief.[49]

In studies that evaluated patients who underwent either major abdominal surgery or total hip arthroplasty, the postoperative use of a 100-mg rectal dose of indomethacin given every 8 hours as an adjunct to morphine was shown to provide superior analgesia than in situations when morphine was used alone.[95,122]

Even though the preemptive use of the NSAIDs remains controversial,[19,38,151] the studies that have been presented and several others (not discussed in this chapter) have demonstrated that multimodal regimens that include the NSAIDs are more likely to be effective when used preemptively and continued during the postoperative period.[19,38,51,140,151]

COX-2 Inhibitors in Perioperative Pain

The identification of the DNA sequence in human tissues for COX-1 in 1991 and COX-2 in 1992[98] led to the belief that drugs that were designed to specifically block COX-2, but not COX-1, would have anti-inflammatory properties that would be as effective and potent as the nonselective NSAIDs, but would have none of their gastrotoxic or bleeding risks.[50] It was believed that the sole inhibition of the COX-2 isoenzyme (by blocking arachidonic acid binding and prostaglandin synthesis [see Figure 21.5]) would avoid inhibition of the synthesis of gastrointestinal PG (thereby avoiding ulcers) and platelet thromboxane (thereby avoiding bleeding).[50]

These discoveries led to the development and the subsequent approval of celecoxib, rofecoxib, and valdecoxib by the US FDA in 1998, 1999, and 2001, respectively. Rofecoxib and valdecoxib have since been voluntarily withdrawn from the market due to safety concerns of an increase risk of cardiovascular events, including heart attack and stroke.[99] Currently, celecoxib is the only COX-2 inhibitor available for use in the U.S. market, but there are other COX-2 inhibitors (eg, etoricoxib, parecoxib, lumiracoxib) that are either undergoing clinical trials or in use in some parts of Europe.

Following the evolution and the general acceptance of the concept of multimodal analgesic therapy, the effort to minimize

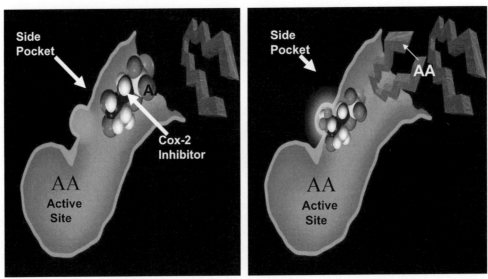

Figure 21.5. COX-2 inhibitors block aracadonic acid (AA) binding and hence PG synthesis. Figure courtesy of Drs Ian Rodger and Raymond S. Sinatra.

the risk of bleeding and bleeding complications, and the risk of gastrointestinal complications that have traditionally been associated with the use of the nonselective NSAIDs, the use of the COX-2 inhibitors became increasingly popular for use as non-opioid adjuvants for minimizing pain during the perioperative period.[55,157] There were many studies that were initiated to evaluate the efficacy of the COX-2 inhibitors, as monotherapy and in combination with other analgesics, for use in surgical pain as a preemptive, postoperative, and/or perioperative analgesic in different types of surgical procedures.[98,157,158] This section of the chapter reviews the efficacy and opiate-sparing effects of the COX-2 inhibitors (including those that are no longer on the market) based on some of the available clinical trials that compare the uses of the COX-2 inhibitors with the other nonselective NSAIDs and other analgesics. A summary of all the clinical trials that were evaluated can be seen in Tables 21.5 to 21.9.

Use of Celecoxib in Surgical Pain

Celecoxib was the first COX-2 inhibitor to be approved for use in the US market and it is currently the only COX-2 inhibitor currently available for use in the United States. This COX-2 inhibitor was approved by the US FDA for the management of the discomfort caused by ankylosing spondylitis, familial multiple polyposis syndrome, juvenile rheumatoid arthritis, osteoarthritis, acute pain, primary dysmenorrhea, and rheumatoid arthritis.[99] In this section, evidence supporting its use and tolerability in acute perioperative pain is discussed (see Table 21.6).

The role and efficacy of the preemptive use of celecoxib in surgical pain has been assessed in clinical trials that involved patients undergoing surgical procedures such as spinal fusion surgery and minor otolaryngologic (ENT) procedures.[71,123,125] In one study that evaluated the use of celecoxib in patients undergoing otolaryngologic surgery, a 200-mg oral dose of celecoxib was found to be comparable to that of a 2-g oral dose of acetaminophen; this dose was not significantly more effective than that of patients who were on placebo in that particular study.[71] However, when the 200-mg dose of celecoxib was added onto a 2-g dose of acetaminophen, it was found to work synergistically with acetaminophen in significantly reducing

pain in patients undergoing ENT procedures.[71] The preemptive use of the same dose of celecoxib was also found to be less effective than an oral dose of 50 mg rofecoxib in patients undergoing spine stabilization surgery.[125] However, in a dose-ranging study that involved ambulatory patients undergoing ENT procedures, the analgesic efficacy of celecoxib has been shown to be dose related and a 400-mg oral dose of this COX-2 inhibitor has been shown to be significantly more effective in relieving severe postoperative pain.[123] The current recommendation for the use of celecoxib as a preemptive analgesic in acute postoperative pain is 400 mg.[123]

The postsurgical utilization of celecoxib has also been assessed in dental pain models and patients undergoing ambulatory orthopedic surgery.[46,58,91] In dental pain, the postsurgical use of 200- and 400-mg oral doses of celecoxib was found to be less effective than a 50-mg dose of rofecoxib and a 400-mg oral dose of ibuprofen; celecoxib proved to be more effective than placebo in all cases.[46,91] The postoperative use of a 200-mg oral dose of celecoxib in orthopedic patients experiencing moderate to severe pain proved to have comparable analgesic efficacy with a single dose of hydrocodone/acetaminophen (10 mg/1000 mg). In that same study, a 200-mg oral dose of celecoxib taken up to 3 times a day (majority of the subjects only required twice daily doses) over a 5-day period demonstrated superior analgesia and tolerability compared with hydrocodone/acetaminophen (10 mg/1000 mg).[58]

Celecoxib has also been assessed perioperatively in patients undergoing spinal fusion surgery. In these studies, a 400-mg oral dose of celecoxib given preoperatively, followed by a postoperative dose of 200 mg every 12 hours for the next 5 days after surgery, showed improved analgesia, a reduction in chronic donor site pain 1 year after surgery, and a significant reduction in opioid use when compared to placebo.[12]

Use of Rofecoxib in Surgical Pain

The FDA initially approved rofecoxib, in 1999, for the relief of osteoarthritis, management of acute pain in adults, treatment of primary dysmenorrhea, and the relief of the signs and symptoms of rheumatoid arthritis. As discussed previously, rofecoxib was

Table 21.5: COX-2 Inhibitors[a]

Generic Name	Brand Name	COX-2/COX-1 Activity	Onset (minutes)	Duration (hours)	Dosage Forms	Suggested Doses for Acute Postoperative Pain[b]	Common Adverse Effects[c]
Celecoxib	Celebrex	8	30–50	4–8	Oral capsule: 100 mg, 200 mg, 400 mg	200–400 mg PO three times a day	Hypertension, peripheral edema, abdominal pain, diarrhea, flatulence, indigestion, nausea, back pain, dizziness, headache, insomnia, pharyngitis, rhinitis, sinusitis, upper respiratory infection, sulfonamide allergy
Rofecoxib	Vioxx	35	30–50	12–24	Oral suspension: 12.5 mg/5 mL, 25 mg/5 mL. Oral tablet: 12.5 mg, 25 mg, 50 mg	25–50 mg PO daily	Hypertension, peripheral edema, abdominal pain, diarrhea, epigastric pain, heartburn, indigestion, nausea, back pain, dizziness, headache, bronchitis, nasopharyngitis, rhinitis, sinusitis, upper respiratory infection, fatigue. Note: Rofecoxib was voluntarily withdrawn from the market because of increased risk for cardiovascular events, including heart attack and stroke
Valdecoxib	Bextra	30	30–40	6–12	Oral tablet: 10 mg, 20 mg	20–40 mg PO daily	Hypertension, peripheral edema, abdominal pain, diarrhea, flatulence, indigestion, nausea, back pain, myalgia, dizziness, headache, sinusitis, upper respiratory infection. Note: Valdecoxib was voluntarily withdrawn from the market because of safety concerns of an increased risk for cardiovascular events, including heart attack and stroke
Parecoxib	Rayzon	Prodrug of valdecoxib	10–15	6–12	Injection powder: 40 mg	Initial dose: 40 mg IV/IM, followed by 20–40 mg every 6–12 hours IV/IM; MAX = 80 mg/day	Peripheral edema, tachycardia, pruritus, ecchymosis, nausea, vomiting, abdominal pain, headache, dizziness, somnolence, rises in serum creatinine and blood urea nitrogen, pharyngitis, higher incidence of sternal wound infection, cardiovascular and cerebrovascular events
Etoricoxib	Arcoxia	106	20–30	≥24	Oral tablet: 60 mg, 90 mg, 120 mg	120 mg PO daily	Nausea, vomiting, diarrhea, heartburn, taste disturbances, decreased appetite, flatulence, headache, dizziness, fatigue, insomnia, myocardial infarction, unstable angina, ischemic stroke, and transient ischemic attacks
Lumiracoxib[a]	Prexige	–	∼38	≥12	Oral tablet: 200 mg, 400 mg	400 mg PO daily	Abdominal pain, myocardial infarction, stroke, cerebrovascular death, severe edema, GI perforation, gastroduodenal ulceration

Abbreviations: PO = by mouth; IV = intravenous; IM = intramuscular.

[a] The table was created based on references from micromedex, lexicomp drugs.

[b] The suggested doses were doses that have been used in clinical trials; they do not necessarily apply to all patients.

[c] Adverse effects reported are a list of only some of the most common adverse effects that have been associated with the drug in question; the table lists neither frequency of occurrence nor all the adverse effects.

Table 21.6: Analgesic Efficacy of Celecoxib

Reference	Dose and Route of Celecoxib (n)	Dose and Route of Comparators (n)	Type of Surgery	Duration/Timing of Dose	Outcome Measures[a]	Analgesic Efficacy Results
71	200 mg PO **C** (28)	**P** (28) 2 g PO **A** (28) 2 g PO **A** + 200 mg PO **C** (28)	ENT	30 to 60 minutes before surgery (1 dose)	1. Percentage of patients with severe postoperative pain	**A + C > C** **A + C > P** **C = P**
125	200 mg PO **C** (20)	**P** (20) 50 mg PO **R** (20)	Spinal fusion	60 minutes before surgery (1 dose)	1. Pain scores (verbal analog pain scale) 2. Morphine use during the first 24 postoperative hours	**R > C > P**
123	200 mg PO **C** (30)	**P** (30) 400 mg PO **C** (33)	ENT	30–45 minutes before surgery	1. Dose of fentanyl required for rescue analgesia in the immediate postoperative period 2. Maximum pain score before rescue with an opioid containing analgesic	400 mg PO **C** > 200 mg PO **C** > **P**
91	200 mg PO **C** (90)	**P** (45) 400 mg PO **C** (151) 50 mg PO **R** (151) 400 mg PO **I** (45)	Oral	Postoperatively as soon as moderate to severe pain	1. Total pain relief and sum of pain intensity difference score over 8 hours and 12 hours 2. Patients' global assessment of study drug at 8 h 3. Time to first dose of rescue medications	**R = I > 400 mg PO C > 200 mg PO C > P** (**R** had a longer duration of action than **I**)
46	200 mg PO **C** (74)	**P** (26) 400 mg PO three times a day **I** (74)	Oral	Postoperatively as soon as moderate to severe pain	1. Onset of pain relief 2. Time to rescue medication	**I > C > P**
58	200 mg PO **C** (141)	**P** (141) 10 mg/ 1000 mg PO **H/A** (136)	Ambulatory orthopedic surgery	Within 24 hours after surgery (single dose)	1. Time specific pain intensity difference 2. Summed pain intensity difference 3. Time to onset of analgesia 4. Time to first use of rescue medication	**C = H/A > P**
58	200 mg PO three times a day PRN **C** (185)	10 mg/1000 mg PO three times a day PRN **H/A** (181)	Ambulatory orthopedic surgery	Taken three times daily from 8 hours after first dose for up to 5 days (multidose)	1. Maximum pain intensity in the past 24 hours for days 2 to 5 2. Number of doses of study medication taken per day on days 2 to 5	**C > H/A**
126	400 mg PO preoperatively, then 200 mg PO every 12 hours postoperatively **C** (40)	**P** (40)	Spinal fusion	1 hour before the induction of anesthesia and every 12 hours after surgery for 5 days	1. Pain scores (verbal rating scale) 2. Morphine use	**C > P**
128	400 mg PO preoperatively, then 200 mg PO every 12 hours postoperatively **C** (40)	**P** (40)	Spinal fusion	1 hour before the induction of anesthesia and every 12 hours after surgery for 5 days	1. Pain scores (verbal rating scale) 2. Morphine use 3. Chronic donor site pain 1 yr after surgery	**C > P**

Abbreviations: **C** = celecoxib; **A** = acetaminophen; **P** = placebo; **H/A** = hydrocodone/acetaminophen; **I** = ibuprofen; **R** = rofecoxib; n = number of patients; PO = by mouth; PRN as needed.

[a] Not all outcome measures are included in this table.

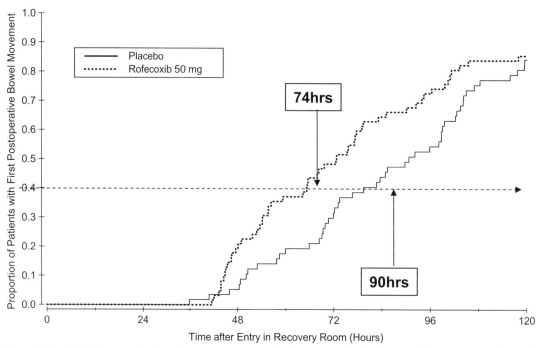

Figure 21.6. Multiple doses of rofecoxib in patients recovering from gynecologic surgery. Rofecoxib group showed a more rapid return to bowel function when compared to placebo group. Sinatra et al.[142]

voluntarily withdrawn from the U.S. market because of concerns that this COX-2 inhibitor could increase the risk of cardiovascular events.[99] Nevertheless, many clinical trials have evaluated the use of rofecoxib in the treatment of acute perioperative pain; therefore, the efficacy of rofecoxib in the treatment of surgical pain is discussed in this section, even though it is no longer in use in the United States (see Table 21.7).

The dose of rofecoxib that has been recommended for the management of acute pain is a daily oral dose of 25 to 50 mg (Table 21.7). As discussed in the previous section, the preemptive use of a 50-mg oral dose of rofecoxib was found to be more effective than a 200-mg oral dose of celecoxib in patients undergoing spine stabilization surgery.[125] The preemptive use of a 50-mg oral dose of rofecoxib has also been studied in surgical procedures like lumbar disk surgery, arthroscopic knee surgery, lower abdominal surgery, abdominal hysterectomy, urologic surgery, and ENT procedures. In ENT and lumbar disk surgery, the preemptive use of rofecoxib provided a significant analgesic benefit and reduced narcotic consumption when compared to placebo.[13,154] The preemptive use of rofecoxib was also shown to be as effective as intravenous ketorolac and more effective with longer duration of postoperative analgesia, and to require less 24-hour need for opioid use than when it is administered postoperatively in patients undergoing arthroscopic knee surgery.[80,127] In patients undergoing abdominal hysterectomy, the preoperative administration of oral rofecoxib provided a significant analgesic benefit and decreased opioid requirements in these patient populations.[76] Rofecoxib's use was also shown to provide an equivalent analgesic effect at a reduced cost when compared to that of intravenous ketoprofen after minor urologic surgical procedures.[20] In patients undergoing tonsillectomy, the preemptive use of rofecoxib in addition to a 1.5-g oral dose of paracetamol showed an analgesic benefit significantly better than when acetaminophen was used alone.[107] In patients who have undergone lower abdominal surgery, the use of a 25- to 50-mg oral sus-

pension of rofecoxib was shown to provide a morphine-sparing effect.[147]

Rofecoxib has also been studied postoperatively in patients undergoing oral surgery and bunionectomy. In oral surgery, a 50-mg oral dose of rofecoxib was found to have greater analgesic efficacy than oral doses of oxycodone/acetaminophen and acetaminophen/codeine but was less effective when compared to an oral dose of 40 mg valdecoxib.[22,23,25,27,54,82] The combination of rofecoxib with acetaminophen in patients undergoing oral surgery has also been shown to have an earlier additive analgesic effect than when rofecoxib was used alone.[22,23,25,27,54,63,82] The postoperative use of rofecoxib have also been found to be more effective than diclofenac in patients who have undergone bunionectomy.[25]

Buvanendran et al and other studies have shown that the perioperative use of 25- to 50-mg doses of rofecoxib is effective in decreasing postoperative pain and the need for analgesic rescue medications in patients undergoing knee replacement, hernia repair, spine, breast, and orthopedic surgery.[18,89,129,131] Sinatra et al[142] evaluated the perioperative use of rofecoxib on pain control and clinical outcomes in patients who underwent and are recovering from gynecologic abdominal surgery. In this study, patients who received rofecoxib required 32% fewer intravenous and oral opioids ($P = .001$) to relieve their pain from days 1 to 5, less sedation, and a 24% reduction in the rate of antiemetic requirement ($P = .37$) over the first 72 hours postsurgery. The rofecoxib group showed a more rapid return to bowel function (see Figure 21.6) with an earlier mean time to first flatus and first bowel movement compared to that of placebo.[142]

Use of Valdecoxib and Its Prodrug Parecoxib in Surgical Pain

The U.S. FDA initially approved valdecoxib in 2001 for the relief of the signs and symptoms of osteoarthritis and rheumatoid

Table 21.7: Analgesic Efficacy of Rofecoxib

Reference	Dose and Route of Rofecoxib (n)	Dose and Route of Comparators (n)	Type of Surgery	Duration/Timing of Dose	Outcome Measures[a]	Analgesic Efficacy Results
154	50 mg PO **R** (30)	**P** (30)	ENT	1 hour before surgery	1. Pain scores 2. Intraoperative fentanyl and postoperative diclofenac requirement	**R > P**
13	50 mg PO **R** (30)	**P** (30)	Lumbar disk surgery	24 hours before surgery then 30 minutes before surgery	1. Total dose of morphine requested during stay in the PACU 2. Number of patients reporting high pain scores	**R > P**
127	preincision dose of 50 mg PO **R** (20)	Postincision dose of 50 mg PO **R** (20) **P** (20)	Arthroscopic knee surgery	Preincision: 1 hour before surgery Postincision: 15 minutes after surgery	1. Pain scores 2. The time to first opioid use 3. 24-hour analgesic use	Preincision **R** > Postincision **R > P**
80	50 mg PO **R** (28)	30 mg IV **kr** (26)	Arthroscopic knee surgery	**R:** 30–60 min before surgery **Kr:** 20 min before end of surgery	1. Proportion of patients reporting pain in the PACU 2. The use of O/A 3. Pain scores 4. Patient satisfaction	**R = Kr**
76	50 mg PO **R** (30)	**P** (30)	Abdominal hysterectomy	1 hour before surgery	1. Pain scores 2. Total and increment tramadol consumption	**R > P**
20	50 mg PO **R** (34)	**Kp** (32)	Urologic surgery	**R:** 1 hour before surgery **Kp:** 24 hours after surgery	1. Need for rescue analgesic medication 2. Pain scores	**R = Kp**
107	50 mg PO **R** + 1.5 g PO **A**	**P** + 1.5 g PO **A**	Tonsillectomy	1.5 hours before surgery	1. Postoperative pain scores 2. Morphine consumption 3. Intraoperative blood loss	**R + A > P + A**
147	50 mg PO **R** (16) (oral suspension)	25 mg PO **R** (16) (oral suspension) **P** (16)	Lower abdominal surgery	1 hour before surgery	1. Effort-dependent pain 2. Postoperative morphine requirement	**R > P**
82	50 mg PO **R** (90)	5 mg/325 mg **O/A** (91) **P** (31)	Oral surgery	Postoperatively as soon as moderate to severe pain	1. Total pain relief over 6 and 4 hours 2. Patient's global assessment of treatment at 6 and 24 hours 3. Onset of analgesic effects	**P**
22	50 mg PO **R** (180)	600 mg/60 mg **A/COD** (180) **P** (30)	Oral surgery	Postoperatively as soon as moderate to severe pain	1. Total pain relief over 6 hours 2. Patient's global assessment 3. Peak pain relief 4. Duration of analgesic effects	**R > A/COD > P**
25	50 mg PO **R** (182)	600 mg/60 mg **A/COD** (180) **P** (31)	Oral surgery	Postoperatively as soon as moderate to severe pain	1. Total pain relief over 6 hours 2. Patient's global assessment 3. Peak pain relief 4. Duration of analgesic effects	**R > A/COD > P**

(continued)

Table 21.7 (*continued*)

Reference	Dose and Route of Rofecoxib (n)	Dose and Route of Comparators (n)	Type of Surgery	Duration/Timing of Dose	Outcome Measures[a]	Analgesic Efficacy Results
23	50 mg PO **R** (121)	50 mg TID **D** (**121**) **P** (63)	Oral surgery	Immediately after surgery	1. Total pain relief over 8 and 24 hours 2. Patient global assessments at 8 and 24 hours	**R > D** **R > P**
54	50 mg PO **R** (82)	40 mg PO **V** (80)	Oral surgery	Within 4 hours after surgery	1. Onset of analgesia 2. Pain intensity levels 3. Pain relief over 24 hours	**V > R > P**
28	50 mg PO **R** (101)	40 mg PO **V** (99) **P** (50)	Oral surgery	Within 4 hours after surgery	1. Onset of analgesia 2. Magnitude of analgesic effect 3. Duration of analgesia	**V > R > P**
63	50 mg PO **R** (40)	50 mg PO **R** + 1 g PO **A** (40) 1 g PO **A** (20) **P** (20)	Oral surgery	Postoperatively as soon as moderate to severe pain occurs	1. Pain intensity 2. Pain relief 3. Global evaluation score 4. Use of rescue medications	**R + A > R > A > P**
43	50 mg PO **R** (85)	100 mg PO **D** (**85**) **P** (82)	Bunionectomy	Postoperatively on study day 1 and subsequent daily doses from days 2 to 5	1. Total pain relief over 8 hours 2. Sum of pain intensity difference 3. Peak pain relief 4. Peak pain intensity difference	**R > D** **R > P**
129	25 mg PO **R** (50)	**P** (50)	Total knee arthroplasty	Daily doses starting 3 days before surgery for 5 days	1. Pain score	**R > P**
18	50 mg PO **R** (35)	**P** (35)	Total knee arthroplasty	Preoperatively 24 hours before surgery, then 1 to 2 hours before surgery, then daily doses for 5 consecutive days after surgery	1. Postsurgical analgesic consumption 2. Pain scores	**R > P**
89	50 mg PO **R** (30)	**P** (30)	Herniorrhaphy	30 to 45 minutes before surgery, then the morning of the first postoperative day	1. Pain scores 2. Need for rescue analgesics	**R > P**
131	Perioperatively: 50 mg PO **R** (180)	Postoperatively: 50 mg PO **R** (180) **P** (180)	Spine, breast or orthopedic surgery	Perioperatively: daily doses at leaset 1 hour before surgery then daily doses 3 days after surgery Postoperatively: daily doses for 3 days after surgery	1. Pain score at rest 2. Morphine consumption	**R > P**

Abbreviations: **R** = Rofecoxib; **A** = acetaminophen; **P** = placebo; **A/COD** = acetaminophen/codeine; **V** = valdecoxib; **R** = rofecoxib; **O/A** = oxycodone/acetaminophen; **D** = diclofenac; **Kr** = ketorolac; **Kp** = ketoprofen; PACU = postanesthesia care unit; PO = by mouth; PRN as needed.

[a] Not all outcome measures have been included in this table.

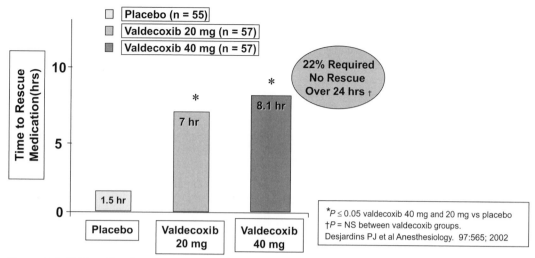

Figure 21.7. Valdecoxib prior to outpatient surgery (bunionectomy); the figure shows a reduction in opioid dose requirement in the 20- and 40-mg doses of valdecoxib, when compared to that of placebo. Desjardins et al (2002).[45]

arthritis and for the treatment of primary dysmenorrhea. The U.S. FDA did not approve its use in the management of acute pain.[55,99] Valdecoxib was, voluntarily withdrawn from the market for the same reasons as rofecoxib.[99] There are, however, many clinical trials that have evaluated the use of valdecoxib and parecoxib for the management of acute surgical pain.[18,25,28,43,89,129,131] This section of the chapter documents the evidence available on the efficacy of valdecoxib and parecoxib for use in the management of surgical pain (see Table 21.8).

Patients undergoing orthopedic surgery (bunionectomy) were randomized to receive valdecoxib (20 mg), valdecoxib (40 mg), valdecoxib (80 mg), or placebo 45–75 minutes prior to surgery. For the primary efficacy end point of time to rescue medication, patients in the valdecoxib 20 mg, 40 mg, and 80 mg groups experienced significantly better pain relief compared with placebo ($P < .05$ for all active treatments vs placebo). There was no difference between valdecoxib 20 mg, 40 mg, or 80 mg (see Figure 21.7; 80 mg data not shown) in the median time to rescue medication. Valdecoxib 40 mg and 80 mg provided significantly better pain relief as measured by pain intensity scores compared with placebo through the 24-hour study period. There was no significant difference between valdecoxib groups from the 4-hour assessment onward. By the end of the 24-hour postoperative period, a significantly greater number of patients in each of the valdecoxib groups remained in the study compared with placebo ($P < .05$ for all active treatments vs placebo).[45]

As discussed in the previous section, the postoperative use of a 50-mg oral dose of valdecoxib was shown to be a superior analgesic when compared to rofecoxib in patients undergoing oral surgery.[54] It was also shown to be equally effective, with a superior duration of analgesia, when compared to oxycodone/acetaminophen.[33] In total knee arthroplasty, valdecoxib provided an effective analgesia and was opioid sparing when used in combination with morphine.[130]

Parecoxib is a water-soluble prodrug of valdecoxib (it is rapidly hydrolyzed in the liver to valdecoxib) and it was developed for parenteral administration. Parecoxib has not been approved for use in the US market, but it is the first injectable COX-2 inhibitor approved for use in Europe for the management of moderate to severe perioperative pain. In an oral surgery pain model, the preemptive use of parecoxib sodium IV doses (20, 40,

and 80 mg) all showed superior analgesic efficacy with opioid-sparing effects over placebo with an analgesic ceiling at 40 mg.[44]

Parecoxib sodium at doses of 20–40 mg has also been shown to be effective in relieving pain and reducing opioid requirements in patients undergoing abdominal surgery and total hip arthroplasty when used postoperatively.[90,152] In oral and gynecologic laparatomy surgery, 20- to 40-mg IV doses of parecoxib sodium was shown to be as effective and better tolerated than parenteral ketorolac tromethamine in relieving postoperative pain.[12,34]

In patients undergoing laparoscopic cholecystetomy, the perioperative use of a 40-mg IV dose of parecoxib followed by a 40-mg oral dose of valdecoxib has been shown to provide greater analgesic efficacy and opioid-sparing benefits than in cases where opioids were used alone.[74]

Use of Etoricoxib in Postsurgical Pain

Although etoricoxib is not available in the US market, it is currently available and in use in some parts of Europe. This section of the chapter evaluates the use and efficacy of etoricoxib in surgical pain (see Table 21.9). In a dose-ranging study that involved patients undergoing dental procedures, a 120-mg oral dose of etoricoxib was shown to be the minimal dose required for use in patients experiencing moderate to severe acute post-operative pain.[94] The analgesic efficacy of etoricoxib has been compared with that of oxycodone/acetaminophen, codeine/acetaminophen, naproxen sodium, and ibuprofen in oral procedures and in orthopedic surgery.[24,63,92,93,121]

In patients undergoing oral surgery, the postoperative use of a 120-mg oral dose of etoricoxib was shown to provide superior analgesic effect and a more rapid and long-lasting effect with significantly lesser adverse effects in most of the studies than when compared to oral doses of 10 mg/650 mg oxycodone/acetaminophen, 400 mg ibuprofen, and 60 mg/600 mg codeine/acetaminophen.[92,93,94,96] Etoricoxib's analgesic efficacy was found to be similar to an oral dose of 550 mg of naproxen sodium.[93] In patients undergoing knee replacement surgery, the postoperative use of a 120-mg oral dose of etoricoxib was found to have similar analgesic effect as an oral dose of 1100 mg of controlled-release naproxen sodium.[121] In all the studies that

Table 21.8: Analgesic Efficacy of Valdecoxib and Parecoxib

Reference	Dose and Route of Valdecoxib or Parecoxib (n)	Dose and Route of Comparators (n)	Type of Surgery	Duration/Timing of Dose	Outcome Measures[a]	Analgesic Efficacy Results
44	40 mg PO **V** (114) 10 mg PO **V** (56) 20 mg PO **V** (113) 80 mg PO **V** (112)	**P** (112)	Oral surgery or bunionectomy	60 to 75 min before surgery	1. Time to rescue medication 2. Proportion of patients requiring rescue medication 3. Pain intensity 4. Patient's global evaluation of study medications	80 mg PO **V** = 40 mg PO **V** > 20 mg PO **V** > 10 mg PO **V** > **P**
44	20 mg IV **PAR** (56) 40 mg IV **PAR** (56) 80 mg IV **PAR** (56)	**P** (56)	Oral surgery	30 to 45 min before surgery	1. Time to rescue medication 2. Proportion of patients requiring rescue medication 3. Patients global assessment 4. Pain intensity	**PAR** > **P** (analgesic ceiling at 40 mg)
33	20 mg PO **V** (52) 40 mg PO **V** (50)	10 mg/1000 mg **O/A** (51) **P** (52)	Oral surgery	Postoperatively as soon as moderate to severe pain	1. Pain intensity difference 2. Time to onset of analgesia 3. Duration of analgesia	**V** = **O/A** > **P** (V has a superior duration of action)
130	20 mg PO twice a day **V** + morphine (69) 40 mg PO twice a day **V** + **M** (70)	**P** + **M** (70)	Orthopedic surgery	Postoperatively as soon as patient can tolerate PO meds, then every 12 hours up to 36 hours	1. Cumulative amount of morphine given over 48 hours 2. Pain intensity 3. Patient's evaluation of medication	**V** + **M** > **P** + **M**
152	20 mg IV **PAR** (19) 40 mg IV **PAR** (18)	**P** (18)	Abdominal surgery	Postoperatively at time of first analgesic request, then 12 and 24 hours after surgery	1. Postoperative opioid analgesic requirement 2. Pain scores 3. Pain relief scores	40 mg IV **PAR** = 20 mg IV **PAR** > **P**
90	20 mg IV **PAR** (67) 40 mg IV **PAR** (64)	**P** (70)	Total hip arthroplasty	Postoperatively at time of first analgesic request, then 12 and 24 hours after surgery	1. Total morphine used 2. Pain relief 3. Pain intensity 4. Time to last dose of morphine 5. Global evaluation rating	**PAR** > **P**
34	40 mg IV **PAR** (51) 40 mg IM **PAR** (50) 20 mg IV **PAR** (50) 20 mg IM **PAR** (51)	**P** (51) 60 mg IM **Kr** (51)	Oral surgery	Postoperatively as soon as moderate to severe pain	1. Time specific pain intensity difference 2. Time to onset of analgesia 3. Time to use of rescue medication	40 mg IV/IM **PAR** = **Kr** > **P**
12	20 mg IV **PAR** (39) 40 mg IV **PAR** (38)	30 mg IV **Kr** (41) 4 mg IV **M** (42)	Gynecologic surgery	Postoperatively as soon as moderate to severe pain after discontinuing PCA morphine	1. Onset of analgesia 2. Time to rescue medications 3. Pain intensity difference	40 mg IV **PAR** = 20 mg IV **PAR** = 30 mg IV **Kr** > **M** > **P**
74	Perioperatively: 40 mg IV **PAR** followed by 40 mg PO **V** (134)	**P** (129)	Laparoscopic cholecystectomy	Preoperatively: 40 mg IV **PAR** 30–45 min before induction of anesthesia then 40 mg PO **V** 6–12 h after **PAR**: Postoperatively: 40 mg PO daily for days 1–4, then 40 mg PO PRN days 5–7	1. Amount of fentanyl consumed 2. Pain scores	**PAR/V** > **P**

Abbreviations: **V** = valdexoxib; **PAR** = parecoxib; **O/A** = oxycodone/acetaminophen; **P** = placebo; **Kr** = ketorolac; **H/A** = hydrocodone/acetaminophen; **I** = ibuprofen; **R** = rofecoxib; PO = by mouth; IV = intravenous; IM = intramuscular; **M** = morphine; PRN = as needed.

[a] Not all outcome measures have been included in this table.

have been evaluated, etoricoxib has proved to have superior analgesic efficacy when compared to placebo.[24,92,93,94,121]

LUMIRACOXIB

Lumiracoxib is a novel COX-2 inhibitor that is in use in some parts of Europe. It has been described as being distinct from other COX-2 inhibitors and has been shown to demonstrate a 24 hour analgesic efficacy when taken once daily, even though it has a short mean plasma half-life of only 4 hours. Lumiracoxib will not be discussed in detail at this time because of its novel nature and also for the fact that few studies have compared its efficacy with other analgesics.[26]

SAFETY AND TOLERABILITY OF THE NSAIDS AND COX-2 INHIBITORS

Unless there is a major contraindication for the use of the NSAIDs, they are generally favored for the management of mild to moderate postoperative pain and as adjuncts for use with other analgesics in moderate to severe postoperative pain.[2,151] The lack of sedation and respiratory depression, low abuse potential, and little to no interference with bowel or bladder function constitute some of the major advantages associated with the use of the NSAIDs.[151] The NSAIDs' inhibition of the COX-1 enzyme may lead to renal toxicity, platelet dysfunction with bleeding disorders, and gastrointestinal toxicity, including serious complications such as gastroduodenal ulcerations and bleeding.[151]

As previously stated in this chapter, the COX-2 inhibitors were developed to provide safer alternatives to the nonspecific NSAIDs without compromising efficacy.[151] Most of the studies that have been evaluated have shown the efficacy of this class of drugs in postoperative pain management. However, there have been emerging controversies regarding the potential adverse cardiovascular risks associated with the use of the COX-2 inhibitors and whether these compounds truly overcome the perceived limitations associated with the use of the NSAIDs.[2,50,150,151] Even among the COX-2 inhibitors, whether the dosing, the duration of drug exposure, and relative degree of selectivity attained may contribute to varying degrees or differences in adverse effects or whether true COX-2 independent effects may be involved, is still not very well established.[64]

Hematologic and Cardiovascular Effects of the NSAIDs versus the COX-2 Inhibitors

The aggregation and hemostasis of the platelets depend on the ability of the platelets to generate thromboxane A_2 from prostaglandin H_2. Platelets are known to contain primarily the COX-1 isoform of the cyclooxygenase enzyme but no COX-2.[5] The nonselective NSAIDs, capable of inhibiting both COX-1 and COX-2, are therefore known to impair the ability of the platelets to aggregate and therefore increase the risk of bleeding.[55] However, several clinical trials have shown that the COX-2 inhibitors do not have much effect on platelets, and so they do not increase the risk of bleeding. [55]

In a study that compared the platelet function and bleeding time in elderly and nonelderly volunteers, a 40-mg twice-daily IV dose of parecoxib sodium given for 8 days compared with a 15- to 30-mg intravenous dose of ketorolac given for 5 days

was shown to have no effect on platelet function. Ketorolac, however, significantly and profoundly reduced thromboxane A_2 in all cases.[109] Other studies have also shown that the COX-2 inhibitors like valdecoxib and celecoxib have no effect on platelet function.[64,83,84,109]

Even though it has been stated and shown in some studies that the nonselective NSAIDs affects platelet aggregation and increases the risk of bleeding,[55,64,83,84,109] in most of the studies that were evaluated in this chapter and many other studies regarding the perioperative use of NSAIDs compared to placebo or other control groups, the incidence of bleeding was not significantly different from placebo or the other comparators in most of the NSAIDs that were assessed.[123] The current recommendation for the use of celecoxib as a preemptive analgesic in acute postoperative pain is 400 mg followed by 200 mg BID.[123]

Few other drugs have generated as much attention and controversy as the introduction and withdrawal from general use of rofecoxib followed by valdecoxib in the U.S. market.[6] Now, the FDA requires a black box warning stating the possibility of adverse cardiovascular effects to be labeled on all NSAIDs, including the COX-2 inhibitors. It has been hypothesized that the COX-2 inhbitors, in inhibiting COX-2 activity, causes an alteration in the balance between prostacyclin I_2 and thromboxane A_2.[6,55] Prostacyclin I_2 has been shown to be the predominant cyclooxygenase product in the endothelium.[6,55] It inhibits platelet aggregation, causes vasodilation, and prevents the proliferation of vascular smooth muscle cells.[6,55,64] Therefore, inhibiting prostacyclin I_2's effects permits unopposed thromboxane A_2 production, which potentiates platelet aggregation, thrombosis, and vasoconstriction.[6,55,64] Because data from the rofecoxib gastrointestinal (GI) outcome research study (VIGOR) was published with an 0.4% incidence of myocardial infarction in the rofecoxib group as compared to an 0.1% incidence in the naproxen group,[17,106] the discussion about the cardiovascular risk of the COX-2 inhibitors have become very popular. Several clinical, epidemiological, and metaanalysis studies have since demonstrated increased risk of myocardial infarction, heart failure, and hypertension in people who have frequently used rofecoxib in high doses.[6,64] However, the decision that led to the withdrawal of rofecoxib from the market was based on data from a 3-year clinical trial that was designed to evaluate the effect of rofecoxib in preventing the recurrence of colorectal polyps in patients with a history of colorectal adenomas. In this study, there was an increased relative risk of confirmed cardiovascular events like stroke and heart attacks beginning after 18 months of treatment in patients taking rofecoxib as compared to placebo.[133] There also have been other studies with celecoxib, parecoxib, valdecoxib, and etoricoxib that have shown an increased risk of cardiovascular events like stroke, myocardial infarction, and sometimes hypertension associated with the use of these drugs.[5,32,110,149]

There are other studies with the COX-2 inhibitors that did not show any significant increase in cardiovascular effects as compared to their comparators.[48,97,143] Some have assumed that the cardiovascular effects caused by the COX-2 inhibitors is a "class effect," whereas others have presented arguments favoring the opinion that the cardiovascular effects of the COX-2 inhibitors would most likely depend on the dosing, the duration of drug exposure, and relative degree of selectivity among the various COX-2 inhibitors.[55,64] Most of the clinical trials involving the COX-2 inhibitors and NSAIDs were not specifically designed to address the cardiovascular effects of these drugs and are underpowered; hence, most of the results are not convincing or conclusive.[55,64]

Gastrointestinal Toxicity of the NSAIDs versus the COX-2 Inhibitors

Prostaglandins play a very important role in maintaining the integrity of the GI mucosa and only COX-1 is present in the normal GI mucosa. The nonselective NSAIDs, which inhibit COX-1 as well as COX-2, are therefore known to induce GI toxicity, and their gastrotoxic effects are known to be one of the most common drug-related serious adverse events in most countries. Its been shown that one in 1200 users of nonselective NSAIDs die from GI bleed within 2 months of starting the drug, 1 of 150 users of nonselective NSAIDs will develop a bleeding complication, whereas 1 in 5 will have an asymptomatic ulcer visible on endoscopy in that time span.[55,64] It has been estimated that over 16 500 people of the over 100 000 patients in the United States with NSAID-induced GI toxicity that are hospitalized because of this adverse effects, result in mortality from GI complications.[55,64]

The selective COX-2 inhibitors promised fewer gastrotoxic effects but similar efficacy in pain control to that of the nonselective NSAIDs because of their minimum to no influence on the COX-1 isoform.[55,64] The COX-2 inhibitors have more or less held their expectation of better GI toxicity compared to that of the nonselective NSAIDs.[17,137,143] There are studies that have also shown that even with the short-term use, nonselective NSAIDs are associated with a higher incidence of GI ulcers compared with the selective COX-2 inhibitors and placebo.[60]

Renal Effects of the NSAIDs versus the COX-2 Inhibitors

It is known that prostaglandins play a very important role in renal function by affecting blood flow, glomerular filtration, natriuresis, and antidiuretic hormone secretion.[55,115] It has also been very well documented that nonselective NSAIDs inhibit the production of such prostaglandins and cause nephrotoxicity when used alone or in combination with other nephrotoxic agents. This therefore leads to renal complications like acute renal failure, hyperkalemia, water and sodium retention, nephrotic syndrome, edema, hypertension, and interstitial nephritis.[55,115]

The COX-2 enzyme has been implicated in the maintenance of renal blood flow, the mediation of renin release, and the regulation of sodium excretion.[55,115] COX-2 inhibitions may, therefore, briefly decrease urine sodium excretion and hence cause urinary retention or edema in some people and induce mild to moderate elevation of blood pressure.[55,115] In cases where considerable intravascular volume depletion and/or renal hypoperfusion have occurred, the use of agents that interfere with COX-2 activity (such as NSAIDs and COX-2 inhibitors) could severely compromise renal blood flow and glomerular filtration rates.[55,115] Patients with severe preexisting renal impairment or high-risk patients like those who are volume depleted or are at risk for severe volume depletion should avoid NSAIDs, including COX-2 inhibitor use, or should be closely monitored if they should end up using NSAIDs or COX-2 inhibitors.[55,115]

Bone and Wound Healing Effects of the NSAIDs versus the COX-2 Inhibitors

Some studies have attempted to explain the effects of the NSAIDs on bone and wound healing.[66] The mechanism by which the NSAIDs exert their effects on the bone has been attributed to several factors, including inhibition of boneforming cells at the

end-ostial bone surfaces, reduction of immune and inflammatory responses, and inhibition of prostaglandin synthesis.[87] Even though the mechanism of action by which the NSAIDs exert their effects is not fully known or understood, many have stated that the COX-2 enzyme most likely plays a significant role in bone healing. Retrospective studies and animal model studies have been used to show that NSAIDs affect bone osteogenesis and bone fusion success rates during bone repair.[41,55,59,65] In some of these studies, the investigators demonstrated that even the short-term use of the NSAIDs could significantly affect spinal fusion.[59] There is, however, an 8-week study involving the use of celecoxib, indomethacin, or placebo, in rabbit models that showed that the COX-2 inhibitors do not have a deleterious effect on the healing of intertransverse process fusions in rabbits as compared to indomethacin.[87] In summary, the effects of COX-2 inhibition on wound/bone healing are not yet fully understood.

USE OF ACETAMINOPHEN IN POSTSURGICAL PAIN

Acetaminophen was first used in medicine in 1883, but gained widespread acceptance only after 1948, when investigators concluded that another popular analgesic drug at that time, acetanilide (discovered in 1886), was toxic. Acetaminophen had already been discovered to be an active metabolite of acetanilide in 1899 (note the derivation for the trademarked version of acetaminophen: N-ace(tyl)-p-aminoph(enol)-Tylenol).[14,70,117,136] In 1955, McNeil laboratories introduced an elixir for children that contained acetaminophen as its sole active ingredient, and, since then, acetaminophen has become one of the most widely used analgesics of our time and it is currently the active ingredient in over 300 prescription and over-the-counter (OTC) medications.[14,86,117,136] Acetaminophen is known to have a well-established safety profile. At recommended doses, it is not associated with the increase incidence of nausea, vomiting, ileus, and respiratory depression associated with opioids or the deleterious gastrointestinal, hematological, renal, and cardiovascular effects associated with the NSAIDs, including the COX-2 inhibitors. Hepatotoxicity is relatively rare, but acetaminophen has been found to have a narrow therapeutic window; therefore, even a modest overdose of the drug has resulted in severe liver damage.[9,39,138] Acetaminophen also has a well-established analgesic profile with a proved record in the management of postoperative pain, alone or in combination.[27,39,118]

The WHO has recommended it to be used as the first-line medication for mild, moderate, or severe pain and to add opioids and other analgesics as the pain remains persistent or increases (see Figure 21.3). This multimodal approach has been adopted in the European Union and has effectively resulted in a 33% decrease in opioid use and its adverse effects. Intravenous acetaminophen (IV APAP) is available in the European Union since 2002 and is marketed by Bristol-Myers Squibb. Cadence Pharmaceuticals acquired the United States and Canadian rights in 2006 and is currently conducting FDA phase 3 trials.

Acetaminophen is available in oral, rectal, and intravenous formulations (see Table 21.10). There is also an intravenous prodrug of acetaminophen (propacetamol) that is rapidly hydrolyzed to acetaminophen in the blood by the enzymatic actions of esterases. This section of the chapter focuses on the various acetaminophen formulations (including propacetamol) and their analgesic efficacy in multimodal analgesia in patients undergoing surgical procedures. This section reviews the use of

Table 21.9: Analgesic Efficacy of Etoricoxib

Reference	Dose and Route of Etoricoxib (n)	Dose and Route of Comparators (n)	Type of Surgery	Duration/Timing of Dose	Outcome Measures[a]	Analgesic Efficacy Results
94	60 mg PO **E** (75) 120 mg PO **E** (76) 180 mg PO **E** (74) 240 mg PO **E** (76)	**P** (49) **I** (48)	Oral surgery	Postoperatively as soon as moderate to severe pain	1. Total pain relief over 8 hours 2. Sum of pain intensity difference over 8 hours 3. Patient's global evaluation 4. Median time to onset of pain relief 5. Peak pain relief 6. Duration of analgesia	120 mg PO **E** = 180 mg PO **E** = 240 mg PO **E** > **I** > **P**
24	120 mg PO **E** (100)	**P** (25) 10 mg/ 650 mg **O/A** (100)	Oral surgery	Postoperatively as soon as moderate to severe pain	1. Total pain relief over 6 hours 2. Patient's global assessment of response to therapy 3. Onset, peak, and duration of analgesia 4. Rescue opioid analgesic used	**E** > **O/A** > **P**
92	120 mg PO **E** (100)	10 mg/650 mg **O/A** (102) 60 mg/600 mg **COD/A** (50) **P** (50)	Oral surgery	Postoperatively as soon as moderate to severe pain	1. Overall analgesic effects 2. Total pain relief over 6 hours 3. Patient global evaluation 4. Time to onset 5. Duration of analgesic effect	**E** > **O/A E** > **COD/A E** > **P**
93	120 mg PO **E** (50)	550 mg PO **N** (51) 60 mg/600 mg **COD/A** (50) **P** (50)	Oral surgery	Postoperatively as soon as moderate to severe pain	1. Total pain relief over 8 hours 2. Sum of pain intensity difference over 8 hours 3. Patient's global evaluation 4. Onset, peak, and duration of analgesia	**E** > **P E** > **COD/A E** = N
55	120 mg PO **E** (50)	1100 mg PO **N** (51) (day 1 only) **P** (50)	Orthopedic surgery	Postoperatively as soon as moderate to severe pain	1. Total pain relief over 8 hours 2. Sum of pain intensity difference over 8 hours 3. Patient's global evaluation at 8 and 24 hours 4. Percentage of patients using rescue medication 5. Time to use of rescue medication	**E** = **N** (day 1) **E** > **P** (day 1–7)

Abbreviations: **E** = etoricoxib; **N** = naproxen; **COD/A** = codeine/acetaminophen; **P** = placebo; **O/A** = oxycodone/acetaminophen; PO = by mouth.

[a] Not all outcome measures listed in literature are included in this table.

acetaminophen in acute pain by mouth and rectal administration and parenteral infusion. For simplicity of understanding, when oral acetaminophen is discussed, the term *acetaminophen* will be used; when intravenous acetaminophen is discussed, the term *paracetamol* will be used, although pharmacologically those compounds are interchangeable – just different preparations and vehicle. It will start with meta-analyses and systematic reviews to place the more recent studies into perspective.

In 1996, de Craen et al[40] performed a systematic review of the literature in the safety and efficacy of acetaminophen/codeine combinations versus acetaminophen alone. This extensive review concluded that there was a small, but significant, difference between the analgesia of acetaminophen alone and acetaminophen with codeine, single-dose studies show a slightly increased analgesic effect when codeine is added to acetaminophen. In contrast, Hyllested et al,[70] in a qualitative review, concluded that acetaminophen is a viable alternative to the NSAIDs, especially because of the low incidence of adverse effects, and should be the preferred choice in high-risk patients. It may be appropriate to combine acetaminophen with NSAIDs, but this was not the focus of the review. In a more recent review, Remy et al[124] revisited the effects of acetaminophen on morphine side effects and consumption after major surgery in a metaanalysis of randomized controlled trials that led to the conclusion that acetaminophen combined with PCA morphine induced a significant morphine-sparing effect, but did not change the incidence of morphine-related adverse effects in the postoperative period. Since this review, a significant, multicenter, phase 2 trial that involved 150 subjects comparing paracetamol, IV propacetamol, and placebo concluded that paracetamol (1 g), when administered over a 24-hour period in patients with moderate to severe pain after orthopedic surgery, provided rapid and effective analgesia with a very favorable safety and tolerability profile.[144] Additionally, paracetamol or propacetamol reduced the need for rescue doses of PCA morphine during the initial 6-hour efficacy evaluation and over the 24-hour evaluation. Intravenous APAP also may also have contributed to fewer adverse events compared to the placebo group, challenging the meta-analysis data discussed earlier in this section.[124,144]

Oral and Rectal Acetaminophen in Postsurgical Pain

The use of oral and rectal acetaminophen in multimodal analgesic therapy has been assessed in several surgical procedures, and some of these studies have already been discussed in previous sections, so they will not be discussed in great detail in this section.

In patients who underwent open reduction and internal fixation as a result of acute limb fractures, the use of a 1-g oral dose of acetaminophen given every 4 hours (6 g/d) as an adjuvant to morphine PCA was shown to be very beneficial with significant improvement in pain scores, time on PCA, morphine consumption, and patient satisfaction when compared to the use of morphine alone.[139] In patients who have undergone abdominal hysterectomy on PCA morphine, the adjuvant use of a 1.3-g dose of acetaminophen given rectally after wound closure, then 8 and 16 hours after surgery, was compared to 50-mg rectal doses of diclofenac or placebo. In that study, the investigators were able to show that the magnitude of the morphine-sparing effect of acetaminophen suppositories were comparable to diclofenac and could be an efficacious adjuvant analgesic in controlling perioperative pain.[29] In cardiac surgery, the use of diclofenac alone or its combined use with rectal acetaminophen was also

shown to have significant opioid-sparing effects and improvement in pain relief.[49] In patients who have undergone dental surgery, the use of a single postoperative oral dose of 1.5 g of acetaminophen given in combination with a 50-mg dose of rofecoxib (a COX-2 inhibitor) was shown to improve analgesic effect compared to the use of rofecoxib alone in the early postoperative period, but after 3 hours following administration, analgesic efficacy between those analgesics were similar to, but better than, the use of paracetamol as a monotherapy in that particular group of patients.[63] Naesh et al[107] were also able to show that the preemptive use of a 1.5-g dose of acetaminophen given in combination with a 50-mg dose of rofecoxib resulted in improved analgesic benefit in the early postoperative period in patients undergoing tonsillectomy.

A systemic review of randomized controlled trials compared the efficacy and safety of paracetamol with and without codeine in postoperative pain (eg, post dental extraction, postsurgical or postpartum pain). In this analysis, the authors were able to show that the use of acetaminophen alone resulted in significant analgesic effect and, if combined with codeine, there was an additional benefit in analgesia.[105]

Thus, the evidence shows that for adults, even large doses of rectal acetaminophen may not provide any added benefit over NSAIDs. Pediatric patients may benefit from 30–40 mg/kg of rectal acetaminophen suppositories administered intraoperatively to augment postoperative analgesia. Additionally, the discomfort of placement and negative psychological effects may minimize its use, except in countries (such as Australia), where this practice may be more accepted and commonplace.

Propacetamol in Postsurgical Pain

Propacetamol is an acetaminophen prodrug that is supplied as powder to be dissolved in saline or glucose solutions immediately before infusion. It has been shown that the hydrolysis of a 2-g dose of propacetamol is equivalent to 1-g intravenous paracetamol. Propacetamol was frequently used in many European countries during the times when there was no intravenous paracetamol yet available (see Table 21.11).[103,145]

In oral surgery, the use of a 2-g intravenous dose of propacetamol infused over 15 minutes was shown to be superior over the recommended dose of 1 g in patients reporting moderate to severe pain after surgery.[75] Aken et al also showed that in patients who have undergone oral surgery, an intravenous dose of 2 g propacetamol followed by a 1-g dose has a better tolerability and a significant analgesic effect that is indistinguishable from the analgesia that is provided by a 10-mg intramuscular dose of morphine.[154] In patients who have undergone knee ligamentoplasty or spinal fusion surgery, a 2-g intravenous dose of propacetamol given every 6 hours as an adjunct to PCA morphine was shown to be useful and safe, with a significant decrease in morphine consumption.[42,65] In patients who have undergone total hip replacement or gynecologic surgery, the use of a 2-g intravenous dose of propacetamol as an adjunct to PCA morphine was found to show similar analgesic efficacy to 15–30 mg of an intravenous dose of ketorolac given postoperatively.[142,156]

Intravenous Acetaminophen (Paracetamol) in Postsurgical Pain

Based on samples of clinical trials that have been presented in the previous section, it is obvious that propacetamol has a proved efficacy and general safety when used in surgical

Table 21.10: Acetaminophen and Propacetamol Preparations and Dosing

Generic Name	Brand Name(s)[a]	Dosage Forms[b]	Suggested Doses in Acute Pain[c]	Common Adverse Effects[d]
Acetaminophen, paracetamol, APAP, others	Tylenol, others	Oral capsule: 81 mg, 160 mg, 325 mg, 500 mg, 650 mg Oral elixir: 125 mg/5 mL, 160 mg/5 mL Oral liquid: 160 mg/5 mL Oral powder for solution: 950 mg Oral solution: 325 mg/12.5 mL, 160 mg/5 mL, 81 mg/2.5 mL, 125 mg/3.75 mL, 500 mg/15 mL, 325 mg/5 mL, 500 mg/5 mL, 81 mg/0.8 mL, 160 mg/mL Oral suspension: 160 mg/5 mL, 81 mg/0.8 mL Oral syrup: 160 mg/5 mL Oral tablet: 81 mg, 160 mg, 325 mg, 500 mg, 650 mg Oral tablet, chewable: 81 mg, 160 mg Oral tablet, disintegrating: 81 mg Oral tablet, extended release: 650 mg Rectal suppository: 81 mg, 125 mg, 325 mg, 650 mg	Mild to moderate pain: 650 mg orally every 4 hours as needed, max: 4 gm/day Mild to moderate pain: 650 mg rectally every 4 to 6 hours as needed, maximum of 6 suppositories/24 hours	Rash, gastrointestinal hemorrhage, hepatotoxicity, nephrotoxicity, pneumonitis
Intravenous Paracetamol	Perfalgan, Acetavance	Injection: 10 mg/mL Solution for infusion	Acute pain: 1 gm IV every 4 hours; Max: 4 g/d	Hepatotoxicity
Propacetamol	Pro-dafalgan	No longer on the market	It has been given intramuscularly or intravenously in usual doses of 1 to 2 g every 4 hours, up to 4 times daily if necessary, to a maximum dose of 8 g daily, for the treatment of pain	Contact dermatitis

[a] Not all brand names are listed.

[b] Dosage forms are based on information given in micromedex and/or used in clinical trials.

[c] Doses for acute pain are those that have been suggested in micromedex and/or used in clinical trials. Doses listed do not necessarily apply to all patients, recommended doses in clinical practice should depend on the clinician's best judgment and should be patient specific.

[d] The table does not give a full list of all the adverse effects that have been reported, only some of the most common adverse events that have been reported in clinical trials are stated in this section.

APAP = N-acetyl-p-aminophenol (acetaminophen).

procedures either alone or as an adjunct to other analgesics. Unfortunately, it is associated with pain at the intravenous injection site or along the vein where its infusion is taking place.[103,145] There have also been reports of contact dermatitis in health care professionals handling the drug. This is important, because the drug comes in a powdered form and must be reconstituted into solution before usage; this increases the risk for contact dermatitis and the possibility for errors. Intravenous acetaminophen was recently developed, and this particular formulation does not require reconstitution, which therefore limits the risk of errors that occurs from reconstitution.[103,145] It is also not associated with injection site pain or contact dermatitis, and, in the development program, a 1-g dose of intravenous paracetamol has been shown to be equivalent to the 2-g dose of propacetamol (see Table 21.10).[103,145]

In patients who have undergone oral surgery, complaining of moderate to severe pain, the use of a 1-g intravenous dose of paracetamol was compared to that of a 2-g dose of propacetamol and with placebo. In this study, both active treatment groups showed a comparable efficacy and a significantly longer duration of analgesia and better patients's global evaluation than when compared with placebo. The incidence of local pain at

infusion sites was found to be significantly less frequent with the intravenous paracetamol group than when compared with propacetamol.[103] Sinatra et al[144] also assessed the efficacy and safety of a 1-g intravenous dose of paracetamol compared to a 2-g intravenous dose of propacetamol and with placebo in patients undergoing major orthopedic surgery. In this study, both active treatments showed comparable efficacy in pain relief, median time to morphine rescue, and morphine consumption and was significantly different from that of placebo. Drug-related adverse events, which were mostly local site reactions, was significantly lower in the intravenous paracetamol group compared to the propacetamol group (see Table 21.11).

SUMMARY AND CONCLUSION

The current recommendation for the preemptive use of the NSAIDs is controversial, and it is still not a universally accepted form of managing postoperative pain. However, the studies that have been presented have demonstrated that multimodal regimens that include the NSAIDs are more likely to be effective when used preemptively and continued during the postoperative period. There are studies that have also shown that even

Table 21.11: Use of Acetaminophen in Surgical Pain

Ref	Dose and Route of Acetaminophen (n)	Dose and Route of Comparators (n)	Type of Surgery	Duration/Timing of Dose	Outcome Measures[a]	Analgesic Efficacy Results[b]
139	1 g PO every 6 hours **A** + PCA morphine (28)	**P** + PCA morphine (33)	Orthopedic surgery	Postoperatively: 1 g acetaminophen or placebo every 4 hours for 72 hours	1. Total morphine consumption 2. Satisfaction with analgesia Pain scores 3. Duration of PCA use 4. Incidence of nausea and sedation	**A** + PCA morphine > **P** + PCA morphine
63	1 g PO **A** + 50 mg PO **R** (40) 1 gm PO **A** + **P**	**P** + 50 mg PO **R** (40)	Dental surgery	Postoperatively: immediately after moderate to severe pain	1. Pain intensity 2. Pain relief 3. Global evaluation score 4. Use of rescue medications 5. Adverse effects	1st 1.5 h: **A** + **R** > **R** > **A** After 3 hours: **A** + **R** = **R** > **A**
107	50 mg PO **R** + 1.5 g PO **A** (20)	**P** + 1.5 g PO **A** (20)	Tonsillectomy	Preoperatively: 1.5 hours before surgery	1. Postoperative pain scores 2. Morphine consumption 3. Intraoperative blood loss	**R** + **A** > **P** + **A** (early postoperative period)
29	1.3 g PR **A** + PCA morphine (24)	50 mg PR **D** + PCA morphine (20) **P** + PCA morphine (21)	Abdominal Hysterectomy	Postoperatively: immediately after wound closure, then 8 and 16 hours after surgery	1. Pain score 2. Level of sedation 3. Morphine consumption 4. Incidence of vomiting	**A** = **D** > **P**
49	100 mg PR **D** + 1 g PR **Acet** (17) 100 mg PR **D** (17)	1 g PR **Acet** (20)	Cardiac surgery	Postoperatively, 2 h after surgery: **D** – every 18 h after surgery for 24 h **Acet**- every 6 h after surgery for 24 h	5. Visual analog scale pain score 6. Morphine consumption 7. Sedation	**D** + **Acet** = **D** > **Acet**
75	2 g IV **PROP** (132) 1 g IV **PROP** (132)	**P** (33)	Dental surgery	Postoperatively: immediately after patients report moderate to severe pain	1. Pain intensity 2. Pain relief scores 3. Time to request rescue medications 4. Adverse effects	2 gm IV **PROP** > 1 gm IV **PROP** (no significant difference in adverse effects)
68	2 g IV **PROP** followed by 1 g IV (31)	10 mg IM morphine (30) **P** (34)	Dental surgery	Postoperatively: immediately after patients report moderate to severe pain	1. Pain intensity score 2. Pain intensity difference 3. Pain relief scores 4. Proportion of patients requiring rescue medications 5. Time to request rescue medications	**PROP** > morphine > **P**
42	2 g every 6 h IV **PROP** + PCA morphine (30)	**P** + PCA morphine (30)	Orthopedic surgery	Postoperatively: immediately after surgery	1. Pain scores 2. Morphine consumption 3. Global efficacy score 4. Adverse effects	**PROP** > **P**
65	2 g every 6 h IV **PROP** for 3 days + PCA morphine (21)	**P** (21)	Spinal fusion surgery	Postoperatively: every 6 hours for 3 days after surgery	1. Pain relief 2. Opioid analgesic consumption 3. Degree of sedation	**PROP** > **P**
142	2 g IV **PROP** + PCA morphine (57)	15 mg IV **K** + PCA morphine (28) 30 mg IV **K** + PCA morphine (27) **P** (52)	Orthopedic surgery	Postoperatively: on the first morning after major joint replacement surgery	1. Pain intensity difference 2. Pain relief intensity difference 3. Time to onset of analgesia 4. Opioid consumption	**PROP** = **K** > **P**
156	2 gm IV **PROP** + PCA morphine (87)	30 mg IV **K** + PCA morphine (89)	Gynecologic surgery	Postoperatively: at tracheal extubation and 6 hours postextubation	1. Total dose of morphine 2. Pain intensity 3. Global efficacy 4. Adverse effects	**PROP** = **K** (propacetamol had excellent tolerability results)
103	1 g IV **PARA** (51)	2 g IV **PROP** (51) **P** (50)	Oral surgery	Postoperatively: immediately after patients report moderate to severe pain	1. Pain relief 2. Maximum pain relief 3. Pain scores 4. Adverse effects	**PARA** = **PROP** > **P**
145	1 g IV **PARA** (49)	2 g IV **PROP** (50) **P** (52)	Major orthopedic surgery	Postoperatively: immediately after patients report moderate to severe pain at 6-hour intervals	1. Pain intensity 2. Pain relief 3. Morphine use 4. Adverse effects	**PARA** = **PROP** > **P**

Abbreviations: **A** or **Acet** = oral paracetamol or acetaminophen; **P** = Placebo; PCA = patient-controlled analgesia; **R** = rofecoxib; PR = per rectum; **D** = diclofenac; **PROP** = propacetamol; PO = orally; IV = intravenous injection; IM = intramuscular injection; **K** = ketorolac; **PARA** = intravenous acetaminophen or paracetamol.

[a] Not all outcome measures listed in literature are included in this table.

[b] Analgesic efficacy results presented in table are a general summary of author(s)' conclusions.

[c] Data taken from references 17, 20, 21, 27, 50, 51, 89.

with short-term use, nonselective NSAIDs are associated with a higher incidence of GI ulcers compared with the selective COX-2 inhibitors and placebo. Patients with severe preexisting renal impairment, or high-risk patients like those who are volume depleted or are at risk for severe volume depletion, should avoid NSAIDs, including COX-2 inhibitor use, or should be closely monitored if they should be treated with NSAIDs or COX-2 inhibitors. The effects of COX-2 inhibition on wound/bone healing are not yet fully understood. Integrating these conclusions with the available data leads to the following recommendations: use of celecoxib as a preemptive analgesic in acute postoperative pain, at the dose of 400 mg. This should be continued postoperatively for up to a week. With regard to adverse effects, most of the clinical trials involving the COX-2 inhibitors and NSAIDs were not specifically designed to address the cardiovascular effects of these drugs and are underpowered; hence, most of the results pertaining to these adverse effects are not convincing or conclusive. Patients with suspected cardiac or renal disease should any avoid long-term use of these drugs without intensive medical monitoring. Also, COX-2 inhibitors should not be assumed to have antiplatelet effects, so all deep vein thrombosis (DVT)/atrial fibrillation prophylaxis must be continued with other medications.

This chapter reviewed the relevant pharmacology and clinical trials validating the use of NSAIDs, COX-2 inhibitors, and APAP in perioperative pain. Each class and each particular drug within the class has advantages and disadvantages, but the overriding themes of multimodal therapy, to minimize the adverse effects of opioids, and preemptive analgesia, to minimize the needed doses of opioids, cannot be disputed. The challenge is in the exact regimen to use in a particular case. One strategy is to consider use of the NSAIDs or COX-2 inhibitors preoperatively, because most of these are only available in an oral preparation. These can be continued postoperatively once oral intake has resumed. To this can be added intravenous paracetamol (available in the EU and application applied for in United States), perioperatively, maximizing the dose to 4 g per 24 hours. It can be discontinued when the patient can again take oral medications. Clearly, caution must be exercised in the use of the NSAIDs or COX-2 inhibiors in patients with medical issue that obviate their use, and the same in patients with severe liver disease for the APAP. However, the large majority of patients would experience relief of pain with less opioid use and fewer adverse effects of the opioids. Additional concerns of postoperative bleeding, gastrointestinal adverse effects, and the complicating factors surrounding need for DVT prophylaxis and prevention of pulmonary embolism makes this equation challenging. However, the fact that there is a probability that NSAIDs might have some effects on platelets may make some in this class ideal for pain control and DVT prophylaxis, although this has yet to be studied in large studies designed to look at this specific issue. This may be an advantage over the COX-2 inhibitors, in that they possess little or no platelet aggregation blocking effects and may require separate anti–deep vein thrombosis and antipulmonary embolism therapy that is already prescribed with separate classes of drugs.

Future work should focus on use of the NSAIDs and possibly COX-2 inhibitors for perioperative pain, minimizing the use of opioids and benefiting from the possibilities of DVT prophylaxis (or, in the case of COX-2 inhibitors, allowing for separate noninterfering prophylaxis). APAP, with an intravenous form available, may provide immediate perioperative alternatives to opioids and provide pain relief with minimal adverse events, where

other forms of sedation are required, such as endoscopy, minor dermatologic/plastics procedures, dental procedures, pediatric procedures, and emergency settings, like sprained ankle. In summary, the 3 classes of drugs may in fact serve to make the WHO pyramid, with use of acetaminophen at all levels of pain, with addition of opioids, into a multimodal approach, using NSAIDs and COX-2 inhibitors when patients can take oral medications, and adding the paracetamol for periods when patients are unable to tolerate oral medications. All would likely minimize the perioperative use of opioids and their multiple adverse events.

REFERENCES

1. Akca T, Colak T. The effect of preoperative intravenous use of tenoxicam: a prospective, double-blind, placebo-controlled study. *J Invest Surg.* 2004;17:333–338.
2. Agency for Health Care Policy and Research. *Acute Pain Management: Operative for Medial Procedures and Trauma.* Rockville, MD: US Department of Health and Human Services; 1992. Publication 92-0032.
3. Alexander R, El-Moalem HE, Gan TJ. Comparison of the morphine-sparing effects of diclofenac sodium and ketorolac tromethamine after major orthopedic surgery. *J Clin Anesth.* 2002;14(3):187–192.
4. Angle PJ, Halpern SH, Leighton BL, et al. A randomized controlled trial examining the effect of naproxen on analgesia during the second day after delivery. *Anesth Analg.* 2002;95:741–745.
5. Arber N, Eagle CJ, Spicak J, et al. Celecoxib for the prevention of colorectal adenomatous polyps. *N Engl J Med.* 2006;355:885–895.
6. Armstrong PW. Balancing the cyclooxygenase portfolio. *Cal Med Assn J.* 2006;174(11):1581–1582.
7. Aubrun F, Langeron O, Heitz D, et al. Randomized, placebo-controlled study of the postoperative analgesic effects of ketoprofen after spinal fusion surgery. *Acta Anesthesiol Scand.* 2000;44:934–939.
8. Bandolier: Independent evidence-based healthcare. www.ebandolier.com. Accessed 1/7/2007.
9. Bannwarth B, Pehourcq F. Pharmacologic rationale for the clinical use of paracetamol: pharmacokinetic and pharmacodynamic issues. *Drugs.* 2003;63:2–5.
10. Barber FA, Gladu DE. Comparison of oral ketorolac and hydrocodone for pain relief after cruciate ligament reconstruction. *J Arthros Rel Surg.* 1998;14(6):605–612.
11. Barden J, Edwards J, Moore RA, et al. Single dose oral diclofenac for postoperative pain. *Cochrane Database Syst Rev.* 2004;2:CD004308.
12. Barton SF, Langeland FF, Snabes MC, et al. Efficacy and safety of intravenous parecoxib sodium in relieving acute postoperative pain following gynecologic laparatomy surgery. *Anesthesiology.* 2002;97:306–314.
13. Bekker A, Cooper PR, Frempong-Boadu A, et al. Evaluation of preoperative administration of the cyclooxygenase-2 inhibitor rofecoxib for the treatment of postoperative pain after lumbar disc surgery. *Neurosurg.* 2002;50:1053–1058.
14. Bertolini A, Ferrari A, Ottani A, et al. Paracetamol: new vistas of an old drug. *CNS Drug Rev.* 2006;12(3–4):250–275.
15. Blackburn A, Stevens JD, Wheatley RG, et al. Balanced analgesia with intravenous ketorolac and patient-controlled morphine following lower abdominal surgery. *J Clin Anesth.* 1995;7:103–108.
16. Boccara G, Chaumeron A, Pouzeratte Y, et al. The preoperative administration of ketoprofen improves analgesia after laparoscopic cholecystectomy in comparison with propacetamol or postoperative ketoprofen. *Br J Anaesth.* 2005;94:347–351.

17. Bombardier C, Laine L, Reicin A, et al. Comparison of upper gastrointestinal toxicity of rofecoxib and naproxen in patients with rheumatoid arthritis. VIGOR Study Group. *New Engl J Med.* 2000;343:1520–1528.

18. Buvanendran A, Kroin JS, Tuman KJ, et al. Effects of perioperative administration of a selective cyclooxygenase 2 inhibitor on pain management and recovery of function after knee replacement. *JAMA.* 2003;290:2411–2418.

19. Cabell CA. Does ketorolac produce preemptive analgesic effects in laparoscopic ambulatory patients? *J Am Assn Nurse Anesth.* 2000;68:343–349.

20. Cabrera MC, Schmied S, Derderian T, et al. Efficacy of oral rofecoxib versus intravenous ketoprofen as an adjunct to PCA morphine after urologic surgery. *Acta Anesth Scand.* 2004;48:1190–1193.

21. Cepeda MS, Carr DB, Miranda N, et al. Comparison of morphine, ketorolac, and their combination for postoperative pain: results from a large randomized, double blind trial. *Anesthesiology.* 2005;103:1225–1232.

22. Chang DJ, Bird SR, Bohidar NR, et al. "Analgesic efficacy of rofecoxib compared with codeine/ acetaminophen using a model of acute dental pain." *Oral Surg Oral Med Oral Pathol Oral Radiol Endod.* 2005;100:E74–E80.

23. Chang DJ, Desjardins PJ, Chen E, et al. Comparison of the analgesic efficacy of rofecoxib and enteric-coated diclofenac sodium in the treatment of postoperative dental pain: a randomized, placebo-controlled clinical trial. *Clin Ther.* 2002;24:490–503.

24. Chang DJ, Desjardins PJ, King TR, et al. The analgesic efficacy of etoricoxib compared with oxycodone/acetaminophen in acute postoperative pain model: a randomized, double-blind clinical trial. *Anesth Analg.* 2004;99:807–815.

25. Chang DJ, Fricke JR, Bird SR, et al. Rofecoxib versus codeine/ acetaminophen in postoperative dental pain: a double-blind, randomized, placebo- and active comparator-controlled trial. *Clin Ther.* 2001;23:1446–1455.

26. Chan VW, Clark AJ, Davis JC, et al. The post-operative analgesic efficacy and tolerability of lumiracoxib compared with placebo and naproxen after total knee or hip arthroplasty. *Acta Anesthesiol Scand.* 2005;49:1491–1500.

27. Charlton JE. Treatment of postoperative pain. In: Giamberardino MA, ed. *Pain 2002 – An Updated Review: Refresher Course Syllabus.* Seattle, WA: IASP Press; 2002:351–355.

28. Christensen KS, Cawkwell GD. Valdecoxib versus rofecoxib in acute postsurgical pain: results of a randomized controlled trial. *J Pain Symptom Manage.* 2004;27:460–470.

29. Cobby TF, Crighton IM, Kyriakides K, et al. Rectal paracetamol has a significant morphine-sparing effect after hysterectomy. *Br J Anaesth.* 1999;83(2):253–256.

30. Code E, Yip R, Rooney M, et al. Preoperative naproxen sodium reduces postoperative pain following arthroscopic knee surgery. *Can J Anaesth.* 1994;41(2):98–101.

31. Comfort KV, Code WE, Rooney ME, et al. Naproxen premedictation reduces tubal ligation pain. *Can J Anaesth.* 1991;39(4):349–352.

32. Curtis SP, Ng J, Yu Q, et al. Renal effects of etoricoxib and comparator nonsteroidal anti-inflammatory drugs in clinical trials. *Clin Ther.* 2004;26:70–83.

33. Daniels SE, Desjardins PJ, Talwalker S, et al. The analgesic efficacy of valdecoxib vs. oxycodone/acetaminophen after oral surgery. *J Am Dent Assoc.* 2002;133:611–621.

34. Daniels SE, Grossman EH, Kuss ME, et al. A double blind, randomized comparison of intramuscularly and intravenously administered parecoxib sodium versus ketorolac and placebo in a post-oral surgery pain model. *Clin Ther.* 2001;23:1018–1031.

35. Dahl JB, Kehlet H. Non-steroidal anti-inflammatory drugs: rationale for use in severe postoperative pain. *Br J Anaesth.* 1991;66:703–712.

36. Dahl V, Hagen IE, Sveen AM, et al. High-dose diclofenac for postoperative analgesia after elective cesarean section in regional anaesthesia. *Int J Obst Anesth.* 2002;11:91–94.

37. Dahl V, Raeder JC. Non-opioid postoperative analgesia. *Acta Anaesthesiol Scand.* 2000;44:1191–1203.

38. Danou F, Praskeva A, Vassilakopoulos T, et al. The analgesic efficacy of intravenous tenoxicam as an adjunct to patient-controlled analgesia in total abdominal hysterectomy. *Anesth Analg.* 2000;90:267–276.

39. Day RO, Graham GG, Whelton A. The position of paracetamol in the world of analgesics. *Am J Ther.* 2000;7:51–54.

40. de Craen AJ, Di Giulio G, Lampe-Schoenmaeckers JE, et al. Analgesic efficacy and safety of paracetamol-codeine combinations versus paracetamol alone: a systemic review. *Br Med J.* 1996;313:321–325.

41. Deguchi M, Rapoff A, Zdebick T. Posterolateral fusion for isthmic spondylolisthesis in adults: a study of fusion rate and clinical results. *J Spinal Disord.* 1998;11:459–464.

42. Delbos A, Boccard E. The morphine-sparing effect of propacetamol in orthopedic postoperative pain. *J Pain Symptom Manage.* 1995;10:279–286.

43. Desjardins PJ, Black PM, Daniels S, et al. A randomized controlled study comparing rofecoxib, diclofenac sodium, and placebo in post-bunionectomy pain. *Curr Med Res Opin.* 2004;20(10):1523–1537.

44. Desjardins PJ, Grossman EH, Kuss ME, et al. The injectable cyclooxygenase-2 specific inhibitor parecoxib sodium has analgesic efficacy when administered preoperatively. *Anesth Analg.* 2001;93:721–727.

45. Desjardins PJ, Shu VS, Recker DP, et al. A single preoperative oral dose of valdecoxib, a new cyclooxygenase-2 specific inhibitor, relieves post-oral surgery of bunionectomy pain. *Anesthesiology.* 2002;97:565–573.

46. Doyle G, Jayawardena S, Ashraf E, et al. Efficacy and tolerability of nonprescription ibuprofen versus celecoxib for dental pain. *J Clin Pharm.* 2002;42:912–919.

47. Edwards JE, Loke YK, Moore RA, et al. Single dose piroxicam for acute post-operative pain. *Cochrane Database Syst Rev.* 2000;4:CD002762.

48. Farkough ME, Kirshner H, Harrington RA, et al. Comparison of lumiracoxib with naproxen and ibuprofen in the therapeutic arthritis research and cardiovascular outcome: randomized controlled trial. *Lancet.* 2004:364–384.

49. Fayaz MK, Abel RJ, Pugh SC, et al. Opioid-sparing effects of diclofenac and paracetamol lead to improved outcomes after cardiac surgery. *J Cardiothorac Vasc Anesth.* 2004;18(6):742–747.

50. Feldman M, Mcmahon A. Do cyclooxygenase-2 inhibitors provide benefits similar to those of traditional NSAIDs, with less gastrointestinal toxicity? *Ann Intern Med.* 2000;132:134–143.

51. Filos KS, Vagianos CE. Pre-emptive analgesia: how important is it in clinical reality? *Eur Surg Res.* 1999;31:122–132.

52. Fletcher D, Zetlaoui P, Monin S, et al. Influence of timing on the analgesic effect of intravenous ketorolac after orthopedic surgery. *Pain.* 1995;61 (1995):291–297.

53. Fourcade O, Sanchez P, Kern D, et al. Propacetamol and ketoprofen after thyroidectomy. *Eur J Anaesthesiol.* 2005;22:373–377.

54. Fricke J, Varkalis J, Zwillich S, et al. Valdecoxib is more efficacious than rofecoxib in relieving pain associated with oral surgery. *Am J Ther.* 2002;9:89–97.

55. Gajraj NM, Joshi GP. Role of cyclooxygenase-2 inhibitors in postoperative pain management. *Anesthesiology Clin N Am.* 2005;23:49–72.

56. Gillberg LE, Harsten AS, Stahl LB. Preoperative diclofenac sodium reduces post-laparoscopy pain. *Can J Anaesth.* 1993;40(5):406–408.

57. Gilron I, Milne B, Hong M. Cyclooxygenase-2 inhibitors in postoperative pain management: current evidence and future decisions. *Anesthesiology.* 2003;99:1198–1208.

58. Gimbel JS, Brugger A, Zhao W, et al. Efficacy and tolerability of celecoxib versus hydrocodone/acetaminophen in the treatment of pain after ambulatory orthopedic surgery in adults. *Clin Ther.* 2001;23:228–241.

59. Glassman SD, Rose SM, Dimar JR, et al. The effect of postoperative non-steroidal anti-inflammatory drug administration on spinal fusion. *Spine.* 1998;23:834–838.

60. Goldstein J, Kivitz A, Verburg K, et al. A comparison of the upper gastrointestinal mucosal effects of valdecoxib, naproxen, and placebo in elderly subjects. *Aliment Pharmacol Ther.* 2003;18:125–132.

61. Gotcche PC. Extracts from clinical evidence: non-steroidal anti-inflammatory drugs. *Br Med J.* 2000;320:1058–1061.

62. Gramke H, Petry JJ, Durieux ME, et al. Sublingual piroxicam for postoperative analgesia: preoperative versus postoperative administration: a randomized, double-blind study. *Anesth Analg.* 2006;102:755–758.

63. Haglund B, Von Bultzingslowen I. Combining paracetamol with a selective cyclooxygenase-2 inhibitor for acute pain relief after third molar surgery: a randomized, double-blind, placebo-controlled study. *Eur J Oral Sci.* 2006;114:293–301.

64. Hermann M, Ruschitzka F. Cardiovascular risk of cyclooxygenase-2 inhibitors and non-steroidal anti-inflammatory drugs. *Ann Med.* 2007;39:18–27.

65. Hernandez-Palazon J, Tortosa JA, Martinez-Lage JF, et al. Intravenous administration of propacetamol reduces morphine consumption after spinal fusion surgery. *Anesth Analg.* 2001;92:1473–1476.

66. Ho M, Chang j, Wang Y, et al. Anti-inflammatory drug effects on bone repair and remodeling in rabbits. *Clin Orthop.* 1995;13:270–278.

67. Hsu H-W, Cheng Y-J, Chen L-K, et al. Differential analgesic effect of tenoxicam on wound pain and uterine cramping pain after cesarean section. *Clin J Pain.* 2003;19:55–58.

68. Hugo V, Thys L, Veekman L, et al. Assessing analgesia in single and repeated administration of paracetamol for postoperative pain: comparison with morphine after dental surgery. *Anesth Analg.* 2004;98:159–165.

69. Hutchison GL, Crofts SL, Gray IG. Preoperative piroxicam for postoperative analgesia in dental surgery. *Br J Anaesth.* 1990;65:500–503.

70. Hyllested M, Jones S, Pedersen JL, et al. Comparative effect of paracetamol, NSAIDs or their combination in postoperative pain management: a qualitative review. *Br J Anaesth.* (2002) 88(2):199–214.

71. Issioui T, Klein KW, White PF, et al. The efficacy of premedication with celecoxib and acetaminophen in preventing pain after otolaryngologic surgery. *Anesth Analg.* 2002;94:1188–1193.

72. Jin F, Chung F. Multimodal analgesia for post-operative pain control. *J Clin Anesth.* 2001;13:524–531.

73. Joshi GP, Viscusi ER, Gan TJ, et al. Effective treatment of laparoscopic cholecystectomy pain with intravenous followed by oral COX-2 specific inhibitor. *Anesth Analg.* 2004;98:336–342.

74. Joshi GP, White PF. Management of acute and postoperative pain. *Curr Opin Anaesthesiol.* 2001;14:417–421.

75. Juhl GI, Norholt SE, Tonnesen E, et al. Analgesic efficacy and safety of intravenous paracetamol (acetaminophen) administered as a 2 gm starting dose following third molar surgery. *Eur J Pain.* 2006;10:371–377.

76. Karamanlioglu B, Turan A, Memis D, et al. Preoperative oral rofecoxib reduces postoperative pain and tramadol consumption in patients after abdominal hysterectomy. *Anesth Analg.* 2004;98:1039–1043.

77. Kehlet H, Jorgen DB. The value of multimodal or balanced analgesia in postoperative pain treatment. *Anesth Analg.* 1993;77:1048–1056.

78. Kelly DJ, Ahmad M, Brull JS. Preemptive analgesia I. Physiological pathways and pharmacological modalities. *Can J Anaesth.* 2001;48(10):1000–1010.

79. Kelly DJ, Ahmad M, Brull S. Preemptive analgesia II: recent advances and current trends. *Can J Anaesth.* 2001;48(11):1091–1101.

80. Kim JT, Sherman O, Cuff G, et al. A double-blind prospective comparison of rofecoxib vs ketorolac in reducing postoperative pain after arthroscopic knee surgery. *J Clin Anesth.* 2005;17:439–443.

81. Kissin I. Preemptive analgesia. *Anesthesiology.* 2000;93(4):1138–1143.

82. Korn S, Vassil TC, Kotey PN, et al. Comparison of rofecoxib and oxycodone plus acetaminophen in the treatment of acute pain: a randomized, double-blind, placebo-controlled study in patients with moderate to severe postoperative pain in the third molar extraction model. *Clin Ther.* 2004;26:769–778.

83. Leese PT, Hubbard RC, Karim A, et al. Effects of celecoxib, a novel cyclooxygenase-2 inhibitor, on platelet function in healthy adults: a randomized controlled trial. *J Clin Pharmacol.* 2000;40(2):124–132.

84. Leese PT, Recker DP, Kent JD. The COX-2 selective inhibitor, valdecoxib does not impair platelet function: results of a randomized controlled trial. *J Clin Pharmacol.* 2003;43(5):504–513.

85. Lepri A, Sia S, Catinelli S, et al. Patient controlled analgesia with tramadol versus tramadol plus ketorolac. *Minerva Anestesiol.* 2006;72:59–67.

86. Loder E. Fixed drug combination for the acute treatment of migraine: place in therapy. *CNS Drugs.* 2005;19(9):769–784.

87. Long J, Lewis S, Kuklo T, et al. The effects of cyclooxygenase-2 inhibitors on spinal fusion. *J Bone Joint Surg Am.* 2002;84:1763–1768.

88. Lu C, Liu J, Lee M, et al. Preoperative cotreatment with dextromethorphan and ketorolac provides an enhancement of pain relief after laparoscopic-assisted vaginal hysterectomy. *Clin J Pain.* 2006;22:799–804.

89. Ma H, Tang J, White PF, et al. Perioperative rofecoxib improves early recovery after outpatient herniorrhaphy. *Anesth Analg.* 2004;98:970–975.

90. Malan TP Jr, Marsh G, Hakki SI, et al. Parecoxib sodium, a parenteral cyclooxygenase-2 inhibitor, improves morphine analgesia and is opioid sparing following total hip arthroplasty. *Anesthesiology.* 2003;98:950–956.

91. Malmstrom K, Daniels S, Kotey P, et al. Comparison of rofecoxib and celecoxib, two cyclooxygenase-2 inhibitors, in postoperative dental pain: a randomized, placebo- and active comparator- controlled clinical trial. *Clin Ther.* 1999;21:1653–1663.

92. Malmstrom K, Ang J, Fricke JR, et al. The analgesic efficacy of etoricoxib relative to that of two opioid-acetaminophen analgesics: a randomized controlled single-dose study in acute dental impaction pain. *Curr Med Res Opin.* 2005;21(1):141–149.

93. Malmstrom K, Kotey P, Coughlin H, et al. A randomized double-blind, parallel-group study comparing the analgesic effect of etoricoxib to placebo, naproxen sodium, and acetaminophen with codeine using the dental impaction model. *Clin J Pain.* 2004;20:147–155.

94. Malmstrom K, Sapre A, Couglin H, et al. Etoricoxib in acute pain associated with dental surgery: a randomized, double blind, placebo and active comparator-controlled dose-ranging study. *Clin Ther.* 2004;26(5):667–669.

95. Mason L, Edwards J, Moore RA, et al. Single dose indomethacin for the treatment of acute post-operative pain. *Cochrane Database Syst Rev.* 2004;18:CD004308.

96. Mason L, Edwards JE, Moore RA, et al. Single dose naproxen and naproxen sodium for acute post-operative pain. *Cochrane Database Syst Rev.* 2004;18(4):CD004308.

97. Matsumoto AK, Melian A, Mandel DR, et al. A randomized, controlled, clinical trial of etoricoxib in the treatment of rheumatoid arthritis. *J Rheumatol.* 2002;29:1623–1630.

98. McCrory CR, Lindahl SG. Cyclooxygenase inhibition for postoperative analgesia. *Anesth Analg.* 2002;95:169–176.

99. Vioxx [package insert]. Whitehouse Station, NJ: Merck & Co. Inc.; 2003.

100. Michaloliakou C, Chung F, Sharma S. Preoperative multimodal analgesia facilitates recovery after ambulatory laparoscopic cholecystectomy. *Anesth Analg.* 1996;82:44–51.

101. Mixter CG, Meeker LD, Gavin TJ. Preemptive pain control in patients having laparoscopic hernia repair: a comparison of ketorolac and ibuprofen. *Arch Surg.* 1998;133:432–437.

102. Moiniche S, Kehlet H, Dahl J. A qualitative and quantitative systematic review of preemptive analgesia for postoperative pain relief: the role of timing of analgesia. *Anesthesiology.* 2002;96:725–741.

103. Moller LP, Juhl GI, Payen-Chanpenois C, et al. Intravenous acetaminophen (paracetamol): comparable analgesic efficacy, but better local safety than its prodrug, propacetamol, for postoperative pain after third molar surgery. *Anesth Analg.* 2005;101:90–96.

104. Moore A, Collins S, Carroll D, et al. Paracetamol with and without codeine in acute pain: a quantitative systemic review. *Pain.* 1997;70:193–201.

105. Moore A, McQuay H. *Bandoliers's Little Book of Making Sense of the Medical Evidence.* New York, NY: Oxford University Press; 2006.

106. Mukherjee D, Nissen S, Topol E. Risk of cardiovascular events associated with selective COX-2 inhibitors. *JAMA.* 2001;286:954–959.

107. Naesh O, Niles LA, Gilbert JG, et al. A randomized, placebo-controlled study of rofecoxib with paracetamol in early post-tonsillectomy pain in adults. *Eur J Anaesthesiol.* 2005;22:768–773.

108. Norman PH, Daley MD, Lindsey RW. Preemptive analgesic effects of ketorolac in ankle fracture surgery. *Anesthesiology.* 2001;94(4):1–7.

109. Noveck R, Laurent A, Kuss M, et al. The COX-2 specific inhibitor, parecoxib sodium, does not impair platelet function in healthy elderly and non-elderly individuals. *Clin Drug Invest.* 2001;211:465–476.

110. Nussmeir NA, Whelton AA, Brown MT, et al. Complications of the COX-2 inhibitors parecoxib and valdecoxib after cardiac surgery. *New Engl J Med.* 2005;352:1081–1091.

111. O'Hanlon JJ, Muldoon T, Lowry D, et al. Improved postoperative analgesia with preoperative piroxicam. *Can J Anaesth.* 1996;43(2):102–105.

112. Ong CK, Lirk P, Seymour R, et al. The efficacy of preemptive analgesia for acute postoperative pain management: a meta-analysis. *Anesth Analg.* 2005;100:757–773.

113. Ong KS, Tan JM. Preoperative intravenous tramadol versus ketorolac for preventing postoperative pain after third molar surgery. *Int J Oral Maxillofac Surg.* 2004;33:274–278.

114. Ong KS, Seymour RA, Chen FG, et al. Preoperative ketorolac has a preemptive effect for postoperative third molar surgical pain. *Int J Oral Maxillofac Surg.* 2004;33:771–776.

115. Perazella M, Tray K. Selective cyclooxygenase-2 inhibitors: a pattern of nephrotoxicity similar to traditional non-steroidal anti-inflammatory drugs. *Am J Med.* 2001;111:64–69.

116. Plummer JL, Owen H, Ilsley AH, et al. Sustained-release ibuprofen as an adjunct to morphine patient-controlled analgesia. *Anesth Analg.* 1996;83:92–96.

117. Prescott LF. Paracetamol: past, present, and future. *Am J Ther.* 2000;7(2):143–147.

118. Prescott LF. Pharmacological actions and therapeutic use of paracetamol. In: *Paracetamol (Acetaminophen): A Critical Bibliographic Review.* London: Taylor & Francis; 1996:197–539.

119. Rautoma P, Santanen U, Avela R, et al. Diclofenac premedication but not intra-articular ropivacaine alleviates pain following daycase knee arthroscopy. *Can J Anesth.* 2000;47(3):220–224.

120. Rautoma P, Santanen U, Perhoniemi V, et al. Preoperative diclofenac is a useful adjunct to spinal anesthesia for day-case varicose vein repair. *Can J Anesth.* 2001;48(7):661–664.

121. Rasmussen GL, Malmstrom K, Bourne MH, et al. Etoricoxib provides analgesic efficacy to patients after knee or hip replacement surgery: a randomized, double-blind, placebo controlled study. *Anesth Analg.* 2005;101:1104–1111.

122. Reasbeck PG, Rice ML, Reasbeck JC. Double-blind controlled trial of indomethacin as an adjunct to narcotic analgesia after major abdominal surgery. *Lancet.* 1982;2(8290):115–118.

123. Recart A, Issioui T, White PF, et al. The efficacy of celecoxib premedication on postoperative pain and recovery times after ambulatory surgery: a dose ranging study. *Anesth Analg.* 2003;96:1631–1635.

124. Remy C, Marret E, Bonnet F. Effects of acetaminophen on morphine side-effects and consumption after major surgery: meta-analysis of randomized controlled trials. *Br J Anaesth.* 2005;94(4):505–513.

125. Reuben SS, Bhopatkar S, Maciolek H, et al. The preemptive analgesic effect of rofecoxib after ambulatory arthroscopic knee surgery. *Anesth Analg.* 2002;94:55–59.

126. Reuben SS, Connelly NR. Postoperative analgesic effects of celecoxib or rofecoxib after spinal fusion surgery. *Anesth Analg.* 2000;91:1221–1225.

127. Reuben SS, Ekman EF, Raghunathan K, et al. The effect of cyclooxygenase-2 inhibition on acute and chronic donor-site pain after spinal fusion surgery. *Reg Anesth Pain Med.* 2006;31:6–13.

128. Reuben SS, Ekman EF. The effect of cyclooxygenase-2 inhibition on analgesia and spinal fusion. *J Bone Surg Am.* 2005;87:536–542.

129. Reuben SS, Fingeroth R, Krushell R, et al. Evaluation of the safety and efficacy of the perioperative administration of rofecoxib for total knee arthroplasty. *J Arthroplasty.* 2002;17:26–31.

130. Reynolds LW, Hoo Rk, Brill RJ, et al. The COX-2 specific inhibitor, valdecoxib, is an opioid sparing analgesic in patients undergoing total knee arthroplasty. *J Pain Symptom Manage.* 2003;25:133–141.

131. Riest G, Peters J, Weiss M, et al. Does perioperative administration of rofecoxib improve analgesia after spine, breast and orthopaedic surgery? *Eur J Anesth.* 2006;23:219–226.

132. Robinson CM, Christie J, Malcolm-Smith N. Nonsteroidal anti-inflammatory drugs, perioperative blood loss, and transfusion requirement in elective hip arthroplasty. *J Arthroplasty.* 1993;8:607–610.

133. Rofecoxib APPROVE study results and their implications. Paper presented at: the American College of Rheumatology 68th Annual Scientific Meeting; October 16–21, 2004; San Antonio, TX.

134. Rosaeg OP, Krepski B, Cicutti N, et al. Effect of preemptive multimodal analgesia for arthroscopic knee ligament repair. *Reg Anesth Pain Med.* 2001;26:125–130.

135. Rumack BH. Acetaminophen misconceptions. *Hepatology.* 2004;40:10–15.

136. Schnitzer TJ, Burnmester GR, Mysler E, et al. Comparison of lumiracoxib with naproxen and ibuprofen in the Therapeutic Arthritis Research and Gastrointestinal Event Trial (TARGET), reduction in ulcer complications: randomized controlled trial. *Lancet.* 2004;364:665–674.

137. Schiodt FV, Rochling FA, Casey DL, et al. Acetaminophen toxicity in an urban county hospital. *New Engl J Med.* 1997;337:1112–1117.

138. Schug SA, Sidebotham DA, McGuinnety M, et al. Acetaminophen as an adjunct to morphine by patient-controlled analgesia in the management of acute postoperative pain. *Anesth Analg.* 1998;87:368–372.

139. Senturk M, Ozcan PE, Talu GK, et al. The effects of three different analgesia techniques on long-term postpost-thoracotomy pain. *Anesth Analg.* 2005;94:11–15.

140. Sevarino FB, Sinatra RS, Paige D, et al. Intravenous ketorolac as an adjunct to patient-controlled analgesia (PCA) for management of postgynecologic surgical pain. *J Clin Anesth.* 1994;6:23–27.

141. Silverstein FE, Faich G, Goldstein JL, et al. Gastrointestinal toxicity with celecoxib vs nonsteroidal anti-inflammatory drugs for osteoarthritis and rheumatoid arthritis: the CLASS study: a randomized controlled trial. Celecoxib Long-term Arthritis Safety Study. *JAMA.* 2000;284:1247–1255.

142. Sinatra RS, Boice JA, Loeys TL, et al. Evaluation of the effect of perioperative rofecoxib treatment on pain control and clinical outcomes in patients recovering from gynecologic abdominal surgery: a randomized double-blind, placebo-controlled clinical study. *Reg Anesth Pain Med.* 2006;31:134–142.

143. Sinatra RS. Role of COX-2 inhibitors in the evolution of acute pain management. *J Pain Symptom Manage.* 2002;24:S18–S27.

144. Sinatra RS, Jahr JS, Reynolds LW, et al. Efficacy and safety of single and repeated administration of 1 gram intravenous acetaminophen injection (paracetamol) for pain management after major orthopedic surgery. *Anesthesiology.* 2005;102(4):822–831.

145. Sinatra RS, Shen QJ, Halaszynski T, et al. Preoperative rofecoxib oral suspension as an analgesic adjunct after lower abdominal surgery: the effects on effort-dependent pain and pulmonary function. *Anesth Analg.* 2004;98:135–140.

146. Slappendel R, Weber EWG, Bugter MLT, et al. The intensity of preoperative pain is directly correlated with the amount of morphine needed for postoperative analgesia. *Anesth Analg.* 1999;88:146–148.

147. Smith LA, Carroll D, Edwards JE, et al. Single-dose ketorolac and pethidine in acute postoperative pain: systemic review with meta-analysis. *Br J Anaesth.* 2000:8448–8458.

148. Solomon SD, Mcmurray JJ, Pfeffer MA, et al. Cardiovascular risk associated with celecoxib in a clinical trial for colorectal adenoma prevention. *N Engl J Med.* 2005;352:1071–1080.

149. Souter JA, Fredman B, White PF. Controversies in the perioperative use of nonsteroidal antiinflammatory drugs. *Anesth Analg.* 1994;79:1178–1190.

150. Stephens J, Laskin B, Pashos C, et al. The burden of postoperative pain and the role of the COX-2 specific inhibitors. *Rheumatology.* 2003;42(suppl.3):iii40–iii52.

151. Tang J, Li S, White PF, et al. Effect of parecoxib, a novel intravenous cyclooxygenase type-2 inhibitor, on the postoperative opioid requirement and quality pain control. *Anesthesiology.* 2002;96:1305–1309.

152. Tramer MR, Williams JE, Carroll D, et al. Comparing analgesic efficacy of non-steroidal anti-inflammatory drugs given by different routes in acute and chronic pain: a quantitative systemic review. *Acta Anaesthesiol Scand.* 1998;42:71–79.

153. Turan A, Emet S, Karamanlioglu, et al. Analgesic effects of rofecoxib in ear-nose-throat surgery. *Anesth Analg.* 2002;95:1308–1311.

154. Vandermeulen EP, Akent HV, Scholtest JL, et al. Intravenous administration of tenoxicam 40 mg for postoperative analgesia: a double-blind, placebo-controlled multicentre study. *Eur J Anesthesiol.* 1997;14:250–257.

155. Varrassi G, Marinangeli F, Agro F, et al. A double-blinded evaluation of propacetamol versus ketorolac in combination with patient-controlled analgesia morphine: analgesic efficacy and tolerability after gynecologic surgery. *Anesth Analg.* 1999;88:611–616.

156. White PF. The changing role of non-opioid analgesic techniques in the management of postoperative pain. *Anesth Analg.* 2005;101 (2005):S5–S22.

157. White PF, Joshi GP, Carpenter RL, et al. A comparison of oral ketorolac and hydrocodone/acetaminophen for analgesia after ambulatory surgery: arthroscopy verus laparoscopic tubal ligation. *Anesth Analg.* 1997;85:37–43.

158. Yeh CC, Wu CT, Lee MS, et al. Analgesic effects of preincisional administration of dextromethorphan amd tenoxicam following laparoscopic cholecystectomy. *Acta Anaesthesiol Scand.* 2004;48:1049–1053.

159. Zhou TJ, Tang J, White P. Propacetamol versus ketorolac for treatment of acute postoperative pain after total hip or knee replacement. *Anesth Analg.* 2001;92:1569–1575.

22

Perioperative Ketamine for Better Postoperative Pain Outcome

Manzo Suzuki

Controlling acute postoperative pain remains a challenge; amelioration of pain affects not only postoperative mobility and mortality, but also the incidence of chronic pain after surgery. Tissue injury from surgery leads to release of inflammatory mediators that activate peripheral nociceptors. Nociceptive information travels thorough A-δ and C fibers to the spinal dorsal horn and creates a reduction in the threshold for activation in the dorsal horn, which is called central sensitization. *N*-methyl-D-aspertate (NMDA) receptors are located presynaptically, and postsynaptically the increase nociceptive pain transmission and play a crucial role in the development of central sensitization. Ketamine, a phencyclidine derivative that possesses a substantial analgesic effect, has been used for intravenous (IV) anesthesia for more than 3 decades. In recent years, hundreds of articles have emphasized the analgesic, preemptive, and antihyperalgesic effects of ketamine.[1] However, from the standpoint of improving pain outcome, the clinical use of ketamine is still controversial. Evidence from several studies strongly suggests that the effect of ketamine appears to depend on the type and duration of surgery, impact on nociception by surgical manipulation, type of basic pain treatment, and duration and amount of ketamine administered. By using ketamine effectively, we may reduce the pain score after surgery, decrease morphine consumption, and reduce the incidence of long-term persistent pain after major surgery. In this chapter, I describe the method for effective administration of ketamine to improve outcome with regard to pain.

BASIC POINTS FOR KETAMINE ADMINISTRATION

Pharmacokinetics of Ketamine

An understanding of the pharmokinetics of ketamine is very important when examining the literature on the effect of ketamine. Figure 22.1 shows changes in blood concentration of ketamine following either a single injection of 125 μg/kg or 250 μg/kg.[2] The blood concentration of ketamine decreases in 2 phases: rapid distribution (alpha phase) and slow elimination (beta phase), with the half-life in the alpha phase being

16 minutes and that in the beta phase 180 minutes. After a single injection of 125 or 250 μg/kg, blood concentration of ketamine decreases below 100 ng/mL within 30 minutes. This pattern of change in ketamine concentration is a key point in its effective use, as the change indicates the difficulty in maintaining the blood concentration above 100 ng/mL with a single injection, especially in a narrow range, such as from 100 to 200 ng/mL.

Analgesic and Side Effects of Ketamine

Ketamine may produce antinociception through interaction with the spinal μ-receptor, NMDA receptor antagonism, and descending pain inhibitory pathways.[3] The affinity of ketamine for NMDA receptors was shown to be more than one order of magnitude higher than that for μ-receptors.[4] The analgesic effect of ketamine is dose dependent. An analgesic effect alone is present at a blood concentration of 150 ng/mL.[5] However, as is well known, the psychedelic side effects of ketamine that are manifested as an emergence phenomenon occur around a blood concentration of 200–300 ng/mL.[6,7] These side effects include hypnosis, dreaming, and perceptual feelings. Ketamine at blood concentrations of 50–200 ng/mL has been shown to produce drowsiness. Considering the rapid distribution of ketamine in the alpha phase, the therapeutic range of ketamine as an analgesic without side effects is very narrow. These pharmacokinetics and side effects prohibit us from using ketamine as the sole analgesic. One study demonstrated an analgesic effect of ketamine at a higher dose (>200 ng/mL) during surgery, but this effect was limited to approximately 4 hours after termination of ketamine infusion.[8] Changes in blood concentration of ketamine after a single injection, constant infusion, and single injection followed by constant administration are presented in Figure 22.1. It is not difficult to keep the blood concentration of ketamine below 100 ng/mL, especially below 50 ng/mL, because of the slow elimination half-life.

Preemptive Analgesic Effect of Ketamine

Intraoperative administration of ketamine is used to prevent the development of opioid-induced hyperalgesia. Preemptive

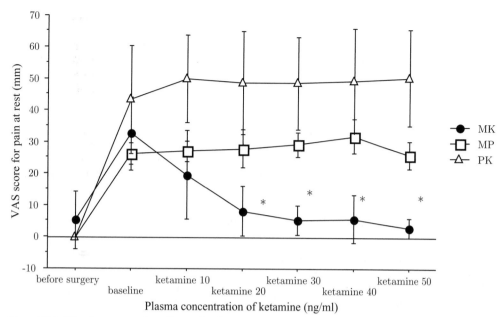

Figure 22.1: Blood concentration of ketamine that potentiates epidural morphine- and bupivacaine-induced analgesia is presented. Group MP (open boxes) and group MK (filled circles) received epidural morphine 2.5 mg and bupivacaine at the end of anesthesia. Group MP received various doses of placebo, whereas group MK received various doses of ketamine. More than 20 ng/mL blood concentration of ketamine significantly potentiates epidural morphine and bupivacaine analgesia. Please note that the pain scores in groups MP and MK before ketamine administration (baseline) were approximately 30 mm (0 00 mm).

analgesia is defined as an antinociceptive treatment begun before surgery to prevent the establishment of central sensitization caused by incisional injury.[9] Ketamine had been expected to demonstrate a preemptive effect. However, a recently published quantitative review denied the presence of a preemptive effect by ketamine.[10] However, another report demonstrated the preemptive effect of ketamine by showing prevention of hyperalgesia induced by an opioid given during surgery.[11] Opioids are routinely administered during surgery for pain control and stabilize hemodynamic control. Animal studies show that NMDA receptor antagonists, such as ketamine, dizocilpine (MK-801), and dextromethorphan suppress the activation of NMDA receptors and inhibit the development of opioid-induced hyperalgesia and opioid tolerance.[12,13] There is a possibility that opioid induces hyperalgesia in a dose-dependent manner.[14] Results of a study using remifentanil during surgery in humans suggest that ketamine administration prevents the development of opioid-induced hyperalgesia.[15]

Enhancement of Opioid-Induced Analgesia: Postoperative Infusion of Ketamine

Animal studies suggest that an NMDA receptor antagonist can potentiate the antinociceptive properties of opioids.[16] Although the results were inconsistent, ketamine coadministered with morphine may provide superior analgesia with a lower incidence of morphine-induced side effects. No study has determined the blood concentration of ketamine required to potentiate IV opioid-induced analgesia. In an investigation of the infusion of ketamine after surgery, the blood concentration was kept over 100 ng/mL.[17] However, maintaining the blood concentration at this level often induces hypnosis, and may interfere

with fast recovery, rehabilitation, and discharge (I received complaints from a surgeon when I administered these doses [about 100 ng/mL] of ketamine, thus I determined the blood concentrations of ketamine to potentiate epidural morphine-induced analgesia). The blood concentration of ketamine to potentiate opioid-induced analgesia may vary according to the route of administration and kind of opioid.[18,19] The maximal blood concentration may be 100 ng/mL after surgery, which may possibly interfere with rapid recovery and rehabilitation.

That these studies failed to demonstrate the efficacy of ketamine in patients who received patient-controlled anesthesia (PCA) morphine indicates that patients who received ketamine infusion displayed significant somnolence induced by both PCA morphine and ketamine infusion.[20,21] From these studies, I speculate that patients who received ketamine infusion could not push the delivery button because of sleepiness. Patients who receive ketamine and are awake may feel pain to the same degree as ketamine-untreated patients. The infusion rate is crucial in postoperative ketamine infusion and easily can be changed to maintain patients' consciousness. As shown in a review article, a dose of ketamine over 30 mg per 24 hours does not result in a dose-dependent morphine-sparing effect.[22] This coincides with the results of our study that presented the dose-independent effect of ketamine potentiating epidural morphine-induced analgesia.[19] Ketamine can be administered intraoperatively, postoperatively, or both. The timing and amount of administration of ketamine depends on the expectation of the ketamine effect (ie, reduced pain in the postanesthesia care unit [PACU], decreased morphine consumption in the wards, reduced persistent pain), not the expectation of the analgesic effect. We should obtain and maintain this optimal blood concentration at times when we desire an antihyperalgesic effect of ketamine.

Importance of Dose of Opioid to Provide Analgesia

Results of an animal study suggested the ratio between the dose of ketamine or other NMDA receptor antagonists and dose of opioid required to relieve pain.[23] The failure of an experimental study to demonstrate a synergistic effect between ketamine and alfentanyl indicates the presence of a specific relationship between dosages of ketamine and opioids.[24] We demonstrated that very low-dose ketamine (approximately 20 ng/mL) potentiates epidural morphine and bupivacaine analgesia.[19] However, this does not imply that this dose of ketamine potentiates the action of larger doses of morphine or other opioids. We must consider that the patients who received epidural morphine and bupivacaine alone (without ketamine) had a relatively low pain score (VAS < 3). I now speculate that if we administer a larger dose of opioid, a larger dose of ketamine might be required to potentiate or prevent the development of opioid-induced hyperalgesia (Figure 22.1). There seems to be a balance between dosages of opioid and ketamine. The dose of ketamine has limitations because of ketamine-induced side effects. Thus, it is important to obtain a lower pain score by lower dosages of opioid. We must remember that low-dose ketamine potentiates opioid-induced analgesia. Adequate analgesia by an opioid or another agent should be present before administration of ketamine. In the case of postoperative management after highly nociceptive procedures, the use of epidural administration of opioid or concomitant use of epidural local anesthesia, that is, a peripheral nerve block, may be important.

PRACTICAL ADMINISTRATION OF KETAMINE IN PERIOPERATIVE PERIOD

Ketamine Administration for Ambulatory Surgery (Excluding Ear, Nose, and Throat Surgery)

Over 60% of surgeries are now performed in an ambulatory setting. Despite improved analgesics and sophisticated drug delivery systems, surveys indicate that over 80% of patients experience moderate to severe pain postoperatively.[25] Pain is the most common cause of hospital admissions or emergency room visits after discharge. Ambulatory surgery is performed under general anesthesia using short-acting analgesics (eg, remifentanil, alfentanil) or inhalational or intravenous anesthesia with rapid emergence (eg, sevoflurane and propofol). Some institutions add peripheral nerve block at the beginning of surgery and perform "balanced analgesia" using acetaminophen, nonsteroidal anti-inflammatory drugs (NSAIDs), and peripheral nerve block. Because of quick recovery from anesthesia, the patient requires pain medicine soon after the surgery. For slight pain, acetaminophen and/or NSAIDs may be effective; however, for moderate to severe pain, an opioid should be administered. Even though peripheral nerve block was administered, rescue opioids should be given after a relatively highly invasive procedure.[26,27] Excess use of opioids induces problems such as nausea and vomiting, which can be another cause for hospital stay. After pain control by IV analgesics, oral pain medication should be started. The purpose of ketamine administration in this type of surgery is prevention of opioid-induced hyperalgesia through administration of opioids during surgery (eg, remifentanil) and potentiation of morphine-induced analgesia in the PACU without delayed recovery from general anesthesia, thus reducing the number of hospital admissions of these patients.

In outpatient surgery, coadministration of ketamine (0.075 mg/kg or 0.1 mg/kg) and morphine (0.1 mg/kg) at the end of surgery resulted in a very high quality of analgesia during PACU phase 1 and phase 2.[28] Because no intraoperative fentanyl had been given, the authors speculate that the effect of ketamine may be related to potentiating analgesia in the PACU. Usually, 1–5 µg/kg of fentanyl may be given during surgery. After surgery, incremental administration of IV morphine and/or IV NSAIDs may be given. Ketamine (0.1 mg/kg–0.2 mg/kg), given at the induction of anesthesia, may prevent opioid-induced hyperalgesia, and, after the surgery, the ketamine remaining in the body (even though at low blood concentration) may enhance analgesia by morphine administered in the PACU. According to discharge criteria in an ambulatory setting, oral pain medication will be given after pain has been treated to achieve a sufficiently low level that can be treated by oral medication. Beneficial effects of ketamine have been observed even after hospital discharge. Intraoperative ketamine administration (0.15- to 0.25-mg/kg bolus) provides a better postoperative outcome in knee arthroplasty, hernia repair, and laparoscopic gynecological surgery, even after discharge.[29–31] No study has shown the effect of ketamine combined with peripheral nerve block in ambulatory surgery. Whether ketamine is given during general anesthesia or during "balanced analgesia" using peripheral nerve block, 0.1–0.25 mg/kg of ketamine at the induction of anesthesia may provide beneficial effects and improve pain outcome. Dosage of ketamine can be decided according to the information shown in Figure 22.1. For short procedures (extracting a screw or hard wires, biopsy, etc), 0.1–0.15 mg/kg may be sufficient and, for relatively longer procedures, 0.25 mg/kg can be administered. Peripheral nerve block should be administered so that the postoperative morphine dose can be reduced.

In the case of surgery that is unexpectedly completed within a short period, it is possible that the blood concentration of ketamine will remain relatively high at the emergence of anesthesia. Before anesthesia, a benzodiazepine, such as midazolam (1–2 mg), should be given. However, even though benzodiazepine has been administered, hallucination can be evoked when ketamine is provided while the patient is awake.[10] With regard to blood concentration after administration of ketamine (0.25 mg/kg), blood concentration will decline to around 20 ng/mL 60 minutes after administration (Figure 22.1). When ketamine is administered at the induction of anesthesia, there is a small possibility of inducing a psychotomimetic side effect.

Remifentanil-Induced Hyperalgesia and Preventive Effect of Ketamine

Remifentanil is a newly developed ultra-short-acting opioid. An experimental study indicated that a relatively large dose of remifentanil induces acute opioid tolerance.[32] In abdominal surgery, intraoperative infusion of ketamine (0.2 mg/kg/h) prevents high-dose remifentanil- (0.4 µg/kg/min) induced hyperalgesia. Area of hyperalgesia and postoperative morphine consumption were reduced by intraoperative ketamine infusion (0.2 mg/kg/h)[15] in addition to remifentanil infusion. Low-dose ketamine infusion was shown to enhance remifentanyl-induced analgesia and reduce remifentanil consumption during surgery as well as reduce the degree of hyperalgesia.[33] Thus far, the minimum blood concentration of ketamine to prevent hyperalgesia induced by remifentanil or to potentiate remifentanil analgesia has not been determined. However, remifentanil-induced hyperalgesia or tolerance has been observed only when relatively high doses of remifentanil are given. As noted in the next section, in a short procedure such as an ear, nose, and throat surgery (ENT) case, a relatively low dose of remifentanil is given and no anitihyperalgesic effect of ketamine is observed.

Ketamine in Ambulatory ENT Surgery

Ear, nose, and throat surgery is also performed in an ambulatory setting. Adult ENT surgery, especially tonsillectomy, is painful. Recently, remifentanil-inhalational anesthesia or remifentanil-propofol anesthesia has been indicated.[34] Consequently, the question has arisen as to whether ketamine may be beneficial in ambulatory ENT surgery. However, several clinical studies failed to demonstrate a preemptive, antihyperalgesic, or morphine-sparing effect of ketamine.[34–36] One reason is that, only a small dose of remifentanil was given, and it may be that the pain pathway during and after surgery is through the pharyngeal nerve, not through spinal gray matter. Although there is no evidence that opioid-induced hyperalgesia is provoked only in spinal gray matter, the spinal cord may play a crucial role in the development of opioid-induced hyperalgesia. I believe there is a small possibility of development of opioid- (remifentanil) induced hyperalgesia in this kind of surgery.

Ketamine as Adjunct to Sedative during Local Anesthesia (MAC Setting)

Several minor procedures such as breast biopsy and minor plastic surgery are performed under local anesthesia (monitored anesthesia care, [MAC]). Sedative and supplemental analgesics are used to improve patients' comfort. Coadministration of ketamine and propofol reduces the incidence of movement of patients at the injection of local anesthetics.[37] This combination does not induce respiratory depression. A study by Mortero demonstrated that coadministration of ketamine (0.25 mg/kg/h = 100 ng/mL) and propofol (2 mg/kg/h) reduced pain after discharge and cut down the use of oral pain medication at home, improved mood, and provided earlier recovery of cognitive function.[37] High doses of ketamine induce hypnosis and vomiting after recovery, which interferes with quick discharge.[38] Ketamine dosages should be limited to subhypnotic and subanalgesic levels (100 ng/mL blood concentration). Bolus administration should be avoided because an MAC setting involves a very short procedure; 0.20–0.25 mg/kg/h (without bolus) is sufficient to improve the postoperative condition after MAC. When propofol is being administered, patient's vital signs and discomfort should be monitored. Some reports cite administration of a mixture of ketamine and propofol; however, such a mixture could possibly result in a much higher concentration of ketamine[38] and ketamine-induced side effects if care is not taken by anesthesiologists to consider the amount of ketamine is being administered (see Figure 22.1[C]). If a ketamine-propofol mixture is administered, a high infusion rate should be avoided (Figure 22.1[C]). Sole administration of ketamine (0.2 mg/kg/h) may be better to avoid ketamine-induced side effects. Monitoring the brain such as by the bispectral index (BIS) or an entropy monitor is commonly used to measure the level of sedation during local anesthesia. During propofol or sevoflurane anesthesia, ketamine administration (0.4–05 mg/kg) paradoxically increases the BIS value.[39,40] When a relatively higher dose of ketamine has been administered, a possibility of dissociation between the level of sedation and the BIS value is suspected. However, the effect of low-dose ketamine infusion (0.1–0.2 mg/kg/h) on the BIS value during propofol infusion has not been studied.

Ketamine for Patients Admitted after Surgery (Major Orthopedic Surgery, Open Cholecystectomy, Gynecologic Laparotomy)

Such surgery is performed on the basis of postoperative admission of the patient, with the patient staying in a hospital for at least 24 hours after surgery. We have two options for the use of ketamine: intraoperative or both intra- and postoperative. Results of a study demonstrating the beneficial effect of ketamine administration (0.15 mg/kg) before surgical incision or at the end of anterior cruciate ligament repair suggest that even a single injection of this dose of ketamine has a morphine-sparing effect or prevents opioid-induced hyperalgesia from the opioid given during surgery, but this dose of ketamine does not reduce the pain score after surgery.[41] Intraoperative and postoperative ketamine infusion (100 and 50 ng/mL blood concentration, respectively) combined with continuous femoral nerve block reduces postoperative morphine consumption.[42] Both of these studies emphasized that patients who received ketamine had superior knee flexion with less pain during rehabilitation. Even if there is no reduction in pain immediately after surgery, reduction in pain during the subacute phase and facilitation of rehabilitation may be beneficial. Ketamine should be administered 0.1–0.15 mg/kg before surgical incision followed by 0.15 mg/kg/h during surgery and 0.05–0.1 mg/kg/h after surgery.

INTRAVENOUS PCA

PCA with opioid is a popular method of delivering postoperative pain relief. Coadministration of ketamine and morphine may provide synergistic analgesia and reduce the incidence of opioid-induced side effects. For effective analgesia and avoidance of side effects, the ratio of morphine to ketamine may be important. Sveticic et al[43] investigated the optimal ratio of morphine and ketamine and the lockout interval to obtain the synergistic effect of both drugs. Possibly, the best combination of morphine with ketamine is a ratio of 1:1, and a lockout interval of 8 min after spinal or hip surgery is recommended. This was not a randomized controlled study, but the pain score after surgery was less than 3 and morphine consumption after surgery was approximately 3 mg/h. However, in a randomized controlled trial of major abdominal surgery, the pain score and morphine consumption did not differ between patients who were coadministered ketamine and morphine, and those who were only given morphine via PCA; the pain score in both groups was more than 3 and more than 3 mg/h of morphine was delivered via PCA. Cognitive function was worse in those coadministered these agents. Coadministration of ketamine and morphine after a major procedure may increase the possibility of ketamine-related side effects such as somnolence because of high doses of both drugs[44]; with such coadministration, there is the possibility that the ketamine blood concentration may reach an unexpected level. Coadministration of morphine and ketamine (1:1) has a limited possibility of improving pain control in low invasive procedures. The effect of coadministration of ketamine and morphine via PCA has been demonstrated in very minor invasive procedures.[45]

KETAMINE FOR MAJOR SURGERY

Major surgery, including upper abdominal surgery, thoracotomy, and breast surgery, induces high nociceptive input from a broad section of spinal nerve and visceral components. Inappropriate pain management after such surgery induces dramatic changes in peripheral and central pain processing; that is, pain occurs that does not require further noxious stimulation, so-called secondary hyperalgesia. Both peripheral and central pain sensitization increases postoperative pain, disability from pain, and impaired rehabilitation. Early ambulation and movement to reduce the incidence of pulmonary complications lead to a dynamic or effort-dependent pain. Consequently, after these procedures, high doses of opioids may be administered intravenously or epidurally. The purposes of ketamine administration for these procedures are to (1) reduce pain, facilitate rehabilitation, and lessen the possibility of pulmonary complications; (2) lessen the dose of IV opioid and the incidence of opioid-related side effects; and (3) reduce the incidence of opioid-induced hyperalgesia and decrease the incidence and severity of postoperative persistent pain.

Administration of Ketamine for Postoperative Pain Management after Major Abdominal Surgery

Maneuvers for major abdominal surgery include nociception for a broad section of spinal and supraspinal nerves. Completion of such surgery takes from a few to several hours and high nociception persists during this interval. Consequently, high doses of opioid may be given during surgery. Ketamine should be administered continuously during and after surgery. Aida et al[46] demonstrated that relatively low doses of ketamine (blood concentration = 120 ng/mL) during surgery combined with epidural morphine infusion produced superior postoperative analgesia and reduced epidural morphine consumption postoperatively compared with epidural morphine alone. In a study in which ketamine was infused only after surgery, the pain score was not reduced in patients receiving ketamine infusion compared with patients treated with PCA morphine alone.[47] Only morphine consumption is reduced in ketamine-treated patients.[47,48] Katz et al[49] did not demonstrate a preemptive effect of low-dose ketamine (=60 ng/mL) coadministered with fentanyl in a short- and long-term postoperative period. An animal study indicated the possibility of a competitive relationship between ketamine and fentanyl in μ-opioid receptors.[18] Epidural administration of morphine is preferable, because it has a 4 times higher potency than intravenous morphine. It is preferable that intravenous ketamine infusion and epidural morphine be given at the beginning of induction of anesthesia.

PREVENTION OF POSTOPERATIVE LONG-TERM PERSISTENT PAIN

Long-term persistent pain has gained attention as a postoperative adverse outcome.[50] Activation of spinal NMDA-receptors

through C-fiber input generated by tissue trauma has a crucial role in central sensitization and evokes persistent pain. Perioperative pain management is signified as having an important role in preventing the development of long-term persistent pain.[51] From the standpoint of opioid-induced hyperalgesia, reduction in the amount of postoperative opioids may also contribute to a reduction in long-standing persistent pain. Preventive analgesia is a perioperative pain management strategy to avoid development of such pain. The hypothesis that intraoperative low-dose ketamine will reduce both short-term and long-term postoperative pain has been proposed. Some studies have shown such beneficial effects of ketamine administration, whereas others have not.

De Kock et al[52] showed that intraoperative ketamine infusion of 100 ng/mL, but not a lower dose (=50 ng/mL), reduced postoperative morphine consumption in surgical patients who had received epidural anesthesia with bupivacaine-sufentanil-clonidine. Also, they found that a significant reduction in the amount of morphine leads to a reduction in residual pain 1 year after the surgery. The importance of the basic pain regime in addition to the administration of low-dose ketamine was noted by Lavand'home et al.[53] They found that when comparing ketamine infusion as an adjunctive to epidural analgesia with that as an adjunctive to intravenous opioid, the latter provides a better analgesic outcome. For a significant preemptive (preventive = avoidance of persistent pain) effect of ketamine in major surgery, basic pain management is important. Epidural anesthesia using local anesthetics and opioid, especially morphine, may be best combination.

KETAMINE INFUSION FOR THORACIC SURGERY

Maneuvers for thoracotomy involve cutting ribs, retracting the pleura and chest wall, and placing an indwelling intercostal trocar in VATs. These manipulations damage intercostal nerves directly and activate C-fiber afferents, which may cause a significant change in peripheral and central nervous systems. Chronic pain after thoracotomy is believed to be of neuropathic origin.[54] Even after completion of surgery, an inflammatory mediator around the skin incision may initiate the development of peripheral and central sensitization. Chronic postthoracotomy pain syndrome is defined as pain that recurs or persists along a thoracotomy scar at least 2 months following a surgical procedure.[55] The incidence is 44% to 67%, but the pain is severe only in 25% of those patients. Patients who developed chronic postthoractomy pain had expressed the presence of severe pain after surgery. Management of acute pain is important to prevent the development of chronic postthoracotomy pain.[56] Epidural analgesia is the mainstay of postthoracotomy pain management.[57,58] Long-term use of ketamine after surgery may be beneficial to reduce the incidence of chronic postoperative pain.[59] However, respiratory complications immediately after surgery are worrisome, and efforts should be made to prevent such complications. Dosages of opioid and ketamine should be limited as much as possible while still treating the pain. The blood concentration of ketamine required to potentiate epidural morphine and bupivacaine analgesia is 20–30 ng/mL. Intra- and postoperative infusion of very low-dose ketamine (20 ng/mL) combined with epidural morphine and ropivacaine resulted in a lower pain score and few patients required rescue pain

A

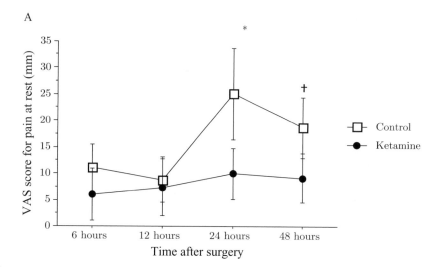

B

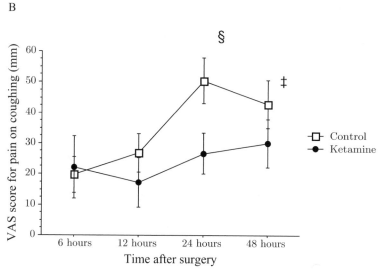

Figure 22.2: The effect of low-dose ketamine (0.05 mg/kg/h, filled circles) with epidural morphine (3 mg/d) and ropivacaine 0.15% (3 mL/h) is presented. When basic pain treatment is adequate (open box) and very low-dose ketamine is sufficient to potentiate analgesia (filled circles), the pain score of the ketamine-treated patients is nearly zero, whereas that of the ketamine-untreated patients is 3.

medication after surgery. This low dose may be effective only when the pain is relatively relieved by epidural analgesia (VAS < 3–4 without ketamine; Figure 22.2).[59] Low-dose ketamine infusion may decrease the pain score (Figure 22.2). Patients who received low-dose ketamine infusions had a lower pain score even 3 months after surgery than those who did not receive such infusions (Figure 22.3). Considering the relatively smooth change in ketamine blood concentration through changes in the infusion rate (Figure 22.3[A]), we can administer ketamine at a relatively high infusion rate and change the infusion rate at the end of surgery. Thus, I advocate an infusion rate for ketamine of 0.2 mg/kg/h during surgery and to change the rate to 0.05 mg/kg/h at the end of surgery. We are using an epidural infusion pump for ketamine because of its low price and ease of portability (Figure 22.3[B]). We are using an infusion pump during surgery followed by use of a disposable epidural infusion pump.

EPIDURAL ADMINISTRATION OF KETAMINE

Although there is a high possibility of psychotomimetic side effects induced by intrathecal administration of ketamine, the direct analgesic effect or enhancement of epidural morphine-induced analgesia by epidural ketamine administration has been investigated.[60,61] Ketamine administered in the epidural space moves smoothly into the systemic circulation. Although the plasma half-life of ketamine administered in the epidural space is longer than that of ketamine administered intravenously, the dose and method of administration (injection or infusion) should be decided according to nociceptive input and length of surgery. Sole administration of ketamine (1 mg/kg) into the epidural space brings about preemptive analgesia and a morphine-sparing effect in thoractomy.[63] Coadministration of ketamine and morphine continuously into the epidural space provides analgesia superior to that of morphine alone.

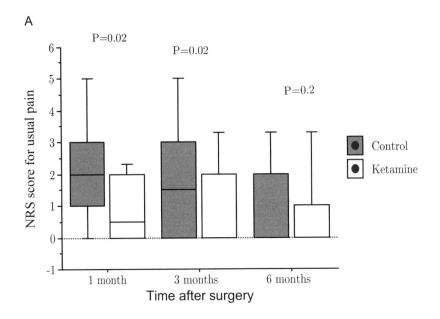

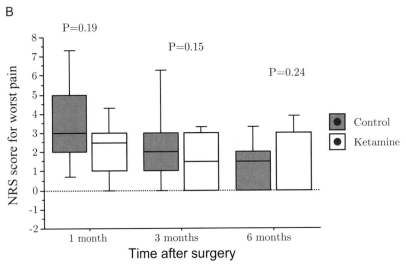

Figure 22.3: The effect of ketamine on persistent pain is presented at 3 months after surgery (A). Usual pain is lower in patients administered perioperative ketamine (blank columns) than in ketamine-untreated patients (filled columns).

In addition, multimodal analgesia by epidural bupivacaine, morphine, and ketamine provides better pain relief. Although the mechanism of the antagonism of spinal NMDA receptors by epidural administration of ketamine is not known, smooth movement of epidurally administered ketamine into the systemic circulation suggests that epidural ketamine possesses both spinal and supraspinal effects. Dosage of ketamine administered into epidural space is from 5% to 10% that of intravenously administered dosages (0.25 mg/kg/d). Higher doses of epidural ketamine may induce a psychotomimetic side effect.

KETAMINE FOR AMPUTATION

Incidence of phantom limb pain after amputation is reported to be 49% to 88%.[64] Its origin is believed to be neuropathic. Because long-term persistent pain is related to the pain just after the surgery, which is called stump pain, a question arises about the use of ketamine to prevent phantom limb pain.[65] Some reports show the effect of ketamine infusion to treat already established phantom limb pain.[66] Only one study, in which relatively high doses of ketamine were administered during and after surgery under general anesthesia, denies the contribution of ketamine infusion to prevent the development of phantom limb pain.[67]

CONCLUSION

How to use perioperative ketamine effectively is described. There is variety in how much ketamine should be used and how it can be used. Its usage depends on nociception and length of the surgical maneuver, and what we expect from its use. An important point is adequate analgesia through basic pain management. Ketamine can be a good adjunct to relatively well-treated pain, but it should not be used as rescue for inadequate analgesia.

PANELS

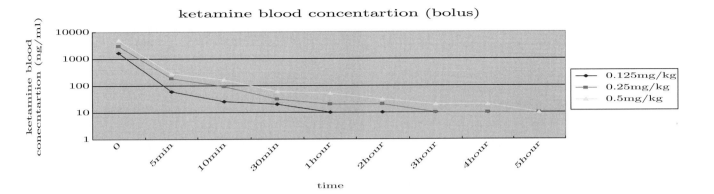

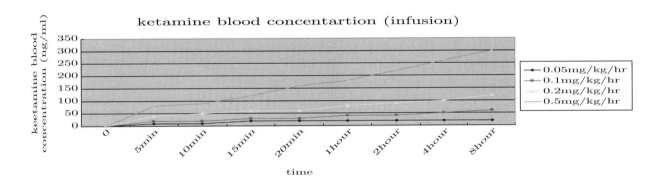

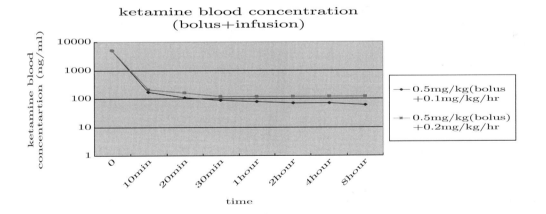

Panel A

Changes in blood concentration of ketamine over time after bolus, infusion, or bolus followed by constant infusion is demonstrated

Image to understand the balance between nociception and the effect of ketamine

| • Nociception
• Dose of opioid | Anti-hyperalgesic of ketamine |

Increased nociception and/or increased dose of opioid may reduce the anti-hyperalgesic effect of ketamine

Panel B

Important points for when to withdraw the effect of ketamine

• Higher dose of ketamine does not induce high quality of analgesia
• Avoid higher dose of opioid as possible
• Multimodal analgesia
• Adequate analgesia by basic pain regime

Panel C

Ketamine for ambulatory surgery

For short procedure (length of surgery 0.5-1h)

Ketamine 0.1-0.15 mg/kg at anesthesia induction

+

fentanyl

For relatively long procedure (length of surgery 1-2 h)

Ketamine 0.2-0.25 mg/kg at anesthesia induction

+

fentanyl

Panel D

Ketamine is NOT recommended for

● Ear, nose, and throat surgery, and maxillofacial surgery

● Use as co-administrator with opioid via patient controlled analgesia (PCA)

Panel E

No mixture ketamine and propofol

Example
Ketamine and propofol mixture
Ketamine(10 mg/ml)*5 ml+propofol (10 mg/ml)*45 ml
=ketamine(1 mg/ml)+propofol(9 mg/ml)
　　　Example: patient of 60 kg, 3 ml/kg/hr infusion
　　　18 ml/hr=ketamine 18 mg/hr=0.3 mg/kg/hr
In case of 5 ml/kg/hr infusion　30 ml/hr=ketamine
　　30 mk/kg/hr=0.5 mg/kg/hr
According to panel A, 0.5 mg/kg/hr of ketamine infusion
　　makes blood concentration of 200 ng/ml at 90
　　minutes.
Thus in this mixture, 5 ml/kg/hr is maximum rate.
　　Infusion rate of mixture should be considered
　　according to possible ketamine administration rate.

Panel F

Intraoperative ketamine infusion

Intraoperative administration of ketamine
Ketamine should be administered by infusion pump.
Ketamine injection 0.5 mg/kg followed by 0.2-0.25
　　mg/kg/hr (terminateat the end of surgery).
Co-administer epidural morphine (3 mg followed by
　　1 mg/hr) + bupivacaine 0.5 % 5-10 ml incremently)
　　during surgery. Postopertaive administration of
　　epidural morphine and bupivacaine by PCEA or
　　infusion (set to deliver epidural morphine 5-
　　10 mg/day and bupivacaine 0.0675%-0.125%,
　　3-5 ml/hr)

Panel G

Postoperative ketamine infusion

Postoperative ketamine infusion
Using multi rate setting epidural infusion pump. Select flow
　　rate from 2, 3 and 5 ml/hr.
Example
Weight=60 kg. Primary infusion rate 3 ml/hr for 70 hr.
　　Ketamine infusion 0.15 mg/kg/hr. (60 ng/ml)
Total amount of infusion: 3*70=210 ml
Ketamine 70 (hr)*60 (kg)*0.15=630 mg ; 63 ml
Mixture is 63 ml of ketamine (10 mg/ml)+147 ml of saline
As shown in Panel A, even after a 5 hour infusion of
　　ketamine, reduction in rate of infusion reset to low blood
　　concentration level within 1 hour. Thus, using multirate
　　pump we can easily change the dose of ketamine when
　　the patients were somnolence.

Panel H

REFERENCES

1. Schmidt RL, Sandler AN, Katz J. Use and efficacy of low-dose ketamine in the management of acute postoperative pain: a review of current techniques and outcomes. *Pain*. 1999;82:111–125.

2. Clements JA, Nimmo WS. Pharmacokinetics and analgesic effect of ketamine in man. *Br J Anaesth*. 1981;53:27–30.

3. Pekoe GM, Smith DJ. The involvement of opiate and monoaminergic neuronal system in the analgesic effects of ketamine. *Pain*. 1982;12:57–73.

4. Smith DJ, Azzaro AJ, Zaldivar SB, Palmer S, Lee HS. Properties of the optical isomers and metabolites of ketamine on the high affinity transport and catabolism of monoamines. *Neuropharmacology*. 1981;20:392–396.

5. Clements JA, Nimmo WS, Grant IS. Bioavailability, pharmacokinetics and analgesic activity of ketamine in humans. *Br J Anaesth*. 1981;53:27–30.

6. Suzuki M, Tsueda K, Lansing P, et al. Midazolam attenuates ketamine-induced abnormal perception and thought process but not mood changes. *Can J Anesth*. 2000;47:866–874.

7. Bowdle TA, Radant AD, Cowley DS, et al. Psychedelic effects of ketamine in human volunteers: relationship to steady-state plasma concentrations. *Anesthesiology*. 1998;88:82–88.

8. Bilgin H, Ozcan B, Bilgin T, et al. The influence of timing of systemic ketamine administration on postoperative morphine consumption. *J Clin Anesth*. 2005;17:592–597.

9. Kissin I. Preemptive analgesia. *Anesthesiology*. 2002;93:1138–1143.

10. Elia N, Tramer MR. Ketamine and postoperative pain- a quantitative systemic review of randomized trials. *Pain*, 2005;113:61–70,

11. Roytblat L, Korotkoruchko A, Katz J, et al. Postoperative pain: the effect of low-dose ketamine in addition to general anesthesia. *Anesth Analg*. 1993;77:1161–1165.

12. Trujillo KA, Akil H. Inhibition of opiate tolerance by noncompetitive N-methyl-D-aspertate receptor anatagonist. *Brain Res*. 1994;633:178–188.

13. Mao J, Price DD, Mayer DJ. Mechanisms of hyperalgesia and morphine tolerance: a current view of their possible interactions. *Pain*. 1995;62:259–274.

14. Célèrier E, Rivat C, Jun Y, et al. Long-lasting hyperalgesia induced by fentanyl in rats. *Anesthesiology*. 2000;92:465–472.

15. Jory V, Richebe P, Guignard B, et al. Remifentanil-induced postoperative hyperalgesia and its prevention with small-dose ketamine. *Anesthesiology*. 2005;103:147–155.

16. Baker AK, Hoffman VLH, Meert TF. Dextromethorphan and ketamine potentiate the antinociceptive effects of μ- but not δ- or κ-opoid agonists in a mouse model of acute pain. *Pharmacol Biochem Behav*. 2002;74:73–86.

17. Stabhaug A, Brevik H, Eide PK, Kreuen M, Foss A. Mapping of punctuate hyperalgesia around a surgical incision demonstrates that ketamine is a powerful suppressors of central sensitization to pain following surgery. *Acta Anaesthesiol Scand*. 1997;41:1124–1132.

18. Hoffman VLH, Baker AK, Vercauteren MP, Adriaensen HF, Meert TF. Epidural ketamine potentiates epidural morphine but not fenanyl in acute nociception in rats. *Eur J Pain*. 2003;7:121–130.

19. Suzuki M, Kinoshita T, Kikutani T, et al. Determining plasma concentration of ketamine that enhances epidural bupivacaine-and-morphine-induced analgesia. *Anesth Analg*. 2005;101:777–784.

20. Ilkjaer S, Nikolajsen L, Hansen TM, Wernberg M, Brenum J, Dahl JB. Effect of i.v. ketamine in combination with epidural bupivacaine or epidural morphine on postoperative pain and wound tenderness after renal surgery. *Br J Anaesth*. 1998;81:707–712.

21. Edwards ND, Fletcher A, Cole JR, Peacock JE. Combined infusions of morphine and ketamine for postoperative pain in elderly patients. *Anesthesia*. 1993;48:124–127.

22. Bell RF, Dahl JB, Moore RA. Kalso E. Peri-operative ketamine for acute-post-operative pain: a quantitative and qualitative systematic review (Cochrane review). *Acta Anaesthesiol Scand*. 2005;49:1405–1428.

23. Price DD, Mayer DJ, Mao J, Caruso FS. NMDA-receptor antagonists and opioid receptor interactions as related to analgesia and tolerance. *J Pain Symptom Manage*. 2000;S7–S11.

24. Sethna NF, Liu M, Gracely R, Bennett GJ, Max MB. Analgesic and cognitive effects of intravenous ketamine-alfentanil combinations versus either drug alone after intradermal capsaicin in normal subjects. *Anesth Analg*. 1998;86:1250–1256.

25. Shang AB, Gan TJ. Optimising postoperative pain management in the ambulatory patient. *Drugs*. 2003;63:855–867.

26. Ben-David B, Schmaleberger K, Chelly JE. Analgesia after total knee arthroplasty: is continuous sciatic blockade needed in addition to continuous femoral nerve blockade? *Anesth Analg*. 2004;98:747–749.

27. Mcnamee DA, Parks L, Milligan KR. Post-operative analgesia following total knee replacement: an evaluation of the addition of an obturator nerve block to combined femoral and sciatic nerve block. *Acta Anaesthesiol Scand*. 2002;46:95–99.

28. Suzuki M, Tsueda K, Lansing PS, Tolan MM, et al. Small-dose ketamine enhances morphine-induced analgesia after outpatient surgery. *Anesth Analg*. 1999;89:98–103.

29. Menigaux C, Guinard B, Fletcher D, Sessler DI, et al. Intraoperative small-dose ketamine enhances analgesia after outpatient knee arthroscopy. *Anesth Analg*. 2001;93:606–612.

30. Palvin DJ, Horvath KD, Palvin EG, Sima K. Preincisional treatment to prevent pain after ambulatory hernia surgery. *Anesth Analg*, 2003;97:1627–1632.

31. Kwok RFK, Lim J, Chan MTV, Gin T, Chiu WKY. Preoperative ketamine improves postoperative analgesia after gynecologic laparoscopic surgery. *Anesth Analg*. 2004;98:1044–1049.

32. Koppert W, Sittl R, Scheuber K, Alsheimer M, Schmeltz M, Schüttler J. Differential moduration of remifentanil-induced analgesia and postinfusion hyperalgesia by s-ketamine and clonidine in humans. *Anesthesiology*. 2003;99:152–159.

33. Guinard B, Coste C, Costes H, et al. Supplementing desflurane-remifentanil anesthesia with small-dose ketamine reduces perioperative opioid analgesia requirements. *Anesth Analg*. 2002;95:103–108.

34. Ganne O, Abisseror M, Menault P, et al. Low-ketamine failed to spare morphine after a remifentanil-based anaesthesia for ear, nose and throat surgery. *Eur J Anaesth*. 2005;22:426–430.

35. Lebrun T, Elstraete ACV, Sandefo I, Polin B, Pierre-Louise L. Lack of a pre-emptive effect of low-dose ketamine on postoperative pain following oral surgery. *Can J Anaesth*. 2006;53:146–152.

36. Elstraete ACV, Lebrun T, Sandefo I, Polin B. Ketamine does not decrease postoperative pain after remifentanil-based anaesthesia for tonsillectomy in adults. *Acta Anaesth Scand*. 2004;48:756–760.

37. Mortero RF, Clark LD, Tolan MM, et al. The effect of a small-dose ketamine on propofol sedation: respiration, postoperative mood, perception, cognition and pain. *Anesth Analg*. 2001;92:1465–1469.

38. Shyamala B, Michail A, Melissa S, Thomas W, Anthony I. The use of ketamine-propofol combination during monitored anesthesia care. *Anesth Analg*. 2000;90:858–862.

39. Hirota K, Kubota T, Ishihara H, Matsuki A. The effects of nitrous oxide and ketamine on the bispectral index and 95% spectral edge frequency during propofol-fentanyl anaesthesia. *Eur J Anaesth*. 1999;16:779–783.

40. Hans P, Dewandre PY, Brichant JF, Bonhomme V. Comparative effects of ketamine on bispectral index and spectral entropy

of the electroencephalogram under sevoflurane anaesthesia. *Br J Anaesth.* 2005;94:336–340.

41. Menigaux C, Fletcher D, Dupont X, et al. The benefits of intraoperative small-dose ketamine on postoperative pain after anterior cruciate ligament repair. *Anesth Analg.* 2000;90:129–135.

42. Adam F, Chauvin M, Manoir B, et al. Small-dose ketamine infusion improves postoperative analgesia and rehabilitation after total knee arthoroscopy. *Anesth Analg.* 2005;100:475–480.

43. Sveticic G, Gentilini A, Eichenberger U, Luginbül M, Curatolo M. Combinations of Morphine with ketamine for patient controlled analgesia. A new optimization method. *Anesthesiology.* 2003;98:1195–1205.

44. Reeves M, Lindholm DE, Myles PS, Fletcher H, Hunt JO. Adding ketamine to morphine for patient-controlled analgesia after major abdominal surgery: a double-blinded randomized controlled trial. *Anesth Analg.* 2001;93:116–120.

45. Javery KB, Ussery TW, Steger HG, Colcrough GW. Comparison of morphine and morphine with ketamine for postoperative amalgesia. *Can J Anaesth.* 1996;43:212–215.

46. Aida S, Yamakura T, Baba H, Taga K, Fukuda S, Shimoji K. Preemtive analgesia by intravenous low-dose ketamine and epidural morphine in gastrectomy. *Anesthesiology.* 2002;92:1624–1630.

47. Guillow N, Tanguy M, Seguin P, Branger B, Campion JP, Mallédant Y. The effects of small-dose ketamine on morphine consumption in surgical intensive care unit patients after major abdominal surgery. *Anesth Analg.* 2003;97:843–847.

48. Adriaenssen G, Vermeyen KM, Hoffman VLH, Mertens E, Adriaensen HF. Postoperative analgesia with i.v. patient-controlled morphine: effect of adding ketamine. *Br J Anaesth.* 1999;83:393–396.

49. Katz J, Schmid R, Snijdelaar DG, Coderre TJ, McCartney CJL, Wowk A. Pre-emptive analgesia using intravenous fentanyl plus low-dose ketamine for radical prostatectomy under general anesthesia dose not produce short-term or long-term reductions in pain and analgesic use. *Pain.* 2004;110:707–718.

50. Perkins FM, Kehlet H. Chronic pain as an outcome of surgery. *Anesthesiology.* 2000;93:1123–1133.

51. Pogatzki-Zahn EM, Zahn PK. From preemptive to preventive analgesia. *Curr Opin Anaesthesiol.* 2006;19:551–555.

52. De Kock M, Lavand'homme P, Waterloos H. 'Balanced analgesia' in the perioperative period: is there a place for ketamine? *Pain.* 2001;92:373–380.

53. Lavand'homme P, De Kock M, Waterloos H. Intraoperative epidural analgesia combined with ketamine provides effective preventive analgesia in patients undergoing major digestive surgery. *Anesthesiology.* 2005;103:813–820.

54. Rogers ML, Duffy JP. Surgical aspects of chronic postthoracotomy pain. *Eur J Cardiothorac Surg.* 2000;18:711–716.

55. Erdek MA, Staats PS. Chronic pain and thoracic surgery. *Thorac Surg Clin.* 2005;15:123–130.

56. Katz J, Jackson M, Kavanagh BP, Sandler AN. Acute pain after thoracic surgery predicts long-term post-thoracotomy pain. *Clin J Pain.* 1996;12:50–55.

57. Tippana E, Nilsson E, Kalso E. Post-thoracotomy pain after thoracic epidural analgesia: a prospective follow-up study. *Acta Anaesthesiol Scand.* 2003;47:433–438.

58. Şentürk M, Ozcan PE, Talu GK, et al. The effects of three different analgesia tecvhniques on long-term postthoracotomy pain. *Anesth Analg.* 2002;94:11–15.

59. Suzuki M, Haraguchi S, Sugimoto K, et al. Low-dose intravenous ketamine potentiates epidural analgesia after thoracotomy. *Anesthesiology.* 2006;105:111–119.

60. Tan PH, Kuo MC, Kao PF, Chia YY, Liu K. Patient-controlled epidural analgesia with morphine or morphine plus ketamine for post-operative pain relief. *Eur J Anaesthsiol.* 1999;16:820–825.

61. Chia YY, Liu K, Liu YC, Chang HC, Wong CS. Adding ketamine in a multimodal patient-controlled epidural regimen reduces postoperative pain and analgesic consumption. *Anesth Analg.* 1998;861:1245–1249.

62. Pedraz JL, Lanao JM, Calvo MB, Muriel C, Haernández-Arbeiza J, Dominguez-Gil A. Pharmacokinetic and clinical evaluation of ketamine administered by i.v. and epidural routes. *Int J Clin Pharmacol Ther Toxicol.* 1987;25:77–80.

63. Ozyaclin NS, Yucel A, Camlica H, Dereli N, et al. Effects of preemptive ketamine on sensory changes and postoperative pain after thoracotomy: comparison of epidural and intramuscular routes. *Br J Anaesth.* 2004;93:356.

64. Kooilman CM, Pijkstra PU, Geertzen JHB, Elzinga A. Schans CP. Phantom pain and phantom sensations in upper limb amputations: an epidemiological study. *Pain.* 2000;87:33–41.

65. Nikolajsen L, Jensen TS. Phantom limb pain. *Br J Anaesth.* 2001;87:107–116.

66. Nikoljsen L, Hansen CL, Nielsen J, et al. The effect of ketamine on phantom pain: a central neuropathic disorder maintained by peripheral input. *Pain.* 1996;67:69–77.

67. Hayes C, Armstrong-Brown A, Burstal R. Peroperative intravenous etamine infusion for the orevention of persistent post-amputation pain: a randomized, controlled trial. *Anaesth Intensive Care.* 2004;32:330–338.

23

Clinical Application of Glucocorticoids, Antineuropathics, and Other Analgesic Adjuvants for Acute Pain Management

Johan Raeder and Vegard Dahl

The opioids are among the oldest of pain relievers known to mankind, and they remain the cornerstone for acute pain management in patients with moderately severe to severe symptoms. Their benefits include a rapid onset of action, no upper limit of efficacy, many modes of administration, and low cost. Well-known side effects such as nausea, vomiting, pruritus, constipation, and respiratory depression limit their use and may impose significant morbidity. Most opioids have a high degree of first-pass metabolism in the liver making oral dosing unpredictable. Opioid-induced sedation and anxiolysis may be of benefit in some situations; but these effects are unreliable and some patients may experience excessive obtundation, sleep apnea, airway obstruction, confusion, and impaired cognition. Whereas opioids may be titrated to effectively relieve pain at rest, they are not as efficient at controlling incident pain during mobilization. This limitation may be problematic in settings where patients require physiotherapy or physical activity during rehabilitation and recovery. Further, the opioids may disturb the natural pattern of sleep, with reduced fraction of REM sleep after dosing and catch-up, and restless nights later on.

Although tolerance and dependency are well-recognized problems with continued opioid use, the development of hyperalgesia or reduced threshold for discomfort from pain stimuli has only recently become recognized as a clinical concern. Such hyperalgesia has been reported after just a few hours of exposure. Opioids also have negative effects on the immune system, which may be unfavorable for debilitated patients in intensive care settings, and they do not seem to protect against development of chronic pain in the same way as some other analgesics may do.

PRINCIPLES FOR EMPLOYING NONOPIOID ANALGESICS

Acute pain reflects potential or established tissue damage. It is now recognized that acute pain is mediated by peripheral nociceptors, which are stimulated by traumatic and inflammatory mechanisms. The best way to treat acute pain is to minimize tissue injury and prevent or reduce the inflammatory and neuropathic stimulation. Administration of nonopioid analgesics/adjuvants can reduce inflammatory responses and peripheral neuropathic sensitization, thereby minimizing nociceptive pain and opioid dose requirements. Prophylactic, preventative measures designed to minimize tissue injury (noninvasive surgery) and inflammation (nonsteroiday anti-inflammatory drugs [NSAIDs] and other anti-inflammatory agents) are important in this context. The importance of gentle and minimally traumatic surgery should also be mentioned; for example, endoscopic procedures are associated with significantly less tissue injury and are generally less painful than open invasive surgery. Also, nonpharmacological measures to further reduce tissue damage, inflammation, and nerve stimulation should be provided, particularly when the pain-provoking process is ongoing. Examples are limb elevation, compression, and localized cooling to reduce inflammation and edema.

Analgesics have variable sites of activity and can interact with receptors, local and humoral mediators in injured tissues, or on nerves and nerve endings that transmit nociceptive stimuli to the central nervous system (Figure 23.1). Analgesics are also effective to modulate the pain impulse at the level of the spinal cord and also at cortical level. This chapter will focus on the role of glucocorticoids, antineuropathics and other analgesics as nonopioid analgesics.

GLUCOCORTICOIDS

Overview

The glucocorticoids are naturally occurring hormones, with a diurnal variation in circulating levels with mobilization and increased circulating levels during trauma and stress (Figure 23.2). Typically about 25–50 mg of cortisone is secreted during a normal 24-hour period.[1] The clinical analgesic effect of stress hormones have long been acknowledged,[2,3] for instance, during combat situations where the pain threshold seems to be significantly elevated, possibly partly from glucocorticoids and other

Table 23.1: Why Administer Nonopioids Analgesics and Analgesic Adjuvants

Opioid sparing
  Fewer opioid-induced side effects
    Constipation
    Nausea
    Respiratory depression
    Sedation
    Sleep apnea
    Sleep disturbance
    Pruritus

Improved analgesia
  Opioids less effective during movement/mobilization
  Delayed and restrictive opioid dosing in clinical practice

Impact on pain mechanisms
  Blocking wind-up, sensitization, hyperalgesia
  Limiting development of chronic pain?

stress hormones. It has also been shown that animals with elevated levels of endogenous glucocorticoids experience less pain than others.[4]

Although the mechanism of action of most analgesics has been elucidated, many were first used empirically, and their efficacy was never tested in large-scale controlled trials. In this regard, therapeutic benefits associated with glucocorticoids have not been studied as other newer analgesic drugs have been studied for regulatory approval. At the present time, there is little incentive for the pharmaceutical industry to develop patents and market higher priced glucocorticoid drugs. Also, the fear of side effects and the lack of exact knowledge of their analgesic mechanisms have limited the introduction of this class into routine clinical use. However, this lack of interest may be challenged as ongoing research is performed on membrane-bound glucocorticoid receptors and more selective and potentially safer steroid agonists.[5] Potential analgesic benefits of glucocorticoids are outlined in Table 23.2.

Effect Mechanisms

Glucocorticoids act by binding to a class of nuclear receptors (corticosteroid receptors). On binding to the receptor transfer (chaperone) protein, the drug-receptor complex diffuses into the nucleus of the cell and binds to deoxyribonucleic acid (DNA), initiating production of proteins and enzymes with subsequent clinical effects (Figure 23.3).[6–8] Traditional pharmacokinetic parameters are not appropriate for describing glucocorticoid pharmacodynamics, because genetic activation is associated with significant latency to effect. For this reason, onset is typically delayed, with maximum glucocorticoid effects observed after 3–4 hours or more.[8–10] For the same reason, the duration of clinical effect is prolonged and does not correlate with plasma

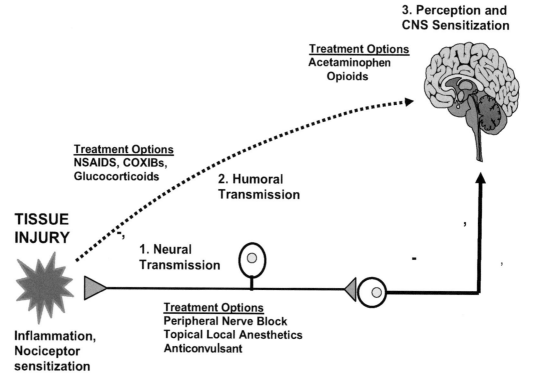

Figure 23.1: Neural and humoral mechanisms underlying pain perception and central sensitization. The central nervous system is sensitized by (1) neural transmission of noxious impulses and (2) humoral transmission of noxious mediators, including cytokines, interleukins, TNF-α, and prostanoids. Neural transmission can be attenuated by neural blockade, epidural analgesia, and antineuropathic agents, whereas administration of NSAIDs, COX-2 inhibitors, and glucocorticoids may reduce local inflammation and humoral induced aspects of central sensitization.

Table 23.2: Corticosteroid Clinical Actions

Anti-inflammatory

Antiedema

Analgesia

Antiemesis

Antipyretic

Euphoria

Alertness

Increased energy

Restless

Increased appetite

concentrations of drugs. In general, effects on cellular processes will continue for hours to days, despite complete clearance of drugs from plasma.

Some direct cellular membrane effects of glucocorticoids have also been suggested.[5] The rapid membrane stabilization from glucocorticoids during anaphylactoid reactions and a study by Romundstad et al,[11] showing analgesic effect within 1 hour of administration, are clinical supportive of these non-DNA-mediated effects of glucocorticoids.

Molecular Actions of Glucocorticoids

The family of steroid molecules includes potent hormones necessary for normal homeostasis and growth of the human body.[3]

The glucocorticoids have virtually no sex hormonal effects, but some of them may still have a slight mineral-corticoid effect (Table 23.3), resulting in renal sodium and water retention.[12] There are also some reports of increased blood sugar levels, especially in diabetic patients.[13] The major effects of the glucocorticoid subclass of steroid hormones are linked to the inflammatory response, including inhibition of inflammatory gene expression and stimulation of anti-inflammatory gene expression. Important mediators include cyclooxygenase 2 (COX-2) inhibition,[14] TNF inhibition, and leukocyte inhibition, both in the peripheral injured tissue, as well as in the spinal dorsal horn and central nervous system. As a part of this general anti-inflammatory action, glucocorticoids also have direct effects on blood capillaries, with decreased permeability and reduced vasodilatation.

A general anti-inflammatory action may be very important for pain reduction per se by reducing local tissue pressure and limiting the release of potent pain mediators. The glucocorticoids have also been shown to have direct effects on pain neurons and receptors. They reduce neuropeptide release, inhibit signal transmission in C fibers, and stimulate the secretion of endogenous endorphins.

Clinical Actions of Glucocorticoids

The well-known clinical effects of glucocorticoids include anti-inflammation, antiedema, antiallergic, and antipyrexia. Also analgesia and antiemetic effects[15] are well documented, although the mechanisms, especially of antiemesis, is less well understood. The glucocorticoids frequently induce a slight feeling of euphoria and alertness (Table 23.2).[16] The patient may sometimes describe a sensation of more "energy" when these drugs are used and also increased appetite may be beneficial in this setting. However, there are also reports of restlessness, dysphoria,

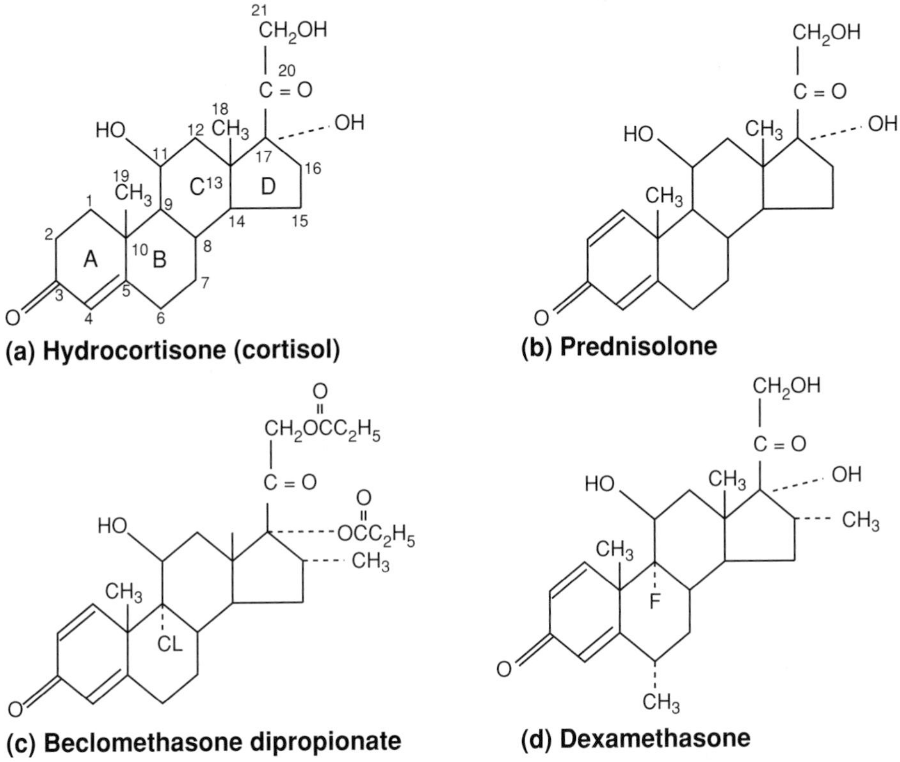

Figure 23.2: The chemical structures of glucocorticoids and other steroid hormones.

Table 23.3: Steroid Pharmocokinetic/Dynamic Characteristics

Drug	Half Life (hours)	Equivalent Dose (mg)	Anti-Inflammatory Potency	Mineral Corticoid Potency	Na+ Retaining Potency
Short acting					
Hydrocortisone	8–12	20	1	1	1
Cortisone	8–12	25	0.8	0.8	0.8
Intermediate					
Prednisolone	18–36	5	4	0.8	0.8
Prednisone	18–36	5	4	0.8	0.8
Methylprednisone	18–36	4	5	0.5	0.8
Triamcinolone	18–36	4	5	0	0
Long acting					
Dexamethasone	36–54	0.75	25	0	0

Note: Endogenous cortisone production: 25–50 mg/d ≈ 1–2 mg dexamethasone. Modified from from: Salerno A, Hermann R. *J Bone Joint Surg.* 2006:88:1361–1372.[12]

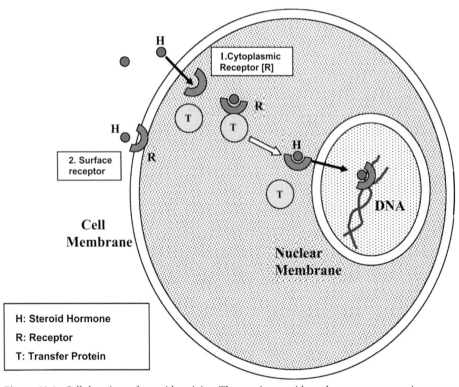

Figure 23.3: Cellular sites of steroid activity. The corticosteroid nuclear receptor requires many steps and significant time (hours to days) to initiate effects. Steroid hormones (H) cross the cell membrane and bind to a cytoplasmic receptor (R). A transfer protein (T) binds to the receptor hormone complex and guides it to the nuclear membrane. The transfer protein then decouples from the receptor, and the receptor hormone complex attaches to and influences specific genetic targets (DNA). Inhibition of inflammatory gene expression and stimulation of anti-inflammatory expression is mediated by selective synthesis of m-RNA and specific proteins/enzymes. Direct steroid effects at the cell membrane occur sooner (minutes to hours).

Table 23.4: Steroid Side Effects

Dermatological	Endocrine
Skin thining	Diabetes
Alopecia	Adrenal-pituitary insufficiency
Hirsuitism	
Acne	
Striae	
Bone	Gastrointestinal
Osteoporosis	Gastritis
Avascular necrosis	Peptic ulcer disease
	Bowel perforation
Muscle	Neuropsychiatric
Myopathy	Euphoria
Renal	Dysphoria
Fluid volume shifts	Psychosis
Hyperkalemia	Insomnia
Cardiovascular	Reproductive
Hypertension	Amenorrhea
Cardiomyopathy	Infertility
Immunological	
Increased risk of infection	
Herpes zoster	

and even rare cases of abrupt psychosis[17] when glucocorticoids are used in the postoperative setting. Less postoperative shivering have been observed and a lower incidence of cardiac arrhythmias has been demonstrated in some but not all studies.[16]

With prolonged use of these drugs there is a very long list of negative effects, from a generalized reduction in tissue growth, decreased cellular activation, and wound healing. The clinical manifestations may be wound dehiscence, nonunion of fractures, gastric ulceration and perforation, skin vulnerability and wound formation, and poor infection control. Also hormonal side effects may develop, such as moon face, sexual hormone dysfunction, mental disturbances, and hyperglycemia. Adverse events associated with long term glucocorticoid exposure are outlined in Table 23.4.

Clinical Analgesic Action

The postoperative analgesic effect of glucocorticoids has been well documented[2,3,9,11,18–24] Compared with other analgesics, the onset of clinical effect is generally delayed. In our experience, no analgesic effect is evident during the first 4 hours following administration of dexamethasone (16 mg) to patients recovering from breast surgery. This correlates with previous reports of delayed onset of effect. Aasboe et al[9] were not able to demonstrate any analgesic effect from bethamethasone (12 mg) until 3 hours postoperatively. In a laparoscopic surgical trial, Coloma et al[10] found that the antiemetic effect of dexamethasone was

more pronounced after discharge than in the immediate 3 hours postoperatively. Alternatively, Romundstad et al[21] reported that the onset of postsurgical analgesia provided by intravenous (IV) methylprednisolone (125 mg) was evident at 60 minutes after administration.[21] This is in accordance with experimental and clinical evidence suggesting that glucocorticoids may have rapid and direct, nongenomic actions on cellular membranes.[8]

The duration of analgesia of a single dose of IV glucocorticoids may be prolonged. Romundstad and coworkers[11] found that a single dose of methylprednisolone (125 mg) provided measurable analgesic effects for 3 days. Similarly, Bisgaard et al[20] reported that a single dose of dexamethasone (8 mg) significantly reduced pain intensity up to 1 week following laparoscopic surgery. The plasma elimination half-life of dexamethasone is only about 6 hours,[25] thus there seems to be ongoing drug effects for a significant period after drug clearance from the plasma.

The optimal dose of a glucocorticoid for analgesia has not been established in double blind placebo controlled trials. Similarly the effective dose of dexamethasone for the prevention of post operative nausea and vomiting ranges from 2.5 to 8 mg.[26,27] For augmentation of analgesia, a dose of dexamethasone (4 mg) resulted in less inhibition of prostanoids and less effective analgesia after dental surgery than ketorolac (30 mg).[28] Bisgaard et al[20] reported that an 8-mg dose of dexamethasone was sufficient for pain relief. Dexamethasone has also been tested out for local application as endoalveolar powder or local infiltration in wisdom tooth surgery.[29] However, the dose used was 4–10 mg, and a systemic effect cannot be ruled out in this experimental design. In another dental surgery study, 8 mg dexamethasone was found to be more efficient than 4 mg, but increasing the dose to 16 mg provided no further improvement in pain relief.[30] The dose of glucocorticoid used in the studies from Romundstad's group[11,21] is more generous, as the 125-mg methylprednisolone dose they employed is equivalent to 25 mg of dexamethasone.[12] Olstad and Skjelbred[31] also reported that 84 mg methylprednisolone administered over 4 days was effective for postdental surgery pain.

Although glucocorticoids have been shown to inhibit the COX-2 enzyme system, much like NSAIDs, they also have hormonal effects and act on a variety of other enzyme systems. Thus, it is of interest to elucidate how the analgesic effect compares with other analgesics in placebo-controlled models: Olstad and Skjelbred[31] studied the effect of betamethasone versus paracetamol during a 4-day study and found a tendency of paracetamol to be more analgesic during the 3–4 hours after administration, whereas betamethasone was best during days 3 and 4. Romundstad et al found that the analgesic effect of a single prophylactic 125-mg dose of methylprednisolone was equivalent to parecoxib (40 mg) during a 6-hour study period, with significantly less nausea and sedation.[21] These authors also evaluated the effectiveness of methylprednisolone (125 mg) versus ketorolac (30 mg) given for postoperative pain. They found that both drugs provided equivalent and effective analgesia during the first 24 hours. Patients treated with ketorolac experienced a more rapid onset of analgesia, whereas those treated with methylprednisolone required significantly less rescue analgesics during postoperative days 2 and 3.[11]

An important question that must be answered is whether the glucocorticoids provide measurable analgesic effects when given alone and whether they provide additive analgesic effects when administered with other analgesics.[18,32,33] In Bisgaard's et al study,[20] the analgesic effect of dexamethasone (8 mg) was in addition to a regimen of local wound anesthesia, paracetamol, and ketorolac. These analgesics were also given to the placebo patients. Similarly, in the study performed by Romundstad and colleagues,[21] the analgesic effect of a glucocorticoid was in addition to that provided by local anesthesia, paracetamol, and codeine.[19] Coloma et al supplied ketorolac and local anaesthesia to all patients for baseline analgesia. Several studies have been designed to test the specific analgesic effects of a glucocorticoid plus an NSAID or COX-2 selective inhibitor (coxib). In one such study of postdental surgery pain, Bamgbose et al[23] added dexamethasone (8 mg) to diclofenac and reported improved pain score at 48 hours with the combination. In a similar clinical model, Moore et al[34] found that dexamethasone (10 mg) added to rofecoxib (50 mg) provided superior pain relief for up to 24 hours than either drug administered alone.[35] Lin and coworkers[24] found that patients treated with the combination of prednisolone (10 mg) plus diclofenac experienced significant reductions in gingival swelling following dental surgery.[24]

Other Clinical Effects and Side Effects

Glucocorticoids may also have beneficial effects on postoperative nausea and vomiting (PONV),[15,36] alertness, appetite, and mood.[16] Potential negative effects include hyperglycemia,[13] flushing, restlessness, impaired wound healing, gastrointestinal ulceration, and increased infection risk.[37] Increased alertness has also been described[20,38] and may result in potential benefits in more rapid clear-headed recovery and discharge. Adverse effects are unlikely following single-dose administration but may increase with repeated doses.[21,36,38]

In a meta-analysis of side effects after single-dose administration by Henzi et al,[36] no significant side effects were demonstrated in the 17 studies of 941 patients receiving dexamethasone. Even more impressive is the absence of side effects revealed in the meta-analyses of a much higher dose of methylprednisolone (ie, 15–30 mg/kg) used for chest trauma care.[37] In more than 2000 patients from 51 single studies, the only significant effect found was an improvement of pulmonary function with glucocorticoid.[37] However, there have been scattered reports of psychotic reactions after a single, high-dose administration of glucocorticoids.[17,39] Also, in a study of dexamethasone (10 mg), a mean 32% increase in postoperative blood sugar was noted, although no placebo group was included.[13]

Glucocorticoids

The glucocorticoids have an postoperative analgesic effect with delayed onset of 1–4 hours and prolonged duration for at least 1–3 days after a single IV dose. The analgesic peak potency seems to be comparable to the effects provided by optimal doses of NSAIDs and paracetamol. The combination of a glucocorticoid plus NSAIDs provides additive anti-inflammatory effects and analgesia. In addition, the glucocorticoids may offer a safe and useful substitute for patients with known contraindications to NSAIDs (asthma, allergy, renal failure, bleeding tendency).

There seem to be no differences in the effect of different glucocorticoids, although very few comparative studies on equipotent doses of different drugs have been done. From a theoretical point of view, dexamethasone may be the most appropriate choice. This drug has no mineralocorticoid effect and has the most prolonged duration of effect after a single dose.[12] The opti-

mal dose of dexamethasone that can be recommended remains unclear and varies according to the location and severity of the surgery. With dexamethasone, reliable analgesic effects have been demonstrated with 8–16 mg after surgery of moderate invasiveness; however, it remains to be determined whether higher doses may be more effective and more long lasting, especially because there are minimal adverse events even with very high doses.[37] There is a need for studies examining the effects of glucocorticoids after major surgery and large-scale studies to unearth any possible rare side effects, with better sensitivity and statistical power.

MEMRANE STABILIZING DRUGS: ANTINEUROPATHICS

Calcium Channel Blockers: Gabapentin and Pregabalin

Pregabalin and gabapentin are γ-aminobutyric acid (GABA) analogs with antiepileptic, analgesic, and anxiolytic activities. Pregabalin was developed as a follow-up compound to gabapentin and is the S-enantiomer of racemic 3-isobutyl GABA. Pregabalin has a more predictable dose-effect relationship, a more prolonged duration of effect, and an improved side-effect profile. Pregabalin has demonstrated efficacy at doses 2 to 4 times lower than gabapentin and seems to have a higher affinity to the binding site at the α_2-δ subunit. Pregabalin and gabapentin work by modulating the presynaptic release of exitatory neurotransmitters like glutamate, substance P, and norepinephrine. They bind selectively to the α_2-δ subunit of voltage-sensitive calcium channels.[40] The action of these compounds seems to be restricted to neurons and they have minor effects on blood pressure and heart rate.[41] Gabapentin and pregabalin modulate the release of sensory neuropeptides but only under conditions corresponding to inflammation-induced sensitization of the spinal cord. Gabapentin has a well-established role in the treatment of chronic pain conditions,[42] especially in neuropathic pain such as postherpetic neuralgia and diabetic neuropathy.[43] Pregabalin has also shown to be effective in alleviating pain in chronic, neuropathic pain conditions.[44–46]

Pregabalin and gabapentin have also been shown to have analgesic, antineuropathic, and opioid-sparing effects in acute pain. Although acute pain is predominately nociceptive in nature, prolonged central sensitization with some degree of hyperalgesia will occur following trauma, thus there is a rational reason for administering gabapentin and pregabalin in acute pain. Further, surgical trauma commonly involves damage to small nerve fibers and neurons, which also explains the activity of these agents in acute pain and their potential efficacy during the initial development of neuropathic pain.

In a systematic review of randomized controlled trials, a single dose of gabapentin (1200 mg or less) given preoperatively significantly reduced pain intensity and opioid consumption for the first 24 hours after surgery.[52] Time to first request for rescue analgesia was also prolonged in subgroups receiving 1200 mg. Multiple dosing preoperatively and/or continued use postoperatively did not reduce VAS scores further. Gabapentin also reduced postoperative pain and vomiting; the mechanism probably reflects the significant reduction in opioid consumption.[47] In a study of gabapentin alone (1800 mg) or in combination with rofecoxib for 3 days after hysterectomy, the combination of was superior to any of the drugs alone or placebo. However, at this dose sedation was more frequent in the gabapentin groups.[48]

Thus far, few studies have been published on acute pain treatment with pregabalin. In a molar extraction dental pain model, 300 mg of pregabalin given after surgery significantly reduced postoperative pain as measured by pain relief and pain intensity difference. A 300-mg dose was more efficacious than 50 mg pregabalin. Pregabalin was comparable to ibuprofen (400 mg) and significantly superior to placebo.[49] Side effects such as dizziness, somnolence, and vomiting were more frequent in the 300-mg group. Reuben and coworkers[50] found that pregabalin (150 mg) given preoperatively and repeated after 12 hours reduced pain and opioid consumption after spinal fusion surgery. They also found that the combination of pregabalin plus the selective COX-2 inhibitor celecoxib (200 mg) provided even better analgesia, reduced the need for IV patient-controlled anesthesia (PCA) morphine by 70%, and was associated with fewer side effects than placebo or either drug alone.[50]

In conclusion, a preoperative dose of either 1200 mg gabapentin or 150 mg pregabalin will reduce postoperative pain intensity and opioid consumption with few side effects. The reduction in opioid dose requirement might decrease associated side effects like nausea and vomiting. The combination of pregabalin plus a nonsteroidal anti-inflammatory drug seems advisable as it would block both neuropathic and inflammatory components of acute pain.

Sodium Channel Blockers: Lidocaine and Mexilitine

Sodium channels are universally located on neurons and nerve fibers, being responsible for the propagation of an action potential along the cell membrane. A complete reversible block of these channels can stop the nerve impulse, which is thought to be the major mechanism for the common use of local anesthetics. For obvious reasons, a complete and generalized sodium channel block, as may be accomplished by the tetrodotoxin of the Japanese puffer fish, may be lethal. However, there are also sodium channels in the periphery that are resistant to this toxin, and these have been shown to be of importance in conditions of neuropatic pain.[51] Systemic low concentrations of lidocaine, and the oral analog mexilitine, act on these channels. They have been shown to be efficient analgesics in neuropatic pain syndromes, such as diabetic neuropathy[52] and reflex sympathetic dystrophy syndrome.[53,54] Action on receptors of G-protein type and N-methyl-D-aspartic acid (NMDA) type have been suggested as the analgesic mechanisms of these drugs.[55] The prolonged analgesic effect is thought to be caused by inhibition of spontaneous impulse generation in injured nerves and ganglion neurons proximal to injured nerve segments.

Efforts to produce drugs that act more specifically on the tetrodotoxin channels are ongoing,[56] but so far clinical trials have not been published. However, there are some studies showing significant effects on postoperative pain from intravenous lidocaine administration.[51,55,57,58] Although the clinical analgesic effect seem to be modest, it was significant and opioid sparing when added to paracetamol and NSAID.[55] Two studies have shown that continuous infusion of lidocaine improves bowel function after surgery,[51,59] Kaba et al[55] have recently shown that the use of systemic lidocaine facilitates acute rehabilitation after laparascopic surgery. Nevertheless, many questions regarding optimal use of these agents and this analgesic principle remain unanswered. For example, what is the optimal dose of lidocaine? What is the optimal timing and duration of infusion? Will other local anesthetics be good alternatives? What is the potential of using oral alternatives (ie, mexilitine) instead or in addition? Will new, more specific, drugs have better clinical potential?

α_2-ADRENERGIC RECEPTOR AGONISTS

The α_2-receptor agonists have sedative, anxiolytic, analgesic, and hemodynamic properties.[32] They decrease sympathetic tone and attenuate the neuroendocrine and hemodynamic response to anesthesia and surgery. They reduce opioid and anesthetic requirements in the perioperative setting and provide measurable analgesia. In humans, α_2 adrenoceptors are located in the dorsal horn of the spinal cord and in several areas of the brain. There are at least 3 different subtypes of the α_2-adrenergic receptor, 2A, 2B, and 2C. Different subtypes may mediate antinociception and sedation separately and be a target for further drug refinement in this class.[60] Sedation is one major effect or side effect of α_2 agonists, and dexmedetomidine has recently been approved by the Food and Drug Administration (FDA) for use as a sedative in the intensive care units. For specific pain treatment the use of high doses of α_2 agonists is limited by their sedative/anesthetic properties, probably by action in the locus coeruleus. Sedation after epidural administration of clonidine reflects a substantial systemic absorption.

The current α_2 agonists used in pain management are clonidine, tizaninidne, dexmedetomidine, and epinephrine. These compounds have different partial agonist properties; dexmedetomidine with a selectivity ratio of 1600:1 for α_2:α_1, clonidine with 200:1, and epinephrine with 1:1. New agonists like radolmidine with high α_2 selectivity are currently being investigated in animal models. They have a better pharmacokinetic profile with less rapid distribution within the central nervous system and may have a potential of analgesia with less central nervous side effects.[61]

Intrathecally administered α_2 agonists produce antinociception in much lower doses than when administered systemically, thus indicating that the main site for analgesia is in the neuraxis.[62] Clonidine is used as a coanalgesic in neuraxial blockades.[62] When administered epidurally or intrathecally, α_2 agonists have synergistic action with opioids. An epidural bolus administration of the combination of fentanyl and clonidine will reduce the analgesic dose of each component by approximately 60%.[68] Clonidine will also enhance and prolong the effect of local anesthesia intrathecally.[64,65] Epinephrine is widely used as an epidural adjunct for postoperative pain relief, the effect being known for more than 50 years.[66] A mixture of 1 μg/mL epinephrine, together with 2 mg/mL bupivacaine and 1 μg/mL fentanyl, is well documented for synergistic epidural pain relief with minor incidence of motor block or hemodynamic instability.[67] Dexmedetomidine and other agonists also have analgesic properties when administered systemically. Dexmedetomidine at dose ranges from 0.5 μg/kg IV to 2.5 μg/kg intramuscularly (IM) or orally results in significant analgesia with few side effects.[5,6] Dexmedetomidine is also highly efficacious when adminstered intrathecally or epidurally in animal models, but its use spinally in humans is still experimental.

Local administration of α_2 agonists at the site of trauma seems to have analgesic properties,[68,69] possibly by a reduction in norepinephrine release in the terminal nerve endings. There is also evidence of additional analgesia when added to local anaesthesia in peripheral nerve blocks or intravenous regional anaesthesia.[62,70]

In acute pain treatment, the use of α_2-receptor agonists either in low dose systemically or as an adjuvant epidurally or intrathecally is highly beneficial. Its synergistic action with opioids and local anesthesia will reduce the doses needed of each drug, thus reducing the possible side effects. The development of less lipid-soluble agonists and a better understanding of the different subtypes of the α_2 receptors will probably result in an extended use of selective α_2 agonists.

OTHER ANALGESIC ADJUVANTS

Cannabinoids

The discovery of the cannabinoid receptors, CB_1 and CB_2 and their endogeneous ligands, has resulted in an extensive research and the development of several cannabinoid receptor agonists and antagonists. Numerous animal studies have demonstrated analgesic and antihyperalgesic properties of both plant-derived and synthetic cannabinoids. Cannabinoids produce antinociception in acute pain models in animals.[71] However, the number of clinical trials investigating their acute analgesic effect on humans is limited and the results are mixed. Nabilone, a synthetic cannabinoid, had no or negative effect on pain scores in patients undergoing major surgery.[72] In a multicenter dose escalation study, 10–15 mg of an oral cannabis extract (cannador) resulted in a dose-related reduction in rescue analgesia requirements in a postoperative pain model.[73] Buggy et al[74] found no effect of 5 mg tetrahydrocannabinol in a double-blinded, placebo-controlled study in women after hysterectomy. Drowsiness and cardiovascular events such as tachycardia, bradycaria, and hypotension are known possible side effects of cannabinoids.[75] In conclusion, further studies are needed to evaluate the possible beneficial role of cannabinoids in the acute pain setting.

Nicotine

As pain generation and mediation may be inhibited by acetylcholine action, there has been some interest into looking at the antinociceptive effect of different cholinergic agonists.[76,77] Nicotine has been one potential agonist candidate, readily available in tablets and skin pads. It has been shown that regular nicotine users (ie, smokers) may have more postoperative pain than nonsmokers,[78,79] especially when they have to abstain from smoking.[80] In a study of uterine surgery, Flood and Daniel[81] showed that a single dose of nasal nicotine just after end of uterine surgery resulted in lower pain scores during 24 hours, without any side effects. However, thus far few studies have been done on nicotine analgesia in the clinical setting.

Neostigmine

Another analgesic is to enhance endogenous acetylcholine levels by using neostigmine.[82] Neostigmine is an inhibitor of the acetylcholinesterase enzyme, thus providing higher concentra-

tions of acetylcholine in the synaptic area. One problem that has limited the exploitation of this analgesic mechanism has been the high incidence of nausea that results from neostigmines' activity in the brainstem emesis center. Nausea is most prominent when neostigmine is given intrathecally, whereas epidural or peripheral administration is associated with a gradual dose-response curve for emetic side effects.[83] Neostigmine provides useful analgesic effects with epidural or caudal routes of administration, whereas the analgesic effects of intra-articular and intravenous administration are not universally apparent.[83–86] It has also being questioned whether there is any physiologic reason to believe in a role of acetylcholine in pain mechanisms outside the central nervous system,[87] suggesting that any effect seen from topical administration may be a central one.

Magnesium

A magnesium ion plug normally maintains the NMDA receptor ion channels in the resting state. Dissociation of magnesium ions is believed to be a mandatory first step that activates these NMDA receptors and enhances pain transmission and sensitization. Receptor antagonists such as ketamine block NMDA activation; however, another way to limit activity is to rapidly replace the magnesium ion block by having increased concentrations of magnesium in the extracellular environment. Indeed, there are numerous clinical studies showing that infusion of magnesium in the perioperative phase has an additive analgesic action.[88–92] There are several negative studies as well.[93,94] Positive effects have been demonstrated after various types of surgery: gynecological, prostate, cardiac, ear/nose/throat, and cholecystectomy. Typically, 20–50 mg/kg magnesium sulfate is given slowly by the start of anesthesia, followed by infusion of 10–20 mg/kg/h for up to 1–3 days. In a dose-finding study Seyhan et al[90] found 40 mg/kg bolus followed by 10 mg/kg/h for 4 hours to be the optimal dose, with no more analgesia by doubling the infusion rate. Some studies have also shown prolonged (ie, until next morning) postoperative efficacy by utilizing a single bolus dose, without the need for infusion.[92,95] Topical administration has also been shown to be safe and effective in patients recovering from knee surgery[96] and intravenous regional anesthesia.[97] In one study looking specifically on magnesium in addition to ketamine for tonsillectomies, there was no analgesic effect of either drug nor of the combination.[93]

Nonpharmacological Approaches

Nonpharmacological measures may be valuable supplements in the treatment of acute pain. Acupuncture and transcutaneaus electrical nerve stimulation (TENS) have been scientifically proven for analgesia.

Psychoprophylaxis (ie, preoperative psychological preparation for a surgical procedure) is also an interesting option in the nonpharmacological approach to optimal pain treatment. Thorough communication with information, both by the surgeon and anesthetist, about the surgical procedure, anesthesia technique, and pain treatment reduces anxiety and stress. It has been known for decades that psychoprophylaxis reduces the need for postoperative analgesics.[98] In a more recent study, Doering et al[99] investigated the use of the preoperative presentation of a videotape showing a patient undergoing total hip replacement surgery. This prophylactic procedure significantly reduced the

Table 23.5: A Balanced Approach to Postoperative Pain Medication

Preoperatively
  Paracetamol (1.5–2 g orally; 40–50 mg/kg children)
  Coxib/NSAID orally
  Pregabalin/gabapentin

Perioperatively
  Local anesthesia, when possible
  Dexamethasone (8 mg IV)
  (paracetamol + NSAID/coxib if not given pre-op)

Postoperatively, in hospital
  Continue local anesthetic infusion
  Fentanyl if needed
  Top-up dose of ketorolac
  Continue pregabalin/gabapentin
  Continue paracetamol every 6 hours

At home, phase I:
  Paracetamol (1 g × 4)
  NSAID/Coxib (× 1–3, depending on drug)
  If needed, oxycodone (fast or slow release) on top

At home, phase II
  Paracetamol
  NSAID/coxib, if needed

perioperative anxiety level and the need for postoperative analgesic medication in patients undergoing hip surgery.

THE CLINICAL APPLICATION OF NONOPIOIDS: PUTTING IT ALL TOGETHER

Unlike opioids, most nonopioid analgesics and adjuvants have a maximal ceiling effect and a delayed onset of action. Further, there is evidence to suggest that many of these drugs, especially local anesthetics, ketamine, NSAIDs/coxibs, and glucocorticoids, have a preemptive or preventive effect,[100] thus there is rationale to administer these agents as early as possible prior to or during exposure to trauma. In this section we have not included most of the "new" analgesic options described above. This is mainly because of lack of extensive documentation of clinically relevant additive effect on top of established multimodal care, but also because of incomplete documentation on optimal dosing and risk of rare side effects. These issues may change rapidly during the next few years. Also, there may be good reason to encourage clinicians to test out some of these modalities, especially in patients where standard opioid-based regimens prove to be suboptimal. Preferably, such testing should be done in controlled studies, to contribute to the development of sound, scientific knowledge on practical use of these agents.

We have included the glucocorticoids in our basic regimens, as we feel the evidence is adequate for making general recommendations. The optimal dose and duration of a ketamine infu-

sion needs to be resolved. With the calcium blockers, systemic local anesthetics, and cannabinoids we think the evidence generally is too sparse at the moment to justify general recommendations.

Acute Postoperative Pain

The cornerstones are paracetamol/acetaminophen and NSAIDs/coxibs to all patients, unless contraindicated, and local anesthesia whenever feasible; in all wounds and even better as dedicated nerve or plexus blocks (Tables 23.5 and 23.6).

Preoperatively

Paracetamol and an NSAID/coxib should be given 1 hour or more prior to a procedure to ensure an empty stomach before anesthetic induction and systemic absorption. Oral paracetamol/acetaminophen should be administered as a 1- to 2-g dose for average adults; in case of body weight less than 60 kg or age above 70 years the dose should be reduced to 1.5 g. Paracetamol is also available in the European Union (EU) as a rapidly disintegrating tablet. The rapidly disintegrating tablets have a peak serum concentration as soon as 27 minutes after ingestion compared with 45 minutes for ordinary tablets.[105] Rectal administration of paracetamol/acetaminophen should be reserved in cases of noncompliance or nonaccessability of the oral route. The rectal administration of acetaminophen has a delayed onset of action with lower, delayed peak plasma levels. In the pediatric population the initial dose is 50–60 mg/kg. NSAIDs, such as diclofenac (50 mg), naproxen (500 mg), or ibuprofen (800 mg), should also be given orally at least 1 hour before surgery; again, dose reduction should be undertaken in small adults and elderly patients (>70 years). In children, ibuprofen or diclofenac are licensed down to 1 year of age in many countries, with a typical dose being 15–20 mg/kg (ibuprofen) or 2–3 mg/kg (diclofenac). As the coxibs seem to carry no more cardiovascular risks than most traditional NSAIDs, such as diclofenac or ibuprofen, the threshold for using a coxib instead of NSAID should be rather low. The potential advantage of the coxibs in the perioperative period is their lack of effect on platelets. Celecoxib is well documented in starting dose of 400 mg followed by 200 mg twice daily. In the EU, etoricoxib is approved for use and doses of 120 mg can provide up to 24 hours of safe and effective analgesia in uncompromised patients.

If oral medication preoperatively is not feasible or practical (eg, too short time delay before start of anesthesia, gastric suction needed), the starting dose of IV paracetamol or NSAID (ie, ketorolac or parecoxib in case of coxib) may alternatively be given IV shortly after induction of anesthesia. Intravenous paracetamol/acetaminophen is readily available and widely administered in the EU. It is undergoing final FDA trials and is not currently available for use in the United States. There are reasons to believe that the IV paracetamol starting dose also should be 2 g instead of the recommended 1-g dose commonly used. For ketorolac or parecoxib the starting dose will typically be 30 and 40 mg, respectively. Parecoxib is not available in the United States.

Peroperatively, Early Phase

After establishment of the IV line in the OR, certainly glucocorticoids are recommended to be administrated as early as possible because of their slow onset of clinical action. However, injection

Table 23.6: Present Status of Nonopioid Adjuvants in Acute Pain

Drug (class)	Effect on Acute Pain	Side Effects	Toxicity	Documentation on Dosing	Documentation on Clinical Usefulness
Paracetamol	+	Few	Toxic with overdose	++	++
NSAID	++	Some	Low	++	+++
Coxib	++	Few	Low	+	++
Local anesthesia	++	Few	Cardio/CNS toxicity	++	+++
Glucocorticoids[a]	+ (+)	0 → many	Chronic use	?	+
Gabapentin/pregabalin	(+)	Few	Cardiovascular	+	+
IV lidocaine (mexilitine)	(+)	Few	Dose dependent	(+)	(+)
Ketamine	++	Psychogenic	Small	(+)	+ (?)
Magnesium	(++)	Dose dependent	Cardiovascular	?	(+)
α_2 block	+	Some	Dose dependent	+	+
Cannabinoids	+	Psychogenic	Low	?	?
Nicotine	+ / ?	Some	Cardiovascular	?	?
Neostigmine	+	Nausea	Dose dependent	?	?

Key: ? = questionable/unknown; + = positive; ++ = very positive; ( ) = disputed or controversial.

[a] Glucocorticoids have a slow, but definite effect on acute pain, with no side effects after single dose and numerous effects with continued use.

of the common solvent in the dexamethasone preparations may result in perineal and genital itching. For this reason, dexamethasone, in typical doses (8 mg for minor surgery, 16 mg for major surgery in adults, and 0.25–0.5 mg/kg in children), is best given after induction or slowly injected after start of sedation in awake patients receiving regional anesthesia. If the surgeon approves of the use of local anesthesia infiltration prior to the initiation of surgery,[100] Lidocaine (5–10 mg/mL) has a rapid onset and, with epinephrine added, the duration is moderately prolonged and hemostasis is improved. Nevertheless, bupivacaine (2.5 mg/mL) is the preferred agent for prolonged postoperative analgesia (up to 10–15 hours). Care should always be taken to avoid high doses and systemic toxicity. If a dose of more than 40 mL (of the 2.5 mL/mg solution) is needed, the infiltration should be with the less toxic levobupivacaine (2.5 mg/mL) or ropivacaine (2–5 mg/mL) instead. If high doses of remifentanil are used intraoperatively (ie, more than 0.3 μg/kg/min or plasma target of more than 7–8 ng/mL for more than 2–3 hours), there are data suggesting development of postoperative hyperalgesia, possibly by NMDA receptor activation. The best documented way of blocking this hyperalgesia is to employ a low-dose infusion of ketamine (ie, 1–2 μg/kg/min) perioperatively and for some hours postoperatively. There is also evidence to suggest that general anesthesia with potent inhalational agents or nitrous oxide will attenuate remifentanil hyperalgesia. Also perioperative administration of NSAIDs or coxibs may also blunt this hyperalgesia.

Postoperatively in the PACU/Hospital

In this phase, there will be an IV line for drug administration and qualified nurses caring for the patients, thus allowing for individualized care of the patient. Still, medications with paracetamol (1 g every 6 hours in adults; 25–30 mg/kg every

6 hours in children) and NSAID/coxib (prescription doses and intervals) should be used as baseline, prophylactic medications. In case of pain, an extra IV dose of ketorolac should be considered (see previously), also if parecoxib was given peroperatively a repeated dose may be considered after 4–6 hours. When patients are still in pain, add small, titrated doses of opioid. Fentanyl (1–2 μg/kg) is a good routine opioid; with a fairly rapid onset of action within 3–4 minutes and limited duration of action, there is reduced risk of overdosing and subsequent nausea or somnolence. Recent evidence suggests that oxycodone may be a better alternative for visceral pain, because of some action on the κ-receptors in addition to primary μ-receptor effects.

Postoperatively at Home or without IV Access at Hospital Ward/Hotel

Whereas the glucocorticoids are recommended only as a single dose preoperatively with potential effect for 2–3 days, the dosing of paracetamol and NSAID/coxib should be repeated on a round the clock basis throughout this phase of recovery. Typically, NSAIDs or coxibs may be dosed for 1, 3, 5, or 10 days based on expected duration of pain after the procedure in question, whereas paracetamol should be used for the whole period of postoperative pain, extending up to 1–2 weeks or more. If additional analgesia is needed, oral oxycodone is an effective alternative. Sustained release oxycodone in an appropriate dose may be useful for moderate to severe pain supplemented with immediate release oxycodone for breakthrough.

Other Types of Acute Pain

Many of the same principles and drugs as used for postoperative acute pain should be valid in other contexts of acute pain;

such as occupational trauma, sports injury, neurologic pain, inflammatory pain, and so on. However, these conditions are usually not planned or predicted, so the option of pretreatment is usually not applicable. Still, the concept of rapid and adequate relief of pain with a multimodal nonopioid regimen is valid. The indication for an IV line should be considered; although impractical and painful for insertion, it may be necessary if the pain is severe with subsequent stop or delay in gastric emptying, making the oral route unpredictable. Nonpharmacological measures should also be in focus; the ICE principle (from sports medicine) may apply to all kind of pain caused by external trauma:

I = cooling via ice, ice-spray, or cold water
C = compression; elastic bandage, taping and also other measures of keeping the injuried place immobilized to avoid edema, hematoma, and further tissue injury
E = elevation; mostly to reduce the edema and pressure but also to facilitate venous blood drainage.

Oral paracetamol, possibly in a rapidly disintegrating formula, may be a primary drug option, supplemented with an NSAID whenever paracetamol is judged to have insufficient analgesic effect alone. In case of bleeding or hematoma formation, there is a good theoretical rationale for using a coxib instead, although there are no good clinical studies available justifying this selection. When there is an inflammatory component to the pain mechaonism (eg, gout, dysmenorrheal, animal bite, infection), NSAIDs can be useful not only as an analgesic but also as a means to reduce the edema and inflammatory process causing the pain.

Finally, glucocorticoids may be added in cases where prolonged analgesic/anti-inflammatory effects are required. An alternative to IV dexamethasone may be oral prednisolone in a 50– to 100-mg dose. If the pain is caused by an infection, steroid should probably be withheld; however, the appropriate use of antibiotics or antiviral drugs (eg, with herpes) is important as both adjuvant and causal therapy. Specific neurologic acute pain, such as migraine and neurogenic pain, are beyond the scope of this chapter but specific pain medications are available and should be employed for these conditions.

CONCLUSIONS

This chapter introduced several analgesic options commonly employed in the EU that may be considered for use in patients receiving multimodal analgesic regimens for acute pain management. The guiding principal is to reduce opioid dosing for acute pain as much as possible by using nonopioids and adjuvants in maximum tolerable doses, in a stepwise fashion, according to intensity of the pain stimulus. In a clinical context, single perioperative doses of glucocorticoid, paracetamol/acetaminophen, and α_2-δ antagonists should be considered and administered in appropriate patients. In combination with standardized regional analgesia, NSAIDs or COX-2 inhibitors, and limited doses of opioid, the overall quality of pain management, rehabilitation, and return to functionality can be optimized while patient safety is maintained.

REFERENCES

1. Buchman AL. Side effects of corticosteroid therapy. *J Clin Gastroenterol.* 2001;33:289–294.
2. Skjelbred P, Lokken P. Post-operative pain and inflammatory reaction reduced by injection of a corticosteroid: a controlled trial in bilateral oral surgery. *Eur J Clin Pharmacol.* 1982;21:391–396.
3. Holte K, Kehlet H. Perioperative single-dose glucocorticoid administration: pathophysiologic effects and clinical implications. *J Am Coll Surg.* 2002;195:694–712.
4. Zhang RX, Lao L, Qiao JT, et al. Endogenous and exogenous glucocorticoid suppresses up-regulation of preprodynorphin mRNA and hyperalgesia in rats with peripheral inflammation. *Neurosci Lett.* 2004;359:85–88.
5. Dallman MF. Fast glucocorticoid actions on brain: back to the future. *Front Neuroendocrinol.* 2005;26:103–108.
6. Barnes PJ. Molecular mechanisms and cellular effects of glucocorticosteroids. *Immunol Allergy Clin North Am.* 2005;25:451–468.
7. Falkenstein E, Tillmann HC, Christ M, et al. Multiple actions of steroid hormones–a focus on rapid, nongenomic effects. *Pharmacol Rev.* 2000;52:513–556.
8. Song IH, Buttgereit F. Non-genomic glucocorticoid effects to provide the basis for new drug developments. *Mol Cell Endocrinol.* 2006;246:142–146.
9. Aasboe V, Raeder JC, Groegaard B. Betamethasone reduces postoperative pain and nausea after ambulatory surgery. *Anesth Analg.* 1998;87:319–323.
10. Coloma M, White PF, Markowitz SD, et al. Dexamethasone in combination with dolasetron for prophylaxis in the ambulatory setting: effect on outcome after laparoscopic cholecystectomy. *Anesthesiology.* 2002;96:1346–1350.
11. Romundstad L, Breivik H, Niemi G, et al. Methylprednisolone intravenously 1 day after surgery has sustained analgesic and opioid-sparing effects. *Acta Anaesthesiol Scand.* 2004;48:1223–1231.
12. Salerno A, Hermann R. Efficacy and safety of steroid use for postoperative pain relief: update and review of the medical literature. *J Bone Joint Surg.* Am 2006;88:1361–1372.
13. Hans P, Vanthuyne A, Dewandre PY, et al. Blood glucose concentration profile after 10 mg dexamethasone in non-diabetic and type 2 diabetic patients undergoing abdominal surgery. *Br J Anaesth.* 2006;97:164–170.
14. O'Banion MK, Winn VD, Young DA. cDNA cloning and functional activity of a glucocorticoid-regulated inflammatory cyclooxygenase. *Proc Natl Acad Sci USA.* 1992;89:4888–4892.
15. Apfel CC, Korttila K, Abdalla M, et al. A factorial trial of six interventions for the prevention of postoperative nausea and vomiting. *N Engl J Med.* 2004;350:2441–2451.
16. Halvorsen P, Raeder J, White PF, et al. The effect of dexamethasone on side effects after coronary revascularization procedures. *Anesth Analg.* 2003;96:1578–1583, table.
17. Fleming PS, Flood TR. Steroid-induced psychosis complicating orthognathic surgery: a case report. *Br Dent J.* 2005;199:647–648.
18. White PF. The role of non-opioid analgesic techniques in the management of pain after ambulatory surgery. *Anesth Analg.* 2002;94:577–585.
19. Coloma M, Duffy LL, White PF, et al. Dexamethasone facilitates discharge after outpatient anorectal surgery. *Anesth Analg.* 2001;92:85–88.
20. Bisgaard T, Klarskov B, Kehlet H, Rosenberg J. Preoperative dexamethasone improves surgical outcome after laparoscopic

cholecystectomy: a randomized double-blind placebo-controlled trial. Ann Surg 2003;238:651–660.

21. Romundstad L, Breivik H, Roald H, et al. Methylprednisolone reduces pain, emesis, and fatigue after breast augmentation surgery: a single-dose, randomized, parallel-group study with methylprednisolone 125 mg, parecoxib 40 mg, and placebo. *Anesth Analg.* 2006;102:418–425.

22. Afman CE, Welge JA, Steward DL. Steroids for post-tonsillectomy pain reduction: meta-analysis of randomized controlled trials. *Otolaryngol Head Neck Surg.* 2006;134:181–186.

23. Bamgbose BO, Akinwande JA, Adeyemo WL, et al. Effects of co-administered dexamethasone and diclofenac potassium on pain, swelling and trismus following third molar surgery. *Head Face Med.* 2005;1:11.

24. Lin TC, Lui MT, Chang RC. Premedication with diclofenac and prednisolone to prevent postoperative pain and swelling after third molar removal. *Zhonghua Yi Xue Za Zhi (Taipei).* 1996;58:40–44.

25. O'Sullivan BT, Cutler DJ, Hunt GE, et al. Pharmacokinetics of dexamethasone and its relationship to dexamethasone suppression test outcome in depressed patients and healthy control subjects. *Biol Psychiatry.* 1997;41:574–584.

26. Liu K, Hsu CC, Chia YY. The effect of dose of dexamethasone for antiemesis after major gynecological surgery. *Anesth Analg.* 1999;89:1316–1318.

27. Lee Y, Lai HY, Lin PC, et al. A dose ranging study of dexamethasone for preventing patient-controlled analgesia-related nausea and vomiting: a comparison of droperidol with saline. Anesth Analg. 2004;98:1066–1071, table.

28. Dionne RA, Gordon SM, Rowan J, et al. Dexamethasone suppresses peripheral prostanoid levels without analgesia in a clinical model of acute inflammation. *J Oral Maxillofac Surg.* 2003;61:997–1003.

29. Graziani F, D'Aiuto F, Arduino PG, et al. Perioperative dexamethasone reduces post-surgical sequelae of wisdom tooth removal. A split-mouth randomized double-masked clinical trial. *Int J Oral Maxillofac Surg.* 2006;35:241–246.

30. Numazaki M, Fujii Y. Reduction of postoperative emetic episodes and analgesic requirements with dexamethasone in patients scheduled for dental surgery. *J Clin Anesth.* 2005;17:182–186.

31. Olstad OA, Skjelbred P. Comparison of the analgesic effect of a corticosteroid and paracetamol in patients with pain after oral surgery. *Br J Clin Pharmacol.* 1986;22:437–442.

32. Dahl V, Raeder JC. Non-opioid postoperative analgesia. *Acta Anaesthesiol Scand.* 2000;44:1191–1203.

33. Kehlet H, Jensen TS, Woolf CJ. Persistent postsurgical pain: risk factors and prevention. *Lancet.* 2006;367:1618–1625.

34. Moore PA, Brar P, Smiga ER, Costello BJ. Preemptive rofecoxib and dexamethasone for prevention of pain and trismus following third molar surgery. *Oral Surg Oral Med Oral Pathol Oral Radiol Endod.* 2005;99:E1–E7.

35. Karst M, Kegel T, Lukas A, et al. Effect of celecoxib and dexamethasone on postoperative pain after lumbar disc surgery. *Neurosurgery.* 2003;53:331–336.

36. Henzi I, Walder B, Tramer MR. Dexamethasone for the prevention of postoperative nausea and vomiting: a quantitative systematic review. *Anesth Analg.* 2000;90:186–194.

37. Sauerland S, Nagelschmidt M, Mallmann P, Neugebauer EA. Risks and benefits of preoperative high dose methylprednisolone in surgical patients: a systematic review. *Drug Saf.* 2000;23:449–461.

38. Ahn JH, Kim MR, Kim KH. Effect of i.v. dexamethasone on postoperative dizziness, nausea and pain during canal wall-up mastoidectomy. *Acta Otolaryngol.* 2005;125:1176–1179.

39. Ferris RL, Eisele DW. Steroid psychosis after head and neck surgery: case report and review of the literature. *Otolaryngol Head Neck Surg.* 2003;129:591–592.

40. Zareba G. Pregabalin: a new agent for the treatment of neuropathic pain. *Drugs Today (Barc).* 2005;41:509–516.

41. Fink K, Dooley DJ, Meder WP, et al. Inhibition of neuronal Ca(2+) influx by gabapentin and pregabalin in the human neocortex. *Neuropharmacology.* 2002;42:229–236.

42. Fehrenbacher JC, Taylor CP, Vasko MR. Pregabalin and gabapentin reduce release of substance P and CGRP from rat spinal tissues only after inflammation or activation of protein kinase C. *Pain.* 2003;105:133–141.

43. Wiffen PJ, McQuay HJ, Edwards JE, Moore RA. Gabapentin for acute and chronic pain. *Cochrane Database Syst Rev.* 2005;CD005452.

44. Bennett MI, Simpson KH. Gabapentin in the treatment of neuropathic pain. *Palliat Med.* 2004;18:5–11.

45. Dworkin RH, Corbin AE, Young JP, Jr, et al. Pregabalin for the treatment of postherpetic neuralgia: a randomized, placebo-controlled trial. *Neurology.* 2003;60:1274–1283.

46. Freynhagen R, Strojek K, Griesing T, et al. Efficacy of pregabalin in neuropathic pain evaluated in a 12-week, randomised, double-blind, multicentre, placebo-controlled trial of flexible- and fixed-dose regimens. *Pain.* 2005;115:254–263.

47. Ho KY, Gan TJ, Habib AS. Gabapentin and postoperative pain: a systematic review of randomized controlled trials. *Pain.* 2006;126:91–101.

48. Gilron I, Orr E, Tu D, et al. A placebo-controlled randomized clinical trial of perioperative administration of gabapentin, rofecoxib and their combination for spontaneous and movement-evoked pain after abdominal hysterectomy. *Pain.* 2005;113:191–200.

49. Hill CM, Balkenohl M, Thomas DW, et al. Pregabalin in patients with postoperative dental pain. *Eur J Pain.* 2001;5:119–124.

50. Reuben SS, Buvanendran A, Kroin JS, Raghunathan K. The analgesic efficacy of celecoxib, pregabalin, and their combination for spinal fusion surgery. *Anesth Analg.* 2006;103:1271–1277.

51. Groudine SB, Fisher HA, Kaufman RP, Jr, et al. Intravenous lidocaine speeds the return of bowel function, decreases postoperative pain, and shortens hospital stay in patients undergoing radical retropubic prostatectomy. *Anesth Analg.* 1998;86:235–239.

52. Jarvis B, Coukell AJ. Mexiletine. A review of its therapeutic use in painful diabetic neuropathy. *Drugs.* 1998;56:691–707.

53. Challapalli V, Tremont-Lukats IW, McNicol ED, et al. Systemic administration of local anesthetic agents to relieve neuropathic pain. *Cochrane Database Syst Rev.* 2005;CD003345.

54. Kalso E. Sodium channel blockers in neuropathic pain. *Curr Pharm Des.* 2005;11:3005–3011.

55. Kaba A Laurent SR, Detroz BJ, et al. Intravenous lidocaine infusion facilitates acute rehabilitation after laparoscopic colectomy. *Anesthesiology.* 2007;106:11–18.

56. Akada Y, Ogawa S, Amano K, et al. Potent analgesic effects of a putative sodium channel blocker M58373 on formalin-induced and neuropathic pain in rats. *Eur J Pharmacol.* 2006;536:248–255.

57. Koppert W, Weigand M, Neumann F, et al. Perioperative intravenous lidocaine has preventive effects on postoperative pain and morphine consumption after major abdominal surgery. *Anesth Analg.* 2004;98:1050–1055.

58. Fassoulaki A, Patris K, Sarantopoulos C, Hogan Q. The analgesic effect of gabapentin and mexiletine after breast surgery for cancer. *Anesth Analg.* 2002;95:985–991.

59. Rimback G, Cassuto J, Tollesson PO. Treatment of postoperative paralytic ileus by intravenous lidocaine infusion. *Anesth Analg.* 1990;70:414–419.

60. Buerkle H, Yaksh TL. Pharmacological evidence for different alpha 2-adrenergic receptor sites mediating analgesia and sedation in the rat. *Br J Anaesth.* 1998;81:208–215.

61. Xu M, Kontinen VK, Kalso E. Effects of radolmidine, a novel alpha2-adrenergic agonist compared with dexmedetomidine in different pain models in the rat. *Anesthesiology.* 2000;93:473–481.

62. Singelyn FJ, Dangoisse M, Bartholomee S, Gouverneur JM. Adding clonidine to mepivacaine prolongs the duration of anesthesia and analgesia after axillary brachial plexus block. *Reg Anesth.* 1992;17:148–150.

63. Eisenach JC, D'Angelo R, Taylor C, Hood DD. An isobolographic study of epidural clonidine and fentanyl after cesarean section. *Anesth Analg.* 1994;79:285–290.

64. Bonnet F, Brun-Buisson V, Saada M, et al. Dose-related prolongation of hyperbaric tetracaine spinal anesthesia by clonidine in humans. *Anesth Analg.* 1989;68:619–622.

65. Liu S, Chiu AA, Neal JM, et al. Oral clonidine prolongs lidocaine spinal anesthesia in human volunteers. *Anesthesiology.* 1995;82:1353–1359.

66. Priddle HD, Andros GJ. Primary spinal anesthetic effects of epinephrine. *Curr Res Anesth Analg.* 1950;29:156–162.

67. Niemi G, Breivik H. Adrenaline markedly improves thoracic epidural analgesia produced by a low-dose infusion of bupivacaine, fentanyl and adrenaline after major surgery. A randomised, double-blind, cross-over study with and without adrenaline. *Acta Anaesthesiol Scand.* 1998;42:897–909.

68. Davis KD, Treede RD, Raja SN, et al. Topical application of clonidine relieves hyperalgesia in patients with sympathetically maintained pain. *Pain.* 1991;47:309–317.

69. Gentili M, Juhel A, Bonnet F. Peripheral analgesic effect of intra-articular clonidine. *Pain.* 1996;64:593–596.

70. Memis D, Turan A, Karamanlioglu B, et al. Adding dexmedetomidine to lidocaine for intravenous regional anesthesia. *Anesth Analg.* 2004;98:835–840.

71. Pertwee RG. Cannabinoid receptors and pain. *Prog Neurobiol.* 2001;63:569–611.

72. Beaulieu P. Effects of nabilone, a synthetic cannabinoid, on postoperative pain. *Can J Anaesth.* 2006;53:769–775.

73. Holdcroft A, Maze M, Dore C, et al. A multicenter dose-escalation study of the analgesic and adverse effects of an oral cannabis extract (Cannador) for postoperative pain management. *Anesthesiology.* 2006;104:1040–1046.

74. Buggy DJ, Toogood L, Maric S, et al. Lack of analgesic efficacy of oral delta-9-tetrahydrocannabinol in postoperative pain. *Pain.* 2003;106:169–172.

75. Notcutt W, Price M, Miller R, et al. Initial experiences with medicinal extracts of cannabis for chronic pain: results from 34 'N of 1' studies. *Anaesthesia.* 2004;59:440–452.

76. Decker MW, Rueter LE, Bitner RS. Nicotinic acetylcholine receptor agonists: a potential new class of analgesics. *Curr Top Med Chem.* 2004;4:369–384.

77. Vincler M. Neuronal nicotinic receptors as targets for novel analgesics. Expert *Opin Investig Drugs.* 2005;14:1191–1198.

78. Creekmore FM, Lugo RA, Weiland KJ. Postoperative opiate analgesia requirements of smokers and nonsmokers. *Ann Pharmacother.* 2004;38:949–953.

79. Woodside JR. Female smokers have increased postoperative narcotic requirements. *J Addict Dis.* 2000;19:1–10.

80. Marco AP, Greenwald MK, Higgins MS. A preliminary study of 24-hour post-cesarean patient controlled analgesia: postoperative pain reports and morphine requests/utilization are greater in abstaining smokers than non-smokers. *Med Sci Monit.* 2005;11:CR255–CR261.

81. Flood P, Daniel D. Intranasal nicotine for postoperative pain treatment. *Anesthesiology.* 2004;101:1417–1421.

82. Eisenach JC. Muscarinic-mediated analgesia. *Life Sci.* 1999;64:549–854.

83. Habib AS, Gan TJ. Use of neostigmine in the management of acute postoperative pain and labour pain: a review. *CNS Drugs.* 2006;20:821–839.

84. Gentili M, Enel D, Szymskiewicz O, et al. Postoperative analgesia by intraarticular clonidine and neostigmine in patients undergoing knee arthroscopy. *Reg Anesth Pain Med.* 2001;26:342–347.

85. McCartney CJ, Brill S, Rawson R, et al. No anesthetic or analgesic benefit of neostigmine 1 mg added to intravenous regional anesthesia with lidocaine 0.5% for hand surgery. *Reg Anesth Pain Med.* 2003;28:414–417.

86. Alagol A, Calpur OU, Usar PS, et al. Intraarticular analgesia after arthroscopic knee surgery: comparison of neostigmine, clonidine, tenoxicam, morphine and bupivacaine. *Knee Surg Sports Traumatol Arthrosc.* 2005;13:658–663.

87. Schafer M. Analgesic effects of neostigmine in the periphery. *Anesthesiology.* 2000;92:1207–1208.

88. Tramer MR, Schneider J, Marti RA, Rifat K. Role of magnesium sulfate in postoperative analgesia. *Anesthesiology.* 1996;84:340–347.

89. Bhatia A, Kashyap L, Pawar DK, Trikha A. Effect of intraoperative magnesium infusion on perioperative analgesia in open cholecystectomy. *J Clin Anesth.* 2004;16:262–265.

90. Seyhan TO, Tugrul M, Sungur MO, et al. Effects of three different dose regimens of magnesium on propofol requirements, haemodynamic variables and postoperative pain relief in gynaecological surgery. *Br J Anaesth.* 2006;96:247–252.

91. Steinlechner B, Dworschak M, Birkenberg B, et al. Magnesium moderately decreases remifentanil dosage required for pain management after cardiac surgery. *Br J Anaesth.* 2006;96:444–449.

92. Tauzin-Fin P, Sesay M, Ort-Laval S, et al. Intravenous magnesium sulphate decreases postoperative tramadol requirement after radical prostatectomy. *Eur J Anaesthesiol.* 2006;23:1055–1059.

93. O'Flaherty JE, Lin CX. Does ketamine or magnesium affect post-tonsillectomy pain in children? *Paediatr Anaesth.* 2003;13:413–421.

94. Paech MJ, Magann EF, Doherty DA, et al. Does magnesium sulfate reduce the short- and long-term requirements for pain relief after caesarean delivery? A double-blind placebo-controlled trial. *Am J Obstet Gynecol.* 2006;194:1596–1602.

95. Levaux C, Bonhomme V, Dewandre PY, et al. Effect of intra-operative magnesium sulphate on pain relief and patient comfort after major lumbar orthopaedic surgery. *Anaesthesia.* 2003;58:131–135.

96. Bondok RS, El-Hady AM. Intra-articular magnesium is effective for postoperative analgesia in arthroscopic knee surgery. *Br J Anaesth.* 2006;97:389–392.

97. Turan A, Memis D, Karamanlioglu B, et al. Intravenous regional anesthesia using lidocaine and magnesium. *Anesth Analg.* 2005;100:1189–1192.

98. Egbert LD, Battit GE, Welch CE, Bartlett MK. Reduction of postopeative pain by encouragement and instruction of patients: a study of doctor-patient rapport. *N Engl J Med.* 1964;270:825–827.

99. Doering S, Katzlberger F, Rumpold G, et al. Videotape preparation of patients before hip replacement surgery reduces stress.
Psychosom Med. 2000;62:365–373.

100. Ong CK, Lirk P, Seymour RA, Jenkins BJ. The efficacy of preemptive analgesia for acute postoperative pain
management: a meta-analysis. *Anesth Analg,* 2005;100:757–
773.

101. Rygnestad T, Zahlsen K, Samdal FA. Absorption of effervescent
paracetamol tablets relative to ordinary paracetamol tablets in
healthy volunteers. *Eur J Clin Pharmacol.* 2000;56:141–143.

Nonpharmacological Approaches for Acute Pain Management

Stefan Erceg and Keun Sam Chung

Pain is defined by the International Association for the Study of Pain as an unpleasant sensory and emotional experience associated with actual or potential tissue damage.[1] It is a subjective experience that develops differently for each individual through life experiences. The pathophysiological mechanisms of pain and sites of pain processing are continually being elucidated and are discussed in other chapters of this textbook. Concepts underlying pain perception include the following: peripheral and central sensitization, higher cortical recognition/interpretation, descending inhibition, and sympathetic responses. A basic understanding of these concepts is the key to better appreciating traditional and nontraditional analgesic techniques.

With the now widely accepted multimodal approach to pain management, our focus must expand to include techniques beyond the strictly Western-based pharmacologic approach to the treatment of pain. A fine balance should be achieved between the use of pharmacologic management and nontraditional nonpharmacologic techniques. Observations made during the 1980s found the approach to analgesia needed to be reexamined. The success of the World Health Organization (WHO) in setting guidelines for pain management was based on the administration of appropriate pharmacologic agents for each level of pain severity. The WHO analgesic ladder provided an impetus for the use of opiate analgesics as the foundation of pain management. This goal was successfully met as evidenced by the fact that opioid sales in the United States, recorded in morphine equivalents, increased from 76,747.0 mg in 1999 to 134,792.7 mg in 2002.[2] It should not be forgotten that the WHO guidelines clearly supported the use of nonopioid analgesics and nonpharmacologic techniques; however, these options are rarely used in optimal fashion.

Opioid monotherapy is associated with significant annoying and occasional life-threatening adverse events. Opioids produce dose-dependent respiratory depression because of impairment of the respiratory center's capnic drive. The medullary cough center may also be affected by opioid usage, leading to increased risk of aspiration. Opioids, such as morphine and fentanyl, are associated with confusion, cognitive dysfunction, increased sedation, and respiratory depression. Such morbidity is particularly troublesome in elderly patients, and may increase morbidity and interfere with activities of daily living. The gastrointestinal effects of morphine and its cousins appear to be dose related and quite varied. Gastrointestinal motility and genitourinary dysfunction often develop from the use of opioid medications. Lower esophageal sphincter relaxation increases the risk for aspiration, whereas the increased tone combined with the decreased propulsive activity of the bowel often leads to constipation. By far, one of the most undesirable effects of opioids involves their activity at the chemoreceptor trigger zone that produces a high risk for nausea and vomiting. Opioid analgesics are also frequently diverted and abused. The Drug Abuse Warning Network published a report in 2006 with data collected from a national sample of general, nonfederal hospitals emergency department (ED) visits. Of the nearly 1.3 million ED visits, the nonmedical use of prescription pharmaceuticals such as opiates, benzodiazepines, and muscle relaxants accounted for nearly half a million. In fact, 31.9% of these visits involved the nonmedical abuse of opiates[3] (Table 24.1).

The National Survey on Drug Use and Health report, published in the same year by Substance Abuse and Mental Health Services Administration, further highlights the methods used to obtain pharmaceuticals for nonmedical purposes, at least by young adults aged 18–25 years. Although the vast majority of cases indicated that the drug in question was obtained free from a friend or relative (53%), the second most common source of nonmedically abused prescriptions were obtained from a physician (12.7%) (Figure 24.1).[4] Regardless of the resource used by individuals to obtain the medications, the stark reality of opiate abuse remains.

A final complication associated with opioid analgesics is termed opioid-induced hyperalgesia (OIH). This well-accepted hyperesthetic phenomenon results in a paradoxically increased sensitivity to painful stimuli. OIH may be differentiated from the development of tolerance by progressive increases in pain intensity despite adequate advancement in dosing. The etiology of OIH is undoubtedly multifactorial; however, researchers have strongly implicated a central role for NMDA receptor activation.[5]

Table 24.1: Emergency Department Visits Involving the Nonmedical Use of Opiates

Drug	Estimated Visits		95% Confidence Interval	
	Number	Percentage	Lower Bound	Upper Bound
Opiates/opioids	158,281	31.9	131,292	185,270
Hydrocodone/combos	42,491		31,831	53,151
Oxycodone/combos	36,559		28,964	44,154
Methadone	31,874		23,752	39,996

Note: Data adapted from the Drug Abuse Warning Network reports of approximately one-half million emergency department visits involving nonmedical use of prescription pharmaceuticals in 2004.

NONPHARMACOLOGIC THERAPY

If our goal is to provide the most effective form of treatment with the least number of associated risks, we must integrate all of our methods of analgesia. Just as the use of multiple classes of analgesic drugs reduces the dosage and side effects of each drug, inclusion of adjuvant nonpharmacologic analgesic techniques could further diminish cumulative analgesic dose, thereby increasing patient safety. Moreover, the majority of nonpharmacologic techniques are predominantly side effect free. Decreasing our exposure should also reduce the incidence of annoying and life-threatening adverse effects, decrease risks of opioid diversion and abuse, and lower the prevalence of opioid induced hyperalgesia. The beneficial contribution provided by nonpharmacologic analgesics should not be overlooked.

Many nonpharmacologic analgesic techniques were spawned from Eastern medicine practices and have yet to gain wide acceptance in the Western medical world. However, it is a burgeoning component of alternative medicine, becoming quite popular with patients. The largest impediments to the incorporation of these techniques in the field of pain management include unfamiliarity, production pressure, and lack of well-developed studies to prove their validity. Unfortunately, because of the nature of many of these interventions, standard Western study models are often difficult to design.

Holistic medicine is one of the uniting themes throughout a large proportion of the proposed mechanisms for many of today's most popular nontraditional, nonpharmacologic anal-

gesics. It is a concept that focuses on the patient as the sum of his or her parts. All of the different parts of the body, including the mind, are interconnected. Pathology involving one part of the body, consequently, will affect other parts of the body. Therefore, to properly treat a patient, one must view the patient as a complex milieu. No form of analgesia illustrates this concept better than the practice of acupuncture.

Beyond the concept of holistic medicine, the fields of acupuncture, acupressure, moxibustion, cupping, transcutaneous electrical nerve stimulation (TENS), and percutaneous electrical nerve stimulation (PENS) (electroacupuncture) have additional similarities. Although acupuncture, acupressure, and moxibustion all developed from ancient, Eastern Asian folk medicine practices; TENS and PENS had a more Western development with its early progenitors found in practices dating back to ancient Grecian times. The underpinning that connects all of these therapies involves the use of subnoxious to noxious stimuli at discrete locations to produce counter irritation and a state of heightened analgesia.

ACUPUNCTURE

Acupuncture was probably first used more than 3000–4000 years ago. The *Huang Di Nei Jing* (*The Yellow Emperor's Classic of Internal Medicine*), initially compiled approximately 400–100 BC, is one of the earliest texts to describe the technique of acupuncture.[6,7] Since its inception, it has grown in popularity with more than 10 million treatments annually in the United

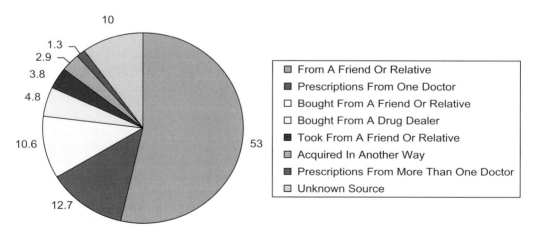

Figure 24.1: Percentages of reported method of acquiring prescription pain medicines for nonmedical use in the past year for 18- to 25-year-olds.

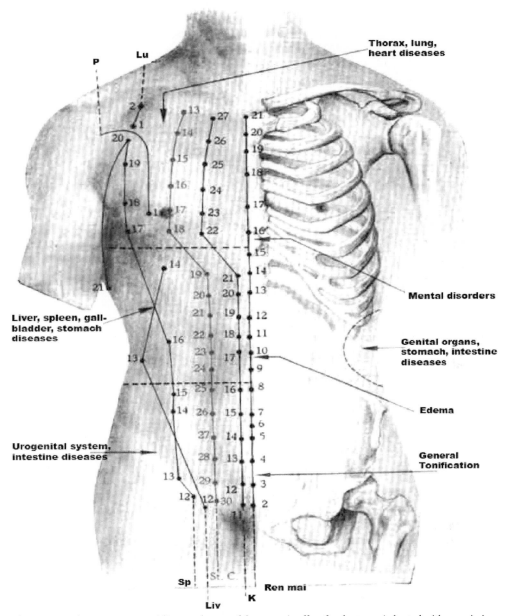

Figure 24.2a: Acupuncture meridians and areas of therapeutic effect for the torso (adapted with permission from Shmuel Halevi).

States.[8] The modern-day embracement of this practice appears to owe thanks to the governmental support, it received under the regime of Mao Zedong in the late 1940s and early 1950s. The practice spread in earnest to Western countries approximately 20 years later, with the growth of US international politics. Its popularity appears to have blossomed out of various reports indicating its effectiveness for surgical anesthesia. Currently, the practice of acupuncture has become so highly regarded, that the Food and Drug Administration (FDA), National Institutes of Health (NIH), and WHO have all given their stamp of approval for its use.[6]

Acupuncture is based on an overall theme of interconnectedness. The philosophy postulates that one energy source permeates the universe and all things within it. This flow remains in a state of perpetual balance between the forces of yin and yang. The energy flow, or qi, travels along pathways known as meridians. In fact, the body is composed of a series of meridians interconnecting the various parts of the body and in continuance with the rest of the universe. Fourteen traditional meridians have been described along with more than 360 specific acupuncture points. If any obstruction should occur along one of the body's meridians, the qi will no longer flow and pathology will develop. (Figures 24.2[a] and 24.2[b] illustrate meridians and areas of treatment for the torso and head.)

Various acupuncture points between these meridians exist on the body, and it is here that the application of needles has its effect. Stimulation of these points is achieved through continual or periodic twirling or flicking of the needles to produce afferent stimuli. The acupuncture points are stimulated to relieve the blockage obstructing the flow of qi through the body. Once this is achieved, balance is returned, and symptoms subsequently resolve.[6,8] Acupuncturists verify accurate placement of needles

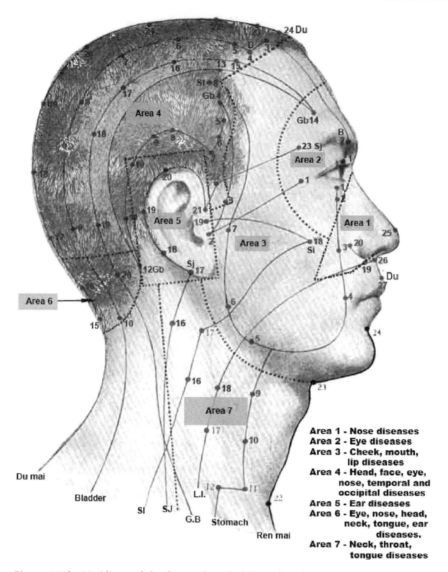

Figure 24.2b: Meridians of the face and neck (adapted with permission from Shmuel Halevi).

Area 1 - Nose diseases
Area 2 - Eye diseases
Area 3 - Cheek, mouth, lip diseases
Area 4 - Head, face, eye, nose, temporal and occipital diseases
Area 5 - Ear diseases
Area 6 - Eye, nose, head, neck, tongue, ear diseases.
Area 7 - Neck, throat, tongue diseases

by the presence of cutaneous hyperemia (de qi phenomenon), which is believed to be mediated by local and humorally released mediators (Figure 24.3).

From its early introduction into Western medicine, clinical researchers have found it difficult to comprehend the mystical nature of acupuncture and have sought to prove or disprove the validity of this technique. Fortunately, the situation has been improved through the keen interest of the Western medical community. Various acupuncture enthusiasts have attempted to explain its mechanism of action; however, only a few of these proposals appear to have withstood the test of time. In 1965, Melzack and Wall introduced the gate control theory, and it was subsequently used to explain a possible mechanism for acupuncture's analgesic qualities.[9] According to their theory, noxious stimulation of A-β sensory fibers sends afferent impulses to the dorsal horn of the spinal cord that inhibit the transmission of pain impulses along the smaller A-δ and C fibers. This theory, along with others, proposed that neural pathways instead of mysterious meridians were involved. This then provided the necessary scientific basis to encourage greater acceptance of acupuncture in the Western world.

Building on this theoretical base, more recent studies have started to explore the neurohumoral contributions of acupuncture. Based on the observation that analgesia produced by acupuncture has a slow onset that outlasts the period of stimulation, humoral mechanisms have been proposed.

Early studies in animals, and later in humans, using opiate antagonists have clearly provided evidence to support the hypothesis that acupuncture is at least partially attributable to the release of endogenous opioids.[10-12] Mayer's team explored the effectiveness of acupuncture after exposure to naloxone, an opioid-specific antagonist. Although their subjects experienced approximately 27% improvement in their pain threshold, these effects were virtually negated after administration of naloxone.[13] Elevation of β-endorphins were also noted in a cohort of males undergoing major abdominal surgery. The results were noted after only 5 minutes post stimulation, but it is somewhat difficult to ascribe them to only acupuncture therapy.[14] Unfortunately, the researcher had exposed the treatment group to both acupuncture and TENS; however, most experts believe these two forms of counter irritation likely have similar mechanisms.

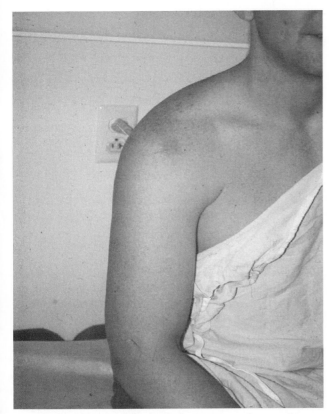

Figure 24.3: Example of the de qi phenomenon, a hyperemic reaction used by acupuncturists to verify accurate placement of needles.

Other investigators have also remarked on possible endorphin-related effects of acupuncture; however, this research has not been without its detractors. Apparently, some researchers have found no correlation between acupuncture therapy and the levels of certain endogenous opioids. Tempfer et al[15] found in their study, of 80 matched prenatal females, no significant increase in β-endorphin levels relative to controls despite the reduction in labor duration. Although their study supports the use of acupuncture during labor, the mechanism by which it works is brought into question.

It would seem difficult to ignore the possible contribution of endogenous opioids, because tolerance and opioid antagonism have both been reported with the use of acupuncture. However, it is difficult to make this assumption in light of published findings to the contrary. It may simply be because of the methodology of studies performed or, more likely, it is a mystery that has yet to be fully uncovered. More research continues to explore the possibility that other endogenous opioids or neurotransmitters may be involved in the analgesic response to acupuncture therapy. Some studies have postulated highly complex interaction between numerous central nervous system (CNS) pathways and various neural and humoral transmitters. One recommended review article of such studies published in 1987 attempts to dissect through the nearly insurmountable literature on this topic. After careful review, one can surmise that numerous CNS loci are linked to acupuncture-induced analgesia and that a number of various endorphins (met-enkephalin, dynorphins, β-endorphins, etc) and neurotransmitters (serotonin and norepinephrine) serve as signals between these systems.[12]

Recent advancements in brain imaging, such as positron emission tomography (PET) and functional magnetic resonance imaging (fMRI), have led to a deeper exploration into the possible mechanisms at work in acupuncture-induced analgesia. Multiple studies have identified purported complex neural systems involved in acupuncture analgesia. These studies have implicated areas such as the hypothalamus, cerebellar vermis, arcuate cingular cortex (ACC), prefrontal cortex, periaqueductal grey, hippocampus, and somatosensory areas I and II as being involved. Although it is recognized that placebo intervention may stimulate some of these brain regions, the degree of stimulation and locale specificity does differ.[16,17]

Although many researchers have proposed different tantalizing explanations for acupuncture's mechanism, no definitive conclusion has yet been made. The mechanism is likely a combination of the aforementioned pathways. Recently, a more eclectic and unified theory on acupuncture's mechanism has been proposed. The noxious stimulus of needles stimulates type I, II, and A-δ afferent nerves, whose impulses reach the anterolateral tract of the spinal cord, producing an increased release of enkephalins and dynorphins. These endogenous opioids then block the ascension of additional pain signals along the spinothalamic tract. Furthermore, acupuncture needles also activate descending inhibitory pathways via increased activity of both norepinephrine and serotonin. Finally, acupuncture stimulates the pituitary-hypothalamic complex, leading to an increased release of β-endorphins.[6] It is likely a complex interplay of neural and humoral mechanisms that produce the analgesic properties of acupuncture therapy.

NIH, WHO, and the FDA have endorsed, regulated, and permitted compensation for the practice of acupuncture for certain maladies. However, this path to acceptance has not been unhindered. Unfortunately, the plethora of studies performed, to date, have uncovered many conflicting results and conclusions. According to some authors, this is because of a placebo effect or the difficulty in designing appropriate studies to adequately test acupuncture's proposed analgesic properties. Nevertheless, today acupuncture is regarded as having greater analgesic effects than can be accounted for by placebo.[10] Some authors even account for the benefits of placebo effect, while clearly showing an improvement on placebo analgesic effect with the inclusion of acupuncture.[11] These results find continuing support with more recent studies using PET and fMRI to identify significant differences between the central neural pathways stimulated or inhibited by acupuncture in comparison to sham acupuncture.[16,17] Undoubtedly, this is an area of research that will provide further elucidation of not only the efficacy of acupuncture but also its etiology.

Acupuncture has found its greatest support in the treatment of both acute and chronic pain syndromes, yet its application in postoperative analgesia has yet to be fully embraced. Some small advances have been made with the NIH Consensus Development Panel's (NIHCDP) support for the clinical efficacy of acupuncture for the relief of postoperative dental pain.[18] Only recently, the clinical practice of postoperative acupuncture analgesia yielded quality research to support its use.

ACUPUNCTURE FOR POSTOPERATIVE PAIN

A well-designed clinical trial by Kotani and colleagues[19] evaluated the effectiveness of acupuncture for postoperative pain. This

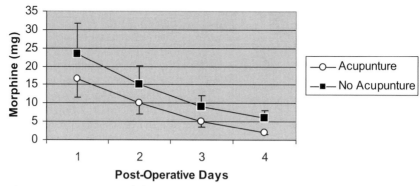

Figure 24.4: Postoperative daily consumption of morphine in patients after upper abdominal surgery. Only days 2 through 4 were deemed statistically significant. (Adapted with permission from Kotani et al, 2001.)[19]

randomized double-blinded controlled trial used both subjective and objective end points to elucidate the effectiveness of acupuncture in the relief of pain. It explored the use of acupuncture versus sham/control for postoperative analgesia in patients undergoing lower and upper abdominal surgery. The control group was designed to prevent the common bias produced by the placebo effect, as the needles were positioned, but never inserted in the control group. All patients received standardized anesthesia as well as identical postoperative analgesic orders. Although initial pain ratings were similar on postop day one, a significant improvement over the control group was noted on day two in the acupuncture group. Moreover, the consumption of morphine analgesia postoperatively was reduced by 50% in the acupuncture group on days 1–4[19] (Figures 24.4 and 24.5). Their objective measurements of plasma cortisol and epinephrine concentrations revealed a greater increase in the control group relative to the treatment group. These studies provide both strong subjective and objective data for the effectiveness of acupuncture in postoperative pain control.

A common theme found in many acupuncture analgesia trials is a lack of improvement in verbal or visual pain intensity scores. Too often, when used as sole end points, these results can be misleading. When taken together with pharmacologic analgesic consumption, an obvious trend is seen. This is no more clearly illustrated than in the work by Lao et al[20] in study published in 1999 that showed, despite insignificant differences in subjective pain reporting, there was a very significant improvement in analgesic consumption, time to first pain medication request, and duration of pain-free period among the acupuncture group. Furthermore, they compared acupuncture therapy to sham acupuncture, which did not require the insertion of needles.

The results, of Lao's work, were recently echoed in an article published by Usichenko and colleagues in the *Canadian Medical Association Journal* in early 2007. The study involved a much larger sample of patients using acupuncture and noninvasive sham acupuncture. Once again, the results showed that analgesic medication consumption was lower in acupuncture patients, despite no difference in patient reported pain scores.[21] Another important aspect of both of these clinical trials was the fact that both employed a certified, licensed acupuncturist, which unfortunately has been an overlooked variable in earlier studies. These two articles helped to eliminate the confounder that any noxious counterstimulus, regardless of its physical location, can produce an analgesic-like effect.

Acupuncture, unlike some of the other modalities of nonpharmacologic analgesia discussed in this chapter, has succeeded in garnering enough attention to stimulate rigorous investigation into its effectiveness and physiologic basis. Fortunately, this interest has translated into significant evidence to support acupuncture's postoperative analgesic properties. Similar interest appears to be producing resurgence in other forms of nonpharmacologic analgesia as well.

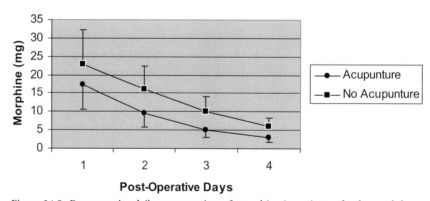

Figure 24.5: Postoperative daily consumption of morphine in patients after lower abdominal surgery. Only days 2 through 4 were deemed statistically significant. (Adapted with permission from Kotani et al, 2001.)[19]

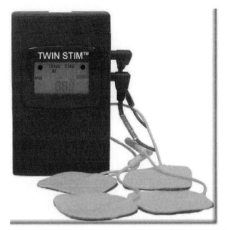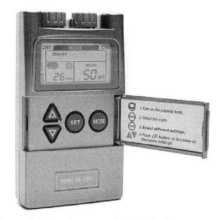

Figure 24.6: Two examples of commercially available and approved TENS devices.

TRANSCUTANEOUS ELECTRICAL NERVE STIMULATION

TENS and PENS are two therapeutic modalities similar to acupuncture that have been receiving considerably more interest over recent years. As mentioned earlier in this chapter, these modalities were likely borne out of ancient Greek medicinal practices. However, they appear to have matured along with acupuncture in Eastern medical practices. Both techniques are based on the practice of counter-irritation and probably have similar if not identical mechanisms. A large number of approved TENS devices are available on the market, with many different capabilities. Two representative units are displayed in Figure 24.6. The units come in a variety of shapes/sizes and with buttons/switches to adjust stimulation parameters. All include a pulse generator, an amplifier, and electrodes. The pulse generator/amplifier is about the size of a small radio and generally comes with a carrying case that can be worn on a belt. The signal produced by the pulse generator can be manually amplified to overcome the impedance among the electrodes, subcutaneous tissues, and peripheral nerves. Therapeutic effectiveness is individualized by the patient and practitioner by adjusting the amplitude of the current from 0 to 50 mA. Other variables that influence efficacy include the pulse width (generally 50–250 μsec) and frequency or number of impulses per second (hertz). Frequencies greater than 100 Hz are perceived as "buzzlike" and most patients prefer rates of 30–60 Hz. In acupuncture-like TENS, patients generally prefer higher amplitude/low frequency (1–2 Hz), which is perceived as a "ticking" stimulus.

Investigation into the etiology of TENS-induced counter-irritation seems to have progressed along a tract parallel to that of acupuncture. Early studies focused on the contribution of endogenous on TENS- and PENS-mediated analgesia. Studies by both Pomeranz and Chiu[11] and Mayer et al[10] clearly demonstrate the analgesic reversing effect of naloxone on animals and humans receiving electroacupuncture (EA).[10,11] In fact, recent literature shows the ability of naloxone to cancel the inhibitory effect of electroaccupunture on sympathetic cardiovascular reflexes, as well.[22,23] Objective results, such as increased levels of endorphins in cerebral spinal fluid of subjects exposed to low-frequency EA, have been reported.[22] Given the quality of these results, it is difficult to rule out the role of endogenous opioids in electrical counter-irritation techniques.

Investigators began to theorize early that more than one mechanism could be involved in the analgesia produced by electrical counter-irritation. By using other neural and humoral transmitter inhibitors, researchers have shown that other substances are involved in the analgesic properties of PENS and TENS. Serotonin is one such hormone. It has been implicated in the development of analgesia with the use of high-frequency electroacupuncture. The reversal of EA's analgesic effect by parachlorophenylalanine and not naloxone gives the impression that high-frequency EA and low-frequency EA may have somewhat different mechanisms.[24,25] A few more recent studies appear to confirm this assertion. Naloxone-reversible analgesia is seen in both high- and low-frequency EA. However, the reversibility appears to be complete only in the low-frequency group, whereas the high-frequency group undergoes only partial reversibility.[25] Further research may have even implicated the specific opiate receptors involved in both low- and high-frequency TENS.

Animals studies focusing on the ventral rostral medulla, an area of the brain believed to contain a dense supply of opiate receptors, have shown some fascinating results in regard to both μ- and δ-opiate receptors. Through the use of naltrindole, a δ_2-receptor antagonist, and naloxone, researchers are believed to have found a predominant role for δ_2-opiate receptors with the use of high-frequency TENS. Low-frequency TENS, once again, appears to be mediated through μ-receptors.[26] Enough evidence currently exists to produce a fairly persuasive argument for supraspinal endogenous opiate activity as at least one of the mechanisms of electrical counter-irritation therapies. However, a fair number of studies do raise the question as to what the other mechanisms might be.

A recent randomized controlled trial using both acupoint-specific locations as well as remote dermatomes provided positive results with only the classical acupuncture points. The authors claim this clearly indicates that production of endogenous opioids cannot be the only mechanism by which percutaneous neuromodulation therapy (PNT) operates. Their presumption is based on the belief that endogenous opiates will be released by any noxious stimulus regardless of its location on the human body. Instead, they postulate roles for direct spinal pain-modulating pathways, neural gating mechanisms, and even placebo responses. On the basis of this trial, one may also conclude not only that the frequency may play a critical role in PNT analgesia, but also that the physical location of the applied

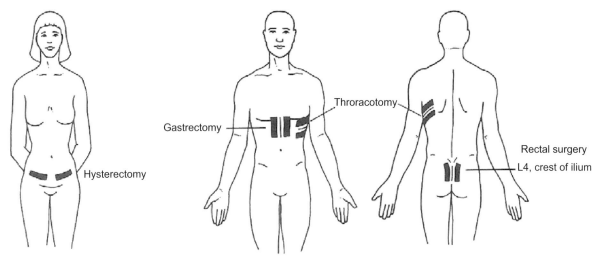

Figure 24.7: TENS electrode pad placement for several types of surgical incisions. Electrodes are generally applied in the operating room by the surgeon or anesthesiologist on completion of the procedure. The electrodes are placed parallel to incision, approximately 2 cm from the edge of the wound, and covered with sterile dressing. (McCaffery M, Beebe A. Pain: a clinical manual for nursing practice. St Louis, MO: Mosby; 1989.)

stimulus is also critical for its effectiveness.[27] The only reality one may be certain of, in regard to the mechanism of electrically applied counterirritant analgesia, is that a final story has yet to be written. Undoubtedly, additional studies will continue to elucidate the mechanism of this analgesic therapy and it will likely be a composite of many, if not all, of the aforementioned proposals.

The efficacy of electrical counter-irritation as a postoperative analgesic modality has, like its cousin, only recently begun to receive support from the Western medical world through the development of well-designed clinical studies. For optimal effectiveness, stimulating electrodes should be closely applied parallel to the surgical incision (Figure 24.7). Many studies clearly report significant improvement in analgesia through the reduction of pharmacologic analgesic requirements[28–32] (Figure 24.8). Reductions of up to 61% in morphine requirements have been recorded in some trials.[28] In fact, significant differences have been seen in total opiate consumption as well as time to first analgesic request.[28,29] One study found that the use of TENS lengthens the time of analgesic request from 38 ± 18 minutes to 581 ± 86 minutes after video-assisted thoracoscopy procedures[29] (Table 24.2).

Interestingly, either the effect on subjective patient-reported pain scores were not end points in some of these studies or no significant benefit was observed. As previously mentioned, if patients report similar levels of pain relief, yet their pharmacologic analgesic consumption differs, then one may conclude a significant effect has taken place.

Some researchers, however, further stipulate that the level of relief seen with either pharmacologic or nonpharmacologic means must be significantly different to that of a strict noninterventional control group. Constructing trials with this parameter in mind is somewhat impractical, as noninterventional control groups are commonly considered unethical. A few authors further refine their outcomes to indicate that the therapeutic effect of TENS and PENS may occur only in specific subsets of postoperative patients. It has been asserted that only patients suffering from either mild or moderate levels of discomfort and pain may receive significant relief through the use of electrical counter-irritation therapies.[29]

A growing amount of evidence suggests that TENS and PENS are useful, yet underappreciated, forms of analgesia. Their acceptance has been seen in a wide array of chronic pain-related maladies, but they have yet to achieve a foothold in the

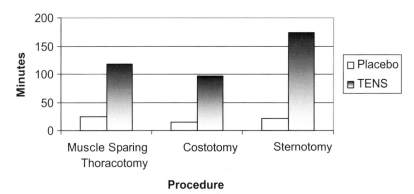

Figure 24.8: Improved analgesic effects as indicated by lengthened time to first postoperative analgesic request (adapted with permission from Benedetti et al 1997).[29]

Table 24.2: Significant Improvements in PCA Demands and Morphine Consumption in Both High and Low Frequency TENS Compared with Controls[a]

	Control Group	Sham EA	Low-Frequency EA	High-Frequency EA
Time to first postoperative dose of pethidine (minutes)	10.6 ± 5.9	18.0 ± 7.9	27.9 ± 12.3	28.1 ± 13.8
PCA demands in the first 24 hours				
1–8 hours	9.0 ± 3.6	7.0 ± 3.6	5.1 ± 4.0	3.3 ± 3.2
8–16 hours	8.2 ± 5.3	5.8 ± 3.8	4.0 ± 2.6	2.8 ± 2.1
16–24 hours	3.2 ± 2.4	3.3 ± 2.1	2.6 ± 2.1	1.8 ± 1.6
Total dosage in 24 hours	20.5 ± 9.2	16.1 ± 7.4	11.7 ± 7.1	7.9 ± 5.9
Morphine delivered (mg)				
1–8 hours	16.1 ± 7.1	12.9 ± 6.6	9.2 ± 7.1	6.1 ± 5.9
8–16 hours	15.5 ± 9.4	10.8 ± 7.7	7.6 ± 5.4	5.4 ± 3.8
16–24 hours	6.5 ± 4.8	6.6 ± 4.1	5.0 ± 4.2	3.5 ± 3.2
Total morphine in 24 hours	38.1 ± 16.0	30.2 ± 14.4	21.8 ± 14.7	15.0 ± 10.7

[a] Adapted with permission from Lin et al (2002).[28]

realm of postoperative analgesia. Their efficacy as an adjunct to pharmacologic medicines has been shown after a wide range of operative situations, from thoracic surgery to gynecological procedures.[28,32] Their relative absence of any significant side-effect profile further strengthens the argument for their inclusion in appropriately selected populations of postoperative patients. Moreover, the usage of TENS and PENS therapies may enable practitioners to decrease their reliance on pharmacologic agents, thereby reducing the subsequent side effects/risks of those medicines.

With a thorough review of the literature, one is quickly confronted with various parameters that may affect the quality of analgesia provided by electrically induced counterirritation therapies. Amplitude and frequency of the electrical stimulus, location of the applied contacts, duration of therapy, temporal onset relative to surgical procedure, surgical procedure performed, number of interventions, level of expertise of the practitioner, and patient demographic, seem to all play an integral role in the success of not only TENS and PENS but also acupuncture. These variables undoubtedly create hurdles for researchers to overcome in the design of their clinical trials. However, in controlling for and standardizing these variables we will be able to develop a better model to support the usage of these therapies for the treatment of acute, chronic, and postoperative pain.

MAGNETISM

Magnetic therapy is a burgeoning business in the field of analgesia. It has generated a lot of public interest with annual sales in the billions of dollars.[33] It has been postulated that all materials organic or inorganic possess a potential to be affected by magnetic forces. The very nature of atomic structure with its balance of positive and negative forces makes magnetic therapy a very intriguing proposition. After all, if animals are capable of using electromagnetic fields as means of orientation and navigation, is it not possible that magnetic fields may be involved in other areas of life? [34] Some researchers ascribe potential opioid pathway modulation to the use of magnetic field therapy. Unfortunately, the literature has yet to bear any conclusive evidence of analgesic properties of this type of therapy in humans. Application of magnet therapy is depicted in Figure 24.9.

As with many other nonpharmacologic antinociceptive techniques, many variations of magnetic therapy exist. In basic terms, magnetic therapy may be applied in either a static or dynamic fashion. These terms describe the use of solid magnets and exposure to magnetic fields, respectively. Furthermore, the location of the applied magnets, the duration of contact, and their strength may affect their efficacy. Magnetic fields also may vary in their frequency, orientation, and duration.

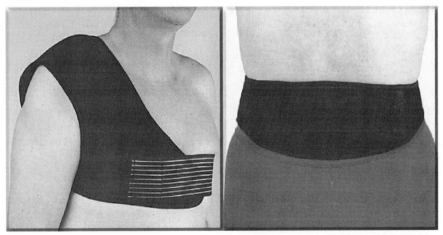

Figure 24.9: Examples of static magnet application via wraps to the shoulder and lower back.

A recent randomized double blinded study reported little benefit in the use of static magnet therapy in the postoperative population. It utilized solid magnets placed around incisional sites for 2 hours postoperatively with the outcome measures of verbal pain scale scores and opioid requirement. Their study revealed no benefit in either outcome relative to the sham control group.[33] Unfortunately, the availability of additional credible RCTs using static magnetic therapy are minimal at best.

Our literature search did locate numerous studies on the analgesic/antinociceptive effect of magnetic field therapy. However, articles pertaining to the use of magnetic fields in humans are lacking, although some of the initial studies are promising. Initial trials in this area incorporated the use of relatively simple forms of magnetic field application. Recent studies have begun to explore the effect of much more complex magnetic field patterns and their effect on living subjects.

Martin et al[35] investigated the effect of complex magnetic burst field application on electrical and thermal noxious stimuli in rats. The results of their trial showed that after 30 minutes of exposure to burst field magnetic therapy that a level of analgesia equivalent to 4 mg/kg of morphine was produced.[35] Moreover, the administration of naloxone to their test subjects appeared to abolish this improvement in latency duration. Therefore, they concluded that the use of magnetic fields was associated with an analgesic response, which is most likely mediated, the endogenous endorphin pathways. Whether this form of intervention may be suitable for humans and has any sustainability has yet to be adequately explored.

A more recent study[36] explored the effect of low-frequency magnetic fields on tail flick latency periods with the additional outcome measure of endorphin, substance P, and serotonin levels in the brain. Another unique feature of the study is the use of continuous low-frequency magnetic therapy over a period of 14 days. Their findings did reveal a positive effect on tail flick latencies of approximately 5 seconds, but only on days 3 and 4. The effect did not carry over the entire 14-day period. Elevated levels of β-endorphins, serotonin, and substance P were also noted.[36] Their data appear to provide some validity to the analgesic effects of magnetic therapy. In addition, it also seems to indicate a more complex integrated mechanism for this proposed form of analgesia, resembling that of the other forms of nonpharmacologic analgesia.

Magnetic field therapy, although fascinating, has not yet matured to the point where it can be actively supported as a modality of postoperative analgesia. Some of the aforementioned studies do indicate a promising future for this field; however, not enough conclusive evidence has been produced. Until the appropriate studies in humans have been performed, this form of therapy will remain investigational. Moreover, a practical, clinical application of this therapy appears to be difficult to implement.

THERAPEUTIC TOUCH AND MASSAGE

Massage, osteopathic manipulations, chiropractic manipulations, and therapeutic touch (TT) are some of the various physical activities believed to be capable of providing significant pain relief. Each of these techniques involves human to human contact that may provide physical stimulation or relaxation as well as psychological benefits not often described in Western medical literature. Such qualities may attest to the usefulness of these therapies or raise a degree of suspicion regarding their benefit over placebo therapies. None of these therapies illustrates this point any more than the field of therapeutic touch.

Therapeutic touch is a practice sometimes mistakenly referred to as the laying of hands, used to achieve a heightened state of well-being. Practitioners of therapeutic touch describe it as assessing and redirecting patients' energy field via the movements of one's hands across the body as the patient maintains a state of meditation.[37] Images of divine intervention and up-tempo eulogies often spring forth with just the thought of such lines of therapy. Is there any scientific basis for this line of therapy, or are there any substantial studies to prove the efficacy of these practices?

The practice of therapeutic touch was developed in earnest by Kunz and Krieger in 1972. Unlike the religious practice of the laying of hands, no overlying religious context or physical contact is necessarily used. Not unlike ancient Eastern acupuncture, TT is thought by some to be based on the concept of unitary human beings. This theory attempts to describe a series of energy fields that are intertwined with each other between humans and their environment. The practice of therapeutic touch is designed to help regulate the proper ebb and flow of energy between the patient and his or her environment.[37] Similarly to acupuncture, any disruption of the natural energy flow between the patient and the environment may produce a painful experience.

Some supporters of therapeutic touch have described the experience of pain to be partially potentiated by a negative physiological response to stressful stimuli. The autonomic nervous system reacts to noxious stimuli by producing a fight or flight response that leads to elevations in blood pressure and heart rate as well as generalized skeletal muscle tension. The platform, thus far, seems reasonable. After adequately assessing the energy field by the passing of his hands above the patient, a practitioner then redirects the energy to depleted areas restoring the overall flow. Although the concepts of TT seem to mimic those of other forms of nonpharmacologic analgesia, no detailed scientific explanation has been provided. Obviously, this is a fundamental weakness for this form of therapy to gain acceptance in the Western medical world; however, this does not by any means indicate that it has no beneficial effect. Therapeutic touch simply has not received the level of attention and investigation necessary to conclusively support its use.

As to the efficacy of this mode of analgesia, very few clinical trials have been developed to draw strong support in the field of postoperative analgesia. The majority of articles on TT have been simple case reports describing potential positive effects after the use of therapeutic touch. Of the few randomized clinical trials performed, the level of methodological errors is high.[38] Understandably, TT would be a difficult practice to standardize, particularly with no detailed mechanism yet elucidated; however, basic study constructs such as standardized anesthesia, acceptable end points, and minimization of other confounders should be achievable. Until adequate and repeatable trials are published, no declaration of acceptance for this form of therapy can be made in the area of postoperative analgesia.

Massage therapy is a long-standing practice designed to help alleviate physical and psychological tension, stress, and discomfort. The mechanism behind it has also yet to be elucidated, but some speculate it works through the physical stimulation of afferent receptors to modify either ascending pain transmission or descending inhibitory pain pathways. Its use has become very widespread, and is even incorporated into the sports medicine programs, rehabilitation programs, and various other forms of

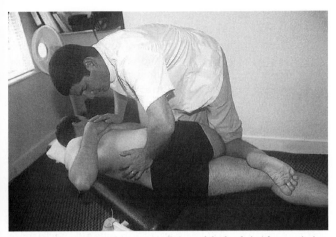

Figure 24.10: Osteopathic manipulation of the back (with permission from Vickers and Zollman 1999).[62]

occupational therapy. Unfortunately, as a means of postoperative analgesia, massage therapy has yet to yield a substantial collection of supporting studies. During our literature review only a few well-performed clinical trials were unearthed.

As with many other nonpharmacologic forms of analgesia, study design is fraught with difficulty in providing a suitable control group. If one uses no intervention, the possibility of placebo effect can be far too strong of a confounder. Sham interventions are undoubtedly the correct form of control group to choose; however, designing the sham group is extremely difficult. Significant attempts have been made to eliminate the uncertainty that plagues nonstandardized interventions. Using mechanical massage devices instead of human touch helps to ensure that the intervention being studied is uniform between patients. Results of this are fairly convincing, showing significant reductions in not only analgesic consumption but also subjective pain reporting scores. Although these positive findings are most notable during postoperative days 2–5, no significant difference has been found in the duration of hospital stay.[39] Whether this form of therapy could be regarded as cost effective in a postoperative setting has not been determined. The results, however, are still intriguing, if only from an academic standpoint.

Other studies, unfortunately, contest these results. Some clinical trials have found little to no benefit in the use of massage therapy in the postsurgical setting. A recent, randomized controlled trial exploring the benefits between massage therapy and simple pharmacologic intervention failed to uncover any significant benefits to massage over the short postoperative period.[40] Moreover, no alterations in objective measures, such as autonomic vital signs or serum cortisol levels, were detected. The study, however, contained some significant flaws in its design. By failing to incorporate sham controls, the role for a placebo effect cannot be ruled out. Also, these patients began with very low reported pain score levels. Any significant benefit seen with such low baseline scores would be difficult to assess.[40] This particular form of therapy may yet become used more as a postoperative analgesic adjunct; however, until sufficient scientific data to warrant its acceptance is provided, it cannot be recommended as such. In fact, until cost-benefit analyses are performed, it is unlikely to be incorporated into common practice, despite any future positive results.

Osteopathic manipulation (OMT) is a form of treatment championed by osteopathic medical schools and practitioners

alike. Once again, osteopathic medicine uses a holistic approach to provide medical therapy for a vast array of ailments. The underlying basis of osteopathic medicine involves the concept of the body as a sum of its parts. A derangement to any of its parts produces a structural abnormality that leads to suffering. Particular focus is placed on the musculoskeletal system, which makes up about two-thirds of the body. Osteopathic physicians (DO) believe that symptoms often develop from underlying musculoskeletal problems that may be relieved through the use of osteopathic manipulative therapy (Figure 24.10).

Similar, perhaps, in some ways to massage and chiropractic therapy, osteopathic manipulation utilizes a hands-on technique to apply pressure, stretching, and resistance to joints and muscles. Through these exercises, the DO hopes to alleviate tension and pain to restore the body's natural function. Critical to the success of OMT is the relief of underlying discomfort and pain. The application of this therapy to postoperative pain has been investigated through the use of randomized, controlled clinical trials. Many studies conclude that manipulations may be used as successful adjuncts to standard pharmacologic analgesics.

The development of a surgically amenable illness is often accompanied by the physiological derangements of inflammation, musculoskeletal tension, and heightened responses to pain. These processes are undoubtedly partial justification for the use of preemptive analgesia. Not only should you avoid the development of such conditions after an invasive surgical procedure, but many of these symptoms may exist secondary to the development of the very pathology that requires surgical intervention.[41] Consequently, with improved analgesia, rehabilitation will be hastened and hospital stay will subsequently be decreased.[42]

When comparing the use of OMT to sham treatment, results have shown reduced blood morphine concentrations, indicating a decrease requirement for opiate analgesics among those supplemented with manipulations.[41] Results such as these seen in patients after total abdominal hysterectomies are quite impressive. The reason is that objective measures are reported, instead of patient reported use of narcotics, which helps to eliminate reporting bias. Other studies have found success with the use of osteopathic-like practices of pressure friction and stretching techniques for thoracotomy patients who were unable to find satisfactory relief with the use of oral analgesics. The small study of postthoracotomy patients showed reductions in visual analog pain scores from 10 to as little as 2.[43] As with trials performed on the use of electrical counterirritation, benefits are seen in reduced reliance on pharmacologic agents. Like TENS/PENS, this does not necessarily translate into significant reductions in subjectively reported pain scales; however, reductions in opioid dose requirements observed with OMT attest to its analgesic benefits. Despite the growing success of this school of medicine, the dearth of literature regarding the use of osteopathic manipulative therapy for postoperative analgesia is surprising. Further studies showing repeatable benefits, performed after different surgical operations and among different demographics, will, of course, provide additional confirmation and support for the use of OMT as a postoperative nonpharmacologic analgesic.

HYPNOSIS

Many forms of nonpharmacologic therapy rely on physical contact to produce alterations or to modulate the pain pathway. Other techniques focus on the use of the mind and senses to produce a heightened state of analgesia. Hypnosis is loosely defined as an altered state of awareness. This may include a highly suggestible state and an intensely relaxed state of being. Hypnosis may be achieved through both pharmacologic and nonpharmacologic means. The term *hypnosis* frequently is used in a generic sense without differentiating among various subgroups such as therapeutic suggestion and mental imagery. Hypnosis, mesmerism, therapeutic suggestion, mental imagery, and relaxation techniques have been used to assist in surgical procedures well before the development of the pharmacologically based practice of anesthesia. These techniques, however, have since been relegated as mystical practices that are incapable of matching the effectiveness of modern-day pharmacologic agents. Whether these techniques are difficult to employ, effective only in select populations, or inadequate as sole anesthetic therapies should not deter a capable practitioner from using these methods to augment their patient's medical therapy. The decision to use any of these techniques should be based solely on the anticipated beneficial effect it may achieve in the patient in question.

No consensus currently exists on the possible mechanisms underlying the effects of hypnosis. It is likely a central neurological process involving higher center interpretation of stimuli. In regard to analgesia, it may involve a reinterpretation of a noxious stimulus to no longer be recognized as harmful or it may involve the interference of the transmission of such noxious stimuli to the conscious mind. With the advent of functional imaging techniques such as PET and fMRI, more light is being shed on possible avenues of activity within the brain during hypnosis therapy. Regions of the brain noted to show increased activity during noxious stimulation include both thalami and caudate nuclei. The left insula and anterior cingulate cortex are also implicated through detection of increased cerebral blood flow. Hypnosis appears to affect cerebral blood flow, primarily in the anterior cingulate cortex (ACC). Therefore, it is reasonable to assume that the ACC plays a key role in the analgesic effects seen with hypnosis.[44] Furthermore, it has been postulated that this area may be specifically linked to the affective response to painful stimuli.

As to whether there are any beneficial effects, with the use of hypnosis therapy, the literature is conflicting at best. Depending on the particular mode of hypnotic therapy used, there are as many studies to indicate positive, as well as negative, results. Presurgical relaxation therapy has been found to provide significant decreases in postoperative analgesic requirements as well as reduced hospitalization.[45] However, these results were not replicated in a recent study by Gavin et al. The single blinded randomized controlled trial compared postoperative pain intensity scores and opioid usage after lumbar and cervical spine surgery. They found that morphine dose requirements were in fact higher in the relaxation group.[46]

Trials involving patients receiving hypnosis are somewhat more promising than those involving relaxation therapy. Unfortunately, study design is less than optimal as many claim that for hypnotherapy to be successful, patients must be susceptible. This often prevents the random allocation of the intervention being studied. Moreover, the nature of the intervention often precludes the ability to create blinded patients. Regardless, a number of well-designed cohort studies have produced good results with the use of hypnosis for control of intraoperative and postoperative analgesia. Hypnosis has been used as a primary anesthetic technique during thyroid and various forms of plastic surgery. In fact, it has been found to be more effective than midazolam/alfentanil combinations for plastic surgery. One

Belgian study produced results showing a median alfentanyl consumption of 10.2 μg/kg/h when hypnosis was used compared to 15.5 μg/kg/h without it. The intensity of subjective pain reporting was also notably less in the hypnosis group during, as well as after, surgery.[47] Self-induced hypnotic states have also been used during radiologic procedures. Intraoperative requirements for midazolam and fentanyl were reduced by half in the hypnosis treatment group compared to controls.[48] A novel study of hypnosis during orthopedic hand surgery also produced complementary results with the use of hypnosis. Using standardized hypnotic scripts, the patients achieved improved analgesia over a 3-day postoperative period. Moreover, the investigatory team measured not only subjective intensity pain scale scores, but also subjective affective pain scale scores. In other words, the patients were asked to qualify their pain intensity in terms of how tolerable that particular level of pain was. The results indicated a more demonstrable improvement in affective pain scores compared to pain intensity scores.[49] Such results provide clues that hypnosis may not simply alter nociceptive transmission, but, instead, may affect the way our higher centers interpret the signal.

Some proponents indicate that children may be the best demographic in which to employ hypnosis. Given that children are much more suggestible than adults, it is reasonable to assume they may more easily be placed into a state of hypnosis. Although I have not uncovered a comparative study between adult and children populations, the use of hypnosis in children has provided as promising results as those in adults. One recent randomized control trial resulted in decreased pharmacologic analgesic consumption when hypnosis was given preoperatively.[50]

Unfortunately, conclusions regarding the effectiveness of therapeutic suggestion are, once again, less convincing. While in combination with strict hypnotic therapy, therapeutic suggestion has produced substantial improvements over controls.[47] However, these improvements in pain scores and narcotic usage have not necessarily been repeated with the use of only therapeutic suggestion. In fact, multiple well-designed randomized control trials have failed to show any improvement over control groups with the use of therapeutic suggestion.[51–53] Therapeutic suggestion comes in two flavors, intraoperative and preoperative. These two forms of interaction rely on different levels of consciousness or memory. It is believed that intraoperative awareness may in some ways be a function of implicit memory. Implicit memory occurs on a subconscious level, which the patient is not aware of during its formation but is able to recall at a later time. Explicit memory is the type of memory with which most of us are familiar. Although the concept of implicit memory has been suggested, no definitive proof has yet been provided to validate its existence. However, some of these studies provide hints of its existence with proper identification of cues related to the suggested material. Despite the questionable capability of the human mind to comprehend intraoperative applied aural stimuli, therapeutic suggestion has not been shown to be of significant benefit in either a preoperative or intraoperative setting.[53] Without the use of a hypnotic state, therapeutic suggestion appears to be an insufficient means of analgesia to recommend based on the current literature.

MUSIC THERAPY

Another form of therapy, designed to incorporate higher center sensory input to modulate pain perception, is music therapy.

Music therapy has been widely studied as an adjuvant to the pharmacologic therapy for the treatment of both pain and anxiety. In fact, many authors have theorized that it is music's effect on anxiety levels that leads to its beneficial effects on pain. Music may provide a useful distraction to help lure a patient away from focusing on his or her pain. It can provide a calming sensation that may help diminish the level of muscular tension a patient experiences, thereby attenuating aggravating factors that would lead to higher levels of pain.[54]

As mentioned, the studies utilizing this nontraditional, non-pharmacologic form of analgesia have been less than ideal. Only recently has there been a push for more standardization to adequately evaluate the effectiveness of music therapy. Nilsson, et al.[55] have attempted to provide some standardization in the type of music therapy provided. Based on studies initially reported by Unestahl in 1970 and White in 2000, their conclusion was that for music therapy to be beneficial, it must produce a sense of relaxation. They propose that this is best achieved by using soft, instrumental melodies with slow flowing rhythms that duplicate a pulse rate of 60–80 beats per minute. This conclusion has been echoed by other authors, who theorize that this form of music stimulates the autonomic production of endorphins by the pituitary gland.[56] Yet another study, published in 1999, demonstrated that the usage of binaural beats to produce hemispheric synchronization markedly reduces the fentanyl requirements of patients under general anesthesia.[57] Whether these musical parameters are correct remains to be borne out in further studies, as other investigators believe the greatest effect of music on one's state of mind is achieved through patients' own musical selection.[58,59] It may be that the empowerment given to patients to select their own musical ambience might increase their level of control, therein reducing their level of anxiety. Unfortunately, there is no current consensus on what type of music is best suited to help reduce pain in the postoperative period.[55] Regardless, standardization of the musical intervention should be a primary goal of additional studies to ensure that results of any future research may be comparable. With comparable investigations, more weight will be lent to this form of intervention as a useful adjunct in the treatment of postoperative pain.

Nilsson, et al.[55,60] have also explored other qualities of music therapy, which will undoubtedly help standardize the intervention. Their work on the timing of music therapy has produced results that indicate no difference between the implementation of music intraoperatively or postoperatively. This, of course, relies on acceptance of the concept of implicit memory. In light of their results, it appears that music therapy may not work solely by providing a distracting stimulus. However, music as a nonpharmacologic analgesic does not lose any ground as an effective therapy on this basis; the etiology of its effect is simply brought into question.

Overall, many of the studies we reviewed showed significant reductions in either subjective reported pain scale scores and/or reductions in the use of opiates. The use of both subjective and objective outcomes is important in the evaluation of the effectiveness of nontraditional analgesic interventions. Standardization of anesthetic technique and exclusion/inclusion criteria are other areas of study design that give these articles particular robustness. The possible beneficial effects of music therapy far outweigh the cost of implementing such techniques, and with a lack of any adverse effects, it seems reasonable for this form of therapy to be added to any postoperative patients analgesic regimen.

Table 24.3: Use of Complementary Medicine Worldwide Gathered from Surveys Taken from 1987 to 1996[a]

Country	Seeing a Practicioner	Using Any Form of Complementary Treatment
United Kingdom	10.5% in past year	33% ever
Australia	20% in past year	46% in past year
United States	11% in past year	34% in past year
Belgium	24% in past year	66%–75% ever
France	No data	49% ever
Netherlands	6%–7% in past year	18% ever
West Germany	5%–12% in past year	20%–30% ever

[a] Adapted with permission from Zollman and Vickers (1999).[62]

CONCLUSIONS

We reviewed the most commonly used nontraditional, non-pharmacologic analgesic techniques; however, those discussed are by no means all inclusive. Numerous other nonpharmacologic techniques exist and are in the process of being studied. Undoubtedly, more analgesic therapies will be developed in the future as well. To become accepted as viable medical techniques, each must be shown to produce effective results with equal or less risk relative to current methods of analgesia. These techniques must also be practical and cost-effective to employ. Some of the aforementioned therapies qualify on the basis of these criteria and should be incorporated into daily practice as either monotherapy or as nonpharmacological adjuvants to conventional analgesic therapy. Others have failed to meet sufficient criteria to be recommended for use as common postoperative analgesic remedies. Their current failure, however, does not necessarily mean they cannot one day be refined or shown to be successful adjuncts to a growing armamentarium of nonpharmalogic analgesic treatments.

Patient acceptance of nonpharmacologic methods of analgesia appears to be growing far more quickly than the clinicians' willingness to practice it. A recent prospective study found that various alternative nonpharmacologic techniques for pain management were used by between 13% and almost 60% of patients.[61] The *British Medical Journal* has published a wide array of articles exploring the use of complementary medicine. One such article, using compiled data from other studies published from 1987 to 1996 (Table 24.3), also found the use of complementary medicine to range between 18% and 75%, depending on the geographical setting.[62]

With the provision of various complementary nonpharmacolog, anxiolytic, and analgesic techniques, patients have been noted to not only utilize them, but also to experience a heightened sense of well-being with a decreased reliance on intravenous opioid use. An apparent divide among the research community, the clinical practice community, and patients appears to exist. Additional research is necessary. However, enough research exists for the limited use of some of these techniques. Yet, most of these techniques have failed to gain widespread acceptance in the Western medical world. With the growing desire among patients to explore the use of nonpharmacologic adjuncts, the medical community should be encouraged to oblige. The provision of improved objective and subjective analgesia while reducing the reliance on pharmacologic agents clearly upholds the principle cornerstone of multimodal analgesia.

APPENDIX

TENS Contraindications and Precautions

- Electrodes should not be placed over the carotid sinuses (anywhere on the front of the neck should be avoided). Stimulation in this area can cause hypotension and risk of laryngeal spasm.
- Electrodes should not be placed over areas that are numb or have altered sensation. There is a risk of skin irritation and sensation signals will not be sent back to the brain.
- Electrodes should not be placed over bony prominences, broken or irritated skin, varicose veins, or directly over open wounds or recent scars. They should not be placed transcerebrally (on each temple), on the front of the neck (because of the risk of acute vasovagal induced hypotension), or on or near the trigeminal nerve if the patient has a history of herpes zoster.
- There is a significant risk that TENS will interfere with the action of a cardiac pacemaker if the electrodes are applied above the waist and clearance from a cardiologist is recommended. TENS is safe for use in pacemaker patients who require use of electrodes below the waist.
- For patients with impaired comprehension and/or who are unable to use the TENS machine, a partner/caregiver may take responsibility following education and instruction in use of TENS.
- Pregnancy – manufacturers do not recommend use of TENS in pregnancy. Although there is no research to support the claim that TENS could cause miscarriage, it would not be ethical to presume it does not. Advice and approval should be sought from patient's obstetrician prior to application.
- Epilepsy – it is unclear whether TENS can induce seizures because of the electrical activity. Patients with epilepsy can have a trial under supervision and if beneficial take TENS home to use when another person is present.
- The TENS unit should not be activated for long periods, as there is an increased risk of sensitizing skin.
- The patient should be aware there is a small risk of sensitivity to the electrodes.

REFERENCES

1. Merskey H, Bogduk N, eds. *IASP Task Force on Taxonomy: Classification of Chronic Pain.* 2nd ed., Seattle, WA: IASP Press; 1994.
2. Paulozzi LJ, Budnitz DS, Xi Y. Increasing deaths from opioid analgesics in the united states. *Pharmacoepidemiol Drug Saf.* 2006;15:618–627.
3. Vickers A, Zollman C. ABC of complementary medicine. the manipulative therapies: Osteopathy and chiropractic. *BMJ.* 1999;319:1176–1179.
4. The NSDUH report patterns and trends in nonmedical prescription pain reliever use: 2002 to 2005, 2007.
5. Angst MS, Clark JD. Opioid-induced hyperalgesia: a qualitative systematic review. *Anesthesiology.* 2006;104:570–587.
6. Chernyak GV, Sessler DI. Perioperative acupuncture and related techniques. *Anesthesiology.* 2005;102:1031–1049; quiz 1077–1078.
7. Lin YC. Perioperative usage of acupuncture. *Paediatr Anaesth.* 2006;16:231–235.
8. Bueno EA, Mamtani R, Frishman WH. Alternative approaches to the medical management of angina pectoris: Acupuncture, electrical nerve stimulation, and spinal cord stimulation. *Heart Dis.* 2001;3:236–241.
9. Wall P, Melzack R, eds. Textbook of Pain. Edinburgh: Churchill and Livingstone; 1984.
10. Mayer DJ, Price DD, Rafii A. Antagonism of acupuncture analgesia in man by the narcotic antagonist naloxone. *Brain Res.* 1977;121:368–372.
11. Pomeranz B, Chiu D. Naloxone blockade of acupuncture analgesia: endorphin implicated. *Life Sci.* 1976;19:1757–1762.
12. He LF. Involvement of endogenous opioid peptides in acupuncture analgesia. *Pain.* 1987;31:99–121.
13. Stoelting RK. Opiate receptors and endorphins: Their role in anesthesiology. *Anesth Analg.* 1980;59:874–880.
14. Kho HG, Kloppenborg PW, van Egmond J. Effects of acupuncture and transcutaneous stimulation analgesia on plasma hormone levels during and after major abdominal surgery. *Eur J Anaesthesiol.* 1993;10:197–208.
15. Tempfer C, Zeisler H, Heinzl H, Hefler L, Husslein P, Kainz C. Influence of acupuncture on maternal serum levels of interleukin-8, prostaglandin F2alpha, and beta-endorphin: A matched pair study. *Obstet Gynecol.* 1998;92:245–248.
16. Dhond RP, Kettner N, Napadow V. Do the neural correlates of acupuncture and placebo effects differ? *Pain.* 2007;128:8–12.
17. Shen J. Research on the neurophysiological mechanisms of acupuncture: Review of selected studies and methodological issues. *J Altern Complement Med.* 2001;7(suppl 1):121–127.
18. Mayer DJ. Acupuncture: an evidence-based review of the clinical literature. *Annu Rev Med.* 2000;51:49–63.
19. Kotani N, Hashimoto H, Sato Y, et al. Preoperative intradermal acupuncture reduces postoperative pain, nausea and vomiting, analgesic requirement, and sympathoadrenal responses. *Anesthesiology.* 2001;95:349–356.
20. Lao L, Bergman S, Hamilton GR, Langenberg P, Berman B. Evaluation of acupuncture for pain control after oral surgery: A placebo-controlled trial. *Arch Otolaryngol Head Neck Surg.* 1999;125:567–572.
21. Usichenko TI, Lysenyuk VP, Groth MH, Pavlovic D. Detection of ear acupuncture points by measuring the electrical skin resistance in patients before, during and after orthopedic surgery performed under general anesthesia. *Acupunct Electrother Res.* 2003;28:167–173.
22. Ho WK, Wen HL. Opioid-like activity in the cerebrospinal fluid of pain patients treated by electroacupuncture. *Neuropharmacology.* 1989;28:961–966.
23. Chao DM, Shen LL, Tjen-A-Looi S, Pitsillides KF, Li P, Longhurst JC. Naloxone reverses inhibitory effect of electroacupuncture on sympathetic cardiovascular reflex responses. *Am J Physiol.* 1999;276:2127–2134.
24. Cheng RS, Pomeranz B. Electroacupuncture analgesia could be mediated by at least two pain-relieving mechanisms; endorphin and non-endorphin systems. *Life Sci.* 1979;25:1957–1962.
25. Lee JH, Beitz AJ. Electroacupuncture modifies the expression of c-fos in the spinal cord induced by noxious stimulation. *Brain Res.* 1992;577:80–91.
26. Kalra A, Urban MO, Sluka KA. Blockade of opioid receptors in rostral ventral medulla prevents antihyperalgesia produced by transcutaneous electrical nerve stimulation (TENS). *J Pharmacol Exp Ther.* 2001;298:257–263.

27. White PF, Craig WF, Vakharia AS, Ghoname E, Ahmed HE, Hamza MA. Percutaneous neuromodulation therapy: Does the location of electrical stimulation effect the acute analgesic response? *Anesth Analg.* 2000;91:949–954.

28. Lin JG, Lo MW, Wen YR, Hsieh CL, Tsai SK, Sun WZ. The effect of high and low frequency electroacupuncture in pain after lower abdominal surgery. *Pain.* 2002;99:509–514.

29. Benedetti F, Amanzio M, Casadio C, et al. Control of postoperative pain by transcutaneous electrical nerve stimulation after thoracic operations. *Ann Thorac Surg.* 1997;63:773–776.

30. Bjordal JM, Johnson MI, Ljunggreen AE. Transcutaneous electrical nerve stimulation (TENS) can reduce postoperative analgesic consumption. A meta-analysis with assessment of optimal treatment parameters for postoperative pain. *Eur J Pain.* 2003;7:181–188.

31. Gejervall AL, Stener-Victorin E, Moller A, Janson PO, Werner C, Bergh C. Electro-acupuncture versus conventional analgesia: A comparison of pain levels during oocyte aspiration and patients' experiences of well-being after surgery. *Hum Reprod.* 2005;20:728–735.

32. Hamza MA, White PF, Ahmed HE, Ghoname EA. Effect of the frequency of transcutaneous electrical nerve stimulation on the postoperative opioid analgesic requirement and recovery profile. *Anesthesiology.* 1999;91:1232–1238.

33. Cepeda MS, Carr DB, Sarquis T, Miranda N, Garcia RJ, Zarate C. Static magnetic therapy does not decrease pain or opioid requirements: A randomized double-blind trial. *Anesth Analg.* 2007;104:290–294.

34. Prato FS, Robertson JA, Desjardins D, Hensel J, Thomas AW. Daily repeated magnetic field shielding induces analgesia in CD-1 mice. *Bioelectromagnetics.* 2005;26:109–117.

35. Martin LJ, Koren SA, Persinger MA. Thermal analgesic effects from weak, complex magnetic fields and pharmacological interactions. *Pharmacol Biochem Behav.* 2004;78:217–227.

36. Bao X, Shi Y, Huo X, Song T. A possible involvement of beta-endorphin, substance P, and serotonin in rat analgesia induced by extremely low frequency magnetic field. *Bioelectromagnetics.* 2006;27:467–472.

37. Samarel N. Therapeutic touch, dialogue, and women's experiences in breast cancer surgery. *Holist Nurs Pract.* 1997;12:62–70.

38. Ramnarine-Singh S. The surgical significance of therapeutic touch. *AORN J.* 1999;69:358–369.

39. Le Blanc-Louvry I, Costaglioli B, Boulon C, Leroi AM, Ducrotte P. Does mechanical massage of the abdominal wall after colectomy reduce postoperative pain and shorten the duration of ileus? results of a randomized study. *J Gastrointest Surg.* 2002;6:43–49.

40. Taylor AG, Galper DI, Taylor P, et al. Effects of adjunctive Swedish massage and vibration therapy on short-term postoperative outcomes: A randomized, controlled trial. *J Altern Complement Med.* 2003;9:77–89.

41. Goldstein FJ, Jeck S, Nicholas AS, Berman MJ, Lerario M. Preoperative intravenous morphine sulfate with postoperative osteopathic manipulative treatment reduces patient analgesic use after total abdominal hysterectomy. *J Am Osteopath Assoc.* 2005;105:273–279.

42. Nicholas AS, Oleski SL. Osteopathic manipulative treatment for postoperative pain. *J Am Osteopath Assoc.* 2002;102:5–8.

43. Hirayama F, Kageyama Y, Urabe N, Senjyu H. The effect of postoperative ataralgesia by manual therapy after pulmonary resection. *Man Ther.* 2003;8:42–45.

44. Faymonville ME, Laureys S, Degueldre C, et al. Neural mechanisms of antinociceptive effects of hypnosis. *Anesthesiology.* 2000;92:1257–1267.

45. Lawlis GF, Selby D, Hinnant D, McCoy CE. Reduction of postoperative pain parameters by presurgical relaxation instructions for spinal pain patients. *Spine.* 1985;10:649–651.

46. Gavin M, Litt M, Khan A, Onyiuke H, Kozol R. A prospective, randomized trial of cognitive intervention for postoperative pain. *Am Surg.* 2006;72:414–418.

47. Faymonville ME, Fissette J, Mambourg PH, Roediger L, Joris J, Lamy M. Hypnosis as adjunct therapy in conscious sedation for plastic surgery. *Reg Anesth.* 1995;20:145–151.

48. Lang EV, Benotsch EG, Fick LJ, et al. Adjunctive nonpharmacological analgesia for invasive medical procedures: A randomised trial. *Lancet.* 2000;355:1486–1490.

49. Mauer MH, Burnett KF, Ouellette EA, Ironson GH, Dandes HM. Medical hypnosis and orthopedic hand surgery: Pain perception, postoperative recovery, and therapeutic comfort. *Int J Clin Exp Hypn.* 1999;47:144–161.

50. Lambert SA. The effects of hypnosis/guided imagery on the postoperative course of children. *J Dev Behav Pediatr.* 1996;17:307–310.

51. Dawson P, Van Hamel C, Wilkinson D, Warwick P, O'Connor M. Patient-controlled analgesia and intra-operative suggestion. *Anaesthesia.* 2001;56:65–69.

52. Lebovits AH, Twersky R, McEwan B. Intraoperative therapeutic suggestions in day-case surgery: Are there benefits for postoperative outcome? *Br J Anaesth.* 1999;82:861–866.

53. Van Der Laan WH, van Leeuwen BL, Sebel PS, Winograd E, Baumann P, Bonke B. Therapeutic suggestion has not effect on postoperative morphine requirements. *Anesth Analg.* 1996;82:148–152.

54. Good M, Anderson GC, Stanton-Hicks M, Grass JA, Makii M. Relaxation and music reduce pain after gynecologic surgery. *Pain Manag Nurs.* 2002;3:61–70.

55. Nilsson U, Rawal N, Enqvist B, Unosson M. Analgesia following music and therapeutic suggestions in the PACU in ambulatory surgery; a randomized controlled trial. *Acta Anaesthesiol Scand.* 2003;47:278–283.

56. Hatem TP, Lira PI, Mattos SS. The therapeutic effects of music in children following cardiac surgery. *J Pediatr (Rio J).* 2006;82:186–192.

57. Kliempt P, Ruta D, Ogston S, Landeck A, Martay K. Hemispheric-synchronisation during anaesthesia: A double-blind randomised trial using audiotapes for intra-operative nociception control. *Anaesthesia.* 1999;54:769–773.

58. McCaffrey RG, Good M. The lived experience of listening to music while recovering from surgery. *J Holist Nurs.* 2000;18:378–390.

59. Koch ME, Kain ZN, Ayoub C, Rosenbaum SH. The sedative and analgesic sparing effect of music. *Anesthesiology.* 1998;89:300–306.

60. Nilsson U, Rawal N, Unestahl LE, Zetterberg C, Unosson M. Improved recovery after music and therapeutic suggestions during general anaesthesia: A double-blind randomised controlled trial. *Acta Anaesthesiol Scand.* 2001;45:812–817.

61. Tracy S, Dufault M, Kogut S, Martin V, Rossi S, Willey-Temkin C. Translating best practices in nondrug postoperative pain management. *Nurs Res.* 2006;55:S57–S67.

62. Zollman C, Vickers A. ABC of complementary medicine: users and practitioners of complementary medicine. *BMJ.* 1999;319:836–838.

25

Opioid-Related Adverse Effects and Treatment Options

Kok-Yuen Ho and Tong J. Gan

Acute pain is common and occurs most often in the immediate postoperative period. Acute nonsurgical pain related to burns injury, trauma, sickle cell crisis, ureteric colic, and acute pancreatitis are also commonly encountered in the hospital. The role of opioids in acute pain management is well established. The high efficacy profile and selectivity of potent opioids provides effective management of severe postsurgical pain, particularly in settings where nonopioid pain relievers are inadequate (refer to Chapter 15, *Clinical Application of Epidural Analgesia*). In general, opioids share a collection of annoying to serious adverse effects and potentially life-threatening complications (Table 25.1). In general, the higher the dose of opioid administered, the greater the incidence and severity of adverse effects. However, there are interindividual variations and some patients may be exquisitely sensitive to the class in general, whereas others develop more side effects with one particular opioid compared to another. Opioid pharmacotherapy therefore requires careful drug selection and dose titration to achieve a satisfactory balance between analgesia and adverse effects.

With greater understanding of their pharmacokinetics and pharmacodynamics, opioids have been administered via different routes to achieve greater efficacy in treating pain (Table 25.2). Consequently, there is also a difference in the type and incidence of adverse effects associated with the various routes of administration.

CARDIOVASCULAR ADVERSE EFFECTS

In general, opioids, particularly rapid-acting lipophilic agents, exhibit vagomimetic effects that tend to slow heart rate. The major exception to this rule is meperidine, which, because of intrinsic antimuscarinic properties, can increase resting heart rate. Administration of large doses of morphine induces a reduction in sympathetic nervous system tone.[1] This results in venous pooling with a consequent decrease in venous return, cardiac output, and blood pressure. Patients are generally asymptomatic when lying supine in bed, but present with postural hypotension and/or syncope when asked to stand.

Morphine causes myocardial depression by producing bradycardia, probably by stimulation of the vagal nuclei in the medulla. It also acts directly on the sinoatrial node and atrioventricular node to slow conduction of cardiac impulses.

Morphine indirectly produces hypotension through the release of histamine.[2] The severity and incidence of morphine-induced histamine release is variable among individuals. Avoiding rapid administration of morphine, maintaining patient in a supine position, and optimizing intravascular volume can attenuate the reduction in blood pressure secondary to histamine release. Pretreatment with H1 and H2 histamine receptor antagonists is also protective against the hemodynamic changes seen with morphine administration, even though histamine release is unaffected.[3] The administration of fentanyl or sufentanil is not associated with histamine release.

With opioid doses commonly used for pain management, hypotension is uncommon. Hypotension after opioid administration is more likely in patients with high sympathetic tone, for example, patients in pain or with poor cardiac function. It is also seen in patients with hypovolemia.

RESPIRATORY ADVERSE EFFECTS

Opioids affect the respiratory system in a dose-dependent manner. Direct action on μ-receptors in the brainstem produces depression of ventilation.[4] Decrease in respiratory rate and tidal volume are common with standard therapeutic doses. Opioids are also known to depress the ventilatory response to hypercapnia, leading to a raised resting end tidal carbon dioxide level.[5,6] Opioid-mediated respiratory depression has been linked to central nervous system (CNS) penetration of drug, binding to μ_1-receptors in the brainstem, and inhibition of cells in the pneumotaxic and apneustic centers. Lipophilic opioids rapidly penetrate CNS and inhibit respiratory drive within seconds to minutes following administration. In general, peak CNS levels of lipophilic opioids and respiratory depressant effects correlate with peak plasma concentrations. In contrast, morphine has difficulty traversing the blood-brain barrier, and its entrance

Table 25.1: Classification of Opioid-Related Adverse Effects

Cardiovascular	Bradycardia
	Hypotension
	Myocardial depression
Respiratory	Decrease respiratory rate and tidal volume
	Respiratory depression/arrest
Neurological	Excessive sedation
	Delirium/euphoria
Gastrointestinal	Delayed gastric emptying
	Nausea and vomiting
	Constipation/ileus
Genitourinary	Urinary retention
Dermatological	Pruritus and anaphylaxis

Table 25.2: Routes of Opioid Administration

Oral (cost-effective, least dose efficient)

Sublingual and buccal (rapid onset)

Rectal (greater dose efficiency than oral)

Transdermal (delayed onset, not for acute pain)

Subcutaneous (more rapid onset than oral, less painful)

Intramuscular (can be painful)

Intravenous
    Bolus dosing
    Continuous infusion
    Patient-controlled analgesia (PCA)

Inhalational
    Nasal (in development)
    Pulmonary (in development)

Neuraxial
    Epidural
    Intrathecal

into, and exit from, the brain are delayed. As a result of this prolonged CNS transfer half-life, morphine's respiratory depressant effects may persist for many minutes to hours, despite significant declines in plasma concentrations.[5,6] Risk factors for opioid-mediated respiratory depression, including patient, caregiver, and drug-related variables, are outlined in Table 25.3.

Neuraxial administration of opioids has the same, or possibly, greater risk of respiratory depression. A multicenter trial involving 14 000 patients showed that the incidence of respiratory depression was between 0.25% and 0.40% after epidural morphine, with all occurrences within 12 hours of administration.[7] Intrathecal morphine administration was shown to produce a diminished ventilatory response to hypoxia of the same magnitude as an equianalgesic dose of intravenous morphine, but the duration of respiratory depressant risk is longer lasting (more than 8 hours).[8] Risk factors for neuraxial opioid-induced respiratory depression are similar to that outlined for parenteral and oral dosing. Additional risk factors with neuraxial doses of morphine include prolonged Trendelenberg positioning following intrathecal dosing and epidural administration via high thoracic catheters.[7]

Opioid-induced respiratory depression can be blunted with amphetamines and mixed agonist antagonists such as nalbuphine and reversed with opioid antagonists, including naloxone or naltrexone. The dose of naloxone should be titrated according to the patient's response. Initially, intravenous naloxone in increments of 0.1–0.2 mg can be administered every 3–5 minutes, as needed, until return of adequate alertness or respiratory rate. Repeat doses of naloxone or naloxone infusions may be required as the duration of action of the opioid outlasts that of the antagonist. Prophylactic infusion of naloxone 40–100 μg/h may also be employed to prevent the worst aspects of respiratory depression in high-risk patients. Excessive doses of naloxone (ie, greater than 800 μg) may reverse opioid-mediated analgesia. High doses and rapid reversal may also precipitate rebound hypertension, tachycardia, pulmonary edema, nausea, and vomiting. If naloxone does not improve the level of consciousness, the caregiver should assume that the patient is markedly hypercarbic and acidotic and initiate ventilatory resuscitation. A continuous intravenous infusion of naloxone

can then be used. Additional discussion regarding the respiratory adverse effects of opioids may be found in Chapter 15.

GASTROINTESTINAL ADVERSE EFFECTS

Opioid-induced bowel dysfunction is a term used to describe a constellation of symptoms including delayed gastric emptying, increased gastroesophageal reflux, bloating, nausea, vomiting, and constipation.[9] Bowel dysfunction can occur after surgery, especially when surgery involves manipulation or resection of the gut. This is further worsened with the use of opioids for analgesia. In patients taking opioids for chronic nonmalignant pain, the incidence of bowel dysfunction is as high as 40%.[10] μ-receptors are found in the central and peripheral nervous system. The effect of opioids on the gastrointestinal (GI) tract is mediated centrally as well as peripherally because both parenteral and epidural morphine influence GI motility.[11] Opioids decrease the peristaltic contractions of the small and large intestines thereby allowing greater absorption of water from the intestinal contents and inhibiting GI motility.[12] Opioids also play a direct role in decreasing GI secretions.[13] With a longer intestinal transit time, there is formation of hard dry stools as well as constipation. There is evidence that μ-receptors are found in the myenteric and submucosal plexi of the small and large intestines and that opioid-induced bowel dysfunction is peripherally mediated.[14] Peripherally acting opioids, such as loperamide, that do not cross the blood-brain barrier have been demonstrated to increase GI transit time.[15]

Gastric emptying is similarly delayed and this is mediated through the vagus nerve.[16] The tone of the pyloric sphincter, ileocecal valve, and anal sphincter are also increased. With a delay in gastric emptying, the risk of aspiration is greater. Intravenous metoclopramide has been shown to be an effective drug for improving gastric emptying in patients receiving opioid therapy.[17]

Table 25.3: Risk Factors for Opioid-Mediated Respiratory Depression

Excessive dose

Extremes of age

Pulmonary disease

Morbid obesity

Sleep apnea

Renal failure (accumulation of active metabolites)

Hepatic failure (accumulation of free drug)

Coadministration of other central acting agents (benzodiazepines, antihistamines, anticholinergics)

Alterations in the blood-brain barrier (tumor, infection, pharmacological agents)

Coadministration of parenteral and neuraxial opioids

Improper use of patient-controlled analgesia ("proxy dosing," dose misprogramming, and use of basal infusions)

Genetic sensitivity (polymorphisms of μ-receptors, CSF transporter molecules, catechol-*O*-methyltransferase, and metabolic enzymes)

Table 25.4: Medications for Treating Opioid-Induced Constipation

Fiber bulking agents
   Methylcellulose PO 1–3 times per day
   Psyllium PO 15–60 g/d

Stool softeners
   Docusate sodium PO 100–400 mg 1–2 times per day

Laxatives
   Bisacodyl PO 10 mg 1–3 times per day
   Senna PO 2–4 tablets 1–2 times per day

Osmotics
   Magnesium citrate PO 10–15 g per day
   Lactulose PO 10–15 mL 2–3 times per day

Peripheral opioid antagonists
   Methylnaltrexone
   Alvimopan

Abbreviation: PO = per oral.

Patients usually do not develop tolerance to constipation and, therefore, constipation should be managed actively. Therapeutic goals should include maximizing stool volume, keeping stools softer and enhancing intestinal peristaltic movement.[10] Fiber bulking agents, stool softeners, laxatives, and osmotic agents can be prescribed to treat constipation (Table 25.4). The efficacy of bulk-forming agents such as methylcellulose and psyllium in treating constipation has been well established.[18,19] These agents work by retaining water in the stools so it is important that patients receive adequate oral hydration. Stool softeners, such as docusate sodium, work by lowering the surface tension of hard, dry stools to allow greater penetration of water. It has also been shown to directly stimulate contraction of the colon and rectum. Bisacodyl and senna are laxatives that stimulate peristalsis and improve GI motility. Osmotic agents such as magnesium citrate, sorbitol, and lactulose draw water into the stools by osmosis and improve laxation. In certain situations, an enema may be useful when defecation has not occurred for more than 5 days.

Since the early 2000s, there has been growing interest in the role of peripheral opioid μ-receptor antagonists in treating postoperative ileus and chronic constipation. Peripherally acting opioid antagonists (eg, methylnaltrexone and alvimopan) do not cross the blood-brain barrier, but can attenuate the delay in gastric emptying or intestinal transit.[16] They are also effective in reversing opioid-induced bowel dysfunction.[20]

Methylnaltrexone, a quaternary derivative of naltrexone, blocks peripheral effects of opioids.[21] Central analgesic effects are spared because methylnaltrexone has low lipid solubility and does not cross the blood-brain barrier.[22] Intravenous (IV) methylnaltrexone (0.3 mg/kg) was able to reverse morphine-induced delay in gastric emptying in volunteers.[23] Yuan et al[24] demonstrated in a randomized, double-blind placebo-controlled trial that IV methylnaltrexone reduced orocecal transit time in patients on chronic methadone therapy. This group of patients also had an immediate laxation response after methylnaltrexone administration with no evidence of opioid withdrawal symptoms. Methylnaltrexone given as an oral dose of up to 3.0 mg/kg similarly improved GI motility and alleviated opioid-induced constipation.[25] A recent phase II trial examining intravenous methylnaltrexone for accelerating recovery of GI function in patients undergoing segmental colectomy via laparotomy demonstrated an improvement of 27 hours in mean time to GI recovery, measured by first toleration of solid food or first bowel movement, whichever occurred first. This was accompanied by a shorter time to eligibility for hospital discharge in the methylnaltrexone group compared with the placebo group.[26] To date, two large-scale phase III trials involving more than 100 patients each showed that subcutaneous methylnaltrexone could be successfully administered to treat opioid-induced constipation.[27,28]

Alvimopan is a peripherally restricted specific μ-opioid receptor antagonist.[29,30] In a human volunteer study, it effectively prevented morphine-induced increase in GI transit time.[31] Alvimopan also shortened the time to laxation after treatment and increased stool weight and number of bowel movements in patients on chronic methadone therapy.[32,33] In the postoperative setting, alvimopan was effective in accelerating the return of bowel function after abdominal surgery.[34,35] Webster and colleagues[36] conducted one of the largest randomized, double-blind, placebo-controlled trials involving 522 subjects taking opioids for noncancer pain. A dose of alvimopan (0.5 mg twice a day) was well tolerated, with increased weekly spontaneous bowel movements and reduced straining and incomplete evacuation. There was also no evidence of reversal of opioid analgesia.[36] However, further clinical studies of alvimopan have been suspending because of a possible increase in cardiovascular morbidity in exposed subjects.[31,37]

OPIOID-INDUCED NAUSEA AND VOMITING

The development of nausea and vomiting is mediated through opioid receptors in the chemoreceptor trigger zone (CTZ) and the emetic center in the brainstem (Figure 25.1). The CTZ is located on the floor of the fourth ventricle and has unique attributes. This neural region lies outside the blood-brain barrier

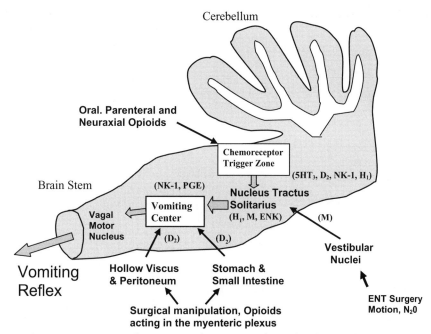

Figure 25.1: Nausea and vomiting pathways: sites of opioid and visceral stimulation.

and is exposed to and responds to opioids in the systemic circulation. Opioids also sensitize the vestibular system such that patient movement may trigger nausea and vomiting. Nausea and vomiting is further aggravated by delayed gastric emptying as well as constipation caused by opioid therapy. The incidence of nausea and vomiting appear to be similar among the opioids, including morphine, meperidine, fentanyl, sufentanil, and alfentanil.[38]

Nausea and vomiting may be seen in one-fourth of patients receiving opioids.[39] In the postoperative setting, the incidence of postoperative nausea and vomiting (PONV) for all surgeries and patient populations ranges between 25% and 30%. Severe, intractable PONV is estimated to occur in 0.18% of all patients.[40] The use of opioids may increase the risk of PONV by more than 4-fold.[41] In addition, there are many other factors that can increase the risk of PONV (Table 25.5).[42] The greater the number of drug, patient, and surgical-related risk factors, the higher the percentage incidence of PONV (Figure 25.2).[42,43]

Administration of a regional anesthetic technique has advantages over a general anesthetic as nitrous oxide, volatile anesthetic gases, and opioids are avoided. If opioids are administered with local anesthetic agents into the epidural or intrathecal space, PONV can still occur. The high incidence of nausea and vomiting seen with neuraxial morphine is related to cephalad cerebral spinal fluid (CSF) flow with transport of morphine molecules to the CTZ. Seventeen percent of patients who had received epidural morphine reported nausea and vomiting after surgery.[45] Therefore, using highly lipophilic opioids such as fentanyl or sufentanil can reduce cephalad spread and lower the risk of emesis.[46]

Postoperative pain prolongs gastric emptying time and contributes to emesis after surgery. A multimodal approach using a combination of systemic opioids, nonsteroidal anti-inflammatory drugs (NSAIDs), neuraxial blocks, regional nerve blocks, and local infiltration of the surgical wound can reduce postoperative pain. Such an approach also will ensure that the lowest possible dose of opioid is given to achieve adequate analgesia as opioids cause PONV.

PONV remains an important cause for poor patient satisfaction (Table 25.5). PONV also results in increased costs of personnel, drug acquisition, materials, prolonged recovery room stay, and unanticipated hospital admission.[47] It is therefore imperative to prevent or treat nausea and vomiting effectively.

Receptors such as the 5-hydroxytryptamine type 3 (5-HT$_3$), dopamine type 2 (D$_2$), and neurokinin-1 (NK-1) are found in the CTZ. The nucleus tractus solitarius has high concentrations of enkephalin, histaminergic (H$_1$), and muscarinic (M) receptors

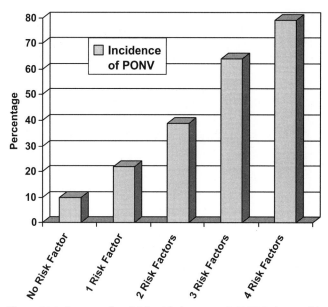

Figure 25.2: Impact of multiple risk factors on PONV. Primary risk factors for PONV: (1) postoperative opioids, (2) history of motion sickness or PONV, (3) female sex, and (4) nonsmoker. Modified from Gan TJ et al (2003).[42]

Table 25.5: Risk Factors for Postoperative Nausea and Vomiting (PONV)[40,43,44]

Patient factors

Female

History of motion sickness or PONV

Nonsmoker

Anxiety

Concurrent therapy (chemotherapy, radiation therapy)

Pregnancy

Surgical factors

Type of surgery (laparoscopy, gynecologic, ENT, strabismus, and breast surgery)

Long duration of surgery

Anesthetic factors

Inhalational anesthetic agents (nitrous oxide, volatile anesthetics)

Opioids

High dose neuromuscular reversal agents (>5 mg neostigmine)

Poorly controlled pain

(Figure 25.1). These receptors transmit messages to the emetic center when stimulated. NK-1 receptors were also recently discovered in the emetic center.[48,49] These receptors are therefore the targets for antiemetic therapy.

Traditional antiemetic drugs used for treating nausea and vomiting include the anticholinergics (scopolamine), antihistamines (diphenhydramine, dimenhydrinate), and antidopaminergics (droperidol, prochlorperazine, and metoclopramide) (Table 25.6). However, many of these are associated with undesirable side effects, including restlessness, dry mouth, sedation, hypotension, dystonia and extrapyramidal symptoms, and even QT prolongation.

Serotonin (5-HT$_3$) antagonists belong to a separate class of antiemetics that can effectively treat opioid-induced nausea and vomiting.[50] Dexamethasone also is an effective antiemetic.[51] Its mechanism of action may be related to the inhibition of prostaglandin synthesis and the stimulation of endorphin release, resulting in mood elevation and a sense of well-being. In PONV studies, dexamethasone (5–10 mg IV) has been demonstrated to have antiemetic efficacy.[52,53] Aprepitant is an NK-1 receptor antagonist that has been used effectively for the prevention of postoperative nausea and vomiting.[54] NK-1 receptor antagonists have also been shown to be efficacious in the treatment of established PONV after gynecologic surgery.[55] Metoclopramide (10 mg IV) can be used for increasing gastric transit, but it is not an effective antiemetic at this dose, although higher doses of 20 mg IV may be more effective.

Combination therapy has been shown to be superior to monotherapy for treatment of nausea and vomiting. The presence of multiple emetic receptors in the emetic center, CTZ, and their association supports the practice of using more than one antiemetic drug. The combination of a 5HT$_3$-receptor antagonist with either droperidol or dexamethasone is superior to using only a 5HT$_3$-receptor antagonist, droperidol, or dexamethasone as the sole agent.[57–59] It also appeared that droperidol has greater efficacy against nausea, whereas ondansetron has better antiemetic properties.[60] Patients with or who will be exposed to multiple risk factors for PONV should receive combination

Table 25.6: Antiemetic Drug Dosing and Timing[a]

Class	Drugs	Dosage	Timing
Anticholinergic	Scopolamine[b]	Transdermal patch	4 hours prior to surgery
Antihistamine	Dimenhydrinate	IV 1–2 mg/kg (up to 12.5 mg) or PO 50–100 mg	As required
	Promethazine	IV 6.25–12.5 mg	At end of surgery
Antidopaminergic	Droperidol[c]	IV 0.625–1.25 mg	At end of surgery
	Prochlorperazine	IV 5–10 mg or PO 10 mg	At end of surgery
	Metoclopramide[d]	10–20 mg	During/after surgery
Antiserotoninergic	Ondansetron	IV 4 mg	At end of surgery
	Dolasetron	IV 12.5 mg	At end of surgery
	Granisetron	IV 0.35–1 mg	At end of surgery
Steroids	Dexamethasone[e]	IV 4–5 mg	Prior to induction
NK-1 antagonist	Aprepitant[f]	PO 40 mg	4 hours prior to surgery

[a] Modified from Gan et al (2007).[56]

[b] Useful for treating neuraxial opioid induced vertigo and nausea, not recommended in elderly and cognitively impaired.

[c] Not recommended in patients with Parkinson's disease.

[d] Avoid in patients with surgical anastomosis.

[e] Clear with surgical staff; may affect immune function and wound healing.

[f] As effective as ondansetron, prolonged duration of effect permits preoperative dosing.

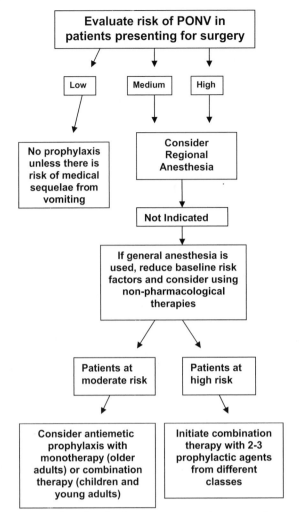

Evaluate risk of PONV in patients presenting for surgery

Low | Medium | High

No prophylaxis unless there is risk of medical sequelae from vomiting

Consider Regional Anesthesia

Not Indicated

If general anesthesia is used, reduce baseline risk factors and consider using non-pharmacological therapies

Patients at moderate risk

Patients at high risk

Consider antiemetic prophylaxis with monotherapy (older adults) or combination therapy (children and young adults)

Initiate combination therapy with 2-3 prophylactic agents from different classes

Figure 25.3: Algorithm for the management of postoperative nausea and vomiting. Modified from Gan TJ et al (2003)[42] and Apfel CC et al (1999).[43]

therapy from at least two different classes for antiemetic prophylaxis. Patients at low risk of PONV may not require prophylactic antiemetics and can be treated postoperatively if they have nausea and vomiting. A treatment algorithm for limiting PONV is described in Figure 25.3.

Opioid antagonists (eg, naloxone and nalmefene) in small doses have also been demonstrated to reduce opioid-related nausea and vomiting. In one study involving patients undergoing total abdominal hysterectomy, a low-dose IV infusion of naloxone at 0.25 μg/kg/h effectively reduce postoperative nausea and vomiting.[61] A separate study showed that a single IV dose of nalmefene of 15–25 μg administered at the end of surgery reduced the need for antiemetic therapy in patients receiving IV PCA morphine after lower abdominal surgery.[62]

GENITOURINARY ADVERSE EFFECTS

Bladder detrusor muscle relaxation occurs with either intravenous or neuraxial administration of opioids.[63–65] As a consequence of the decrease in bladder tone, an increase in maximal bladder capacity occurs with urinary retention. At the same time, an increase in vesicle sphincter tone because of opioids also contributes to voiding difficulty.[66] Urinary retention was reversible with a single dose of naloxone (0.01 mg/kg IV).[67] Methylnaltrexone (0.3 mg/kg IV) was able to reverse opioid-induced bladder dysfunction as well. The efficacy of methylnaltrexone also proved that opioid-induced bladder dysfunction was peripherally mediated.[67] When severe or distressing urinary retention remains, catheterization or discontinuation of opioid therapy may be required.

NEUROLOGICAL ADVERSE EFFECTS

Opioids produce a variety of CNS effects, including sedation, cognitive impairment, and neuroexcitation. Sedation is a common side effect of opioid therapy. It is also a useful early indicator of the development of respiratory depression. Regular monitoring of sedation scores is therefore mandatory in all patients receiving opioids for acute pain management. In the presence of concomitant usage of CNS depressant drugs, such as benzodiazepines, antidepressants, anticonvulsants, or skeletal muscle relaxants, the incidence of sedation is markedly increased.

Neuroexcitatory features may range from delirium to grand mal seizurelike activity.[68–70] Delirium is characterized by a global disorder of cognition and consciousness. Meperidine was particularly associated with delirium because of its anticholinergic activity. Normeperidine, the breakdown product of meperidine, has also been reported to produce seizures at high concentrations.[71] Accumulation of breakdown metabolites of morphine in patients with renal impairment may also lead to postoperative delirium.

Sleep disturbances, including reduction in rapid eye movement (REM) and slow wave sleep, as well as vivid dreams, can occur with postoperative opioid therapy.[38] Doctors managing acute pain with opioids should be aware of the risk factors that may predispose a patient to delirium. These include patient age, comorbidities, and drug interactions (Table 25.7).

DERMATOLOGICAL ADVERSE EFFECTS

Cutaneous changes, such as erythema and urticaria, can result from opioid-induced histamine release. Pruritis, in the absence of urticaria, can occur with both systemic and neuraxial administration of opioids. The incidence of pruritis is higher with epidural or intrathecal morphine administration and, notably, it is most commonly seen in obstetric patients. It usually affects the face, neck, and chest in this population. The incidence has been reported to be as high as 80%.[72] Pruritis is in fact the most common side effect associated with intrathecal opioid administration.[73] The incidence among the different intrathecal opioids (morphine, fentanyl, and sufentanil) appears to be similar.[74,75]

The pathogenesis of pruritis remains unclear and therefore anti-itch therapies have lagged behind treatments for other opioid-related adverse effects. Previously, it was believed that opioid-induced histamine release or spinal modulation of nociceptive afferent input led to spinal and trigeminal interpretation of such information as pruritis.[76] Animal studies published later showed that μ-receptors at the level of the medullary dorsal horn

Table 25.7: Risk Factors for Development of Delirium

Patient Factors	Advanced Age
	Preexisting cognitive dysfunction
	Renal impairment
	Hypercalcemia
	Sepsis
	Dehydration
	Hypoxia
	Poorly controlled pain
	Bladder distention
Drug interactions	Benzodiazepines
	Opioids (particularly κ agonists)
	Anticholinergics
	Residual volatile anesthetics

Table 25.8: Approaches to Managing Opioid-Related Adverse Effects

Reducing opioid dose (IV PCA and epidural PCA bolus dose)

Addition of a nonopioid analgesics (multimodal analgesia)

Prophylatic administration of antiemetics in at risk populations

Assess and aggressively manage adverse effects symptomatically

Consider opioid rotation

Switch route of administration

Further development and use of peripheral acting opioid antagonists (alvimopan, methylnaltrexone)

Further development and use of opioid analgesics with low adverse event profiles such as tapentadol, (combined μ agonist/ norepinephrine reuptake inhibitor) and DPI-3290 (combined δ-/μ-agonists)

were responsible for pruritis and that its manifestation was not histamine mediated.[77,78] It now appears that a distinct spinothalamic pathway exists for itch – one that is separate from the pain and temperature spinothalamic tracts.[79] Opioid agonists reduce tonic inhibition of these itch-specific pathways, allowing spontaneous activity of central itch neurons.[80] The reversibility of pruritis with naloxone also supports a mechanism that is mediated through opioid receptors.

Various drugs have been used to treat pruritis, but none abolishes it completely. Traditionally, antihistamines have been used to treat this side effect but their poor efficacy can be explained by the absence of histamine-mediated pruritis. The continued use of antihistamines and the purported effectiveness may be related to the sedative effects of this class of drugs.

The only effective treatment of pruritis appears to be naloxone. Other drugs that have been used to treat pruritis include serotonin antagonists, propofol, and NSAIDs. True allergy or anaphylactic reactions to opioids are rare. In general, opioids cause histamine release and patients may manifest signs and symptoms, including urticaria, pruritis, sneezing, and exacerbation of asthma. These are not considered allergic reactions. Such reactions can usually be prevented or treated with antihistamine agents such as diphenhydramine (25–50 mg orally).

FUTURE DEVELOPMENTS

Allyl-2,5-dimethyl-1-piperazines have been of interest as analgesic agents for the management of moderate to severe pain. One of these agents, DPI-3290, has been examined in animal studies.[81,82] It is a combined δ- and μ-receptor opioid receptor agonist. When compared with strong opioids such as morphine and fentanyl, DPI-3290 had equivalent antinociceptive efficacy, but produced less respiratory depression.[81] DPI-125 is another novel mixed δ- and μ-opioid receptor agonist that has successfully completed a phase 1 clinical trial for its IV formulation. Preclinically, DPI-125 has shown similar efficacy to morphine and fentanyl, with the potential for reduced respiratory depression, emesis, and addiction over those agents.

A final analgesic in late stage development that has a lower incidence of adverse events is tapentadol. This combination μ-receptor agonist/catecholamine reuptake inhibitor provides analgesic efficacy similar to oxycodone, but with a lower incidence of nausea and vomiting in acute pain trials and a reduced risk of constipation following chronic exposure.

The continued development of these drugs in human trials in the future shows great promise. An opioid analgesic that is as potent as the currently available strong opioids, such as morphine and fentanyl, whereas devoid of adverse effects like nausea, vomiting, and respiratory depression, will have an important role in acute pain management.

CONCLUSION

The side-effect profiles of equianalgesic doses of opioids are similar, but there are interpatient variations in the occurrence and severity of these adverse effects. A generalized approach that may be recommended to minimize morbidity and improve patient satisfaction includes reduction in opioid exposure and aggressive treatment of adverse events (Table 25.8).

The use of nonopioid analgesics, including acetaminophen (paracetamol), NSAIDs, and cyclooxygenase type 2 inhibitors, in postoperative pain management is well established.[83] These drugs exert either an additive or synergistic effect when given in combination with opioids. At the same time, they reduce total opioid requirement (opioid-sparing effect), along with its associated adverse effects. There is also evidence to suggest that coxib-/NSAID-mediated inhibition of prostaglandin E synthesis in the brainstem and medulla may directly reduce nausea and vomiting responses. A multimodal approach to acute pain management, therefore, allows lower doses of different analgesics to be used while reducing the side effects associated with each of them.[84] Opioid rotation, or switching from one opioid to another, may be helpful if the side effects experienced with one particular opioid are too distressing. Patients may tolerate one opioid better than another.

Opioid-related adverse effects are commonly seen during acute pain management. With greater understanding and knowledge of the etiology of unwanted side effects of opioids, and with the ability to administer opioids via various routes into the body, it may be possible to reduce the incidence and severity of side effects, whereas maintaining or enhancing the efficacy of opioids. Currently, however, a potent μ-opioid receptor agonist will be associated with adverse effects as discussed in this chapter – with respiratory depression being the most feared and lethal complication. Developments in finding drugs that potentiate opioid analgesia without increasing the risk of opioid-induced respiratory depression are already ongoing[85] and opioids that work on other receptor subtypes (eg, δ and κ) may also reduce some of the μ related opioid side effects.

REFERENCES

1. Lowenstein E, Whiting RB, Bittar DA, et al. Local and neurally mediated effects of morphine on skeletal muscle vascular resistance. *J Pharmacol Exp Ther*. 1972;180:359–367.

2. Rosow CE, Moss J, Philbin DM, Savarese JJ. Histamine release during morphine and fentanyl anesthesia. *Anesthesiology*. 1982;56:93–96.

3. Philbin DM, Moss J, Akins CW, et al. The use of H1 and H2 histamine antagonists with morphine anesthesia: a double-blind study. *Anesthesiology*. 1981;55:292–296.

4. Atcheson R, Lambert DG. Update on opioid receptors. *Br J Anaesth*. 1994;73:132–134.

5. Weil JV, McCullough RE, Kline JS, Sodal IE. Diminished ventilatory response to hypoxia and hypercapnia after morphine in normal man. *N Engl J Med*. 1975;292:1103–1106.

6. Martin WR. Pharmacology of opioids. *Pharmacol Rev*. 1983;35:283–323.

7. Rawal N, Arner S, Gustafsson LL, Allvin R. Present state of extradural and intrathecal opioid analgesia in Sweden: a nation-wide follow-up survey. *Br J Anaesth*. 1987;59:791–799.

8. Bailey PL, Lu JK, Pace NL, et al. Effects of intrathecal morphine on the ventilatory response to hypoxia. *N Engl J Med*. 2000;343:1228–1234.

9. Kurz A, Sessler DI. Opioid-induced bowel dysfunction: pathophysiology and potential new therapies. *Drugs*. 2003;63:649–671.

10. Thomas J. Opioid-induced bowel dysfunction. *J Pain Symptom Manage*. 2008;35:103–113.

11. Thorn SE, Wattwil M, Lindberg G, Sawe J. Systemic and central effects of morphine on gastroduodenal motility. *Acta Anaesthesiol Scand*. 1996;40:177–186.

12. Yukioka H, Tanaka M, Fujimori M. Recovery of bowel motility after high dose fentanyl or morphine anaesthesia for cardiac surgery. *Anaesthesia*. 1990;45:353–356.

13. De Luca A, Coupar IM. Insights into opioid action in the intestinal tract. *Pharmacol Ther*. 1996;69:103–115.

14. Sternini C, Patierno S, Selmer IS, Kirchgessner A. The opioid system in the gastrointestinal tract. *Neurogastroenterol Motil*. 2004;16S:3–16.

15. Basilisco G, Camboni G, Bozzani A, et al. Oral naloxone antagonizes loperamide-induced delay of orocecal transit. *Dig Dis Sci*. 1987;32:829–832.

16. Murphy DB, Sutton A, Prescott LF, Murphy MB. A comparison of the effects of tramadol and morphine on gastric emptying in man. *Anaesthesia*. 1997;52:1224–1229.

17. McNeill MJ, Ho ET, Kenny GN. Effect of i.v. metoclopramide on gastric emptying after opioid premedication. *Br J Anaesth*. 1990;64:450–452.

18. Ashraf W, Park F, Lof J, Quigley EM. Effects of psyllium therapy on stool characteristics, colon transit and anorectal function in chronic idiopathic constipation. *Aliment Pharmacol Ther*. 1995;9:639–647.

19. Snape WJ, Jr. The effect of methylcellulose on symptoms of constipation. *Clin Ther*. 1989;11:572–579.

20. Becker G, Galandi D, Blum HE. Peripherally acting opioid antagonists in the treatment of opiate-related constipation: a systematic review. *J Pain Symptom Manage*. 2007;34:547–565.

21. Yuan CS, Israel RJ. Methylnaltrexone, a novel peripheral opioid receptor antagonist for the treatment of opioid side effects. *Expert Opin Investig Drugs*. 2006;15:541–552.

22. Yuan CS. Methylnaltrexone mechanisms of action and effects on opioid bowel dysfunction and other opioid adverse effects. *Ann Pharmacother*. 2007;41:984–993.

23. Murphy DB, Sutton JA, Prescott LF, Murphy MB. Opioid-induced delay in gastric emptying: a peripheral mechanism in humans. *Anesthesiology*. 1997;87:765–770.

24. Yuan CS, Foss JF, O'Connor M, et al. Methylnaltrexone for reversal of constipation due to chronic methadone use: a randomized controlled trial. *JAMA*. 2000;283:367–372.

25. Yuan CS, Foss JF. Oral methylnaltrexone for opioid-induced constipation. *JAMA*. 2000;284:1383–1384.

26. Viscusi ER, Rathmell J, Fichera A, et al. A double-blind, randomized, placebo-controlled trial of methylnaltrexone (MNTX) for post-operative bowel dysfunction in segmental colectomy patients. *Anesthesiology*. 2005;103:A893.

27. Slatkin N, Karver S, Thomas J. A Phase III double-blind, placebo-controlled trial of methylnaltrexone for opioid-induced constipation in advanced illness (MNTX 302). *Digest Dis Week*. 2006:686e.

28. Thomas J, Lipman A, Slatkin N, et al. A phase III double-blind placebo-controlled trial of methylnaltrexone (MNTX) for opioid-induced constipation (OIC) in advanced medical illness (AMI). *Proc Am Soc Clin Oncol*. 2005;23:8003.

29. Camilleri M. Alvimopan, a selective peripherally acting mu-opioid antagonist. *Neurogastroenterol Motil*. 2005;17:157–165.

30. Neary P, Delaney CP. Alvimopan. *Expert Opin Investig Drugs*. 2005;14:479–488.

31. Liu SS, Hodgson PS, Carpenter RL, Fricke JR, Jr. ADL 8–2698, a trans-3,4-dimethyl-4-(3-hydroxyphenyl) piperidine, prevents gastrointestinal effects of intravenous morphine without affecting analgesia. *Clin Pharmacol Ther*. 2001;69:66–71.

32. Paulson DM, Kennedy DT, Donovick RA, et al. Alvimopan: an oral, peripherally acting, mu-opioid receptor antagonist for the treatment of opioid-induced bowel dysfunction – a 21-day treatment-randomized clinical trial. *J Pain*. 2005;6:184–192.

33. Schmidt WK. Alvimopan (ADL 8-2698) is a novel peripheral opioid antagonist. *Am J Surg*. 2001;182:27S–38S.

34. Delaney CP, Wolff BG, Viscusi ER, et al. Alvimopan, for postoperative ileus following bowel resection: a pooled analysis of phase III studies. *Ann Surg*. 2007;245:355–363.

35. Herzog TJ, Coleman RL, Guerrieri JP, Jr, et al. A double-blind, randomized, placebo-controlled phase III study of the safety of alvimopan in patients who undergo simple total abdominal hysterectomy. *Am J Obstet Gynecol*. 2006;195:445–453.

36. Webster L, Jansen JP, Peppin J, et al. Alvimopan, a peripherally acting mu-opioid receptor (PAM-OR) antagonist for the treatment of opioid-induced bowel dysfunction: Results from a randomized, double-blind, placebo-controlled, dose-finding study in subjects taking opioids for chronic non-cancer pain. *Pain* 2008;137:428–440.

37. Gonenne J, Camilleri M, Ferber I, et al. Effect of alvimopan and codeine on gastrointestinal transit: a randomized controlled study. *Clin Gastroenterol Hepatol*. 2005;3:784–791.

38. Coda BA. Opioids. In: Barash PG, Cullen BF, Stoelting RK, eds. *Clinical Anesthesia*. 4th ed. Philadelphia, PA: Lippincott Williams & Wilkins, 2001; 345–375.

39. Cepeda MS, Farrar JT, Baumgarten M, et al. Side effects of opioids during short-term administration: effect of age, gender, and race. *Clin Pharmacol Ther*. 2003;74:102–112.

40. Watcha MF, White PF. Postoperative nausea and vomiting. Its etiology, treatment, and prevention. *Anesthesiology.* 1992;77:162–184.

41. Junger A, Hartmann B, Benson M, et al. The use of an anesthesia information management system for prediction of antiemetic rescue treatment at the postanesthesia care unit. *Anesth Analg.* 2001;92:1203–1209.

42. Gan TJ, Meyer T, Apfel CC, et al. Consensus guidelines for managing postoperative nausea and vomiting. *Anesth Analg.* 2003;97:62–71.

43. Apfel CC, Laara E, Koivuranta M, et al. A simplified risk score for predicting postoperative nausea and vomiting: conclusions from cross-validations between two centers. *Anesthesiology.* 1999;91:693–700.

44. Cheng CR, Sessler DI, Apfel CC. Does neostigmine administration produce a clinically important increase in postoperative nausea and vomiting? *Anesth Analg.* 2005;101:1349–1355.

45. Reiz S, Westberg M. Side-effects of epidural morphine. *Lancet.* 1980;2:203–204.

46. Borgeat A, Ekatodramis G, Schenker CA. Postoperative nausea and vomiting in regional anesthesia: a review. *Anesthesiology.* 2003;98:530–547.

47. Hill RP, Lubarsky DA, Phillips-Bute B, et al. Cost-effectiveness of prophylactic antiemetic therapy with ondansetron, droperidol, or placebo. *Anesthesiology.* 2000;92:958–967.

48. Rigby M, O'Donnell R, Rupniak NM. Species differences in tachykinin receptor distribution: further evidence that the substance P (NK1) receptor predominates in human brain. *J Comp Neurol.* 2005;490:335–353.

49. Saito R, Takano Y, Kamiya HO. Roles of substance P and NK(1) receptor in the brainstem in the development of emesis. *J Pharmacol Sci.* 2003;91:87–94.

50. Gan TJ. Selective serotonin 5-HT3 receptor antagonists for postoperative nausea and vomiting: are they all the same? *CNS Drugs.* 2005;19:225–238.

51. Henzi I, Walder B, Tramer MR. Dexamethasone for the prevention of postoperative nausea and vomiting: a quantitative systematic review. *Anesth Analg.* 2000;90:186–194.

52. Wang JJ, Ho ST, Lee SC, et al. The use of dexamethasone for preventing postoperative nausea and vomiting in females undergoing thyroidectomy: a dose-ranging study. *Anesth Analg.* 2000;91:1404–1407.

53. Wang JJ, Ho ST, Liu YH, et al. Dexamethasone reduces nausea and vomiting after laparoscopic cholecystectomy. *Br J Anaesth.* 1999;83:772–775.

54. Gan TJ, Apfel CC, Kovac A, et al. A randomized, double-blind comparison of the NK1 antagonist, aprepitant, versus ondansetron for the prevention of postoperative nausea and vomiting. *Anesth Analg.* 2007;104:1082–1089.

55. Diemunsch P, Schoeffler P, Bryssine B, et al. Antiemetic activity of the NK1 receptor antagonist GR205171 in the treatment of established postoperative nausea and vomiting after major gynaecological surgery. *Br J Anaesth.* 1999;82:274–276.

56. Gan TJ, Meyer TA, Apfel CC, et al. Society for Ambulatory Anesthesia guidelines for the management of postoperative nausea and vomiting. *Anesth Analg.* 2007;105:1615–1628.

57. Habib AS, El-Moalem HE, Gan TJ. The efficacy of the 5-HT3 receptor antagonists combined with droperidol for PONV prophylaxis is similar to their combination with dexamethasone. A meta-analysis of randomized controlled trials. *Can J Anaesth.* 2004;51:311–319.

58. Lopez-Olaondo L, Carrascosa F, Pueyo FJ, et al. Combination of ondansetron and dexamethasone in the prophylaxis of postoperative nausea and vomiting. *Br J Anaesth.* 1996;76:835–840.

59. Wu O, Belo SE, Koutsoukos G. Additive anti-emetic efficacy of prophylactic ondansetron with droperidol in out-patient gynecological laparoscopy. *Can J Anaesth.* 2000;47:529–536.

60. Henzi I, Sonderegger J, Tramer MR. Efficacy, dose-response, and adverse effects of droperidol for prevention of postoperative nausea and vomiting. *Can J Anaesth.* 2000;47:537–551.

61. Gan TJ, Ginsberg B, Glass PS, et al. Opioid-sparing effects of a low-dose infusion of naloxone in patient-administered morphine sulfate. *Anesthesiology.* 1997;87:1075–1081.

62. Joshi GP, Duffy L, Chehade J, et al. Effects of prophylactic nalmefene on the incidence of morphine-related side effects in patients receiving intravenous patient-controlled analgesia. *Anesthesiology.* 1999;90:1007–1011.

63. Drenger B, Magora F. Urodynamic studies after intrathecal fentanyl and buprenorphine in the dog. *Anesth Analg.* 1989;69:348–353.

64. Malinovsky JM, Le Normand L, Lepage JY, et al. The urodynamic effects of intravenous opioids and ketoprofen in humans. *Anesth Analg.* 1998;87:456–461.

65. Rawal N, Mollefors K, Axelsson K, et al. An experimental study of urodynamic effects of epidural morphine and of naloxone reversal. *Anesth Analg.* 1983;62:641–647.

66. Dray A. Epidural opiates and urinary retention: new models provide new insights. *Anesthesiology.* 1988;68:323–324.

67. Rosow CE, Gomery P, Chen TY, et al. Reversal of opioid-induced bladder dysfunction by intravenous naloxone and methylnaltrexone. *Clin Pharmacol Ther.* 2007;82:48–53.

68. Haber GW, Litman RS. Generalized tonic-clonic activity after remifentanil administration. *Anesth Analg.* 2001;93:1532–1533.

69. Mets B. Acute dystonia after alfentanil in untreated Parkinson's disease. *Anesth Analg.* 1991;72:557–558.

70. Parkinson SK, Bailey SL, Little WL, Mueller JB. Myoclonic seizure activity with chronic high-dose spinal opioid administration. *Anesthesiology.* 1990;72:743–745.

71. Armstrong PJ, Bersten A. Normeperidine toxicity. *Anesth Analg.* 1986;65:536–538.

72. Harrison DM, Sinatra R, Morgese L, Chung JH. Epidural narcotic and patient-controlled analgesia for post-cesarean section pain relief. *Anesthesiology.* 1988;68:454–457.

73. Ko MC, Naughton NN. An experimental itch model in monkeys: characterization of intrathecal morphine-induced scratching and antinociception. *Anesthesiology.* 2000;92:795–805.

74. Dahl JB, Jeppesen IS, Jorgensen H, et al. Intraoperative and postoperative analgesic efficacy and adverse effects of intrathecal opioids in patients undergoing cesarean section with spinal anesthesia: a qualitative and quantitative systematic review of randomized controlled trials. *Anesthesiology.* 1999;91:1919–1927.

75. Nelson KE, Rauch T, Terebuh V, D'Angelo R. A comparison of intrathecal fentanyl and sufentanil for labor analgesia. *Anesthesiology.* 2002;96:1070–1073.

76. Scott PV, Fischer HB. Intraspinal opiates and itching: a new reflex? *Br Med J (Clin Res Ed).* 1982;284:1015–1016.

77. Thomas DA, Williams GM, Iwata K, et al. The medullary dorsal horn: a site of action of morphine in producing facial scratching in monkeys. *Anesthesiology.* 1993;79:548–554.

78. Thomas DA, Williams GM, Iwata K, et al. Multiple effects of morphine on facial scratching in monkeys. *Anesth Analg.* 1993;77:933–935.

79. Andrew D, Craig AD. Spinothalamic lamina I neurons selectively sensitive to histamine: a central neural pathway for itch. *Nat Neurosci.* 2001;4:72–77.

80. Schmelz M. A neural pathway for itch. *Nat Neurosci.* 2001;4:9–10.

81. Gengo PJ, Pettit HO, O'Neill SJ, et al. DPI-3290 [(+)-3-((alpha-R)-alpha-((2S,5R)-4-Allyl-2,5-dimethyl-1-piperazinyl)-3-hyd roxybenzyl)-N-(3-fluorophenyl)-N-methylbenzamide]. II. A mixed opioid agonist with potent antinociceptive activity and limited effects on respiratory function. *J Pharmacol Exp Ther.* 2003;307:1227–1233.

82. Gengo PJ, Pettit HO, O'Neill SJ, et al. DPI-3290 [(+)-3-((alpha-R)-alpha-((2S,5R)-4-allyl-2,5-dimethyl-1-piperazinyl)-3-hyd roxybenzyl)-N-(3-fluorophenyl)-N-methylbenzamide]. I. A mixed opioid agonist with potent antinociceptive activity. *J Pharmacol Exp Ther.* 2003;307:1221–1226.

83. Dahl V, Raeder JC. Non-opioid postoperative analgesia. *Acta Anaesthesiol Scand.* 2000;44:1191–1203.

84. Kehlet H, Dahl JB. The value of "multimodal" or "balanced analgesia" in postoperative pain treatment. *Anesth Analg.* 1993;77:1048–1056.

85. Dahan A, Kest B. Recent advances in opioid pharmacology. *Curr Opin Anaesthesiol.* 2001;14:405–410.

26

Respiratory Depression: Incidence, Diagnosis, and Treatment

Dermot R. Fitzgibbon

The overall effectiveness of any analgesic technique depends on the adequacy of pain relief that can be provided and the incidence of side effects or complications. Opioids represent the major class of analgesics for treating severe and unremitting pain and are widely used in the treatment of pain associated with surgery or chronic conditions. Most modern postoperative analgesic techniques incorporate the administration of neuraxial opioids (with or without local anesthetic) or systemic (usually by patient-controlled analgesia [PCA]) routes. Although opioid administration is generally considered safe on surgical wards,[1,2] respiratory depression associated with opioids occur and have the potential for major morbidity and even mortality. Serious complications or deaths from opioid-induced respiratory depression are rare, but the risk is not zero, and a death or neurologic injury for a patient with an otherwise treatable illness is tragic. In July 2000, the Joint Commission on Accreditation of Health Care Organizations (JCAHO) developed new standards to create higher expectations for the assessment and management of pain in hospitals and other health care settings in the United States.[3] In response, many institutions implemented treatments guided by patient reports of pain intensity indexed with a numerical scale. Vila et al[4] reported that the incidence of opioid oversedation per 100,000 inpatient hospital days increased from 11.0 pre–numeric pain treatment algorithm (NPTA) to 24.5 post–NPTA (*P* <.001). Of these patients, 94% had a documented decrease in their level of consciousness preceding the event. Although there was an improvement in patient satisfaction, the authors reported a greater than 2-fold increase in the incidence of opioid oversedation adverse drug reactions after implementation of NPTA. Before experiencing an opioid oversedation adverse drug reaction (ADR), the recorded numerical pain scores varied widely suggesting that the coexistence of pain is not necessarily protective against this complication or that opioid use is driven by factors other than just pain.[5] Concerns regarding opioid overdose and death are not limited to the inpatient perioperative setting. Prescription drug overdose deaths are rising in the United States and worldwide as both the medical and nonmedical use of prescription drugs, particularly opioids, increases.[6] Paulozzi et al[7] reported that, between 1999

and 2002, opioid analgesic poisoning surpassed cocaine and heroin poisoning as the most frequent type of drug poisoning found on death certificates. Franklin et al[8] reported an increase in prescription-related opioid deaths, from 1995 to 2002, in patients receiving opioids for chronic noncancer pain. White and Irvine[9] reviewed the mechanisms of fatal opioid overdose and, although our understanding of the pharmacological basis of opioid-induced respiratory depression has advanced, further research in this area is warranted. This chapter reviews our current understanding of opioid-induced respiratory depression.

DEFINITION AND INCIDENCE OF OPIOID-INDUCED RESPIRATORY DEPRESSION IN THE PERIOPERATIVE PERIOD

The term *respiratory depression* has no clear definition despite a significant proportion of studies using the term, but not defining it.[10] Of the studies that attempt to define respiratory depression, the incidence of opioid-induced respiratory depression is difficult to compare because of variability in the definitions used. Respiratory depression is most often defined by a reduction in respiratory rate (eg, <8 breaths per minute, <10 breaths per minute) or by a decrease in the rate and depth of breathing from baseline. It typically does not take into account hypoventilation resulting from shallow breathing or ineffective respirations resulting from sedation, although increased level of sedation has been used.[11] Respiratory depression has also been defined by decreases in oxygen (O_2) saturation as measured by pulse oximetry or by partial pressure of carbon dioxide (CO_2) greater >50 mm Hg. Finally, respiratory depression may also be defined as a critical incident when intervention, such as an opioid antagonist (naloxone), was needed.

Sedation occurs frequently in the postoperative period and can cause concern. In postoperative opioid-naïve patients, sedation has been reported to occur in up to 83% of those receiving intramuscular morphine.[12] Excessive sedation may be considered to be a clinical sign of impending respiratory depression[13] although the evidence for this is scant in the literature. Sedation

Table 26.1: Incidence of Mild and Excessive Sedation by Analgesic Technique (IM, IV PCA, Epidural)[a]

Parameter	Analgesic Technique	Total Number of Patients	Sedation Mean (%)	Sedation 95% CI
Mild sedation	All	9451	23.9	23.0%–24.8%
	IM	352	53.7	48.3%–59.0%
	IV PCA	1822	56.5	54.2%–58.8%
	Epidural	7277	14.3	13.5%–15.1%
Excessive sedation	All	15 522	2.6	2.3%–2.8%
	IM	1528	5.2	4.1%–6.4%
	IV PCA	3763	5.3	4.6%–6.4%
	Epidural	10 231	1.2	0.9%–1.4%

[a] Material, modified with permission, from Dolin SJ, Cashman JN. Tolerability of acute postoperative pain management: nausea, vomiting, sedation, pruritis, and urinary retention. Evidence from published data. *Br J of Anaes*, 2005;95:584–591.[15]

may be defined as "somnolence" or "sleepy;" and when defining sedation, the degree of arousal should also be included. A sedation scale for monitoring patients receiving parenteral or neuraxial opioids was developed by Ready et al.[2] The ability to monitor for opioid-induced sedation is considered important and is routinely used by Acute Pain Services.[14] The incidence of opioid-induced sedation is dependent on the analgesic technique employed. Dolin and Cashman[15] examined the incidence of opioid-induced sedation for common analgesic techniques used for postoperative pain management (Table 26.1). Mild sedation is common (incidence 24%), but it is probably of little clinical significance alone; although it may be distressing for the patient. Excessive sedation is less common with an incidence of 2.6%. Intramuscular (IM) opioid analgesia and IV PCA are associated with a similar incidence of sedation, whereas epidural analgesia is associated with the lowest incidence of sedation.[15]

The incidence of respiratory depression is indicative of the safety of an analgesic technique that incorporates opioid use. Data from most audits suggest that the incidence of opioid-induced respiratory depression from PCA use range from 0.1% to 0.8%.[16–22] Audits of large numbers of adult patients have shown that the risk of respiratory depression is increased (overall ranges from 1.1% to 3.9%) when a background infusion is used with a PCA.[18–20,23] When epidurals are used for postoperative pain relief, the incidence of respiratory depression depends to some extent on whether an opioid has been used in addition to the local anesthetic. Several large prospective studies on epidural opioid-only administration indicate that the incidence of respiratory depression varies between 0.2% and 1.2% of patients.[2,24,25] This may be lower than the incidence with PCA, although the two have not been formally compared. Cashman and Dolin[26] examined the evidence from published data on the safety of three analgesic techniques (IM, PCA, and epidural opioids) after major surgery (Table 26.2). Cohort studies, case controlled studies, and audit reports as well as randomized controlled clinical trials were included in this analysis. Case reports were not included. The criteria used to define respiratory depression included ventilatory frequency, percutaneous O_2 saturation, arterial blood gas analysis, and the need to administer respiratory stimulants. Of these, ventilatory frequency was the most frequently used criterion. A ventilatory frequency of less than 10 breaths per minute was the most common threshold figure. When pulse oximetry was used to identify respiratory depression, an O_2 saturation of less than 90% was most commonly reported, although other end points such as saturations of less than 95%, 85%, or even 80% were also used. In contrast, arterial blood gas analysis, being relatively invasive, was much less frequently used. When blood gas analysis was used, a partial pressure of CO_2 greater >50 mm Hg was the most frequently used end point. The overall mean (95% CI) incidence of respiratory depression of the three analgesic techniques was 0.3 (0.1%–1.3%) using requirement for naloxone as an indicator, 1.1 (0.7%–1.7%) using hypoventilation as an indicator, 3.3 (1.4%–7.6%) using hypercarbia as an indicator, and 17.0 (10.2%–26.9%) using O_2 desaturation as an indicator. For IM opioid analgesia, the mean (95% CI) reported incidence of respiratory depression varied between 0.8 (0.2%–2.5%) and 37.0 (22.6%–45.9%) using hypoventilation and O_2 desaturation, respectively, as indicators. For PCA, the mean (95% CI) reported incidence of respiratory depression varied between 1.2 (0.7%–1.9%) and 11.5 (5.6%–22.0%), using hypoventilation and O_2 desaturation, respectively, as indicators. For epidural analgesia, the mean (95% CI) reported incidence of respiratory depression varied between 1.1 (0.6%–1.9%) and 15.1 (5.6%–34.8%), using hypoventilation and O_2 desaturation, respectively, as indicators. The parameter used to define respiratory depression has a major influence on the incidence of depression and clearly suggests that using O_2 desaturation as the sole parameter tends to overestimate the incidence.

Early reports of 0.5- and 1.0-mg doses of intrathecal morphine to postsurgical cancer patients resulted in 15–22 hours of analgesia without respiratory depression or somnolence.[27] However, others reported an unacceptably high frequency of delayed respiratory depression, although the morphine doses used were extremely large (2–15 mg).[28,29] Subsequently, small or "minidose" morphine (<1.0 mg) was reported to be effective for managing acute postoperative pain after a variety of surgeries and to do so without any evidence of respiratory depression.[30] The administration of morphine by the intrathecal route has been associated with delayed onset respiratory depression.[29,31,32] Intrathecal morphine produces a dose-related respiratory depression.[31] Peak depression occurs between 3.5

Table 26.2: Reported Incidence of Respiratory Depression by Analgesic Technique (IM, IV PCA, Epidural) as Indicated by Ventilatory Frequency, O$_2$ Saturation, PaCO$_2$, and Naloxone Use[a]

Parameter	Analgesic Technique	Total Number of Patients	Respiratory Depression Mean (%)	95% CI
Ventilatory frequency	All	29,607	1.1	0.7%–1.7%
	IM	1590	0.8	0.2%–2.5%
	IV PCA	6922	1.2	0.7%–1.9%
	Epidural	21,035	1.1	0.6%–1.9%
O$_2$ saturation	All	1516	17.0	10.2%–26.9%
	IM	246	37.0	22.6%–45.9%
	IV PCA	707	11.5	5.6%–22.0%
	Epidural	563	15.1	5.6%–34.8%
PaCO$_2$	All	3170	3.3	1.4%–7.6%
	IM	1508	1.3	0.7%–2.3%
	IV PCA	301	1.3	0.2%–7.7%
	Epidural	1361	6.0	2.1%–15.6%
Naloxone use	All	55,404	0.3	0.1%–1.3%
	IM	71	1.4	0.1%–12.7%
	IV PCA	4691	1.9	1.9%–2.0%
	Epidural	50,642	0.1	0.1%–0.2%

[a] Material, modified with permission, from Cashman JN, Dolin SJ. Respiratory and haemodynamic effects of acute postoperative pain management: evidence from published data. *Br J of Anaes*, 2004;93:212–223.[26]

to 12 hours post injection.[31,33,34] The incidence of respiratory depression ranges from 0.03% to 7%.[14,35] The coadministration of parenteral opioids concomitantly with spinal opioids has been regarded as a significant risk factor for the development of respiratory depression.[13] However, Gwirtz et al[36] reported on the routine use of IV opioids administered concomitantly by PCA to approximately 6000 major urologic, orthopedic, general/vascular, thoracic, and gynecologic patients who also received intrathecal morphine without incurring respiratory depression, and suggested that judicious parenteral opioid supplementation is a safe and reasonable practice.

ANATOMY AND PHYSIOLOGY OF RESPIRATION

In contrast to the internally controlled rhythmicity of the heart, respiration is entirely dependent on external input from the central nervous system (CNS). Although there are influences from cortical and other regions, control of breathing is localized principally to the brain stem. Respiratory neurons are concentrated in two distinct medullary regions: the dorsal respiratory group (DRG) in the ventrolateral nucleus of the solitary tract and the ventral respiratory group (VRG) in the ventrolateral medulla (Figure 26.1). The VRG has been further divided into a caudal, intermediate, rostral, pre-Bötzinger, and Bötzinger complex. A third less well characterized respiratory group is situated in the medial parabrachial nucleus and in the Kölliker-Fuse nucleus; this group is now termed the *pontine respiratory group* (PRG), formerly termed the *pneumotaxic center*. The DRG and VRG contain output of bulbospinal neurons, many of which have

medullary arborizations.[37] It appears that the central respiratory rhythm generator is located within subregions of the VRG.[38,39] Efferent fibers emanating from the VRG innervate the muscles of respiration. Thus, the VRG is likely to be involved in shaping motor output rather than being the source of the rhythmic pattern. VRG neurons are also influenced by innervation from the pons. Although pontine regions are not essential for respiratory rhythm, they may play some role in influencing the timing of the different phases.

Generation of respiratory rhythm requires phasic activation and inhibition. The major neurotransmitters and receptors mediating each of these processes have been identified. Within the VRG, excitation is mediated via excitatory amino acid acting on glutamate receptors,[39] whereas inhibition is glutamate mediated, via γ-aminobutyric acid (GABA) acting on GABA receptors.[41,42] Glutamate acts primarily at non-*N*-methyl-D-aspartic acid (NMDA) receptors within the network to generate respiratory rhythm in neonatal in vitro preparations, but it may also engage NMDA receptors in mature, intact animals. There is evidence for roles for both NMDA and non-NMDA receptors in the control of respiration in the DRG, VRG, and pons.[40,43] GABA receptors are found in relatively high density in the DRG and VRG. Glycine may also play some role in producing inhibition in these centers.[41]

Adjustments in the rate and pattern of breathing occur in response to input from peripheral sources. The stretch receptors, which provide information on the degree of inflation of the lungs, form one such source. Stretch receptors respond to inflation with input to the DRG via the vagus nerve. Chemoreceptors, which respond to changes in blood gases, are located in the carotid and aortic bodies. Specialized cells in these zones

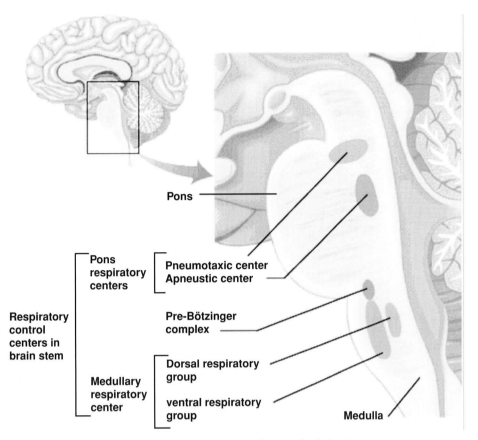

Figure 26.1: Respiratory control centers in the brain.

are stimulated by a decrease in O_2 and, to a lesser extent, by an increase in CO_2 or a decrease in pH. Like the stretch receptors, projections from the peripheral chemoreceptors eventually terminate in the DRG. Inputs from the chemoreceptors can be considered the main "drivers" of respiration.

MECHANISMS OF OPIOID-INDUCED RESPIRATORY DEPRESSION

Respiratory depression may be considered a failure to respond adequately to hypercapnia or hypoxia.[45] Normally, the dominant control of ventilation is mediated through an increase in $PaCO_2$, which strongly stimulates central chemoreceptors leading to increased ventilation. Opioid-induced respiratory depression is characterized by a dose-related, naloxone-reversible depression of resting minute ventilation with proportional reduction of tidal volume, decreased PaO_2 and pH, increased $PaCO_2$, and decreased ventilatory drive stimulated by hypercapnia and hypoxia.[46,47] The effects of opioids on respiration are listed in Table 26.3.

Opioids decrease respiration by both central and peripheral actions. The central depressant effects are because of decreases in spontaneous respiratory unit activity and possibly suppression of recurrent excitation by glutamatergic inputs within the primary respiratory network.[42] This central mechanism involves the suppression of baseline inspiratory neuronal activity and possibly the blunting of glutamate-evoked increases in inspiratory drive. Whether opioids merely decrease background neuronal activity so that stimulus-evoked increases are propor-

Table 26.3: Effects of Opioids on Respiration

Shift apneic threshold to right

Flatten slope of CO_2-response curve

Blunt increase of minute ventilation to hypoxia

Decrease minute ventilation

Increase $PaCO_2$

Cause irregular breathing patterns

tionally smaller or whether opioids modulate the release or post-synaptic processing of glutamate is not clear.

Opioid-induced respiratory depression is caused by μ-, κ-, and δ-receptor activation within the brainstem.[48–52] The molecular mechanism by which morphine affects respiration was elucidated in a study using mice that lacked the μ-opioid receptor.[53–55] These findings confirm that μ-opioid receptors are the essential targets of opioid analgesic and respiratory responses and that these responses are inseparable. In the brainstem, the rostral ventrolateral medulla (considered to be an important area for respiratory rhythm generation)[56,57] may be the target area for opioid-induced respiratory depression. Opioid receptors are also found in central respiratory centers. Both μ- and δ-receptors are located in these regions. This suggests that opioid peptides such as β-endorphin and metenkephalin may have an important physiological role in respiration.[58] However, despite the profound effect of exogenously administered opioids and the presence of opioid receptors at high concentrations on respiratory neurons there is, as yet, no clear role for endogenous

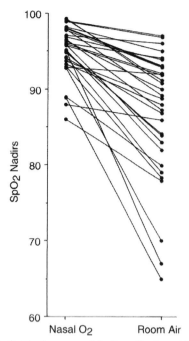

Figure 26.2: Individual nocturnal SpO_2 nadirs breathing O_2 supplemented air the first postoperative night and room air the second night (n = 32) (a). Figure reproduced with permission, from Stone JG, Cozine KA, Wald A. Nocturnal oxygenation during patient-controlled analgesia. *Anesthesia and Analgesia*, 1999;89:104–110 (Fig. 4, p. 107).[70]

opioid peptides in normal control of respiration.[59,60] Kappa receptor agonists either produce no effect on respiration or cause a mild respiratory stimulation.[61] Within the system controlling respiration described above there are several sites at which opioid drugs may produce an effect.[62] At each of these sites, the action of opioids is to depress neuronal activity. At chemoreceptors the inhibitory activity of opioids appears to be mediated principally by μ-opioid receptors and results in diminished sensitivity to changes in O_2 and CO_2. Opioids may particularly affect the magnitude of the response to increased CO_2. The effects of exogenous opioids on respiration include changes in both tidal volume and respiratory frequency. The nature of the effect depends in part on the concentration of the opioid. Low concentrations appear to have effects mainly on tidal volume, whereas at higher concentrations both tidal volume and respiratory frequency may be affected.[60]

The production of respiratory rhythm relies on excitatory and inhibitory neurotransmitter systems, which mediate fast synaptic responses in the CNS. Excitation is mediated via the excitatory amino acid glutamate, whereas inhibition is mediated via GABA receptors through which benzodiazepines and barbiturates act to magnify the degree of neuronal inhibition. Opioid peptides decrease activity because of a reduction in glutamate-induced excitation Morphine reduces CO_2 responsiveness and respiratory frequency. The dose-dependent effect may appear in the postoperative period with subsequent bradypnea and desaturation.[63,64] Bradypnea may also lead to hypercapnia and, eventually, apnea. Such effects precipitate myocardial hypoxia and cardiac arrhythmias.[65] Opioid-induced hypoventilation is not always obvious in patients receiving supplemental O_2 postoperatively.[66,67]

Opioids cause hypoventilation and decrease the ventilatory response to both hypercapnia and hypoxemia.[68,69] Stone et al[70]

studied the prevalence and severity of nocturnal hypoxemia in 32 postoperative patients receiving morphine PCA. On the first postoperative night with patients breathing supplemental O_2, the nocturnal mean SpO_2 was 99% $\pm$ 1%, and 94% $\pm$ 4% ($P < .001$), and only 4 patients had periods of hemoglobin desaturation <90% (Figure 26.2). In contrast, breathing only room air the subsequent night the mean SpO_2 was lower (94% $\pm$ 4%; $P < .001$) than the previous night, and hypoxemia occurred more frequently and was more severe: 18 patients experienced episodes of $SpO_2 < 90\%$, 7 patients experienced episodes of $SpO_2 < 80\%$, and 3 patients experienced episodes of $SpO_2 < 70\%$. One patient required resuscitation for profound bradypnea and cyanosis, but none suffered permanent sequelae.

Measurement of Opioid-Induced Respiratory Depression

Opioid-induced respiratory depression has been quantified by comparing the slope and intercept (apneic threshold) of CO_2-response curves (Figure 26.3),[72–74] measurement of minute ventilation during room air breathing, challenges such as the addition of CO_2 to inspired air,[75,76] or the administration of hypoxic mixtures and measurement of $PaCO_2$ concentrations before, during, and after opioid administration.

Bailey et al[77] studied the influence of intrathecal versus intravenous morphine on the ventilatory response to sustained isocapnic hypoxia in healthy volunteers. Depression of the ventilatory response to hypoxia after the administration of intrathecal morphine was similar in magnitude to, but longer lasting (>12 hours) than, after the administration of an equianalgesic dose of intravenous morphine. This indicates that opioids affect ventilatory control via central and not peripheral sites. This study also suggests the modulation of the secondary slow ventilatory decline during hypoxic exposure by opioid receptor activation.

Measuring respiratory parameters during spontaneous breathing demonstrates that administration of opioids is accompanied by a decrease in total minute ventilation with an increase in

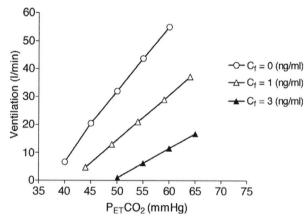

Figure 26.3: CO_2 response curve simulated with the model at three different fentanyl concentrations. Data points were obtained by applying different step increases in end tidal PCO_2 ($P_{ET}CO_2$) from its resting value, and considering the value of ventilation reached in steady-state conditions (ie, after the transient response to $P_{ET}CO_2$ increase was exhausted) (a). Figure reproduced with permission from Magosso E, Ursino M, van Oostrom JH. Opioid-induced respiratory depression: a mathematical model for fentanyl. *IEEE Transact Biomed Eng*, 51(7): 1115–1128 (Fig. 4, p. 1120).[71]

end tidal PCO_2 ($P_{ET}CO_2$).[78-80] Responsiveness to CO_2 is widely used for evaluation of drug-induced respiratory depression. It is well established that the ventilatory response to CO_2 is attenuated in presence of opioids: the slope of the CO_2-response curve is depressed, and the zero intercept is shifted to higher CO_2 tension values.[74,78,79,81,82] Most methods for assessing opioid-induced respiratory depression consist of measuring ventilatory responsiveness to CO_2[78,81] or hypoxia.[69,78,83]

Irregular breathing patterns after opioid administration have been described in children.[84] Bouillon et al[85] demonstrated a method to quantify the increase in respiratory variability caused by opioids. They demonstrated that the time course of respiratory variability measured as $Qeff_{20}$ of tidal volume parallels that of minute ventilation and that it correlates with the severity of respiratory depression. Furthermore, they observed that clinically obvious irregular breathing after the administration of opioids was a sign of severe respiratory depression. Opioids apparently not only change the set point for $PaCO_2$, but also impaired the function of respiratory centers involved in rhythm generation.

Regardless of the route of administration, continuous infusions of opioids given by either fixed or variable rates are associated with a high incidence of respiratory abnormalities.[63,86,87] Disturbances in respiratory pattern, with apneas and slow respiratory rates, exist independently of other abnormalities, such as reduced alveolar ventilation,[64] especially in elderly persons.[88] A number of authors[89-91] have found that normal respiratory rates may coexist with marked respiratory depression, limiting the sensitivity of the respiratory rate in clinical assessment. Irregularities of respiratory pattern are associated with opioid analgesia after major surgery and may contribute to patient hypoxia, apneas, and cardiovascular deterioration.[63] Sleigh[92] demonstrated in patients who underwent major surgery that short central apneas are common in the early postoperative period, are not easy to detect without continuous respiratory monitoring, and are not predictable using the commonly quoted clinical factors (patient age, drowsiness, route of administration of opioids, or even opioid dose) and that the only way to identify the subgroup of patients at risk is direct observation of their breathing pattern. There is neurophysiological evidence to suggest that respiratory drive and the generation of respiratory pattern are functionally separate.[93] Because of this discrepancy, attempts to assess the effects of drugs on respiration should not rely solely on the ventilatory response to hypercarbia but should include both direct measurement of respiratory pattern, and other ways of assessing respiratory drive, such as resting $P_{ET}CO_2$ levels and mean inspiratory flow rates.

INFLUENCE OF SLEEP DISTURBANCE ON OPIOID–INDUCED RESPIRATORY DEPRESSION

Both anesthesia and surgery affect the architecture of sleep (Table 26.4). The potential adverse effects of parenteral opioid therapy used in the perioperative setting have been emphasized especially in patients with sleep apnea.[94-97] Taylor et al[97] reported that the first 24 hours after surgery represents a high-risk period for a respiratory events (defined as <10 breaths/minute) and/or a decrease in O_2 saturation (<90%) that was reversed by naloxone) in patients who received

Table 26.4: Effects of Major Surgery and IV Opioids on Sleep[a]

Major Surgery	IV Opioids
Decreased REM sleep	Decreased REM sleep
Decreased slow wave sleep	Decreased slow wave sleep
Increased stage 2 (non-REM) sleep	Increased stage 2 (non-REM) sleep
Decreased total sleep time	

Note: Changes are most profound on postoperative nights one and two with subsequent rebound on following nights. Material, modified with permission, from Knill RL, Moote CA, Skinner MI, Rose EA. Anesthesia with abdominal surgery leads to intense REM sleep during the first postoperative week. *Anesthesiol*, 1990;73:52–61.[106]

[a] Material, modified with permission, from Shaw I, Lavigne G, Mayer P, Choinière M. Acute intravenous administration of morphine perturbs sleep architecture in healthy pain–free young adults: a preliminary study. *Sleep*. 2005;6:677–682.[109]

opioid therapy. Of the 62 patients identified, 77.4% (48 of 62) had a respiratory event at 24 hours or less after the end of surgery, and of those 56.5% (35 of 62) had an event at 12 hours or less with a median onset time of 10 hours. Although no deaths were reported, 5 patients had a full code called. Sleep may be associated with increased upper airway resistance, obstructive sleep apnea (OSA) syndrome, alveolar hypoventilation, and central apnea, including Cheyne-Stokes breathing pattern.[98] Restoration of ventilation and prevention of asphyxia is dependent on the interaction of peripheral chemoreceptors (carotid body) mediated through the carotid sinus nerve, mechanoreceptors in the chest wall and lungs mediated through the vagus nerve, and central respiratory controllers located in the brainstem. The carotid bodies appear to be responsible for immediate breath-by-breath dynamic control, whereas the central brainstem controllers establish the baseline minute ventilation and respond relatively slowly to changes in CO_2 levels. The coordinated contraction of the tongue (especially the genioglossus) and pharyngeal musculature helps to maintain airway patency and prevent snoring or inspiratory collapse of the airway.[99,100]

Microdialysis delivery of of morphine to the hypoglossus nucleus in Wistar rats produced a naloxone-reversible, dose-dependent increase in acetylcholine release. Acetylcholine decreases tongue tone. Sleep and opioids separately, and in concert, depress genioglossus and pharyngeal muscle tone and diminish airway protective reflexes. In REM sleep, the neural drive to the pharyngeal muscles is at a minimum, and the atonia of antigravity muscles predisposes the patient to airway instability, causing episodic hypoxemias.[101] The effect of sleep deprivation on upper airway muscle function is of concern. A lower threshold for upper airway collapse, presumably resulting from reduced genioglossus muscle activity,[101] has been reported following complete sleep deprivation for one night.[102]

Sleep cycle disruption by opioids is recognized in the substance abuse literature, and clinical data implicate opioids as a potential contributor to postoperative sleep disruption.[103,104] Multiple brain mechanisms contribute to sleep disruption caused by opioids.[105] Profound alterations in sleep patterns occur during the first 1–6 nights after major abdominal surgery.[104] The clinical consequences of suppression of REM sleep and slow wave sleep (SWS) with subsequent rebound in the postoperative period is unknown. However, postoperative rebound of REM sleep in the middle of the first postoperative week may contribute to the development of sleep-disordered breathing and nocturnal hypoxemia.[106,107] Episodic hypoxemia is more frequent during periods of REM rebound than during other stages in the postoperative period.[107] Borgbjerg et al[108] demonstrated that both pain stimulation and morphine administration altered the threshold of the respiratory centre to CO_2 stimulation. Dahan et al[5] noted that severe respiratory depression is possible despite the occurrence of severe pain. Furthermore, when postoperative patients cycle between awake and sleep states, they may be in pain and breathing while awake, but severely respiratory depressed when asleep. During these sleep/sedated periods, respiratory depression may even increase to values much less than 40% of control (40% of control is equivalent to an increase of 10–15 mm Hg $P_{ET}CO_2$ together with a reduction of minute ventilation by 40%-50% in spontaneously breathing patients not stimulated by CO_2), or patients may even stop breathing completely.

Shaw et al[109] reported that clinical doses of intravenous morphine (0.1 mg/kg) in human volunteers altered sleep architecture, as demonstrated by reductions in slow wave sleep (75%), REM sleep (5%), and by a 15% increase in non–rapid-eye-movement (NREM) stage 2 sleep. Postoperative rebound of REM sleep may contribute to the development of sleep-disordered breathing and nocturnal episodic hypoxemia.[107] Sleep itself is affected by opioids in the postoperative period; rapid eye movement is nearly eliminated, and slow wave activity is severely suppressed.[106] Sleep also becomes fitful and fragmented, and patients often display erratic breathing patterns.[63,106,110,111] These nocturnal episodes of abnormal ventilation are similar in character to those seen in individuals with sleep apnea and are accompanied by profound hypoxemia.[63,110,111]

Catley and colleagues[63] studied patients during the first 16 hours after open cholecystectomy or total hip replacement. They found, primarily during the first 8 hours after operation, a high frequency of episodic O_2 desaturation associated with disturbances in ventilatory pattern, namely obstructive apneas, paradoxical breathing, and periods of slow ventilatory rate. In the immediate postoperative period, in the recovery area, residual effects of general anesthesia together with morphine administration may be a primary cause of ventilatory disturbance. In the late postoperative period in the surgical ward, however, the main reason for ventilatory disturbances is probably a sleep disturbance with rebound of REM sleep on the second and third postoperative nights.[104,107,108] Catley et al[63] found significantly more ventilatory arrhythmias and episodic desaturations in patients receiving IV morphine compared with local anesthetic regimens for pain relief. Ventilatory disturbances are not uncommon in the late postoperative period in the general surgical ward, where patients are usually without intensive monitoring. Rosenberg et al[112] have shown that a high proportion of the apneas and hypopneas was associated with episodic hypoxemia and that ventilatory disturbances were not uncommon on the second and third postoperative nights in patients undergoing major abdominal surgery.

In all cases of sleep-disordered breathing, the control of breathing may be compromised by medications such as sedatives, hypnotics, and opioids. Table 26.5 lists the effects on respiration noted by Farney et al[113] in patients receiving sustained-release opioids. Thresholds for breathing abnormalities may be

Table 26.5: Breathing Patterns with Opioid Use[a]

Apnea duration and severity of hypoxia worse during NREM vs REM sleep

Ataxic (Biot) breathing pattern during NREM

   Irregular respiratory pauses

   Gasping without periodicity

Recurrent and prolonged episodes (>5 minutes) of obstructive hypoventilation

   Nasal CPAP typically ineffective

[a] Material, modified with permission, from Farney RJ, Walker JM, Cloward TV, Rhondeau S. Sleep–disordered breathing associated with long-term opioid therapy. *Chest.* 2003;123:632–639.[113]

chosen on the basis of common practice in clinical somnography and the report of the American Academy of Sleep Medicine Task Force.[114] Apnea was defined as a pause in airflow for at least 10 seconds. Hypopnea was defined as a decrease in airflow of at least 50% less than average amplitude for at least 10 seconds with a decrease in SpO_2 of at least 5%. The respiratory disturbance index (RDI) was defined as the sum of the number of apneas and hypopneas divided by the recording time (units of events per hour).

MONITORING

The causes of respiratory failure may be obstructive, central, or a combination of both. Clinically, respiratory activity includes such descriptors as respiratory rate and depth, as well as quantifiable information about the degree of gas exchange taking place. The ideal respiratory monitor would provide continuous information about all these variables in a nonobtrusive fashion. In some ways, the dedicated, qualified human observer comes close to the ideal monitor, being responsive to several variables related to respiratory activity, intelligent, selective, adaptive, contactless, fast responding, technology independent, and immune to irrelevant disturbances. Human observation of respiratory rate is time-consuming, and the result is not always accurate. Observing the movement of the abdomen and rib cage gives a subjective clinical estimation of the tidal volume, but there is a tendency to overestimation that could be dangerous at low tidal volume. The indirect means for an unaided observer to estimate respiratory gas exchange, by observing skin color variations and the like, are even more imprecise and subjective. The need for objective and reliable monitoring equipment is obvious. In addition to measuring relevant variables, thus providing adequate information, it is important that the rate of false alarms or, even worse, false nonalarms is minimized.

Monitoring respiratory activity in clinical practice introduces a number of problems that do not exist in a laboratory-like or operating room setting. In addition, clinical monitoring of opioid-induced respiratory depression is likely to require several different variables, including respiratory rate, tidal volume, apnea events, pattern of respiration, and blood gas concentration estimates. Folke et al[115] reviewed noninvasive monitoring in medical care and Table 26.6 lists the categories of sensing principles cited for respiratory monitoring devices and methods. Table 26.7 lists a summary of current methods of detecting

Table 26.6: Categories of Sensing Principles for Respiratory Monitoring Devices and Methods

Category	Typical Measured Quantity	Typical Sensor Position
Movement, volume, and tissue composition detection	Electromyography, abdomen and thoracic circumference, impedance or blood volume	Abdomen and chest wall
Airflow sensing	Respiratory gas flow	Nasal/oral area
Blood gas measurement	Arterial gas concentration	Peripheral organ or nasal/oral area

Table 26.7: Current Methods of Detecting Opioid-Induced Respiratory Depression[a]

Method	Primary Measures	Sensitivity[b]	Specificity[c]	Reliablity[c]	Response Time	Frequency of Measurement	Cost	Comments
Clinical observation	Oxygenation and ventilation	Variable	Variable	Variable	Variable	Intermittent	Variable	Depends on observer skill and observation frequency
Chest wall impedance	Ventilation	Low	Low	Low	Moderate	Contnuous	Modest	May be nonspecific in airway obstruction
Respiratory rate	Ventilation	Low	Moderate	Moderate	Moderate	Intermittent/ continuous	Variable	May not be helpful in patients with obstructive sleep apnea (OSA)
Tidal volume	Ventilation	Moderate	Moderate	Low	Moderate	Continuous	Modest	Unreliable technology
SpO_2 (Without supplemental FIO_2)	Oxygenation	Low	Moderate	High	Slow	Continuous	Modest	Desaturation may be late and then very rapid
Venous blood gas	Oxygenation and ventilation	High	Modest	High	Slow	Intermittent	High	Depends on prior clinical observation or fortuity
Arterial blood gas	Oxygenation and ventilation	Very High	Very High	Very High	Slow	Intermittent	High	Depends on prior clinical observation or fortuity
Minute ventilation	Ventilation	Moderate	Moderate	Low	Moderate	Continuous	Modest	Unreliable technology
SpO_2 (without supplemental FIO_2)	Oxygenation and ventilation	High	High	High	Fast	Continuous	Modest	Alveolar gas equation predicts a drop in SpO_2 even with modest hypoventilation
$PETCO_2$ (unintubated)	Ventilation	Moderate	High	Moderate	Fast	Continuous	Modest	High $PaCO_2$ significant but dependent on sampling; underestimates $PaCO_2$. Some believe only reliable as measure of respiratory rate
$PETCO_2$ (intubated)	Ventilation	Very high	Very high	High	Fast	Continuous	Modest	Not viable option on ward

[a] Table, reproduced with permission, from Weinger MB. Dangers of postoperative opioids: APSF workshop and white paper address, prevention of postoperative respiratory complications. *Anesthesia Patient Safety Foundation Newsletter*, 2006;21(4):61, 63–7 (Table 1, p. 65).[116]

opioid-induced respiratory depression. If one considers that respiratory depression may be primarily considered as a failure to respond adequately, on a moment-to-moment basis, to hypercapnia or hypoxia, then clinically the detection of hypercapnia appears to be the best method for monitoring of respiratory depression.

Measurement of CO_2 and O_2 concentration in the expired air is the only direct way to confirm satisfactory gas exchange on a breath-by-breath basis. Capnography, the continuous measurement of the partial pressure of CO_2 in respiratory gas, has become the standard of care for monitoring intubated patients in the operating room. CO_2 monitors measure gas concentration or partial pressure using one of two configurations: mainstream or sidestream. Mainstream devices measure respiratory gas directly inline, with the sensor located on the airway adapter in the patient's breathing circuit. Sidestream devices measure respiratory gas remotely by aspirating a small sample of gas from the breathing circuit through tubing to a sensor located inside the monitor. Significant and troublesome technical problems have limited the effective use of capnography and restricted its clinical applications in the past. These problems include interference with the sensor by condensed water and patient secretions in both mainstream and sidestream devices, cross sensitivity with anesthetic gases in conventional CO_2 sensors, lack of ruggedness for intra- and interhospital transport, inability to use with nonintubated patients (mainstream), and falsely low $P_{ET}CO_2$ readings.

Microstream capnography features low flow rates, reduced dead space, lack of moisture-associated occlusion problems, and low power consumption.[117] Furthermore, it can be used reliably in both intubated and nonintubated patients. Capnography is based on the principle that CO_2 molecules absorb infrared radiation (IR) at specific wavelengths. Microstream technology is built on a unique approach to IR emission. Laser-based technology (ie, molecular correlation spectroscopy) is used to generate an IR emission that precisely matches the absorption spectrum of the CO_2 molecule. The high emission efficiency and extreme CO_2 specificity and sensitivity of the emitter-detector combination allows for an extremely short light path that allows the use of a very small sample cell (15 μL). This in turn permits the use of a very low flow rate (50 mL/min) without compromising accuracy or response time. The microstream capnometer provides a more accurate end tidal CO_2 partial pressure measurement in nonintubated, spontaneously breathing patients than conventional sidestream capnometers, allowing for adequate monitoring of the respiratory function in nonintubated patients.[118] Microstream technology has been incorporated into a broad range of patient-monitoring architectures from stand-alone units to multiparameter monitors. For nonintubated patients, nasal and combined oral-nasal cannulae accommodate mouth and nose breathers (Figure 26.4).

Role of Pulse Oximetry for Monitoring

Profound hypoventilation with the development of CO_2 narcosis can cause coma, respiratory arrest, and circulatory failure.[119] Although pulse oximetry is used widely to monitor arterial blood oxygenation, it is possible that pulse oximetry can be used to detect abnormalities in ventilation by quantifying changes in SpO_2.[120] However, there are limitations in using pulse oximetry for monitoring ventilatory status particularly when supplemen-

tal O_2 is administered.[66,67] Fu et al[121] advocate the application of supplemental O_2 only in patients who are unable to maintain an acceptable SpO_2 while breathing room air. In patients able to maintain SpO_2 90% on an FIO_2 of 0.21, pulse oximetry monitoring during room air breathing is a useful tool to assess ventilation, without the need for capnography or arterial blood gas analysis. Pulse oximetry during room air breathing also will be useful in guiding and/or limiting the administration of opioids and other respiratory depressant drugs. Assessment of ventilatory abnormalities in patients receiving neuraxial and parenterally administered opioids could be achieved with pulse oximetry but only during room-air breathing.[121] The decision to administer supplemental O_2 should not be based on routine practice but should entail consideration of the risk of masking undetected hypoventilation, or mismatching of ventilation and perfusion, in accordance with the patient's need for increased SpO_2. If persistent, decreased SpO_2 may indicate the need for arterial blood analysis to determine if the arterial hypoxemia is due to hypoventilation or mismatching of ventilation and pulmonary perfusion. Pulse oximetry primarily has been used to assess oxygenation but not ventilation.

Role of Respiratory Rate in Monitoring

The advantages of using respiratory rate in defining respiratory depression are that the method is simple and noninvasive and the patient is not inconvenienced. Many authors consider respiratory rate to be an inadequate index of ventilatory depression.[34,45,61,122] After administration of intrathecal morphine, respiratory rate does not necessarily correspond with opioid dose, hypoxemia, or depressed ventilatory response to CO_2 stimulation.[89,123] Conversely, patients with low respiratory rates may compensate adequately to keep $PaCO_2$ levels within normal limits.[124] Furthermore, the use of respiratory rate may be a poor indicator of impending apnea.[45] Consequently, respiratory rate should not be used alone to define opioid-induced respiratory depression.

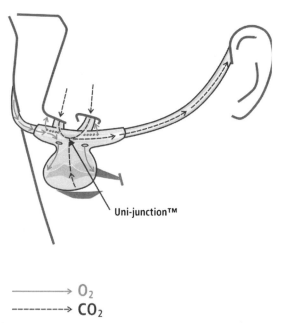

Uni-junction™

$\longrightarrow$ O_2

$----\rightarrow$ CO_2

Figure 26.4: Continuous $P_{ET}CO_2$ monitoring, cannula system.

Table 26.8: Sedation Scale

Score	Level of Consciousness	Degree of Arousal
0	Normal level	Easily aroused
1	Intermittently sleepy	Easily aroused
2	Frequently sleepy	Easily aroused
3	Frequently sleepy	Not easily aroused
S	Normal sleep	Easily aroused

Table 26.9: Risks Factors for Opioid-Induced Respiratory Events

Continuous opioid infusions

Age

Upper abdominal surgery

Sleep apnea

Concurrent use of CNS depressants

Impaired organ function

PCA pump errors

Obesity

ROLE OF SEDATION SCORES

Among morphine-induced side effects, sedation occurs in up to 60% of cases during morphine titration and represents a common cause of discontinuation of titration for reasons of safety.[125] Several behavioral scales assess depth of sedation. Among them, the Ramsay score (RS) is a validated and widely used technique.[126] The components of this scale are somewhat subjective and prone to observer bias. The use of this scale is easy, for it does not require any device, but its accuracy in detecting deep sedation is questionable during the early postoperative period.[127] Most sedation assessment tools incorporate monitoring level of consciousness and the degree of ability to arouse. Table 26.8 lists one example of an assessment tool.

PREDICTING OPIOID-INDUCED RESPIRATORY EVENTS IN THE POSTOPERATIVE SETTING

Preventing adverse events associated with patient therapies is a primary concern in any health care environment. Intravenous PCA is an established method to manage acute postoperative pain, supported by favorable efficacy and patient preference data. PCA pumps were developed to provide safe self-administration of opioids. PCA administration of opioids is perceived as being safer with fewer logistic problems in monitoring and general patient than other techniques such as IM administration of opioids or neuraxial opioid use.[128] Schug and Torrie[20] analyzed safety outcome in 3016 consecutive postoperative patients treated by an Acute Pain Service and concluded that, although potentially serious complications without sequelae were discovered in 0.53% of patients, the incidence was similar for techniques of systemic opioid administration and continuous regional analgesia. Flisberg et al[1] monitored 2696 postoperative patients for efficacy of pain relief and adverse effects of postoperative epidural and intravenous analgesia. Patients receiving IV opioids demonstrated a higher incidence of serious adverse events (sedation and respiratory depression).

Despite apparent advantages, the use of IV PCA for management of acute postoperative pain is associated with a number of unique safety concerns that arise as a result of the inherent technical complexity of the technique. Although medication errors involving opioid analgesics can occur in any setting, when combined with a PCA device, the potential for patient harm as a result of opioid overdose is significant. Issues related to the safe introduction of PCA opioid administration have been known since the early 1990s.[19] Problems were encountered with slow respiratory rate, monitoring, equipment function, and ward management. In general, factors increasing the potential for respiratory depression may be considered as patient related and technique related. Essential to safe administration of opioids in the perioperative period is the identification of higher risk patient groups. Although multiple factors can contribute to respiratory compromise, particular attention should be paid to certain patient-related factors, including concomitant use of a background infusion, physician- or nurse-administered boluses, concomitant administration of sedative or hypnotic medications, renal failure/insufficiency, and preexisting respiratory insufficiency or sleep apnea syndrome.[63,91,129] Sidebotham et al[21] noted in postoperative patients who experienced hypoxemia and respiratory depression that virtually all had 1 of 3 risk factors: bolus dose by PCA greater than 1 mg morphine, age greater than 65 years, or intraabdominal surgery. Factors related to technique include operator error, inadequate patient teaching, PCA by proxy, equipment failure, and concomitant use of a continuous infusion particularly in opioid-naïve patients. Risk factors for opioid administration are listed in Table 26.9.

In November 2001, The Commonwealth of Massachusetts Medical Society Patient Care Assessment Committee reported on unexpected deaths of patients who were receiving PCA. In some of the cases, analgesia was being used for postoperative pain management, whereas others involved patients being treated for management of other causes of chronic or acute pain. Most of the events occurred within the first 10 hours of analgesia administration and many occurred during the late evening or night. The majority of the incidents involved women. Nearly all of the patients had medical conditions or physical traits, such as obesity, asthma, sleep apnea, or nasopharyngeal swelling, which potentially increased their risks for respiratory complications. The cause of death was never conclusively determined in any of these cases. In two incidents, questions were raised about whether potentially additive effects of intraoperative or supplemental medications, such as opioids, benzodiazepines, sedatives, hypnotics, or antihistamines, were adequately considered when the PCA was ordered. Among the recommendations were the following:

- Adequate assessment by the prescribing physician of any potential risks for respiratory depression or compromise and consideration of that risk when determining the loading and maintenance dosage for PCA
- Consideration of intraoperative medications and other medications that the patient received or is receiving prior to calculating the loading or maintenance dosage for PCA, including

Table 26.10: APSF Recommendations to Prevent Opioid-Induced Respiratory Depression[a]

Health care providers should have "zero tolerance" for respiratory morbidity and mortality associated with opioid use in the postoperative period, because these events should be completely preventable.

Although there are limitations to existing monitoring technologies for detecting opioid-induced respiratory depression, the use of continuous monitoring of oxygenation (generally pulse oximetry) and of ventilation in nonventilated patients receiving PCA, neuraxial opioids, or serial doses of parenteral opioids, is recommended.

Although pulse oximetry will monitor oxygenation during PCA, it may have reduced sensitivity, as a monitor of hypoventilation, when supplemental oxygen is administered. When supplemental oxygen is indicated, monitoring of ventilation may warrant the use of technology designed to assess breathing or estimate arterial carbon dioxide concentrations. Continuous monitoring is most important for the highest risk patients, but depending on clinical judgment, should be applied to other patients. In particular, continuous monitoring should be strongly considered in any patient with significant OSA receiving PCA or neuraxial opioids.

Even the best monitoring system will be of limited value if the response to the incipient event is ineffective. When the monitoring system alarms, the message must rapidly get to a clinician capable of responding in a timely and appropriate manner. Because staffing constraints necessitate only intermittent presence of clinicians at the bedside of unintubated postoperative patients receiving parenteral opioids, reliable alerting methods (eg, audible alarms, central stations, pagers, etc) are required. Moreover, the responding clinician must be trained to effectively recognize opioid-induced respiratory depression and to intervene appropriately. A mechanism must be in place to allow a bedside clinician to rapidly call for additional help if needed. To effectively manage rare cases of opioid-induced respiratory arrest, the facility must have a well-trained rapid response (or code) team.

A widespread program should be initiated to educate providers and patients about the risks of life-threatening respiratory depression associated with the postoperative use of parenteral opioid analgesics.

[a] Material, modified with permission, from Weinger MB. Dangers of postoperative opioids: APSF workshop and white paper address, prevention of postoperative respiratory complications. *Anesthesia Patient Safety Foundation Newsletter*, 2006;21(4):61, 63–7.[116]

any opioids, benzodiazepines, sedatives, hypnotics, or antihistamines
- Consideration of the patient's nighttime needs and nighttime medications when adjusting the analgesia, with special emphasis on continuous infusion rates
- A requirement that the order form for PCA not be filled by pharmacy unless all sections are completed
- A system for double checking the drug being used for analgesia, the PCA pump setting, and the dosage
- Appropriate levels of assessment, monitoring, and documentation of vital signs, oxygen saturations, sedation levels, and degree of pain, particularly immediately following initiation of PCA and during nighttime hours, including the use of apneic alarms on high-risk patients
- The immediate availability of oxygen for all patients receiving PCA
- The immediate availability of an opioid reversal agent for emergency use in the event of potential oversedation
- If an adverse event occurs, procedures for determining whether the pump was functioning properly and whether the concentration of the drug and rate of administration were as ordered

In spite of almost 2 decades of experience with PCA use, problems persist with opioid-induced respiratory depression. Of concern, even with proper patient selection and appropriate PCA orders, some patients may develop respiratory depression. Regardless of modern advances in technology, such as Microstream capnography, the key to early detection and appropriate treatment remains the provision of adequate in-service education of the nursing staff and clear monitoring policies on patient care units. The ability to recognize signs and symptoms

of oversedation and to respond rapidly is crucial to those caring for patients receiving opioid analgesia, as is the ability to distinguish overdosage from other possible causes of the adverse event, such as pulmonary, neurologic, or cardiovascular complications. Medical and nursing staff must be vigilant for and discriminate between normal sleep and excessive sedation or coma. Although it may not be necessary to wake sleeping patients, it is necessary to determine that they are readily aroused. If sleeping patients do not respond normally to the noise of the nurse in the room or to light touch, it is necessary to stimulate the patient more vigorously and to ensure that the patient can, in fact, be easily awakened. Traditional monitoring parameters of opioid-induced respiratory depression such as respiratory rate may not be adequately sensitive or specific for detection of impending problems. Catley et al[63] noted that patients on IV PCA may experience multiple episodes of hypoxemia not associated with decrease of respiratory rate. Ongoing education should be provided to medical and nursing staff about PCA, including associated risks, policies and procedures for administration, and recognition and treatment of signs and symptoms of complications. Recommendations by the Anesthesia Patient Safety Foundation (APSF) for the prevention of opioid-induced respiratory depression are listed in Table 26.10.

CONCLUSIONS

Postoperative respiratory events are complex and multifactorial. Although opioid administration is frequently implicated in such events, surgical factors, including persistent and significant disturbances in normal sleep patterns, also contribute to unexpected events. Serious complications or deaths from opioid-induced respiratory depression are rare, but the risk is not zero and as such, all patients receiving opioids for perioperative pain management should be monitored for this complication. Opioids cause hypoventilation and decrease the ventilatory response to both hypercapnia and hypoxemia. They also make patients drowsy, and CO_2 retention occurs even during unmedicated sleep. In addition, opioids alter the rhythmicity and pattern of breathing. Appropriate monitoring of patients continues to be the key to early detection and prevention of opioid-induced respiratory depression.

REFERENCES

1. Flisberg P, Rudin A, Linner R, Lundberg CJ. Pain relief and safety after major surgery: a prospective study of epidural and intravenous analgesia in 2696 patients. *Acta Anaesthesiologica Scand.* 2003;47:457–465.

2. Ready LB, Loper KA, Nessly M, Wild L. Postoperative epidural morphine is safe on surgical wards. *Anesthesiology.* 1991;75:452–456.

3. Phillips DM. JCAHO pain management standards are unveiled: Joint Commission on Accreditation of Healthcare Organizations. *JAMA.* 2000;284:428–429.

4. Vila H, Jr, Smith RA, Augustyniak MJ, et al. The efficacy and safety of pain management before and after implementation of hospital-wide pain management standards: is patient safety compromised by treatment based solely on numerical pain ratings? *Anesth Analg.* 2005;101:474–480.

5. Dahan A, Romberg R, Teppema L, Sarton E, Bijl H, Olofsen E. *Simultaneous measurement and integrated analysis of analgesia and respiration after an intravenous morphine infusion. Anesthesiology.* 2004;101:1201–1209.

6. Mueller MR, Shah NG, Landen MG. Unintentional prescription drug overdose deaths in New Mexico, 1994–2003. *Am J Prev Med.* 2006;30:423–429.

7. Paulozzi LJ, Budnitz DS, Xi Y. Increasing deaths from opioid analgesics in the United States. *Pharmacoepidemiol Drug Saf.* 2006;15:618–627.

8. Franklin GM, Mai J, Wickizer T, Turner JA, Fulton-Kehoe D, Grant L. Opioid dosing trends and mortality in Washington State workers' compensation, 1996–2002. *Am J Ind Med.* 2005;48:91–99.

9. White JM, Irvine RJ. Mechanisms of fatal opioid overdose. *Addiction (Abingdon, England).* 1999;94:961–972.

10. Ko S, Goldstein DH, VanDenKerkhof EG. Definitions of "respiratory depression" with intrathecal morphine postoperative analgesia: a review of the literature. *Can J Anesth.* 2003;50:679–688.

11. Grace D, Fee JP. A comparison of intrathecal morphine-6-glucuronide and intrathecal morphine sulfate as analgesics for total hip replacement. *Anesth Analg.* 1996;83:1055–1059.

12. Forrest WH, Jr, Brown BW, Jr, Brown CR, et al. Dextroamphetamine with morphine for the treatment of postoperative pain. *New Engl J Med.* 1977;296:712–715.

13. Ready LB, Oden R, Chadwick HS, et al. *Development of an anesthesiology – based postoperative pain management service. Anesthesiology.* 1988;68:100–106.

14. Rawal N, Allvin R. Epidural and intrathecal opioids for postoperative pain management in Europe: a 17-nation questionnaire study of selected hospitals. Euro Pain Study Group on Acute Pain. *Acta Anaesthesiol Scand.* 1996;40:1119–1126.

15. Dolin SJ, Cashman JN. Tolerability of acute postoperative pain management: nausea, vomiting, sedation, pruritus, and urinary retention. Evidence from published data. *Br J Anaesth.* 2005;95:584–591.

16. Ashburn MA, Love G, Pace NL. Respiratory-related critical events with intravenous patient – controlled analgesia. *Clin J Pain.* 1994;10:52–56.

17. Etches RC. Respiratory depression associated with patient-controlled analgesia: a review of eight cases. *Can J Anesth.* 1994;41:125–132.

18. Fleming BM, Coombs DW. A survey of complications documented in a quality-control analysis of patient-controlled analgesia in the postoperative patient. *J Pain Symptom Manage.* 1992;7:463–469.

19. Notcutt WG, Morgan RJ. Introducing patient – controlled analgesia for postoperative pain control into a district general hospital. *Anaesthesia.* 1990;45:401–406.

20. Schug SA, Torrie JJ. Safety assessment of postoperative pain management by an acute pain service. *Pain.* 1993;55:387–391.

21. Sidebotham D, Dijkhuizen MR, Schug SA. The safety and utilization of patient – controlled analgesia. *J Pain Symptom Manage.* 1997;14:202–209.

22. Wheatley RG, Madej TH, Jackson IJ, Hunter D. The first year's experience of an acute pain service. *Br J Anaesth.* 1991;67:353–359.

23. Silvasti M, Rosenberg P, Seppala T, Svartling N, Pitkanen M. Comparison of analgesic efficacy of oxycodone and morphine in postoperative intravenous patient-controlled analgesia. *Acta Anaesthesiol Scand.* 1998;42:576–580.

24. Scott NB, James K, Murphy M, Kehlet H. Continuous thoracic epidural analgesia versus combined spinal/thoracic epidural analgesia on pain, pulmonary function and the metabolic response following colonic resection. *Acta Anaesthesiol Scand.* 1996;40:691–696.

25. Stenseth R, Sellevold O, Breivik H. Epidural morphine for postoperative pain: experience with 1085 patients. *Acta Anaesthesiol Scand.* 1985;29:148–156.

26. Cashman JN, Dolin SJ. Respiratory and haemodynamic effects of acute postoperative pain management: evidence from published data. *Br J Anaesth.* 2004;93:212–223.

27. Wang JK, Nauss LA, Thomas JE. Pain relief by intrathecally applied morphine in man. *Anesthesiology.* 1979;50:149–151.

28. Davies GK, Tolhurst-Cleaver CL, James TL. Respiratory depression after intrathecal narcotics. *Anaesthesia.* 1980;35:1080–1083.

29. Gjessing J, Tomlin PJ. Postoperative pain control with intrathecal morphine. *Anaesthesia.* 1981;36:268–276.

30. Abboud TK. Mini-dose intrathecal morphine for analgesia following cesarean section. *Anesthesiology.* 1988;69:805.

31. Jacobson L, Chabal C, Brody MC. A dose–response study of intrathecal morphine: efficacy, duration, optimal dose, and side effects. *Anesth Analg.* 1988;67:1082–1088.

32. King HK, Tsai SK. Delayed respiratory depression following repeated intrathecal low dose morphine. *Anaesth Intensive Care.* 1985;13:334–335.

33. Cousins MJ, Mather LE. Intrathecal and epidural administration of opioids. *Anesthesiology.* 1984;61:276–310.

34. Etches RC, Sandler AN, Daley MD. Respiratory depression and spinal opioids. *Can J Anesth.* 1989;36:165–185.

35. Gustafsson LL, Schildt B, Jacobsen K. Adverse effects of extradural and intrathecal opiates: report of a nationwide survey in Sweden. *Br J Anaesth.* 1982;54:479–486.

36. Gwirtz KH, Young JV, Byers RS, et al. The safety and efficacy of intrathecal opioid analgesia for acute postoperative pain: seven years' experience with 5969 surgical patients at Indiana University Hospital. *Anesth Analg.* 1999;88:599–604.

37. Ezure K. Synaptic connections between medullary respiratory neurons and considerations on the genesis of respiratory rhythm. *Prog Neurobiol.* 1990;35:429–450.

38. Onimaru H, Homma I. Respiratory rhythm generator neurons in medulla of brainstem-spinal cord preparation from newborn rat. *Brain Res.* 1987;403:380–384.

39. Smith JC, Ellenberger HH, Ballanyi K, Richter DW, Feldman JL. Pre-Botzinger complex: a brainstem region that may generate respiratory rhythm in mammals. *Science.* 1991;254:726–729.

40. Pierrefiche O, Schmid K, Foutz AS, Denavit-Saubie M. Endogenous activation of NMDA and non–NMDA glutamate receptors on respiratory neurones in cat medulla. *Neuropharmacology.* 991;30:429–440.

41. Haji A, Takeda R, Remmers JE. Evidence that glycine and GABA mediate postsynaptic inhibition of bulbar respiratory neurons in the cat. *J Appl Physiol.* 1992;73:2333–2342.

42. Bonham AC. Neurotransmitters in the CNS control of breathing. *Respir Physiol.* 1995;101:219–230.

43. Fung ML, Wang W, St John WM. Involvement of pontile NMDA receptors in inspiratory termination in rat. *Respir Physiol.* 1994;96:177–188.

44. Pierrefiche O, Foutz AS, Champagnat J, Denavit-Saubie M. NMDA and non–NMDA receptors may play distinct roles in timing mechanisms and transmission in the feline respiratory network. *J Physiol.* 1994;474:509–523.

45. Camporesi EM, Nielsen CH, Bromage PR, Durant PA. Ventilatory CO2 sensitivity after intravenous and epidural morphine in volunteers. *Anesth Analg.* 1983;62:633–640.

46. Nagashima H, Karamanian A, Malovany R, et al. Respiratory and circulatory effects of intravenous butorphanol and morphine. *Clin Pharmacol Ther.* 1976;19:738–745.

47. Popio KA, Jackson DH, Ross AM, Schreiner BF, Yu PN. Hemodynamic and respiratory effects of morphine and butorphanol. *Clin Pharmacol Ther.* 1978;23:281–287.

48. Ballanyi K, Lalley PM, Hoch B, Richter DW. cAMP-dependent reversal of opioid- and prostaglandin-mediated depression of the isolated respiratory network in newborn rats. *J Physiol.* 1997;504(1):127–134.

49. Greer JJ, Carter JE, al-Zubaidy Z. Opioid depression of respiration in neonatal rats. *J Physiol.* 1995;485(3):845–855.

50. Suzue T. Respiratory rhythm generation in the in vitro brain stem–spinal cord preparation of the neonatal rat. *Physiol.* 1984; 354:173–183.

51. Tabatabai M, Kitahata LM, Collins JG. Disruption of the rhythmic activity of the medullary inspiratory neurons and phrenic nerve by fentanyl and reversal with nalbuphine. *Anesthesiology.* 1989;70:489–495.

52. Takita K, Herlenius EA, Lindahl SG, Yamamoto Y. Actions of opioids on respiratory activity via activation of brainstem mu-, delta- and kappa-receptors: an in vitro study. *Brain Res.* 1997;778:233–241.

53. Dahan A, Sarton E, Teppema L, et al. Anesthetic potency and influence of morphine and sevoflurane on respiration in mu–opioid receptor knockout mice. *Anesthesiology.* 2001;94:824–832.

54. Romberg R, Sarton E, Teppema L, Matthes HW, Kieffer BL, Dahan A. Comparison of morphine-6-glucuronide and morphine on respiratory depressant and antinociceptive responses in wild type and mu-opioid receptor deficient mice. *Br J Anaesth.* 2003;91:862–870.

55. Sarton E, Teppema L, Nieuwenhuijs D, Matthes HW, Kieffer B, Dahan A. Opioid effect on breathing frequency and thermogenesis in mice lacking exon 2 of the mu-opioid receptor gene. *Adv Exp Med Biol.* 2001;499:399–404.

56. Ballanyi K, Onimaru H, Homma I. Respiratory network function in the isolated brainstem–spinal cord of newborn rats. *Prog Neurobiol.* 1999;59:583–634.

57. Hilaire G, Duron B. Maturation of the mammalian respiratory system. *Physiol Rev.* 1999;79:325–360.

58. Morin-Surun MP, Boudinot E, Fournie-Zaluski MC, Champagnat J, Roques BP, Denavit-Saubie M. Control of breathing by endogenous opioid peptides: possible involvement in sudden infant death syndrome. *Neurochem Int.* 1992;20:103–107.

59. Bianchi AL, Denavit-Saubie M, Champagnat J. Central control of breathing in mammals: neuronal circuitry, membrane properties, and neurotransmitters. *Physiol Rev.* 1995;75:1–45.

60. Santiago TV, Edelman NH. Opioids and breathing. *J Appl Physiol.* 1985;59:1675–1685.

61. Shook JE, Watkins WD, Camporesi EM. Differential roles of opioid receptors in respiration, respiratory disease, and opiate-induced respiratory depression. *Am Rev Respir Dis.* 1990;142:895–909.

62. Yeadon M, Kitchen I. Opioids and respiration. *Prog Neurobiol.* 1989;33:1–16.

63. Catley DM, Thornton C, Jordan C, Lehane JR, Royston D, Jones JG. Pronounced episodic oxygen desaturation in the postoperative period: its association with ventilatory pattern and analgesic regimen. *Anesthesiology.* 1985;63:20–28.

64. Sandler AN. Opioid-induced respiratory depression in the postoperative period. *Anesthesiol Clin North Am.* 1989;7(1):193–210.

65. Rosenberg J. Hypoxaemia in the general surgical ward: a potential risk factor? *Eur J Surg.* 1994;160:657–661.

66. Davidson JA, Hosie HE. Limitations of pulse oximetry: respiratory insufficiency – a failure of detection. *Br Med J (Clin Res Ed).* 1993;307:372–373.

67. Hutton P, Clutton-Brock T. The benefits and pitfalls of pulse oximetry. *Br Med J (Clin Res Ed).* 1993;307:457–458.

68. Berkenbosch A, Teppema LJ, Olievier CN, Dahan A. Influences of morphine on the ventilatory response to isocapnic hypoxia. *Anesthesiology.* 86:1342–1349.

69. Weil JV, McCullough RE, Kline JS, Sodal IE. Diminished ventilatory response to hypoxia and hypercapnia after morphine in normal man. *New Engl J Med.* 1975;292:1103–1106.

70. Stone JG, Cozine KA, Wald A. Nocturnal oxygenation during patient–controlled analgesia. *Anesthesia and Analgesia.* 1999;89:104–110.

71. Magosso E, Ursino M, van Oostrom JH. Opioid-induced respiratory depression: a mathematical model for fentanyl. *IEEE Transact Biomed Eng.* 2004;51(7):1115–1128.

72. Forrest WH, Jr, Bellville JW. The effect of sleep plus morphine on the respiratory response to carbon dioxide. *Anesthesiology.* 1964;25:137–141.

73. Romagnoli A, Keats AS. Comparative respiratory depression of tillidine and morphine. *Clin Pharmacol Ther.* 1975;17:523–528.

74. Scamman FL, Ghoneim MM, Korttila K. Ventilatory and mental effects of alfentanil and fentanyl. *Acta Anaesthesiol Scand.* 1984;28:63–67.

75. Bragg P, Zwass MS, Lau M, Fisher DM. Opioid pharmacodynamics in neonatal dogs: differences between morphine and fentanyl. *J Appl Physiol.* 1995;79:1519–1524.

76. Glass PS, Iselin-Chaves IA, Goodman D, Delong E, Hermann DJ. Determination of the potency of remifentanil compared with alfentanil using ventilatory depression as the measure of opioid effect. *Anesthesiology.* 1999;90:1556–1563.

77. Bailey PL, Lu JK, Pace NL, et al. Effects of intrathecal morphine on the ventilatory response to hypoxia. *New Engl J Med.* 2000;343:1228–1234.

78. Cartwright P, Prys-Roberts C, Gill K, Dye A, Stafford M, Gray A. Ventilatory depression related to plasma fentanyl concentrations during and after anesthesia in humans. *Anesth Analg.* 1983;62:966–974.

79. Hill HF, Chapman CR, Saeger LS, et al. Steady-state infusions of opioids in human. II. Concentration-effect relationships and therapeutic margins. *Pain.* 1990;43:69–79.

80. Mildh LH, Scheinin H, Kirvela OA. The concentration-effect relationship of the respiratory depressant effects of alfentanil and fentanyl. *Anesth Analg.* 2001;93:939–946.

81. Berkenbosch A, Olievier CN, Wolsink JG, DeGoede J, Rupreht J. Effects of morphine and physostigmine on the ventilatory response to carbon dioxide. *Anesthesiology.* 1994;80:1303–1310.

82. Harper MH, Hickey RF, Cromwell TH, Linwood S. The magnitude and duration of respiratory depression produced by fentanyl and fentanyl plus droperidol in man. *J Pharmacol Exp Ther.* 1976;199:464–468.

83. Santiago TV, Johnson J, Riley DJ, Edelman NH. *Effects of morphine on ventilatory response to exercise. J Appl Physiol.* 1979;47:112–118.

84. Barbour SJ, Vandebeek CA, Ansermino JM. Increased tidal volume variability in children is a better marker of opioid-induced respiratory depression than decreased respiratory rate. *J Clin Monitor Comput.* 2004;18:171–178.

85. Bouillon T, Bruhn J, Roepcke H, Hoeft A. Opioid–induced respiratory depression is associated with increased tidal volume variability. *Eur J Anaesthesiol.* 2003;20:127–133.

86. Sandler AN, Stringer D, Panos L, et al. A randomized, double-blind comparison of lumbar epidural and intravenous fentanyl infusions for postthoracotomy pain relief: analgesic, pharmacokinetic, and respiratory effects. *Anesthesiology.* 1992;77:626–634.

87. Wheatley RG, Somerville ID, Sapsford DJ, Jones JG. Postoperative hypoxaemia: comparison of extradural, i.m. and patient-controlled opioid analgesia. *Br J Anaesth.* 1990;64:267–275.

88. Arunasalam K, Davenport HT, Painter S, Jones JG. Ventilatory response to morphine in young and old subjects. *Anaesthesia.* 1983;38:529–533.

89. Bailey PL, Rhondeau S, Schafer PG, et al. Dose-response pharmacology of intrathecal morphine in human volunteers. *Anesthesiology.* 1993;79:49–59.

90. Boylan JF, Katz J, Kavanagh BP, et al. Epidural bupivacaine-morphine analgesia versus patient-controlled analgesia following abdominal aortic surgery: analgesic, respiratory, and myocardial effects. *Anesthesiology.* 1998;89:585–593.

91. Etches RC, Sandler AN, Lawson SL. A comparison of the analgesic and respiratory effects of epidural nalbuphine or morphine in postthoracotomy patients. *Anesthesiology.* 1991;75:9–14.

92. Sleigh JW. Postoperative respiratory arrhythmias: incidence and measurement. *Acta Anaesthesiol Scand.* 1999;43:708–714.

93. Feldman JL, Smith JC, Ellenberger HH, et al. Neurogenesis of respiratory rhythm and pattern: emerging concepts. *Am J Physiol.* 1990;259:879–886.

94. Boushra NN. Anaesthetic management of patients with sleep apnoea syndrome. *Can J Anesth.* 1996;43:599–616.

95. Keamy MF, 3rd, Cadieux RJ, Kofke WA, Kales A. The occurrence of obstructive sleep apnea in a recovery room patient. *Anesthesiology.* 66:232–234.

96. Rennotte MT, Baele P, Aubert G, Rodenstein DO. Nasal continuous positive airway pressure in the perioperative management of patients with obstructive sleep apnea submitted to surgery. *Chest.* 1995;107:367–374.

97. Taylor S, Kirton OC, Staff I, Kozol RA. Postoperative day one: a high risk period for respiratory events. *Am J Surg.* 2005;190:752–756.

98. Guilleminault C, Stoohs R, Clerk A, Simmons J, Labanowski M. Excessive daytime somnolence in women with abnormal respiratory efforts during sleep. *Sleep.* 1993;16:137–138.

99. Oliven A, Schnall RP, Pillar G, Gavriely N, Odeh M. Sublingual electrical stimulation of the tongue during wakefulness and sleep. *Respir Physiol.* 2001;127:217–226.

100. Skulsky EM, Osman NI, Baghdoyan HA, Lydic R. Microdialysis delivery of morphine. *Sleep.* 2007;30(5):566–573.

101. Cherniack NS. Respiratory dysrhythmias during sleep. *New Engl J Med.* 1981;305:325–330.

102. Series F, Roy N, Marc I. Effects of sleep deprivation and sleep fragmentation on upper airway collapsibility in normal subjects. *Am J Respir Crit Care Med.* 1994;150:481–485.

103. Lamberg L. Chronic pain linked with poor sleep; exploration of causes and treatment. *JAMA.* 1999;281:691–692.

104. Rosenberg-Adamsen S, Kehlet H, Dodds C, Rosenberg J. Postoperative sleep disturbances: mechanisms and clinical implications. *Br J Anaesth.* 1996;76:552–559.

105. Lydic R, Baghdoyan HA. Sleep, anesthesiology and the neurobiology of arousal state control. *Anesthesiology.* 2005;103:1268–1295.

106. Knill RL, Moote CA, Skinner MI, Rose EA. Anesthesia with abdominal surgery leads to intense REM sleep during the first postoperative week. *Anesthesiology.* 1990;73:52–61.

107. Rosenberg J, Wildschiodtz G, Pedersen MH, von Jessen F, Kehlet H. Late postoperative nocturnal episodic hypoxaemia and associated sleep pattern. *Br J Anaesth.* 1994;72:145–150.

108. Borgbjerg FM, Nielsen K, Franks J. Experimental pain stimulates respiration and attenuates morphine-induced respiratory depression: a controlled study in human volunteers. *Pain.* 1996;64:123–128.

109. Shaw I, Lavigne G, Mayer P, Choinière M. Acute intravenous administration of morphine perturbs sleep architecture in healthy pain-free young adults: a preliminary study. *Sleep.* 2005;6:677–682.

110. Jones JG, Jordan C, Scudder C, Rocke DA, Barrowcliffe M. Episodic postoperative oxygen desaturation: the value of added oxygen. *J R Soc Med.* 1985;78:1019–1022.

111. Rosenberg J, Pedersen MH, Gebuhr P, Kehlet H. Effect of oxygen therapy on late postoperative episodic and constant hypoxaemia. *Br J Anaesth.* 1992;68:18–22.

112. Rosenberg J, Rasmussen GI, Wojdemann KR, Kirkeby LT, Jorgensen LN, Kehlet H. Ventilatory pattern and associated episodic hypoxaemia in the late postoperative period in the general surgical ward. *Anaesthesia.* 1999;54:323–328.

113. Farney RJ, Walker JM, Cloward TV, Rhondeau S. Sleep-disordered breathing associated with long-term opioid therapy. *Chest.* 2003;123:632–639.

114. Force AAoSMT. Sleep-related breathing disorders in adults: recommendations for syndrome definition and measurement techniques in clinical research: the Report of an American Academy of Sleep Medicine Task Force. *Sleep.* 1999;22:667–689.

115. Folke M, Cernerud L, Ekstrom M, Hok B. Critical review of non–invasive respiratory monitoring in medical care. *Med Biol Eng Comput.* 2003;41:377–383.

116. Weinger MB. Dangers of postoperative opioids: APSF workshop and white paper address, prevention of postoperative respiratory complications. *Anesthesia Patient Saf Found Newslett.* 2006;21(4):61:63–67.

117. Colman Y, Krauss B. Microstream capnograpy technology: a new approach to an old problem. *J Clin Monitor Comput.* 1999;15:403–409.

118. Casati A, Gallioli G, Passaretta R, Scandroglio M, Bignami E, Torri G. End tidal carbon dioxide monitoring in spontaneously breathing, nonintubated patients: a clinical comparison between conventional sidestream and microstream capnometers. *Minerva Anestesiol.* 2001;67:161–164.

119. Sieker HO, Hickam JB. Carbon dioxide intoxication: the clinical syndrome: its etiology and management with particular reference to the use of mechanical respirators. *Medicine.* 1956;35:389–423.

120. Downs JB. Prevention of hypoxemia: the simple, logical, but incorrect solution. *J Clin Anesth.* 1994;6:180–181.

121. Fu ES, Downs JB, Schweiger JW, Miguel RV, Smith RA. Supplemental oxygen impairs detection of hypoventilation by pulse oximetry. Chest. 2004;126:1552–1558.

122. Rawal N, Wattwil M. Respiratory depression after epidural morphine: an experimental and clinical study. *Anesth Analg.* 1984;63:8–14.

123. Johnson A, Bengtsson M, Soderlind K, Lofstrom JB. Influence of intrathecal morphine and naloxone intervention on postoperative ventilatory regulation in elderly patients. *Acta Anaesthesiol Scand.* 1992;36:436–444.

124. Boezaart AP, Eksteen JA, Spuy GV, Rossouw P, Knipe M. Intrathecal morphine: double-blind evaluation of optimal dosage for analgesia after major lumbar spinal surgery. *Spine.* 1999;24:1131–1137.

125. Aubrun F, Monsel S, Langeron O, Coriat P, Riou B. Postoperative titration of intravenous morphine. *Eur J Anaesthesiol.* 2001;18:159–165.

126. Ramsay MA, Savege TM, Simpson BR, Goodwin R. Controlled sedation with alphaxalone–alphadolone. *Br Med J.* 1974;2:656–659.

127. Paqueron X, Lumbroso A, Mergoni P, et al. Is morphine–induced sedation synonymous with analgesia during intravenous morphine titration? *Br J Anaesth.* 2002;89:697–701.

128. Walder B, Schafer M, Henzi I, Tramer MR. Efficacy and safety of patient-controlled opioid analgesia for acute postoperative pain: a quantitative systematic review. *Acta Anaesthesiol Scand.* 2001;45:795–804.

129. Looi-Lyons LC, Chung FF, Chan VW, McQuestion M. Respiratory depression: an adverse outcome during patient controlled analgesia therapy. *J Clin Anesth.* 1996;8:151–156.

Acute Pain Management in Special Patient Populations

27

The Acute Pain Management Service: Organization and Implementation Issues

Paul Willoughby

Acute pain management remains challenging in hospitals throughout the world. Over the past few decades, management has advanced from intermittent dosing of intramuscular narcotics to implementation of multimodal analgesia, including the use of continuous administration of local anesthetics via peripheral nerve catheters. In many institutions, evaluation and management of patients' pain has changed from being primarily the patient's surgeon/physician responsibility to the integration of an Acute Pain Service (APS) or Acute Pain Management Service (APMS) team providing the care in conjunction with the surgeon/physician. Despite the increase in APS/APMS and the advent of the concept of multimodal analgesia and proliferation of guidelines for acute pain management,[1-3] postoperative pain continues to be problem.[4] The reasons for this are unclear, but they are certainly in part because of the fact that implementing change can take a long time. The purpose of this chapter is to provide strategies for organization and implementation of an APMS using basic business management methods. The reader is also referred to Chapter 28 (*Acute Pain Management in the Community Hospital Setting*).

ORGANIZATIONAL ROLE OF APMS IN A HOSPITAL SETTING

Organization cannot make a genius out of an incompetent; even less can it, of itself make the decisions which are required to trigger the necessary action. On the other hand, disorganization can scarcely fail to result in inefficiency and can easily lead to disaster. Organization makes more efficient the gathering and analysis of facts, and the arranging of the findings of experts in logical fashion. Therefore organization helps the responsible individual make the necessary decision, and helps assure that it is satisfactorily carried out.

Dwight D. Eisenhower

Dwight D. Eisenhower changed the way the presidential office was managed. He created a White House chief-of-staff, a cabinet secretariat, a congressional liaison function, and a press office. He applied the military administrative principles he had learned in the army to the oval office. In many ways, organizing an APMS is similar. Although some may view the APMS as a minor part of a department of anesthesiology, it actually has far-reaching effects within a hospital. As opposed to operating room anesthesiologists, the APMS team will be known throughout the hospital. The APMS will be involved not only in the evaluation and management of patients but also with hospital policies and the daily management of pain by other surgeons/physicians. The APMS will be involved in the practice of physicians, surgeons, medical students, nurses, pharmacists, patient relations, presurgical testing centers, outpatient follow-up, patient relations, quality assurance, and the financial management of the hospital. It can do so only by being highly organized.

TYPES OF ORGANIZATIONS

When establishing an APMS, the scope of practice needs to be assessed (Table 27.1). Depending on the scope of practice, staffing can either be large or small. At a minimum, all hospitals must have one person with the responsibility of an APMS. The primary role is to educate and enforce the Joint Commission on Accreditation of Health Care Organization (JCAHO) requirements for pain management standards[5] and other hospital policies and nursing education. In small hospitals, it may be one nurse administrator or nurse practitioner. In larger, academic settings, the team can be larger and integrate more functions (Table 27.2).

For the most part, anesthesiologists usually lead the APMS in large centers. After all, anesthesiologists manage pain in the operating room and provide interventional therapy in the outpatient setting. Depending on how the anesthesiology group is organized, the APMS may be led by anesthesiologists who specialize in chronic pain management. In this case, catheters are often placed by a team of regional anesthesiologists who manage intraoperative care but transfer postoperative care to the APMS. In the past, this was the most likely scenario. However,

Table 27.1: Scope of Practice of the Acute Pain Management Service

IV PCA

Epidurals

Single-dose intrathecal morphine

Peripheral nerve catheters

Regional anesthesiology

Acute pain consults

Chronic pain consults

Oncological pain management

Interventional pain management

Intrathecal pumps

Dorsal column stimulators

End of life care

Oral medication management

Hospital policies

Hospital formulary

Outpatient management

Psychological treatments

Physical therapy

Table 27.2: Potential Members of an Acute Pain Management Service

Anesthesiologist

Nurse practitioner

Nurse

Physician Assistant

Resident

Psychiatrist

Psychologist

Neurologist

Pharmacist

Physical therapist

with the expansion of services offered in the outpatient pain setting and the increase in patient loads inside the hospital, chronic pain management and acute pain management can be separate divisions. Thus, a regional anesthesiologist team may also be the physicians managing the postoperative care. In this case, chronic pain management issues inside the hospital are often referred to a chronic pain management specialist and the regional anesthesiologists manage acute pain and postoperative care. In a private practice setting, this split of services is more likely to occur where chronic pain management is not part of the anesthesiology group. Regardless of the delegation of duties, it is important to provide both acute and chronic pain management services for the hospital.

Nursing is a key component to any APMS. One of the first to fully implement an APMS with patients managed by nurses using protocols was at Thomas Jefferson University (Philadelphia, PA, USA) by Dr Eugene Viscusi (personal communication). During the resident shortage of the mid-1990s, acute pain services in academic settings lost the ability to utilize residents for postoperative coverage after hours. Under this scenario, it became popular to implement a nurse-based, protocol-driven acute pain service. As adversity brings opportunity, using nurses created new benefits. Instead of having a continuous group of residents who are trained and then move on, the APMS became a group of stable professionals who, through repetition, become more competent. Patient care becomes more streamlined. Consistency of care and a communication within the hospital personnel improved. Indeed much is written about the nursing role on APMS with much success.[6]

Using nurse practitioners existed prior to utilizing nurses. Nurse practitioners can prescribe medications, whereas nurses cannot. They have received more training and experience in the evaluation and clinical management of patient care. Nurse practitioners on the APMS often are the nursing administrators, educators, and managers of the service. They communicate with the nursing department of the hospital and provide a key role in the establishment of policies and quality assurance issues. The nursing leaders of the APMS play a vital role in educating nurses within the hospital. Acute pain management involves not only the evaluation and pharmacological management but also the complexity of equipment involved with peripheral nerve catheters, epidural catheters, and interventional pain management; it is vital to have a nursing resource for teaching floor nurses about the care of patients who have undergone these procedures. Although physician assistants can also be used instead or with nurse practitioners, physician assistant's practices are sometimes limited and their orders may need to be cosigned by a physician.

Nursing education can expand to improving the organization of the service. In the European model,[12] there are pain resource nurses on every floor for every shift in the hospital. The same model is used in the United States. A pain resource nurse on each floor for each shift can be helpful in the management of difficult patients and the setup and troubleshooting of specialized equipment. This model is for other specialty areas such as infection control and fire marshal.

The psychological aspects of acute pain management cannot be overlooked. Psychological and coping factors can have a magnifying effect on the perception of pain. Patients with overriding psychological conditions or addictions will need special attention. A psychiatrist or psychologist can be an important resource for an APMS. Occasionally a psychiatrist who specializes in pain management may lead the team. At the very least, it is important that an APMS develops a good relationship with a psychiatrist or psychologist for referral and consultation. A psychiatrist specializing in addiction or an addictionologist is particularly important resource when issues of addiction are suspected or diagnosed. The nurses and nurse practitioners on the APMS should be familiar with the care of patients with anxiety and substance abuse.

Pharmacists can play a vital role on an APMS. Their knowledge of medications can be very educational in an academic setting. They are helpful in adjusting hospital formulary and in constructing medication paradigms for treatments. The pharmacy is involved in the delivery of medications to patients. When medications are not available, analgesic gaps can occur. A

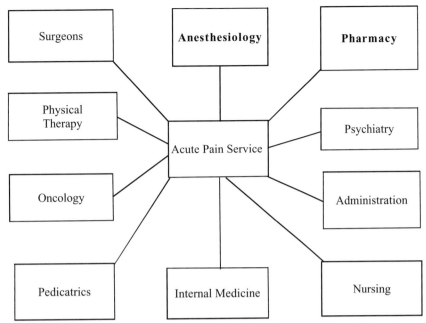

Figure 27.1: Relationships between the APMS and other departments within the hospital.

pharmacist can help in proper labeling of medications and develop simplification of infusions to prevent confusion. Pharmacy departments provide the critical safety net to guard against medication errors, drug interactions, and other medication safety protocols.

In the United States, hospitals and anesthesiology groups are organized in functional organizational structure or, if the group is large, a divisional structure. Lines of responsibility and reporting are clearly defined in a mostly vertical pattern. The divisional structure has replication of duties, but is necessary because of the larger size and subspecialized nature of its members. In Europe, where hospitalists are used more frequently for inpatient care, a functional structure for an acute pain service is also used. Surgeons frequently perform only the surgery and turn over the postoperative care to the hospitalists. Primary care physicians in Europe often do not admit or follow their patients when they are in the hospital. Having physicians who are present on certain floors by shift allows one to educate, communicate, and develop protocols more easily.

The Europeans have criticized the United States methods of organization of the APMS as expensive and requiring more personnel. However, in the United States the pain management team does not have the luxury of hospitalists present on each floor. Instead, numerous physicians and surgeons manage their patients throughout the hospital. There is far more physician autonomy and customer loyalty for their surgeon/physician in the United States. Moreover, although some floors may concentrate on a particular type of patient or service, patients can be located on any floor if a shortage of hospital beds occurs. Thus, in the United States, the APMS functions more in a matrix pattern than a functional or divisional structure in a hospital and anesthesiology group (Figure 27.1). Thus, the APMS functions outside lines of responsibility and must rely on developing good relationships with each division inside the hospital or anesthesiology group to achieve its goals. The APMS manages the patient's pain control for surgeons, internists, oncologists, pediatricians, and so on. Physical therapy has functional goals

for patients, which need to be considered. Having medications arrive safely and timely for patients requires discussions with pharmacy. However, internally, the APMS usually has a functional structure (Figure 27.2).

The matrix organization often exists inside an anesthesiology group that is organized in a functional or divisional structure. Teams and divisions have been created in many groups to manage patients undergoing cardiac surgery, neurosurgery, pediatrics, obstetrics, orthopedic surgery, and so on. The APMS often manages the postoperative pain of these patients, whereas other anesthesiologists provide their intraoperative care. Thus the APMS can only educate but otherwise has little influence on the intraoperative patient care performed by other anesthesiologists. This shared responsibility for an individual patient's care rarely occurs among the other anesthesiology divisions.

The difficulties in creating change in practice become even more apparent when implementing regional anesthesiology into acute pain management. There is a shortage of regional anesthesiologists in the United States. In academic centers alone, a survey performed in 2005 demonstrated that another 250 regional

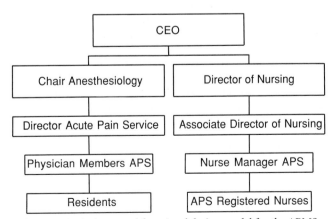

Figure 27.2: An improved functional design model for the APMS.

Table 27.3: Goals of the Acute Pain Management Service

Patient care

Education

Research

Financial

Community Service

Table 27.4: Standardized Treatment Plan for Total Knee Arthroplasty

Patients meet with APMS nurses, orthopedic floor nurses, and physical therapists preoperatively to discuss their care

Patients receive oxycodone CR (10–20 mg PO) preoperatively

Femoral nerve catheter placed in the block area and loaded with ropivacaine (0.5%)

Spinal or general anesthesiology intraoperatively

Ketorolac (15 mg IV) every 6 hours intraoperatively or before spinal anesthesiology wears off

Femoral nerve catheter maintained for until 5 P.M. next day with a ropivacaine (0.2%) infusion

Oxycodone CR (10–20 mg PO) every 12 hours

Oxycodone (5–10 mg PO) every 4 hours PRN for breakthrough pain

Ketorolac (15 mg IV) every 6 hours for 48 hours

Substitute celecoxib (200 mg twice a day) for 48–72 hours if the patient is at risk for or is experiencing poor hemostasis

Consider pregabalin (100–150 mg twice a day) for 72 hours

Cryotherapy to knee

Passive range of motion started day of surgery

Patient ambulated next day

Discharge to inpatient rehabilitation in 48 hours or for home rehabilitation in 72 hours

Abbreviations: PO = per oral; PRN = as needed.

---

anesthesiologists would be necessary to fully staff these training programs. Although many anesthesiologists would prefer regional anesthesiology for themselves, most would not perform it for their patients because of lack of skill and comfort performing the procedures.

There are two methods of integrating regional anesthesiology into acute pain management. The ruthless method involves simply firing every anesthesiologist who does not wish to change practice. Although efficient, this method is not always practical when the group wishes to maintain their staff or when the majority of cases are performed under general anesthesiology. In this case the group would need to hire trained staff and create a regional anesthesiology/acute pain management division within the department that may require specialty call and salary adjustment. This division will operate as a matrix within the group unless acute pain management is placed at a higher level within the organization. Another alternative would be to create a committee with all of the divisional directors or their representatives that focuses purely on the implementation and improvement of acute pain management in the operative setting.

DEVELOPING GOALS AND OBJECTIVES

Goals and objectives for achieving the goals has become the preferred administrative method for setting priorities and measuring outcomes. Goals should be clearly stated and then objectives can be instituted to measure the achievement of the goals. The goals we use at our hospital are listed in Table 27.3.

The patient care must be the highest priority when establishing goals for the APMS. Education is also important to improving patient care. Although epidural analgesia, patient-controlled analgesia, and peripheral nerve catheters improve comfort, one cannot utilize these methods if the hospital staff does not know how to manage them. The nurse practitioner/manager is instrumental in negotiating these policies and standards of care through the various committees or the hospital and then educating the nurse educators and staff.

The patient care and education goals are thus interconnected. The scope of patient care for an inpatient APMS will range from preoperative care through postoperative care as per JCAHO requirements.[5] Patients will need to be educated often in the surgeon's office and in a preadmission testing facility. In the hospital, patients can be identified from the operative schedule and if they are present in the hospital, they can be met the night before and a treatment plan can be created with their input.

Treatment plans need to be created with surgeons, physicians, physical therapists, and nurses. The main goal of analgesia is to have the patient regain normal function with a minimal amount of side effects. With that goal in mind, an example of a multimodal analgesia and treatment plan is listed in Table 27.4.

Research is an important factor in academic centers and for some private practices. It may provide notoriety and financial resources for an acute pain service. Financial implications will be discussed later in the chapter. Community service is an important part of marketing your services and is discussed later. In the private practice setting, research and community service are often considered a lower priority than the financial aspects.

COMMUNICATION

Avenues of communication for identifying patients for painful procedures or with specific conditions need to be created. As the APMS is ubiquitous in the hospital, the nurses need to have a way of reaching an APMS member when problems or questions arise. The leader of the APMS needs to develop systems of communication with surgeons, physicians, and nurses. A specific pager or phone should be available 24 hours a day, 7 days a week, for consultation and response. A backup plan, in case the pager or phone is not functioning, should be in place. To maintain or establish credibility, response times need to be established for certain conditions and situations. Priority must be placed on emergency situations. In our institution all patients must be seen within 2 hours of being called.

The booking area for the operating room schedule facilitates this communication as well. After treatment plans have been created and agreed on by surgeons, patients can either be scheduled with an APMS consult or simply be identified from the schedule based on prior agreement with the surgeon and then scheduled for postoperative epidural analgesia, regional anesthesiology, or peripheral nerve catheter placement.

MARKETING

Nothing is worse than having a patient arrive for a painful, surgical procedure and not having been informed prior to arrival in the operating suite of the effective techniques available for relieving their pain. It produces undo stress and can become litigious if a complication occurs. After developing treatment plans, educational materials, such as pamphlets, need to be created that explain the care the patients can receive. The surgeons and preadmission testing personnel need to be aware to discuss these treatments. Whenever possible, the APMS staff themselves should meet with the patients. The best patient marketing actually occurs in the surgeons' waiting room. When patients who are there for postoperative visits talk to each other and praise the quality of care, or critique the lack thereof, the preoperative patients listen.

Community service is also a part of marketing. Participating in community events such as state fairs or health fairs is educational for patients and they will seek out your care. Community lectures are also helpful.

The APMS should establish a presence in the hospital. Even if there are no patients on a particular ward, walking through the ward and conversing with the nurses often brings up questions of improving a particular patient's care or other situations. Then, when another occasion arises, the ward nurses will suggest to the physician that perhaps they should contact the APMS for assistance.

Education is an important part of marketing your services. Providing education opportunities to medical students, nursing students, residents, attending and administrative staff is an easy way to increase the APMS notoriety. These educational opportunities include lectures, journal clubs, committees, participation on rounds, and social occasions. JCAHO mandates creating pamphlets concerning patients' rights to pain management.[5] It is also a perfect opportunity to advertise the unique treatments available by a modern APMS.

Overall, the best marketing is achieved through good results. When the surgeons, physicians, nurses, administrators, and patients see the improved results of modern acute pain management techniques and care, they will seek out the APMS for the treatments that are offered.

HUMAN RESOURCE MANAGEMENT

Once the scope of practice for the APMS is delineated, the leader of the team will need to gather staff so that the work can be accomplished. Although physicians are not trained in medical school to be managers, human resource management is an important and often undervalued aspect of managing an APMS.

Negotiations will need to take place with the entity that will be employing the staff (hospital or anesthesiology group). Certainly no work (epidurals, peripheral nerve catheters, or consults) should take place until the staff are hired and a start date is agreed on. If in the negotiations for staff the hospital or group declines to hire what is needed for the scope of practice desired,

then the scope of practice should be decreased. Compromises in the quality of care will only cause the service to gain a bad reputation and eventually collapse.

What do employees look for in a job? Although priorities vary, most employees look for growth potential, upward mobility, and having an input on the work being performed, a good work environment, income, and lifestyle. It is important to make it clear to the potential employee how each of these aspects will be present on the APMS.

For anesthesiologists joining the pain management service, all of the above are easily accomplished. Regional anesthesiology is one of the fastest growing subspecialties and the skills obtained are highly marketable. For nurses, the APMS also offers a wide variety of growth opportunities. Upward mobility is possible because the work of the APMS is hospital-wide and all the members gain notoriety.

Maintaining a good work environment is important. Screening for malcontents and argumentative people is crucial. Rules of behavior should be set prior to employment. The leader of the APMS will need to listen often and intervene when relationships issues arise. Having meetings with the APMS staff will allow the staff members to identify problems and design mutually agreed upon solutions that are practical. In this way all of the staff will have the opportunity to provide input to their jobs and improve their work environments at the same time. These meeting also accomplish the goals of quality improvement, developing research ideas and implementing new methods of pain management.

Unfortunately, the income potential for an APMS member is about the same as that of any other anesthesiology or nursing professional. The economics of the APMS are discussed later. However, when negotiating with the group or hospital, it is important to maintain salaries and bonuses commensurate with other anesthesiology subspecialties, especially if call is involved.

Lifestyle issues are important and are an increasing factor in medicine and nursing. Many physicians and nurses are in two-income families with children. Child care, family issues, and staff health issues will arise. Employees will ask to work certain hours to accommodate their lifestyles. Nurturing a team concept, recognizing the importance of lifestyle of the employee, and being open about the hours and expectations when hiring will help with the management of lifestyle issues.

Most managers would plan a full-time equivalent (FTE) as 200 days per year. However, as the APMS is usually a small team, more staff will be necessary to insure coverage. Developing relationships with other nurses in the hospital to offer overtime when sick calls or disability occur can aid in staffing. Having other anesthesiologists rotate through the APMS will allow for better flexibility and backup if a sick call or other reason for absence occurs.

When hiring staff, there are three sources of information: curriculum vitae (resume), interview, and recommendations. Standards for job qualifications and a rating system for evaluation of applicants are necessary. A quantitative system for qualitative evaluation will aid in clarifying the qualities and expectations of the potential employee and conform to equal employment opportunity requirements.

The physician leader should be a person of character who has the appropriate knowledge, experience, and background. Leadership skills and managerial experience are paramount and should be part of the quantitative evaluation. As the leader will need to make change, personality and communication skills are also important. In an academic center, it is desirable for the APMS director to be experienced in pain research and be a recognized leader in acute pain management.

In some setting, nurses may be unionized and/or seniority can take priority. Sometimes the APMS leader will have little input into who is hired. Therefore, requiring that the nurses have a background in intensive care or postanesthesia recovery is necessary to obtain the desired qualities of an APMS nurse.

When evaluating the curriculum vitae, evaluate job continuity and longevity. Everyone is allowed one occasion of brief employment. Sometimes jobs do not work out well. However, a pattern of jobs that last less than 6 months to a year is a negative. Many nurses change jobs every 3 years within an institution and that is perfectly acceptable. Many enjoy growing in their profession.

The purpose of an interview is to evaluate the ability of the employee to interact with the employer and current staff. To determine the qualities of the potential employee the following questions might be asked: How well will this person interact with personnel and patients? How well will they interact with the managers? What is their body language saying? Do they give positive responses? Do they give negative responses (would they then talk negatively about the service)? What are they looking for in their employment?

The interview also gives the potential employee the opportunity to learn what is expected of them. This is important because the job may not be quite what they expected and they may be better suited for other employment.

Recommendations can be variable depending on the source. If they are from a good source they can be very helpful. However, if a manager wishes to have an employee move to a new job, a glowing recommendation may aid them in their cause, but not help you find a good employee. Letters of recommendation can also become litigious and need to be interpreted accordingly. A letter simply outlining someone's duties is a bad indicator of work performance. Conversely a letter that has the words outstanding and excellent used frequently is a good indicator of a potentially good employee.

Hiring the right staff is very important to creating a strong APMS. They should be team players with enough intelligence and a firm commitment to getting the job done right. Pain management in the hospital requires superior interpersonal skills.

After hiring the staff, they will need to be trained. Usually they will need a period of time with someone expert before working solo. This period can be highly variable depending on the previous level of experience. Having guidelines/protocols available for the agreed-on management of patients' conditions is necessary to aid in the education. For the most part, employees will work their hardest in the beginning of their employment. So gradually moving them into a job often gives the impression that their performance expectations are low. It is a difficult balance of education and developing experience. Having mentors available for guidance and answering questions will help balance inexperience with autonomy.

Periodic evaluation and feedback are a necessary part of human resource management. Specific criteria for performance and grading need to be established and periodically reevaluated. It is an increasingly common practice to perform 360-degree evaluations so that the people the employee interacts with also can help in this input. For the most part, it is always best to praise in public and criticize in private. Pathways for dealing with troublesome employees with counseling need to be established. Although no one enjoys terminating employment, it is sometimes necessary. In this case, fair documentation of evaluation of all employees will help avoid any union grievances and aid in legal matters.

OPERATION AND PRODUCTION MANAGEMENT

Efficiency and hospital flow are an increasingly important aspect of acute pain management. Before establishing an APMS, one must survey the territory. The processes of how a patient moves through the system need to be evaluated. When integrating acute pain procedures, consideration should be given for incorporating time for evaluation of patients and performance of procedures. Although most surgeons appreciate the benefits of regional analgesia, many are concerned when it interferes with their operative start times.[15] Having patients arrive earlier for procedures and establishing a separate block area (Figure 27.3) can improve efficiency.[16] Thus, the decrease in wake-up times with regional anesthesiology can be more fully appreciated and overall operating room time may decrease. Although many argue that another case cannot often be added to the schedule by decreasing operating room time, decreasing operating room time will increase surgeon and anesthesiologist job satisfaction by allowing them to leave earlier.

Using maximal evaluation and procedure times is better than using mean times for scheduling patient arrival times in the block area. Although it is inconvenient for the patient to wait, it improves operating room flow and surgeon satisfaction. It also allows for anesthesiologists who are just starting to perform new techniques or for residents to perform the procedures in a less stressful environment than the operating room with a pacing surgeon present. Providing the patient with the ability to wait with relatives or companions in the block area before and after the procedure can decrease the anxiety of waiting. Other distractions such as televisions or providing magazines are helpful.

The block area needs to be equipped with all of the medications and equipment for the safe practice of regional anesthesiology. Standard ASA monitors should be available. Adequate lighting and privacy should be maintained. Medications for performance of blocks and rescue medication including a stocked and checked code cart need to be present. Suction, oxygen, intubating equipment, and ventilatory equipment need to be available. Proper needles and ancillary equipment such as neurostimulators, ultrasound, or fluoroscopy should have a proper place in the block area. Sedative and anxiolytics can be brought in from a secure location. Finally, it may be prudent to have a supply of intralipids readily available to reverse accidental local anesthetic cardiotoxicity.

The patient flow through the postanesthesia care unit to the floor or intensive care unit should be evaluated. Processes such as completion of postoperative pain orders and evaluation and treatment of patients with agreements on intervention need to be established.

When the patient reaches the floor or intensive care unit, treatment plans such as physical therapy and feeding need to be incorporated to maximize the benefits of regional analgesia. Discharge planning is an important part of the process and

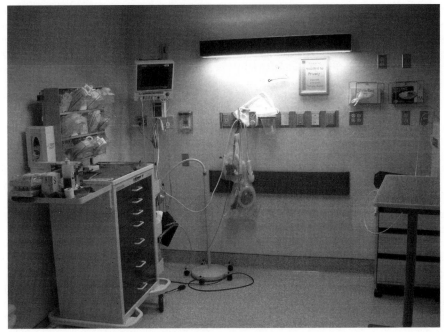

Figure 27.3: A dedicated regional/neuraxial block area.

communication with the primary services on conversions in pain management therapy need to implemented smoothly to avoid analgesic gaps. Medication flow from the pharmacy is another important aspect of avoiding analgesic gaps. Thus, treatment plans need to be established to improve patient flow through the hospital as well as to provide outstanding care.

Documentation plays a vital role in this process. Prewritten order sheets for patient-controlled analgesia (PCA), epidural analgesia, peripheral nerve blocks and catheters, ketamine infusions, procedures notes,[17] and follow-up daily management notes are important parts of improving efficiency and communication (see the appendix for standardized orders for IV PCA, neuraxial analgesia, continuous neural blockade, and IV ketamine). Standardized orders allow for consistency of care, improved communication, and a decrease in errors.

Periodic audits and quality assurance mechanisms need to be established. This provides the service with the ability to critically evaluate the effectiveness, side effects, and complications of the various treatments. The typical process consists of establishment of processes, implementation of processes, audit of processes, re-evaluation of treatment methods, and back to establishment of improved processes. Typical indicators for measurement include numerical pain scores, ability to ambulate, discharge times, naloxone usage, and patient satisfaction. The latter can be measured through surveys handed to patients or through an outside agency.

The Harvard Business School teaches their students to use the 7 Ms of production and operation management[18] to improve an operation. These 7 Ms are as follows: man- and womanpower, materials, machines, managers, messages, methods, and money. It is an easy pneumonic to remember when evaluating any process. These can be applied to improving efficiency of the APMS and hospital patient flow. There are always different solutions for every problem. Finding the best solution for any hospital will involve teamwork, communication, and an appreciation for what is practical.

ECONOMICS

The U.S. medical establishment is based on capitalism. Thus, if physicians wish to have an income, they must generate it. Although many academic institutions will state that the APMS and regional analgesia procedures do not have to be profitable, so long as they provide good care and an educational experience for their residents, it is always desirable to be in the position of generating income for the group. Hospitals are also concerned with being financially solvent.

Economic considerations involve improving assets (income, good will) and decreasing expenses (hospital stay, complications, operating room efficiency, staff, materials, infrastructure, etc). Thus, the financial benefits of improving patients' pain come from two sources: income from procedures and consultation and by decreasing overall hospital costs.

Regional analgesic techniques are billable so long as they are considered as for postoperative analgesia and not as the true anesthetic. The procedures are best documented on a separate form from the anesthetic record.[19] A copy of this record should be sent to the billing office as insurance companies frequently request documentation prior to payment.

Most of the regional analgesic techniques are listed under surgical codes. This has created a rather confusing situation where many carriers will not allow anesthesiologists to bill for these regional techniques while supervising another room or billing for time. This has caused many practices to either not venture into performing regional analgesic techniques or needing to assign extra staff at an increased cost to their departments.

Single injections of long-acting medications generally receive[67] 5–6 units and catheters receive 12–14 units (Viscusi, personal communication). However, these rates are negotiable with private insurance carriers. As the pain management physician is usually not involved with the negotiations, rates are often undernegotiated. This process is part of the reason for the exodus of chronic pain management physicians from anesthesiology groups, where units for surgical anesthesiology are negotiated at the same time as reimbursement for interventional pain therapies. Because their reimbursement rates are no longer being negotiated with typical anesthesiology units, they are able to secure better contracts as a separate entity. It is important that reimbursement rates are evaluated prior to initiation of a regional analgesia service and then periodically to obtain appropriate reimbursement for these procedures.

The outpatient arena presents other financial challenges. Many carriers will not reimburse for regional techniques if the procedure is not preapproved. This creates bureaucratic hurdles that in effect limit patient access to these pain-relieving procedures.

If the pain service is also going to perform consultations in the hospital, appropriate codes must also be used. These involve evaluation and management (E&M) codes, which have unique rules. Basically, the proper code is based on the level of decision making involved in the evaluation and management of the patient. The more complicated the pain management, the more evaluation and management are needed and the higher the code. As always, more documentation is needed with higher codes. Codes change and the ICD 10 codes will be arriving soon after submission of this chapter.

The value of goodwill is always difficult to document in a spreadsheet and is thus often overlooked. An APMS improves patient satisfaction in a variety of ways. Providing regional analgesia via epidural, single shot peripheral nerve block, or peripheral nerve catheters are associated with improved patient satisfaction. Being available to provide consultation and management for the most difficult patients in the hospital satisfies not only the patients, but also the nursing and physician staff who attend to them.

GOVERNMENTAL ASPECTS

The government has influence on the practice of medicine. In the United States, the state government influences practices through state specific laws and regulations that define educational requirements and determine scope of practice. For example, in New York State, there has been extensive lobbying by the cancer organizations to have mandatory education in pain management for all physicians ending with a test to demonstrate that the knowledge has been obtained. In Louisiana, nurse anesthetists have tried to increase their scope of practice to include pain management procedures.

On the federal level, CMS (Centers for Medicare and Medicaid Services) determines the rates and rules regarding the practice of pain management as well as for the rest of medicine. With the development of peripheral nerve catheters, CMS has changed our normal way of billing when compared to epidural management. For epidural management, an anesthesiologist can bill for the daily management of the catheter. For peripheral nerve catheters, CMS has placed a 10-day global care addendum to the placement of the catheter. Thus peripheral nerve catheters are treated like procedures of our surgical colleagues who have their postoperative care bundled into the procedural fee and we cannot bill for daily management.

Modifiers can be used when a different procedure is necessary for patient care (a patient who has suffered a multiple traumatic event requires a brachial plexus catheter and then a few days later requires a sciatic catheter for a different operation)

but these should be used with caution as they serve as "red flags" for automated audits. The use of modifiers to simply uncouple bundled aspects of a procedure should never be used.

Physicians have input in these matters through their state and national society associations. For antitrust reasons they cannot boycott or discuss specific fee amounts; however, they do provide recommendations through the *Relative Value Guide.* Recommendations for reimbursement are forwarded for consideration to CMS and insurance companies, but CMS and insurance companies are not under any obligation to accept or implement them.

The leader of the APMS is obliged to stay current and should become involved in their national and state societies. Through these societies, the practice of acute pain management and the care of our patients can be improved.

THE FUTURE

It is important to be prepared for changes in pain treatments. Business models that work today are obsolete tomorrow. In the past, placing an intravenous line was considered a medically invasive procedure only to be performed by a physician. Today, it is basic nursing care. Nurses in England have already started to venture into femoral nerve blocks for patients with fractured hips. In the future, PCA machines may be replaced by credit card-sized analgesic pumps. Peripheral nerve catheters could be replaced by long-acting local anesthetics or other unknown medications. Ultrasound is revolutionizing the performance of regional anesthesiology and could move regional anesthesiology as a subspecialty of anesthesiology to a procedure taught to other areas of medicine.

The business of acute pain management presented in this chapter will change over time. Scope of practice is constantly changing. Many of the managerial aspects will not and can be applied to other areas of our practice.

REFERENCES

1. Practice guidelines for acute pain management in the perioperative setting. A report by the American Society of Anesthesiologists Task Force on Pain Management, Acute Pain Section. *Anesthesiology.*1995;1071–1081.
2. An updated report by the American Society of Anesthesiologists Task Force on Acute Pain Management. *Anesthesiology.* 2004;100:1573.
3. *Acute pain management: operative or medical procedures and trauma.* Agency for Health Care Policy and Research Clinical practice guidelines number. US Department of Health and Human Service, Publication #92–0032. Rockville, MD: AHCPR Publications, 1992.
4. Apfelbaum JL, Chen C, Mehta SS, Gan TJ. Postoperative pain experience: results from a national survey suggest postoperative pain continues to be undermanaged. *Anesth Analg.* 2003;92(2):534–540.
5. Joint Commission on the Accreditation of Health Care Organizations. *Accreditation Manual for Hospitals.* Oakbrook Terrace, IL: JCAHO; 2001.
6. McDonnel A, Nicholl H, Read S: Acute Pain Teams in England: current provision and their role in postoperative pain management. *J Clin Nurs.* 2003;12:387–393.

7. Coleman S, Booker-Milburn J. Audit of postoperative pain control: influence of a dedicated acute pain nurse. *Anaesthesia.* 1996;51:1093–1096.

8. Bardiau F, Braeckman M, Seidel L, et al. Effectiveness of an acute pain service in a general hospital. *J Clin Anesth.* 1999;11:583–589.

9. Musclow SL. A community hospital acute pain service. *Can Nurs.* 2005;101(9):29–33.

10. Gordon DB, Pellino TA, Enloe MG, Foley DK. A nurse-run inpatient pain consultation service. *Pain Manage Nurs.* 2000;1(2):29–33.

11. Musclow SL, Sawhney M, Watt-Watson J. The emerging role of advanced nursing practice in acute pain management throughout Canada. *Clin Nurse Spec.* 2002;16(2):63–67.

12. Rawal N. Organization, function, and implementation of acute pain service. *Anesthesiol Clin North Am.* 2005;23(1):211–225.

13. Neal JM, Kopacz DJ, Liguori GA, Beckman JD, Margett MJ. The training and careers of regional anesthesia fellows: 1983–2002. *Reg Anesth Pain Med.* 2005;30(3):226–232.

14. Smith MP, Sprung J, Zura A, Mascha E, Tetzlaff JE. A survey of exposure to regional anesthesia techniques in American anesthesia residency training programs. *Reg Anesth Pain Med.* 1999;24(1):11–16.

15. Oldman M, McCartney CJ, Leung A, et al. A survey or orthopedic surgeon's attitudes and knowledge regarding regional anesthesia. *Anesth Analg.* 2004;5:1486–1490.

16. Armstrong KP, Cherry RA. Brachial plexus anesthesia compared to general anesthesia when a block room is available. *Can J Anaesth.* 2004;51(1):41–44.

17. Gerancher JC, Viscusi ER, Ligouri GA, et al. Development of a standardized peripheral nerve block procedure note form. *Reg Anesth Pain Med.* 2005;30(1):67–71.

18. Kelly FJ, Kelly HM. *What They Really Teach You at the Harvard Business School.* New York, NY: Warner Books; 1986: 137.

19. Liu SS, Wu CL. The effect of analgesic technique on postoperative patient outcomes including analgesia: a systemic review. *Anesth Analg.* 2007;105(3):789–808.

20. Shapiro A, Zohar E, Kantor M, Memrod J, Fredman B. Establishing a nurse-based, anesthesiologist supervised inpatient acute pain service: experience of 4,617 patients. *J Clin Anesth.* 2004;16(6):415–420.

21. Sartain JB, Barry JJ. The impact of an acute pain service on postoperative pain management. *Anaesth Intensive Care.* 1999;27(4):375–380.

22. Tighe SO, Bie JA, Nelson RA, Skues MA. The acute pain service: effective or expensive care? *Anaesthesia* 1998;53(4): 397–403

23. Luscombe FE, Wallace L, Williams J, Griffiths DP. A district general hospital pain management programme: first year experiences and outcomes. *Anaesthesia.* 1995;50(2):114–117.

24. Werner M, Selholm L, Rotbell-Nielsen P, et al. Does an acute pain service improve postoperative outcome? *Anesth Analg.* 2002;95:1361–1372.

25. Layzell M. Pain management: setting up a nurse-led femoral nerve block service. *Br J Nurs.* 2007;16(12):702–705.

26. Viscusi ER, Reynolds l, Tait S, Melson T, Atkinson LE. An iotophoretic fentanyl patient-activated analgesic delivery system for postoperative pain: a double-blind, placebo-controlled trial. *Anesth Analg.* 2006;102(10):188–194.

27. Stone MB, Price DD, Wang R. Ultrasound-guided supraclavicular block for the treatment of upper extremity fractures, dislocations, and abscesses in the ED. *Am J Emerg Med.* 2007;25(4):472–475.

Appendices

ACUTE PAIN SERVICE
INTRAVENOUS PATIENT CONTROLLED
ANALGESIA (PCA)
STANDARD ORDER FORM

DOSE RANGES ARE PROVIDED AS GUIDELINES. INDIVIDUAL PATIENTS MAY NEED DOSING OUTSIDE RANGE.

ALLERGIES: PATIENT WEIGHT (required for pediatric patient):

Agent (circle one, cross out 2)	Morphine 1 milligram/mL	Hydromorphone (DILAUDID) 2 milligrams/mL Normal Saline	Fentanyl 50 Micrograms/mL	RN Initial
1. Demand Dose	_____ mg (1-2.5 mg)	_____ mg (0.3-0.7 mg)	_____ micrograms (10-30 micrograms)	
2. Lockout interval	_____ minutes (5-15 minutes)	_____ minutes (5-15 minutes)	_____ minutes (5-15 minutes)	
3. Continuous rate	_____ mg/hr (0.5-1 mg/hr) (Caution in opioid naïve patients)	_____ mg/hr (0.1-0.4 mg/hr) (Caution in opioid naïve patients)	_____ micrograms/hr (10-30 micrograms /hr) (Continuous rate may be necessary)	
4. Four hour limit If 4 hour limit reached, assess patient, and call Acute Pain Service (APS).	No / Yes _____ mg	No / Yes _____ mg	No / Yes _____ micrograms	
5. Loading Dose (At initiation therapy or additional analgesia during therapy)	_____ mg (2-3 mg) Q _____ minutes Maximum _____ mg	_____ mg (0.5-1 mg) Q _____ minutes Maximum _____ mg	_____ micrograms (25-100 micrograms) Q _____ minutes Max. _____ micrograms	
6. Inadequate Analgesia May increase demand dose ONCE by this amount if VAS > 4/10 AND OAAS SEDATION SCORE >3/5.	_____ mg	_____ mg	_____ micrograms	
7. When initiating PCA, Document vital signs, pain score, sedation score (OAAS) every 15 minutes for 1 hour. **Respiratory rate, pain score and sedation score (OAAS) must be monitored every 2 hours for 18 hours then every 4 hours while on PCA.**				
8. With Loading Dose, Syringe change, or Setting change: monitor respiratory rate, pain score, sedation score (OAAS) every 15 minutes for 30 minutes, then every 4 hours while on PCA.				
MD/LIP/NP Signature:		ID#:	Date:	Time:
Nurse Signature:		ID#:	Date:	Time:

PAGE 1 OF 2   AN2C002 (9/06)
SCAN WHITE COPY TO PHARMACY AND PLACE IN PATIENT CHART
YELLOW: ACUTE PAIN SERVICES

Appendix 1: Standardized orderset for IV PCA.

CONTINUOUS PERIPHERAL NERVE AND PLEXUS ANALGESIA ORDERS
☐ Postoperative Orders

DATE / TIME	ORDERS: **MUST** INCLUDE PHYSICIAN'S SIGNATURE AND ID#	INITIALS / ID #
	1. _____ mg of Bupivacaine / Ropivacaine with _____ in _____ mL of preservative free normal saline.	
	a. Basal/Continuous infusion Rate:_____mL/hr.	
	b. PCA dose: _____ mL.	
	c. Delay / Lockout interval: _____min.	
	d. Maximum dose in 1 hour: _____mL.	
	e. Initial loading dose: _____ mL	
	2. Monitor VS, level of sedation and pain score q 15 min x 4; Subsequent to initiation, document pain score q4hrs and vital signs per primary service for the duration of therapy.	
	3. Maintain an intravenous access.	
	4. Keep O_2 setup and ambu bag at bedside.	
	5. Call Acute Pain Service (APS) for:	
	a. Inadequate analgesia.	
	b. Displacement or disconnection of catheters.	
	c. Removal of catheters when discontinuing treatment.	
	6. Stop Infusion and Call APS and the Primary Service for signs of local anesthetic toxicity:	
	a. Hypotension (Systolic less than 90)	
	b. confusion/lightheadedness	
	c. tinnitus	
	d. visual disturbances	
	e. paraesthesia	
	Acute Pain Service may be reached: Short range: 8393 Long range: 733-6016 In emergency and if no response to above, call the Anesthesia Coordinator 4-7481 or call 4-2444 and ask for the Anesthesia Attending.	
	_____ MD/LIP/NP Signature ID# Date Time	
	_____ Nurses Signature ID# Date Time	

DISTRIBUTION: WHITE- MEDICAL RECORDS

AN2C015 (3/02)

Appendix 5: Standardized orderset for continuous peripheral nerve and plexus analgesia.

**REGIONAL BLOCK
SEDATION AND ANALGESIA
RECORD**

PRE-PROCEDURE

Date:_____ Time:_____

For MD to complete:

ASA Class (circle one): I II III IV V

Please check when complete:

☐ Regional Anesthesia Consent Form Completed   ☐ Anesthesia pre-operative evaluation

☐ Surgical Consent Reviewed

Regional Anesthesia Procedure:_____

Attending MD Signature:_____ ID#:_____

For RN/MD monitor to complete:

NPO since:_____ BP:_____/_____ Pulse:_____ Resp:_____ Body Weight:_____kg

Allergies:_____

Aldrete Score

Activity	Respirations	Circulation BP is	Consciousness	Color
2 = Moves 4 limbs	2 = Deep breaths/coughs freely	2 = 20mmHg baseline	2 = Fully awake	2 = Pink
1 = Moves 2 limbs	1 = Dyspnea/Limited breathing	1 = 21-50mmHg baseline	1 = Arousable on calling	1 = Pale/dusky
0 = Moves 0 limbs	0 = Apneic	0 = 51mmHg baseline	0 = Not Responding	0 = Cyanotic
ACTIVITY +	RESPIRATIONS +	CIRCULATION +	CONSCIOUSNESS +	COLOR = TOTAL

Monitors: ☐ Cardiac   Safety precautions: ☐ Fall precautions band applied

☐ Pulse Oxymetry   ☐ Siderails Up

☐ B/P

☐ IV_____ O₂ Therapy (circle): No Yes – Amount via:_____

Comments:

RN/MD Monitor Signature:_____ Title:_____ ID#:_____

SIDE 1 OF 2   AP2C001 (1/07)

Appendix 6: Standardized orders for regional analgesia and sedation.

North Shore LIJ *Huntington Hospital*
North Shore-Long Island Jewish Health System

Name:
DOB: Age: Sex:
Acct#:   Religion:
MR#:
Attending MD:
Admitted on:

PAIN MANAGEMENT ORDER SHEET
INTRAVENOUS PCA

(Recommended for patients over 40 kg)

Allergies: _____ Height: _____ Weight: _____ lb _____ kg ☐ Actual ☐ Estimated

Pregnant: ☐ Yes ☐ No   Breast Feeding: ☐ Yes ☐ No

DATE: _____ TIME: _____

1. **SELECT** drug therapy **(ONE DRUG <u>ONLY</u>):** If questions, please contact **prescriber**

☐ <u>MORPHINE 5 mg/mL</u>	☐ <u>HYDROMORPHONE 1 mg/mL</u>	☐ <u>FENTANYL 50mcg/mL</u>
Loading dose (2-5mg) _____ mg	**Loading dose (0.3-0.5mg)** _____ mg	**Loading dose (25-75mcg)** _____ mcg
☐ One dose <u>only</u>	☐ One dose <u>only</u>	☐ One dose <u>only</u>
☐ Repeat X ___ , ___ minutes apart	☐ Repeat X _____ , ___ minutes apart	☐ Repeat X _____ , _____ minutes apart
PCA dose (1-2mg) _____ **mg**	**PCA dose (0.2-0.4mg)** _____ **mg**	**PCA dose (10-25mcg)** _____ **mcg**
Lockout interval (5-15 min)____ minutes	Lockout interval (5-15 min) _____ minutes	Lockout interval (5-15 min) _____ minutes
Continuous rate (1-2mg/hr) ____ **mg/hr**	**Continuous rate (0.2-0.4mg/hr)** ____ **mg/hr**	**Continuous rate (10-25mcg/hr)**____ **mcg/hr**
Total dose _____ mg in 4 hrs (50 mg maximum)	Total dose _____ mg in 4 hrs (10 mg maximum)	Total dose _____ mcg in 4 hrs (500 mcg maximum)

2. **SUPPORTIVE** therapy medication(s) while on PCA.
   For itching: Naloxone (Narcan®) 0.1mg SC q 2h PRN

   For nausea: Ondansetron (Zofran®) 4mg IVP q 6h PRN
   If ineffective after 20 minutes call anesthesiologist/prescriber

   ☐ Oxygen via nasal cannula at _____ L/min

3. While on PCA **NO** sedatives, opioids or other respiratory depressants are to be given, <u>except</u> by order of an anesthesiologist.

4. **MONITOR** vital signs (BP, HR, RR), sedation level, pain level and pump settings and document:
   a. q 1 hour X 2, then q 4 hours
   b. q 4 hours for duration of PCA.
   c. q 1 hour X 2 after **any change,** then q 4 hours

5. **RESCUE: If respiratory rate falls below 6 per minute with changes in level of sedation:**
   a. Stop PCA infusion pump
   b. Give naloxone (Narcan®) 0.2 mg IVP, may repeat X 1 in 5 minutes if RR remains below 6 per minute.
   c. Call prescriber <u>immediately.</u>

6. **OTHER** instructions: _____
   _____

Signature: _____ # _____ Beeper # _____

Orders verified by: _____ RN _____ RN

1PO

Rev. 4/07   #1-369

Figure 28.5: IV PCA order sheet.

North Shore LIJ Huntington Hospital
North Shore-Long Island Jewish Health System

Name:
DOB: Age: Sex:
Acct#:   Religion:
MR#:
Attending MD:
Admitted on:

PAIN MANAGEMENT ORDER SHEET
EPIDURAL INFUSION

Allergies: _____   Pregnant: ☐Yes ☐ No   Breast Feeding: ☐ Yes   ☐ No

Height: _____   Weight: _____ lb _____ kg ☐ Actual ☐ Estimated

Date: _____   **Time:** _____

1. The patient has an **epidural catheter** in place, which is to be handled only by an anesthesiologist. Patient has received:

Drug(s):_____   Time:_____   Date:_____

2. **SELECT** drug therapy (**ONE** preservative free drug **ONLY**) and initiate via **Infusion Pump**

Morphine 50 mcg/mL +	**Hydromorphone 10 mcg/mL+**	**Fentanyl 4 mcg/mL +**
bupivacaine 0.04%	bupivacaine 0.04%	bupivacaine 0.04%
Continuous Rate: _____ mL/hr	**Continuous** Rate: _____ mL/hr	**Continuous** Rate: _____ mL/hr
Demand Dose (PCEA):	**Demand** Dose (PCEA):	**Demand** Dose (PCEA):
☐ 3mL every 10 minutes	☐ 3mL every 10 minutes	☐ 3mL every 10 minutes
☐ 5mL every 10 minutes	☐ 5mL every 10 minutes	☐ 5mL every 10 minutes
☐ 5mL every 15 minutes	☐ 5mL every 15 minutes -	☐ 5mL every 15 minutes
☐ ____ mL every ____ minutes	☐ ____ mL every ____ minutes	☐ ____ mL every ____ minutes

3. **SUPPORTIVE THERAPY** medication(s) while on epidural
    For itching: Naloxone (Narcan®) 0.1 mg SC q 2h PRN
    For nausea: Ondansetron (Zofran®) 4 mg IVP q 6 h PRN. If ineffective after 20 minutes call anesthesiologist .
    ☐ Oxygen via nasal cannula at _____ L/min

4. **MAINTAIN** IV saline lock for duration of epidural infusion.

5. **RESCUE** If Respiratory Rate (**RR) falls below 8/minute** with changes in sedation level.
    a. Stop infusion pump
    b. Give naloxone (Narcan®) **0.2 mg** IVP, may repeat X 1, in 5 minutes if RR remains below 8/min
    c. Call anesthesiologist immediately

6. **MONITOR** vital signs (BP, HR, RR), sedation level, pain level and pump settings and document on PMFS:
    a. q 15 MINUTES X 1 hour, then
    b. q 2 hour for duration of infusion

7. **NO** sedatives, opioids or other respiratory depressants are to be given, except by order of an anesthesiologist.

8. **CALL** anesthesiologist if patient has:
    a. Change in level of sedation, lethargy, increased somnolence.
    b. Systolic BP less than 90
    c. Evidence of airway obstruction, change in respiratory pattern, decrease in respiratory effort, respiratory rate less than 10/min.
    d. Complains of weakness or numbness in lower extremities, pain, urinary retention, severe itching, severe nausea or vomiting

9. **CHECK** and document patient's ability to maintain motor function in lower extremities.
    Patient may ambulate only under the following circumstances:
    a. Have a surgical order to ambulate.
    b. Registered nurse assesses the patient and verifies absence of residual weakness or motor block.
    c. Patient is able to stand without assistance
    d. Patient must be assisted by RN or LPN while ambulating

10. **NOTIFY** anesthesia if anticoagulants, thrombolytics, anti-platelets or IIb IIIa inhibitors are ordered by another physician prior to administration.

> DO NOT administer enoxaparin (Lovenox®) or any LMW heparins until 12 hours after epidural catheter is discontinued.
> Notify anesthesia before IV or SC heparin therapy is started.
> Notify anesthesia if warfarin (Coumadin®) is ordered after the day of surgery.

11. **CONTACT** anesthesiologist on call if primary anesthesiologist is unavailable (after 8 pm, on weekends & holidays).

Signature: _____   # _____ Beeper #: _____

Orders verified by: _____   RN _____   RN

1PO

#1-371   Rev. 4/07

Figure 28.6: Epidural infusion order sheet.

North Shore LIJ *Huntington Hospital*
North Shore-Long Island Jewish Health System

PAIN MANAGEMENT ORDER SHEET
CONTINUOUS REGIONAL ANALGESIA

Name:
DOB: Age: Sex:
Acct#:   Religion:
MR#:
Attending MD:
Admitted on:

Allergies: _____

Height: _____

Weight: _____lb _____ kg ☐ Actual ☐ Estimated

Pregnant: ☐Yes   ☐ No   Breast Feeding: ☐ Yes   ☐ No

Date: _____ Time: _____

1. **Catheter site:**
   ☐ Axillary   ☐ Femoral
   ☐ Infraclavicular   ☐ Popliteal
   ☐ Interscalene   ☐ Psoas
   ☐ Fascia iliac   ☐ Other (specify): _____

2. **ENSURE** that catheter site, infusion and tubing (no ports) are clearly labeled.
   Catheter positioned at _____ cm at skin.
   DO NOT MANIPULATE catheter.

3. **DRUG:**
   ☐ Ropivacaine (Naropin®) 0.2% (2mg/mL)
   ☐ Other: _____ .

4. **DOSING:**
   ☐ Manual Loading (**by anesthesiologist only**): Dose _____ mL
   ☐ Continuous Infusion via pump: Rate _____ mL/hr (Max. 25mL/hr).
   ☐ Titrate: _____
   ☐ Other: _____

5. **MAINTAIN** IV access during drug administration (Saline lock).

6. **MONITOR** and document data as per Pain Management Flowsheet q 4 hours.

7. **Additional** pain management:
   ☐ PCA (see PCA order sheet).
   Other: _____

8. **CALL** anesthesiologist if patient has:
   a. Inadequate pain relief.
   b. Signs of toxicity (e.g. ringing in the ears, perioral numbness or tingling, change in sedation level or mental changes).
   c. SBP above _____ or below _____; sustained heart rate above _____ bpm or below_____ bpm.
   d. Kinking or dislodgment of catheter.
   e. Catheter site problems (e.g. leaking, edema, erythema and/or signs of infection).
   f. Lower Extremity Motor Block; **score of 2 or above** on the 0-3 Bromage scale.

9. **CONTACT anesthesiologist on call,** for any problems (Ext. **2491** or **2353**) if primary anesthesiologist is unavailable (after 8 pm, on weekends & holidays).

10. **AMBULATE** Patient may ambulate only under the following circumstances:
    a. Have a physician's order to ambulate.
    b. Registered nurse assesses the patient and verifies absence of residual weakness or motor block.
    c. Patient is able to stand without assistance.
    d. Patient **must be assisted** by RN, LPN or P.T. while ambulating.

Signature: _____ # _____ Telephone # _____ Beeper # _____

Orders verified by: _____ RN _____ RN

IPO

#1-370   Rev. 4/07

Figure 28.7: Regional analgesia order sheet.

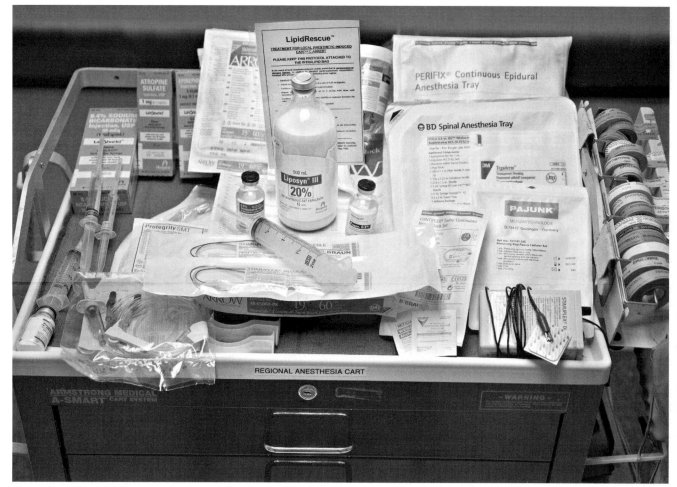

Figure 28.8: Photo of the contents of a typical regional anesthesia cart. The cart includes, catheters, stimulators, local anesthetic solutions, gowns, gloves, and prep solutions. Of importance, the cart is also stocked with resuscitative medications and intralipid solution for emergency treatment of bupivacaine/ropivacaine cardiotoxicity.

The anesthesiology-based options available can be considered through a spectrum of complexity (Figure 28.9). A brief consideration of the more commonly encountered modalities is presented below from a community practice perspective.

LOW COMPLEXITY

Low complexity options represent the ultimate in physician-directed, nurse-administered pain management. Intravenous patient-controlled analgesia (IV-PCA), a relatively simple modality, constitutes the analgesia default mode. Intravenous PCA should be sufficiently established at virtually all institutions to be

---

Low Complexity
   Intravenous PCA

Moderate Complexity
   Single-dose intrathecal opiates
   Single-dose epidural opiates
   Single-injection nerve blocks

High Complexity
   Continuous epidural analgesia
   Continuous perineural analgesia

Figure 28.9: Anesthesia-based pain management options.

able to be initiated and maintained by nurses without hands-on interaction by physicians.

Intravenous PCA[25]

The availability and ease of IV PCA has helped make it one of the most widely used methods for acute pain management. Intravenous PCA is generally safe and effective, with its primary disadvantage being a heavy reliance on opiates (with expected side effects). Although many agents have been used by this route, morphine is probably most commonly employed, with fentanyl an attractive alternative if metabolites are a concern. Meperidine use, with possible accumulation of normeperidine, is generally discouraged and should be reserved for patients intolerant to other options. The addition of continuous background infusions is associated with a marked increase in the risk of respiratory depression and should therefore be reserved for opioid-tolerant patients. Despite the commonplace use of IV PCA by many specialties, anesthesiologists are encouraged to cultivate a detailed knowledge of this approach to ensure maximal patient benefit.[26] Recommended doses for PCA are presented in Figure 28.10.

Recently, transdermal fentanyl PCA systems have been developed and may have desirable advantages over traditional intravenous PCA, particularly when employed with continuous regional analgesia.[27] By using this small device, the need for two

Drug	Demand Dose	Lockout (min)	Continuous Basal
Morphine	1–2 mg	6–10	0–2 mg/hr
Fentanyl	20–50 μg	5–10	0–60 μg/hr
Hydromorphone	0.2–.04 mg	6–10	0–0.4 mg/hr
Meperidine	10–20 mg	6–10	0–20 mg/hr

Figure 28.10: Suggested IV PCA regimens.

cumbersome infusion devices that interfere with ambulation, is obviated.

MODERATE COMPLEXITY

Modalities considered to be of moderate complexity encompass a wide range of options. They can be distinguished from low-complexity approaches by the requirement for hands-on initiation (which also implies some degree of operator dependence) and from high-complexity approaches by their limited duration of action. Appropriate management of these options requires a higher level of assessment skills by nursing personnel than low-complexity options.

Single-Dose Intrathecal Opiates[28]

Usually used in addition to single-dose spinal local anesthetics, intrathecal opiates are capable of providing significant analgesic effects. Because of its prolonged effect (up to 24 hours), preservative-free morphine is most commonly employed for postoperative analgesia. The limitations of this option are the risks of spinal anesthesia (postdural puncture headache, etc) as well as dose-related opioid-mediated side effects. The ideal dose of morphine used for intrathecal analgesia will depend on the specific surgical procedure and patient population. Efforts to determine the optimal intrathecal morphine dose in specific clinical settings have commonly sought the best balance between analgesic efficacy and side effects (notably nausea, pruritis and delayed respiratory depression). The risk of delayed respiratory depression mandates close patient observation and limits the use of intrathecal morphine to inpatients.

Although continuous epidural analgesia has been successfully used for many lower abdominal or lower extremity surgeries, single-dose subarachnoid opiates often presents a more practical approach to pain relief in the community practice setting, especially when patients are expected to be able to tolerate oral analgesics within 24 hours (such as cesarean delivery, abdominal hysterectomy, radical prostatectomy, or total hip/knee arthroplasty).

Single-Dose Epidural Opioids

Similar to subarachnoid opiates, epidural opiates may result in prolonged analgesia after a single administration. However, single-injection epidural opioids are uncommonly utilized in modern practice and perhaps most often administered just prior to discontinuing a continuous epidural catheter. Similar to intrathecal dosing, optimal doses of epidural opioids depend on the specific surgical procedure and patient population. Once again, dose-related opioid-mediated side effects (including respiratory depression) are limitations of this option.

An extended duration version of single dose epidural morphine is currently available (DepoDur), and has been demonstrated to provide epidural analgesia for 48 hours.[29] Although limited studies have favorably compared this novel delivery of morphine to other opiate regimens, it may be most reasonably utilized in low dose as the opiate component of a multimodal analgesic approach.

Single-Injection Nerve Blocks[30]

Single-injection nerve blocks may block peripheral nerves or nerve plexuses. The widespread application of single-injection peripheral nerve/plexus blocks for postoperative pain control is arguably the greatest advance in pain management during the past decade. Single injections of long-acting local anesthetics can provide a reasonably extended duration of pain relief without opioid-related side effects (femoral block with 25 mL bupivacaine [0.25%] + epinephrine [1:200 000], for example, has a duration of action of 23.2 ± 7 hours).[31] Addition of adjuncts such as preservative-free clonidine (at doses up to 150 μg) to local anesthetics may further prolong the action of single injection blocks.[32] The primary disadvantages of single injection blocks are the production of motor blockade and potential injury of an insensate limb. Although all perineural injections have an inherent risk of neuropathy, this feared complication has generally been demonstrated to be temporary and rare.[33]

In the community practice setting, single-injection techniques have obvious appeal and may be more appropriate than continuous options in many clinical circumstances. Single-injection femoral nerve block, for example, has been demonstrated to provide significant pain relief following total knee arthroplasty and, in this situation, may be more practical than continuous femoral block as hospital length of stay and long-term functional recovery appear to be similar between the two approaches.[34]

HIGH COMPLEXITY

All continuous techniques should be considered to be of high complexity and have been demonstrated to be capable of providing superior levels of pain control over prolonged periods of time. The addition of patient-controlled bolus features may further improve patient satisfaction and decrease the total amount of drug administered. Despite these advantages, it must be acknowledged that, when compared to single-injection techniques, continuous techniques require special supplies, take longer to perform, are more operator-dependent to initiate, and are more labor intensive to maintain. Indwelling catheters are also associated with mechanical problems, infectious risks, and concerns regarding coagulation status (particularly in the case of epidural catheters). Appropriate management of high-complexity options requires a specialized level of nursing education and assessment skills. In the community practice setting, continuous techniques are best used selectively and reserved for situations requiring treatment of severe pain for significantly longer than 24 hours.

Continuous Epidural Analgesia[35]

Continuous epidural analgesia has been demonstrated to provide superior pain relief, especially during movement (eg, coughing), in many clinical circumstances and is associated with some improved clinical outcomes. Its use is particularly appropriate for major thoracic and upper abdominal surgeries. Epidural infusions result in segmental analgesia in the vicinity of the catheter, with optimal catheter placement corresponding to the dermatomal distribution of the patient's pain. Limitations of continuous epidural analgesia include adverse effects of both local anesthetics (hemodynamically significant sympathectomy, motor block) and opioids (pruritis, nausea, respiratory

Local Anesthetic		+	Opioid	Concentration
Bupivacaine	0.04–0.125%		Fentanyl	4–6 µg/ml
Ropivacaine	0.0625–0.2%		Morphine	40–60 µg/ml
			Hydromorphone	8–12 µg/ml

Examples: Bupivacaine 0.0625% + Fentanyl 5 µg/ml
Bupivacaine 0.05% + Hydromorphone 10 µg/ml

Epidural infusion solutions usually consist of a fixed combination of local anesthetic and opioid. Whereas any number of combinations are possible, some general rules are:
*Lower concentrations of bupivacaine or ropivacaine are commonly used with lumbar catheters because of the possibility of lower extremity weakness.
*Continuous infusion rates are dependent on the catheter site, with higher infusion rates required for lumbar (6–18 ml/hr) than thoracic catheters (4–12 ml/hr).
*For patient-controlled epidural analgesia (PCEA), background infusion rates are usually decreased by around 30% and bolus demand volumes are 30%–50% of the hourly rate (usually 3–5 ml with a lockout interval of 10–15 minutes).
*Patients intolerant of opiates can be placed on an epidural infusion of local anesthetic alone.

Figure 28.11: Suggested regimens for continuous epidural infusions.

depression). However, dilute combinations employing both local anesthetics and opioids are routinely utilized to minimize side effects and maximize benefits. Serious risks of continuous epidural analgesia are rare, but include epidural hematoma and infection. The combined spinal-epidural technique is a variation on simple continuous epidural analgesia and can compensate for the delayed onset seen with initiation of epidural analgesia alone.

In the community practice setting, a compelling justification for continuous epidural analgesia can be made in specific situations where multiple significant benefits have been demonstrated, such as abdominal aortic surgery.[36] Recommended doses and infusion rates for continuous epidural analgesia is presented in Figure 28.11.

Continuous Perineural Analgesia[37]

Continuous perineural analgesia, directed toward peripheral nerves or plexuses, can be utilized to provide targeted long-lasting pain control with minimal adverse effects.[38] As with single-injection nerve blocks, the major advantage of continuous blocks is their nonopiate mechanism of action. Despite the use of dilute solutions of local anesthetics for continuous techniques, motor blockade is still frequently encountered and should be anticipated. Continuous perineural analgesia is frequently associated with minor adverse events (notably including accidental withdrawal of the catheter) and bacterial colonization, but infrequently with serious complications.[39] Although experience is limited, continuous peripheral nerve blocks have also recently been demonstrated to be safe and effective when used in the outpatient setting.[40] At present, many anesthesiologists in community practice have limited experience with these newer techniques, and continuous peripheral nerve blocks are only sporadically used outside of academic settings. However, practitioners intimidated by these techniques should take heart in the fact that most institutions have "cleared" the technically larger hurdle of continuous epidural analgesia. Recommended doses and infusion rates for continuous perineural analgesia is presented in Figure 28.12.

Agent	Concentration	Manufacturers' recommended Maximum 24-hour dose
Bupivacaine	0.125%	400 mg
Ropivacaine	0.2%	770 mg

Peripheral nerve blocks are usually established with large volumes of local anesthetic (20–40 ml) prior to initiating continuous perineural infusions.

Four approaches to most continuous perineural blocks are commonly described:
*Continuous infusion: 5–7 ml/hr
*Continuous infusion + patient-controlled bolus: 3 ml/hr + 4–5 ml bolus (30 minute lockout)
*Patient-controlled bolus only: 5–10 ml (60 minute lockout)
*Physician-controlled bolus: 15 ml every 8 hours

Notes: 1. Higher concentrations of local anesthetic (eg, bupivacaine 0.25%) are used for the physician-controlled bolus.
2. Lower concentrations of local anesthetic (eg, ropivacaine 0.1%) are commonly used if the preservation of motor function is desired.
3. An exception to the volumes shown above is continuous femoral block, where larger volumes are used for continuous infusions (7–12 ml/hr), continuous infusion + patient-controlled bolus (5 ml/hr + 5–7 ml bolus), patient-controlled bolus only (8–10 ml), and physician-controlled bolus (20 ml).

Figure 28.12: Suggested regimens for continuous perineural blocks.

The Pragmatic Approach to Regional Techniques in Community Practice

Given the options presented earlier, it is readily apparent that the successful performance of regional techniques is critical to an anesthesia-based acute pain service. Yet the realities of modern community practice can often make these techniques seem impractical, if not impossible, to put into practice. The keys to successfully performing and expanding the use of these techniques in the community environment can be summarized as follows:

Operate within the Comfort Zone

Each institution has its own comfort zone that, although capable of being expanded, should not be violated. The overzealous forcing of change is rarely sustainable, as lasting change will only take hold through popular support. The evolution of acute pain management, with the integration of new modalities, usually necessitates an incremental culture change. This progression must be accompanied by appropriate communication and education.

In general, and especially with new approaches to acute pain, it is ideal that these modalities require minimal attention outside of the operating room and normal working hours. The concomitant provision of IV PCA, in particular, has proved to be a major consolation when initiating more advanced nonopioid pain management modalities (ie, single-injection or continuous nerve blocks). The patient-titrated nature of IV PCA has the advantages of minimizing nursing care, whereas being capable of independently providing adequate postoperative analgesia. The extent of IV PCA use (or, more accurately, the extent to which it was not used) also to some degree reflects the efficacy of nonopioid techniques being simultaneously utilized.

Operating within the comfort zone also means that practitioners should strive to gain sufficient experience with single-injection options before taking on continuous techniques and develop familiarity with pain management innovations in inpatients before extending their use to ambulatory patients.

Learn in a Logical Progression

Because few practitioners have advanced skills in all types of regional techniques, using these modalities in acute pain management requires a lifelong commitment to further learning. It is easy to appreciate that some regional procedures (eg, spinal anesthesia) are more readily mastered than others. With this thought in mind, the full spectrum of regional techniques has been stratified into basic, intermediate, and advanced categories.[41] An awareness of this classification can help practitioners develop further competence and confidence with more advanced regional techniques in a logical progression.

Anesthesiologists should liberally utilize regional techniques in appropriate clinical situations, not just when it is crucial that they work. Proficiency with manual skills is developed through practice, and skills learned with one block will generally build confidence with all regional procedures. A brief review of anatomy, block technique, side effects, and potential complications should precede every regional block as practitioners strive to solidify their knowledge base.

Ultrasound guidance of regional anesthesia is currently an area of intense interest and appears to offer unique advantages over traditional paresthesia or nerve-stimulating techniques.[42] The literature suggests that this technology may be capable of improving the efficiency and efficacy of regional blocks. Despite the fact that the vast majority of anesthesiologists in community practice are untrained in ultrasound use, proficiency may be quickly attained through one of many hands-on courses currently offered by recognized experts. However, it must be stated that, at this time, the clinical utility of this technology in the community practice setting is largely unproved and can realistically provide only limited returns for those already proficient in regional anesthesia. Although community hospital practitioners are encouraged to investigate the relative value of ultrasound guidance in their own hands, they are at the same time advised to avoid reliance on such a high-tech approach to what are truly basic techniques.

Be Cost-Conscious

Anesthesiologists must be knowledgeable regarding the hospital cost of supplies and consistently choose cost-efficient means of providing pain control. Although few supplies are essential, practitioners are faced with a number of important choices whenever regional techniques are contemplated. For example, either nonstimulating or comparatively expensive stimulating catheters may be utilized for continuous femoral nerve block after total knee arthroplasty, yet the evidence would indicate that the two appear to be equally effective.[43] Costs may also be reduced through the use of a prep sponge and sterile towel pack instead of a commercially manufactured block tray, choosing bupivacaine over ropivacaine as circumstances permit, and using reusable pumps as opposed to disposable infusion devices.

In this era of cost containment, the conscious and purposeful choice of supplies can help to justify the more frequent use of regional techniques. Furthermore, the economical use of equipment may also make practitioners less hesitant to appropriately abandon a difficult (ie, time-consuming and possibly futile) block procedure.

Avoid Delays

The production pressures mentioned above require that practitioners ensure that regional techniques not be perceived as a cause of delays. On the contrary, a systematic multimodal approach to acute pain management, which includes regional analgesia, should be viewed as the ideal strategy to improve efficiency through "fast-tracking" (bypass of phase 1 recovery) and speeding discharge readiness.[44]

When performing regional blocks, anesthesiologists should develop a reasonable degree of clock consciousness and may find it a useful exercise to occasionally time themselves. As a general rule, single-injection techniques should be able to be completed within 10 minutes and continuous techniques within 15 minutes. Practitioners who are unable to perform regional techniques within these parameters should strive to improve their skills when extra time can be afforded easily (such as before the first case of the day).

Performing blocks preoperatively (as in a block room or area) or postoperatively (in the PACU) is often more expeditious than in the operating room (Figure 28.1). The first case of the day generally presents an ideal opportunity to perform blocks in a preoperative area. Preoperative performance also allows for greater "soak time" and evaluation of block effects. Although many published studies compare regional techniques against general anesthesia, regional blocks are usually best considered as being complementary to a general anesthetic. A planned "light general" is not viewed as a compromise to regional anesthesia and can compensate for delays in onset and occasional failures. Although rightly considered to be a significant component of a balanced anesthetic, regional techniques are most appropriately perceived as being utilized primarily for postoperative analgesia.

Finally, practitioners must have a realistic perspective on abandoning frustrating unsuccessful efforts at regional block in a timely manner. Although beneficial in many respects, regional techniques are rarely essential for patient care, and stubbornly persisting with attempts at regional anesthesia in difficult situations is seldom in the best interests of the patient. Refer to Box 1 for tips that help make regional-based analgesia succeed.

Box 1 Clinical Tips
Suggestions to Avoid Delays with Regional Anesthesia Procedures

- Be consistently clock conscious (i.e. be aware of how long specific blocks usually take and how this compares with the present attempt)
- Perform blocks outside of the operating room
- Perform some blocks postoperatively
- Plan on combining regional techniques with general anesthesia
- Reasonably abandon difficult attempts at regional analgesia

---

DOCUMENTATION

Proper documentation is an essential component of modern medical care. Documentation of pain management techniques primarily serves as a basic communication tool between anesthesiologists and all other members of the care team. However, the ramifications of accurate descriptions of interventions performed for the management of pain extend well beyond the clinical setting and are of obvious importance as legal records and to satisfy billing and regulatory requirements.

Most institutions require that patients provide written informed consent for anesthesia care that is separate from surgical care. Practitioners may wish to obtain additional consent for pain management procedures, which can be considered apart from surgical anesthesia care. Procedures performed for postoperative pain are considered separate from the anesthesia care provided for surgery. As such, these procedures should be documented on a form separate from the anesthesia record. These interventions can essentially be divided into two categories: central neuraxial techniques and peripheral nerve blocks, with either further divided into single-injection or continuous techniques. The key elements to a standardized peripheral nerve block procedure note form have been described and analyzed.[45] Dedicated procedure notes have been developed for both neuraxial[46] and peripheral nerve blockade,[45] which can be readily combined into a single form (Figure 28.2).

Finally, the importance of documentation in the context of reimbursement cannot be overstated. Several aspects of the procedure note are specifically included to address reimbursement issues. Namely the form should specifically state that the procedure was performed for the purpose of postoperative analgesia (not surgical anesthesia), the indication for pain control (ie, the location of pain being treated rather than the surgical procedure performed), and that anesthesia-based pain management has been requested by the attending surgeon (some have advocated obtaining the surgeon's signature on this form to more fully document this request). Although the issue of reimbursement

for pain management services involves a multitude of variables and is beyond the scope of this discussion, it is fair to state that proper reimbursement begins with proper documentation.

FOLLOWING THROUGH ON AN ACUTE PAIN MANAGEMENT COURSE

Proper follow-through is a duty of ownership and critical to the long-term success of any patient care program. Efforts by anesthesiologists that clearly extend to the conclusion of care are necessary to maximize benefits and minimize risks associated with acute pain management and will ensure the highest levels of satisfaction from both patients and surgeons.

Follow-Through for Outpatients

Adequate analgesia is an obvious prerequisite for ambulatory surgery, where inadequate pain control has been shown to be a common reason for prolonged postoperative stays and unanticipated admissions. Furthermore, it is essential to anticipate pain-related issues that may become evident following discharge in ambulatory patients, as inadequate pain management has been shown to be a leading and preventable cause for readmissions.[47]

Successfully caring for patients on an ambulatory basis requires that an individualized plan be devised for the ongoing multimodal management of pain. Outpatients should be provided written instructions concerning further out-of-hospital management of their pain[3] (eg, oral analgesics), precautions regarding the care of an insensate limb (if they have had regional blocks), and a 24-hour telephone contact number should they have any problems or concerns (Figure 28.3). Patients discharged with continuous perineural infusions must have explicit instructions regarding the care of an indwelling catheter and should be capable of discontinuing the catheter at home without necessarily returning for personal medical attention.

Each institution must establish a system for follow-up with outpatients. A brief telephone call 24 to 72 hours postoperatively, usually by a nurse, is generally sufficient. General questions regarding patient satisfaction with intraoperative anesthesia and postoperative analgesia should be asked and any degree of patient dissatisfaction promptly passed on to the department of anesthesiology through established channels. The essence of these follow-up efforts should be documented and maintained by the department of quality management for a reasonable period of time (but does not necessarily need to be placed in the patient's permanent medical record). If efforts by telephone are unsuccessful, a card may be sent by mail to the patient explaining that reasonable attempts were made to establish routine postoperative follow-up by telephone and encouraging the patient to provide feedback regarding their perioperative experience either by telephone or in writing.

Follow-Up for Inpatients

Hospitalized patients, by virtue of their higher acuity of illness and injury, may stand to benefit the most from the effective management of pain through minimizing complications and possibly preventing chronic pain. Following up on inpatients is a primary function of an acute pain service. It has been repeatedly acknowledged that there is no consensus regarding the optimal structure or function of an acute pain service.[48] In the diverse reality of community practice, an acute pain service may take many forms but must at least consist of involved physician (eg, anesthesia) and nursing personnel.

Nurses are at the core of inpatient follow-up and are empowered to assume the leading role in assessing and treating postoperative pain. Regular assessment of pain, commonly every 4 hours using a 0–10 pain rating scale, is noted on pain assessment flow sheets that serve to track the "fifth vital sign" (ie, pain) over time and record responses to treatment (Figure 28.4). Multimodal treatment of pain based on scores >4 is usually included in standing pain management orders. This approach has been used successfully in many practice settings and shown to result in improved pain control and patient satisfaction but can also be associated with an increased incidence of opioid-induced oversedation.[49] This oversedation is usually preceded by a gradual decrease in the patient's level of consciousness, which underscores the critical importance of frequent clinical assessment by nursing.

Written orders are necessary to enable nurses to assume the leading hands-on role in the treatment of acute postoperative pain. Orders should be devised for each of the three basic anesthesia-based modalities: intravenous PCA, central neuraxial techniques (subarachnoid and epidural), and peripheral nerve/plexus blocking techniques (Figures 28.5, 28.6 and 28.7, respectively). Dedicated orders are recommended for each approach as this provides the clearest direction to nursing staff and serves to emphasize important difference between central and peripheral techniques, such as anticoagulation issues and the addition of other analgesics. Orders should allow for prudent adjustments of each of the primary modalities as well as provide direction for the addition of supplemental or adjunctive measures.

With the exception of patients receiving IV PCA, all patients enrolled in the acute pain service must be seen by anesthesia staff on a daily basis. This visit serves as a single-time assessment of pain management as well as an important opportunity to interact with nursing staff. A proactive effort to address any nursing-related concerns regarding pain management at this time can alleviate a number of night and cross-coverage issues. Anesthesiologists should also use postoperative visits as a means of extracting the greatest amount of experience from each pain management intervention (eg, the efficacy and duration of single-injection blocks). Documentation of daily pain management follow-up should be placed in the patient's chart as well as submitted for billing purposes. One successful approach to the various documentation requirements has been the development of a carbon copy peel-and-stick form, where the procedure with billing codes is documented at the top, a self-adhesive daily "SOAP" format note can be placed in the progress notes, and the carbon copy is submitted for billing purposes (Figure 28.13). Alternatively, using an index card system, notes may be written directly in the patient's chart and, at the conclusion of pain service involvement, the updated index card submitted for billing of daily pain management.

Although the acute pain service in many community practice settings is not a formal, distinct entity, prompt 24-hour coverage is essential. Instructions for appropriate contact of anesthesia personnel should be included in all pain management orders. An acute pain service beeper can help maintain continuity of communication within a system. If in-house anesthesia coverage is available, then an on-call physician manages overnight pain-related issues. If in-house overnight coverage is not available, then a mechanism that provides for off-hour patient evaluation needs to be devised. One solution is to specifically train selected night-shift nursing personnel to evaluate and troubleshoot common issues concerning acute pain management (for continuous epidurals, for example, this would include occlusion alarms, catheter disconnections, and evaluation of skin entry sites).

Management of Complications

The ideal management of complications begins with the tacit acknowledgement that complications are inevitable. Having realistic preoperative discussions with patients regarding potential complications, obtaining meaningful written informed consent, and keeping accurate records comprise the foundations of appropriately dealing with adverse events.

One goal of any anesthesia-based acute pain service should be to promptly and directly deal with any adverse outcomes potentially related to pain management. Certain complications should be anticipated and managed proactively. All opiate-based modalities should include standing orders for intravenous naloxone to be administered by nursing in the event of significant respiratory depression. Making contact with patients, either personally or by telephone, into a routine part of postoperative care will help to ensure the consistent and early discovery of any complications. Patients whose analgesic care included subarachnoid opiates, for example, should be specifically asked about the presence of postural headache symptoms. If any potential complications of acute pain management are first encountered by nursing personnel, they should be reported without delay to designated anesthesia personnel (as well as to the surgeon's office).

A detailed discussion of the multitude of possible complications associated with acute pain management is beyond the scope of this chapter. Because appropriate management of complications will depend on individual circumstances, it is critical that each be personally evaluated. Fortunately, most potential adverse events are rare and/or self-limiting. In the unlikely event of a serious complication, cultivating a professional relationship with a department of neurology can help to facilitate prompt consultations and referrals.

To a degree that would be considered appropriate, anesthesiologists are encouraged to stay involved in the care of any patients suffering adverse outcomes secondary to pain management efforts. It should be emphasized that taking an active interest in potential complications does not imply fault or negligence by anesthesiologists, but reinforces the commitment to quality health care and serves to legitimize the pain service in the eyes of other medical professionals. Continued personal communication with the patient helps to reinforce the desired message of genuine concern.

The complete management of complications secondary to pain management requires that all occurrences be compulsively included in quality improvement efforts (discussed in the following sections).

Quality Improvement

A process for quality improvement (QI), also commonly referred to as quality management (QM), is a fundamental requirement of all health care organizations. Although QI for the department of anesthesiology largely concerns the operative period, in the case of an anesthesiology-based acute pain service it must extend through the entire duration of management. Quality improvement efforts allow for clinically significant data concerning pain management to be collected and monitored with the goal of improving performance and enhancing patient safety.

HUNTINGTON HOSPITAL
ACUTE PAIN MANAGEMENT SERVICE

_____ PCA
_____ E P I
_____ CRA

Surgeon: _____

Diagnosis code: _____

Anesthesiologist: _____

Operation: _____

ROOM NO.

Date of service: _____

HUNTINGTON HOSPITAL ACUTE PAIN MANAGEMENT SERVICE: THERAPY INITIATION
CHECK ONE:

☐ I. V. PCA	☐ EPIDURAL/NEURAXIAL	☐ PERIPHERAL NERVE BLOCK

CPT: 01997
 	
 INITIAL SETTINGS:
 	
 ☐ MSO₄ ☐ Dilaudid
 	
 Continuous Rate: _____ mg./hr.
 	
 Demand Dose _____ mg.
 	
 Lockout Interval _____ Min.
 	
 4 Hr. Dose Limit _____
	CPT ☐ Thoracic 62318 + 99231
	      ☐ Lumbar 62319 + 99231
	 ☐ Postop Pain Rx only (Daily Mgmt.) 01996
	 ☐ Postop Visit (Single Shot) 99231
	 ☐ Blood Patch 62273
	 INITIAL SETTINGS:
	 ☐ Continuous Rate:____ml./hr./Titrate ___ to ___
	 Bupivacaine: _____ % Ropivacaine _____ %
	 + Fentanyl ___ mcg./ml., Dilaudid ___ mcg./ml.
	 or Duramorph ___mcg./ml.
	 ☐ PCEA Dose _____ ml. Delay _____ Min.
	 ☐ Other:
		Brachial Plexus ☐ Single shot 64415 ☐-59
		      ☐ Continuous 64416 ☐-22
		 Sciatic ☐ Single shot 64445
		      ☐ Continuous 64446
		 Femoral ☐ Single shot 64447
		      ☐ Continuous 64448
		 Psoas ☐ Continuous 64449
		 Bolus _____ ml. Continuous Rate: _____ ml./hr.
		 Ropivacaine _____ % Other _____
		 During Placement: ☐ Yes ☐ No Heme ☐ Yes ☐ No Paresthesia
		 ☐ Yes ☐ No Pain on Injection ☐ Yes ☐ No Low Resistance to Inj.
		 PCRA Dose _____ ml. Delay _____ Min.

☐ Procedure Explained to Patient Including Risks/Benefits/Alternatives. Patient Consents to Procedure.

POSTOP DAY # ____

Date:_____

Time: _____

Provider
Signature: _____

HUNTINGTON HOSPITAL · ACUTE PAIN MANAGEMENT SERVICE

SUBJECTIVE:_____

OBJECTIVE: Pain Score: _____ /10

     ☐ PCA ☐ Epidural ☐ Peripheral nerve block ☐ Single shot neuraxial

     ☐ Vital signs stable ☐ Alert & oriented ☐ No motor/sensory block ☐ Nausea ☐ Pruritis ☐ Headache

     ☐ Bromage Score _____

ASSESSMENT/PLAN: ☐ Continue current Rx ☐ Catheter removed, tip intact ☐ Further pain Rx plan _____

COMMENTS: _____

POSTOP DAY # ____

Date:_____

Time: _____

Provider
Signature: _____

HUNTINGTON HOSPITAL · ACUTE PAIN MANAGEMENT SERVICE

SUBJECTIVE:_____

OBJECTIVE: Pain Score: _____ /10

     ☐ PCA ☐ Epidural ☐ Peripheral nerve block

     ☐ Vital signs stable ☐ Alert & oriented ☐ No motor/sensory block ☐ Nausea ☐ Pruritis ☐ Headache

     ☐ Bromage Score _____

ASSESSMENT/PLAN: ☐ Continue current Rx ☐ Catheter removed, tip intact ☐ Further pain Rx plan _____

COMMENTS: _____

POSTOP DAY # ____

Date:_____

Time: _____

Provider
Signature: _____

HUNTINGTON HOSPITAL · ACUTE PAIN MANAGEMENT SERVICE

SUBJECTIVE:_____

OBJECTIVE: Pain Score: _____ /10

     ☐ PCA ☐ Epidural ☐ Peripheral nerve block

     ☐ Vital signs stable ☐ Alert & oriented ☐ No motor/sensory block ☐ Nausea ☐ Pruritis ☐ Headache

     ☐ Bromage Score _____

ASSESSMENT/PLAN: ☐ Continue current Rx ☐ Catheter removed, tip intact ☐ Further pain Rx plan _____

COMMENTS: _____

FORM 1-324 (REV. 3/04)

66653 · PHYSICIANS' RECORD COMPANY · BERWYN, IL · 800-323-9268

= peel and stick on chart

Figure 28.13: Peel and Stick Initiation/Encounter Form. This sticker includes all the ICD codes and is applicable for IV PCA, continuous epidural, and both single-injection and continuous peripheral nerve blocks. It also includes a small box to document and bill for a blood patch. After you have initiated the intervention, you then have 3 separate stickers in SOAP format to use for daily follow-up. Most continuous infusions (both continuous epidural and peripheral nerve) are pulled after 3 days. When complete, send the back (carbon copy) to the insurance carrier because all the CPT and ICD codes are included.

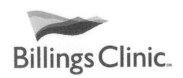

Billings Clinic ℠

Patient Identification

Outpatient Postoperative Contact Form

Patient Information
(to be completed upon entry into Outpatient Surgery)

Date: _____   Address: _____
                                                                    _____

Procedure: _____   Telephone: _____

Anesthesiologist: _____   Parents: _____

Telephone Interview

Date/Time of Callback: _____

Did you have any problems after leaving the hospital?
(i.e. pain control, nausea/vomiting, incision site drainage/bleeding, fever, bowel/bladder etc.)
_____
_____
_____

Did you meet and talk with your anesthesiologist before surgery?
_____

Do you have any other questions, comments, or suggestions?
_____
_____
_____
_____

Actions

Actions taken by RN:
_____
_____
_____
_____
_____

☐ Unable to contact by telephone. Card sent to address above on _____
                                                                                                   (date)

RN: Signature _____   Printed Name _____

Figure 28.14: Outpatient Contact form. At Huntington Hospital and Billings Clinic, ambulatory nurses call the patients the next day and communicate directly to the anesthesia department if there is an untoward event. In addition, the anesthesia department has formulated a postprocedure patient log form that is given to all of the surgeons and is a way for us to track/manage complications directly from the referring doctors' office.

The American Society of Anesthesiologists Web site is an excellent resource regarding quality improvement (www.asahq.org). The Quality Management Template found at the ASA Web site, developed by ASA committees and provided without charge, serves as an indispensable guide to implementing a quality improvement program in any practice setting.[50]

The ready availability of occurrence reporting forms is a key element in the consistent self-reporting of adverse events. For cases in the operating room, reporting forms are often attached to the anesthesia record. Similarly, anesthesia-specific incident reporting forms should be immediately at hand as nurses and anesthesiologists are engaged in following through on an acute pain management plan (Figure 28.14). Although occurrence forms are usually completed manually, if large amounts of data will require analysis it is advisable that these forms be capable of being scanned. A number of computer-ready process improvement tracking tools are commercially available, with several examples provided in the ASA's Quality Management Template. Although self-reporting of adverse outcomes has inherent weaknesses, it has been shown to be more reliable than medical chart review or incident reports and tends to be successful in environments where it is perceived that participation may result in improved patient care.[51]

Finally, it is essential that one member of the department of anesthesiology assume the leadership role regarding quality improvement. This individual is responsible for assuring the consistent reporting of sentinel events (a significant limitation of self-reporting), managing the appropriate analysis of data (usually consisting of at least some type of peer review), and overseeing the adoption of appropriate measures to improve performance and safety.

CONCLUSION

Anesthesiologists currently have the understanding, as well as the pharmacologic and technological tools necessary, to successfully control postoperative pain in private practice settings; however, inadequate analgesia continues to be a prominent medical issue. Meeting the challenges of acute pain management in modern community practice requires a comprehensive appreciation of the entire process, physician leadership, and an organizational commitment. Primarily through the coordinated efforts of anesthesiology and nursing staff, a culture of consistent and efficient pain management can be established in any practice setting.

REFERENCES

1. Rathmell JP, Wu CL, Sinatra RS, et al. Acute post-surgical pain management: a critical appraisal of current practice. *Reg Anesth Pain Med.* 2006;31:1–42.
2. Apfelbaum JL, Chen C, Mehta SS, et al. Postoperative pain experience: results from a national survey suggest postoperative pain continues to be undermanaged. *Anesth Analg.* 2003;97:534–540.
3. McGrath B, Elgendy H, Chung F, et al. Thirty percent of patients have moderate to severe pain 24 hr after ambulatory surgery: a survey of 5,703 patients. *Can J Anesth.* 2004;51:886–891.
4. Kopacz DJ, Neal JM. Regional anesthesia and pain medicine: residency training – the year 2000. *Reg Anesth Pain Med.* 2002;27:9–14.
5. Hadzic A, Vloka JD, Kuroda MM, et al. The practice of peripheral nerve blocks in the United States: a national survey. *Reg Anesth Pain Med.* 1998;23:241–246.
6. Abouleish AE, Prough DS, Whitten CW, et al. Comparing clinical productivity of anesthesiology groups. *Anesthesiology.* 2002;97:608–615.
7. Oldman M, McCartney CJL, Leung A, et al. A survey of orthopedic surgeons' attitudes and knowledge regarding regional anesthesia. *Anesth Analg.* 2004;98:1486–1490.
8. Gaba DM, Howard SK, Jump B. Production pressure in the work environment. California anesthesiologists' attitudes and experiences. *Anesthesiology.* 1994;81:488–500.
9. Matthey PW, Finegan BA, Finucane BT. The public's fears about and perceptions of regional anesthesia. *Reg Anesth Pain Med.* 2004;29:96–101.
10. Rupp T, Delaney KA: Inadequate analgesia in emergency medicine. *Ann Emerg Med.* 2004;43:494–503.
11. Foss NB, Kristensen BB, Bundgaard M, et al. Fascia iliaca compartment blockade for acute pain control in hip fracture patients. *Anesthesiology.* 2007;773–778.
12. Guay J. The benefits of adding epidural analgesia to general anesthesia: a metaanalysis. *J Anesth.* 2006;20:335–340.
13. Ballantyne JC, Carr DB, de Ferranti S, et al. The comparative effects of postoperative analgesic therapies on pulmonary outcome: cumulative meta-analysis of randomized, controlled trials. *Anesth Analg.* 1998;86:598–612.
14. Stadler M, Schlander M, Braeckman M, et al. A cost-utility and cost-effectiveness analysis of an acute pain service. *J Clin Anesth.* 2004;16:159–167.
15. Armstrong KPJ, Cherry RA. Brachial plexus anesthesia compared to general anesthesia when a block room is available. *Can J Anesth.* 2004;51:41–44.
16. Weinber GL. Lipid infusion resuscitation for local anesthetic toxicity; proof of clinical efficacy. *Anesthesiology.* 2006;105:7–8.
17. Rosenblatt MA, Abel M, Fischer GW, Itzkovitch CJ, Eisenkraft JB. Sucessful use of a 20% lipid emulsion to resuscitate a patient after a presumed bupivacaine-related cardiac arrest. *Anesthesiology.* 2006;105:217–218.
18. Litz RJ, Popp M, Stehr SN, Koch T. Successful resuscitation of a patient with roivacaine-induced asystole after axillary plexus block using lipid infusion. *Anaesthesia.* 2006;61:800–801.
19. Practice guidelines for acute pain management in the perioperative setting: an updated report by the American Society of Anesthesiologists Task Force on Acute Pain Management. *Anesthesiology.* 2004;100:1573–1581.
20. Schug SA, Manopas A. Update on the role of non-opioids for postoperative pain treatment. *Best Pract Res Clin Anaesthiol.* 2007;21:15–30.
21. Lennon RL, Horlocker TT. *Mayo Clinic Analgesic Pathway: Peripheral Nerve Blockade for Major Orthopedic Surgery.* London, UK: Taylor & Francis; 2006.
22. Kehlet H, Wilkinson RC, Fischer HBJ, et al. PROSPECT: evidence-based, procedure-specific postoperative pain management. *Best Pract Res Clin Anaesthiol.* 2007;21:149–159.
23. Liu SS, Richman JM, Thirlby RC, et al. Efficacy of continuous wound catheters delivering local anesthetic for postoperative analgesia: a quantitative and qualitative systematic review of randomized controlled trials. *J Am Coll Surg.* 2006;203:914–932.
24. Gupta A, Bodin L, Holmstrom B, et al. A systematic review of the peripheral analgesic effects of intraarticular morphine. *Anesth Analg.* 2001;93:761–770.
25. Grass JA: Patient-controlled analgesia. *Anesth Analg.* 2005; 101:S44–S61.
26. Macintyre PE. Intravenous patient-controlled analgesia: one size does not fit all. *Anesthesiology Clin N Am.* 2005;23:109–123.
27. Power I. Fentanyl HCl iontophoretic transdermal system (ITS): clinical application of iontophoretic technology in the management of acute postoperative pain. *Br J Anaesth.* 2007;98:4–11.

28. Rathmell JP, Lair TR, Nauman B: The role of intrathecal drugs in the treatment of acute pain. *Anesth Analg.* 2005;101:S30–S43.

29. Holt DV, Viscusi ER, Wordell CJ. Extended-duration agents for perioperative pain management. *Curr Pain Headache Rep.* 2007;11:33–37.

30. Klein SM, Evans H, Nielsen KC, et al. Peripheral nerve block techniques for ambulatory surgery. *Anesth Analg.* 2005;101:1663–1676.

31. Mulroy MF, Larkin KL, Batra MS, et al. Femoral nerve block with 0.25% or 0.5% bupivacaine improves postoperative analgesia following outpatient arthroscopic anterior cruciate ligament repair. *Reg Anesth Pain Med.* 2001;26:24–29.

32. Murphy DB, McCartney CJL, Chan VWS. Novel analgesic adjuncts for brachial plexus block: a systematic review. *Anesth Analg.* 2000;90:1122–1128.

33. Auroy Y, Benhamou D, Bargues L, et al. Major complications of regional anesthesia in France: the SOS Regional Anesthesia Hotline Service. *Anesthesiology.* 2002;97:1274–1280.

34. Salinas FV, Liu SS, Mulroy MF. The effect of single-injection femoral nerve block versus continuous femoral nerve block after total knee arthroplasty on hospital length of stay and long-term functional recovery within an established clinical pathway. *Anesth Analg.* 2006;102:1234–1239.

35. Richman JM, Wu CL. Epidural analgesia for postoperative pain. *Anesthesiol Clin N Am.* 2005;23:125–140.

36. Nishimori M, Ballantyne JC, Low JHS. Epidural pain relief versus systemic opioid-based pain relief for abdominal aortic surgery (Cochrane Reviews). The Cochrane Library:Issue 3, 2006.

37. Boezaart AP. Perineural infusions of local anesthetics. *Anesthesiology.* 2006;104:872–880.

38. Richman JM, Liu SS, Courpas G, et al. Does continuous peripheral nerve block provide superior pain control to opioids? A meta-analysis. *Anesth Analg.* 2006;102:248–257.

39. Capdevila X, Pirat P, Bringuier S, et al. Continuous peripheral nerve blocks in hospital wards after orthopedic surgery. A multicenter prospective analysis of the quality of postoperative analgesia and complications in 1,416 patients. *Anesthesiology.* 2005;103:1035–1045.

40. Ilfeld BM, Enneking FK. Continuous peripheral nerve blocks at home: a review. *Anesth Analg.* 2005;100:1822–1833.

41. Hargett MJ, Beckman JD, Liguori GA, et al. Guidelines for regional anesthesia fellowship training. *Reg Anesth Pain Med.* 2005;30:218–225.

42. Marhofer P, Chan VWS. Ultrasound-guided regional anesthesia: current concepts and future trends. *Anesth Analg.* 2007;104:1265–1269.

43. Hayek SM, Ritchey RM, Sessler D, et al. Continuous femoral nerve analgesia after unilateral total knee arthroplasty: stimulating versus nonstimulating catheters. *Anesth Analg.* 2006;103:1565–1570.

44. White PF, Kehlet H, Neal JM, et al. The role of the anesthesiologist in fast-track surgery: from multimodal analgesia to perioperative medical care. *Anesth Analg.* 2007;104:1380–1396.

45. Gerancher JC, Viscusi ER, Liguori GA, et al. Development of a standardized peripheral nerve block procedure note form. *Reg Anesth Pain Med.* 2005;30:67–71.

46. Viscusi ER, Gerancher JC, Weller R, et al. Not documented? Not done! A proposed procedure note for neuraxial blockade. American Society of Regional Anesthesia and Pain Medicine 30th Annual Spring Meeting and Workshops Abstract 68, April 21–24, 2005.

47. Coley KC, Williams BA, DaPos SV, et al. Retrospective evaluation of unanticipated admissions and readmissions after same day surgery and associated costs. *J Clin Anesth.* 2002;14:349–353.

48. Rawal N. Organization, function, and implementation of acute pain service. *Anesthesiology Clin N Am.* 2005;23:211–225.

49. Vila H, Smith RA, Augustyniak MJ, et al. The efficacy and safety of pain management before and after implementation of hospital-wide pain management standards: is patient safety compromised by treatment based solely on numerical pain ratings? *Anesth Analg.* 2005;101:474–480.

50. Committee on Performance and Outcomes Measurement (CPOM), Committee on Quality Management and Departmental Administration (QMDA): Quality Management Template, http://www.asahq.org/quality/qmtemplate013105.pdf. 2004.

51. Katz RI, Lagasse RS. Factors influencing the reporting of adverse perioperative outcomes to a quality management program. *Anesth Analg.* 2000;90:344–350.

Ambulatory Surgical Pain: Economic Aspects and Optimal Analgesic Management

Tariq M. Malik and Raymond S. Sinatra

Approximately 73 million surgeries are performed annually in the United States,[1] with nearly 70% of the procedures performed in ambulatory settings.[2] This trend from inpatient to outpatient recovery has been spurred by economic factors as well as improved surgical and anesthetic techniques. The national health expenditure, which stood at 1.3 trillion dollars in the year 2000, is projected to grow at an average annual rate of roughly 7% throughout this decade. From 1991 to 2002, outpatient costs grew at rate of 12.1% faster than every other category. From 1981 to 2000, based on national health expenditure accounts data, hospital-based outpatient costs increased by 922%, whereas those for inpatient hospital services increased 121%. These unexpected findings underscore the importance of controlling expenses in ambulatory surgical centers.[3]

Factors responsible for increased ambulatory surgical cost include surgical complications, anesthetic related complications, and patient-related issues. Because of technical and pharmacological improvements in surgical and anesthetic care, ambulatory surgical mortality and morbidity is no different from that observed with procedures requiring inpatient recovery. In one study of 38,598 patients followed for 30 days, there were only 4 deaths, of which 2 were because of motor vehicle accidents, and 31 major morbidities (0.08%).[4] Vila and coworkers[5] reported a mortality rate of 0.78 in 100,000 procedures in the ambulatory setting. However, mortality and morbidity is more a measure of patient health status and other variables than a measure of health care quality the patient has received.

The major postsurgical milestone following ambulatory surgery is the return to preoperative functional status and quality of life. Of the many variables that increase hospital cost and affect patient satisfaction the most important are pain control, postoperative nausea and vomiting (PONV), return to functionality, and prolonged hospital stay. Because ambulatory surgery is performed in many settings, including hospitals, surgery centers, specialized clinics, and office practices, the American Society of Anesthesiologists (ASA) Committee on Ambulatory Surgical Care, and the Task Force on Office-Based Anesthesia developed

a list of outcome indicators of which pain control has major importance.[6]

PAIN FOLLOWING AMBULATORY SURGERY

Poorly controlled pain is among the most commonly observed complication following ambulatory surgery.[7] This distressing adverse event is responsible for high patient dissatisfaction, increased morbidity, and increased hospital readmission (Figure 29.1). The negative consequence of ineffective pain control are many and include deep vein thrombosis, coronary ischemia, poor wound healing, and chronic postsurgical pain[7,8] Chronic postoperative pain is a serious yet, until recently, underrecognized clinical entity. Its incidence varies from 10% to 50% after common ambulatory procedures such as groin hernia repair and breast surgery.[9] Persistent pain is characterized as severe and disabling in 2%–10% of these cases.[10] In addition to these medical issues, there are the economic costs of prolonged hospital stay, long-term analgesic dependency, hospital readmission, multiple clinic visits, and reduced patient functionality. The economic burden of chronic pain that develops following acute trauma in patients 30 years of age and younger approaches $1 million.[11]

In an effort to underscore the significance of optimal pain control, the Agency for Health Care Policy and Research issued guidelines for acute pain management in 1992[12,13] and The Joint Commission on the Accreditation of Health Care Organizations (JCAHO) incorporated new standards for pain control in 2001.[14] However, analgesic undermedication and severe postoperative pain remains a common problem. In ambulatory settings, postoperative pain control remains suboptimal as traditional techniques such as intravenous patient-controlled anesthesia (IV PCA) and neuraxial opioids cannot be provided, and prescriptions for oral analgesics are often inadequate or poorly tolerated. In a study of 175 patients recovering from ambulatory surgery, 60% described their pain intensity at 24 hours as moderate to severe.[15] Moderate to severe pain delayed postanesthesia care unit (PACU) discharge by 54 minutes and,

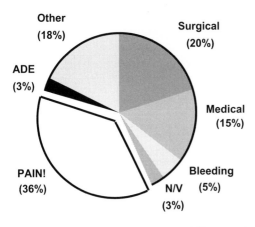

ADE = adverse drug event; N/V = nausea/vomiting.

Figure 29.1: Unanticipated ambulatory surgical admissions: pain versus other causes. From Coley KC, Williams BA, Da Pos SV, Chen C, Smith R. Retrospective evaluation of unanticipated admissions after same day surgery and associated costs. *J Clin Anesth.* 2002:14:349–353.[30]

following discharge, diminished activities of daily living and affected sleep in 33% and 46% of patients, respectively.[15] Pain was found to be most severe after microdiscectomy, open hernia repair, laparoscopic procedures, and some forms of plastic surgery.[15,16] Persistent pain was reported in 74% of patients 2 weeks after uneventful ambulatory surgery. Of these, 25% reported severe pain at some point during recovery, whereas 12% rated their average pain as severe.[17] McGrath and coworkers[18] reported a 30% incidence of moderate to severe pain at 24 hours after ambulatory surgery. They also found that microdiscectomy, lap cholecystectomy, orthopedic surgeries, groin surgery, and groin hernia repair was associated with the highest pain intensity at 24 hours (Figure 29.2). Findings similar to McGrath were reported by Rawal and colleagues,[19] who found that 35% of patients experienced severe pain during the first 48 hours following ambulatory surgery with 20% suffering sleep disturbance because of pain. Despite this high incidence of poorly controlled pain, 95% of patients expressed very high global satisfaction scores.

Despite the supposed transient nature of the ambulatory surgical pain, studies designed to assess return to preoperative functional status found that many patients suffered from functional distress, and only 22% were able to return to part time or full work by postoperative day 7.[20,21] This finding raises the question of whether ambulatory surgery is truly cost-effective or are the costs being diverted from hospital to patients and/or their employers.

In an outcome study based on questionnaires filled out prior to surgery and then 24 hours, 48 hours, and 7 days later, 40% of the patients reported moderate to severe pain during the first 24 hours after hospital discharge.[23] Poor pain control in the PACU was the best indicator of pain severity after discharge. About 25% of patients contacted a health care provider because of pain at home. A significant number of patients (33% to 51%) reported that instructions about pain control were either unclear or nonexistent on several aspects. Thirty-two percent of the patients took no pain medication in the first 24 hours after discharge even though 46% of those patients rated their pain above 4 on the visual analog scale (VAS).[23] More surprising was

the finding that 80% of the participants were satisfied overall with their pain treatment.

Pain following ambulatory surgery is also responsible for increased PACU stay. Poorly controlled pain prolongs PACU stay by 32% or an average of 54 minutes.[22,23] Prolongation in stay contributes to increased ambulatory surgical expense; however, the major cost saving measure is to cut PACU nursing staff. Such cuts may not occur until peak patient load in PACU is reduced by 25% or more. Nevertheless delayed time to discharge requires greater nursing time and supervision and decreases overall patient satisfaction.[23–25]

Poorly controlled pain is also responsible for unanticipated hospital visits or admissions after ambulatory surgery. Gold and coworkers[25] reported an incidence of 1.03%, that being 100 unanticipated admissions of 9616 ambulatory cases, most being related to poor pain control, bleeding, or PONV. Twersky et al[26] reported that the incidence of return to hospital within 30 days following ambulatory surgery was 2.9%, with severe pain being the third most common reason. A similar prospective study reported by Fortier and coworkers[27] found that the rate of unanticipated hospital admission was 1.42%. PONV and poorly controlled pain accounted for 14% and 12.1%, respectively, of unanticipated readmissions. Of pain-related readmissions, 60% were associated with ambulatory orthopedic procedures. In a Norwegian evaluation of ambulatory surgical outcomes, the incidence of readmission was 1.5% and, as might be expected, 20% were related to inadequate analgesia. In children, the unanticipated admission rate was 2.2% and the most common reasons for admission were, again, pain, nausea, surgical complication, or more extensive surgery.[28]

From an economic standpoint, readmission for poor pain control increases overall hospital costs.[28,29] In another cost-benefit analysis Coley and coworkers[30] found readmission rate of 1.5% following ambulatory surgery, with severe pain being responsible for hospital admission in 38% of the cases (117 of 303 patients readmitted). Most of these patients returning with inadequate pain control were recovering from orthopedic surgery. The overall cost of readmission for severe pain was $218,756 with mean charges per patient amounting to $1869 (±$4,553).[29,30]

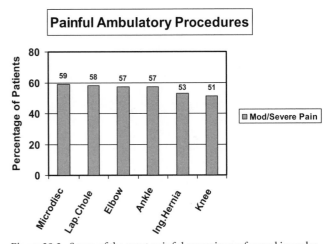

Figure 29.2: Seven of the most painful surgeries performed in ambulatory settings. In a survey of 5073 patients, 30% reported moderate to severe pain 24 hours after ambulatory surgery. From McGrath B et al. *Can J Anesth.* 2004;51(9):886–891.[18]

Table 29.1: Factors Responsible for Moderate to Severe Pain Following Ambulatory Surgery

---

Excessive pain in PACU (intraoperative analgesic deficit, discontinuance of baseline COX-2 inhibitor and opioid analgesics)

Pain during transport or following home discharge

Overreliance on opioid monotherapy and PRN analgesic dosing

Excessive and poorly treated nausea and vomiting

Abrupt transition from neural blockade to oral analgesics

Technology failures (Catheter dislodgement with Painbuster™ Pumps)

Not recognizing and compensating for opioid tolerance

Analgesic gaps responsible for inadequate analgesia and related complications following ambulatory procedures are presented in Table 29.1.

IMPROVING PAIN CONTROL FOLLOWING AMBULATORY SURGERY

Improved Patient Education

For most patients, uncontrolled pain is their main concern following ambulatory surgery. They have many misconceptions about using opioids for pain control, namely fear of side effects and possible addiction.[23,31–33] A large number experience opioid-associated side effects (25% or more) such as nausea, sedation, and dysphoria, which influence and limit their use of postoperative analgesics.[31,32] Others consider pain a necessary evil. In one survey, 82% of the people agreed that pain is severe after major surgery, yet, 46% of the people agreed that they would rather suffer pain than complain about it.[31] One way to improve ambulatory surgical pain control is to increase patient education. Preoperative education has shown to decrease patient anxiety and postoperative pain.[32–34] Patients should be informed about expected intensity of pain, duration of pain, and duration of functional limitation. Differences in choice of postoperative pain control should also be discussed and benefits versus risks of analgesic techniques that can reduce pain intensity should be explained.[34] Patients should be provided with clear instructions about medications, their side effects, and a contact number in case questions arise at home. Marquardt and Razia[32] reported that written instructions designed to guide patients on how to adjust analgesic doses in response to increasing pain intensity significantly improved pain control and sleep pattern for the first 3 days following ambulatory surgery. Goldsmith and Safran[33] found that Web-based pain management information provided to patients prior to ambulatory procedures significantly reduced postoperative pain intensity scores. Follow-up phone calls can also improve patient satisfaction and reduce the need for hospital readmission. In a pediatric study, parents were interviewed over the phone 24 hours after surgery to assess the adequacy of pain control in their children. These authors concluded that with proper education parents can manage their child's pain very well at home and most of them appreciated the phone call and found it very helpful.[35]

Preoperative (Preventative) Analgesia

Preventative analgesia describes a presurgical dosing scheme having the potential to prevent sensitization of peripheral and central pain pathways.[36,37] Such sensitization and associated hyperalgesia increase acute pain intensity and analgesic dose requirements. Although the usefulness of preventative analgesia was clearly established in experimental studies, clinical trials employing presurgical dosing of opioid analgesics were unable to detect significant advantages.[37] In contrast, several studies employing nonsteroidal anti-inflammatory drugs (NSAIDs), cyclooxygenase 2 (COX-2) inhibitors (coxibs), and local anesthetic blockade have demonstrated that analgesic administration before the incision clearly reduced the intensity of postprocedure pain.[38,39,40] In ambulatory settings, discontinuation of COX-2 inhibitors should be avoided as these agents effectively reduce postsurgical pain and opioid dose requirements, yet do not influence platelet function or increase postoperative bleeding.[39]

Multimodal Therapy

Like other forms of trauma, ambulatory surgical pain is a combination of nociceptive and neuropathic injury and response. Although opioids remain the foundation of pain management, overreliance on this class of analgesics commonly results in dose-dependent side effects.[41,42] These adverse events may diminish the potential advantages of outpatient surgery by increasing the need to treat symptoms, prolonging hospital stay, and increasing the number of unanticipated admissions. Despite adequate opioid prescription, many patients experience ineffective postoperative analgesia and report dissatisfaction with therapy because of three principal factors.

First, opioid monotherapy may not control all aspects of postsurgical pain, particularly if the primary noxious stimulus is inflammatory or neuropathic in nature. Second, outpatient administration of opioids is often limited and occasionally discontinued entirely because of intolerable adverse effects such as nausea, vomiting, and sedation. Third, because of fears of addiction/dependence among patients and physicians alike, a large number of same-day surgical prescriptions are for less-regulated opioids such as codeine and hydrocodone. These agents are incorrectly perceived to have lower abuse/diversion risks and are often ineffective and have high adverse event profiles. For these reasons, we recommend that the choice and dose of opioid analgesic be prescribed according to expected intensity of the postsurgical pain stimulus and, unless contraindicated, supplemented with regional blockade and nonopioid analgesics.

Multimodal or balanced analgesic techniques employ two or more analgesics or modalities that work by different mechanisms or at different sites in the nervous system to improve overall effectiveness.[42,43] For example, administering multiple doses of an NSAID in combination with an opioid reduces postoperative pain while at the same time decreases opioid consumption and dose-related adverse events.[44,46] Currently, the Agency for Healthcare Research and Quality and the ASA Task Force on Acute Pain Management recommend the use of multimodal analgesia.[47,48] Reuben and coworkers[49] evaluated the benefits of multimodal analgesia for patients recovering from anterior cruciate ligament reconstruction performed in an ambulatory surgical center. In this large 1200-patient randomized controlled trial, patients received a standardized general anesthetic and a prescription for oxycodone for postoperative pain relief. Patients in the preemptive multimodal group received a COX-2 inhibitor for 48 hours prior to surgery, a femoral nerve block prior to surgery, and intra-articular bupivacaine, morphine, and clonidine on completion of the procedure. Patients randomized to the preemptive multimodal analgesic group benefited from improved pain control that more than justified its labor intensiveness. These patients experienced less pain, required dramatically less opioid analgesic (fentanyl), and experienced less nausea and vomiting in the PACU ($P < .01$). They also benefited from a more rapid time to PACU discharge, required less oxycodone following discharge, and reported lower pain intensity scores during home recovery. Improvements in acute pain intensity were associated with additional long-term benefits, including less pain 6 months postsurgery, a more rapid return to functionality, and a lower incidence of patellofemoral complications at 1-year follow-up ($P < .01$). A less complicated, multimodal protocol provided similar improvements in pain control for patients recovering from arthroscopic knee surgery. Brill and Plaza[50] found patients receiving intra-articular clonidine and ketorolac post procedure, reported lower pain intensity scores, and required less opioid analgesic following home discharge.

Other multimodal evaluations using single doses of gabapentin, clonidine, and coxibs have demonstrated similar opioid-sparing effects and reductions in pain intensity scores following inpatient and same-day surgery.[51,54] These studies, however, were underpowered to demonstrate significant reductions in nausea and vomiting, bowel dysfunction, and other opioid-associated adverse effects as a result of decreased consumption. A larger, well-controlled multimodal protocol employing pre- and postsurgical doses of a coxib in patients recovering from abdominal gynecological surgery reported a 30% reduction in overall opioid requirement and clinically significant reductions in sedation scores. Of importance, were findings that bowel sounds and return to solid diet occurred 10 and 14 hours sooner ($P > .01$) in the multimodal group.[55] Additional benefits of NSAIDs and coxibs in ambulatory surgical settings are discussed in sections that follow.

Opioid Analgesics

Opioids remain the therapeutic foundation for managing moderate to severe postoperative pain. Although opioids are titrated typically to alleviate pain at rest, pain during movement or activity (eg, coughing or ambulating) may be more difficult to control and has a greater impact on postsurgical recovery.[56] In ambulatory surgery effective pain relief can be obtained with skillful intraoperative use of fentanyl, alfentanil, and, in more painful procedures, hydromorphone. Fentanyl bolus (1–2 μg/kg) administered at the start of the case can be used as a sole agent or can be later supplemented with hydromorphone or morphine. Alfentanil is often administered as a bolus dose and then continued as an infusion. This method of administration is useful for maintaining a constant level of analgesia, especially for monitored anesthesia care, which then can be easily reversed at the end of the case. In more extensive procedures, morphine or hydromorphone can be titrated as required later in the case. Hydromorphone has high analgesic potency and, in our experience, has a more rapid onset and cleaner adverse event profile than morphine.[56] Hydromorphone is administered in selective painful surgeries and for patients with opioid dependencies.

Newly released opioids tested in ambulatory settings include combination oxycodone plus ibuprofen (combunox) and immediate release oxymorphone (Opana IR). Gimbel and coworkers[57] evaluated immediate release oxymorphone for mild to moderate pain following ambulatory knee arthroscopy. Among 122 patients evaluated, those treated with oxymorphone IR (5 mg) reported greater pain relief compared with the placebo group during the first 8 hours following surgery. More placebo patients (48.4%) required rescue medication than oxymorphone IR-treated patients (16.7%). No oxymorphone IR-treated patients discontinued because of adverse events (AEs) or experienced serious adverse events.

Opioid plus acetaminophen compounds, including oxycodone plus APAP and hydrocodone plus APAP, provide superior pain relief than either opioid alone and are routinely provided for pain control following outpatient surgery. A new oral preparation containing (Combunox, 400 mg) provides central opioid-mediated analgesia as well as peripheral anti-inflammatory effects. In a randomized trial of patients recovering from ambulatory orthopedic surgery,[58,59] pain relief provided by combunox was more rapid in onset than ibuprofen alone (22 minutes vs 39 minutes, $P < .05$) and of longer duration than oxycodone alone (5.2 hours vs 2.3 hours, $P < .05$). The combination tablet was associated with significantly less nausea than oxycodone alone. This reduction in the incidence of nausea and vomiting may have been related to an overall reduction in oxycodone requirements, however the authors speculated that inhibition of CNS prostaglandin synthesis by ibuprofen may provide an additional reason.[59] Recommended oxycodone (5 mg) and ibuprofen dosing for moderate to severe pain following ambulatory surgery is 1 tablet every 6 hours for the short-term management of acute pain; that is no more than 7 days.[58,59]

Nonsteroidal Anti-Inflammatory Drugs

NSAIDs provide highly effective anti-inflammatory and central analgesic effects that are useful for patients suffering acute and chronic pain. NSAIDs provide analgesia by inhibiting cyclooxygenase and blocking peripheral and central production of prostaglandins. The effectiveness of NSAIDs following ambulatory surgery has been well documented.[60–62] The clinician may base the selection of the most appropriate NSAID on clinical experience, potential side effects, and cost. Ketorolac is commonly used as it is available as an injectable analgesic that can be administered either in the operating room or PACU on completion of uncomplicated cases.[63] Intramuscular ketorolac (30–60 mg) produces analgesia of the quality and duration achieved with 12 mg of parenteral morphine. Primary or adjunctive use of ketorolac can significantly reduce opioid requirements in patients recovering from orthopedic, gynecological, and general surgery.[60,64,65] O'Donavan and coworkers[60] reported that patients treated with ketorolac following uncomplicated outpatient hemorrhoidectomy reported lower pain scores and experienced less PONV and urinary retention than patients treated with morphine. Of importance, patients in the toradol group experienced less constipation, an adverse event that can potentially complicate recovery from this procedure. Early experience using relatively high doses of ketorolac (60-mg load, followed by 30 mg every 6 hours) was associated with increased surgical bleeding. Follow-up trials[64,65] found that lower doses ranging from 15 mg to as little as 7.5 mg provided measurable opioid sparing and possibly less risk of clinically significant bleeding. These doses may be employed during surgical closure in patients without NSAID contraindications or significant intraoperative bleeding.

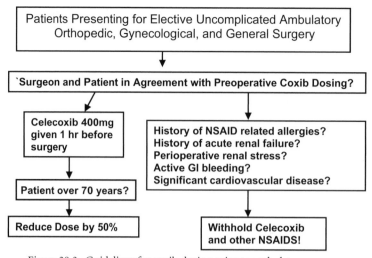

Figure 29.3: Guidelines for coxib dosing prior to ambulatory surgery.

Cox-2 Inhibitors *(Coxibs): Indications for Ambulatory Surgery*

Although lacking some of the troublesome side effects of opioids, nonselective NSAIDs may affect platelet function and increase risks of surgical bleeding. For this reason, coxibs are attractive opioid-sparing alternatives. Clinical studies have demonstrated that COX-2-selective inhibitors offer analgesic equivalency to NSAIDs, provide effective control of postoperative pain, and reduce postoperative opioid requirements. Recent concerns regarding the long-term cardiovascular safety of COX-2 inhibitors, including the voluntary withdrawal of rofecoxib (Vioxx, Merck Inc) in 2004 and valdecoxib (Bextra, Pfizer), have dramatically reduced prescriptions for this class in the United States and Canada. Although parecoxib, lumiracoxib, and celecoxib are available for use in the European Union and South America, only celecoxib (Celebrex) is approved for postoperative pain control in the United States. Nonetheless, celecoxib has been well studied, is effective, and remains available for acute pain management.[66]

The benefits of perioperative COX-2 inhibitors for ambulatory surgical pain were demonstrated by Gimbel and coworkers,[67] who compared celecoxib (200 mg twice a day) with hydrocodone (10 mg) plus acetaminophen for pain control in 416 patients recovering from outpatient orthopedic surgery. Patients in both groups reported similar pain relief scores; however, those treated with hydrocodone plus acetaminophen required more rescue analgesic and were troubled by a higher incidence of adverse events, particularly nausea, vomiting, and sedation (89%) than those treated with celecoxib (43%) over the 5-day study period.

In a second ambulatory surgical study, Gan et al[68] evaluated 223 patients recovering from laproscopic cholecystectomy. Patients were treated with IV parecoxib (40 mg) or placebo prior to surgery and oral valdecoxib (40 mg) daily for the next week. Following discharge, patients were followed by telephone and utilized pain diaries. These authors found that patients treated with parecoxib/valdecoxib required significantly less fentanyl and experienced less nausea and were discharged from the hospital sooner than patients treated with placebo. At home, patients required significantly less rescue opioid (vicodin) and were less likely to call back health care providers or return to the hospital. With regard to return to functionality, patients treated with valdecoxib benefited from significant advancement in time to light activity in home, light activity outside home, and return to normal activity.

Perioperative administration of celecoxib has not been shown to decrease cardiovascular safety[66]; however, like any COX inhibitor, dosing should be limited or withheld in patients at risk for renal failure. Recommended dosing of celecoxib for postoperative pain management is 400 mg followed by 200 mg on day 1, and 200 mg twice a day for the next 7 days as required. Celecoxib dosing guidelines employed at Yale-New Haven Hospital are presented in Figure 29.3.

Adjuvant Analgesics

Anticonvulsant-Type Analgesics

In addition to their antineuropathic effects, anticonvulsants such as gabapentin and pregabalin potentiate opioid-based analgesia while at the same time providing measurable opioid-sparing effects. They also minimize the development of secondary hyperalgesia following surgery.[52,54,69] Gabapentin and pregabalin exerts their effect by binding to the α_2-δ subunit[2] of the N-type calcium channels in the central nervous system (CNS) neurons. Although not approved for acute pain management, they have been advocated, and can contribute to, multimodal analgesia by enhancing the analgesic effect of opioids, NSAIDs, and COX-2 inhibitors.

In a same-day hospital discharge setting, Dirks and coworkers[70] evaluated in double-blind fashion the effects of gabapentin (1200 mg) or placebo given 1 hour preop to patients undergoing unilateral radical mastectomy. Intravenous PCA morphine consumption and pain intensity during rest and movement were measured postoperatively. Patients in the gabapentin group required 53% less morphine (placebo: 29 [21–23] mg; gabapentin: 15* [10–19] mg) and reported lower incident pain intensity scores. Patients treated with gabapentin were troubled by more sedation and light headedness, but experienced less nausea. It is likely that increased levels of sedation were related to the relatively large dose of gabapentin used in this clinical trial.

Seib and Paul[71] recently published a meta-analysis of 8 randomized, placebo-controlled trials that examined the effect of preoperative gabapentin administration on postoperative pain control. The authors concluded that patients who received preoperative gabapentin had significantly lower pain scores and opioid consumption during the first 24 hours after surgery. Treatment with gabapentin did not reduce the incidence of opioid-related adverse effects. The most common adverse effect of gabapentin in this analysis was sedation, with the highest incidence reported at the initiation of therapy (Figure 29.1). The new derivative, pregabalin, has greater bioavailability and a shorter time to achieve analgesic effect. Reuben and coworkers[72] examined the effectiveness of pregabalin alone and combined with celecoxib for postoperative analgesia. The combination of pregabalin and celecoxib, administered before and 12 hours after spinal fusion surgery, significantly reduced pain at rest and during movement, opioid consumption, and nausea in the first 24 hours after surgery when compared with placebo. The incidence of sedation was significantly lower in the subjects who received celecoxib or the combination of celecoxib and pregabalin when compared with subjects who received placebo (10% vs. 50%, $P < .008$.

In ambulatory settings, administration of gabapentin (300–600 mg) or pregabalin (75 mg) with celecoxib (400 mg) 2 hours prior to surgery should be considered as a relatively safe method to reduce opioid exposure while maintaining highly effective analgesia. Large randomized controlled trials are needed to determine the optimal dose, dosing regimen, and surgical population that could achieve the greatest benefit.

Ketamine

There is a good evidence that low-dose ketamine can contribute to improving postoperative pain management when used as an adjunct to opioids or local anesthetic-based analgesia.[73–75] Ketamine has shown to be of value in the management of pain following orthopedic surgery and for managing severe pain in patients with high-grade opioid tolerance. A single intraoperative injection of ketamine (0.15 mg/kg) improved analgesia and passive knee mobilization 24 hours after outpatient arthroscopic anterior cruciate ligament surgery and was not associated with dysphoria or confusion. It also improved the postoperative functional outcome after outpatient knee arthroscopy.[74,75]

IV Acetaminophen

Intravenous acetaminophen (paracetamol, ProDalfgan, Acetavance) has been used in Europe for over 15 years with over 35 million patients treated. It is available as a new nonirritating buffered 100-mL solution and is currently under phase III investigation in the United States. Injectable acetaminophen derivatives offer advantages over opioids as they are associated with little to no risk of nausea, vomiting, sedation, ileus, or respiratory depression. They also offer advantages over ketorolac in that there is little to no risk of platelet inhibition, gastrointestinal (GI) ulceration, GI bleeding, or renal toxicity.

In clinical trials the analgesic efficacy of intravenous acetaminophen (IV APAP) was found to be equivalent to an earlier developed injectable acetaminophen preparation (IV propacetamol) and IV ketorolac (30 mg).[76,77] In a randomized, double-blinded, controlled trial, Sinatra and coworkers[77] evaluated the safety and efficacy of IV APAP and IV propacetamol in patients recovering from from total hip and knee replacement surgery. Patients treated with IV APAP (4 g/day) required 28% less morphine and reported lower pain intensity scores than those treated with placebo

Clinical applications for IV APAP in ambulatory surgery would include patients at risk for opioid-associated respiratory depression, nausea, and ileus and patients with visceral pain following ureteral, tubal, or uncomplicated laproscopic surg-

eries. In addition, patients recovering from orthopedic surgery, including noncemented prostheses and spinal fusion, could benefit from improved pain control and opioid sparing following presurgical coadministration of IV APAP with COX-2 inhibitors. IV APAP dose is 1 g every 6 hours, which should be reduced or avoided in patients with hepatic disease.

Finally, it should be remembered that oral acetaminophen is the least expensive and one of the safest analgesics that can be used to potentiate opioid and NSAID-based analgesia. Watcha and colleagues[78] found that oral acetaminophen provided measurable analgesic effects but was less effective than either celecoxib or rofecoxib for outpatient otolaryngologic surgery. In a similar outpatient trial, premedication with celecoxib (200 mg) plus acetaminophen (2 g) combination was significantly more effective than placebo or either drug alone in reducing pain intensity and opioid requirements. Satisfaction with analgesic therapy was highest in the combination group.[79]

Regional Blockade

Local anesthetics are widely administered in ambulatory settings using techniques such as local injection into the wound, field block, and peripheral nerve/plexus block. Single-injection techniques employing prolonged duration local anesthetics provide short-term analgesic benefits that are superior to those of general anesthesia; however, most patients report increasing pain intensity during the first 24 hours following surgery and many require significant doses of opioid analgesics during the first 5–7 days of recovery.[56,61,80,81] Nevertheless analgesic and economic benefits provided by single-injection techniques are worth consideration, particularly for painful outpatient procedures. In a large clinical trial both femoral-sciatic and femoral nerve block were superior to opioid-based analgesia for complex outpatient knee surgery.[80] Patients treated with nerve block reported significantly lower pain scores and benefited from a 2.5-fold reduction in need for hospital readmission. Of importance, was the finding that the less complicated and time-consuming femoral nerve was equally effective as the femoral sciatic block.

Continuous wound and perineural infusions of local anesthetic are increasingly employed following ambulatory surgery as they provide prolonged analgesia that may be maintained on discharge to home.[81–83] Continuous infusion of bupivacaine (0.5%) or ropivacaine (0.2%) at 2–4 mL/h administered using an ON-Q elastomeric pump provides safe and effective therapy for ambulatory surgical pain management. Such therapy has been evaluated for pain control following open inguinal hernia repair, arthroscopic orthopedic, and breast reconstructive surgeries.[81–86]

Effective pain control is essential to successfully perform arthroscopic shoulder surgery such as arthroscopic rotator cuff repairs, subacromial decompressions, and capsular reefings in an outpatient setting. Continuous infusion of bupivacaine into the wound is effective during the first 48 hours, when pain intensity and opioid requirements are highest. Once initiated, preemptive neural blockade provides analgesic effects that linger even after the infusion is discontinued.[82,83]

Capdevila and coworkers[81] employed a perineural PCA technique for pain management following outpatient orthopedic shoulder and foot surgeries. They reported that the technique that used a disposable elastomeric infusion device was safe, effective, and adaptable for home use. Patients self-administering ropivacaine (0.2%) bolus in addition to a basal infusion, experienced superior pain relief and functionality, required less opioid rescue, and reported greater satisfaction that others treated with either a perineural basal infusion of ropivacaine or opioid-based analgesia.

Concerns have been raised regarding the potential complications of placing a catheter beneath the operative site for infusion of local anesthesia plus epinephrine; however, no apparent increase in infection or ischemic risk has been detected.[87] Potential drawbacks of the ON-Q infusion system or other elastomeric devices includes its high cost and frequent seepage of blood-stained anesthetic fluid into the wound dressing. Refer to Chapter 19 for a detailed overview of local anesthetic blockade for patients recovering from ambulatory surgery.

Nonpharmacologic Methods

Nonpharmacologic methods for the management of postoperative pain include acupuncture, electrical stimulation, hypnosis, and the use of music during surgery. However, further research regarding the efficacy of these techniques is warranted to elucidate their effectiveness in ambulatory settings. Improved postoperative pain control through innovation and creativity may improve compliance, functionality, and patient satisfaction.[88]

ACUPUNCTURE

Acupuncture is now accepted as a complementary analgesic treatment that has been employed for postoperative pain management. Electrical stimulation of acupoints (electroacupuncture) increases the effects of acupuncture. Recently, an auricular electroacupuncture device, the P-Stim, has become available. Clinical studies in outpatients have investigated the P-Stim in chronic musculoskeletal pain and its use for minor surgery. In chronic cervical or low back pain, auricular electroacupuncture was more effective than conventional auricular acupuncture.[89] The results in acute pain were controversial. Auricular

electroacupuncture reduced pain and remifentanil consumption during oocyte aspiration when compared with conventional auricular acupuncture or a sham treatment.[90] However, after third molar tooth extraction, auricular electroacupuncture and auricular acupuncture failed to reduce either postoperative pain or analgesic consumption.[91] A final study, performed in patients recovering from ambulatory orthopedic surgery, found the technique to be minimally effective.[92] Further large-scale studies are required to evaluate the analgesic efficacy of auricular electroacupuncture.[93]

Transcutaneous Electrical Nerve Stimulation

Transcutaneous electrical nerve stimulation (TENS) has been used to treat chronic pain syndromes and has been reported to be of some utility in the treatment of postsurgical pain.[94–97] TENS utilizes a battery powered stimulator to stimulate large caliber nerve fibers in regions adjacent to the site of surgery. By varying stimulation strength and frequency, noxious processing in the spinal dorsal horn is suppressed and pain perception reduced. In a double-blinded evaluation, TENS applied postoperatively after shoulder surgery clearly reduced analgesic consumption in the first 72 hours.[96] Furthermore, there was a significant difference in the pain intensity scores in the active TENS group. The authors concluded that TENS applied postoperatively is an effective, simple modality with few side effects. Bjordal and coworkers[97] performed a meta-analysis of randomized controlled trials to determine whether TENS and acupuncture-like TENS (ALTENS) reduce analgesic consumption following surgery. Twenty-one trials involving 1350 patients were identified. The authors found that patients treated with TENS/ALTENS consumed 26.5% (range 6%–51%) less analgesic than those treated with placebo. Further reductions were noted in 11 studies using strong subnoxious stimulation with adequate frequency. In these trials the weighted reduction in analgesic consumption was 35.5% (range 14%–51%) less than

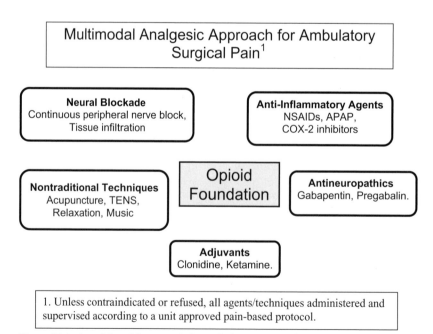

Figure 29.4: A multimodal approach for ambulatory surgical pain management. Multimodal employs a variety of agents and techniques to block pain perception at different sites in the nervous system.

Table 29.2: Guidelines for Optimizing Pain Control Following Ambulatory Surgery

Is the patient already in pain or have an opioid dependency?

Maintain baseline NSAIDs or coxib (Celecoxib) as well as opioids preoperatively; if concerned about hemostasis, consider switching NSAIDs to celecoxib 5–7 days prior to surgery; ensure that the patient takes his or her standard opioid dose on the morning of surgery

Can the procedure be performed with neural blockade?

Consider skin infiltration with bupivacaine; also nerve, plexus, intra-articular, and neuraxial blocks with IV sedation as required

Analgesics that can be given prior to or during the procedure

Use celecoxib (400 mg) 2 hours prior to surgery; patients at risk for developing neuropathic pain may be given gabapentin (600 mg) or pregabalin (100 mg) 2 hours prior to surgery. Also consider IV ketamine (0.15–0.25 mg/kg) for these patients as well as opioid-dependent and hyperalgesic patients; consider clonidine patch (0.2 mg/h) in opioid intolerant patients; carefully titrate opioids (fentanyl for most patients; however, we prefer hydromorphone for more painful surgeries), consider IV acetaminophen 1 g (when and where available), finally, consider intra-articular morphine (0.5–1 mg) and ketorolac (2.5–5 mg) following knee arthroscopy.

Analgesics that can be given on completion of surgery

Wound infiltration with bupivacaine or ropivacaine, continuous wound infiltration with bupivacaine (0.25%) using On-Q painbuster infusion pump; consider IV ketorolac (7.5–15 mg) on completion of uncomplicated surgery: judicious use of fentanyl or hydromorphone on emergence from anesthesia.

Analgesics for use in the ambulatory PACU

Titrate IV fentanyl or hydromorphone, initiate oral opioids (oxycodone, hydrocodone); consider oxymorphone (10–20 mg) or combination oxycodone plus ibuprofen for more painful surgeries. Consider IV ketorolac and acetaminophen if not given intraoperatively; ice pack arthroscopic procedures.

Analgesics for home discharge

Continue celecoxib (200 mg twice a day) or switch to NSAIDs (diclofenac, naproxen sodium) for 5–7 days. Restart baseline NSAIDs or celecoxib in arthritic or other patients dependent on this class of analgesic. Provide oral opioids (oxycodone, hydrocodone) as required. For more painful surgeries consider oxycontin (10–20 mg twice a day) for up to 7 days plus immediate release opioids as required; also consider oxymorphone IR (10–20 mg) and combination oxycodone plus ibuprofen. Maintain continuous wound infiltration (bupivacaine [0.25%]) 2–4 days using On-Q painbuster infusion pump; consider gabapentin/pregabalin in patients at risk for neuropathic pain; consider clonidine patch and TENS for patients intolerant of opioids.

---

placebo. In ambulatory settings, similar analgesic dose reductions may be beneficial in patients intolerant of opioids and others at risk for opioid-induced ileus.[97]

An overview of pharmacologic and nonpharmacologic and interventional techniques that may be employed to complement opioid-based analgesia and further optimize outpatient pain management is depicted in Figure 29.4.

Protocol-Based Pain Control

In an effort to avoid analgesic gaps, caregivers should consider pain treatment protocols based on patient related and procedure related factors. A treatment protocol that we employ to minimize ambulatory surgical pain is presented in Table 29.2. Identifying painful procedures, procedures with a high rate of progression to persistent pain, highly anxious patients with low pain thresholds, and those with ongoing chronic pain and opioid dependencies will help individualize analgesic treatment plans to optimize postoperative analgesia and increase satisfaction. For example, opioid-dependent and anxiety-disturbed patients should be instructed to take their baseline medications the morning of surgery. Chronic arthritic patients may be instructed to switch from nonspecific NSAIDs to a COX-2 inhibitor 5–7 days prior to surgery to prevent a flare in disease symptoms, but not interfering with platelet function or increasing risk of postoperative bleeding.[98] Patients taking celecoxib may be

instructed to double their dose from 200 to 400 mg the morning of surgery.

Risk factors linked to the development of persistent pain include individuals presenting for open hernia repair, axillary dissections, mastectomy, and plastic surgical flaps. Persistent pain is more commonly observed in younger patients with ongoing or preceding pain at the site of surgery and in individuals with psychosocial abnormalities and specific genetic susceptibilities.[10] Lopez et al[99] employed a previously developed list of painful procedures[18] and an aggressive procedure-related analgesic protocol to treat pain in an ambulatory setting. By using these tools, 86% of patients reported pain scores of less than 3 following discharge. PROSPECT is a European project that provides evidence-based pain management recommendations for patients undergoing common surgical procedures. The information is available at Web site (www.postoppain.org). The ASRA is developing similar evidence based screening and treatment guidance protocols under the name Acute Postoperative Pain (POP) initiative (www.acutepop.org).

CONCLUSION

Optimizing pain management in patients recovering from ambulatory surgery is generally given less attention than that provided to those requiring in-hospital recoveries as the procedures are perceived as being less painful. Nevertheless, a significant number of ambulatory surgical patients experience moderate to severe pain either because prescriptions were inadequate or side effects related to opioid monotherapy resulted in patient self-underdosing. These analgesic gaps have a significant impact on patient well-being and overall medical costs, as they are associated with increased patient returns to hospital and hospital readmission for severe pain or nausea and vomiting related to opioid exposure.[100] Economic costs related to impaired rehabilitation, and delayed functionality and return to work, are also significant, albeit more difficult to calculate. Improved patient and caregiver education, preoperative analgesic dosing, and an aggressive multimodal approach that combines pharmacotherapy as well as alternative medical techniques may help optimize ambulatory pain management, whereas reducing opioid-related adverse events. In the near future, novel analgesics and analgesic delivery systems may further improve ambulatory surgical pain management. Transdermal iontophoretic fentanyl PCA (Ionsys), intranasal fentanyl, and morphine delivery systems may be more effective and better tolerated than oral opioids for analgesia following home discharge. Liposomal pastes incorporating local anesthetics may be able to provide sustained (72 hour) and effective perineural or injury site analgesia without the need for catheters and elastomeric infusion pumps. Peripheral κ receptor agonists may provide effective relief of gynecological surgical pain and other forms of visceral pain, without adverse CNS effects. Dual acting analgesics that have moderate opioid efficacy and central adrenergic analgesic effects (tapentadol) have been found to provide analgesic effects similar to more potent opioids but with a lower adverse event profile. Finally, injectable acetaminophen and parenteral diclofenac offer potential safety advantages over ketorolac and may soon be approved for use in the United States. Both of these analgesics should be well suited for intraoperative and PACU analgesia.

REFERENCES

1. Fast stats. National Center for Health Statistics Web site available at www.cdc.gov/nchs/fastats.

2. SMG forecast of surgical volume in hospital/ambulatory settings 1994–2001.Chicago: SMG Marketing Group, Inc 1996.

3. Koening L, Hearle K, Seigel JM, et al. Drivers of expenditure growth in outpatient care services. *Am J Managed Care.* 2003;9:SP25–SP33.

4. Warner MA, Shields SE, Chute CG. Major morbidity and mortality within 1 month of ambulatory surgery and anesthesia. *JAMA.* 1993;270:1437–1441.

5. Vila H, Soto R, Cantor AB, Mackey D. Comparative outcomes analysis of procedures performed in physician offices and ambulatory centers. *Arch Surg.* 2003;138:991–995.

6. Available at ASA website at www.asahq.org/ publicaionsAnd Services/outcomeindicators.pdf.

7. Carr DB, Goudas LC. Acute Pain. *Lancet.* 1999;353:2051–2058.

8. Breivik H. postoperative pain management: why is it difficult to show that it improves outcome? *Eur J Anaesthesiol.* 1998;15:748–751.

9. Visser JE. Chronic post surgical pain: epidemiology and clinical implications for acute pain management. *Acute Pain.* 2006;8:73–81.

10. Kehlet H, Jensen TS, Woolf CJ. Persistent postsurgical pain: risk factors and prevention *Lancet.* 2006;367:1618–1625.

11. Cousins MJ, Power I, Smith G. Pain: a persistent problem. *Reg Anesth Pain Med.* 2000;25:6–21.

12. Acute Pain Management: operative or medical procedures and trauma I. Agency for Health Care Policy and Research. *Clin Pharma.* 1992;11:309–331.

13. Acute Pain Management: operative or medical procedures and trauma II. Agency for Health Care Policy and Research. *Clin Pharma.* 1992;11:391–414.

14. Pain management standards. Available at: www.jcaho.org/ accredited=organizations/hopitals/standards/revisons/index. htm.

15. Pavlin DJ, Chen C, Penaloza BS, Buckley PF. A survey of pain and other symptoms that affect the recovery process after discharge from an ambulatory surgery center. *J Clin Anesth.* 2004;16(3):200–206.

16. Shaikh S, Chung F, and Imarengiaye C, et al. Pain, nausea, vomiting and ocular complications delay discharge following ambulatory microdiscectomy. *Can J Anaesth.* 2003;50:5:514–518.

17. Rocchi A, Chung F, Forte L. Canadian Survey of post surgical pain and pain medication experience. *Can J Anesth.* 2002;49:10;1053–1056.

18. McGrath B, Chung F, and Elgendy H, et al. Thirty percent of patients have moderate to severe pain 24 hr after ambulatory surgery: a survey of 5073 patients. *Can J Anesth.* 2004; 51(9):886–891.

19. Rawal N, Hylander J, Nydhal PA, Olofsson I, Gupta A. Survey of postoperative analgesia following ambulatory surgery. *Acta Anaesthesiol Scan.*1997;41:1017–1022.

20. Swan BA, Maislin G, Traber K. Symptom distress and functional status changes during the first seven days after ambulatory surgery. *Anesth Analg.* 1998;86:739–745.

21. Mattila K, Toivonen J, Janhunen L, Rosenberg PH, Hynynen M. Postdischarge symptoms after ambulatory surgery: first week incidence, intensity, and risk factors. *Anesth Analg.* 2005;101:1643–1650.

22. Chung F, Mezei G. Factors contributing to prolonged hospital stay after ambulatory surgery. *Anesth Analg.* 1999;89:1352–1359.

23. Beauregard L, Pomp A. Chioniere: severity and impact of pain after day-surgery. *Can J Anesth.* 1998:45:304–311.

24. Dexter F, Tincker J. Analysis of strategies to decrease postanesthetic care unit costs. *Anesthesiology.* 1995;82:1534–1535.

25. Gold BS, Kitz DS, Lecky JH. Neuhaus: unanticipated hospital admission following ambulatory surgery. *JAMA.* 1989;262:3008–3010.

26. Twerksy R, Fishman D, Homel P. What happens after discharge? Return visits after ambulatory surgery. *Anesth Analg.* 1997:84:319–324.

27. Fortier J, Chung F, Su J. Unanticipated admission after ambulatory surgery: a prospective study. *Can J Anesth.* 1998;45:612–619.

28. Awad T, Moore M, Rushie C, Elburki A, Obrein K, Warde D. Unplanned hospital admission in children undergoing day case surgery. *Eur J Anesth.* 2004;21:379–383.

29. Williams B, Kentor ML, Vogt MT, et al. Economics of nerve block pain management after anterior cruciate ligament reconstruction. *Anesthesiology.* 2004;100:697–706.

30. Coley KC, Williams BA, Da Pos SV, Chen C, Smith R. Retrospective evaluation of unanticipated admissions after same day surgery and associated costs. *J Clin Anesth.* 2002:14;349–353.

31. Scott NB, Hodson M. Public perception of postoperative pain and its relief. *Anesthesia.* 1997;52:438–442.

32. Marquardt HM, Razis PA. Prepacked take home analgesia for day case surgery. *Br J Nurs.* 1996;5:1114–1118.

33. Goldsmith DM, Safran C. Using web to reduce postoperative pain following ambulatory surgery. *Proc AMIA Symp.* 1999;780–784.

34. Hekmat N, Burke M, Howell SJ: Preventive pain management in the postoperative hand surgery patient. *Orth Nurs.* 1994:13:3.

35. Jonas DA. Parent's management of their child's pain in the home following day surgery. *J Child Health Care.* 2003;7(3):150–162.

36. Kissin I Preemptive analgesia. *Anesthesiology.* 2000;93:1138–1143.

37. Woolf CJ, Chong MS. Preemptive analgesia-treating postoperative pain by preventing the establishment of central sensitization. *Anesth Analg.* 1993;77:362–379.

38. Moiniche S, Kehlet H, Dahl JB. A qualitative and quantitative systematic review of preemptive analgesia for postoperative pain relief: the role of timing of analgesia. *Anesthesiology.* 2002;96:725–741.

39. Reuben SS, Bhopatkar S, Maciolek H, et al. The preemptive analgesic effect of rofecoxib after ambulatory arthroscopic knee surgery. *Anesth Analg.* 2002;94:55–59.

40. Ejlersen E, Andersen HB, Eliasen K, Mogensen T. A comparison between pre- and postincisional lidocaine infiltration on postoperative pain. *Anesth Analg.*1992;74:495–498.

41. Philip BK, Reese PR, Burch SP. The economic impact of opioids on postoperative pain management. J Clin Anesth. 2002;14:354–364.

42. Sinatra RS. Role of cox-2 inhibitors in the evolution of acute pain management. *J Pain Symptom Manage.* 2002;24(1S):18–27.

43. Kehlet H, Dahl JB. The value of "multimodal" or "balanced analgesia" in postoperative pain treatment. *Anesth Analg.* 1993;77:1048–1056.

44. Neligan PJ, Cunningham AJ. The multimodal approach to pain in ambulatory anesthesia. *Curr Anesthesiol Rep.* 2000;2:320–326.

45. Buvanendran A, Kroin JS, Tuman KJ, et al. Effects of perioperative administration of a selective cyclooxygenase 2 inhibitor on pain management and recovery of function after knee replacement: a randomized controlled trial. *JAMA.* 2003;290:2411–2418.

46. Watcha MF, White PF. Post operative nausea and vomiting: its etiology, treatment and prevention. *Anesthesiology.* 1992;77:162–184.

47. United States Acute Pain Management Guideline Panel. Acute pain management: operative or medical procedures and trauma. Pub. no. 92-0032. Rockville, MD: United States Department of Health and Human Services, Public Health Service Agency for Health Care Policy and Research; 1992.

48. Ashburn MA, Caplan RA, Carr DB, et al. Practice guidelines for acute pain management in the perioperative setting: an updated report by the American Society of Anesthesiologists Task Force on Acute Pain Management. *Anesthesiology.* 2004;100:1573–1581.

49. Reuben SS, Gutta SB, Maciolek H, Sklar J, Redford J. Effect of initiating a preventative multimodal analgesic regimen upon long-term patient outcomes after anterior cruciate ligament reconstruction for same-day surgery: a 1200-patient case series. Acute Pain. 2005;7:65–73.

50. Brill S, Plaza M. Intra-articular administration of clonidine and ketorolac for pain control following knee arthroscopy. *Can J Anaesth.* 2004;51:975–978.

51. Segal IS, Jarvis DJ, Duncan SR. Clinical efficacy of oral-transdermal clonidine combinations during the perioperative period. *Anesthesiology.* 1991;74:220–205.

52. Hurley RW, Chatterjea D, Rose Feng M, Taylor CP, Hammond DL. Gabapentin and pregabalin can interact synergistically with naproxen to produce antihyperalgesia. *Anesthesiology.* 2002;97:1263–1273.

53. Gilron I, Orr E, Tu D, O'Neill JP, Zamora JE, Bell AC. A placebo-controlled randomized clinical trial of perioperative administration of gabapentin, rofecoxib and their combination for spontaneous and movement-evoked pain after abdominal hysterectomy. *Pain.* 2005;113:191–200.

54. Dahl JB, Mathiesen O, Moiniche S. Protective premedication: an option with gabapentin and related drugs? A review of gabapentin and pregabalin in the treatment of post-operative pain. *Acta Anesthesiol Scand.* 2004;48:1130–1136.

55. Sinatra RS, Boice J, Jahr J, Cavanaugh J, Reicin J. Multiple doses of rofecoxib in patients recovering from gynecological surgery: effects on pain intensity, morphine consumption, and bowel function. *Reg Anesth Pain Med.* 2006;31:134–142.

56. Sinatra RS, Torres J, Bustos AM. Pain management after major orthopaedic surgery: current strategies and new concepts. *J Am Acad Orthop Surg.* 2002;10:117–129.

57. Gimbel JS, Walker D, Ma T, Ahdieh H. Efficacy and safety of oxymorphone immediate release for the treatment of mild to moderate pain after ambulatory orthopedic surgery. *Arch Phys Med Rehab.* 2005;86:2284–2289.

58. Combunox [package insert]. St Louis, MO: Forest Pharmaceuticals, Inc.; 2004.

59. Litkowski LJ, Christensen SE, Adamson DN, et al. Analgesic efficacy and tolerability of oxycodone 5 mg/ibuprofen 400 mg compared with those of oxycodone 5 mg/acetaminophen 325 mg and hydrocodone 7.5 mg/ acetaminophen 500 mg in patients with moderate to severe postoperative pain: a randomized, double-blind, group study in a dental pain model. *Clin Ther.* 2005;27:418–429.

60. O'Donavan S, Ferrara A, Larach S, Williamson P. Intraoperative use of Toradol facilitates outpatient hemorrhoidectomy. *Dis Colon Rectum.* 1994;37:739–799.

61. White PF. The role of non-opioid analgesic techniques in the management of pain after ambulatory surgery. *Anesth Analg.* 2002;94:577–585.

62. Marret E, Kurdi O, Zufferey P, Bonnet F. Effects of nonsteroidal antiinflammatory drugs on patient-controlled analgesia morphine side effects: meta-analysis of randomized controlled trials. *Anesthesiology.* 2005; 102:1249–1260.

63. Reinhart D. Minimising the adverse effects of ketorolac. *Drug Safety.* 2000;22:487–497.

64. Reuben SS, Connelly NR, Steinberg RB. Dose response of ketorolac as an adjunct to PCA morphine. *Anesth Analg.* 1998;87:98–102.

65. Sevarino FB, Sinatra RS, Paige D, et al. The efficacy of intramuscular ketorolac in combination with intravenous PCA morphine for postoperative pain relief. *J Clin Anesth.* 1992;4:285–288.

66. Caldwell B, Aidington S, Weatherall M, et al. Risk of cardiovascular events and celecoxib: a systematic review and meta-analysis. *J R Soc Med.* 2006;99:132–140.

67. Gimbel JS, Brugger A, Zhao W, et al. Efficacy and tolerability of celecoxib versus hydrocodone/acetaminophen in the treatment of pain after ambulatory orthopedic surgery in adults. *Clin Therapeut.* 2001;23:228–241.

68. Gan TJ, Joshi GP, Viscusi E, et al. Preoperative parenteral parecoxib and follow-up oral valdecoxib reduce length of stay and improve quality of patient recovery after laparoscopic cholecystectomy surgery. *Anesth Analg.* 2004;98:1665–1673.

69. Hurley RW, Cohen SP, Williams KA, Rowlingson AJ, Wu CL. The analgesic effects of perioperative gabapentin on postoperative pain: a meta-analysis. *Reg Anesth Pain Med.* 2006;31:237–247.

70. Dirks J, Freensberg BB, Christensen D, et al. A randomized study of the effects of single dose gabapentin versus placebo on postoperative pain. *Anesthesiology.* 2003;97:560–564.

71. Seib RK, Paul JE. Preoperative gabapentin for postoperative analgesia: a meta-analysis. *Can J Anesthes.* 2006;53:461–469.

72. Reuben SS, Buvanendran A, Kroin JS, Raghunathan K. The analgesic efficacy of celecoxib, pregabalin and their combination for spinal fusion. *Anesth Analg.* 2006;103:1271–1276.

73. Subramaniam K, Subramaniam B, Steinbrook RA. Ketamine as adjuvant analgesic to opioids: a quantitative and qualitative systematic review. *Anesth Analg.* 2004;99:482–495.

74. Menigaux C, Fletcher D, Dupont X, Guignard B, Guirimand F, Chauvin M. The benefits of intraoperative small-dose ketamine on postoperative pain after anterior cruciate ligament repair. *Anesth Analg.* 2000;90:129–135.

75. Menigaux C, Guignard B, Fletcher D, Sessler DI, Dupont X, Chauvin M. Intraoperative small-dose ketamine enhances analgesia after outpatient knee arthroscopy. *Anesth Analg.* 2001;93:606–612.

76. Moller PL, Juhl GI, Payen-Champenois C, Skoglund LA. Intravenous acetaminophen: comparable analgesic efficacy but better safety than its prodrug, propacetamol for postoperative pain after third molar surgery. *Anesth Analg.* 2005;101:90–96.

77. Sinatra R, Jahr J, Reynolds L, et al; Efficacy and safety of single and repeated doses of 1 gram acetaminophen injection (paracetamol) for pain management after major orthopedic surgery. *Anesthesiology.* 2005;102:822–831.

78. Watcha M, Issioui T, Klein K, et al. Cost and effectiveness of rofecoxib, celecoxib and acetaminophen for preventing pain after ambulatory otolaryngologic surgery. *Anesth Analg.* 2003;96:987–994.

79. Issioui T, Klein K, White PF, et al. (The efficacy of premedication with celecoxib and acetaminophen in preventing pain after otolarygologic surgery. *Anesth Analg.* 2002;94:1188–1193.

80. Williams B, Kentor M, Vogt M, et al. Femoral sciatic nerve blocks for complex outpatient knee surgery are associated with less postoperative pain before same day discharge: a review of 1,200 consecutive cases. *Anesthesiology.* 2003;98:1206–1213.

81. Capdevila X, Dadure C, Bringuier S, et al. Effect of patient controlled perineural analgesia in rehabilitation and pain after ambulatory orthopedic surgery. *Anesthesiology.* 2006;105:566–575.

82. Barbar FA, Herbert MA. The effectiveness of an anesthetic continuous infusion device on postoperative pain control. *Arthroscopy.* 2002;18:76–81.

83. Swenson, JD, et al. Outpatient management of continuous peripheral nerve catheters placed using ultrasound guidance: an experience in 620 patients. *Anesth Analg.* 2006;103(6):1436–1443.

84. Sanchez B, Waxman K, Tatevossian K, et al. Local anesthetic infusion pumps improve postoperative pain after inguinal hernia repair. *Am Surg.* 2004;70:1002–1006.

85. Woods GW, O'Connor DP, Calder CT. Continuous femoral nerve block versus intra-articular injection for pain control after anterior cruciate ligament reconstruction. *Am J Sports Med.* 2006;34:1328–1333.

86. Liu L, Fine NA. The efficacy of continuous infiltration in breast surgery:reduction mammoplasty and reconstruction. *Plast Reconstr Surg.* 2005;115(7):1927–1934.

87. Bergman BD, Hebl JR, Kent J, Horlocker TT. Neurologic complications of 405 consecutive continuous axillary catheters. *Anesth Analg.* 2003;96:247–252.

88. Shang A, Gan TJ. Optimising postoperative pain management in the ambulatory patient. *Drugs.* 2003;63(9):855–867.

89. Sator-Katzenschlager SM, Michalek-Sauberer A. Auricular-electronic acupuncture stimulation device for pain relief. *Acupunct Med.* 2002;20:56–65.

90. Tsen LC. Electro-acupuncture was as efficacious as IV alfentanil for pain control during oocyte retrieval: evidence-based. *Obstet Gynecol.* 2004; 6:120–123.

91. Lao L, Bergman S, Hamilton GR, et al. Evaluation of acupuncture for pain control after oral surgery. *Arch Otolaryngol Head Neck Surg.* 1999;125:567–571.

92. Usichenko TI, Kuchling S, Witstruck T. Auricular acupuncture for pain relief after ambulatory knee surgery: a randomized trial. *Can Med Assoc J.* 2007;176;179–183.

93. Sim CK, Xu PC, Pua HL. Effects of electroacupuncture on intraoperative and postoperative analgesic requirements. *Expert Med Devices.* 2007;4:23–32.

94. Solak O, Turna A, Pekcolaklar A, et al. Transcutaneous nerve stimulation for the treatment of post-thoracotomy pain. *Thorac Cardiovasc Surg.* 2007;55;182–185.

95. Rakel B, Frantz R. Effectiveness of transcutaneous electrical nerve stimulation on postoperative pain with movement. *J Pain.* 2003;8:455–464.

96. Likar R, Moinar M, Pipam W, et al. Postoperative TENS in shoulder surgery. *Schmerz.* 2001;5:158–163.

97. Bjordal JM, Johnson MI, Ljunggreen AE. Transcutaneous electrical nerve stimulation can reduce postoperative analgesic consumption: a meta-analysis. *Eur J Pain.* 2003;7:181–188.

98. Reuben SS, Ekman EF. The effect of cyclooxygenase-2 inhibition on analgesia and spinal fusion. *J Bone Joint Surg.* 2005;87:536–542.

99. Lopez M, Fortuny G, Riera F: Effectiveness of a clinical guide for the treatment of postoperative pain in a major ambulatory surgery unit. *Ambul Surg.* 2001;9:33–35.

100. Hill RP, Lubarsky DA, Phillips-Bute B, et al. Cost effectiveness of prophylactic antiemetic therapy with ondeansetron, droperidol, or placebo. *Anesthesiology.* 2000;92:958–967.

30

Pediatric Acute Pain Management

Giorgio Ivani, Valeria Mossetti, and Simona Italiano

PAIN IN INFANTS, CHILDREN, AND ADOLESCENTS

Pain management in childhood is a theme that only since the early 2000s has assumed a more central role in the current medical practice. Despite the fact that pain is considered to be a universal human experience, the international research regarding pain during the first years of life is limited to a few studies. A review published in 1991[1] revealed that the most frequently administrated therapy to manage postoperative pain in childhood was the intramuscular (IM) administration of opioids, despite the poor efficacy of this method and the obvious psychological consequences as a result of the children's fear of needles. Underestimating the importance of analgesic treatment in childhood can be the result of several causes, not only the poor knowledge of pain treatment and the fear of the pharmacologic side effect in children, such as respiratory depression or addiction, but also the idea that children, especially infants, do not feel pain the way adults do, or, if they do, the consequences of pain suffered during the first age of life are not relevant. Moreover, there is a lack of knowledge of the ways to assess for the presence of pain.

Unrelieved pain has negative physical and psychological consequences.[2] This is the reason why preventing and controlling the acute pain occurrence before, during, and after medical procedures can lead to both short- and long-term benefits. However, the established pain is more difficult to control and often more severe.[3]

Premature infants often undergo painful medical and surgical procedures that can cause pain. Until recently, it was believed that infants are insensitive to pain because of their immature nervous systems. Recent research confirmed the hypothesis that infants and also newborns have nervous systems mature enough to feel pain.[3]

It is clear that pain pathways develop early in the fetus and must be regarded as operational from as early as 18 weeks of gestation.[4] The nature of these pathways are distinct from those of the mature infant. It remains unclear at what stage pain transmission becomes pain sensation for the fetus or preterm infant.

Although this issue will continue to be debated emotionally and philosophically, it is important to be aware of the other important consequences of noxious stimuli and bodily injury: the hemodynamic, inflammatory, and stress responses.[5] Prevention of the undesirable effects of noxious stimulation in the preterm infant with adequate amounts of analgesic and anesthetic drugs reduces both short- and long-term morbidity and at the same time provides adequate analgesia, regardless of any philosophical standpoint.[6] It is unclear if the use of analgesic drugs in the developing infant has long-term effects, but it must be studied carefully to ensure that the drugs themselves do not cause additional problems. In older infants, pain can be identified more easily and it is essential to use appropriate techniques to identify and treat pain promptly. Pain, like hunger, is a nonnegotiable experience for a young child: he or she is either free of pain or has pain that requires immediate attention. More work is needed to develop techniques to identify the onset of pain more rapidly or find techniques that can measure the offset of analgesic drugs. Moreover, the psychological aspects, such as the fact that children, especially if they are very young, cannot understand pain as a part of the healing process, but rather tend to consider suffering as a punishment, makes the effort to overcame pain in children even more important.[7]

Painful procedures in infancy may lead to permanent changes in the pain threshold. Thus, effective pain interventions are needed for premature infants who are now surviving because of medical and technical advances.

PROCEDURE-RELATED PAIN

Managing acute pain in children today means coping not only with the pain caused by the illness itself, but also with pain caused by lumbar punctures, bone marrow aspiration, and bone biopsies. Many procedures related with the medical or surgical treatment can lead to a painful experience for the child, especially because the child is not always able to recognize pain as a part of the therapeutic path. The key to managing procedure-related pain and distress is handling the anticipation.[7] The approach to procedural pain varies according to the anticipated intensity and duration of expected pain, the context and meaning as seen by the child and family, the coping style and temperament of the child, the type of procedure, the child's history of pain, and the family support system. Procedures should be performed or supervised by persons with sufficient technical expertise so that pain is minimized to the greatest extent possible. Children and parents should receive appropriate information about what to expect and how to minimize distress. It is advisable in appropriate situations to have parents prepared with specific ways of comforting their children.

The choice of the treatment approach should meet the child's needs. There are different possibilities to achieve this using the mono or multimodal approach in a graduate range of interventions ranging from deep sedation and anesthesia to strategies aimed at facilitating competent coping with the procedure in ways that enhance self-esteem with little or no pharmacologic support.[8]

Cognitive behavioral strategies that involve the use of relaxation techniques to stimulate the imagination or increase self-control can help reduce pain. Strategies that reduce distress and worry for parents and children have been associated with reductions in children's report of pain sensation and observations of their pain behavior. In a certain number of situations these strategies have significantly reduced the amount of pharmacological support needed to relive the pain, especially for older children and adolescents.[9] Overall, a quiet environment, calm adults, and clear, confident instructions increase the cooperation of the patient and increase the success of the procedure.

Local anesthetics and strategies to soothe and minimize distress should be considered even for simple procedures. Venipuncture and intramuscular injections are considered very stressful in childhood, even if they seem harmless for adults, and must be treated as a form of procedure-related acute pain.[10]

Moreover, some studies have demonstrated that the stress resulting from even short procedures is associated with irritability and feeding disturbances days afterward.[11] This is the reason it is extremely important to adopt measures to alleviate the pain before, during, and after the procedure.

The use of anxiolytics or sedatives alone for painful procedures does not provide analgesia, but makes a child less able to communicate distress. The child still experiences pain during the procedure, and they are no longer able to express their feelings. This can lead to anxiety and distress, even long after the end of the procedure.[12]

There are several nonpharmacologic techniques that can help boost the pain relief effects of drugs. Like pain medicine, each nondrug method works differently for different types of pain. A few of the most useful methods in children are as follows:

- use of heat or cold (check with your child's nurse)
- distraction (music, video games, TV, stories, blowing bubbles, puzzles)
- relaxation (breathing exercises, rocking chair)
- massage (bed bath, gentle back rub, lotion)
- rest (dimming lights and reducing noise, encouraging sleep)
- changing position (use of pillows, sitting up)
- imagination (creating stories, drawing pictures)

When the pain from a procedure is assumed to be severe, the traditional measure may be inadequate to relieve the pain, and the use of pharmacological remedies is needed to bring pain to acceptable levels.[13] When it is necessary to use sedation and analgesia for painful procedures, the guidelines issued by the American Academy of Pediatrics (AAP) should be followed. These guidelines recommend that sedation can be administered by a competent person in a monitored setting with resuscitative drugs and equipment available. The guidelines stipulate that one person is assigned to monitor the child's condition and another qualified person is present to respond to medical emergencies.

OPERATIVE AND POSTTRAUMATIC PAIN

The study of operative and postoperative pain has contributed enormously to the understanding of effective assessment and treatment of pain. This knowledge can be applied to many other areas of pediatric pain management.[14]

Data support the concept that morbidity and mortality can be reduced by good pain treatment.[5] Unrelieved pain after surgery is unhealthy; fortunately, it is preventable or controllable in an overwhelming majority of cases. Some techniques to alleviate pain in the postoperative period are based on typical anesthesiologic approaches (like epidural continuous infusion of local anaesthetic or patient-controlled analgesia [PCA]), but many studies demonstrated also that the use of simple pharmacological support, such as the use of acetaminophen, usable by pediatrician or simply by the parent, can really improve the well-being of the child, especially for short-lasting procedures.[15]

Plans for postoperative pain management should be discussed with the family and generated before surgery.

Postoperative pain is characterized by the following:

- constant surgical-related pain, frequently described as aching in nature and ordinarily near the surgical site
- acute exacerbation of pain added to the pain at rest; usually the result of activities such as coughing, getting out of bed, physiotherapy, and dressing changes
- regularly, it is a self-limiting condition
- usually there is a progressive improvement over a relatively short period

The goal of good postoperative pain management is to rapidly control the pain and avoid the risk of side effects, or overdose. For this to occur, the starting dose should be optimal, and the remaining doses need to be titrated, based on the child's needs. Administration of multiple, small, ineffective doses of analgesic may result in the prolongation of pain, exacerbation of anxiety, and even severe adverse effects of the analgesic, such as respiratory depression.

Early effective treatment is safer and more efficacious than delayed treatment. It results in improved patient comfort and possibly less total analgesic administered. Except in extenuating circumstances, medication should not be given intramuscularly, because it is painful and absorption can be variable. Oral administration is preferred for mild to moderate pain. When the child needs immediate pain relief, intravenous administration is indicated.

Postoperative pain management encompasses the use of different classes of drugs, including opioids and nonopioid analgesics.[16] The use of analgesics such as acetaminophen and nonsteroidal anti-inflammatory drugs (NSAIDs) can reduce the amount of opioid required for postoperative pain management. Even in this situation, the use of opioids in postoperative therapy in children requires a very careful monitoring of the vital signs. The side effects of these drugs, including respiratory depression, can arise at any moment and can lead to serious and, sometimes, irreversible consequences.

As part of the comprehensive assessment and management of trauma, pain should be addressed in the emergency department.[17] Sometimes pain management tends to be underestimated because the emphasis on life support care is primary. In severe trauma, the psychological effect of the injury and the intensive care unit experience necessitate the optimal treatment of pain to reduce the effects of the pain in the acute phase and to reduce symptoms and complications during the acute phase (blood pressure increasing, bleeding, tachycardia, hypovolemic shock) and the delayed consequences such as psychological distress and anxiety.

In an emergency situation, pain may be attributable to a variety of causes.[18] They include the trauma itself, surgical procedures,[19] restricted movement, underlying disease, and the presence of lines, tubes, and drains. Pain treatment, including choice of drug, dosage, route, and mode (continuous vs. intermittent) of administration, must be titrated on the individual patient and analgesics given in the overall context of what is best for the patient. Communication among caregivers and an interdisciplinary approach are helpful. Attention should be paid to optimizing sleep-wake cycles. Sufficient sleep will enable the child to cope better when awake. Prolonged pain may require use of opioids for an extended duration. Dosages should be adjusted to compensate for the development of physical tolerance, and weaning strategies should be used to minimize withdrawal symptoms.

PAIN ASSESSMENT

The difficulty of describing subjective experiences as pain has been an obstacle in the diagnostic phase of the medicine for ages. This is even more difficult for children, especially those who are so young that they do not have the verbal skill necessary to communicate the intensity and the type of their pain.

Many tools have been used to quantify the depth and the kind of pain for adults. Some of these scales have been modified to fit the needs and the communication skill of children and adolescents. The involvement of the family in the self-assessment of pain for children is very important. They can help the child identify his or her pain during and after the treatment.[20] Reliable, valid, and clinically sensitive assessment tools are available for neonates through adolescents.[21]

In a hospital setting, pain and response to treatment, including adverse effects, should be monitored routinely and documented clearly and in a visible place, such as on the vital sign sheet, to facilitate treatment and communication among health care professionals.

To treat pain adequately, ongoing assessment of the presence and severity of pain, and the child's response to treatment is essential. The scale used to assess pain in children classifies pain into two groups. The first group is based on self-assessment and is used for children able to understand and communicate the painful experience in terms of quantification. This way of identifying pain is very useful for children between ages 3 and 7 years and provides information on location, quality, intensity, and tolerability of the pain.

The second group is based on the observation of a behavior; whether the focus is on the child's behavior itself, or on the presence of precise signs and symptoms, such as blood pressure or heart rate.

Accurate acute pain assessment requires consideration of the plasticity and complexity of children's pain perception, the influence of psychological and developmental factors, and the appreciation of the potential severity and specific types of pain experienced. It is very important to understand how pain is not only a physical reflex of a distressful situation, but also an emotional state, influenced by lifestyle, family, and cultural expectations. Trouble can arise when the patient is particularly problematic, as in the case of those who are cognitively impaired, severely emotionally disturbed, or impaired in sensory or motor modalities.

The avoidance of pain begins as early as birth. The helpless newborn's behavior signals the caregivers to remove the cause of pain. As the newborn becomes an infant, he or she learns that crying is not the only possible response to the pain. The infant learns to avoid the potential painful stimuli and to modify his or her behavior so as not to repeat the painful experience. As they develop, young children change their behavior response to painful stimuli, their reporting of pain intensity, their understanding of pain, and they modify their skill in communication of the intensity, quality, and affective dimension of the painful experience.

Self-Assessment of Pain

Faces Pain Scale

This scale (Figure 30.1) is absolutely the most common and probably the easiest to adopt. It has been widely modified and is available in several versions.

The concept is to identify a facial expression that explains the intensity of the pain. Some scales have a smiling face to mean "no pain." This version has recently been criticized because it may lead to overestimation of pain. Children with no pain, but with distress from other sources may be reluctant to choose the smiling face.[22] For this reason, it is preferable to use the scale in which the face with the neutral expression represents "no pain." This scale is very useful for children older than 4 years, even if recent studies have demonstrated that younger children also can be accurate in describing their pain through the faces scale. Additionally, the faces scale is the most preferred scale by children and their parents when compared with other tools.[23]

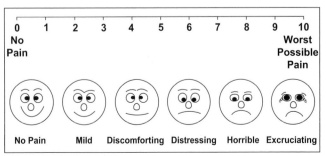

Figure 30.1: Faces Pain Scale.

Numeric Scale

The numeric scale uses a linear horizontal line, with the end points identified as "no pain" and "worst pain." The divisions along the line are marked in numbers and the child can identify the depth of his or her pain using a number between 1 and 10. The use of any numeric scale requires that the child must understand the concept of order, proportionality, (eg, 4 is more than 2) and number. These skills may not be present until age 7 years. Other vertical variations of the numeric scale are the pain thermometer and the pain ladder. With both scales, the higher numbers (like the higher rungs of a ladder) represent a greater degree of pain. Numeric scales have been shown to have a high degree of interrater reliability, validity, and versatility.

1	2	3	4	5	6	7	8	9	10

Word Graphic Rating Scale

This scale is similar to the numeric scale, but it does not require that a child understand numeric order. The child, with or without the help of an adult, is asked to draw a vertical line along this scale to indicate the extent of pain. This scale has the words *no pain* and *worst possible pain* written at each end of the line. The words *little pain*, *medium pain*, and *large pain* are written at fixed intervals along the line. The child should be able to read or to understand the graduality, if the words are read by a parent. This scale is a little more difficult to use in clinical practice, even if it can be quite accurate in describing the intensity of the pain.[24]

NO PAIN	LITTLE PAIN	MEDIUM PAIN	LARGE PAIN	WORST PAIN

Oucher

This scale can be compared to the faces scale for its basic idea; it consists of 2 vertical scales. The first is a photographic scale with 6 different pictures representing a child with expressions of increasing pain. The second is a numerical scale from 0 to 100. Children use the Oucher scale by selecting the number or photograph that most closely represents their pain intensity. Different ethnic versions of the Oucher are available (white, African American, Hispanic, and Asian). To determine if the child has the cognitive ability to use this tool, the child is asked to arrange 6 geometric figures in ascending order of size. The Oucher has been extensively validated with a high degree of correlation between both Oucher scales, the visual analog scales (VAS), and the poker chip tool (PCT).

Poker Chip Tool

This tool uses four red poker chips to quantify pain (some versions include a white chip to represent no pain). The red chips represent pieces of "hurt." One chip is a little bit of hurt, whereas all four chips are the most hurt the child can have. The child is told to select the number of chips that indicate how much pain he/she is experiencing. The poker chip tool has been used with success in children aged 3 to 5 years. Its validity has been established by high correlations in pain ratings assigned using the PCT and the hurt thermometer as well as the PCT and the oucher tool.

Table 30.1: Children and Infants Postoperative Pain Scale (CHIPPS)

Item	Structure	Points
Crying	None	0
	Moaning	1
	Screaming	2
Facial expression	Relaxed/smiling	0
	Wry mouth	1
	Grimace (mouth and eyes)	2
Posture of the trunk	Neutral	0
	Variable	1
	Rear up	2
Posture of the legs	Neutral, released	0
	Kicking about	1
	Tightened legs	2
Motor restlessness	None	0
	Moderate	1
	Restless	2

Pain Descriptors

The pain descriptors, a multidimensional tool developed by Savedra et al includes a body outline, a word graphic rating scale, and a pain descriptor list of 43 words. This tool has been used in 8- to 17-year-old children. They are asked to mark the location of their pain on the body outline, rate the intensity by drawing a line on the word graphic rating scale, and describe the pain by circling appropriate words that describe their pain. This tool offers a comprehensive assessment of pain, but may be cumbersome to use in a busy clinical setting.

Other Self-Report Measures

Studies associating color with the extent of pain have found red and black to be the colors most frequently associated with pain, and yellow, blue, green, and orange to be least frequently associated with pain. In addition to these measures, other ways to get children to self-report or quantify pain include pain interviews, questionnaires, and pain diaries.

Behavioral-Based Scales

These scales are based on the principle that the pain is usually associated with iterative behaviors and are very helpful in quantifying pain in children unable to provide self-report. The real problem is that these behaviors are not always associated with pain, but can be the result of other situations of discomfort, such as anxiety.[25] These scales are useful when the child is too young to express the pain with a self-assessment scale and needs to be more clear or precise in identifying the pain.[26]

When self-report is not possible, interpretation of pain behaviors requires careful consideration of the context of behaviors. There are many scales to quantify the pain by the observation of behaviors or symptoms. Some were created specifically for the pediatric use, and some as a result of the modification of scales for adults.[27]

Children's and Infants' Postoperative Pain Scale

This is a behavior-based scale that is widely used for the assessment of pain in very young children (Table 30.1). The

Table 30.2: Children's Hospital Eastern Ontario Pain Scale (CHEOPS)

Item	Behavioral	Score	Definition
Cry	No cry	1	Child is not crying.
	Moaning	2	Child is moaning or quietly vocalizing silent cry.
	Crying	2	Child is crying, but the cry is gentle or whimpering.
	Scream	3	Child is in a full-lunged cry; sobbing; may be scored with complaint or without complaint.
Facial	Composed	1	Neutral facial expression.
	Grimace	2	Score only if definite negative facial expression.
	Smiling	0	Score only if definite positive facial expression.
verbal	None	1	Child not talking.
	Other complaints	1	Child complains, but not about pain, e.g., "I want to see mommy" of "I am thirsty."
	Pain complaints	2	Child complains about pain.
	Both complaints	2	Child complains about pain and about other things, e.g., "It hurts; I want my mommy."
	Positive	0	Child makes any positive statement or talks about others things without complaint.
Torso	Neutral	1	Body (not limbs) is at rest; torso is inactive.
	Shifting	2	Body is in motion in a shifting or serpentine fashion.
	Tense	2	Body is arched or rigid.
	Shivering	2	Body is shuddering or shaking involuntarily.
	Upright	2	Child is in a vertical or upright position.
	Restrained	2	Body is restrained.
Touch	Not touching	1	Child is not touching or grabbing at wound.
	Reach	2	Child is reaching for but not touching wound.
	Touch	2	Child is gently touching wound or wound area.
	Grab	2	Child is grabbing vigorously at wound.
	Restrained	2	Child's arms are restrained.
Legs	Neutral	1	Legs may be in any position but are relaxed; includes gentle swimming or separate-like movements.
	Squirm/kicking	2	Definitive uneasy or restless movements in the legs and/or striking out with foot or feet.
	Drawn up/tensed	2	Legs tensed and/or pulled up tightly to body and kept there.
	Standing	2	Standing, crouching, or kneeling.
	Restrained	2	Child's legs are being held down.

Note: Recommended for children 1–7 years old; a score greater than 4 indicates pain.

following behaviors are given scores of 0 to 2 as indicators of the level of pain experienced:

- crying
- facial expression
- posture of the trunk
- posture of the legs
- motor restlessness

- verbal expression
- movement of torso
- touching of wound
- movement of legs

A score ranging from 0 to 2 or 1 to 3 is assigned to each activity and the total score ranges from 4 to 13 (Table 30.2).

Children's Hospital Eastern Ontario Pain Scale

This behavioral scale is the most widely used for newborns and infants for the evaluation of acute and chronic pain. It has been used in the intensive care unit (ICU), in the surgery ward for postoperative evaluation, and in the neonatology ward. However, studies have found that the Children's Hospital Eastern Ontario Pain Scale (CHEOPS) may not provide valid indicators of pain intensity after discharge from the postanesthesia care unit (PACU).[28] It is based on observations of these 6 behaviors:

- crying
- facial expression

The Pediatric Pain Profile

This is composed of a set of 20 behaviors such as facial expressions, body movement, tone, social reactions, mood, and consolability. Pain is scored on a 4-point ordinal scale (0–3) based on frequency of occurrence over 5-minute observation periods.

This scale has been studied for children with communication problems but can be enumerated among the scales that are based on behavior. For this reason it is applicable to every child who is not able to describe his or her pain; from those who have impairment problems to those who are very young.[29]

Table 30.3: FLACC Scale

Categories	Scoring		
	0	1	2
Face	No particular expression or smile	Occasional grimace or frown, withdrawn, disinterested	Frequent to constant quivering chin, clenched jaw
Legs	Normal position or relaxed	Uneasy, restless, tense	Kicking, or legs drawn up
Activity	Lying quietly, normal position, moves easily	Squirming, shifting back and forth, tense	Arched, rigid, or jerking
Cry	No cry (awake or asleep)	Moans or whimpers; occasional complaint	Crying steadily, screams or sobs, frequent complaints
Consolability	Content, relaxed	Reassured by occasional touching, hugging, or being talked to, distractable	Difficult to console or comfort

Objective Pain Scale

This scale includes 4 pain behaviors:

- crying
- movement
- agitation
- verbalization

These are added to the monitoring of BP changes to give a physiologic measure of pain. Each of these categories are scored from 0 to 2.

FLACC

The FLACC assessment tool was created to communicate pain in both verbal and preverbal children.

This scale includes 5 categories of behavior, represented by the acronym FLACC:

- face
- legs
- activity
- cry
- consolability

Each category can be scored from 0 to 2, with total scores ranging from 0 to 10. Interrater reliability of the FLACC among 2 observers was established in 30 children in the PACU (r = 0.94). Validity was established by demonstrating an appropriate decrease in FLACC scores after analgesic administration. Also, a high degree of agreement was found between FLACC scores, the PACU nurses global rating of pain, and with objective pain scale scores. The reliability and validity of this tool has been established in diverse settings and in different patient populations (Table 30.3).[28]

There is another group who can experience pain without being able to describe it and to assess its intensity. This group is represented by all the children affected by various forms of cognitive impairment. Their inability to understand their painful experience and to communicate their distress can make it a very difficult situation to cope with for their parents and for the medical team. Moreover, they are subject to more frequent painful experiences than their intact counterparts, because of the diagnostic path and because they incur traumatic events

more easily. The majority of work in pain assessment for the cognitively impaired consists of observation of the frequency of occurrence of core sets of pain behaviors over varied observation periods. More recently, specific tools for assessment of pain in this population have been developed and tested.

The Pain Indicator for Communicatively Impaired Children

Stallard et al[30] identified 6 core pain cues reported by caregivers of children with communicative impairment (CI) as signs of definite or severe pain in their child. These cues include the following:

- crying
- screaming or yelling
- screwed up or distressed looking face
- body appears stiff or tense
- difficult to comfort or console
- flinches if moved or touched

Each of these cues is scored on a 4-point scale, which is based on the frequency of occurrence of the behavior over the observation period. Caregivers of 49 children with severe CI and a chronic serious illness were instructed to complete this scale at home for 1-hour observation periods. They were also instructed to record whether they believed their child was in pain during these periods and rate its severity from 1 to 5. Caregivers reported no significant relationship between crying and the presence of pain, but found that a "screwed up" or distressed looking face had the strongest relationship with the presence of pain. In fact, when facial expression was used alone, it correctly identified 71% of children in pain and 93% of those not in pain with an overall correct classification rate of 87%.

The Non-Communicating Children's Pain Checklist – Postoperative Version (NCCPC-PV)

Breau et al tested the reliability of this checklist of pain behaviors (27 behaviors across 6 categories, including vocal, facial, social, body and limbs, activity, and physiologic signs) in 25 children with severe CI.[31] Each of these behaviors is scored on a scale from 0 to 3 based on the frequency of observation of that behavior over a 10-minute observation period. The scores of all items are summed to provide a total pain score. This study demonstrated good interrater reliability in 4 of the 6 behavior categories and good correlation between Non-Communicating Children's Pain Checklist – Postoperative Version (NCCPC-PV) scores and VAS scores when the same individual assigned both scores. However, no significant correlations were found between NCCPC-PV scores assigned by primary caregivers or a researcher and VAS scores assigned by a bedside nurse who had not used the checklist to assess pain. This suggests a bias when the same individual used both scoring methods. Although this checklist provides a comprehensive pain assessment method for children with CI undergoing surgery, it may be cumbersome for frequent pain assessment in the clinical setting.[31]

The Individualized Numeric Rating Scale

This tool was specifically designed to incorporate parents' knowledge of their cognitively impaired child's pain expression. Parents are asked to score severity of pain behaviors (based on previous painful experiences) on a scale from 0 to 10 using the categories of the FLACC tool. This individualized tool then becomes part of the patient's permanent medical record for use in subsequent hospitalizations. Pain descriptors are added to each patient's individualized numeric rating scale based on observations by nurses.

PHARMACOLOGICAL MANAGEMENT OF ACUTE PAIN IN CHILDREN

Acute pain management encompasses the use of different classes of drugs, including opioids and nonopioid analgesics. A gradual approach, mediated by the kind of surgery or traumatic event and the severity of the estimated pain, can provide a good indication to the class of drug to prescribe. A multimodal approach, based on pharmacologic and nonpharmacologic support is recommended. Overall, regional anaesthesiology is recommended. It is safe and easier to tolerate for the young patients and it has showed a very low amount of side effects, especially when compared with major analgesic drugs, such as opioids. However, the techniques of regional anaesthesia are not always applicable and the use of analgesic medication is mandatory. Using analgesic drugs in children means having a complete knowledge of doses, contraindications, and possible side effects to prevent complications and, managing them if they occur.

Basic elements of pharmacologic treatment include the following:

- type of analgesic
- dose
- timing
- routes of delivery

Acetaminophen

Acetaminophen is the most widely used analgesic to treat mild and moderate pain in children. Acetaminophen's mechanism of action is not yet fully understood. It works as a weak prostaglandin inhibitor by blocking the production of prostaglandins, which are chemicals involved in the transmission of the pain message to the brain. However, a recent study supports that the inhibition of cyclooxygenase in central nervous system may explain most of its analgesic action.[32]

Acetaminophen can be used by patients for whom NSAIDs are contraindicated, including those with asthma or with sensitivity to aspirin. Metoclopramide and domperidone, which are used to relieve the symptoms of stomach disorders, may enhance the effect of acetaminophen and must be used with caution.

Acetaminophen has shown no propensity to be addictive, even after frequent use. Acetaminophen is a valuable central analgesic, but weak peripheral anti-inflammatory agent and also exhibits antipyretic action. It does not inhibit respiration, alter acid base balance, and does not cause gastric irritation or uricosuria.

At recommended therapeutic doses, acetaminophen is a well-tolerated and a safe drug. However, overdose with acetaminophen is particularly dangerous, because it can result in hepatic toxicity. The therapeutic index of acetaminophen is narrow. Doses 5- to 10-fold higher than the normal therapeutic dose may cause severe hepatocellular necrosis. The early symptoms of acetaminophen toxicity may be mild, and often just nausea and vomiting may occur. Therefore, despite any significant early symptoms, all children who have taken an overdose should be treated accordingly. Acetylcysteine should be administered if there are any doubts of overdose.

Acetaminophen is still administered rectally, although suppositories may not be the optimal dosage form. Children dislike suppositories and, therefore, other routes should always be considered in awake children. There is also a great variation in bioavailability of rectal drugs. Hence, the recent launch of intravenous acetaminophen preparation is a welcome addition to the treatment armamentarium. Intravenous preparation allows convenient administration during the perioperative period.

The results of controlled clinical trials show that when using APAP in acute pain management, the initial dose and daily dose for the first few days should be high enough to have the maximal analgesic effect. The first dose should be around 40 mg/kg and the cumulative daily dose 100 mg/kg or less. Higher doses do not improve analgesia and daily doses over 150 mg/kg may cause toxicity. In infants lower doses and/or less frequent administration should be used. In intravenous administration the first dose should be 15–30 mg/kg infused in 15 minutes, followed by 15 mg/kg administered every 6 hours.

Nonsteroidal Anti-Inflammatory Drugs

NSAIDs, with their analgesic, antipyretic, antiplatelet, and anti-inflammatory effects, are a wide group of substances with a similar mechanism of action. Their use has increased in pediatric practice because they are easy to obtain and are relatively safe. Unlike opioids, NSAIDs show no ventilatory side effects and do not cause addiction or other side effects such as nausea, vomiting, urinary retention, constipation, and bile spasm. However, because of the risk of renal (decreased glomerular filtration rate), gastrointestinal (peptic ulcer formation and erosive gastritis), and platelet (decreased function) side effects of nonselective NSAIDs, therapy is usually recommended to be short-term only (72 hours), especially if prescribed around the clock.

NSAIDs should be used with extreme caution in patients with hypovolemia or decreased renal perfusion. Of note, aspirin should not be used because of the possible association with Reye's syndrome after a viral infection. Cyclooxygenase 2 (COX-2) inhibitors, such as celecoxib (Celebrex), may minimize the adverse effects of nonselective NSAIDs, but more long-term pediatric data are needed for safety evaluation.

Table 30.4: Pediatric Doses of Administered NSAIDs

Name of Drug	Single Dose (mg/kg)	Number of Daily Doses	Route of Administration	Maximum Dose/Day
Acetaminophen	20 (first dose)		PO	100 mg/kg
	30	3		
	40 (first dose)		PR	
	30	3		
	15–30 (first dose)	3	IV	
	15	3		
Naproxen	5–10	2–3	PO	20 mg/kg
			PR	
Ibuprofen	5–10	3	PO	30 mg/kg
Diclofenac	1–2	2–3	PO	3 mg/kg
			PR	
Ketorolac	0.3–0.5	3–4	IV	Give no more than 5 days

Abbreviations: PO = per os, PR = per rectum, IV = intravenous.

Their applicability in the pediatric field is wide and includes several pathological situations, such as fever, inflammatory conditions, and peri- and postoperative pain. Pain following surgery is best managed by providing nonopioid analgesics on a regular basis and by preventing the pain from recurring. NSAIDs should be administered before severe pain occurs, because they are more effective in pain prevention than in the relief of established pain. For mild to moderate pain, NSAIDs are appropriate alone.

NSAIDs are expected to have a ceiling on their analgesic effectiveness. As the safety of NSAIDs has not been established, there are only a few studies that have compared different doses of NSAIDs. In children over 6 months of age, some of the older NSAIDs may be used quite safely. Recently, the American Heart Association published an advisory regarding the long-term use of NSAIDs (selective and nonselective), especially at high doses, because of the increased risk of adverse cardiovascular and cerebrovascular effects. In general, the statement concurs with World Health Organization recommendations to start with acetaminophen and nonselective NSAIDs at the lowest efficacious doses for short-term pain relief. For patients requiring long-term or high doses of NSAIDs, adding a proton pump inhibitor can decrease the risk of gastrointestinal (GI) bleeding. If acetaminophen or nonselective NSAIDs are ineffective, not tolerated, or inappropriate, a selective NSAID (cyclooxygenase 2 inhibitor [coxib]) may be recommended. Renal function and blood pressure should be monitored closely. Although these recommendations were based on adult data, similar caution can be applied when recommending NSAID use in pediatric patients with preexisting hypertension, renal disease, or heart failure.

Ibuprofen, diclofenac, ketoprofen, and ketorolac are the most extensively evaluated NSAIDs in children.[33] Ketorolac is the most widely used in our center, at a dose of 0.5 mg/kg taken 3 or 4 times a day. Ketoprofen has been proved to have a substantial analgesic efficacy at a dose as low as 0.3 mg/kg; this dose can be increased to 3 mg/kg without showing remarkable side effects.

Recent data suggest that in children aged 1 to 16 years, the same weight-adjusted doses and dosing intervals for adults may be used. Only a few trials have compared different NSAIDs. There are no major differences in the analgesic action when appropriate doses of each drug are used. However, there may be some differences in the speed of analgesic action because some

NSAIDs enter in to the cerebrospinal fluid (CSF) so readily that allows a rapid central analgesia action.

The combined use of different NSAIDs is not recommended, because this increases the risk of adverse effects, whereas it largely proved the efficacy of the combination of acetaminophen and NSAIDs to manage to acute pain in childhood, not only in the postoperative period. Currently, the use of NSAIDs is not recommended, because of the increased risk of adverse events. Thus, the use of acetaminophen is more widely accepted in this population.

The great advantage of NSAIDs is their anti-inflammatory and antipyretic activities, in addition to the analgesic properties, that makes them the drugs of choice in the postop period. However, these same characteristics can mask the signs and symptoms of a possible postoperative infection. Also, a small percentage of patients can show an increased tendency of post-op bleeding if NSAIDs are administered for the pain management.[35]

Whether NSAIDs differ in the incidence and severity of adverse effects of pain management is open to discussion. A few studies indicate that ketorolac may increase bleeding more so than other NSAIDs, but the evidence is conflicting. NSAIDs are contraindicated in patients in whom sensitivity reactions are precipitated by aspirin (acetylsalicylic acid) or other NSAIDs. They should be used with caution, if at all, in children with liver dysfunction, impaired renal function, hypovolemia, hypotension, coagulation disorders, thrombocytopenia, or active bleeding. In contrast, it seems that most children with mild asthma may use NSAIDs (Table 30.4).[34]

Opioids

The use of opioids in the management of acute pain in children must be considered when the intensity and the duration of the pain does not respond to the other classes of analgesic drugs.

Since the early 2000s the use of weak opioids, like codeine or tramadol, has been used in children. The increase in the knowledge of these medications has reduced the fear of their application in the pediatric field and helped in the recognition and management of side effects, especially the nausea and vomiting, which are surely the most frequent.

Excessive sedation and severe respiratory depression are the most serious adverse effect to opioids. Depth and rate of respiration and level of sedation should be monitored closely and regularly for every child receiving opioids. In postoperative patients sedation can also be attributed to the residual effect of anesthetics. In these cases small pinpoint pupils are a particularly useful clinical sign to distinguish opioid overdose. Naloxone is a specific antidote to opioids. Small intravenous doses (2–5 µg/kg) reverse respiratory depression immediately while preserving the analgesic effect. Because the duration of action of naloxone is short, close monitoring is necessary. The dose should be repeated or continuous infusion should be initiated to ensure safe recovery. The incidence and severity of nausea and vomiting associated with the use of opioids in children varies according to drug and dosage used. The incidence of nausea and vomiting with morphine, buprenorphine, and tramadol is high and up to 50% of children may develop emesis. Nausea and vomiting may occur significantly less often with fentanyl and sufentanil. Recent trials indicate that oxycodone may also induce less nausea and vomiting than morphine. The risk of nausea and vomiting seems to be dose dependent. Morphine doses above 0.1 mg/kg are associated with a greater than 50% incidence of vomiting. With fentanyl at doses of 2 µg/kg or less vomiting rarely occurs. In contrast to dose dependency the risk of nausea and vomiting seems not to vary between different administration routes.

Other adverse effects commonly reported are ileus, constipation, urinary retention, and itching. Itching seems to occur with a higher incidence with epidural opioids. Urinary retention may also occur, therefore, the bladder should always be monitored when opioids are administered to children. Low-dose naloxone infusion may also be used to treat opioid-induced itching and urinary retention.

Weak Opioids

Codeine is a weak opioid drug that binds to µ- and κ-opioid receptors, producing all the effects of the major opioids. It has a low affinity for opioid receptors, resulting in significantly lower analgesic activities compared to morphine (about 1/6th to 1/10th the potency of morphine). It is easily absorbed after oral and intramuscular administration. The primary metabolites, codeine-6-glucuronide, norcodeine, and morphine, and some minor metabolites are excreted in the urine. The average elimination half-life of codeine in children and adults is 2 to 4 hours. Infants have been reported to have a longer half-life, up to 6 hours. The onset of analgesic action with codeine is typically within 30 minutes after oral administration, with a maximum effect at 60 to 90 minutes. The duration of action is approximately 4 to 6 hours. The recommended oral analgesic dose for codeine in children is 0.5 to 1 mg/kg administered every 4 to 6 hours as needed, to a maximum of 60 mg per dose. The same dose may be used for intramuscular or subcutaneous administration, although not commonly used. Codeine is usually combined with acetaminophen; the added analgesic effect is very useful in clinical practice.

Another common weak opioid used in pediatrics to control acute moderate to severe pain is tramadol. Tramadol is a synthetic analgesic that acts centrally by binding to opioid receptors. It works via a tricyclic-like mechanism, inhibiting neuronal reuptake of serotonin and norepinephrine within the central nervous system (CNS).[36] Additionally, tramadol inhibits the reuptake of serotonin and norepinephrine, which is believed to contribute to its analgesic properties. The initial time to achieve the therapeutic response for tramadol is 1 hour. Tramadol is almost completely absorbed and the peak plasma concentrations occur 2 hours after the dose. Thirty percent of tramadol will be excreted in the urine unchanged and 60% of the drug will be excreted in the urine as metabolites. The rest is unidentified or is a metabolite that could not be extracted. Tramadol itself is eliminated via the liver. The half-life of tramadol is 6.3 hours and the half-life of its metabolite, which has a poor analgesic effect, is 7.4 hours. After repeated dosing of tramadol the half-life increases to about 7 hours. The dose for children is 1–2 mg/kg intravenously over 30 minutes. The treatment can be repeated 3 times a day.

As side effects can occur, very careful monitoring of the patient is fundamental. Administering tramadol to children younger than 1 year outside of the ICU is not recommended, because of the more frequent insurgence of respiratory depression.

Vomiting and nausea are more common and a preventive therapy must be considered when tramadol is administered.

Major Opioids

Major opioids, like fentanyl and remifentanil, are reserved for the anesthesiological practice. They have no ceiling for analgesic efficacy, but adverse effects with higher doses limits their use outside OR. Like other opioids, they act through interaction with specific opioid receptors, and also have a dose-dependent analgesic effect. For severe postoperative pain, children should be provided opioids to ensure ongoing effective analgesia. When severe pain is likely to last for a short period, short-acting opioids, like fentanyl, may be used. After major surgery, either continuous infusion of short-acting opioids or opioids with longer half-life, like morphine, are used. During the immediate postoperative period, opioids are often administered by small intravenous boluses to obtain sufficient analgesia. The amount of opioid needed for titration is then used for the selection of further dosage and frequency of administration.

Continuous intravenous infusion of morphine has been used extensively in children after major surgery. Continuous infusion may or may not be more effective or safer than a bolus dose. If continuous infusion of morphine is used the dose should be titrated against each patient's needs to ensure effective and safe analgesia.

There is no justification for intramuscular administration of opioids in children, because intravenous morphine provides better pain relief. Intravenous administration ensures that all the drug enters the circulation without interindividual and interadministrational variation. In addition, fear of needles makes intramuscular injection an undesirable route of administration for children.

Transmucosal route is an attractive method for opioid administration in children. This route avoids first-pass hepatic metabolism and is therefore expected to be more effective than the oral route. Intranasal, sublingual, and buccal administration represents a fast and reliable method of opioid administration. Intranasal administration of fentanyl provides sufficient analgesic serum concentration and clinical efficacy without an increase in adverse effects during brief day-case procedures. Intranasal administration is unpleasant for awake children, but sublingual and buccal administration is more tolerated. Fentanyl and buprenorphine are used for transmucosal administration also in children.

PCA allows the most individualized administration of opioid. After initial titration of a desired level of analgesia,

Table 30.5: Opioid Dosage for Infants and Children

Medication	Route/Method	Dosage
Oxycodone	PO	0.1 mg/kg every 4 hours
Codeine	PO	0.5 to 1 mg/kg every 4 hours
Tramadol	PO	1–2 mg/kg every 8 hours
	IV	
Morphine	Intermittent IV bolus	0.1 mg/kg every 3–4 hours
	Continuous IV infusion	0.03–0.06 mg/kg/h with initial bolus of 0.05 mg/kg
	PO (MSIR)	0.01–0.3 mg/kg every 4 hours
	PCA	0.01 mg/kg bolus
		0.01–0.02 mg/kg every 10 minutes
Fentanyl	Intermittent IV bolus	1–2 μg/kg
	Continuous IV infusion	1–3 μg/kg/h
Remifentanil	Continuous IV infusion	0.125–0.3 μg/kg/min

Abbreviations: PO = per os.

children as young as 5 years old may use a PCA device efficiently. However, in pediatric populations, lack of comprehension and somnolence after surgery limits the maximal utilization of this technique (Table 30.5).

LOCAL ANESTHETICS

Local anesthetics are drugs that reversibly block conduction of neural impulses along central and peripheral pathways. To be effective, local anesthetics must be physically deposited, usually by needles or by indwelling catheter, in the immediate vicinity of the nerves to be blocked. Removal of local anesthetics from the neural tissue results in spontaneous and complete return of nerve conduction with no evidence of structural damage of nerve fibers as a result of the drug's effects. All local anesthetics share a common chemical structure. They are all tertiary amines and weak bases. They are all composed of a lypophilic and hydrophilic portion that are separated by a hydrocarbon chain. The lypophilic portion is composed of an unsaturated aromatic ring, such as para-amino benzoic acid, which is essential for the drug's anesthetic activity. The lypophilic portion is linked to its carbon chain by either an amide or ester bond. The nature of this linkage is the basis for classifying the two major classes of local anesthetic agents used in clinical practice. The final component of the molecule, the hydrophilic end, is a tertiary amine that confers on the molecule the properties of a weak base as well as its water solubility.

The mechanism of action of local anesthetics is similar between adults and children. Local anesthetics bind to sodium channels of the neurons preventing depolarization, thereby blocking nerve impulse conduction. The minimum concentration of local anesthetic necessary to block impulse conduction along a nerve fiber is called the Cm. A variety of factors affect Cm, including fiber size and degree of myelination of the nerve to be blocked, pH, local calcium concentration, and the rate at which a nerve is stimulated. With a lower Cm, less local anesthetic is necessary to block the transmission of pain than

is necessary to produce muscle paralysis. Thus, one can block pain sensation and not block motor function by using dilute concentrations of local anesthetic solution. Concentrated local anesthetic solutions will increase the quality of sensory block only minimally and will increase the incidence of motor blockade and systemic toxicity. Furthermore, because the process of myelination of central nervous system is not completed until 18 months after birth, Cm can be reduced in younger children.[37–40] Newborns and infants, in fact, may develop complete analgesia and even motor blockade when even dilute concentrations of local anesthetics are used.

All the ester local anesthetics are metabolized by plasma cholinesterase. The rapidity of hydrolysis and the ubiquity of cholinesterase in the plasma limits the toxicity and the duration of action of ester local anesthetics. However, because the CSF does not contain cholinesterase, ester local anesthetics deposited in the subarachnoid space will last much longer than if administered in other parts of the body.[41] Neonates and infants up to six months of age have less than half of the adult levels of this plasma enzyme.[42] Clearance may thereby be reduced and the effects of ester local anesthetics prolonged.

Amides are metabolized in the liver in a much more complex and slow manner. Sustained elevation of amide local anesthetic levels and systemic toxicity are more likely than with ester local anesthetics. Additionally, the amide local anesthetics are bound by plasma proteins, particularly α_1 acid glycoprotein, and alterations in the levels of these proteins may lead to systemic toxicity. Neonates and infants younger than 3 months, have reduced liver blood flow and immature metabolic degradation pathways.[43–49] Larger fractions of local anesthetics are unmetabolized and remain active in the plasma of infants. Furthermore, neonates and infants may be at increased risk of toxicity because of lower levels of albumin and α_1 acid glycoproteins, which are essentials for drug binding. This leads to increased concentrations of free drug and potential toxicity, particularly with bupivacaine. However, the larger volume of distribution at steady state found in neonates for these drugs may confer some clinical protection by lowering plasma drug levels.[49–54]

Table 30.6: The Systemic Effects of Local Anesthetics

	Usual Concentration (%)	Usual Dose (mg/kg)	Duration of Effects (hours)
Bupivacaine	0.25–0.5	2	2–4
Ropivacaine	0.2	2–3	2.5–5
Levobupivacaine	0.25–0.5	2–3	3–4

The metabolism of the amide local anesthetic prilocaine is unique in that it results in the production of oxidants (ortho-toluidine) that can lead to the development of methemoglobinemia. Premature and full-term infants have decreased levels of methemoglobin reductase, which make them more susceptible to developing methemoglobinemia.[50] Therefore prilocaine cannot be recommended for use in neonates.

The systemic effects of local anesthetics are determined by the total dose of drug administered and by the rapidity of absorption into the blood. In general, peak absorption of local anesthetic is dependent on the total dosage of drug administered, the volume of solution used, and the site of the block. The order of absorption from highest to lowest is as follows: intercostals, intratracheal, caudal/epidural, brachial plexus, distal, peripheral, subcutaneous. At recommended clinical dosages (Table 30.6), local anesthetic plasma levels usually remain well below toxic concentrations. Toxic effects exist and depend on the rapidity of rise and the total plasma concentration achieved following drug administration. The majority of complications occur from inadvertent intravascular or intraosseous administration. Before injection of local anesthetics, careful aspiration for blood is suggested and the bolus dose should be fractionated and administered slowly over 2–3 minutes while repeating aspiration for blood. Moreover, accurate monitoring of heart rate (rhythm, S-T wave), blood pressure, and respiratory rate are mandatory during delivery of the drug.

In pediatric age groups, local anesthetics like mepivacaine, lidocaine, and bupivacaine are still largely used. Even though adequate dose guidelines are available, case reports on toxic plasma concentrations (mainly concerning bupivacaine) have been described. Recently two new aminoamide local anesthetics, ropivacaine and levobupivacaine, have been introduced and are showing promise in pediatrics. Ropivacaine and levobupivacaine have similar characteristics: both of them are isomers, S-(-) enantiomers, whose main pharmacological aspects, in comparison with the racemic mixture, are the minor cardio and nervous affinity and toxicity and a differential neural blockade with less motor than sensitive block. Looking at the studies in children, some differences appear among ropivacaine, levobupivacaine, and bupivacaine in comparison with adults' results. For ropivacaine the studies confirm an equianalgesic effect of 0.2% solution versus 0.25% bupivacaine. This effect is probably linked to the biphasic vascular action of ropivacaine vasoconstriction at lower concentrations that is no more detectable at higher concentrations. Moreover, this action adds safety delaying the uptake from the action sites.[51–55] For levobupivacaine there are thus far very few studies in children but with data concerning both single-shot and continuous infusion, pharmacokinetics, and dose response. One of the main characteristics of these isomers in children is the reduced motor block: at the end of surgery the motor impairment, even for a short time, is stressful both for children and parents; the use of L-enantiomers reduces this motor block: it is not evident at 0.2%–0.25%, whereas it increases with higher concentrations. Thus, far there are very few studies comparing ropivacaine, levobupivacaine, and bupivacaine;[56–61] the results that are available showed that onset time and analgesic duration were similar, whereas the motor block impairment was statistically longer with bupivacaine in comparison with the two isomers.

ADJUVANTS

Even if the risk of toxicity is significantly reduced with these new local anesthetics, the duration of analgesia is quite similar to that of the other anesthetics. It is preferable to add drugs that have a synergistic action to prolong the analgesic effect without increasing the dose (thus also increasing the risk). Various adjuvants have been added to local anesthetics: opioids are extremely effective as analgesics but their side effects (pruritus, nausea, and vomiting, and especially respiratory depression) could limit their use via neuroaxial administration. Clonidine and ketamine have been used as adjuvants in children showing a better feasibility.

Clonidine

Clonidine, administered neuroaxially, shows a direct pre- and postsynaptic action as a result of activation of α_2 adrenoceptors in the dorsal horn gray matter of the spinal cord. It is also able to reduce the release of substance P. Clonidine potentiates the analgesic effect of local anesthetic and prolongs the duration of anesthesia. Several studies confirmed the efficacy of this adjuvant, which has been considered safe, effective, and cheap.[62–64]

Ketamine

Ketamine is a potent anesthetic whose action develops through the antagonism of N-methyl-D-aspartic acid (NMDA) receptors present at the spinal level and involved in pain modulation. Recently various studies were performed with preservative-free ketamine, both the racemic and the isomeric drug.[65–68] Looking at these studies it seems that a dose of S-ketamine in the range of 0.25–0.5 mg/kg is optimal for prolonging the pain relief given by local anesthetics.

CENTRAL BLOCKS IN CHILDREN

Because regional anesthesia produces profound analgesia with minimal physiologic alterations, it is increasingly being used in children as a component of intra- and postoperative pain management and posttraumatic pain management and for pain that is difficult to treat with systemic narcotics. For example, children who cannot tolerate opioids because of opioid-induced ventilatory depression or who have become tolerant to the analgesic effects of opioids can be made completely pain-free with the use of local anesthetic techniques.

The difference between children and adults is not only in terms of size, but also in the anatomic and physiologic features.

A different approach is needed when performing a block or in drug administration.

Anatomy

The relationship of the termination of the spinal cord and the dural sac to the bony spine varies with age. At birth the cord ends at L3 and the dura at S3, therefore an injury to the spinal cord can occur when a lumbar epidural block is performed even at low levels. As the child grows, the bony structures grow more than the content of the spinal canal. The cord and the dural sac rise to reach their adult level, L1 and S2, respectively, by the end of the first year of life. Moreover, the intercristal line crosses the midline at the L5–S1 space in newborn, whereas it crosses L5 in older children. The elasticity of the spine, the softness of the tissues, and the absence of lumbar lordosis make central blocks easier to perform in children than in adults. Furthermore, up to the age of 6–7 years, the epidural space contains gelatinous fat without much connective tissue, which becomes surrounded by fibrous stalks only in older children, hence catheters can easily be introduced several centimeters.

The amount of CSF in children is double that in adults (4 mL/kg vs 2 mL/kg) and 50% of this can be found in the spinal canal. The effect of this is a higher drug dilution and, in addition to the higher blood flow in children, there is higher uptake and a shorter duration of intrathecal analgesia (60–90 min).

In terms of physiology, the hemodynamic response to sympathetic blockade caused by spinally administered local anesthetics is age dependent. Unlike adults, children up to 8 years of age have little or no change in blood pressure following epidural or intrathecal administration of local anesthetics, even when the block achieved reaches high thoracic levels.

Sedation

In general, children have a fear of needles, and any performance of a block on a screaming, moving child not only is unethical, but also could be dangerous when the needle approaches the delicate nervous structures. It is, therefore, mandatory to associate most regional block procedures with general anesthesia. Performing a block on a deeply sedated child could be dangerous as well: any warning signals that something is going wrong could be easily missed. Therefore, deep anesthesia should be avoided before the performance of a block. A light general anesthesia with spontaneous breathing, without muscle relaxation or injection of narcotic, guarantees immobility and avoids the dangerous untoward effects related to respiratory and circulatory failures. In the meantime the adverse events that could result from a faulty technique, such as excruciating pain or convulsions or tachycardia can be caught.[69]

Caudal Block

The caudal approach to the epidural space is the most commonly used locoregional technique for intra- and postoperative analgesia in pediatric surgery because it is easy and safe. A few important points need to be kept in mind: a caudal block is an epidural block by a sacral approach and therefore requires a sterile technique similar to that for a major block. The position of the spinal cord and the dural sac in the spinal canal varies with age, so even if a caudal approach is used, cord injuries may occur. In newborns and infants the sacral bone is composed mostly of

cartilage and soft bony tissue. It is not surprising that cases of bone and even rectal punctures have been reported performing this kind of block.[43,70–73]

Indications

Single-shot caudal anesthesia is the technique of choice for surgery below T10 lasting no longer than 60–90 minutes. Therefore, it can be performed in surgery for inguinal hernia, hydrocele, testicular torsion, hypospadia, and diseases affecting the pelvis, anorectum, and hips.

Landmarks

The sacral hiatus results from the failure of fusion of the laminae of the last sacral vertebra and tends to close only around 7–8 years of age. It is covered by a thin ligament, the sacrococcygeal ligament, fatty tissue, and the skin. The sacral hiatus is easily detected in the lower posterior part of the sacrum, above the sacrococcygeal joint. It may be represented as the tip of an equilateral triangle turned upside down, where the upper angles are the posterior superior iliac spines. It can also be identified by its palpable margins, formed by the sacral cornua, which are remnants of the lower articular apophyses of the fifth sacral vertebra.

Through the sacral hiatus we enter the sacral canal, the end of the medullary canal. The dural sac extends to S3-S4 at birth, reaching S2 only toward 2 years of age. The distance between dural sac and hiatus varies, but in newborns it is less than 10 mm, thus there is a risk of dural puncture during caudal anesthesia.

Materials

A 19- or 22-guage metallic short beveled needle with a stylet especially designed for caudal use is used.

Single-Shot Technique

The child is first anesthetized or deeply sedated under complete monitoring. The patient is positioned on his or her side with legs and knees flexed at 90°. The sacral hiatus is identified and marked.

Two different techniques can be applied to perform a caudal block in children: the classic and the "no turn" approach. In the classic approach the needle is inserted in the midline at the apex of the sacral hiatus perpendicularly to the sacral plane. A characteristic "pop" is felt when passing the sacrococcygeal ligament. Then the needle is lowered 20° and advanced 2–3 mm to introduce the bevel completely into the sacral canal. To do so might result in puncturing the sacral bone straight to the rectum or puncturing the dural sac, producing a spinal tap.

In the "no turn" technique, described by Ivani, the needle is inserted at a 60° angle to the sacral plane. After crossing the sacrococcygeal ligament, the needle is already within the epidural space and there is no need for further movements.[74]

Whatever the technique used, needle placement should then be checked. This can be done by gently aspirating with a syringe for blood or CSF. If blood or clear fluid is aspirated, the needle should be withdrawn and the procedure started again. Even if this test is negative, it will unfortunately not ensure that the needle is not in a blood vessel or in the dural sac. Therefore, the aspiration test should be repeated often during drug administration and the local anesthetic solution should be injected in small increments. Moreover, an eventual subcutaneous pomphi because of incorrect placement of the needle should also be checked (Figures 30.2–30.6).

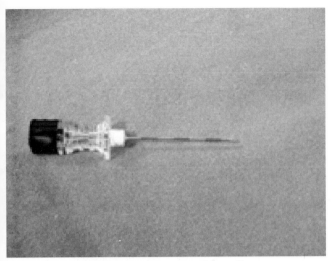

Figure 30.2: Pediatric caudal needle.

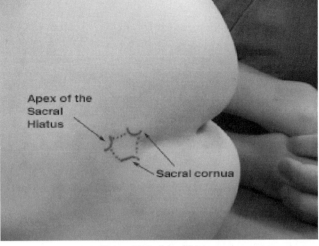

Figure 30.3: Sacral hiatus.

Continuous Technique

It is easy to place a catheter in the sacral canal using a specific epidural catheter passed through a Tuohy needle. Epidural catheter introduced by this route can be easily advanced in the epidural space at very high levels, especially in younger children, because the fatty tissue contained in the epidural space at that age is very thin and loose. However, because of the proximity of the anus, the risk of infection is elevated, therefore a lumbar approach is preferred. Moreover, it is advisable to advance the catheter only 2–3 cm because the risk of kinking and malpositioning increases.[75–78]

Drugs

Ropivacaine (0.2%) for children up to 7 years and levobupivacaine (0.25%) for older children (1 mL/kg) should be used. Clonidine (2 μg/kg) can be used as adjuvant.

Contraindications

The contraindications are few and include infection at the site of puncture, progressive neurological disease, and sacral malformation such as myelomeningocele.

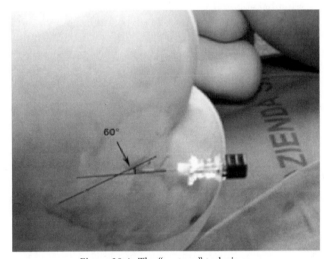

Figure 30.4: The "no turn" technique.

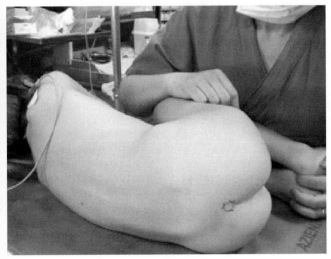

Figure 30.5: Patient positioning.

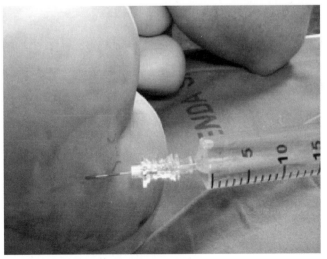

Figure 30.6: Caudal local anesthetic injection.

Complications

The complications are rare and are primarily caused by intravascular or intraosseous injections that lead to systemic toxicity of local anesthetics. Moreover, a subarachnoid injection is possible and it provokes a complete spinal anesthesia. Minor complications are the subcutaneous injection that produces a pomphus or hematoma at the injection site. Complications such as perforation of the rectum or other viscera are exceptional and mainly ascribed to lack of experience.

Epidural Block

The epidural technique in children is quite similar to the technique used in adults. Among the epidural blocks, the lumbar approach is the most commonly used technique in the pediatric population. The level of the block depends on the surgical site, keeping in mind that both single-shot block and placement of the catheter should be performed near the dermatomes that are to be anesthetized.

Indications

A lumbar epidural approach is indicated for all surgical procedures between T5 and S5 in single-shot or continuous infusion. A thoracic approach at the level of T2–T4 is indicated for thoracic surgery, at the level of T6–T8 for upper abdominal surgery, and at the level of T10–T12 for lower abdominal surgery in single-shot or continuous infusion.

Landmarks

As discussed earlier in this chapter, the anatomy of children differs from that of adults in the size and position of the spinal cord and its enveloping structures. At birth the cord ends at L3 and the dura at S3, therefore an injury to the spinal cord can occur when a lumbar epidural block is performed even at low levels. As the child grows, the cord and the dural sac rise to reach their adult level, L1 and S2, respectively, by the end of the first year of life.

The lumbar block is usually performed at the level of L4–L5 or L5–S1, the so-called Taylor's modified level, with a midline approach. The landmark is the intercristal line that crosses the midline at L5–S1 space in the newborn, whereas in older children it crosses L5. The landmark for the thoracic approach is the line joining the inferior angles of the scapulae that cross T7.

Materials

A 19- or 20-guage Tuohy needle should be used.

Single-Shot Technique

The child is first anesthetized or deeply sedated under complete monitoring. The patient is turned on his or her side with legs and knees flexed at 90°. An assistant is standing on the other side of the child and keeps the child's knees in the appropriate position during the procedure.

For lumbar block, using sterile technique, the Tuohy needle is inserted perfectly perpendicular to the axis of the spine in the midline and advanced with the bevel pointing cephalad. After crossing the superficial planes, the stylet is removed and a syringe is connected to the needle. The dorsum of the left hand lies on the child's back and the left fingers direct and advance the needle while, with the right hand, the anesthesiologist holds the syringe for detection of loss of resistance (LOR). The needle travels through the supraspinous ligament, the interspinous

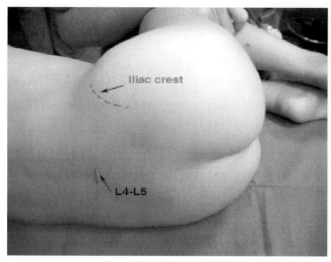

Figure 30.7: Intercristal line.

ligament, and finally the ligamentum flavum, where a distinct loss of resistance is felt. The LOR technique can be performed with air or with saline solution and different opinions support one technique over the other.[79] Air may be useful in newborns and infants to verify eventual accidental puncture of the dura mater. In fact, saline solution may mask reflux of CSF, which at this age does not have the normal pressure as in adults. In addition, saline solution may dilute the small amount of drug used. Of course, it is compulsory not to inject air in the epidural space. The key is to use only 1–1.5 mL of air for the LOR technique without injecting it. The distance from the skin to the epidural space is very short in small children. The Busoni formula may be used to calculate this distance:

$$\text{distance in mm} = (\text{age} \times 2) + 10.$$

After reaching the epidural space, needle placement should then be checked. This can be done by gently aspirating with a syringe for blood or CSF. If blood or clear fluid is aspirated, the needle should be withdrawn and the procedure started again. If this test is negative it will unfortunately not ensure that the needle is not in a blood vessel. Therefore aspiration test should be repeated often during drug administration and the local anesthetic solution should be injected in small increments and thereby serve as many mini test doses (Figures 30.7–30.10).

THORACIC BLOCK

The thoracic technique is the same as that of the lumbar technique, but it is necessary to remember that the spinous processes are more oblique than at cervical and lumbar levels. The epidural space is reduced and the dura mater is much closer to the yellow ligament (Figures 30.11–30.13).

Continuous Technique

When positioning a catheter, the Tuohy needle should be inserted close to the target area to block to avoid excessive postoperative infusion of drug and the risk of kinking and coiling of the catheter.

The short bevel of the pediatric-sized needle is big enough to allow the catheter to enter the epidural space without problems. If there is resistance when the catheter reaches the tip of the needle, however, it could mean that the bevel is lying partly in

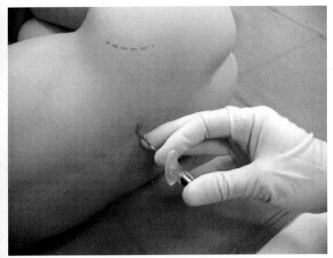

Figure 30.8: Lumbar block.

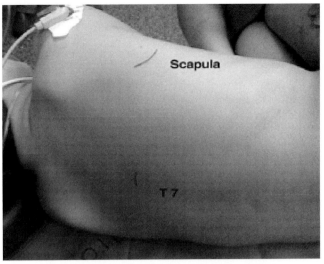

Figure 30.11: Landmark for thoracic epidural block.

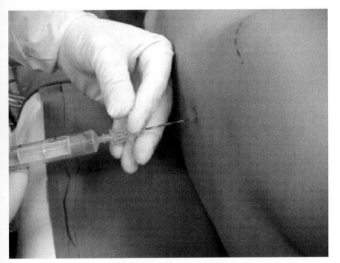

Figure 30.9: Lumbar block. Loss of resistance technique.

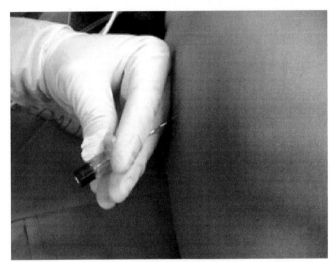

Figure 30.12: Thoracic block.

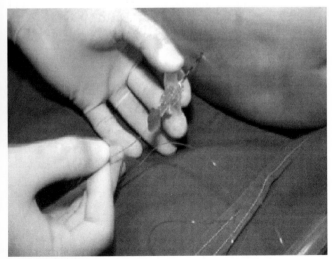

Figure 30.10: Lumbar epidural catheter.

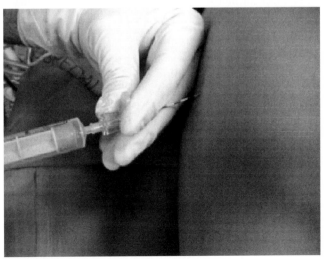

Figure 30.13: Thoracic block. Loss of resistance technique.

the ligamentum flavum. Attempts to force the catheter should be avoided and it is preferable to withdraw the needle and catheter together and try again.

Securing the catheter in place is an important step, we prefer a transparent adhesive drape over the puncture point, also including the initial course of the catheter, to be able to visualize leakage of the infusate at the puncture site.

Drugs

Ropivacaine (0.2%) for children up to 7 years and levobupivacaine (0.25%) for older children should be used in doses of 0.7 mL/kg for lumbar block and 0.5 mL/kg for thoracic block. Clonidine (2 µg/kg) should be used as adjuvant. For continuous infusion, ropivacaine (0.1%) for children up to 7 years levobupivacaine (0.125%) for older children at a dose of 0.3–0.4 mg/kg/h should be used. Clonidine (3 µg/kg/24 h) should be used as an adjuvant.

Contraindications

The contraindications are few and include infection at the site of puncture, coagulation disorders, and progressive neurological disease.

Complications

The complications are rare and include primarily systemic toxicity caused by accidental intravascular injection of local anesthetics and total spinal caused by needle misplacement or by secondary migration of the catheter and by errors in the drug injected or the dose used.

PERIPHERAL NERVE BLOCKS IN CHILDREN

Safety and efficacy have been evidenced in a large survey showing that pediatric regional anesthesia has a low rate of complications and no major sequelae or deaths. Light sedation/anesthesia plus a block offers an optimal pain control throughout surgery and good postoperative analgesia.

Peripheral blocks are increasingly used, but are still less common than central blocks. There were no complications in over 9000 blocks.[80] The advantages of using a peripheral nerve block include the following: major safety, no urinary retention, long-lasting analgesia, and less postoperative analgesia. There is a possible limitation in patients with coagulation problems. There are few disadvantages, which include the following: major technical demand, larger volume of anesthetic solution requested, and longer onset time. Basically, whenever appropriate, a peripheral nerve block is preferable to an axial block.

Even with the mandatory use of a nerve stimulator (NS), the anesthesiologist must have structures such as nerves, veins, and arteries lie in very close proximity to each other. In unexperienced hands, while placing a plexus block, severe injuries can result because of the needle and the small distance between skin nerves. To practice a safe peripheral nerve block it is necessary to do continuous monitoring, use dedicated pediatric tools, and observe drug guidelines strictly. These blocks must be executed by an experienced anesthesiologist in an operating room and with the same monitoring as used for general anesthesia. As with any regional anesthetic technique, an IV line must be in place. Monitoring should include electrocardiogram (ECG), noninvasive blood pressure, pulse oximetry, and capnography if

the child is sedated or anesthetized. All resuscitation drugs and all the equipment required to handle possible complications should be available. Light general anesthesia or deep sedation with spontaneous breathing is used for both single-shot and continuous peripheral blocks.

Indications

For many years, the application of regional anesthetic techniques, especially peripheral nerve blocks, has been restricted to emergency conditions and, occasionally, to patients with specific disorders exposing to potentially severe intra- or postoperative anesthesia-related complications. Currently, the most common indications are for pain management during and after elective surgery. All peripheral nerve blocks used in adults can be used in pediatrics. The commonly performed peripheral blocks in children are the brachial plexus block (parascalene or axillary) for forearm and hand surgery and for revascularization; the femoral nerve block for femoral fractures, femoral osteotomies, and quadriceps muscle biopsy; the fascia iliaca block with the same indications for the femoral nerve block plus the knee surgery; the sciatic nerve block with the lateral approach at the trochanter level for fibular osteotomy, club foot repair, and the removal of plantar foreign bodies; and the sciatic nerve block with the lateral approach at the popliteal level for tibial osteotomy or ankle fractures.

Placement of a reinjection catheter along the nerve path allows for continuous infusion of local anesthetics, which guarantees long-lasting pain relief, the passive and active mobilization of joints, and pain-free dressing of wounds, which in turn favors early and more complete postop recovery.

Contraindications

There are few contraindications to peripheral nerve blocks in children. These include lesions of the skin at the point of injection, a severe generalized infection, an allergy to the local anesthetics (very rare), psychological disorders, and parental denial. The presence of a cast is not a contraindication but needs specific postop monitoring to identify any signs of compression. The management of patients with peripheral neuropathy is a controversial issue because there are no scientific data that suggest that a peripheral nerve block can worsen the illness, but there are always legal problems that could be raised.

Complications

The disadvantages of regional anesthesia are very few if these blocks are performed by an expert anesthesiologist. One of the most frequent complications is an inadequate block. Although side effects are very rare, nerve damage depends in part on the size and type of the needle (only use pediatric set), and also on the pressure of injection of local anesthetic. In fact, if the needle is placed incorrectly, injection of local anesthetic with low pressure can lead to transitory damage of the nerve, whereas if the pressure of the injection is high the nerve will be permanently damaged. Another complication is infection if aseptic rules are not followed. Infection is more frequent when a catheter is left in place for a long time. Another very rare side effect is hematoma, especially from the external jugular vein or axillary artery.

The most harmful side effect associated with the use of this technique is the systemic toxicity of local anesthetics. It may occur after inadvertent intravascular or intraosseous injection or following overdosage. The clinical symptoms and the treatment are the same as in adults. Because the little patient is sedate or under light general anesthesia, it is impossible to recognize the minor initial symptoms of central nervous system toxicity (perioral and lingual paresthesia, dizziness, vertigo), whereas convulsions and cardiovascular signs like ECG anomalies can easily be seen.

Materials

For many years there has been a lack of specific materials to perform PNB in infants and children. A radial artery catheterization set, epidural kit, and peripheral and central venous catheter set have been used for continuous peripheral nerve blocks. These days, for safety, it is mandatory to use dedicated pediatric tools.

A peripheral nerve can be blocked either by infiltrating a local anesthetic within a compartment space through which the nerve runs or by precisely locating the nerve. Compartment blocks, such as intercostal block, intrapleural block, fascia iliaca compartment block, penile block, and so on, depends on the localization of the fascial plane. When the relevant fascia is unique with no underlying vital structure, different needles, such as an IM needle, can be safely used. When there are several fascial planes or there is a danger of damaging important anatomical structures, such as during performance of an ilioinguinal block, only a short beveled or pin-point needle should be selected.

Precise localization of a plexus or a nerve trunk must not be performed by seeking paresthesias with standard IM needles because of a danger of direct nerve damage. Only short-beveled needles that are insulated and connected to a nerve stimulator are suitable. For most peripheral nerve blocks in children, 21-23-gauge and 35- to 50-mm-long needles are used, depending on the type of block and on the age of the child. Eliciting a motor response using a nerve stimulator is the most useful and safe technique for performing a pediatric nerve block.

The plexuses in children are quite superficial, especially the brachial plexus at the axilla. Therefore before introducing the needle, position of the plexus should be detected by use of the transcutaneous technique. This is a simple but very effective method to reduce mistakes during the performance of a peripheral block. This method was published in 2002 by Adrian Bosenberg.[81] The technique, called mapping of the nerves, requires use of the unblunted tip of the negative electrode of the nerve stimulator (NS): after increasing the mA of the NS up to 3 mA or more one can touch the skin close to the nerve plexus, stimulating it until the twitches are elicited, and then reduce the voltage, resulting in detection of the best point to perform the block. In the same year (2002), Urmey and Grossi[82] described the same technique for adults using a device with a needle-through passage, obtaining an even more successful performance. In this case they employed a higher voltage, 4–5 mA, because of the thickness of the skin in adults. In 2003, they described a modified tool for the same technique. More recently new devices have been produced by industrial companies using a penlike stimulator instead of the negative electrode, which allows easier mapping. The NS must be set at 3 mA, 2 Hz, 1 ms (whereas 0.1 ms is usually used for performing the block with the needle); a twitch is elicited by changing the position of the tip of the pen slightly and the best position can be chosen (and the best twitch according to the need of surgery) and marked with a pen. The success rate of a block in children can

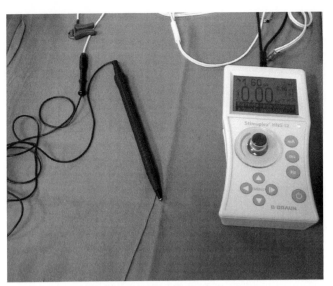

Figure 30.14: ENS and stimulating pen.

be increased, keeping in mind that often one has to deal with malformations, whereby it is hard to find where to place the needle (ie, arthrogriposis).

This technique can be used for the axillary and the parascalene approach of the brachial plexus, the femoral approach, and more distal detection of nerves (ie, popliteal level), including the "small blocks" (Figure 30.14).

After introducing the tip of the needle, connect it to the neurostimulator and set it to stimulate at a frequency of 2 Hz, starting with a current of 1–1.5 mA. Advance the needle until distinct contractions of the nerves to be blocked are noticed. The optimum nerve location is achieved by adjusting the needle so that these contractions are still visible with currents of 0.4 mA. It is now possible to inject the bolus dose of local anesthetic. It is important to remember that nerves are thin and very closely linked to each other without sheaths dividing them. One twitch of a single nerve is enough to administer the drug without using a multiple twitch technique.

Ultrasonography was introduced into anesthesia practice in the mid-1990s. In recent years, however, interest in using this technology to aid in nerve localization has significantly increased.[83,84] Although ultrasound may be useful for nerve localization, one of the main benefits is to provide visualization of the dispersion of local anesthetic within the desired tissue pains. This technology, however, requires significant training and skill to implement it successfully. At the time of the publication of this text, there are relatively few practitioners who are adequately skilled and comfortable with the use of ultrasound in children for peripheral nerve blockade (Figure 30.15 and 30.16).

BRACHIAL PLEXUS BLOCK

Although the interscalene block is often used in adults for most surgical procedures of the shoulder, this approach is used infrequently in children. This is because of the increased incidence of complications associated with the use of the interscalene approach, particularly in children who are under general anesthesia. Therefore, the most common approaches to the brachial

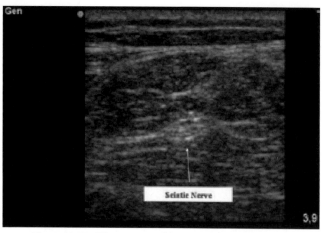

Figure 30.15: Ultrasonographic view of the sciatic nerve.

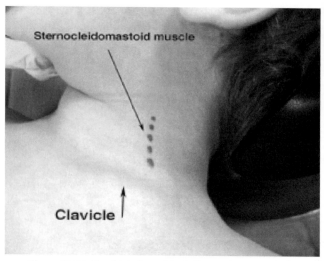

Figure 30.17: Brachial plexus block. Parascalene approach.

plexus in children include the parascalene approach and the axillary approach.

Parascalene Block

In children, this is the easiest and safest approach to the supraclavicular part of the brachial plexus with the aim of penetrating the interscalene space at a distance from the apical pleura, the great vessels and nerve of the neck, the stellate ganglion, and the spinal canal.

This technique provides excellent analgesia to the upper part of the arm, but in 50% of patients the lower branches of the cervical plexus are also blocked.[85–87] It is, therefore, indicated for anesthesia and postoperative analgesia for surgery of the shoulder and of the proximal upper arm, above the elbow, as a single-shot technique or continuous infusion.

Single-Shot Technique

The child lies supine, the head slightly to contralateral side, the arm extended comfortably along the body. The landmarks are the clavicle, the lateral border of the sternocleidomastoid muscle, and the transverse process of C6 (Chassaignac tubercle). An imaginary line is drawn between the Chassaignac's tubercle and the midpoint of the clavicle. A 23-gauge, 35-mm, insulated beveled needle, connected to the nerve stimulator, is introduced

perpendicularly at the junction of the upper two-third and lower one-third of this imaginary line. It is directed in the anteroposterior plane until twitches (contraction of biceps and/or brachial muscle) are obtained.

Possible complications are Horner's syndrome (ptosis of the eye, miosis, anophthalmosis, hyperemia of the conjunctiva, hyperthermia, anhidrosis of the face) by blocking the stellate ganglion; phrenic paresis by blocking of the phrenic nerve (bilateral block should be avoided), puncture of a large blood vessel of the neck (carotid artery and internal jugular vein), or puncture of the vertebral artery, and pneumothorax (Figures 30.17 and 30.18).

DOSAGES

Ropivacaine (0.2%) for children up to 7 years and levobupivacaine (0.5%) for older children (0.5 mL/kg) should be used. Clonidine (2 μg/kg) should be used as an adjuvant.

Continuous Technique

For continuous technique, we prefer to use the Contiplex D set: a 20-gauge, 35- to 55-mm long, short-beveled (15°) conducting needle with a plastic cannula and a 24-gauge, 400-mm-long catheter.

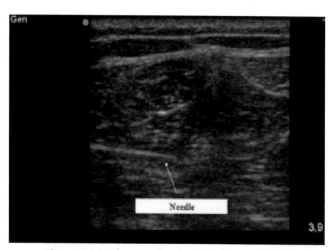

Figure 30.16: Ultrasound-assisted sciatic nerve block.

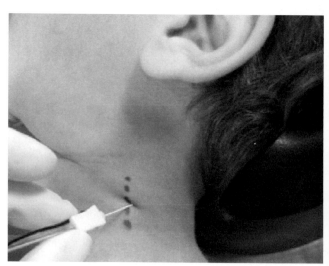

Figure 30.18: Brachial plexus block. Parascalene approach.

After appropriate positioning of the needle to maintain the muscle response with a current of 0.5 mA, the local anesthetic solution is slowly injected after negative aspiration. The needle is then withdrawn from the cannula and the catheter is inserted and left in place. The catheter tip has to be advanced 2 to 3 cm beyond the tip of the cannula, at which point it is removed. The catheter is fixed to the skin with a transparent tape.

DOSAGES

Ropivacaine (0.1%) for children until 7 years old, levobupivacaine (0.125%–0.25%) for older children. A bolus volume (0.5 mL/kg) is used for continuous infusion (0.3 mL/kg/h). Clonidine (3 μg/kg/24 h) is also used as an adjuvant.

Axillary Block

The axillary approach to the brachial plexus is the most commonly used approach in children and adolescents. It is used for procedures on the forearm and the hand. The primary advantage of the axillary approach is the ease of placement and the relatively low risk of complications. There is a 40%–50% chance of missing the musculocutaneous nerve with this approach because of the proximal exit of this nerve from the axillary sheath. While performing a block using this approach, the musculocutaneous nerve should be blocked separately when analgesia of the biceps and anterior forearm is sought.[88,89]

Single-Shot Technique

The child lies supine, with the arm to be blocked abducted at the shoulder and flexed 90° at the elbow so that the wrist is at the same level as the child's head. The landmarks are the axillary artery, the coracobrachialis muscle, and the major pectoralis muscle. Although multiple methods have been reported in adults, the simple common method of using a single injection technique seems to be very effective in children.[90]

The axillary artery should be palpated and followed as high as possible up into the axilla. The site of introduction of the needle (a 23-gauge, 35-mm-long, insulated beveled needle) is just above the axillary artery at an angle of 30° with the tip pointed toward the midpoint of the clavicle. Adjust the position of the needle to maintain the appropriate muscle response with a current of 0.4–0.5 mA. After negative aspiration, the local anesthetic solution is slowly injected. In infants and children it is enough to block just one of the components of the plexus to obtain a complete anesthesia of the hand. The complication rate of the axillary block is virtually nil, whichever technique is used. One complication is a hematoma if the axillary artery is injured or if the puncture is too deep (Figures 30.19 and 30.20).

DOSAGES

Ropivacaine (0.2%) for children up to 7 years and levobupivacaine (0.5%) for older children (0.5 mL/kg) should be used. Clonidine (2 μg/kg) should be used as an adjuvant.

Continuous Technique

The needle is inserted at a 15° angle to the skin to give a minimum of tunnelization of the catheter. It is advanced until it elicits twitches in muscles supplied by 1 of the 3 terminal nerves of the brachial plexus (median, ulnar, or radial). The conducting needle is then removed and the catheter is introduced, through the plastic cannula, 2 cm into the plexus sheath.

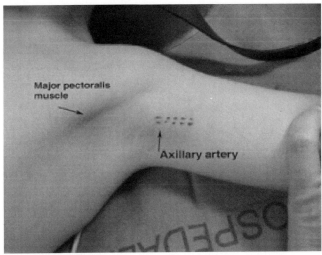

Figure 30.19: Brachial plexus block. Axillary approach.

DOSAGES

Ropivacaine (0.1%) for children until 7 years old levobupivacaine (0.125%–0.25%) for older children should be used. A bolus volume (0.5 mL/kg) is used for continuous infusion (0.3 mL/kg/h). Clonidine (3 μg/kg/24 h) should be used as an adjuvant.

LUMBOSACRAL PLEXUS BLOCK

Femoral Block

This is the most commonly performed lower extremity peripheral nerve block in children. The femoral nerve is located at the level of the crease at the groin, lateral to the pulsation of the femoral artery. This block has a very high success rate, around 100%, without any particular contraindications or side effects. It is used for providing anesthesia and postoperative analgesia to the thigh, the medial aspect of the leg, and the periosteum of the femur as a single-shot technique or continuous infusion.[95–97]

Single-Shot Technique

The technique is similar to that in the adult. The child lies supine, with the thigh slightly abducted, if possible. The

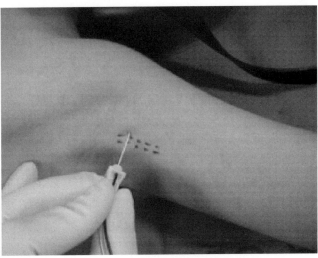

Figure 30.20: Brachial plexus block. Axillary approach.

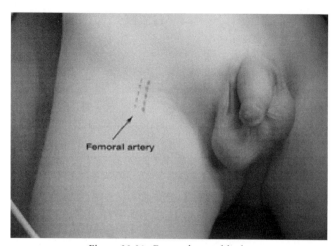

Figure 30.21: Femoral nerve block.

landmarks are the inguinal ligament and the femoral artery. The femoral artery pulse is located and the needle (a 21-gauge, 55-mm-long, insulated beveled needle connected to the nerve stimulator) is inserted vertically 1 cm lower and 1 cm lateral to the pulse. The needle is pointed perpendicularly to the skin in an anteroposterior direction until a motor response of the femoral nerve is elicited: contraction of the quadriceps muscle with the phenomenon of the "dancing patella." Once the location of the needle is stabilized, and after careful aspiration to prevent intravascular injection, local anesthetic solution is injected (Figures 30.21 and 30.22).

DOSAGES

Ropivacaine (0.2%) for children up to 7 years old and levobupivacaine (0.5%) for older children (0.5 mL/kg) should be used. Clonidine (2 μg/kg) should be used as an adjuvant.

Continuous Technique

The block needle is inserted at an angle of 30° to the skin in a cephalad direction, 1–2 cm both distal to the inguinal ligament and lateral to the femoral artery. The needle is advanced until twitches of the quadriceps muscle are obtained. After appropriate positioning of the needle to maintain the muscle response

with a current of 0.5 mA, the local anesthetic solution is slowly injected after negative aspiration. The needle is then withdrawn from the cannula and the catheter is inserted, through the plastic cannula, 2 to 3 cm into the femoral nerve sheath and left in place. The catheter is fixed to the skin with a transparent tape.[94,95]

DOSAGES

Ropivacaine (0.1%) for children up to 7 years old and levobupivacaine (0.125%–0.25%) for older children should be used. A bolus volume (0.5 mL/kg) is used for continuous infusion (0.3 mL/kg/h). Clonidine (3 μg/kg/24 h) should be used as an adjuvant.

Fascia Iliaca Block

The fascia iliaca compartment block is a multiblock technique, with a single injection made just below the fascia iliaca. This covers the psoas muscle and is from which emerge all the terminal nerves of the lumbar plexus. The femoral nerve (100%), the lateral femoral cutaneous, and the obturator nerves (70%–90%) are blocked with this technique.[96]

Single-Shot Technique

The child lies supine with the thigh slightly abducted, if possible. The landmark is the inguinal ligament. The line uniting the pubic spine to the anterior superior iliac spine is divided in three equal parts. A short beveled needle (ie, a caudal needle) is then introduced vertically 0.5–1 cm below the union of the lateral one-third to the medial two-thirds, until two losses of resistance, corresponding to the fascia lata and the fascia iliaca, respectively, are felt. After careful aspiration to prevent intravascular injection, local anesthetic solution is injected (Figure 30.23).

DOSAGES

Ropivacaine (0.2%) for children up to 7 years old and levobupivacaine (0.5%) for older children (0.5 mL/kg) should be used. Clonidine (2 μg/kg) should be used as an adjuvant.

Continuous Technique

The site of puncture is located 1 cm below the junction of the lateral one-fouth of a line drawn from the pubic tubercle to the

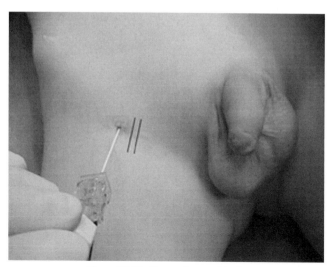

Figure 30.22: Femoral nerve block.

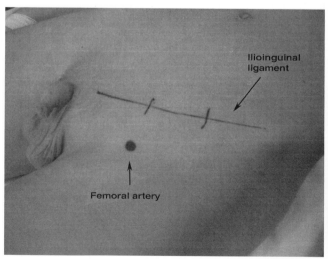

Figure 30.23: Fascia iliaca compartment block.

anterior superior iliac spine. The needle is inserted at an angle of 40° to the skin in a perpendicular direction. It is advanced until two pops (passage through the fascia lata and iliaca) are felt. The catheter is then inserted 3 to 7 cm into the fascial sheath.[97]

DOSAGES

Ropivacaine (0.1%) for children until 7 years old and levobupivacaine (0.125%–0.25%) for older children should be used. A bolus volume (0.5 mL/kg) is used for continuous infusion (0.3 mL/kg/h). Clonidine (3 μg/kg/24 h) should be used.

SACRAL PLEXUS BLOCK

The sacral plexus is represented by the sciatic nerve, which provides the innervation to the posterior thigh and the leg and most of the foot. The medial portion is innervated by the saphenous nerve, a branch of the femoral nerve.

In children, the sciatic nerve is much more superficial than in adults, therefore it is easiest to use the ultrasound technique for this block. The block can be performed at any point from the gluteus to the popliteal fossa. Because the child is sedated it is preferable to perform the lateral approach to the block with the child in the supine position.

There are a number of techniques used in children for sciatic nerve block. One addresses two main methods, the upper lateral approach and the popliteal fossa approach.

Sciatic Block

Lateral Approach

This is an easy block to perform in children under general anesthesia, because it can be performed in the lateral position with no need to mobilize the child. With this approach the child can spontaneously breathe properly. There are no particular contraindications or side effects.[98–101]

A combined sciatic and femoral or saphenous nerve block can be used for most lower extremity surgeries. The total dose of local anesthetic must be reduced for each block.

Single-Shot Technique

The patient is supine, with the leg in a neutral position or rotated slightly inward. The landmark is the greater trochanter of the femur. The needle (a 21-gauge, 55-mm-long or, in larger children, a 20-gauge, 120-mm-long insulated beveled needle) is introduced horizontally 1 to 3 cm below the lateral skin projection of the greater trochanter of the femur. It is advanced, passing below the femur, until the motor response of the foot and toes is elicited. Inversion of the foot indicates blockade of the tibial nerve. If plantar flexion or dorsiflexion are only present, without eversion of the foot, the block can not be complete (Figures 30.24 and 30.25).

DOSAGES

Ropivacaine (0.2%) for children up to 7 years old and levobupivacaine (0.5%) for older children (1 mL/kg) should be used. Clonidine (2 μg/kg) should be used as adjuvant.

Continuous Technique

The block needle is inserted horizontally, perpendicular to the skin. The needle is advanced until twitches of the foot are obtained. After appropriate positioning of the needle, the local

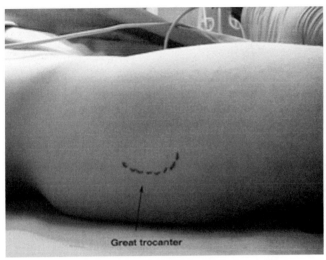

Figure 30.24: Sciatic nerve block. Lateral approach.

anesthetic solution is slowly injected after negative aspiration. The conducting needle is then removed and the catheter is introduced, through the plastic cannula, 2–4 cm into the sciatic nerve sheath and let in place. The catheter is fixed to the skin with a transparent tape.

DOSAGES

Ropivacaine (0.1%) for children up to 7 years old and levobupivacaine (0.125%–0.25%) for older children should be used. A bolus volume (0.5 ml/kg) is used for continuous infusion (0.3 mL/kg/h). Clonidine (3 μg/kg/24 h) should be used as an adjuvant.

Subgluteal Approach

This is a common approach when blocking the sciatic nerve in children. The child may remain in a supine position for this technique, but a prone or side position is also possible. There are no particular contraindications or side effects despite inferior gluteal artery could be punctured. A potential error could be the local anesthetic injection on stimulatory response of the gluteal muscles.

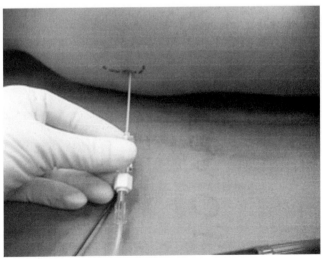

Figure 30.25: Sciatic nerve block. Lateral approach.

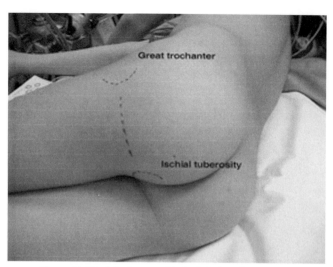

Figure 30.26: Sciatic nerve block. Subgluteal approach.

SINGLE-SHOT TECHNIQUE

The patient is supine with both the hip flexed and the knee flexed at 90° with the aid of a nurse. The landmarks are the greater trochanter of the femur and the ischial tuberosity. Insert the needle perpendicularly to the skin at the midpoint of the line joining the great trochanter with the ischial tuberosity. Connect to the nerve stimulator set at 1.5 mA and 2 Hz, and advance it until the motor response of the foot and toes is elicited. Adjust the position of the needle to maintain the appropriate muscle response with a current of 0.4–0.5 mA. After negative aspiration, slowly inject the local anesthetic solution (Figures 30.26 and 30.27).

DOSAGES

Ropivacaine (0.2%) for children up to 7 years old and levobupivacaine (0.5%) for older children (1 mL/kg) should be used. Clonidine (2 µg/kg) should be used as an adjuvant.

CONTINUOUS TECHNIQUE

The block needle is inserted at 30° to the skin in a caudal cephalad direction. The needle is advanced until twitches of the foot are obtained. After appropriate positioning of the needle,

the local anesthetic solution is slowly injected after negative aspiration. The conducting needle is then removed and the catheter is introduced, through the plastic cannula, 2–4 cm into the sciatic nerve sheath and let in place. The catheter is fixed to the skin with a transparent tape.

DOSAGES

Ropivacaine (0.1%) for children up to 7 years old and levobupivacaine (0.125%–0.25%) for older children should be used. A bolus volume (0.5 mL/kg) is used for continuous infusion (0.3 mL/kg/h). Clonidine (3 µg/kg/24 h) should be used as an adjuvant.

Popliteal Approach

The popliteal fossa block is our preferred method for blocking the sciatic nerve. There are two approaches to the sciatic nerve in the popliteal fossa: a lateral approach and a posterior approach. Because anesthetized children are typically in the supine position, the lateral approach is particularly advantageous.[102–104]

SINGLE-SHOT TECHNIQUE

The child is supine, with the leg in a neutral position or slightly rotated inward, elevated on a pillow at the knee level. The landmarks are the patellar crest, the vastus lateralis muscle, and the tendon of the long head of the biceps femoris muscle. The biceps femoris tendon is identified and the needle (a 21-gauge, 55-mm-long, insulated bevelled needle) is placed between the vastus lateralis and the biceps femoris tendon at an angle of about 30° about 5 to 6 cm above the popliteal crease. A response to nerve stimulation at 0.4 mA, usually plantar or dorsiflexion, confirms the position of the needle (Figures 30.28 and 30.29).

DOSAGES

Ropivacaine (0.2%) for children up to 7 years old and levobupivacaine (0.5%) for older children (0.5 mL/kg) should be used. Clonidine (2 µg/kg) should be used as adjuvant.

CONTINUOUS TECHNIQUE

The needle is introduced exactly as the single-shot technique. After appropriate positioning of the needle to maintain the muscle response with a current of 0.5 mA, the local anesthetic solution is slowly injected after negative aspiration. The conducting needle is then removed and the catheter is introduced, through the plastic cannula, 2 cm into the sciatic nerve

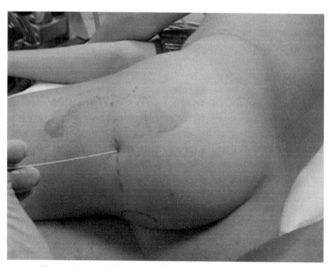

Figure 30.27: Sciatic nerve block. Subgluteal approach.

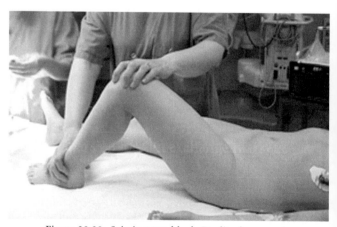

Figure 30.28: Sciatic nerve block. Popliteal approach.

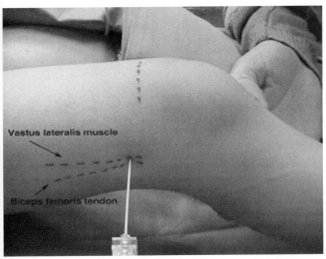

Figure 30.29: Sciatic nerve block. Popliteal approach.

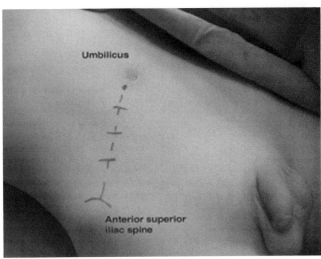

Figure 30.30: Ilioinguinal/iliohypogastric block.

sheath and let in place. The catheter is fixed to the skin with a transparent tape.

DOSAGES

Ropivacaine (0.1%) for children up to 7 years old and levobupivacaine (0.125%–0.25%) for older children should be used. A bolus volume (0.5 mL/kg) is used for continuous infusion (0.3 mL/kg/h). Clonidine (3 μg/kg/24 h) should be used as an adjuvant.

ILIOINGUINAL/ILIOHYPOGASTRIC BLOCK

For most hernia surgeries in children, a caudal block is the block of choice. However, if there is a relative contraindication to a caudal block because of the presence of a sacral dimple or if the child is obese and the caudal space is not easily identified, an ilioinguinal nerve block is utilized. The ilioinguinal and iliohypogastric nerves originate from the T12 (subcostal nerve) and L1 (ilioinguinal, iliohypogastric) nerve roots of the lumbar plexus. These nerves pierce the internal oblique aponeurosis 2 to 3 cm medial to the anterior superior iliac spine. It travels between the internal oblique and the external oblique aponeurosis.[105,106] The simultaneous block of these two nerves provides anesthesia for surgery on the inguinal region including: hernia repair, orchidopexy, and hydrocele.

Technique

The child lies supine. A line is drawn between the umbilicus and anterior superior iliac spine. The line is divided into thirds. The point where the lateral third meets with the medial two-thirds is where the needle is inserted. The needle (short beveled, ie, a caudal needle) is advanced toward the inguinal canal and passed in until a pop is felt, corresponding to the piercing of the superficial layer of the external oblique muscle. Local anesthetic solution is injected into the area after aspiration. Recently, the group of Willschke et al demonstrated with the use of the ultrasound technique that the landmark is more lateral compared to the previous point of injection (less than 1 cm medially to the anterior superior iliac spine). In a double-blinded study, they succeeded in reducing the amount of administered drug in the

ultrasound group (1–2 mL only), with an increase of duration of analgesia.[107,108] Two major complications have been described with this block: undesired femoral nerve block because of the spread of the local anesthetic to the inguinal ligament and the perforation of the bowel wall (Figures 30.30, 30.31, and 30.32).

Dosages

Ropivacaine (0.2%) for children up to 7 years old levobupivacaine (0.5%) for older children (0.2–0.3 mL/kg) should be used. Clonidine (2 μg/kg) should be used as an adjuvant.

PENILE BLOCK

This block is indicated to provide analgesia during and after operations on the penis, such as circumcision and phimosis. It is also suitable for pain management following hypospadia repair. Although it is not sufficient for the surgery itself, caudal anesthesia is preferable.

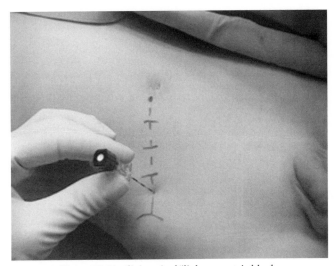

Figure 30.31: Ilioinguinal/iliohypogastric block.

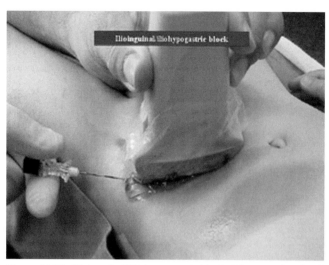

Figure 30.32: Ilioinguinal/iliohypogastric block. Ultrasound-assisted technique.

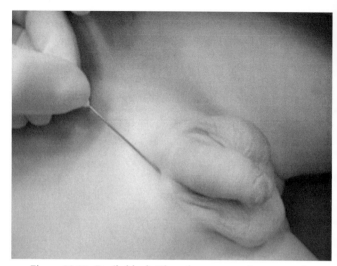

Figure 30.35: Penile block. The subcutaneous ring approach.

Technique

The patient lies on his back. The landmark is the pubic symphysis. The penis is pulled downward and two symmetrical sites for needle insertion are marked, both 0.5–1 cm below the pubic symphysis, lateral to the midline. The short beveled needle (ie, a caudal needle) is then inserted vertically, pointing slightly caudal until there is a loss of resistance when Scarpa's fascia is pierced. The two-injection technique is recommended, because the pubic space is frequently divided into two separate compartments by a medial division. Another very useful technique is the subcutaneous ring approach. It is a very simple and successful technique, using a subcutaneous ring of local anesthetic placed around the base of the penis. In this case, no attempt is made to inject local anesthetic within Buck's fascia. This could avert the risk of compression of the vascular structures when an excessive volume of local anesthetic is injected within the Buck's fascia. The points of injection are 2–3 cm from the base, at 10 and 2 o'clock, in the subcutaneous space, pointing to the base, with the needle raised superficially, injecting a half dose into each side, making a ring of local anesthetic. To complete the ring 1 mL of local anesthetic should be injected at the base of the penis, in the ventral part (Figures 30.33, 30.34, 30.35, and 30.36).

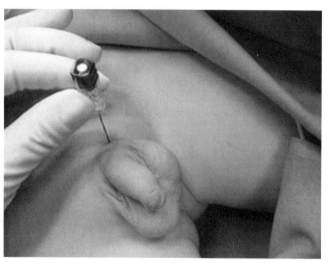

Figure 30.33: Penile block. The subpubic approach.

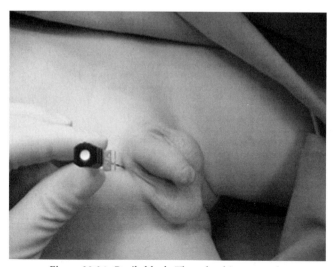

Figure 30.34: Penile block. The subpubic approach.

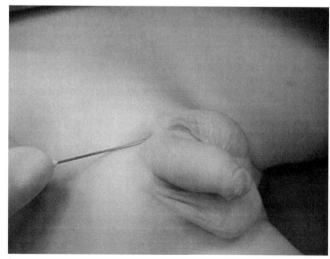

Figure 30.36: Penile block. The subcutaneous ring approach.

Dosages

Ropivacaine (0.2%, 0.1 ml/kg) for children up to 7 years old and levobupivacaine (0.5%) for older children for each side up to a maximum of 5 mL per side should be used. Epinephrine is absolutely contraindicated, because of the risk of ischemia of the dorsal arteries of penis.

REFERENCES

1. Paediatric analgesia. Which drug? Which dose? *Drugs.* 1991; 41(1):52–59.
2. Brobeck E, Marklund B, Haraldsson K, Berntsson L. Stress in children: how fifth-year pupils experience stress in everyday life. *Scand J Caring Sci.* 2007;21(1):3–9.
3. Grunau RE, Whitfield MF, Fay T, Holsti L, Oberlander T, Rogers ML. Biobehavioural reactivity to pain in preterm infants: a marker of neuromotor development. *Dev Med Child Neurol.* 2006;48(6):471–476.
4. Slater R, Boyd S, Meek J, Fitzgerald M. Cortical pain responses in the infant brain. *Pain.* 2006;123(3):332.
5. Oddson BE, Clancy CA, McGrath PJ. The role of pain in reduced quality of life and depressive symptomology in children with spina bifida. *Clin J Pain.* 2006;22(9):784–789.
6. Grunau RE, Holsti L, Peters JW. Long-term consequences of pain in human neonates. *Semin Fetal Neonatal Med.* 2006;11(4):268–275.
7. Jöhr M, Berger TM. Ruesch S. Systemic analgesia adapted to the children's condition. *Ann Fr Anesth Reanim.* 2007;26(6):546–553.
8. Salas Arrambide M, Gabaldón Poc O, Mayoral Miravete JL, Guerrero Pereda R, Amayra Caro I. Psychological intervention for coping with painful medical procedures in pediatric oncology. *An Pediatr (Barc).* 2003;59(1):105–109.
9. Miner JR, Krauss B. Procedural sedation and analgesia research: state of the art. Aca? *Emerg Med.* 2007;14(2):170–178.
10. Lemyre B, Hogan DL, Gaboury I, Sherlock R, Blanchard C, Moher D. How effective is tetracaine 4% gel, before a venipuncture, in reducing procedural pain in infants: a randomized double-blind placebo controlled trial. *BMC Pediatr.* 2007;8:7.
11. Holland JC, Rowland J, Plumb M Psychological aspects of anorexia in cancer patients. *Cancer Res.* 1977;37(7/2):2425–2428.
12. Tsao JC, Lu Q, Kim SC, Zeltzer LK. Relationships among anxious symptomatology, anxiety sensitivity and laboratory pain responsivity in children. *Cogn Behav Ther.* 2006;35(4):207–215.
13. Meyer S, Grundmann U, Gottschling S, Kleinschmidt S, Gortner L. Sedation and analgesia for brief diagnostic and therapeutic procedures in children. *Eur J Pediatr.* 2007;166(4):291–302.
14. Kain ZN, Mayes LC, Caldwell-Andrews AA, Karas DE, McClain BC. Preoperative anxiety, postoperative pain, and behavioral recovery in young children undergoing surgery. *Pediatrics.* 2006;118(2):651–658.
15. Finley GA, McGrath PJ, Forward SP, McNeill G, Fitzgerald P. Parents' management of children's pain following 'minor' surgery. *Pain.* 1996;64(1):83–87.
16. Klein-Kremer A, Goldman RD. Opioid administration for acute abdominal pain in the pediatric emergency department? *Opioid Manag.* 2007;3(1):11–14.
17. Drendel AL, Brousseau DC, Gorelick MH. Pain assessment for pediatric patients in the emergency department. *Pediatrics.* 2006;117(5):1511–1518.
18. Khan AN Msc, Sachdeva S. Current trends in the management of common painful conditions of preschool children in United States pediatric emergency departments. *Clin Pediatr (Phila).* 2007 Jun 19.
19. Shavit I, Keidan I, Augarten A. The practice of pediatric procedural sedation and analgesia in the emergency department. *Eur J Emerg Med.* 2006;13(5):270–275.
20. American Academy of Pediatrics. The assessment and management of acute pain in infants, children, and adolescents. *Pediatrics.* 2001;108(3):793–797.
21. Denecke H, Hunseler C. Assessment and measurement of pain. *Schmerz.* 2000;14(5):302–308.
22. Chambers CT, Hardial J, Craig KD, Court C. Montgomery Faces scales for the measurement of postoperative pain intensity in children following minor surgery. *Clin J Pain.* 2005;21(3):277–285.
23. Bailey B, Bergeron S, Gravel J, Daoust R. Comparison of four pain scales in children with acute abdominal pain in a pediatric emergency department. *Ann Emerg Med.* 2007 Jun 2.
24. LaFleur CJ, Raway B. School-age child and adolescent perception of the pain intensity associated with three word descriptors. *Pediatr Nurs.* 1999;25(1):45–50.
25. Newton JT, Buck DJ. Anxiety and pain measures in dentistry: a guide to their quality and application. *J Am Dent Assoc.* 2000;131(10):1449–1457.
26. Suraseranivongse S, Kaosaard R, Intakong P, et al. A comparison of postoperative pain scales in neonates. *Br J Anaesth.* 2006;97(4): 540–544.
27. Büttner W, Finke W. Analysis of behavioural and physiological parameters for the assessment of postoperative analgesic demand in newborns, infants and young children: a comprehensive report on seven consecutive studies. *Pediatr Anesthes.* 2000;10:303–318.
28. Suraseranivongse S, Santawat U, Kraiprasit K, Petcharatana S, Prakkamodom S, Muntraporn N. Cross-validation of a composite pain scale for preschool children within 24 hours of surgery. *Br J Anaesth.* 2001;87(3):400–405.
29. Hunt A, Wisbeach A, Seers K, et al. Development of the paediatric pain profile: role of video analysis and saliva cortisol in validating a tool to assess pain in children with severe neurological disability? *Pain Symptom Manage.* 2007;33(3):276–289.
30. Stallard P, Williams L, Velleman R, Lenton S, McGrath PJ, Taylor G. The development and evaluation of the pain indicator for communicatively impaired children (PICIC). *Pain.* 2002;98(1–2):145–149.
31. Breau LM, Finley GA, McGrath PJ, Camfield CS. Validation of the Non-communicating Children's. Pain Checklist-Postoperative Version. *Anesthesiology.* 2002;96(3):528–535.
32. Botting R, Ayoub SS. COX-3 and the mechanism of action of paracetamol/acetaminophen. *Prostaglandins Leukot Essent Fatty Acids.* 2005;72(2):85–87.
33. Clark E, Plint AC, Correll R, Gaboury I, Passi B. A randomized, controlled trial of acetaminophen, ibuprofen, and codeine for acute pain relief in children with musculoskeletal trauma. *Pediatrics.* 2007;119(3):460–467.
34. Desikan SR, Meena NG. Do non-steroidal anti-inflammatory drugs increase the risk of bleeding after tonsillectomy? *Arch Dis Child.* 2004;89(5):493–494.
35. Leroy S, Mosca A, Landre-Peigne C, Cosson MA, Pons G. Ibuprofen in childhood: evidence-based review of efficacy and safety. *Arch Pediatr.* 2007;14(5):477–484.
36. Veyckemans F, Pendeville PE. Tramadol for acute postoperative pain in children. *Ann Fr Anesth Reanim.* 2007;26(6):564–569.
37. Anand KJ, Carr DB. The neuroanatomy, neurophysiology, and neurochemistry of pain, stress and analgesia in newborns and children. *Pediatr Clin North Am.* 1989;36:795–822.
38. Anand KJ, Hickey PR. Pain and its effects in the human neonate and fetus. *N Engl J Med.* 1987;317:1321–1329.

39. Murat I, Walker J, Esteve C, Saint Maurice C. Effect of lumbar epidural anaesthesia on plasma cortisol levels in children. *Can J Anesth.* 1988;35:20–24.

40. Murat I, delleur MM, Esteve C. Continuous extradural anaesthesia in children. Clinical and haemodynamic implications. *Br J Anaesth.* 1987;59:1441–1450.

41. Liu Pl, Feldman HS, Giasi R. Comparative CNS toxicity of lidocaine, etidocaine, bupivacaine and tetracaine in awake dogs following rapid intravenous administration. *Anesth Analg.* 1983;62:375–379.

42. Zsigmond EK, Downs JR. Plasma cholinesterase activity in newborns and infants. *Can Anaesth Soc J.* 1989;18:278–285.

43. Yaster M, Maxwell LG. Pediatric regional anesthesia. *Anesthesiology.* 1989;70:324–338.

44. Dalens B. Regional anesthesia in children. *Anesth Analg.* 1989;68:654–672.

45. Rice LJ, Hannallah RS. Local and regional anesthesia. In: Motoyama EK, Davis PJ, eds. Smith's Anesthesia for Infants and Children. St Louis, MO: Mosby; 1990:393–426.

46. Berde CB. Pediatric postoperative pain management. *Pediatr Clin North Am.* 1989;36:921–940.

47. Brown TCK, Shulte-Steinberg O. Neural blockade for pediatric surgery. In: Cousins MJ, Bridenbaugh PO, eds. *Neural Blockade in Clinical Anesthesia and Management of Pain.* Philadelphia, PA: JB Lippincott; 1988:669–692.

48. Yaster M, Maxwell LG. The management of acute pain in children. In: Hoekelman RA, Friedman SB, Nelson NM, Seidel HS, eds. *Primary Pediatric Care.* St Louis, MO: Mosby; 1992:302–317.

49. Lerman J, Strong HA, Le Dez KM. Effects of age on the serum concentration of alpha 1-acid glycoprotein and the binding of lidocaine in pediatric patients. *Clin Pharmacol Ther.* 1989;46:219–225.

50. Feig Sa. Methemoglobinemia. In: Nathan DG, Oski FA, eds. *Hematology of Infancy and Childhood.* Philadelphia, PA: WB Saunders: 1974:378–389.

51. Dalens B, Ecoffey C, Joly A. et al. Pharmacokinetics and analgesic effect of ropivacaine following ilioinguinal/iliohypogastric nerve block in children. *Paediatr Anaesth.* 2011;11:415–420.

52. Hansen TG, Ilett KF, Reid C, et al. Caudal ropivacaine in infants: population pharmacokinetics and plasma concentrations. *Anesthesiology.* 2001; 94:579–584.

53. Habre W, Bergesio R, Johnson C. et al. Pharmacokinetics of ropivacaine following caudal analgesia in children. *Paediatr Anaesth.* 2000;10:143–147.

54. Paut O, Schreiber E, Lacroix F, et al. High plasma ropivacaine concentrations after fascia iliaca compartment block in children. *Br J Anaesth.* 2004; 92:416–418.

55. Rapp HJ, Molnar V, Austin S, et al. Ropivacaine in neonates and infants: a population pharmacokinetic evaluation following single caudal block. *Paediatr Anaesth.* 2004; 14:724–732.

56. Gunter JB, Gregg T, Varughese AM, et al. Levobupivacaine for ilioinguinal/iliohypogastric nerve block in children. *Anesth Analg.* 1999;89:647–649.

57. Ivani G, DeNegri P, Conio A, et al. Comparison of racemic bupivacaine, ropivacaine and levobupivacaine for paediatric caudal anaesthesia: effects on postoperative analgesia and motor blockade. *Reg Anesth Pain Med.* 2002;27:157–161.

58. Chalkiadis GA, Eyres RL, Cranswick N, et al. Pharmacokinetics of levobupivacaine 0.25% following caudal administration in children under 2 years of age. *Br J Anaesth.* 2004;92:218–222.

59. Locatelli B, Ingelmo P, Sonzoni V, et al. Randomized, double-blind, phase III, controlled trial comparing levobupivacaine 0.25%, ropivacaine 0.25% and bupivacaine 0.25% by the caudal route in children. Br J Anaesth Advance Access.

60. Breschan C, Jost R, Krumpholz R, et al. A prospective study comparing the analgesic efficacy of levobupivacaine, ropivacaine and bupivacaine in pediatric patients undergoing caudal blockade. *Ped Anesth.* 2005;15:301–306.

61. Ivani G, L'Erario M, Mossetti V, et al. Ropivacaine vs levobupivacaine in pediatric caudal anesthesia. *Paediatr Anaesth.* 2005;15(6):491–494.

62. Ivani G, De Negri P, Conio A, et al Ropivacaine-clonidine combination for caudal blockade in children. *Acta Anaesth Scand.* 2000;44:446–449.

63. De Negri P, Ivani G, Visconti C, et al. The dose-response relationship for clonidine added to a postoperative continuous epidural infusion of ropivacaine in children. *Anesth Analg.* 2001;93:71–76.

64. Sharpe P, Klein JR, Thompson JP, et al. Analgesia for circumcision in a paediatric population: comparison of caudal bupivacaine alone with bupivacaine plus two doses of clonidine. *Paediatr Anaesth.* 2001;11:695–700.

65. Cooper R. Clonidine in paediatric anaesthesia. *Paediatr Anaesth.* 2000;10:223–224.

66. De Negri P, Ivani G, Visconti C, et al. How to prolong postoperative analgesia after caudal anaesthesia with ropivacaine in children: S-ketamine versus clonidine. *Paediatr Anaesth.* 2001;11:679–683.

67. Lee HM, Sanders GM. Caudal ropivacaine and ketamine for postoperative analgesia in children. *Anaesthesia.* 2000;55:806–810.

68. Marhofer P, Krenn CG, Plochl W, et al. S(+)-ketamine for caudal block in paediatric anaesthesia. *Br J Anaesth.* 2000;84(3):341–345.

69. Krane E, et al. Editorial. *Reg Anaesth Pain Med.* 1998;23(5):433–438.

70. Broadman LM, Hannallah RS, Norden JM, McGill WA. "Kiddie caudals": Experience with 1154 consecutive cases without complications. *Anaesth Analg.* 1987;66:S18.

71. Dalens B, Hasnaoui A. Caudal anaesthesia in paediatric surgery: success rate and adverse effects in 750 consecutive patients. *Anaesth Analg.* 1989;68:83–89.

72. Gunther J. Caudal anaesthesia in children: a survey. *Anaesthesiology.* 1991;75(3A):A936.

73. Broadman L, Ivani G. Caudal block: techniques in regional anaesthesia. *Pain Manage.* 1999;3:150–156.

74. Ivani G. Caudal block: the 'no turn technique.' *Paediatr Anaesth.* 2005;15(1):83–84.

75. Bosenberg AT, Bland BAR, Schulte-Steinberg O, et al. Thoracic epidural anaesthesia via caudal route in infants. *Anaesthesiology.* 1988;69:265–269.

76. Bosenberg AT, Wiersma R, Hadley GP. Oesophageal atresia: caudo-thoracic epidural anaesthesia reduces the need for postoperative ventilatory support. *Paediatr Surg Int.* 1992;7:289–291.

77. Gunter GB, Eng C. Thoracic epidural anaesthesia via caudal approach in children. *Anesthesiology.* 1992;76:935–938.

78. Emmanuel ER. Post-sacral extradural catheter abscess in a child. *Br J Anaesth.* 1994;73:548–549.

79. Scott DB. Identification of the epidural space: loss of resistance to air or saline? *Reg Anesth.* 1997;22(1):1–2.

80. Giaufre E, Dalens B, Gombert A. Epidemiology and morbidity of regional anesthesia in children: a one- year prospective survey of the French-Language Society of Pediatric Anesthesiologists. *Anesth Analg.* 1996;83:904–912.

81. Bosenberg A, Raw R, Boezaart AP. Surface mapping of peripheral nerves in children with a nerve stimulator. *Paediatr Anaesth.* 2002;12(5):398–403.

82. Urmey WF, Grossi P. Percutaneous electrode guidance and subcutaneous stimulating electrode guidance: modifications of the original technique. *Reg Anesth Pain Med.* 2003;28:253–255.

83. Marhofer P, Sitzwohl C, Greher M, Kapral S. Ultrasound guidance for infraclavicular brachial plexus anaesthesia in children. *Anaesthesia.* 2004;59:642–646.

84. Chan VW. Applying ultrasound imaging to interscalene brachial plexus block. *Reg Anesth Pain Med.* 2003;28:340–343.

85. Dalens B, Vanneuville G, Tanguy A. A new parascalene approach to the brachial plexus in children: comparison with the supraclavicular approach. *Anesth Analg.* 1987;66:1264–1271.

86. Vongvises P, Beokhaimook N. Computed tomographic study of parascalene block. *Anaesth Analg.* 1997;84:379.

87. McNeely JK, Hoffman GM, Eckert JE. Postoperative pain relief in children from the parascalene injection technique. *Reg Anaesth.* 1991;16:20.

88. Dalens B. *Regional Anaesthesia in Infants, Children and Adoloscents.* Baltimore, MD: Williams & Wilkins; 1995.

89. Fisher WJ, Bingham RM, Hall R. Axillary brachial plexus block for perioperative analgesia in 250 children. *Paediatr Anaesth.* 1999;9:435.

90. Carre P, Joly A, Cluzel Field B. Axillary block in children: single or multiple injection? *Paediatr Anaesth.* 2000;10(1):35–39.

91. Koo ST, Brown TCK. Femoral nerve block: the anatomical basis for a single injection technique. *Anaesth Intensive Care.* 1983;11:40.

92. Ronchi L, Rosenbaum D, Athouel A, et al. Femoral nerve blockade in children using bupivacaine. *Anaesthesiology.* 1989;70:622.

93. Maccani RM, Wedel DJ, Melton A. Femoral and lateral femoral cutaneous nerve block for muscle biopsies in children. *Paediatr Anaesth.* 1995;5(4):223–227.

94. Tobias JD. Continuous femoral nerve block to provide analgesia following femur fracture in a paediatric ICU population. *Anaesth Intensive Care.* 1994;22(5):616–618.

95. Johnson CM. Continuous femoral nerve blockade for analgesia in children with femoral fractures. *Anaesth Intensive Care.* 1994;22(3):281–283.

96. Dalens B, Vanneuville G, Tanguy A. Comparison of the fascia iliaca compartment block with the 3-in-1 block in children. *Anaesth Analg.* 1989;69:705.

97. Paut O, Sallaberry M, et al. Continuous fascia iliaca compartment block in children: a prospective evaluation of plasma bupivacaine concentrations, pain scores, and side effects. *Anesth Analg.* 2001;92(5):1159–1163.

98. Ichikiyanagi K. Sciatic nerve block: lateral approach with the patient supine. *Anaesthesiology.* 1959;20:601.

99. Gardini R, Waldron BA, Wallace WA. Sciatic nerve block: a new lateral approach. *Acta Anaestesiol Scand.* 1985;29:515.

100. Dalens B, Tanguy A, Vanneuvile G. Sciatic nerve block in children: a comparison of the posterior, anterior and lateral approaches in 180 paediatric patients. *Anaesth Analg.* 1990;70:131.

101. Ivani G, Tonetti F. Postoperative analgesia in infants and children: new developments. *Minerva Anestesiol.* 2004;70(5):399–403.

102. MCLeod DH, Wong DV, et al. Lateral poplieal sciatic nerve block compared with ankle block for analgesia following foot surgery. *Can J Anaesth.* 1995;42:765–769.

103. Vloka JD, Hadzic A, Kitain E. Anatomic considerations for sciatic nerve block in the popliteal fossa through the lateral approach. *Reg Anesth* 1997;84:387–390.

104. Ter Rahe C, Suresh S. Popliteal fossa block: lateral approach to the sciatic nerve. *Tech Reg Anesth Pain Manag.* 2002;6(3):141–143.

105. Hannallah RS, Broadman LM, Belman AB, et al. Comparison of caudal and ilioinguinal/iliohypogastric nerve block for control post-orchidopexy pain in paediatric ambulatory surgery. *Anaesthesiology* 1987;66:832

106. Dalens B. Bloc ilioinguinal et iliohypogastrique chez l'enfant. In: Dartayet B, ed. Paris : MAPAR ; 1997:235.

107. Willschke H, Bosenberg A, Marhofer P, et al. Ultrasonographic-guide? ilioinguinal/iliohypogastric nerve block in pediatric anesthesia: what is the optimal volume? *Anesth Analg.* 2006;102(6):1680–1684.

108. Willschke H, Marhofer P, Bosenberg A, et al. Ultrasonography for ilioinguinal/iliohypogastric nerve blocks in children. *Br J Anaesth.* 2005;95(2):226–230.

31

Acute Pain Management for Elderly
High-Risk and Cognitively Impaired
Patients: Rationale for Regional Analgesia

Thomas M. Halaszynski, Nousheh Saidi, and Javier Lopez

The large number of theories describing the multidimensionality and consequences of the aging process underscore the complexity and difficulty in developing optimal anesthetic and analgesic choices for elderly patients. Despite advances in anesthesia, analgesia, and drug delivery systems, the debate continues as to whether general anesthesia (GA) or neural blockade and regional analgesia is more efficacious and safer in elderly patients, particularly those with clinically significant comorbidities and cognitive deficits. The focus of this chapter is to outline the physiologic and pharmacologic implications of aging on surgical anesthesia and acute pain management, as well as the potential benefits of neural blockade and regional anesthesia (RA) in geriatric and cognitively impaired patients.

Over the past century, remarkable achievements in medicine and public health have made it possible for people to live longer and have more productive lives. Of all the people who have ever lived to age 65 years, more than half are now alive.[1] In the United States, people over the age of 65 years now account for about 13% of the population and this number will increase to about 20% by 2030 as the "baby boomers" continue to age.[1,2] Larger numbers of patients in their 60s are healthier and can anticipate their life expectancy to continue an additional 30 years or longer. At the present time, patients older than 65 years of age account for 49% of all hospital days in U.S. health care institutions.[1] Therefore, physicians can expect to spend a significantly larger portion of their practice dealing with disease management and operative procedures in older adults. Estimates of future health care use suggest that greater than 50% of Americans over 65 years of age will undergo a major surgical procedure.[1,2]

Although age alone has sometimes been thought to be a major predictor of disease, disability, and death; the health status, prognosis, and preferences of care for patients in their 70s, 80s, and 90s varies widely. Advances in both anesthetic and surgical techniques combined with sophisticated perioperative monitoring are primary factors that have contributed to an expanding number of older adults undergoing and successfully recovering from major surgery. In addition, an anesthesia preoperative assessment has proven to be beneficial in identifying specific health care risk factors and potential complications of proposed elective surgical interventions. Preoperative assessments allow perioperative health care plans to be based on the patients' medical history and physiological status, not on age or type of surgical procedure alone. Together, a tailored perioperative management plan focused on optimizing pain control while minimizing therapy-related adverse events can be developed for elderly patients undergoing major surgery.

DEFINITION OF ELDERLY

Defining the term *elderly* involves both chronologic and physiologic components. Literature has divided the elderly population into two separate groups: the "young old" (65 to 80 years of age) and the "older old" (greater than 80 years of age).[2] An issue that arises in describing the elderly population are the discrepancies between chronologic and physiologic age. Chronologic age is the actual number of years an individual has lived. Physiologic age describes functional capacity or reserve of a patients' organ systems defined in pathophysiologic parameters. Physiologic reserve describes the level of functioning of patients' organ systems that allows them to compensate for acute stress and traumatic derangements. Comorbid disease states such as diabetes mellitus, coronary artery disease, arthritis, and renal and pulmonary disease may decrease the physiologic reserve in certain patients, making it more difficult for them to recover from traumatic or surgical injury.

Described from a physiologic viewpoint, human aging can be characterized by progressive reductions in homeostatic reserves of nearly every organ system.[3] Declines in organ function, often referred to as homeostenosis, may become evident by the third decade of life, are often gradual and progressive in nature, and vary in the rate and extent of decline. The compromising function of each organ system generally occurs independently of changes in other organ systems and may be influenced by diet, environmental factors, personal habits, and genetic predisposition. Optimal anesthetic management of elderly patients depends on a knowledge and understanding of normal age related changes in anatomy, physiology, and response

Table 31.1: Anatomical Changes of the Central and Peripheral Nervous System during Normal Aging

Central Nervous System	Peripheral Nervous System
Volume of thalamus and cortical gray matter decreases	Decreases in number and deterioration (atrophy) of large myelinated nerve fibers
Volume of cerebrum, pons, corpus collosum, and cerebellum white matter remains intact (from ages 20–90 years)	Dysfunction of gene expression for protein components of the myelin sheath resulting in detrimental effects of remyelination
Limited loss of neurons (neuronal cell death) in the cerebral cortex (some neocortical areas lose no neurons)	Impairment of oligodendrocyte recruitment and differentiation
Brain cells shrink and brain becomes more compact	Impaired sensory and motor function of the feet
Increased volume of intracranial cerebrospinal fluid low pressure, nonpathological hydrocephalus[103]	Alteration of macrophage inflammatory responses
Possible regional reductions in the neurotransmitters of serotonin, norepinephrine, dopamine, and acetylcholine[1]	Decreased conduction velocity of myelinated nerves (unmyelinated fibers unaffected by aging)
Decreased cerebral blood flow, cerebral metabolic activity, and O_2 consumption	Changes of the senses of touch, taste, hearing, sight, pain (?), but not smell
Degenerative changes in myelin sheaths of nerve fibers	Adaptability to stresses is limited
Loss of nerve fibers from the cerebral white matter	Reduced noradrenergic reuptake yielding a net activation of the sympathetic nervous system
Reactive gliosis and neuronal losses occur in the spinal cord	Dysfunction of homeostatic functions such as heat intolerance, orthostatic hypotension, and intolerance to exercise
Loss of cell bodies and shrinkage/degeneration of nerve fibers in (1) dorsal columns of cervical spine, (2) ventral horn, and (3) gray matter (intermediate) of spinal cord thoracic segments	If the autonomic nervous system is attenuated, then perioperative lability of hemodynamics may be suspected
Atrophy of the cephalic extremity of spinal cord, decreased anteriorposterior diameter and transverse area of cervical spinal cord	Decreased activity of parasympathetic system
Narrowing of the bony spinal canal	

to pharmacologic agents. It is also important to distinguish between normal physiologic alterations of the central nervous system (CNS) and cardiovascular and hepatorenal systems along with disease-related pathophysiologic changes.

EFFECT OF AGING ON THE NERVOUS SYSTEM

Some degree of memory deterioration can be measured in >40% of people older than 60 years of age.[4] The progressive loss of intellectual activity and gradual mental deterioration (senile dementia) occurs in 14% of the population aged 75 years or more. Daily living activities can be dramatically affected by age-related memory decline but is not inevitable. Age-related alterations in nervous system function result from changes in receptors, signal transduction, and homeostatic mechanisms of the CNS. Aging is associated with decreases in cholinergic and dopaminergic neurons, as well as reductions in synaptic contacts and receptors. Deficiencies of acetylcholine, dopamine, and other neurotransmitters as well as extraneuronal accumulation of amyloid underlie neurocognitive dysfunction such as Parkinson's and Alzheimer's dementia. Alterations of brain phospholipid chemistry associated with changes in second messengers, such as diacylglycerol, are also evident.[5]

Normal aging results in biochemical and anatomical changes of the brain and spinal cord and there are qualitative and quantitative influences on the nervous system in the elderly (Table 31.1). Typical age-related anatomical alterations and bio-

chemical changes of the brain and spinal cord include the following: (1) reduced volume of brain mass, decreased neuronal and glial cell arborization, and reduction in neurotransmitter concentrations; (2) reductions in cerebral electrical and metabolic activity; (3) changes in brain nerve fibers; (4) changes within the spinal cord (cervical spinal cord maintains it shape, but decreases in size); and (5) modification of the bony spinal canal. Alterations of functional reserve in the elderly may be reflected as increased susceptibility to postoperative cognitive dysfunction (POCD), delirium, altered pharmacodynamics, and stroke. Changes in the peripheral nervous system (PNS) and CNS may affect functional outcomes from both the perioperative period and later during the recovery phase, and should be considered in a patients' preoperative evaluation. The effect of aging on the functional reserves of the CNS and PNS along with potential surgical and anesthetic ramifications must be considered. Brain sensitivity to anesthetic and analgesic agents increases with age and is unique to each drug.

Overall, cerebral metabolic activity is decreased in older compared to young subjects and may be a result of decreased neurotransmitter concentrations and loss of synaptic contacts. It is possible that degenerative changes of the myelin sheaths in the CNS may lead to cognitive dysfunction through changes in nerve conduction velocity leading to disruption of normal timing of neuronal circuits. Further contribution to cognitive decline is because of the loss of cerebral white matter nerve fibers, resulting in decreased connections between neurons. Although the above-described changes have been identified in the aging brain, the mechanism(s) responsible for diminished functional activity reserve remain unclear. Reductions of brain reserve are portrayed as symptoms and signs of neurological dysfunction, decreases in functional activities of daily living, increased risk of POCD, and increased sensitivity to anesthetic medications. The major signs, symptoms, and changes include altered reflexes, deteriorations of gait and mobility, altered sleep patterns, impairment of memory and intellect, and decrements of the senses (vision, hearing, etc).

Changes that occur in the somatic nervous system component of the PNS with aging include (1) peripheral nerve deterioration, (2) dysfunction of genes responsible for myelin sheath protein components, (3) decreased myelinated nerve fiber conduction velocity, (4) mild motor and sensory discriminatory changes of the feet, and (5) changes of the senses (pain, touch, etc).[6] The autonomic nervous system (ANS) division of the PNS also experiences alterations secondary to the aging process. The ANS (composed of nerves, ganglia, and plexus) dictates most of the involuntary physiological functions of the body through the parasympathetic and sympathetic divisions. Aging of the ANS is characterized by (1) limited adaptability to stress, (2) an overall net activation of the sympathetic nervous system, (3) decreased basal activity of the parasympathetic nervous system, (4) decreased baroreflex sensitivity, and (5) slowing and weakening of homeostatic functions of the ANS.[7]

Aging affects the peripheral nerves of all mammals resulting in deterioration and decreases in the number of myelinated nerve fibers. Aging particularly affects large myelinated fibers, resulting in degrees of atrophy along with degenerative changes of the myelin.[8] Aging processes affect levels of expression for key genes encoding major protein components of the myelin sheath such as (1) proteolipid protein and (2) myelin basic protein. Maintenance of myelin sheath integrity involves continued expression of genes specifically associated with myelin protein production. Restoration of myelin sheaths to demyelinated axons occurs spontaneously in the adult nervous system, but aging has a detrimental effect on the process. Spontaneous remyelination efforts and the rate of reappearance of proteolipids and myelin basic proteins are slowed. In the CNS, oligodendrocyte progenitor recruitment and differentiation are also impaired by age-related declines in remyelination.

Aging induces functional changes by decreasing peripheral myelinated nerve conduction velocity. Older adults have a 10%–30% decrease of efferent motor fiber conduction velocity, but unmyelinated nerves seem to be unaffected. Normal manifestations in patients older than 65 years include some degree of absent ankle reflexes along with mild abnormal sensory and motor symptoms of the feet (ie, absent vibratory sensation of the big toe). Along with aging, patients also experience various changes of the senses: touch may be affected by poor circulation, pain sensitivity may decline, smell is not affected significantly, night-time adaptation and color vision are adversely affected, and various degrees of hearing loss (presbycusis in 13% of population >65 years) occur, as well as a decrease in taste sensitivity.

The aging ANS has reduced autonomic abilities that influence a patients' response to physiologic changes, stresses, surgery, and anesthesia. Increases in sympathetic nervous system activity are organ specific with the gastrointestinal (GI) system and skeletal muscle as targets. Neuronal noradrenergic reuptake is reduced in the elderly resulting in an increased sympathetic tone of the heart and an increase in basal adrenal secretions along with attenuation of adrenal adrenergic secretion in response to stress.[9] There is a loss of beat-to-beat heart rate variability during respiration in the elderly because of reduced respiratory vagal modulation of the resting heart. Findings of decreased baroreflex sensitivity are because of a function of increased arterial stiffness versus aging associated alterations of the ANS. The ANS and its effectors play an important role in responses to hemodynamic challenges. Advancing age could result in an imbalance of homeostatic mechanisms as evidenced by orthostatic hypotension, exercise intolerance, increased upper body sweating, and temperature intolerance that may be evident. Finally, older patients often have cognitive impairments that may not be recognized by some health care providers.[10]

Predictive stroke risk indices use advancing age as an important mediating factor of the 5-year stroke rate. Advancing age is an independent predictor of postoperative stroke, especially subsequent to coronary artery bypass grafting. Increasing age as a risk factor for stroke may be the result of an increased incidence of atherosclerosis or increased susceptibility to ischemia from the aging process. However, how age actually increases the risk of stroke is currently unclear, but the surgical procedure plays an important role in defining the perioperative risk of stroke in the elderly. Cardiac, vascular, orthopedic, and neurosurgical procedures have an increased incidence of perioperative (and microembolic) stroke compared to an incidence of 0.08%–0.2% following general surgery and this risk increases to 2.9% with a prior history of a stroke.

POSTOPERATIVE COGNITIVE DYSFUNCTION

Postoperative cognitive disorders include a broad spectrum of impairments in cognitive function and memory or of consciousness along with deficits in cognition and memory. Cognitive impairment includes acute confusion states and delirium as well as worsening progression of baseline dementia. Abnormal cognitive states in older patients may adversely affect the consistency of obtaining a medical history, negatively affect disposition planning, and complicate the perioperative course and rehabilitation. Acute cognitive impairment can also be an important underlying symptom of sepsis, congestive heart failure, metabolic abnormality, adverse drug effects, or subdural hematoma development.

Studies on POCD have identified that patients 60 years and older are at increased risk of suffering cognitive impairment subsequent to major noncardiac surgery.[11,12] Localized areas of the brain are responsible for cognitive function. For example, the frontal lobe and subcortical network portions control executive function (concentration, self-monitoring, and information processing) and the medial temporal lobe is for memory (learning and remembering). Brain regions associated with cognitive functions differentially change with aberrant brain processes (stoke, dementia) and with the aging process. Therefore, to better understand POCD, determining the type of cognitive change may provide information as to which brain system(s) are vulnerable to adverse events during the perioperative period. This will also have implications toward postsurgical convalescence and rehabilitation.

Cognitive disorders can occur after surgery in which mental function reaches a nadir in the early postoperative period and returns to preoperative levels within 1 week following surgery in the majority of patients. Cognitive dysfunction is common in elderly postoperative patients, but stroke occurs relatively infrequently.[13] A more common occurrence in the postoperative period is the incidence of POCD and postoperative delirium (POD); the most often observed psychiatric conditions of older hospitalized patients. The incidence of POD and POCD may exceed 50% in certain surgical settings such as cardiac and orthopedic (femoral neck fracture repairs) surgeries.[14,15] POD and POCD are the two most common complications in elderly surgical patients and the incidence is higher than other postoperative comorbidities such as respiratory failure and myocardial infarction.[12,16] Definitions of the various cognitive changes and dysfunctions that may be experienced by the elderly surgical patient are presented in Table 31.2.

POD is further characterized by alterations in orientation, consciousness, memory, thought processes, and behavior.[17] Elderly patients generally experience the onset of POD and acute confusion states in the postanesthesia care unit (PACU) or immediately following transport to a postsurgical care unit or intensive care unit (ICU). Although the onset of delirium may be abrupt, delirium can also develops over several hours to days and its course tends to fluctuate.[18] Initial symptoms can often progress and extend into a variety of clinically significant complications, including patient agitation and the subsequent need for sedation, an increased risk of falls, wound seromas, pulled nasogastric tubes and IV catheters, aspiration pneumonia, and increased need for urinary catheters. When the onset of delirium is gradual, patients may experience fatigue, inability to concentrate, irritability, anxiety, and/or depression. Older patients may also have hallucinations, experience vivid and disturbing dreams, or have trouble distinguishing dreams from reality. Although patients may seem lucid at times, their symptoms of delirium are typically worse at night, leading to the colloquial term *sun-downing*.

The perioperative etiology of cognitive dysfunction is multifactorial and may include drug effects, reactions to poorly controlled pain, underlying dementia, hypothermia, and metabolic disturbances. Elderly patients are extremely sensitive to centrally acting anticholinergic agents, opioids, and antihistamines, such as scopolamine, atropine, morphine, vistaril, and diphenhydramine. It is known that antinausea medications such as droperidol, phenergan, and a scopolamine patch can also precipitate acute confusion states, particularly when coadministered with opioid analgesics in the elderly. Specific pain management strategies that rely solely on opioids and other central-acting analgesics may be associated with a higher incidence of POD and POCD. Poorly controlled postoperative pain has also been implicated in development of POD and POCD in the elderly. High pain scores at rest are associated with an increased risk of delirium over the first 3 postoperative days and more effective pain management has been shown to reduce the incidence of POD in the elderly patient.[5,19]

Some geriatric patients suffer prolonged or permanent POCD after surgery and anesthesia. There are studies to suggest that POCD can be detected in 10%–15% of elderly patients >60 years of age for up to 3 months following major surgery.[11,12] The most commonly affected cognitive dysfunction was attention to detail and cognitive speed. In certain settings, such as cardiac and major orthopedic procedures, intraoperative arterial emboli may also be contributory. Elderly patients admitted to the hospital following their surgical procedure appear to have a significantly higher risk for POCD than elderly outpatients.

Although the etiology still remains unclear, both anesthetic and nonanesthetic factors are likely responsible for the development of POCD.

Complications of POD and POCD are significant because adverse outcomes may result in increased length of hospital stay and medical complications, including death and could require discharge to skilled care facilities.[20,21] The economic impact of delirium is considerable as it adds costs to hospitalization and is responsible for billions in additional Medicare charges along with significant health care implications. Because POD and POCD occurs more frequently in the elderly than in younger patients, and given the fact that the elderly surgical population is increasing in number, it is necessary to gain knowledge of these conditions and apply that understanding to the care of these surgical patients. Geriatric patients undergoing certain high-risk types of surgery or those with certain coexisting medical disease(s), patients with preoperative cognitive dysfunction, and patients with advanced age are at higher risk for the development of postoperative cognitive disorders and long-term cognitive dysfunction. Therefore, functional status of the elderly surgical patient may be more relevant than medical morbidity outcomes. Cognitive functioning relates directly to the patient's functional status, which is a determining factor as to whether a patient is discharged to home or will require a skilled care facility for rehabilitation. In addition, functional status serves as a strong predictor of mortality as a result of hospitalization.[22] Especially significant is the understanding that cognitive disorders are independent predictors of short- and long-term outcomes. This adverse event is also associated with an increased incidence of postoperative complications, increased mortality, higher rates of discharge to rehabilitation facilities, and longer lengths of hospital stay, even with adjustments accounting for functional status, age, and comorbidities.[23] Decreased cognitive function diminishes health-related quality of life and is associated with adverse financial and social penalties for patients and their care providers.[24]

Investigations on normal aging show a relationship between abrupt declines in cognitive function with early death in older adults.[24] POCD has also often been associated with cardiac surgery.[25] Another study evaluated cognitive decline in elderly patients (1218 patients 60 years and older) who had major noncardiac surgery and found that 26% of older patients had cognitive dysfunction 1 week postsurgery and 10% had dysfunction 3 months after surgery.[11] Therefore, one risk factor for POCD after major surgery is advancing age, and POCD can affect mortality during the time period following surgery.[11,12]

Older patients with POCD may be at increased risk of death within the first year following surgery. Therefore, efforts should be made to reduce the negative impact on independent factors and predictors of cognitive dysfunction after major surgery. Studies have shown and confirmed that advancing age and lower educational levels are risk factors for development of cognitive decline.[11,12,26] In addition, a history of cerebral vascular injury (with or without impairment) and POCD at hospital discharge had a higher incidence of POCD at 3 months following surgery.[12] These predictors of cognitive dysfunction correlate with an increased risk of early mortality in older patients because (1) patients with POCD at hospital discharge had a higher death rate in the first 3 months after surgery and (2) patients with POCD at discharge with persistence 3 months following surgery were also more likely to die within the year subsequent to surgery.[12]

Table 31.2: Definitions of Cognitive Impairment

Dementia Alzheimer's disease (most common form), vascular dementias, frontal lobe, reversible, senile, Lewy body, and Parkinson-associated	Apathy and personality changes occur early
	Behavioral changes appear as the condition progresses
	Psychotic symptoms are late signs (typically difficult to control)
	Multiple cognitive deficits
	memory impairment* executive decision making
	aphasia inability to think abstractly
	apraxia inability to organize and sequence
	agnosia inability to plan
	(*memory impairment [most prominent] plus at least one of the above must be present)
	Clinical findings are associated with
	problems with social activities
	decline from a previous status
	problems of occupational activities
	Up to 75% of dementia cases are not diagnosed
	Gradual and progressive loss of mental abilities
	thought disturbances
	disorientation
	sensory impairment
	personality changes
	(symptoms may be treated, but not cured)
	Dementia often results in postoperative delirium
Mild cognitive impairment (MCI) (4 subtypes associated with causes of dementia)	Concept to describe transitional level of neurocognitive impairment
	normal aging process
	mild cognitive impairment
	early dementia
	MCI is a predictor of future dementia
	MCI diagnosis results in development of dementia at 12% per year
	Diagnosis by neuropsychological testing and clinical observation
	Divided into 4 subtypes (based on presence of memory impairment plus number of other cognitive domains affected)
	Preoperative MCI may result in postoperative delirium
Postoperative cognitive dysfunction (POCD)	Condition in which patients have difficulty in performing cognitive tasks after surgery that they could perform prior to surgery. Tasks/domains of
	perceiving recognizing sensing
	judging conceiving reasoning
	imagining quality of knowing
	Occurs frequently in and following
	carotid endarterectomy hip fracture repair surgery
	cardiac surgery patients (most frequent)
	Patients are generally alert and oriented
	POCD not yet defined as an objective condition
	True deterioration versus random variation
	International Study of Postoperative Cognitive Dysfunction (ISPOCD)
	developed criteria of POCD from range of above cognitive domains
	based on pre- and postoperative neuropsychological testing scores
	Controversy as to time point when POCD may exist (1 day/1 week/1 year)
	Predictors of POCD 1 week postoperatively include:
	duration of anesthesia age (predictor of POCD at 3 mo.)
	postoperative infection low level of patient education
	pulmonary complications need for a second operation
	Up to 2% of cases of POCD persists >1 year

Delirium	Fluctuating consciousness that develops over hour to days
	Psychiatric diagnosis (inattention is a key feature)
	Altered perception and cognition (not associated with dementia)
	Condition is a result of a general medical condition[102]
	Predictive models (such as impaired vision, dehydration, and severe illness) and interventional strategies exist for delirium in medical patients
	In-hospital predictors of delirium include

bladder catheters	functional status	male sex
malnutrition	infection	depression
3 or more medications	H2 antagonists	age
iatrogenic events	benzodiazepines	opioids
alcohol + drug abuse		

Postoperative delirium (POD)	Not present in immediate postoperative period
	Develops on postoperative days 1–3 and can be sustained >1 week
	Predictors and preoperative factors of POD

anticholinergic drugs	polypharmacy	benzodiazepines
cognitive impairment	advanced age	sleep deprivation
functional impairment	impaired vision	immobility
low serum albumin	impaired hearing	dehydration
glucose abnormalities	ETOH abuse	comorbidities
hip fracture repair	cardiac surgery	eye surgery
aortic aneurysm repair	thoracic surgery	other ortho
intraperitoneal surgery	massive blood loss	hypoxia
electrolyte abnormalities	hypotension	meperidine
postoperative pain at rest		

? age associated central cholinergic deficiency as a positive predictor

Two types of postoperative delirium

    hypoactive form (more common and more commonly overlooked)

    hyperactive type

Confusion Assessment Method tool for clinical diagnosis by assessing

    fluctuating course of an acute change in mental status

    inattention

    altered level of consciousness

    disorganized thinking

(diagnosis of POD when a and b are present with either c or d)

Perioperative use of benzodiazepines are associated with POD

Ill-defined effects of POD on long-term cognitive outcomes

? perioperative haloperidol to decrease duration and severity of POD

Postoperative in-dwelling perineural catheters reduce incidence of POD

POD may indicate symptoms of other complications

sepsis	urinary tract infection
myocardial infarction	stroke
pneumonia	

Emergence delirium	Present on regaining consciousness following general anesthesia
	Common in the pediatric surgical population
	No agreed-on diagnostic criteria (? usefulness of traditional tools)
	Predicts postoperative delirium

PHARMACOKINETIC ALTERATIONS IN THE ELDERLY PATIENT

The aging process can produce pharmacokinetic (the relationship between drug dose and plasma concentration) and pharmacodynamic (the relationship between plasma concentration and clinical effect) alterations. Alterations of clinical response to anesthetic medications in the elderly may be the result of altered pharmacokinetics as well as increases in target organ sensitivity. Physiological changes that accompany aging affect key pharmacologic processes, including drug absorption, distribution, metabolism, and excretion. Some pharmacokinetic alterations are related exclusively to the aging process, whereas other alterations are likely the result of combined effects of age, disease, and environmental influences. Although increasing age is often accompanied by reductions in the physiologic reserve of several organ systems independent of the effects of any disease, these changes are not typically uniform. Consideration of the patients' physiologic status (ie, hydration, nutrition, hepatorenal function, and cardiac output) and its impact on analgesic pharmacokinetics are as important as physiologic age-related changes.

Changes in the body composition associated with aging include an increase in body fat, decrease in the content of total-body water and lean body mass, and a progressive loss of muscle mass (sarcopenia).[27] Muscle mass is reduced by approximately one-third between the ages of 50 and 80 years as a routine component of the aging process.[28] Progressive decreases in total-body water content result in a smaller body central compartment while increases in body fat lead to a greater volume of drug distribution.[29] Increases in body fat and diminished muscle mass are generally more pronounced in older women. The relative increase in body fat and decrease in lean body mass of older patients alters drug distribution such that fat-soluble drugs are more widely distributed.[30] In contrast, the volume of distribution of water-soluble compounds is reduced such that the dose required to reach a target plasma concentration is decreased.

Age-related alterations in renal function lead to clinically significant reductions in the excretion rate of water-soluble drugs and their active metabolites.[31] Renal blood flow and kidney mass, including glomerular number and glomerular tubular length, decrease with age.[32] There is a progressive loss of GFR during the aging process. Renal blood flow (RBF) is maintained up until the fourth decade of life, but is reduced by approximately 10% per decade thereafter. The decline in RBF is associated with a 50% reduction in GFR between the ages of 20 and 90.[33] Blood urea nitrogen (BUN) gradually increases by 0.2 mg/dL per year with aging, but the serum creatinine level is typically unchanged because of a decrease in body muscle mass and reduced creatinine production. Ultimately, reductions of drug clearance results in prolonged duration of action of several opioids and morphine-6-glucoronide. Therefore, elderly patients receiving opioid analgesics should have them administered judiciously, and BUN and creatinine clearance should be monitored throughout the perioperative period.

Plasma binding proteins for the acidic class of drug is albumin and plasma binding proteins for basic type drugs are α_1-acid glycoproteins. Circulating levels of albumin will typically decrease with age, whereas α_1-acid glycoprotein levels usually increase with age. For drugs that bind to serum proteins, equilibrium exists between the bound or ineffective portion and the unbound (free) or effective portion. In addition, reductions in albumin observed during illness further elevate levels of free acidic drugs and may increase risks of toxicity. Basic drugs, such as lidocaine and propanolol, that bind primarily to α_1-acid glycoprotein are less affected by illness. Overall, plasma concentration of free drug correlates well with pharmacologic action.

Because of an increase in hepatic reserve, loss of hepatic function in the elderly is less likely despite decreases in hepatic blood flow and liver cell mass with age.[34] However, the rate of drug biotransformation decreases with age. The liver metabolizes drugs through two different mechanisms, phase I and phase II hepatic metabolism. Phase I metabolism involves drug oxidation and reduction, catalyzed primarily by the cytochrome P450 system within the smooth endoplasmic reticulum of hepatocytes. Phase II hepatic metabolism involves the conjugation of drugs and/or their metabolites into other organic substrates. Drugs that are metabolized through phase I enzymatic activity have prolonged half-lives, because this metabolic activity decreases with age. Opioid analgesics are primarily metabolized in the liver by enzymatic activity (microsomal CYP450-2D6, deaminases, and glucoronidases). Drugs that undergo phase II metabolism are less affected by the aging process and show no evidence of prolonged half-life in older patients. Therefore, because activity of hepatic cytochrome P450-dependent reactions and glucoronidases decrease with age, this may lead to increased risk of toxicity with opioid analgesics.[35]

PHARMACODYNAMIC ALTERATIONS IN THE ELDERLY

Pharmacodynamics will define the biochemical and physiological effects of drugs along with their mechanism of action. Age-related alterations in the number of drug receptors and sensitivity of receptors to specific drugs could influence pharmacodynamics. Elderly patients are generally more sensitive to anesthetics and analgesics. These patients usually require less medication to achieve the desired clinical response and often experience a prolonged duration of effect. Therefore, undesirable hemodynamic consequences may occur more frequently in older patients. For example, a hemodynamic response to intravenous anesthetics may be exaggerated in the elderly as a consequence of decreased myocardial reserve and reduced vasculature compliance. Expected compensatory or reflex responses are often slowed, blunted, or absent because of the physiologic changes associated with normal aging and age-related disease. A reduced or downward adjustment in drug dosage is often required in older patients secondary to the multifaceted causes of altered and often variable pharmacologic effect. However, many of these pharmacodynamic parameters are not well understood, so all drugs administered to older patients should be used with caution because reactions may be variable, different, and with unforeseen consequences and side effects.

In the elderly, anesthetic dosage requirements for local anesthetic minimum concentration (C_m) and GA minimum alveolar concentration (MAC) are reduced, and a longer duration of action may be expected from spinal and epidural anesthetics.[36] A given volume of an epidural local anesthetic tends to result in more cephalad spread and a prolonged duration of motor block in older patients. Recovery time following GA is often prolonged in elderly patients along with evidence of a longer time to recover from its CNS depressive effects. Therefore, prolonged recovery times, potential for mental status changes and negative cognitive effects from GA may be exaggerated in older patients, especially those with underlying cognitive dysfunction.

Elderly patients show lower postoperative pain relief requirements.[37] Opioids are used during anesthesia and for postoperative pain management but may also have a high potential to be problematic for older patients. Enhanced sensitivity to fentanyl, alfentanil, and sufentanil seems to be pharmacodynamic in nature for elderly patients.[29] Opioids have a larger volume of distribution in older patients, yet opioid pharmacokinetics do not appear significantly affected by age. In addition, dose requirements of fentanyl and alfentanil to achieve end-point reductions in the electroencephalogram (EEG) are lower in elderly patients.[29] In a comprehensive review, activity of sufentanil, alfentanil, and fentanyl were found to be about twice as potent in elderly patients.[29] Such findings are related to increased brain sensitivity with advancing age rather than alterations in opioid pharmacokinetics.

Morphine and, to a lesser extent, meperidine are employed for postoperative analgesia. The clearance of morphine is decreased in the elderly and the clearance of morphine-6-glucuronide is critically dependent on renal excretion.[38,39] Patients with renal insufficiency have impaired elimination of morphine-6-glucoronide that may account for enhanced analgesia along with potential for increased adverse events.[40] Meperidine should be avoided in the elderly, because it has a relatively long half-life and its metabolite, normeperidine, has anticholinergic activity that may lead to seizures and predispose patients to cognitive dysfunction.[41,42] Because meperidine is metabolized in the kidneys and dependant on renal function, this may predispose older patients with decreased glomerular filtration rates to the deleterious effects of normeperidine.

Opioid analgesic common complications include nausea and vomiting, sedation, delirium, and respiratory depression. Constipation is also a common side effect of opioids with elderly patients being very susceptible. Sedation and delirium are CNS side effects produced by opiates in older patients and when these symptoms develop, decreasing the opioid dosage or switching to a different opioid may minimize or alleviate these side effects. Another common effect of opioid use is respiratory depression that may be exacerbated in the opiate-naïve and patients with chronic obstructive pulmonary disease (COPD) and sleep apnea.

The volume of distribution for benzodiazepines increase with age and advancing age prolongs its elimination half-life. There is an enhanced pharmacodynamic sensitivity to benzodiazepines in older patients. For example, the elimination half-life of diazepam can be as long as 36–72 hours and elimination half-life of midazolam (requirements are 50% less in elderly patients) can be prolonged from 2.5 to 4 hours.[43]

Local anesthetic (LA) metabolism varies considerably in older patients and is a major factor in selecting a particular agent for use. LA toxicity is related to the free concentration of drug in the plasma and binding of LA to proteins in the serum and to tissue receptor sites reduces the concentration of free drug in the systemic circulation.[44] Amide-linked local anesthetics are degraded by hepatic cytochrome P450 enzymes with the initial reactions involving N-dealkylation and then hydrolysis, so caution should be exercised with amide local anesthetics in elderly patients with hepatic disease. Amide local anesthetics are extensively (55% to 95%) bound to plasma proteins, particularly α_1-acid glycoprotein, and there are factors that may increase (eg, cancer, surgery, trauma, myocardial infarction, smoking, and uremia) or decrease (eg, oral contraceptives) plasma levels of α_1-acid glycoprotein and local anesthetic delivery to the liver. In addition to the age-related changes of protein binding abilities to local anesthetics, elderly patients with reduced cardiac output could result in slow delivery of amide compounds to the liver, thus prolonging their plasma half-lives.

ALTERATIONS IN PAIN PERCEPTION AND DIFFICULTIES ASSESSING PAIN IN THE ELDERLY PATIENT

Clinical studies and experimental evidence provide support that pain perception and reaction to noxious stimulation are reduced in elderly patients.[45,46] However, it is not clear if alterations in pain perception are because of aging processes or age-associated comorbid disease such as diabetes and neuropathy.[47] Controversy exists regarding pain perception in cognitively impaired patients. Pain intensity measurements in patients with moderate to severe cognitive impairment is difficult for pain specialists and geriatricians alike.[48] Nevertheless, basic principles for evaluating pain intensity and relief should remain similar to that employed for other patients.[49] In mildly confused patients, continual pain assessment using descriptor or "faces" scales rather than difficult to comprehend numerical scales should be considered.

There are several general principles that should be practiced when managing perioperative analgesic needs of elderly patients. It is important to reduce the burden of opioids, benzodiazepins, and other CNS depressants by incorporating alternative modalities of analgesia such as central-neuraxial blockade, peripheral nerve and nerve plexus blockade, nonopioid analgesics, and adjuvants. Intravenous patient-controlled analgesia (IV PCA) may be poorly understood and not optimized by elderly patients, and if cognitive dysfunction is evident, then discontinuation of such therapy should be considered. Peripheral nerve blockade (PNB), neuraxial analgesia, nonsteroidal anti-inflammatory drugs (NSAIDs), acetaminophen, and intermittent small doses of IV opioids will enhance analgesia, reduce opioid requirements, and minimize risk of narcotic toxicity. Use of multimodal regimens that include neural blockade is especially important in elderly patients with significant comorbid disease and decreased physiological reserve.[50]

NEURAXIAL REGIONAL ANALGESIA AND PERIPHERAL NERVE BLOCKADE VERSUS OPIOID-BASED ANALGESIA

A general approach to optimize perioperative pain management in geriatric patients is to consider postoperative complications commonly associated with routine surgical procedures to assess any potential benefits associated with PNB and neuraxial regional anesthesia/analgesia (NRA). Neurologic, pulmonary, and cardiovascular complications are among the most common observed in the elderly and occur most frequently in orthopedic and general surgical settings. There are both established and theoretical indications supporting the concept that NRA provides a more effective and safer analgesic option for elderly and cognitively impaired patients, and these are listed in Table 31.3. Nevertheless, it is the lack of consistency within NRA studies that has prevented firm recommendations, indications, and guidelines, about which techniques offer the greatest advantage for elderly and cognitively impaired patients undergoing particular surgical procedures.

Table 31.3: Perioperative Outcomes of Regional Anesthesia and Analgesia

Organ System	Theoretical and Established Benefits of Regional Anesthesia
Central nervous system	Questionable influence on postoperative cognitive function
	Preoperative placement of RA (with or without GA) may provide preemptive analgesia
	Improved functional outcome and less need for psychological rehabilitation
Cardiovascular system	May influence or reduce incidence of myocardial infarction
	Provide more stable perioperative hemodynamics
Respiratory system	When used as primary anesthetic technique, RA can avoid endotracheal intubation and mechanical ventilation
	RA may lead to less respiratory complications (especially if able to avoid GA)
	Preserved respiratory responses to hypercapnia and hypoxia
	Reduced incidence of pneumonia
	Reduced length of intubation time
	Maintenance of functional residual capacity
	Preservation of pulmonary gas exchange
Gastrointestinal system	Reduced risk of postoperative nausea and vomiting (especially when opioid use is reduced or not used perioperatively)
	Reduced incidence of gastrointestinal dysfunction
Endocrine and immune system	May preserve patient immune response
	Maintain glucose homeostasis and tolerance
	Reduce catabolic activity and responses (improve protein economy)
	May suppress stress response of surgery and GA
	Decreased incidence of postoperative infection
Hematologic system	Lowered incidence of venous thromboembolism
	Reduced occurrence (lowers risk) of deep vein thrombosis
	Lowered risk/incidence of pulmonary embolism
	Reduced intraoperative blood loss
	Reduced need for perioperative blood transfusion
	Reduced incidence of graft thrombosis
Other	Possibly improved postoperative recovery profile (especially early)
	Reduced dependence on opioids and opioid-related complications (pulmonary function, GI system, CNS, etc)
	Superior perioperative pain relief (RA anesthesia and analgesia)
	May result in shortening or bypassing the PACU
	May shorten hospital stay (shorter home readiness time), along with reductions in hospital readmissions
	Superior pain management/pain relief may lead to reduced costs and reduction of intensity of medical ancillary provider care
	Improved economics and cost-effectiveness
	Better satisfaction from the patient and patient family
	Overall improved surgical outcomes

Abbreviations: CNS = central nervous system; GA = general anesthesia; GI = gastrointestinal; PACU = postanesthesia care unit; RA = regional anesthesia.

Definitions and descriptions of RA are variable as are definitions of the various techniques of analgesia and anesthesia (Table 31.4). Most clinical investigations use neuraxial anesthesia (with or without analgesia) to mean RA, yet some studies will include peripheral nerve plexus blockade and PNB, LA infiltration, and LA injection to depict RA. In this chapter, NRA will refer to neuraxial regional anesthesia and analgesia (spinal and/or epidural anesthesia and analgesia), PNB will be considered separately, and RA will be used to encompass all non-GA techniques. Perioperative outcomes and clinical outcomes associated with NRA effectiveness, morbidity (traditional and nontraditional complications[51]), and mortality to be

Table 31.4: Techniques of Analgesia and Anesthesia

Regional Anesthesia and Analgesia	With or without other intravenous perioperative medications (analgesics, sedation)
Neuraxial	Spinal (subarachnoid) and/or epidural anesthesia and/or analgesia
	single injection, with or without catheters
	local anesthetic (type, concentration) with or without opioids and other adjuncts
	vertebral level of block placement/initiation
	level of blockade achieved
	length or duration of postoperative anesthesia and analgesia
Peripheral nerve/nerve plexus blockade	Peripheral nerve block
	local anesthetic with or without additives
	single injection or continuous catheter technique
Infiltration/field block	Local anesthetic infiltration/injection (diffusion blockade)
	with or without indwelling catheters
General anesthesia and analgesia	With or without perioperative medications
Anesthesia	Inhalation agents, intravenous agents, and/or total intravenous anesthesia (TIVA)
Analgesia	Systemically administered analgesia with opioids, nonopioids, and other adjuncts
	intramuscular injections
	intravenous boluses
	patient-controlled analgesia (PCA)
	transdermal, mucous membrane and oral routes
Local monitored anesthesia care (LMAC)	LMAC with and/or without intravenous and oral sedatives, hypnotics, analgesics (opioid and nonopioid)

discussed include pain management, functional and economical outcomes, functional health status, quality of life measurements, morbidity (cognitive, CNS, cardiovascular, pulmonary, GI, immune, endocrine, and coagulation), and mortality. With either NRA or PNB, it is important to consider and take into account patient age, anticipated surgical procedure, patient comorbidity(ies), and potential postoperative pain management requirements when deciding on an appropriate choice of anesthetic technique in the elderly.

CHOICE OF ANESTHESIA AND ANALGESIA: IMPACT ON POSTOPERATIVE COGNITIVE FUNCTION IN ELDERLY PATIENTS

Drugs administered to the elderly during the perioperative period may have significant variability, profound influence, and many potential adverse effects on the nervous system. Prior to surgery, a comprehensive perioperative evaluation of the elderly patient should be performed as a multidisciplinary team approach. In addition to assessing vital organ function, the preoperative evaluation should always assess for evidence of any cognitive impairment. Elderly patients often present with age-related changes of the nervous system, and whether these changes are normal or pathologic, they are to be considered in the anesthetic plan and during the selection of appropriate postoperative pain management.

Hypothesis and theory abound that NRA and PNB followed by continuous neural infusion may reduce the incidence of POCD in the elderly.[52] Preliminary outcome studies have noted

such reductions in morbidity when RA was provided to elderly patients undergoing certain surgical procedures (Table 31.5). For example, (1) the incidence of acute postoperative confusion in elderly patients recovering from hip fracture surgery was reduced with RA[53] and (2) elderly patients recovering from high delirium risk surgery (femoral neck fracture repair) performed under spinal anesthesia did not experience clinically significant delirium.[54] It is important to note that these individuals did not receive perioperative premedication or excessive sedation. As discussed, poorly controlled postoperative pain is associated with an increased incidence of cognitive dysfunction.[19] Thus, it would seem prudent to provide optimal pain management and use agents that have fewer adverse events along with medications and medication concentrations yielding minimal influence on cognitive function. This implication is important when considering RA techniques because LA infusions have been shown to provide superior pain control compared to systemic opioids[55] along with reductions in side effects, such as POCD, that have been associated with use of systemic narcotics.[56] In addition, epidural analgesia can reduce the incidence of postoperative pulmonary complications that have shown to be connected with an increased occurrence of POCD.[11,57,58]

Numerous trials examining intraoperative neuraxial anesthesia versus GA have not observed improved preservation of postoperative cognitive function and neuraxial anesthesia has yet been shown to reduce the overall incidence of POCD. There is inconclusive evidence that PNB and continuous regional analgesia are associated with a lower incidence of POCD. Some of the problems evaluating studies that address the issue of cognitive preservation in elderly patients are related to multiple

Table 31.5: Comparing Effects of Regional Anesthesia on Morbidity and Mortality

Positive Conclusions with Regional	Negative Conclusions with Regional	Reference
Reductions of intraoperative blood loss and postoperative thromboemblic events after prostatectomy and hip surgery	No definitive results confirming reductions in CNS, cardiac, respiratory, and GI morbidity	Kehlet (1984)[105]
Diminished incidence of postoperative morbidity		
Decreased incidence of postoperative mortality		
30% reduction in *early* mortality		Atanassoff (1996)[62]
Some benefit on *short*-term survival		

Epidural opioid vs. systemic opioid:
    decreased occurrence of atelectasis
    decreased incidence of pulmonary infections
    increased PaO_2
    decreased overall rate of pulmonary complications
	Epidural opioid vs. systemic opioid: no significant differences in other pulmonary function factors	Ballantyne et al (1998)[57]

Reduced morbidity in patients with neuraxial block:
    decreased incidence of MI (30%)
    decreased incidence of DVT (40%)
    decreased incidence of PE (55%)
    decreased incidence of respiratory depression (59%)
    decreased incidence of pneumonia (39%)
    decreased incidence of blood transfusion (50%)
Overall mortality reduced (33%)
	Most of the study subjects (N = 9559) received single-shot epidural anesthesia
	
	The study subjects (N = 9559) were predominantly orthopedic patients and no significant effects were found in other surgical procedures
		Rodgers et al (2000)[58]

Group 1 – GA + PCA, Group 2 – epidural + GA
Group 2 – epidural + GA:
    reduced ICU stay in abdominal surgical pts
    reduced incidence of major complications in abdominal surgical pts
    shorter intubation time for abdominal surgical pts
    improved pain relief despite reduced analgesic drugs
    reduced mortality in abdominal surgical pts
    improved overall outcome in abdominal surgical pts
	No difference in mortality when all types of abdominal surgeries (4 types) were combined from all subjects (N = 1021)	Park et al (2001)[64]

Patients in the epidural group: better analgesia reduced incidence of postoperative MI significantly reduced postoperative MI in the patients with thoracic epidural analgesia	Results of this meta-analysis did not show statistical significance in mortality of study subjects (N = 1173)	Beattie et al (2001)[66]
Epidural (+ GA) group of patients for AAA had reduced time to extubation compared to the GA only group	Study patients (N = 168) had similar postoperative outcomes related to: morbidity (renal failure, MI, medical costs, reoperation, length of hospital stay, pneumonia) and mortality	Norris et al (2001)[104]
Reduced pulmonary morbidity from epidural opioid analgesia in thoracic surgery patients	No difference in length of hospital stay No change in cardiac morbidity	Kehlet and Holte (2001)[79]
Reduced pulmonary morbidity from epidural (with or without opioid) in abdominal surgical patients	No effects toward POCD	
Reductions of surgical stress response from epidural		
Reductions of thromboembolic problems from epidural		
Reductions of ileus from epidural (without opioids)		
Improved transition to rehabilitation		

Positive Conclusions with Regional	Negative Conclusions with Regional	Reference
Improved oxygen saturation on first postoperative day with RA Reduced incidence of DVT Reduced incidence of mortality at 1 month	No differences for study subjects (N = 2262) in: length of surgery, PE incidence, or length of hospital stay Reduced mortality but not significant statistically	Sharrock (1995)[112]
When RA combined with GA in major abdominal surgery: reduced pulmonary failure and improved pain control	Other morbidity events were not reduced in patients (N = 915) undergoing abdominal surgery with the addition of RA to GA	Rigg et al (2002)[76]
Epidural anesthesia and analgesia had reduced pulmonary failure	No differences in other morbidity events or mortality	Peyton et al (2003)[106]
Preoperative epidural reduced preoperative cardiac events in elderly hip fracture patients (N = 68)		Matot et al (2003)[65]

Epidural compared to parenteral opioids:
 	
    improved analgesia for thoracic surgery
 	
    improved rest and movement pain scores
 	
    improved analgesia for abdominal surgery
 	
    reduced PONV (without epidural opioid)
	Of the 100 study trials, thoracic epidural was similar to the parenteral opioids	Block et al (2003)[55]

Reductions in postoperative MI with thoracic epidural analgesia (meta-analysis, N = 2427)		Beattie et al (2003)[67]
Unadjusted 7- and 30-day mortality reduced in RA (+ GA) compared to GA alone group	No difference in multivariate regression analysis in morbidity and mortality at 7 and 30 days	Wu et al (2003)[107]
Reduced risk of DVT Reduced rate of acute postoperative confusion Reduced mortality at 1 month in 8 of 22 trials (N = 2567)	No difference in mortality in 6 of 22 trials (N = 2567)	Parker et al (2004)[53]
Reduced mortality at 7 and 30 days with postoperative epidural analgesia (N = 12,780)	Incidence of pneumonia increased at 30 days in epidural analgesia group (N = 12,780) Overall, morbidity unchanged (N = 68,723)	Wu et al (2004)[68]

Thoracic epidural + GA in CABG:
 	
    reduced pain and pain scores (also intrathecal group)
 	
    reduced opioid use and requirements
 	
    reduced time to extubation
 	
    reduced risk of respiratory complications
 	
    decreased incidence of dysrhythmias
	No difference in morbidity and mortality of intrathecal RA
	
	No difference in mortality with thoracic epidural
		Liu et al (2004)[108]

Improved cognitive function in first few hours postoperatively	No difference in mental status beyond first few hours postoperatively	Handley et al (1994)[109]; Williams-Russo et al (1995)[59]
Permits increased activity and improved mobility (short- and long-term postoperatively)	Time to first ambulation is not effected	Gottsahalk et al (1998)[110]; Gilbert et al (2000)[111]

Abbreviations: AAA = abdominal aortic aneurysm; CABG = coronary artery bypass grafting; CNS = central nervous system; DVT = deep vein thrombosis; GA = general anesthesia; GI = gastrointestinal; ICU = intensive care unit; MI = myocardial infarction; PCA = patient controlled analgesia; PE = pulmonary embolism; POCD = postoperative cognitive dysfunction; PONV = postoperative nausea and vomiting; RA = regional anesthesia.

design flaws and the methodological variability of clinical trials (Table 31.6). Attempts at interpreting past and current evidence provides conflicting results and even in the hierarchy of evidence, such as meta-analysis of randomly controlled trials and large randomized trials as best evidence, there is lack of data to demonstrate preservation of cognition beyond the first few hours after surgery when selecting NRA and PNB rather than GA.[59,60]

Meta-analysis results may demonstrate significant improvement in mortality when neuraxial blockade is used without GA,[55,58,61] but until POCD predictors and consequences are determined, it will remain difficult to make recommendations for appropriate treatment and prevention of POCD. When POCD has been identified or suspected in a surgical patient, work-up for additional causes of cognitive impairment (ie, Alzheimers',

Table 31.6: Study Design Flaws and Complexity of Conflicting Results

Design Flaws	*Conflicting Results and Methodological Difficulties*
Indiscriminant use and lack of accounting for use of sedative/hypnotic drugs. No controls for preoperative sedation/analgesia in RA patients	Mortality rates are decreasing, necessitating the need for studies that have large numberss of patients (underpowered studies)[112]
Duration of postoperative analgesia must be identified and remains important factor for pain & stress responses, morbidity and mortality	Diverse surgical procedures and heterogeneous patient populations
Diversity of assessment of POCD	Diversity of definitions of POCD and POD
No uniformity of neuropsychological testing	Lack of control of sedation depth may disregard differences between GA & RA[63]
Studies not being double-blinded[30]	Timing of placement of RA (uncontrolled factor)
Diversity on modes of POCD analysis	Lack of routine consideration of different anesthetic techniques: upper vs lower body, anesthesia vs analgesia, RA + GA vs RA, LA alone vs LA + adjuncts
Parenteral use of postoperative sedatives and opioids uncontrolled and indiscriminately used	Vertebral location of RA (thoracic, lumbar, etc)

Abbreviations: GA = general anesthesia; LA = local anesthesia; POCD = postoperative cognitive dysfunction; POD = postoperative delirium; RA = regional anesthesia.

stroke, cerebral hematoma) should be initiated. These patients should be followed closely with subspecialty consultation if necessary and then reassured because POCD does not typically persist (>1 year in 1%–2% of cases). Additional consequences warranting further examination are that symptoms from pain and untoward effects of postoperative medications may result in poor performance in the varied forms of neuropsychological testing. These factors may prove to lead to declines in cognition in the days following major surgery when use of such postoperative medications and pain levels are at there greatest.

CHOICE OF ANESTHESIA AND ANALGESIA: IMPACT ON POSTOPERATIVE CARDIOVASCULAR FUNCTION IN THE ELDERLY

With aging, there are a variety of morphological and functional changes in the cardiovascular system. These changes include reduction in left ventricular compliance, generalized hypertrophy of the left ventricular wall, fibrotic changes in the heart, and decreased myocardial compliance. These changes result in increased stoke volume and elevated diastolic and systolic blood pressure (Table 31.7). Many elderly patients present with cardiac pathology, including moderate to severe coronary artery disease, valvular heart disease, and conduction defects that increases risk of postsurgical morbidity and death. Aging effects on cardiac output have minimal influence in the resting individual, but functional changes become evident with stress. Similar effort dependent stress is observed with negative influences on pulmonary function.

Aging influences on the heart and vascular system have important clinical implications for the treatment of elderly surgical patients and for considerations of postoperative pain management, especially those patients receiving RA. Currently, there is little statistical evidence to suggest differences in cardiovascular outcome and effects on mortality between RA versus GA in the elderly,[62,63] although there have been studies showing a significant benefit for use of RA and its influence on cardiac morbidity and short-term survival (Table 31.5). Even though there is little suggestion and data to indicate a statistically signif-

icant difference in anesthetic technique (RA versus GA) toward the overall incidence of death or major complications; analysis of RA has detected a positive influence on pain management and better outcomes when considering the type of surgery being performed. For example, when epidural anesthesia and analgesia are combined with GA for elective abdominal aortic aneurysm repair, the duration of postoperative tracheal intubation, mechanical ventilation, total ICU stay, and use of resources are reduced. In addition, the quality of postoperative analgesia is improved, whereas the incidence of major complications and death are reduced.[64] Early placement of continuous epidural analgesia in elderly patients for hip fracture surgery versus a regimen of systemic opioids has been associated with a reduced incidence of adverse cardiac events.[65] Therefore, when studies are tailored with consideration for planned surgery, patient comorbid disease(s), and perioperative patient management needs, evidence may then be available to better provide guidelines followed by anesthesia protocols that could affect surgical patient cardiovascular outcomes.

Currently, there remains conflicting results and altering consensus between analgesic technique and cardiac morbidity. However, recent meta-analysis of randomly controlled trials (N = 9559) showed that patients undergoing various orthopedic procedures and receiving neuraxial blockade had a one-third reduction in overall mortality.[58] An additional meta-analysis (N = 2427) found that patients who received epidural anesthesia and analgesia (with or without GA) had a reduced incidence of perioperative myocardial infarction and, in those instances when a thoracic epidural was maintained for analgesia longer than 24 hours, results showed significantly fewer postoperative myocardial infarctions.[66,67] Yet another meta-analysis (N = 68 723) on Medicare patients found the association of a significantly lower odds ratio of death at 7 and 30 days when postoperative epidural analgesia was used.[68]

Perioperative stresses of acute lifestyle disruption, anesthesia, surgery, postoperative pain, and convalescence will activate (to a varying degree) the sympathetic nervous system of the elderly surgical patient. These stresses result in mixed and potentially negative imbalances between myocardial oxygen supply and demand and possibly lead to myocardial ischemia and infarction. Perioperative myocardial infarction and other

Table 31.7: Influence of Age on the Cardiovascular System

Morphological Cardiovascular Changes of Aging	*Functional Cardiovascular Effects of Aging*
Progressive loss of elasticity of large arteries	Increased systolic blood pressure
Generalized hypertrophy of the left ventricular wall	Increased afterload for the left ventricle
	Increased left ventricular end-diastolic volume
Fibrotic changes and diminished elasticity of heart muscle (reduced myocardial compliance)	Cardiovascular system is volume sensitive and volume intolerant
Reduced compliance of left ventricular ejection fraction (LVEF)	Unable to optimally respond to stress (cannot significantly increase LVEF)
Cardiac output is maintained by increasing end diastolic volume	Overall results are an increased stroke volume
Elderly patients may not maintain blood pressure when challenged with minor hypovolemia or added cardiovascular stresses	
Sympathetic blockade from neuraxial anesthesia may lead to hypotension in a setting of hypovolemia	

deleterious cardiovascular events such as congestive heart failure (CHF), sudden death, and cardiac arrhythmias typically occur with increased frequency within the first few days following a surgical intervention[69,70] and patients with a reduced cardiovascular reserve or patients at risk of perioperative myocardial events have a higher incidence of perioperative myocardial ischemia and infarction.[71] Therefore, goals for anesthesia and surgery during the perioperative period would be to reduce or eliminate the many physiologic imbalances and stresses associated with operative interventions to minimize negative cardiovascular effects.

Thoracic epidural analgesia may attenuate adverse cardiovascular pathophysiologic events because neural blockade decreases sympathetic outflow yielding a more favorable balance between myocardial oxygen supply and demand. Reductions in sympathetic activity result in decreased cardiac inotropy and decreased heart rate and blood pressure instability, whereas at the same time increasing coronary blood flow to subendocardial regions at risk for ischemia. There currently remains uncertainty to the statistically proven beneficial influence of postoperative epidural analgesia on the incidence of myocardial ischemia, myocardial infarction, or myocardial malignant arrhythmias (Table 31.5). However, use of thoracic epidural analgesia (not lumbar) has revealed statically significant reductions in ventricular malignant arrhythmias and decreased incidence of postoperative myocardial infarction.[66] Therefore, in the appropriate surgical setting, physiologic benefits of thoracic epidural analgesia can decrease adverse cardiovascular pathophysiologic events such as myocardial infarction in the older surgical candidate.

There is relatively little information or outcome data regarding the benefits of PNB with or without continuous LA infusion on perioperative cardiac morbidity and mortality in the older surgical patient. However, it is likely that adequately controlled postoperative pain could have beneficial cardiovascular effects with regard to development of myocardial dysfunction if catecholamine levels associated with stress and pain of the perioperative period are minimized. Also apparent are benefits of superior analgesia with PNB compared to systemic opioids that may result in reductions or preventions of myocardial sensitization and minimizing the pain induced stressful component associated with surgery.

PNB are used in older surgical patients to provide preemptive analgesia, reduce or avoid the need for GA and its many deleterious effects, and reduce untoward sympathetic stimulations and stress responses associated with surgical interventions. PNB that complement multimodal therapies have been demonstrated to have ameliorative effects on acute pain[72] with resulting potential indirect influence of improvement in anesthesia and surgical management that may lead to a reduction in cardiac morbidity and mortality. An additional important factor to consider is the method used to achieve the necessary duration of postoperative analgesia. Postoperative analgesia is important because pain from surgery, surgical stress responses, and effects from surgery on the cardiovascular system do not subside until a few days following surgery. Therefore, timing and duration of a PNB, achieved with a continuous catheter technique, may provide cardiovascular benefits by reducing surgical pain and associated sympathetic and neuroendocrine stress responses during the postoperative period.

CHOICE OF ANESTHESIA AND ANALGESIA: EFFECT ON POSTOPERATIVE PULMONARY FUNCTION IN THE ELDERLY

Significant perioperative risk among elderly patients is attributable to respiratory compromise and complications. A substantial portion of the risk is explained by both functional and structural changes within the pulmonary system commonly associated with aging (Table 31.8). Reductions in functional residual capacity (FRC) are created by assuming the supine position and under the influence of GA. GA can reduce FRC by 15%–20% and can last 7–10 days following surgery.[73] Older patients undergoing GA are predisposed to atelectasis from the combination of reduced FRC and age-associated increases in closing volume. Vital capacity can be reduced after upper abdominal incisions (25%–50%) and postoperative pain along with systemic opioid analgesics can contribute to a reduction in tidal volume and impair clearing of secretions (altered cough mechanics). Hypoxic pulmonary vasoconstriction (HPV) is adversely affected and maybe abolished during inhalation anesthesia. Blunting of HPV in the elderly during GA causes a greater incidence of intraoperative ventilation perfusion (V/Q) mismatch, and an increased alveolar-to-arterial oxygen gradient. Inhalation anesthesia depresses respiratory responses to hypoxia and hypercarbia and patients receiving inhalation agents commonly require tracheal intubation because of a high incidence of airway obstruction. These negative influences can compromise the usual protective responses of the pulmonary system during the perioperative period and are to be considered in the

Table 31.8: Influence of Aging on the Pulmonary System

Structures	Functional Changes	Results
Conducting airways (nose to respiratory bronchioles)	Changes (minor) of muscle and cartilaginous support Slow loss of elastin, collagen, water content, along with muscle atrophy	May result in dry mouth, snoring, bleeding, and mucosal injury Predisposes to upper airway obstruction
Diameter of trachea and central airways	Increase in size of cartilaginous airways (trachea and bronchi) by 10% Calcification of central airway cartilage Bronchial mucous gland hypertrpophy ? increased compliance of small and large airways	Functional increase in anatomical dead space Airways more prone to compression with forced exhalation Decreased maximum expiratory flow rate Increased residual volume
Upper airway reflexes	Depression of protective airway reflexes (sneezing, coughing, etc) Decreased upper laryngoesophageal sphincter contractile reflex Decreased number and activity of respiratory cilia Coughing reflex impairment	Increased chance of pulmonary aspiration Greater stimulation required to trigger sensory and motor components of airway reflexes
Lung parenchyma, alveolar surface area and elastic recoil	Enlargement of bronchioles and alveolar ducts and shortened alveolar septa Alveolar air decreases as air volume in alveolar ducts increases Reduced surfactant production Lung parenchyma loses elastic recoil Chest wall becomes stiffer	Alveolar surface area decreases (15% by age 70 years) Aging lung: airspace enlargement Flattening of the volume-pressure curve of the lung and less lung compliance
Function of lung defenses	Local defenses (cough, mucocilia) are decreased Humoral defenses (cellular, immune) reduced by decreased T-cell function and regeneration	Failure of T-cell homeostasis
Pulmonary mechanics, chest wall compliance	Calcification of rib cage, vertebral joints, and costal cartilage Osteoporosis and vertebral compromise Altered diaphragm affecting force-generating ability	Chest wall stiffens and decreased chest wall compliance Increase in respiratory work requirements
Respiratory muscles	Decreased strength and speed of skeletal muscle contraction Loss of motor neurons Reduced diaphragm strength Shortened rest-length of inspiratory muscles	Increased oxygen cost of ventilation (especially with stress and physical activity)
Pulmonary vasculature	Reduced volume of pulmonary capillary bed	Increased pulmonary arterial pressure and vascular resistance
Lung volumes and capacities	Increased residual volume because of chest wall stiffness, loss of lung recoil, and decreased muscle strength. Decreased FEV_1	Decreased vital capacity Mild increase of functional residual capacity
Expiratory flow	Decreased elastic recoil pressure	Reduced maximum expiratory flow rate
Gas exchange diffusing capacity	Loss of functional alveolar surface area	Decreased oxygen diffusing capacity Increased arterial-alveolar oxygen gradient
Ventilation/perfusion matching	Premature lung airway closure (occurs in tidal volume range) Inspired air is distributed at apexes rather than lung bases Site where small airways close is shifted distally so airways close at smaller exhaled tidal volume	Reduced capillary oxygen tension of basilar lungs Decreased arterial oxygen tension Increased closing volumes Ventilation-perfusion mismatch
Control of respiration ventilatory responses	Decrement of central and peripheral chemoreceptors	Decreased ventilatory response to hypercapnia and hypoxia Increased sensitivity to narcotic induced respiratory depression Increased disruption of sleep ventilation

elderly surgical candidate during the postoperative period. Negative effects on pulmonary function predispose older patients to atelectasis, increased risk of hypoxemia and pneumonia, V/Q mismatch, and other postoperative pulmonary complications.[74] Therefore, clinicians should titrate analgesic medications carefully and assess patients frequently for evidence of adverse side effects and adequate pain control throughout the perioperative period.

Although NRA is commonly used for older patients, many studies have shown that the anesthetic choice has no significant effect on respiratory perioperative morbidity and mortality within any age group. Intuitively it seems reasonable to believe that elderly patients may benefit from NRA because they can remain minimally sedated while breathing spontaneously, airway manipulation is avoided, postoperative pain control is provided, and recovery from any adverse respiratory influences of inhalation anesthetics/GA is minimized or eliminated (Table 31.5). A multitude of factors influence perioperative outcome and make it difficult to decide which form of anesthesia is most appropriate for a given patient and surgical setting. Therefore, the decision to perform RA must be determined on a case-by-case basis, and consideration of the patient's cardiopulmonary reserve, baseline cognitive function, anesthesiologist expertise, type of surgery, and surgical duration must all be assessed. For example, epidural analgesic techniques may benefit elderly patients undergoing thoracic and upper abdominal surgery because these techniques allow a more rapid restoration of respiratory function with added benefits of decreasing morbidity and hospital stay.[75]

With NRA, airway manipulation is avoided and respiratory parameters of lung volumes, tidal volume, respiration rate, respiratory drive (effort), and end-tidal carbon dioxide concentration are preserved. Unchanged FRC, from baseline, has been observed during spinal and lumbar epidural anesthesia. However, intercostal blocks and cervical or high thoracic epidural blockade can be associated with lung volume reductions secondary to intercostal muscle relaxation. Therefore, choice of anesthesia may affect the degree of pulmonary dysfunction (Table 31.5). Studies have shown that elderly patients undergoing lower extremity orthopedic procedures have fewer hypoxic events with epidural anesthesia (using LA) compared to systemic opioids; GA in older patients results in lower PaO_2 levels (on postop day 1) compared to epidural anesthesia; and respiratory complications are less frequent when comparing GA with postoperative intravenous morphine analgesia versus combined epidural plus GA with postoperative epidural analgesia.[76]

NRA with dilute LA solutions for analgesia may provide a greater safety margin for elderly patients compared to administration of systemic and epidural opioids. Using NRA (without opioids) in the elderly population, especially for patients with severe pulmonary dysfunction, may be more appropriate for postoperative pain relief.[62,77] Oxygen saturation in elderly patients with epidural anesthesia and analgesia without an opioid is typically higher and the use of systemic (and epidural) opioids results in a higher incidence of hypoxic events compared to epidural analgesia with a LA alone.[78] However, overreliance on LA may be associated with a greater incidence and severity of hypotension. In addition, there is a reduced incidence of pulmonary infection, an increase in PaO_2, and an overall decrease in pulmonary complications with epidural LA compared to systemic opioids for postoperative analgesia.[57] However, several meta-analysis have found that reduced atelectasis is observed with epidural opioids compared to systemic opioids (for postoperative analgesia) and that continuous epidural LA or local anesthetic-opioid mixtures resulted in reduced postoperative pulmonary morbidity after major abdominal and thoracic procedures when compared to parenteral opioids.[79]

Another meta-analysis has shown that RA may decrease pulmonary complications because patients receiving epidural analgesia were found to have shortened ICU stays and reduced tracheal intubation times versus patients receiving systemic postoperative opioids for analgesia.[53] A meta-analysis of 141 clinical trials have discovered results showing a 39% reduction in pneumonia and 60% less pulmonary depression with thoracic epidural anesthesia and analgesia versus GA and postoperative patient-controlled analgesia.[58] Therefore, much of the controversy as to why several randomized trials have not demonstrated a statistical advantage to RA in reducing respiratory complications in the elderly is lack of differentiation and uniformity of epidural mixtures, whether an opioid or how much opioid (systemic and/or epidural) was used, the site of surgery, timing and duration of neuraxial anesthesia and analgesia, and vertebral level of neuraxial blockade insertion.

The benefits of PNB on postoperative pulmonary function have not been well studied. However, with utilization of PNB, manipulation of the airway can be avoided, patient lung volumes and function are preserved, and the respiratory drive is minimally (sedation for block placement) or not affected. Given that GA may have greater negative effects on the respiratory system compared to RA, the choice of anesthesia may affect the degree of postoperative pulmonary dysfunction in the elderly. Therefore, any surgery involving the extremities (orthopedic procedures), vascular procedures, skin grafting, and amputations should be considered for a PNB anesthetic. Because the reduction of FRC following GA may persist for up to 10 days following surgery with GA,[74] possibly fewer hypoxic events with PNB using LA compared to systemic opioids after surgery may result. The lower PaO_2 levels[80] and other potential respiratory complications[76] reported with GA may also be minimized or eliminated if the surgical intervention is amendable and a PNB with LA is used versus reliance on postoperative intravenous opioid analgesia.

PNB differ from GA and neuraxial anesthesia/analgesia in terms of influence on the respiratory system. There are few investigations comparing pulmonary morbidity and mortality among GA, neuraxial anesthesia, and PNB, although there are several advantages of PNB to consider for elderly patients, especially in orthopedic procedures. PNB of the lower extremities and neuraxial anesthesia has a positive influence on vascular blood flow. Increased blood flow reduces the incidence of postoperative thromboembolic complications such as deep vein thrombosis (DVT) and pulmonary emboli. By avoiding airway manipulation and preserving respiratory drive, PNB are also associated with a lower incidence of hypercarbia, hypoxia, and pulmonary complications. By minimizing exposure to opioids, PNB and central neuraxial LA blockade may shorten tracheal intubation time and ICU stay when compared to systemic analgesia with opioids.

CHOICE OF ANESTHESIA AND ANALGESIA: EFFECT ON POSTOPERATIVE ENDOCRINE AND IMMUNE FUNCTION

With possible exception of large doses of opioids prior to surgical incision, GA alone cannot prevent stress responses of surgery from being initiated.[81] Some of the metabolic effects of surgical stress are hyperglycemia and overall catabolism. RA may provide the most physiological anesthesia for surgery and theoretically prevent or reduce the surgical stress response (Table 31.5). For example, epidural anesthesia may minimize surgical stress by blocking sympathetic and somatic nervous systems from being activated. Epidural blockade reduces postoperative hyperglycemia and improves glucose tolerance despite plasma insulin concentrations being unchanged.[79] More stable cardiovascular hemodynamics and attenuation of the stress response to surgery has been demonstrated with RA.[82] The metabolic effects of surgical stress, hyperglycemia, and catabolism may predispose patients (especially critically ill patients) to increased morbidity (polyneuropathy, infection, multiorgan dysfunction/failure) and mortality. Plasma glucose normalization and improved glucose tolerance with epidural anesthesia and analgesia can improve perioperative management of optimal glucose control. Epidural anesthesia and analgesia can reduce the catabolic response to surgery and improve on gastrointestinal rehabilitation, economy of proteins, and nutritional status of surgical patients, especially in abdominal surgery.[83]

The communicating capability of circulating immune cells and cytokines of the immune system serve as major defense systems in the human body. However, there are reduced cellular and humoral responses seen throughout the entire immune system and there is a corresponding reduction and deterioration of immune system components with aging. The thymus gland and thymulin secretions undergo an involutionary process and decreased production, respectively, as we age. Hormones responsible for mature T-cell modulation and progenitor phenotypic cell maturation processes are reduced and T-lymphocyte number contribution into circulation is lessened with aging.

Immunological changes of the aging process become evident when older patients become stressed and move away from the homeostatic state. Therefore, measures taken to ensure homeostasis and to reduce surgical stress will help preserve function of the immune system. It has been shown that epidural anesthesia and analgesia can preserve both humoral and cellular immune functions in surgical patients (especially for procedures below the umbilicus).[84] GA may worsen the immunosuppression responses that can occur subsequent to surgery. Both GA and lumbar epidural anesthesia have minor influences on the human immune function in the absence of surgery, but it is with epidural anesthesia and analgesia (with LA) that may decrease the postoperative infectious complications of surgery.[84]

Whether PNB and continuous peripheral catheter infusion techniques blunt the effects of stress on the endocrine and immune system and improve surgical outcomes remains unclear. Many components of the pain pathway are sensitized by painful stimulation and there are a network of theories (immune deficiency, autoimmune, network, etc) to explain the complex interactions of pain and influence on the immune and endocrine systems of all patients. Therefore, attempts to achieve a balanced multimodal anesthetic (along with the theory of preemptive analgesia) may provide a significant role for PNB as an intervention that targets one of the key sites (peripheral nociceptors) along the pain pathway aiding in the prevention of nervous system sensitization and activation of the endocrine system.

In many surgical settings (especially surgery performed on the extremities), superior pain relief provided by PNB may reduce the stress response that could have otherwise been escalated by inadequately controlled pain. Reductions in pain intensity may lead to additional endocrine and immune response benefits, including improved postoperative mood and better sleep after surgery.[85] PNB using LA can also provide preemptive analgesia and postoperative pain management that may reduce the incidence of chronic pain syndromes known to negatively influence the immune system.

CHOICE OF ANESTHESIA AND ANALGESIA: EFFECT ON POSTOPERATIVE OUTCOMES IN ELDERLY PATIENTS

Patient age alone should no longer be considered a key variable in predicting the risks associated with anesthesia and surgery. More important factors and better predictors of outcome for the elderly are their overall physical status, medical history, and disease state or condition. In the absence of significant disease, anesthetic complication rates do not increase dramatically with advancing age. Instead, perioperative risk is directly related to the number of patient comorbidities and extent of existing diseases, evidence of cognitive dysfunction, and medical condition(s) discovered in the preoperative period. Adverse preoperative medical conditions most indicative of the need for concern and predictive of higher surgical risk of perioperative morbidity and mortality are diabetes mellitus, hypertension, and ischemic heart disease.[86] In addition, the extensiveness of surgery, duration, and site of planned or emergency surgery also play important roles as major determinants of perioperative risk. Upper abdominal surgical procedures followed by thoracic and open-heart surgical procedures are associated with the highest morbidity and mortality and pose increased risk for the elderly surgical patient. Therefore, the geriatric patient may be at an increased risk of perioperative morbidity and mortality because of the higher incidence of coexisting disease (four-fifths of older patients have at least 1 complicating condition and one-third have 3 or more coexisting diseases), but additional issues of concern are type, urgency, and potential duration of surgery, which also serve as important predictors of elderly patient outcome.

Postoperative pain management continues to be a problem in the elderly despite advanced understanding of pain management modalities, improved drug delivery systems, and known benefits of optimal analgesia. Studies and surveys of surgical patients have reported varying degrees and intensities of pain following surgery along with reports of inadequate postoperative pain management, sometimes necessitating hospital readmission.[87,88] Part of the problem lies with the fact that caregivers worry about prescribing opioids to elderly patients because of fears of initiating or exacerbating cognitive dysfunction, ileus, addiction, and respiratory depression. These concerns may provide greater justification for employing RA and nonopioid analgesics in the elderly.

Positioning elderly patients for neuraxial anesthetic techniques becomes more difficult with age, creating potential risks for failure or complications. Geriatric individuals often have dorsal kyphosis, resulting in anatomic changes of the thoracic and lumbar vertebral spine. Osteoarthritis changes and calcification of cartilage in elderly individuals often results in an increasing likelihood of the patient to flex at the hips and knees. Compression and distortion of the epidural space is common with advanced age because of degenerative disk and joint changes. The ligamentum flavum changes and may be calcified in which attempts to accomplish an epidural or dural puncture may not be successful. This may occur because needle placement and advancement encounters difficulty in passing through the calcification and may also present obstruction to the intended path or direction of needle insertion causing deviation from a straight path. Bony overgrowth (osteophytes) may limit access to the desired central neuraxial space because of decreased size and/or obstruction of the intervertebral foramina. An anatomical characteristic that may be of aid to gaining access to the epidural or subarachnoid space is the awareness that the largest intervertebral foramen in elderly individuals is the L5–S1 interspace. Therefore, to avoid the technical difficulties caused by ligament calcification and alterations in dorsal vertebrae, a lateral approach ("Taylor" approach) may be employed for subarachnoid or epidural needle/catheter placement in elderly patients.

Continuous neuraxial and PNB techniques can provide targeted pain relief and minimize postsurgical opioid dose requirements. Although these pain management modalities are well tested and generally quite successful, they can be associated with patient safety issues that must be considered. These include patient tampering, need for patients to comprehend the system operation, and adequate patient cognition and psychological ability to play an active role in their own pain management. There are also mechanical issues to consider, including pump programming (failures, pump malfunctions, programming errors), catheter concerns (obstruction, kinks), effect on patient mobility, and concern for postoperative requirements of anticoagulation (increased risk epidural hematoma). These techniques also place a burden on the health care staff for preparation, implementation, and monitoring of the chosen pain management modality. There are staff-related system errors (syringe and drug mix-ups, programming errors) to consider, cost and time allocation of these pain treatment programs, and adverse event monitoring that should be constantly assessed.

A major issue of concern is the portrayal of epidural analgesia as being viewed merely as an alternative to IV opioids or IV PCA, despite evidence to suggest that postoperative regional analgesia results in improved patient perioperative outcomes.[56,57,66,76] This interpretation is unfortunate because various parameters, including choice of analgesic agent(s), vertebral level of catheter placement, duration of epidural analgesia, and so on, will affect both technique efficacy and influence patient outcome. Optimal epidural analgesic effects on postsurgical pain and outcome are gained when the epidural catheter is placed in close proximity to the corresponding dermatome distribution of the surgical incision.[89] There are physiologic benefits in placing epidural catheters at dermatomes (T8–T12) involved with abdominal surgery. Such placement reduces sympathetic inhibition of gastrointestinal tone, increases intestinal blood flow, and facilitates return of gastrointestinal function.[56] High-risk cardiovascular patients presenting for noncardiac thoracic and upper abdominal surgery show benefits from thoracic epidural analgesia. When the epidural catheter more closely corresponds to the surgical incision, the results are attenuation of sympathetic-mediated coronary vasoconstriction and increased coronary blood flow to subendocardial and potentially ischemic areas of the heart, both of which can be supportive of a decreased incidence of myocardial infarction.[66,90] Therefore, the demonstrated benefit of postoperative catheter location, coinciding closely with the surgical area, may show physiologic and analgesic improvement in patient outcome that has not been consistently established with either (1) epidural catheter location

incongruent with the surgical incision or (2) pain management with systemic opioids.

Patients will not receive intended analgesic and physiologic benefit of epidural analgesia if the epidural catheter should become accidentally dislodged or removed prematurely. Postoperative epidural analgesia (not intraoperative epidural anesthesia) appears to minimize the negative influence and incidence of myocardial infarction that coincided with the peak occurrence of myocardial compromise between 24 and 48 hours following surgery.[66,69] Surgical studies that have identified a facilitated return of gastrointestinal function were those in which surgical patients' maintained epidural analgesia for >24 hours postoperatively versus those patients receiving epidural analgesia for less time.[56,91] Therefore, the duration of epidural analgesia is an additional factor influencing patient outcome because the pathophysiologic responses that begin intraoperatively will frequently continue into the postoperative period.

The choice of specific analgesic agents used with epidural analgesia (LA with or without opioids and other adjuncts) will influence patient outcome. Central-neuraxial opioids prove effective in controlling postoperative pain, but only epidural LA have the ability to attenuate and influence adverse pathophysiologic responses that can contribute to perioperative morbidity.[92] Neuraxial LA are effective through prevention of spinal reflex inhibition of diaphragmatic and gastrointestinal function, suppression of responses to surgical stress, and blockade of efferent and afferent nerve signals to and from the spinal cord. In addition, epidural local analgesia used without neuraxial opioids may improve patient outcome as a result of a decreased incidence of respiratory complications and earlier recovery of gastrointestinal motility following abdominal surgery.[57,93]

PNB techniques and the many advantages they provide for the surgical candidate are reemerging into the practice of anesthesia and analgesia (Table 31.9). Success and effectiveness of PNB may be improved when single-shot techniques and catheters are placed using a nerve stimulator and/or under ultrasound guidance. Studies of PNB in the elderly patient are currently limited to small study series and case reports with yet inconclusive evidence of influence on morbidity and mortality. PNB are used as an attempt to reduce perioperative stress responses and in an effort to avoid the need or reduce the potential deleterious effects of GA. Studies have shown that LA used in PNB can ameliorate the negative influence on wound hyperalgesia for several days subsequent to surgery.[94] Therefore, including PNB into the mainstream of multimodal anesthesia care of the elderly surgical patient will allow opioid sparing and permit the proved benefits of LA (regarding sensitization of the nervous system) to become a useful choice in anesthetic care of the elderly.

Reviewing the many benefits associated with PNB is beyond the scope of this chapter; however, Evans et al have provided a review of supportive evidence for the various PNB techniques.[95] The advantages of PNB may be further facilitated with the added benefits and safety profile provided by the use of nerve stimulator evidence and ultrasound guided/directed block placement. Ultrasound-guided PNB placement is also an emerging field and studies are being performed to assess the role it may play in the setting of perioperative pain management in the elderly patient. In addition, more studies are embarking on investigating the use of continuous PNB and nerve plexus catheter techniques to provide postoperative analgesia. The use of continuous catheter techniques may prove to be even more efficacious than

Table 31.9: Comparing Effects of Peripheral Nerve Blocks

Positive Conclusions	Negative Conclusions	Ref. #
Interscalene Nerve Block		
Ideal for analgesia for shoulder and upper arm surgery compared to opioid analgesia	Potential complications 　　local anesthetic toxicity 　　total spinal anesthesia 　　Horner's syndrome 　　diaphragm paralysis (phrenic nerve block, up to 90%)	Kinnard et al (1994)[113]
Delayed time to first PO analgesics		
Reduced total opioid requirements (reduced PONV)		
Improved sleep and postoperative mood		
Preservation of cognitive function		
Supraclavicular Nerve Block		
Consistent, rapid onset of anesthesia of long duration	Potential complications: 　　pneumothorax 　　phrenic nerve block (up to 50%)	Kinnard et al (1994)[113]
Broad upper extremity coverage		
Infraclavicular Nerve Block		
Good analgesic efficacy	Interpreting the response from a nerve stimulator	Desroaches (2003)[114]
Favorable safety profile (low chance of pneumothorax)		
Lower pain scores compared to GA with IV PCA		
Reduced opioid requirement and time to first opioid use		
Easy to maintain catheter insertion site compared to other locations in the brachial plexus		
Axillary Nerve Block		
Favorable safety profile with reduction in pain scores	Septae within the sheath may influence local anesthetic spread and extent of anesthesia	Kinnard et al (1994)[113]
Broad applicability (hand, wrist, forearm)	Maintaining a clean, sterile site	
High patient acceptance with improved PACU profile		
Easy peripheral nerve block to master		
Prolonged analgesia and reduced opioid requirements with addition of adjuvants to solutions		
Sympathectomy from block enhances blood flow		
Lumbar Plexus Block		
Reliable anesthesia of 3 terminal n. of the lumbar plexus (eg, femoral, lateral femoral cutaneous, obturator)	Inconsistent anesthesia of proximal n. (eg, ilioinguinal, iliohypogastric, genitofemoral)	Parkinson et al (1989)[115]
Safe and effective for hip and knee procedures	No long-lasting benefit with single shot (when compared to GA)	
Possible PACU bypass, lower pain scores, decreased PO analgesics (same-day surgery patients) compared to GA	Potential for LA toxicity	
Lower opioid use and lower opioid-related side effects	Risk of epidural spread (up to 15%)	
Combined with sciatic n. block, easier recovery, less opioid use compared to GA in TKA		
Femoral Nerve Block		
Simple technique, excellent analgesia post-knee surgery	Possible inadequate analgesia (because of unblocked sciatic or obturator n.)	Hirst et al (1996)[116]
High patient acceptance, decreased length of hospital stay, lower pain scores compared to GA for knee surgery	Low risk of complications (LA toxicity, vascular puncture, infection, difficult to keep catheter site clean, n. injury)	
Prolong time to first PO analgesic and reduced opioid need		
Reduced incidence of opioid side effects		
Shorter hospital stay compared to GA and IV PCA		
Improved short-term rehabilitation and joint mobility		
Sciatic Nerve Block		
Safe and effective analgesia of foot and ankle surgery	Catheter needed to prolong analgesia	Taboada et al (2004)[117]
Reduced postoperative pain scores and opioid needs	Moderate patient discomfort (needle passes through gluteus muscle)	
Excellent patient satisfaction		
Reduced incidence of phantom limb pain		

Positive Conclusions	Negative Conclusions	Ref. #
Popliteal Fossa Nerve Block		
Preserves hamstring muscle function (easier ambulation)	Sensation to posterior thigh remains	Provenzano et al (2002)[118]
High patient acceptance of both anesthesia and analgesia	Possible difficult positioning of posterior approach	
Lower pain scores, opioid sparing with fewer to no opioid side effects, longer analgesia than ankle/infiltration blocks	Vascular injury/hematoma	
Reduced sleep disturbances	Catheter issues of continuous technique	
Reduced hospital stay and lowered readmission rates		
Paravertebral Nerve Block		
Dense sensory and sympathetic unilateral/segmental block for thoracic, abdominal, inguinal, and breast surgeries	Total spinal	Richardson et al (1999)[119]
Analgesia similar or better than thoracic epidural with equal or better influence on pulmonary function	Paravertebral muscle pain	
Fewer side effects of continuous block versus epidural:	Puncture of the lung or abdominal contents	
reduction of hypotension		
decreased incidence of PONV		
reduced rate of urinary retention		
Lower pain scores and reduced opioid use compared to GA		

Abbreviations: GA = general anesthesia; LA = local anesthetic; n. = nerves; PACU = postanesthesia care unit; PCA = patient controlled analgesia; PO = parenteral; PONV = postoperative nausea and vomiting; RA = regional anesthesia; TKA = total knee arthroplasty.

the historically used single injection technique and achieve prolonged analgesia without reliance on the mainstay of systemic opioids for both in- and outpatient surgical procedures in elderly patients.

RECOMMENDATIONS

Perioperative RA and PNB techniques may positively influence surgical outcome by (1) reducing neuroendocrine stress responses, (2) improving effective pain control, (3) facilitating return of gastrointestinal function (earlier enteral feeding), and (4) encouraging patient mobilization, all of which will play an integral and important role in elderly patients recuperating from major surgery.[96] Optimal pain relief and facilitated return to normal daily functioning of elderly patients is difficult to achieve with analgesic monotherapy because of the possible risks of side effects from reliance on a single agent. The inclusion of RA as part of a multimodal treatment paradigm may further enhance overall physiologic and analgesic benefits in elderly and cognitively impaired patients. Improvement in surgical outcome and convalescence has been reported in the following studies: (1) postoperative regional analgesia as part of a perioperative multimodal approach in patients undergoing abdominal-thoracic esophagectomy can result in a shorter time to patient extubation, earlier return of bowel function, superior analgesia, and earlier fulfillment of discharge criteria of an intensive care unit.[97] (2) Patients participating in a perioperative multimodal pain pathway following major surgery benefited from a diminution in metabolic and hormonal stress, as well as a more rapid return to baseline functionality during convalescence,[98] and (3) patients undergoing colon resection incorporating epidural analgesia and receiving a multimodal

approach to surgical rehabilitation showed a decreased length of hospitalization from 6–10 days to a median of 2 days.[99]

For surgery of the extremities, PNB provides highly effective and site-specific postoperative analgesia with few side effects, particularly when supplemental opioid use is reduced or eliminated. Following major joint surgery, single-injection techniques and continuous PNB offer benefits of enhanced mobilization and rehabilitation along with potential cost savings and outcome improvements. In elderly patients, symptoms of excessive sedation, concentration difficulties and negative cognitive influence commonly observed with opioids may be reduced with PNB techniques along with more rapid return to preoperative baseline functions of ambulation, sleeping, eating, and drinking.

CONCLUSIONS

Elderly patients and those presenting with cognitive deficits for major surgery are at an increased risk for developing postoperative cognitive dysfunction and further reductions in baseline cognition. Anesthetic and analgesic techniques that provide optimal pain control with low side-effect profiles and minimizing opioid analgesic and benzodiazepine exposure should always be considered for elderly and cognitively impaired patients. Such therapy, including RA and PNB techniques, along with incorporation of a multimodal analgesic approach may help in reducing the risk and burden of postoperative delirium and cognitive dysfunction. Moreover, improvements in analgesic efficacy may help attenuate pathophysiologic surgical responses, reduce the length of hospitalization, facilitate patient benefit and satisfaction, and accelerate patient rehabilitation and recovery.[100] Although the many beneficial effects of multimodal analgesia, NRA, and PNB techniques are evident and becoming progressively more recognized, additional research is needed to demonstrate clear evidence of improved outcomes and to further justify there expanded use in elderly surgical patients.

REFERENCES

1. Administration of Aging. A Profile of Older Americans. Washington DC: Department of Health and Human Services; 2000.
2. Schwab CW, Kauder DR. Trauma in the geriatric patient. *Arch Surg.* 1992;127:701.
3. Troncale, JA. The aging process: physiologic changes and pharmacologic implications. *Postgrad Med.* 1996;99:111–114, 120–122.
4. Scott AS. Age-related memory decline. *Arch Neurol.* 2001;58:360–364.
5. Turnheim K. When drug therapy get old: pharmacokinetics and pharmacodynamics in the elderly. *Exp Gerontol.* 2003;38:843–853.
6. Morrison JH, Hof P. Life and death of neurons in the aging brain. *Science.* 1997;278:412–419.
7. Collins KJ, et al. Functional changes in the autonomic nervous responses with aging. *Age Ageing.* 2001;9:17–24.
8. Meier-Ruge W, et al. Age related white matter atrophy in the human brain. *Ann NY Acad Sci.* 1992;673:260–269.
9. Seals DR, Esler MD. Human aging and the sympathoadrenal system. *J Physiol.* 2000;528:407–417.
10. Naughton BJ, Moran MB, et al. Delirium and other cognitive impairment in older adults in an emergency department. *Ann Emerg Med.* 1995;25:751.
11. Moller JT, Cluitmans P, et al. Long-term postoperative cognitive dysfunction in the elderly: ISOPCD study 1. *Lancet.* 1998;351:857–861.
12. Monk TG, Weldon BC, Garvan CW, et al. Predictors of cognitive dysfunction after major noncardiac surgery. *Anesthesiology.* 2008;108:8–17.
13. Kam PC, Calcroft RM. Perioperative stroke in general surgery patients. *Anaesthesia.* 1997;52:879–883.
14. Olfosson B, Lundstrom M, et al Delirium is associated with poor rehabilitation outcome in elderly patients treated for femoral neck fractures. *Scand J Caring Sci.* 2005;19:119–127.
15. Murkin JM, Martzke JS, et al. A randomized study of the influence of perfusion technique and pH management strategy in 316 patients undergoing coronary artery bypass surgery: neurologic and cognitive outcomes. *J Thorac Cardiovasc Surg.* 1995;110:349–362.
16. Lawrence VA, Hilsenbeck SG, et al. Incidence and hospital stay for cardiac and pulmonary complications after abdominal surgery. *J Gen Intern Med.* 1995;10:671–678.
17. Cole MG. Delirium in elderly patients. *Am J Geriatr Psychiatry.* 2004;12:7–21.
18. Tucker J. The diagnosis of delirium and DSM-IV. *Dement Geriatr Cogn Disord.* 1999;10:359–367.
19. Lynch EP, Lazor MA, et al. The impact of postoperative pain on the development of postoperative delirium. *Anesth Analg.* 1998;86:781–785.
20. Zakriya K, Sieber FE, et al. Brief postoperative delirium in hip fracture patients affects functional outcome at three months. *Anesth Analg.* 2004;98:1798–1802.
21. Marcantonio ER, Goldman L, et al. A clinical prediction rule for delirium after elective noncardiac surgery. *JAMA.* 1994;274:134–139.
22. Inouye SK, Peduzzi PN, et al. Importance of functional measures in predicting mortality among older hospitalized patients. *JAMA.* 1998;279:1187–1193.
23. Inuoye SK, Schlesinger MJ, et al. Delirium: a symptom of how hospital care is failing older persons and a window to improve quality of hospital care. *Am J Med.* 1999;106:565–573.
24. Schupf N, Tang MX, et al. Decline in cognitive and functional skills increases mortality risk in nondemented elderly. *Neurology.* 2005;65:1218–1226.
25. Newman MF, Kirchner JL, et al. Neurological Outcome Research Group and the Cardiothoracic Anesthesiology Research Endeavors Investigators: Longitudinal assessment of neurocognitive function after coronary-artery bypass surgery. *N Engl J Med.* 2002;344:395–402.
26. Price CC, Garvan CW, et al. Type and severity of cognitive impairment in older adults after noncardiac surgery. *Anesthesiology.* 2008;108:8–17.
27. Fujita S, Volpi E: Amino acids and muscle loss with aging. *J Nutr.* 2006; 136(suppl 1):277S–280S.
28. Wolfson L, Judge J, et al. Strength is a major factor in balance, gait, and the occurrence of falls. *J Gerontol.* 1995;50:S64–S67.
29. Shafer S. The pharmacology of anesthetic drugs in elderly patients. *Anesthesiol Clin North Am.* 2000;18:1–29.
30. Vestal RE, Dawson GW. *Handbook of the Biology of Aging.* 2nd ed. New York, NY: Van Nostrand Reinhold; 1985;744–819.
31. Cova D, Balducci L, et al. Cancer Chemotherapy in the Older Patient. London/New York, NY: Taylor & Francis, 2004;463–488.
32. Adkins BA, Davies J, et al. The anatomic and physiologic aspects of aging. In: Adkins RB, Jr and Scott HW, Jr, eds. *Surgical Care for the Elderly.* Baltimore, MD: Williams & Wilkins; 1988;10–28.
33. Lubran MM. Renal function in the elderly. *Ann Clin Lab Sci.* 1995;25:122–133.
34. Bender AD. The effect of increasing age on the distribution of peripheral blood flow in man. *J Am Geriatr Soc.* 1965;13:192–198.
35. Carreca L, Balducci M, et al. Cancer in the older patient. *Cancer Treat Rev.* 2005;31:380–402.
36. Vuyk J. Pharmacodynamics in the elderly. *Best Pract Res Clin Anaesthesiol.* 2003;17;207–218.
37. Macintyre PE, Jarvis DA. Age is the best predictor of postoperative morphine requirements. *Pain.* 1996;64:357–364.
38. Baillie SP, Bateman DN, et al. Age and the pharmacokinetics of morphine. *Age Ageing.* 1989;18:258–262.
39. Wolff J, Bisler D, Christensen CB, et al. Influence of renal function on the elimination of morphine and morphine glucuronides. *Eur J Clin Pharmacol.* 1988;34:353–357.
40. Sear JW, Hand CW, Moore RA. Studies on morphine disposition: plasma concentrations of morphine and its metabolites in anesthetized middle-aged and elderly surgical patients. *J Clin Anesth.* 1989;1:164–169.
41. Clark RF, Wei EM, et al. Meperidine: therapeutic use and toxicity. *J Emerg Med.* 1995;13:797–802.
42. Eisendrath SJ, Goldman B, et al. Meperidine-induced delirium. *Am J Psychiatry.* 1987;144:1062–1065.
43. Platten H, Schweizer E, et al. Pharmacokinetics and the pharmacodynamic action of midazolam in young and elderly patients. *Clin Pharm Ther.* 1998;63:552–560.
44. Arthur GR. Pharmacokinetics. In: Strichartz GR, ed. *Handbook of Experimental Pharmacology: Local Anesthetics,* Vol. 81. Berlin: Springer-Verlag; 1987:165–186.
45. Tucker MA, Andrew MF, et al. Age-associated change in pain threshold measured by transcutaneous neuronal electrical stimulation. *Age Ageing.* 1989;18:241–246.

46. Washington LL, Gibson SJ, Helme RD. Age-related differences in the endogenous analgesic response to repeated cold water immersion in human volunteers. *Pain.* 2000;89:89–96.

47. Gibson SJ, Helme RD. Age-related differences in pain perception and reporting. *Clin Geriatr Med.* 2001;17:433–456.

48. Cohen-Mansfield J, Lipson S. Pain in cognitively impaired nursing home residents: How well are physicians diagnosing it? *J Am Geriatr Soc.* 2002;50:1039–1044.

49. Katz PR, Grossberg GT, Potter JF, Solomon DH. *Geriatrics Syllabus for Specialists.* New York, NY: American Geriatrics Society; 2002.

50. Egbert A. Postoperative pain management in the frail elderly. *Clin Geriatr Med.* 1996;12:583–599.

51. Wu CL, Fleisher LA. Outcomes research in regional anesthesia and analgesia. *Anesth Analg.* 2000;91:1232–1242.

52. Mackensen GB, Gelb AW. Postoperative cognitive deficits: more questions than answers. *Eur J Anaesthesiol.* 2004;21:85–88.

53. Parker MJ, Handol HH, et al. Anaesthesia for hip fracture surgery in adults. *Cochrane Database Syst Rev.* 2004;4:CD000521.

54. Inouye SK, Viscoli CM, et al. A predictive model for delirium in hospitalized elderly patients based on admission characteristics. *Ann Intern Med.* 1993;119:474–481.

55. Block BM, Liu SS, et al. Efficacy of postoperative epidural analgesia: a meta-analysis. *JAMA.* 2003;290:2455–2463.

56. Hodgson PS, Liu SS. Thoracic epidural anaesthesia and analgesia for abdominal surgery: effects on gastrointestinal function and perfusion. *Clin Anaesthesiol.* 1999;13:9–22.

57. Ballantyne JC, Carr DB, et al. The comparative effects of postoperative analgesic therapies on pulmonary outcomes: cumulative meta-analysis of randomized controlled trials. *Anesth Analg.* 1998;86:598–612.

58. Rodgers A, Walker N, et al. Reductions of postoperative mortality and morbidity with epidural or spinal anesthesia: results from overview of randomized trials. *Br Med J.* 2000;321:1493.

59. Williams-Russo P, Sharrock NE, et al. Cognitive effects after epidural vs general anesthesia in older adults: a randomized trial. *JAMA.* 1995;274:44–50.

60. Riis J, Lomholt B, et al. Immediate and long term mental recovery from general versus epidural anesthesia in elderly patients. *Acta Anaesthesiol Scand.* 1983;27:44–49.

61. Peters A. Structural changes in the normally aging cerebral cortex of primates. *Prog Brain Res.* 2002;136:455–465.

62. Atanassoff PG. Effects of regional anesthesia on perioperative outcome. *J Clin Anesth.* 1996;8:446–455.

63. Roy RC. Choosing general versus regional anesthesia for the elderly. *Anesthesiol Clin North Am.* 2000;18:91–1104.

64. Park WY, Thompson JS, et al. Effect of epidural anesthesia and analgesia on perioperative outcome: a randomized controlled Veterans Affairs cooperative study. *Ann Surg.* 2001;234:560–571.

65. Matot I, Oppenheim-Eden A, et al. Preoperative cardiac events in elderly patients with hip fracture randomized to epidural or conventional analgesia. *Anesthesiology.* 2003;98:156–163.

66. Beattie WS, Badner NH, et al. Epidural analgesia reduces postoperative myocardial infarction: a meta-analysis. *Anesth Analg.* 2001;93:853–858.

67. Beattie WS, Bander NH, et al. Meta-analysis demonstrates statistically significant reduction in postoperative myocardial infarction with the use of thoracic epidural analgesia. *Anesth Analg.* 2003;97:919–920.

68. Wu CL, Hurley RW, et al. Effect of postoperative analgesia on morbidity and mortality following surgery in Medicare patients. *Reg Anesth Pain Med.* 2004;29:525–533.

69. Mangano DT, Hollenberg M, et al. Perioperative myocardial ischemia in patients undergoing non-cardiac surgery-I: incidence and severity during the 4 day perioperative period. *J Am Coll Cardiol.* 1999;17:843–850.

70. Badner NH, Knill RL, et al. Myocardial infarction after noncardiac surgery. *Anesthesiology.* 1998;88:572–578.

71. Trip MD, Volkert MC, et al. Platelet hyperreactivity and prognosis in survivors of myocardial infarction. *N Engl J Med.* 1990;322:1549–1554.

72. Richman JM, Liu SS, et al. Does continuous peripheral nerve block provide superior pain control to opioids? A meta-analysis. *Anesth Analg.* 2006;102:248–257.

73. Don HF, Wahba M, et al. The effects of anesthesia and 100% oxygen on the functional residual capacity of the lungs. *Anesthesiology.* 1970;32:521–529.

74. Craig DB. Postoperative recovery of pulmonary function. *Anesth Analg.* 1981;60:46–52.

75. Gruber EM, Tschernko EM. Anaesthesia and postoperative analgesia in older patients with chronic obstructive pulmonary disease: special considerations. *Drugs Aging.* 2003;20:347–360.

76. Rigg JR, Jamrozik K, et al. MATS: epidural anaesthesia and analgesia and outcome of major surgery: a randomized trial. *Lancet.* 2002;13:1276–1282.

77. Savas JF, Litwack R, et al. Regional anesthesia as an alternative to general anesthesia for abdominal surgery in patients with severe pulmonary impairment. *Am J Surg.* 2004;188:603–605.

78. Moraca RJ, Sheldon DG, Thirby RC. The role of epidural anesthesia analgesia in surgical practice. *Ann Surg.* 2003;238:663–673.

79. Kehlet H, Holte K. Effect of postoperative analgesia on surgical outcome. *Br J Anaesth.* 2001;87:62–72.

80. Hole A, Terjesen T, et al. Epidural versus general anesthesia for total hip arthroplasty in elderly patients. *Acta Anaesthesiol Scand.* 1980;24:279–287.

81. Desborough JP. The stress response to trauma and surgery. *Br J Anaesth.* 2000;85:109–117.

82. Carli F, Halliday D. Continuous epidural blockade arrests the postoperative decrease in muscle protein fractional synthetic rate in surgical patients. *Anesthesiology.* 1997;86:1033–1040.

83. Holte K, Kehlet H. Epidural anesthesia and analgesia-effects on surgical stress responses and implications for postoperative nutrition. *Clin Nutr.* 2002;21:199–206.

84. Liu S, Carpenter RL, Neal JM, et al. Epidural anesthesia and analgesia: their role in postoperative outcome. *Anesthesiology.* 1995;82:1474–1506.

85. Gilbert TB, Hawkes WG, Hebel JR, et al. Spinal anesthesia versus general anesthesia for hip fracture repair: a longitudinal observation of 741 elderly patients during 2-year follow-up. *Am J Orthop.* 2000;29:25–35.

86. Leung JM, Dzankic S. Relative importance of preoperative health status versus intraoperative factors in predicting postoperative adverse outcomes in geriatric surgical patients. *J Am Ger Soc.* 2001;49:1080.

87. Coley KC, Williams BA, DaPos SV, et al. Retrospective evaluation of unanticipated admissions and readmissions after same day surgery and associated costs. *J Clin Anesth.* 2002;14:349–353.

88. Apfelbaum JL, Cehn C, et al. Postoperative pain experience: results from a national survey suggest postoperative pain continues to be undermanaged. *Anesth Analg.* 2003;97:534–540.

89. Kahn L, Baxter FJ, et al. A comparison of thoracic and lumbar epidural techniquesfor post-thoracoabdominal esophagectomy analgesia. *Can J Anaesth.* 1999;46:415–422.

90. Kock M, Blomberg S, et al. Thoracic epidural anesthesia improves global and regional left ventricular function during stress-induced myocardial ischemia in patients with coronary artery disease. *Anesth Analg.* 1990;71:625–630.

91. Neudecker J, Schwenk W, et al. Randomized controlled trial to examine the influence of thoracic epidural analgesia on postoperative ileus after laparoscopic sigmoid resection. *Br J Surg.* 1999;86:1292–1295.

92. Kehlet H. Modification of responses to surgery by neural blockade: clinical implication. In: Cousins MJ, Bridenbaugh PO, eds. *Neural Blockade in Clinical Anesthesia and Management of Pain.* 3rd ed. Philadelphia, PA: Lippincott-Raven; 1998;129–175.

93. Liu SS, Carpenter RL, et al. Effects of perioperative analgesic technique on the rate of recovery after colon surgery. *Anesthesiology.* 1995;83:757–765.

94. Bugedo GJ, Carcamo CR, et al. Preoperative percutaneous ilioinguinal and iliohypogastric nerve block with 0.5% bupivacaine for post-herniorrhaphy pain management in adults. *Reg Anesth.* 1990;15:130–133.

95. Evans H, Steele SM, et al. Peripheral nerve block and continuous catheter techniques. *Anesthesiol Clin North Am.* 2005;23:141–162.

96. Kehlet H. Multimodal approach to control postoperative pathophysiology and rehabilitation. *Br J Anaesth.* 1997;78:606–617.

97. Brodner G, Pogatzki E, et al. A multimodal approach to control postoperative pathophysiology and rehabilitation in patients undergoing abdominalthoracic esophagectomy. *Anesth Analg.* 1998;86:228–234.

98. Brodner G, Van Aken H, et al. Multimodal perioperative management-combining thoracic epidural analgesia, forced mobilization, and oral nutrition-reduces hormonal and metabolic stress and improve convalescence after major urologic surgery. *Anesth Analg.* 2001;92:1954–1600.

99. Basse L, Jacobsen D, et al. A clinical pathway to accelerate recovery after colonic resection. *Ann Surg.* 2000;232:51–57.

100. Kehlet H, Wilmore DW. Multimodal strategies to improve surgical outcome. *Am J Surg.* 2002;183:630–641.

101. Peters A. Structural changes in the normally aging cerebral cortex of primates. *Prog Brain Res.* 2002;136:455–465.

102. American Psychiatric Association. *Diagnostic and Statistical Manual of Mental Disorders.* 4th ed. Text revision. Washington DC: American Psychiatric Association; 2000.

103. Kehlet H. Influence of regional anesthesia on postoperative morbidity. *Ann Chir Gynaecol.* 1984;73:171–176.

104. Norris EJ, Beattie C, et al. Double-masked randomized trial comparing alternate combinations of intraoperative anesthesia and postoperative analgesia in abdominal aortic surgery. *Anesthesiology.* 2001;95:1054–1067.

105. Lien CA. Regional versus general anesthesia for hip surgery in older patients: does the choice effect outcome? *J Am Geriatr Soc.* 2002;50:191–194.

106. Peyton PJ, Myles PS, et al. Perioperative epidural analgesia and outcome after major abdominal surgery in high-risk patients. *Anesth Analg.* 2003;96:548–554.

107. Wu CL, Anderson GA, et al. Effect of postoperative analgesia on morbidity and mortality after total hip replacement surgery in Medicare patients. *Reg Anesth Pain Med.* 2003;28:271–278.

108. Liu SS, Block BM, et al. Effects of perioperative central neuraxial analgesia on outcome after coronary artey bypass surgery: a meta-analysis. *Anesthesiology.* 2004;101:153–161.

109. Handley GH, Silbert BS, et al. Combined general and epidural anesthesia versus general anesthesia for major abdominal surgery: postanesthesia recovery characteristics. *Reg Anesth.* 1997;22:435–441.

110. Gottschalk A, Smith DS, et al. Preemptive epidural analgesia and recovery from radical prostatectomy: a randomized controlled trial. *JAMA.* 1998;279:1076–1082.

111. Gilbert TB, Hawkes WG, et al. Spinal anesthesia versus general anesthesia for hip fracture repair: a longitudinal observation of 741 elderly patients during 2-year follow-up. *Am J Orthop.* 2000;29:25–35.

112. Sharrock NE, Cazan MG, et al. Changes in mortality after total hip and knee arthroplasty over a ten-year period. *Anesth Analg.* 1995;80:242–248.

113. Kinnard P, Truchon R, et al. Interscalene block for pain relief after shoulder surgery: a retrospective randomized study. *Clin Orthop.* 1994;304:22–24.

114. Desroches J. The infraclavicular brachial plexus block by the coracoid approach is clinically effective: an observational study of 150 patients. *Can J Anaesth.* 2003;50:253–257.

115. Parkinson SK, Mueller JB, et al. Extent of blockade with various approaches to the lumbar plexus. *Anesth Analg.* 1989;68:243–248.

116. Hirst GC, Lang SA, et al. Femoral nerve block: single injection versus continous infusion for total knee arthroplasty. *Reg Anesth.* 1996;21:292–297.

117. Taboada M, Alverez J, et al. The effects of three different approaches on the onset time of sciatic nerve blocks with 0.75% ropivacaine. *Anesth Analg.* 2004;98:242–247.

118. Provenzano DA, Viscusi ER, et al. Safety an efficacy of the popliteal fossa nerve block when utilized for foot and ankle surgery. *Foot Ankle Int.* 2002;23:394–399.

119. Richardson J, Sabanathan S, et al. A prospective, randomized comparison of preoperative and continuous balanced epidural or paravertebral bupivacaine on post-thoracotomy apin, pulmonary function and stress responses. *Br J Anaesth.* 1999;83:387–392.

32

Postcesarean Analgesia

Kate Miller and Ferne Braveman

A commitment to postoperative analgesia has been mandated in the present health care environment. Pain assessment as the fifth vital sign provides the opportunity for us to identify and treat a symptom that has for years been undermanaged.

Intrapartum analgesia has always been an important part of the practice of obstetrical anesthesiology. The cesarean delivery, at 38% of all deliveries, is now the most common surgical procedure in the United States, and thus we must address postpartum/postoperative analgesia as part of our obstetrical anesthesia practice. The goal of intrapartum analgesia has always been to provide safe and efficacious analgesia with minimal effects on the mother, fetus, or course of labor. Postcesarean analgesia must also be safe and efficacious, with minimal effect on the mother's ability to bond with her newborn. The physiologic perturbations associated with pregnancy and the surgical stress and physiologic changes that occur with intra-abdominal surgery affect maternal well-being and postoperative outcome. Pain therapy must take into account all of these variables. Nikolajsen et al[1] has suggested that patients with recall of severe postoperative pain are more likely to experience chronic pain following cesarean delivery. More effective analgesia would thus minimize the occurrence of chronic pain complaints. Women recovering from cesarean section desire to ambulate early and care for their infants. However, because of their wish to bond with their babies, many mothers avoid analgesics that may cause sedation and as a result have a level of pain that impairs mobility. Nursing mothers are concerned about the neonatal effects of medications, especially opioid analgesics that may cross into breast milk. Although not all postcesarean section mothers share such attitudes or anxieties, attention must be given to these issues to facilitate a positive experience for the mother. The goal is to provide effective pain relief that is safe for the mother as well as her baby. It should allow the mother to ambulate, care for her baby, and breastfeed without causing adverse consequences.[2]

Because most cesarean sections in the United States are performed under regional anesthesia, the use of epidural and intrathecal opioids has become a popular means of providing postoperative analgesia. Currently at Yale-New Haven Hospital and in many other teaching institutions, more than 95% of cesarean deliveries are performed with regional anesthesia. A recent survey of type of anesthesia used for cesarean section in the United Kingdom from 1992 to 2002 showed that regional anesthesia was used in 94.9% of elective and in 86.7% of emergent cesarean sections.[2] If present, an indwelling epidural catheter facilitates the administration of epidural opioids for augmentation of anesthesia during cesarean section and for effective control of postsurgical pain.

A survey of anesthesiologists at the 1987 meeting of the Society of Obstetric Anesthesia and Perinatology (SOAP) revealed that greater than 77% utilized epidural opioids, predominantly morphine, fentanyl, or both, for pain relief after cesarean section.[3] Twenty years later, almost all patients receiving regional anesthesia for cesarean delivery receive neuraxial opioids for intraoperative and postoperative analgesia. Spinally administered opioids bind and activate opioid receptors located in the substantial gelatinosa of spinal cord dorsal horn.[4,5] After epidural administration, a small portion of the opioid dose crosses the dura to enter the cerebrospinal fluid (CSF) and then penetrates spinal tissues in amounts proportional to its lipid solubility. The remainder of the dose is absorbed systemically, producing plasma levels comparable to an intramuscular injection and adding to the analgesic effect as the drug is distributed to the central nervous system.

There is no difference in the rate of cesarean section in women receiving neuraxial versus intravenous analgesia during labor.[6] The misconception still exists, however, that neuraxial analgesia increases the risk for cesarean section. The American College of Obstetricians and Gynecologists currently recognizes that there are many techniques for pain relief of parturients, including neuraxial analgesia, and none of them are associated with an increased risk of cesarean delivery when compared to one another or unmedicated labor.[7] The current trend in postcesarean analgesia is to use a multimodal approach. As noted above, most cesarean sections are performed with regional anesthesia and most patients received neuraxial opioids as part of that anesthetic. The addition of other medications with different mechanisms and/or sites of action will create additive or supraadditive effects with a lower incidence of dose-related side effects as the dosage of each drug is lower than if a single drug were used.

The vast majority of patients receive opioid therapy for post-cesarean analgesia – neuraxial and/or parenteral and/or oral. Obviously, those patients who have general anesthesia will not have neuraxial opioids but rather parenteral and/or oral opioid therapy. Nonsteroidal anti-inflammatory drugs (NSAIDs) are often coadministered. Clonidine, metaclopramide, and ondansetron are also used as analgesic adjuvants.

EPIDURAL ANALGESICS

Morphine

Morphine was the first opioid to receive Food and Drug Administration (FDA) approval for epidural and/or intrathecal administration. Morphine is highly ionized and is the least lipid-soluble opioid currently employed in this setting. These qualities create a unique pharmacodynamic profile. Most notably, morphine has a slow onset, often taking 60 to 90 minutes to appreciate peak analgesic effect, and a prolonged duration of action.

Epidurally administered morphine may be an excellent choice for the high-risk obstetric patient. Patients with severe preeclampsia, cardiac disease, and morbid obesity may benefit from the reduced stress and improved pulmonary function that excellent levels of postsurgical analgesia can provide. Rawal and coworkers[8] compared the effects of intramuscular and epidural morphine in 50 "grossly obese" patients recovering from gastric stapling procedures. Patients in the epidural morphine group were more alert, able to walk unassisted sooner, recovered bowel function earlier, and "benefited more from vigorous physiotherapy routine, which resulted in fewer pulmonary complications." No similar study has been performed in morbidly obese obstetric patients, but the use of epidural morphine in this group should provide significant benefits as well.

Fuller and colleagues[9] retrospectively reviewed the records of nearly 5000 patients who received epidural morphine at the conclusion of cesarean section. The average time to first request for additional analgesia was 23.5 hours, but patients differed greatly. The shortest time to supplemental analgesia was 30 minutes, but 8% of patients did not require additional analgesics for over 48 hours. Leicht and colleagues[10] did a comparison of postcesarean section pain relief, side effects, and 24-hour narcotic requirements in two groups of patients receiving epidural morphine. One group was administered morphine as a single 5 mg bolus dose versus a regimen of reduced bolus (2.5 mg) plus continuous infusion (0.5 mg/hour). Patients receiving single 5 mg doses of morphine had a higher incidence of severe nausea and vomiting (17%). Only 50% of patients experienced excellent pain relief, two patients were extremely dissatisfied, and 100% requested supplemental postoperative analgesia. In comparison, the group receiving the 2.5 mg bolus plus continuous infusion noted superior pain relief, a lower requirement for additional analgesics, and no complaints of severe nausea or vomiting. In a randomized dose-response study by Palmer and colleagues,[11] patients received epidural morphine following cesarean section in increments of 1.25, 2.5, 3.75, and 5 mg and were then given intravenous patient-controlled analgesia (IV PCA) for pain relief. As measured by IV PCA use, the quality of analgesia was dose dependent in patients who received up to 3.75 mg of epidural morphine, and there was no difference in the analgesic effect above that dose. The duration of analgesia was 18–26 hours. Although all patients experienced pruritus, this was not related to the dose of morphine received.

Depodur is a sustained-release epidural morphine release preparation. It has shown promise for postoperative analgesia but requires that no other medication be administered through the epidural catheter to protect the integrity of the sustained release preparation. Its role in obstetrics will thus be limited to those receiving CSE, in whom the epidural catheter does not need to be used for anesthesia.[12–14]

The choice of local anesthetic utilized for epidural anesthesia may affect the action of epidural morphine. Kotelko and coworkers[15] studied 276 parturients treated with various local anesthetics plus 5 mg of epidural morphine during cesarean delivery. Of the patients who received 2-chloroprocaine as the primary local anesthetic, "an unexpectedly high proportion (13 of 23) had poor postoperative pain relief, usually lasting less than three hours." The authors speculated that the low pH of the 2-chloroprocaine solution may have been the cause. However, the efficacy of epidural morphine is similar when either unbuffered 2-chloroprocaine (pH < 4.0) or bicarbonate-buffered 2-chloroprocaine (pH approximately 6.17) was used for cesarean section. Hess and colleagues found no effect from chloroprocaine on morphine analgesia.[16] Meagher and coworkers[17] compared the efficacy of 5 mg of epidural morphine for cesarean section when 2% lidocaine with epinephrine (1:200 000) or 0.5% bupivacaine was used. The analgesia obtained by the lidocaine and bupivacaine groups did not differ, and the median time to narcotic supplement was 25 hours.

EPIDURAL ANALGESIA

Lipophilic Opioids

Fentanyl is much more lipid soluble and less ionized than morphine and rapidly penetrates the dura and spinal tissues to find and activate opioid receptors.[4,5] The standard commercial preparation contains no preservative and is suitable for intravenous or epidural use. Epidurally administered fentanyl is frequently employed for intraoperative augmentation of epidural anesthesia and to provide effective but limited duration for postcesarean analgesia. Naulty and coworkers[18] originally reported that fentanyl 50 to 100 μg produced 4 to 5 hours of postoperative analgesia in parturients receiving epidural anesthesia with 0.75% bupivacaine and significantly reduced 24-hour parenteral analgesic requirements. Follow-up studies have been unable to duplicate these results, however, and report postcesarean analgesia lasting up to a maximum of 1 to 2 hours.[19]

Several techniques have been employed to extend fentanyl's relatively short duration of action. The degree to which epidurally administered fentanyl is diluted affects both its onset and duration of action. Both Naulty and coworkers[18] and Robertson and coworkers[20] used total fentanyl volumes of 10 mL. Birnbach and colleagues[21] evaluated the analgesic efficacy of a standardized fentanyl dose (50 μg) that was diluted in 1 to 25 mL of saline solution; total volumes less than 10 mL were associated with a significantly longer onset time. Furthermore, patients who received a 1 to 2 mL total volume frequently failed to develop complete analgesia. Volumes of 20 mL or greater were associated with the longest durations of analgesia, 200 minutes or more. The addition of epinephrine[21] appears to increase the duration of epidural fentanyl analgesia.

Youngstrom and coworkers[22] proposed continuous epidural infusion of fentanyl and epinephrine for postcesarean analgesia. By using a dilute concentration of fentanyl and epinephrine, both opiate and adrenergic-mediated spinal analgesia was effected. Postoperatively, an infusion of 4 μg of fentanyl with 1.6 μg of epinephrine per milliliter, was administered in doses of 10, 15, or 20 mL/h. Patients receiving 15mL/h continuous infusion obtained excellent pain relief and required minimal use of PCA for supplementation of analgesia. The high-dose requirements, that is, 60 to 80 μg/h, and 1500 to 2000 μg/d, underscore the relative inefficiency of fentanyl and other lipophilic opioids when continuously administered via lumbar epidural catheters. Such doses given parenterally provide similar intensities of postsurgical analgesia.[23] One final attempt to extend analgesic duration has been to combine fentanyl with small doses of morphine. Naulty and Ross[24] administered either 5 mg of epidural morphine or 50 μg of epidural fentanyl with 0, 1, 2, or 3 mg of epidural morphine to patients undergoing cesarean section delivery. They noted that the onset of analgesia was significantly more rapid in all patients who received fentanyl. Moreover, patients receiving 3 mg of morphine with fentanyl noted potentiation of analgesia in that duration, and the 24-hour supplemental narcotic dosage was similar to that observed in patients treated with higher doses (5 mg) of morphine alone. These researchers found no respiratory depression in any of the 104 patients evaluated.

Sufentanil is another highly lipid-soluble opioid agonist that provides an extremely rapid onset, usually within 15 minutes of epidural administration. However, dose requirements are much higher than one might expect, given the drug's high potency when compared with fentanyl or morphine. In cesarean section patients, doses of 25 μg of sufentanil produced less than 2 hours of complete analgesia, whereas 50 μg provided only 3 to 4 hours of complete analgesia.[31]

Rosen and coworkers[30] compared the effects of 5 mg of epidural morphine and epidural sufentanil (30, 45, or 60 μg). Sufentanil analgesia lasted only 3.9, 4.5, and 5.6 hours, respectively. In contrast, most patients receiving morphine experienced 26 hours of pain relief. Although generalized pruritus and nausea with vomiting were more common in patients who received morphine, respiratory rates did not differ among any of the treatment groups. Rosen et al concluded that sufentanil "may be superior to morphine for epidural analgesia in clinical settings in which rapid onset is desired." However, the authors cautioned that "if the relatively large doses of sufentanil evaluated in this study are accidentally injected intravenously, there is a high likelihood of adverse effects, particularly respiratory depression." A more rational method of extending the duration of epidural sufentanil analgesia may be accomplished by the addition of small amounts of morphine.[31]

Other opioids that are less commonly employed epidurally include hydromorphone,[32] meperidine,[33] butorphanol, buprenorphine, and methadone.[34,35] Hydromorphone is a hydroxylated derivative of morphine available in preservative-free solution that provides effective epidural analgesia in patients recovering from cesarean section. Chestnut and colleagues evaluated the use of 1.0 mg of hydromorphone in a total 10mL volume given during wound closure in patients who had received epidural anesthesia with either 2% lidocaine with epinephrine 1:200,000 or 0.5% bupivacaine.[32] The mean time to first request for supplemental analgesia was 13.0 ± 12.4 hours, and 92% of patients reported good or excellent pain relief. In another study of patients receiving the same hydromorphone dose, analgesia lasted a median of 19.3 hours. Pruritus was the most common side effect, reported in approximately 50% of patients. Nausea

was also reported frequently. No patient in either group had clinical signs of respiratory depression.

Epidural meperidine provides about 2.5 hours of postoperative pain relief at doses up to 25 mg. Ngan and colleagues found that duration of analgesia is not extended with larger doses.[33] The onset of methadone is faster compared to morphine, but the duration of analgesia is only 4 to 5 hours after a dose of 4 to 5 mg.[34] Diamorphine, or heroin, provides an inconsistent duration of epidural analgesia and is not available in the United States.[35,36]

Epidurally administered mixed agonist-antagonist opioids, including butorphanol, provide intermediate durations of analgesia but are associated with significant sedation secondary to vascular uptake and activation of κ-receptors in the central nervous system. Excessive maternal sedation detracts from the overall mission of epidural analgesia in this clinical setting and often leads to patient dissatisfaction. Nalbuphine, also a mixed agonist-antagonist, has also been found to cause significant sedation.[25] See Tables 32.1 and 32.2 for epidural medications.

Epidural Adjuvant Therapy

The addition of local anesthetics such as bupivicaine and ropivicaine in combination with neuraxial opioids produces an additive and possibly a synergistic effect, allowing for a decreased dose requirement of both classes of drugs, and therefore a decreased potential for side effects associated with each drug.[2]

The addition of clonidine, an α_2-adrenergic agonist, to epidural morphine has been shown to prolong the duration of analgesia after cesarean section as compared with morphine alone. This is attributed to the activation of α-adrenergic receptors in the descending inhibitory pathways of the spinal cord. Capogna and colleagues[37] found that 2 mg of epidural morphine provided analgesia for 6.27 ± 1.6 hours, but adding 75 μg and 150 μg of clonidine increased the time of analgesia to 13.25 ± 3.8 hours and 21.55 ± 6.3 hours, respectively. However, its use is not currently recommended for postcesarean analgesia because of the increased risk for excessive sedation and hypotension.[25]

Epinephrine, an α- and β-adrenergic agonist, also prolongs the duration of analgesia, decreases systemic uptake, and decreases the incidence of side effects attributed to opioids. The mechanism for analgesia is likely its α_2 agonist property. When given with lidocaine, it prolongs and enhances the quality of analgesia.[38]

Side Effects

Administering epidural morphine for postcesarean section analgesia is easy and effective, and perhaps it would be universally popular were it not for troublesome side effects. The most common of these is pruritus. Pruritus occurs more often in obstetric patients than in any other group, ranging from 40% to 90%.[9,15,17] Mild pruritus, usually of the face or chest, is probably even more frequent because patients may not mention it unless directly questioned. Why pruritus occurs is poorly understood, but its occurrence does not appear to be related to excessive histamine release, nor is it thought to be dose related for clinically appropriate doses.[11] Nonetheless, antihistamines may provide some relief, and 12.5 to 25 mg of diphenhydramine is a recommended treatment. Nalbuphine (5 mg IV) will relieve pruritus without reversing analgesia or causing other side effects and is

Table 32.1: Neuraxial Opioid Administration

Opioid	Spinal Bolus (with Intraoperative LA)	Epidural Bolus	PCEA/CI
Morphine	01–0.2 mg (duration: 18–24 hours)	2–5 mg (duration: 18–24 hours)	Loading: 1–3 mg CI: 50 μg/mL @ 6–12 mL/h PCEA: 2–4 mL every 10–15 minutes, 50–60 mL 4-hour lockout
Depodur	Not recommended	10 mg (duration: 24–48 hours)	Not recommended
Meperidine	10 mg (duration: 4 hours)	50 mg (duration: 4 hours)	Not recommended
Hydromorphone	Not recommended	200–300 μg (duration: 8–12 hours)	Loading: 200–300 μg CI: 3–5 μg/mL @ 6–12 mL/h PCEA: 2–4 mL every 4–6 minutes, 50–60 mL, 4-hour lockout
Diamorphine	0.25–1 mg (duration: 6–8 hours)	2–5 mg (duration: 8–12 hours)	Not recommended
Sufentanil	15 μg (duration: 2 hours)	25 μg (duration: 2–3 hours)	Loading: 25 μg CI: 2 μg/mL @ 5–10 mL/h PCEA: 2–4 mL every 4–6 minutes, 40–50 mL, 4-hour lockout
Fentanyl	10 μg (duration: 2 hours)	50 μg (duration: 2–3 hours)	Loading: 50–100 μg CI: (5 μg/mL) @ 10–15 mL/h 40–50 mL, 4-hour lockout
Butorphanol	Not recommended	2–4 mg (duration: 4–6 hours)	Not recommended

Abbreviations: PCEA = patient-controlled epidural analgesia; CI = continuous infusion.

Modified from: Braveman. The Requisites in Anesthesiology: *Postcesarean Analgesia*. 2006.

an excellent first-line choice.[25] A small intravenous bolus, 0.04 to 0.08 mg, of naloxone usually will also improve patient comfort without reversing analgesia. Occasionally, the intensity of itching interferes with sleep. In our experience, severe pruritus is the most frequent cause of patient dissatisfaction with epidurally administered morphine.

Nausea, another common side effect associated with epidural morphine, is attributed to rostral spread of the drug in spinal fluid to higher brainstem nuclei, including the vomiting center and chemoreceptor trigger zone. Nausea and vomiting occurs in 20% to 60% (or 11% to 30% according to others) of postcesarean patients, although the percentage of patients whose symptoms are severe enough to require treatment is lower. In the presence of intractable nausea, a small intravenous bolus of naloxone followed by continuous infusion may be useful. One may conveniently manage a continuous infusion by adding 1 or 2 ampules of naloxone, 0.4 to 0.8 mg, to each liter of the patient's maintenance intravenous fluid. An infusion rate of 125 mL/hour will deliver 50 to 100 μg/hour of naloxone and will usually attenuate the symptoms without significant loss of analgesia. The use of a transdermal scopolamine patch has also been reported to reduce the incidence of nausea and vomiting, particularly during the first 10 hours after cesarean delivery. However, it must be applied a few hours prior to the exposure of epidural morphine to have its desired effect.[27] Ondansetron (4 mg IV) and droperidol (0.625 mg IV) are other effective treatment options.[25] Table 32.3 summarizes treatment for opioid-related side effects.

Reactivation of herpes simplex virus labialis (HSVL) is a more unusual and worrisome side effect of epidural morphine. In a prospective study of 729 patients recovering from cesarean

section, Crone and coworkers[26] reported recurrent oral herpes lesions in 13 of 140 (9.3%) patients treated with epidural morphine but in only 6 of 583 (1.0%) of those who did not receive morphine. The authors proposed that the mechanism responsible for facial pruritus might be involved in reactivating the HSVL, perhaps because of opioid activity within the spinal nucleus of the trigeminal nerve. These researchers found no incidence of primary neonatal HSV infection and did not determine the frequency of maternal asymptomatic oral viral shedding. Similar results were also found by Gieraerts et al[28] in 1987. Of 44 postcesarean patients, 9 of 26 patients who received epidural morphine developed recurrent herpes simplex labialis lesions, as opposed to none of the patients who received intramuscular morphine.[29] Davies and colleagues found an association between the use of parenteral and spinal morphine and reactivation of oral herpes. Spinal morphine was associated with a greater incidence of reactivation. The current opinion on reactivation of herpes is not yet conclusive.

Although rare in comparison with other side effects, respiratory depression is the most feared complication associated with epidural morphine. Fortunately, only 0.2% to 0.3% of obstetric patients have been found to exhibit clinically significant respiratory depression after receiving 5 mg or less of epidural morphine.[25] An early period of respiratory depression occurs 30 to 90 minutes after epidural administration, in association with peak serum morphine concentrations. However, "delayed-onset" respiratory depression resulting from rostral spread of morphine in CSF occurs 6 to 10 hours later. On reaching the fourth ventricle, the drug rapidly equilibrates with intracranial CSF and acts on the medullary respiratory centers to reduce the

Table 32.2: Intrathecal and Epidural Opioids Employed for Postcesarean Delivery Analgesia

	Drug	Dose	Onset (Minutes)	Peak Effect (Minutes)	Duration (Hours)	Advantages	Disadvantages
Epidural analgesia	Morphine	24–5 mg	45–60	90–120	16–24	Long duration	Delayed onset: significant side effects; delayed respiratory depression
	Fentanyl	50–100 μg	10	20	2–3	Rapid onset; few side effects; may be combined with PCA	High dose requirement; short duration
	Sufentanil	25–50 μg	10	15–20	2–4	Rapid onset; may be combined with PCA	High dose requirement; short duration
	Hydromorphone	0.2–0.3 mg	30	45–60	10–18	Long duration; more rapid onset than morphine	Similar side-effect profile to morphine
	Butorphanol	2–4 mg	15	40	2–4	Fairly rapid onset	Excessive sedation
	Meperidine	50 mg	15	30	5–6	Rapid onset; intermediate duration; few side effects; reduces "shaking"	None
	Morphine/ fentanyl	3 mg/50 μg	10	15	12–18	Rapid onset; long duration	Pruritus
	Morphine/ sufentanil	3 mg/20 μg	10	15	12–18	Rapid onset; long duration	Pruritus
	Continuous fentanyl	100 μg bolus 50–60 μg/h	10	20	Indefinite	Rapid onset; long duration; reduced side effects	Labor intensive; requires infusion device; must maintain epidural catheter Cumulative toxicity? High-dose requirement
	Continuous sufentanil	25 μg bolus	10	15	Indefinite	Rapid onset; long duration; reduced side effects	Labor intensive; requires infusion device; must maintain epidural catheter Cumulative toxicity? High-dose requirement
Intrathecal analgesia	Morphine	0.1–0.2 mg	30	60	18–24	Long duration	Significant side effects; delayed respiratory depression
	Fentanyl	10–12.5 μg	5	10	2–3	Rapid onset; few side effects	Short duration
	Sufentanil	5–15 μg	5	10	2–4	Rapid onset; few side effects	Short duration
	Meperidine	10 mg	10	15	5–6	Rapid onset; potentiation of spinal anesthesia	Smooth transition from spinal anesthesia to IV opioid analgesia; may increase intraop nausea and vomiting

ventilatory response to carbon dioxide. This effect may persist for up to 24 hours. The risk is increased at doses of epidural morphine greater than 5 mg, with the concomitant administration of other narcotics, and in the obese population. The treatment of respiratory depression is 0.2 to 0.4 mg of naloxone IV with ventilatory support if necessary. A naloxone bolus followed by continuous infusion appears to reverse the most severe aspects of both early- and late-onset respiratory depression.

Most patients presenting for cesarean section do not have severe underlying pulmonary disease or other risk factors that increase the likelihood of respiratory depression after epidural morphine administration. However, life-threatening respiratory depression has been reported in this "low-risk" population. Fuller's survey revealed a respiratory rate of less than 10 breaths per minute in 2.5 of 1000 patients.[9]

What is the most appropriate method of respiratory monitoring if epidural morphine is to be used routinely in the patient after cesarean section? This question is difficult, and no one solution appears applicable to every institution. In most published studies, hourly monitoring of respiratory rate has been

Table 32.3: Treatment of Side Effects of Neuraxial Opioids

Side Effect	Incidence	Therapy	Dose	Route
Pruritis	40%–60%	Naloxone	0.04–0.08 mg	IV
		Naloxone	400 μg/L in maintainance IVF	IV
		Nalbuphine	5 mg	IV
		Propofol	10 mg	IV
		Diphenhydramine	12.5 to 25 mg	IV
Nausea/vomiting	25%–30%	Cyclizine	50 mg	IV
		Metoclopramide	10 mg	IV
		Ondansetron	4 mg	IV
		Acupressure	at P6 point	
		Dexamethasone	5 to 10 mg	IV
		Promethazine		
		Hydroxyzine		
		Droperidol	0.625 mg	IV
Respiratory depression		Naloxone	0.2–0.4 mg	IV
		Ventilatory support		

IVF = intravenous fluid.

the most commonly used method. However, respiratory depression caused by epidural morphine may develop rapidly once the drug reaches the intracranial CSF, and either hypercapnia or hypoxemia can develop with a respiratory rate of 10 or more. Furthermore, ensuring hourly checks on a busy ward may be difficult, especially during the night shift when many hospitals are short staffed. Apnea monitors may be prone to annoying false alarms, do not detect hypoventilation, and require cooperation from patients and nurses to turn them off during wakefulness or ambulation. Pulse oximetry has the drawback of frequent motion artifact alarms and cannot detect hypercapnia. Vigilant nursing attention to observe inadequate respiratory effort, slow respiratory rate, or unusual somnolence is probably the best form of monitoring, but the hospital that can guarantee such care 24 hours a day outside of the intensive care setting is rare. See Table 32.3 regarding summary of therapeutic interventions for side effects of neuraxial opioids.

No matter which dose regimen is used, managing patients who have received morphine epidurally on a routine postpartum ward presents certain problems. As we have seen, significant percentages of patients require additional analgesia within 12 hours. Should standard doses of opioids be ordered if analgesia is needed within 12 hours of epidural morphine administration or should doses be reduced to avoid any additive risk of respiratory depression from residual epidural activity? No study has addressed this question or whether the onset of pain in an individual patient after cesarean section means that the respiratory depressant effect of the initial epidural dose has completely ceased. Ketorolac tromethamine may be the analgesic of choice in this setting because it augments epidural analgesia without increasing the risk of additive opioid-induced respiratory depression; otherwise, reduced doses of opioids should be available. After 12 hours, "standard" opioid dosing may be safely employed to augment epidural morphine analgesia. The side effects of nausea and pruritus may be severe enough to warrant low-dose naloxone infusions in some patients, but on

many routine care wards, the nursing staff may not wish to assume responsibility for administering such infusions. At the very least, a member of the anesthesia care team must be available at all times to respond if an urgent problem develops in a patient who has received epidural morphine.

Side effects noted with epidural fentanyl include pruritus of the face, chest, or both, seen in up to one-third of patients, as well as occasional nausea.[33,42] Both pruritus and nausea tend to be much milder than that occurring with epidural morphine, are generally self-limited and rarely require treatment. No large published series has addressed the question of whether epidurally administered fentanyl increases the rate of HSVL reactivation in patients after cesarean section. There has also been no evidence indicating that epidural fentanyl may cause "late" respiratory depression beyond the period of its clinical analgesic effect. Although many previously described studies focused on postoperative analgesia, all noted significant intraoperative benefits after epidural administration of fentanyl. In particular, there is a noticeable reduction in visceral discomfort during abdominal manipulation and peritoneal closure. In this regard, Ackerman and coworkers,[29] observed a significant reduction in nausea and vomiting associated with extra-peritoneal uterine closure in patients receiving 50 μg of epidural fentanyl epidurally.

Patients routinely stay in the postanesthesia recovery area for 1 to 2 hours after cesarean section for observation of bleeding and return of function after regional anesthesia. Thus staff members observe them closely for a minimum of 60 minutes after epidural administration of fentanyl. The literature indicates that 1.5 hours should be ample time for any untoward effect to manifest. Most patients do not need additional pain relief until 2 to 3 hours after the end of surgery. Opioid therapy on the postpartum ward may then be provided by intravenous PCA or oral medication combined with other adjuvants (see Multimodal Therapy). A final epidural analgesic that may be considered for patients following cesarean delivery is extended duration morphine (DepoDur). A single epidural dose of DepoDur (10 mg or less) may provide up to 48 hrs of pain relief. The safety and effectiveness of this preparation are discussed in Chapter 20 (Novel analgesics and drug delivery systems).

Intrathecal Analgesia

A large percentage of patients in the United States undergo cesarean section under spinal anesthesia. Thus, intrathecally administered morphine offers an attractive option for long-lasting postoperative analgesia. The clinical use of intrathecal morphine is similar to that of epidural morphine, except that dose requirements are much smaller (0.1 to 0.5 mg). Onset of analgesia, though faster than that observed with epidural dosing, still requires up to 45 to 60 minutes to achieve peak effect, whereas the duration of postoperative pain relief averages 16 to 24 hours.[2,4,39] Early-onset respiratory depression resulting from vascular uptake and delivery to the central nervous system is not seen with intrathecal morphine because of the small dose administered. However, late-onset respiratory depression similar to that observed with epidural dosing may develop 6 to 10 hours after administration, as drug migrates rostrally in the cerebrospinal fluid. Ventilatory response to CO_2 and respiratory rate may require 8 to 12 hours to return to normal.

Chadwick and Ready[40] reviewed their experience with intrathecal and epidural morphine in cesarean section patients. A significantly greater proportion of patients (78%) receiving spinal anesthesia and intrathecal morphine (0.3 to 0.5 mg) experienced 20 or more hours of postoperative analgesia, compared with only 64% of patients who received epidural anesthesia and 3 to 5 mg of epidural morphine. The side effects of pruritus and nausea were similar in the spinal and epidural groups. A respiratory rate less than 11 breaths per minute was present in two patients in each group but did not require intervention.

Other authors have used even smaller doses of intrathecally administered morphine with success. In a double-blinded study, Abouleish and coworkers[41] administered 0.2 mg of morphine or an equal volume of saline solution to 34 patients with their dose of hyperbaric spinal bupivacaine for cesarean section. Patients who received intrathecal morphine required intraoperative opioid supplements less often and in smaller amounts, and their time to first request for additional analgesia after the operation averaged almost 27 hours, compared with only 3 hours for the saline solution group. Pulse oximetry of all patients for 24 hours after the operation showed that both oxygen saturation and respiratory rates were similar. Likewise, neonatal apgar scores, cord blood gases, and neurobehavioral scores in the two groups did not differ. Furthermore, a more recent metanalysis by Dahl and colleagues demonstrated excellent results with 0.1 to 0.2 mg of intrathecal morphine, and no additional pain relief at doses higher than 0.2 mg. The median time to requesting additional analgesia in this study was 27 hours.[42]

Abboud and colleagues[39] studied the ventilatory responses to carbon dioxide in 33 cesarean section patients, who received, in double-blind fashion, either 0.25 mg of morphine, 0.1 mg of morphine, or saline with hyperbaric spinal bupivacaine. All patients in the saline group required 8 mg of subcutaneous morphine within 3 hours of spinal anesthesia. Analgesia lasted a mean of 27.7 hours for patients who received 0.25 mg of morphine and 18.6 hours for those who received 0.1 mg. The authors measured the ventilatory responses to progressive hypercapnia

in all 3 groups at intervals up to 24 hours. Neither the CO_2 response curves, nor the minute ventilation at a $PaCO_2$ of 50 changed significantly over 24 hours for patients in either of the 2 intrathecal morphine groups, but both values were significantly depressed for 3 hours after the administration of subcutaneous morphine to the saline solution group.

On the basis of data verifying the safety and efficacy of low-dose intrathecal morphine for analgesia after cesarean section, this technique is very popular. It seems a dose of 0.2 mg of morphine is ideal for providing 18 to 20 hours of postcesarean analgesia without significant side effects.[25] Respiratory monitoring other than the routine monitoring of vital signs appears to be unnecessary, making low-dose intrathecal administration convenient on postpartum wards. Appropriate education of the nursing staff is extremely important if long-acting intraspinal narcotics are to be used on any routine-care ward and 24-hour in-house anesthesia coverage is a reasonable expectation. If an intrathecal morphine dose larger than 0.5 mg is administered, prudence recommends arranging overnight care in a more supervised setting such as "step-down" unit.

Less information is available concerning the use of sub-arachnoid fentanyl for postoperative analgesia.[43] Palmer and colleagues[44] found that the duration of analgesia was even shorter as opposed to bupivacaine when fentanyl was added to lidocaine. In the usual clinical setting, the effects of intrathecally administered fentanyl wane soon after the patient is discharged from the postanesthesia recovery area. PCA may then be initiated as soon as the patient perceives mild-moderate discomfort. Although effective for intraoperative cesearean pain management, the short duration of postcesarean analgesia limits the usefulness of fentanyl as a postoperative analgesic.[25] Intrathecal sufentanil (2.5 and 5 μg) may result in better analgesia in the first 6 hours postoperatively than fentanyl (10 μg).[46,47] Nevertheless, its short duration limits the usefulness of sufentanil as a postoperative analgesic.

Meperidine has commonly been used in the postcesarean section patient as a parenteral analgesic. Intrathecally administered meperidine is efficacious as a surgical anesthetic. Although meperidine is not approved by the FDA for spinal opioid analgesia, clinical experience indicates that 10 mg of preservative-free meperidine administered intrathecally provides effective post-surgical analgesia of intermediate duration (ie, 5 to 6 hours). Although significant complications have not been reported, potential side effects include pruritus, nausea, vomiting, and urinary retention.

The use of intrathecal nalbuphine is limited by the lack of safety trials in humans, as well as the potential to elicit withdrawal in opioid-dependent patients because of its opioid agonist-antagonist property.[2] It has also been noted to increase nausea.[25] Buprenorphine (0.045 mg) added to bupivacaine spinal results in 6 to 7 hours of effective postcesarean pain relief with a lower incidence of pruritis as compared to morphine.[48]

Continuous intrathecal analgesia has been achieved best with highly lipid-soluble opioids such as fentanyl and sufentanil because of their fast onset and short duration. For example, infusions of bupivacaine (1.5 mg/hour) and fentanyl (15 μg/hour) or sufentanil (2.5 to 5 μg/hour) have been used successfully.[49] The disadvantage is the increased risk for respiratory depression, especially with sufentanil.[50,51] This may require closer monitoring with continuous pulse oximetry, possibly in an intensive care setting. Tables 32.1 and 32.2 summarize intrathecal opioid dosing.

Table 32.4: Maternal Goals after Cesarean Delivery Guide Selection of Opioid and Mode for PCA

Postcesarean Maternal Goal	PCA Opioid and Mode	
	Optimal	Less Optimal
Alertness	PCA meperidine	PCA morphine
Ambulation	PCA + BI morphine	PCA meperidine
Rapid onset of analgesia	PCA oxymorphone	PCA morphine
Sleep	PCA + BI morphine	PCA + BI oxymorphone

Abbreviation: BI = basal infusion; PCA = patient-controlled analgesia.

Intrathecal Adjunct Therapy

Just as clonidine prolongs the duration of analgesia when added to epidural morphine, the addition of 60 μg of clonidine to 100 mcg of morphine in a bupivacaine spinal[52] will prolong the duration of spinal morphine analgesia. Although epinephrine may prolong the effects of intrathecal local anesthetics, it has not been shown to be helpful in postcesarean analgesia when added to 0.2 mg of intrathecal morphine.[53]

Intravenous Patient-Controlled Analgesia

Intravenous patient-controlled analgesia (IV PCA) can be used as the sole method for postoperative pain management, or it can be added as supplemental analgesia to epidural or intrathecal opioid analgesia. Intravenous PCA allows the patient to self-administer a preprogrammed dose of opioid IV at a determined lockout interval, and maximum doses that can be delivered in certain time periods are also preset as an added safety feature. The advantages of this method include improved pain relief, a more consistent blood concentration, and the convenience of bypassing the need for a nurse to administer each dose of pain medication. IV PCA therapy thus eliminates delays related to communication, nursing evaluations and drug preparation. Overall, this results in greater patient satisfaction and better pain relief when compared with intramuscular (IM) opioids.[2,58]

There are a wide variety of opioids that may be administered by intravenous PCA at equipotent dosages to provide equivalent analgesic responses (Table 32.3); however, differences in opioid-specific pharmacokinetics, pharmacodynamics and complications may result in different patient satisfactions. An investigation of PCA with morphine, meperidine, or oxymorphone after cesarean delivery showed that patient groups had similar opioid requirements and achieved equivalent pain relief at rest.[54] However, PCA oxymorphone promoted the most rapid onset of analgesia, whereas patients receiving PCA morphine reported the lowest pain scores beyond 8 hours postoperatively. Meperidine was associated with the most pain during movement, morphine produced the most sedation, and oxymorphone induced the greatest degree of nausea and emesis (Table 32.4). Depending on individual patient risk factors, patient preferences, and efficacy of supplemental medications to prevent or treat complications, each PCA opioid has unique benefits and risks. Using PCA meperidine, parturients with morbid obesity may be reluctant to ambulate and thus increase their risk of deep vein thrombosis and pulmonary embolus; patients with renal insufficiency may accumulate normeperidine and risk develop-

Table 32.5: IV PCA Opioids

Drug	Bolus Dose (mg)	Interval (min)	CI (mg/hr)	4 hr Lockout (mg)
Fentanyl	0.01–0.05	3–5	0.02	≤1
Meperidine	5–10	6	5–10	300
Morphine	1–1.5	6	1–2	30
Hydromorphone	0.1–0.2	6	0.1–0.5	5–10

Source: Braveman. Requisites in Anesthesiology: Postcesarean Analgesia. 2006.

ing neuromuscular tremors or seizures.[55] PCA morphine-related sedation may adversely affect maternal-infant bonding. However, after prolonged course of labor followed by cesarean delivery, parturients may benefit from the sedating properties of PCA morphine postoperatively. Prophylaxis against nausea and emesis might be necessary for patients receiving PCA oxymorphone. Table 32.5 summarizes IV PCA opioid therapeutic options.

Frequent, intermittent activation of the PCA device maintains plasma concentrations of opioids within a narrow therapeutic range to produce a consistent level of analgesia over time. However, during periods of sleep, this plasma opioid level declines because the PCA pump is not activated. As a result, patients may awaken at night because of waning analgesia or may arise early in the morning with normal movement evoking unexpected pain. These problems can be avoided by programming the PCA pump to infuse opioid continuously, in addition to delivering bolus doses in response to patient activation (patient-controlled analgesia + basal infusion, PCA + BI). The use of PCA alone versus PCA + BI has been studied among parturients after cesarean delivery who received either morphine or oxymorphone.[56] Among patients receiving oxymorphone, the addition of a basal infusion to PCA decreased pain scores at rest and with movement, increased the incidence of nausea and emesis, did not increase sedation or produce respiratory depression, and, had no significant effect on patient satisfaction. For patients receiving morphine, the addition of a basal infusion to PCA decreased pain scores with movement, did not significantly increase the incidence of sedation or produce respiratory depression, had no effect on the severity of sedation, and had no effect on satisfaction scores. These results emphasize that although analgesia may be enhanced by adding a basal infusion of opioid, patient satisfaction varies independent of the level of analgesia. Specifically, overall satisfaction remained unchanged because the incidence of adverse side effects was unchanged (sedation) or exacerbated (nausea, emesis). Among postcesarean patients, there are some (as after cesarean hysterectomy) who might benefit by the addition of a basal infusion of opioid, particularly if they experience inadequate analgesia with PCA alone. In those instances, however, close attention must be given toward adequate prophylaxis and treatment of side effects to optimize patient satisfaction. See Table 32.5 to choose the most appropriate opioid to optimize patient satisfaction.

It is evident that many factors contribute to the development of a logical plan for maintaining analgesia by PCA after cesarean delivery, including patient evaluation, opioid drug choice, programming infusion pump modalities, and the prevention and treatment of side effects. In addition, one must recognize that intraoperative anesthetic management also plays a significant role, especially as parturients begin to use the PCA pump.

Intravenous opioidsmust be present in plasma at or above their minimum effective concentrations to produce analgesia. Usual PCA dosing regimens are designed to maintain this plasma level, thus effective analgesic with PCA must be preceeded by an intravenous loading dose of opioid to achieve an initial therapeutic level.

Most parturients after cesarean delivery use PCA to achieve adequate but not exquisite analgesia. In fact, when compared to neuraxial morphine administration, pain relief is less, but satisfaction is greater because of decreased side effects.[58] Limiting self-administered doses tends to reduce the incidence and severity of opioid-related side effects, thus enhancing patient satisfaction. IV PCA may also be initiated as neuraxial opioid effects wane postoperatively, allowing for a smoother transition to postoperative analgesia. On occasion, however, a postcesarean patient may complain of moderate to severe pain despite a loading dose and appropriate use of PCA. Parturients with a recent history of drug abuse (that is, opioids or cocaine) may present in this manner. Among patients with a remote history of drug abuse, inadequate postoperative analgesia may also occur, especially if their usual daily methadone maintenance dose is omitted. Management of such patients should include maintaining a daily methadone dose (oral or parenteral) preadmission and throughout their hospitalization. This will allow normal utilization of PCA opioids after cesarean delivery. The use of opioid antagonists or mixed agonist antagonists must be avoided in these patients so as not to precipitate opioid withdrawal symptoms.[59] One must anticipate increased opioid dose requirements to maintain adequate postoperative analgesia in selected patients.

Multimodal Therapy

Typically, following cesarean delivery oral intake is begun within 12 hours of surgery. Sips of fluids are often tolerated and requested by the patient in the postanesthesia care unit (PACU). Thus, the use of oral analgesics can be an effective, inexpensive, and labor-saving method of achieving postoperative analgesia. Oral therapy with opioid, nonopioid, or opioid/nonopioid combinations has been shown effective for analgesia when administered around the clock (RTC) with additional PRN dosing for breakthrough pain. Therapy is especially efficacious when combined with a single-dose neuraxial opioid. In fact, Davis and colleagues suggest that oral therapy may be associated with better analgesia and fewer side effects than IV PCA therapy.[57] Table 32.6 lists commonly used oral opioid medications.

Because the intensity of postcesarean pain diminishes progressively, IV PCA may also be initiated as neuraxial opioid effects wane, with less risk of a "transitional hiatus" with inadequate analgesia.[58] Ideally, neuraxial opioids should decrease overall opioid requirement during the postoperative period. However, epidural fentanyl does not, as its effects do not last beyond the intraoperative period. Neuraxial opioids with long durations (24 hours) should best promote a smooth transition to postoperative analgesia; however, the duration of analgesia averages only 4 to 6 hours after epidural meperidine, methadone, butorphanol, or buprenorphine. Only intrathecal morphine and epidural hydromorphone or morphine produce 20 to 24 hours of analgesia, and the latter is associated with a 73% incidence of pruritus and 20% incidence of nausea despite prophylaxis. Clearly, reductions in cumulative opioid dose achieved by neuraxial opioids may not reduce the incidence of opioid-related side effects. Despite much larger cumulative amounts of opioid

Table 32.6: Oral Opioid Therapy

Opioid	Dose	Interval (Hour)
Morphine	10–30 mg	3–4
Oxycodone	5–10 mg	3–4
Percocet (oxycodone/ acetaminophen)	*5/325–15/1000*	*3–4*
Hydromorphone	2–6 mg	3–4
Hydrocodone	5–15 mg	4–6
(Lortab) (hydrocodone/ acetaminophen)	*5/500–15/1000*	*4–6*
Vicoprofen (hydrocodone/ ibuprofen)	*7.5/200–15/400*	*4–6*

Source: Braveman. Requisites in Anesthesiology: Postcesarean Analgesia. 2006.

accrued using PCA, compared to neuraxial administration, side effects with PCA are proportionally fewer and seem to be better tolerated.

The use of intramuscular and subcutaneous opioids do not provide the consistent levels of analgesia obtained with the therapies discussed above and are thus not recommended for postcesarean analgesia in 2007.

NSAIDs and COX-2 inhibitors, such as celecoxib, have been helpful in treating visceral pain, such as menstrual cramping, and are useful in a multimodal approach to pain relief in terms of enhancing analgesia and reducing opioid-related side effects. The site of action of these agents is not the opioid receptor. NSAIDs decrease inflammation and prostaglandin release centrally and peripherally. Intramuscular diclofenac (75 mg) or IV ketorolac (15 mg), for example, can be beneficial in women postcesarean, regardless if they had general anesthesia or neuraxial blockade (Table 32.7).[2]

Subcutaneous local wound infiltration with local anesthetics with or without NSAIDs has been used to decrease opioid requirements by blocking pain transmitters.[60] Clonidine administered both neuraxially and orally has also been a useful agent to opioid therapy.[37]

NEONATAL CONSIDERATIONS

Maternal use of parenteral opioids after cesarean delivery carries the potential risk for central nervous system depression in the fetus or neonate, secondary to opioid distribution via the placental circulation or breast milk, respectively. The incidence and severity of opioid-related depression is difficult to assess. Evaluation of the fetus in utero is usually limited to fetal heart rate pattern, fetal movements (including breathing patterns), and scalp capillary blood gas analysis. These measurements may reveal fetal distress but are not diagnostic for or predictive of opioid-related depression.

After cesarean delivery, PCA, in addition to its maternal effects, may also produce neonatal manifestations if the mother is breastfeeding. Thus, the maternal option to nurse should be a routine part of the evaluation of parturients who are scheduled for cesarean delivery and who elect to receive PCA for postoperative pain relief.

After clamping of the umbilical cord, any opioids administered intravenously to the mother must take a circuitous

Table 32.7: Nonopioid Therapy

Drug	Dose	Route	Interval (Hours)	Comments
Ketorolac	15 mg	IV/IM	4–6	Avoid NSAIDs in patients with hepato-renal disease, severe preeclampsia, and those with coagulation disorders and/or postsurgical bleeding.
Diclofenac	75 mg	IM	12	Avoid NSAIDs in patients with hepato-renal disease, severe preeclampsia, and those with coagulation disorders and/or postsurgical bleeding.
	100 mg	PR	8	
Ibuprofen	400 mg	PO	3–4	First dose 3 hours postoperative
Celecoxib	200 mg	PO	12	Does not affect platelet function
Clonidine	60–150 μg	Spinal	Single dose	Multimodal therapy with spinal opioid provides 6 hrs of analgesia.
				Higher doses (alone or with opioid) have unacceptable incidences of side effects.
	150–300 μg	Epidural	Single dose	Continuous infusion necessary for sustained analgesia.
				In combination with opioids, clonidine will prolong the duration of analgesia.
	4 μg/kg	PO	Single dose	Give 1 hour preoperatively
Bupivacaine	Varies	Skin infiltration	–	Can be administered via a SQ infusion pump (On-Q)

Abbreviations: IV = intravenous; IM = intramuscular; PR = per rectum; PO = per os.

Source: Requisites in Anesthesiology: Postcesarean Analgesia, Ferne Braveman, M.D., 2006.

pathway through maternal breast milk and neonatal gastrointestinal tract to the neonatal circulation. Regulatory mechanisms in this pathway are complex. First, maternal uptake of opioid during PCA utilization depends on the degree of postcesarean pain, its duration, and the level of maternal tolerance to pain. As a result, opioid concentrations in maternal plasma reflect the need for postoperative analgesia over time. Second, plasma opioids will distribute into and out of the breast milk tissue compartment. Influx and efflux depend on many factors, including regional blood flow, lipid solubility, milk solubility, and maternal metabolic and excretory pathways. Third, neonatal ingestion relies on the adequacy of both maternal lactation and infant sucking. Fourth, to enter the neonatal circulation, opioids must undergo gastrointestinal absorption (which is enhanced by greater lipid solubility) and venous drainage through the liver (exposing opioids to possible first-pass metabolism). Fifth, the degree to which opioids persist in the neonatal circulation (and may depress central nervous system functions) depends on their biodegradation and elimination pathways (notably in hepatic and renal systems).

Because this pathway is so complex, it is difficult to predict opioid-specific effects on neonatal neurobehavioral. However, applied opioid biochemistry may form a basis for a few common principles. Given the same requirement for postcesarean analgesia and sufficient time to achieve equilibrium between maternal plasma and breast milk, parturients using different PCA opioids will accumulate opioids in breast milk with equivalent potencies.[61,62] Neonatal gastrointestinal absorption of ingested opioids will be greater with more lipid-soluble opioids and opioid metabolites. Finally, if neonates cannot adequately detoxify or secrete certain opioids (notably those that require renal excretion), neonatal CNS depression is more likely to occur.

To detect neonatal CNS depression in this setting is not difficult. In a study of intravenous fentanyl for postcesarean analgesia, it was noted that among a group of 9 infants, 1 (who was nursing) developed recurrent apnea and cyanosis requiring cardiopulmonary resuscitation and naloxone.[63] Intensive follow-up observation revealed no intrinsic imbalance in respiratory control, but quantitation of fentanyl in maternal breast milk or neonatal serum were not performed. It is not surprising that a serum concentration of fentanyl producing maternal analgesia may (through that circuitous pathway through breast milk) also produce neonatal apnea, especially since fentanyl is very highly lipid soluble. However, fentanyl (like butorphanol), in small doses via epidural catheter (for analgesia during cesarean delivery), elicits no decrement in neonatal respiratory function.

Detecting more subtle neurologic depression among nursing neonates requires one or more neurobehavioral exams as performed by trained and certified personnel. Furthermore, to determine why this depression occurs requires quantitation of opioid concentrations in relevant tissue compartments. One study utilized both these approaches to assess the incidence, severity, and cause of neonatal depression among infants of nursing parturients who used PCA meperidine or PCA morphine after cesarean delivery.[62] Neonates in the morphine group were significantly more alert and significantly more responsive to human orientation cues than neonates in the meperidine group on their third day of life. Decrements in alertness and human orientation seen with meperidine not only reflect opioid-related neonatal depression, but may also inhibit normal maternal-infant bonding interactions.

To approach an understanding of the cause of these opioid-specific effects, breast milk specimens were obtained at intervals throughout the 4-day hospitalizations and analyzed for meperidine, morphine, and their metabolites.[61] Beyond 48 hours postpartum, normeperidine concentrations in breast milk exceeded meperidine concentrations by a 3:1 ratio, whereas morphine and morphine-3-glucuronide accrued in equal concentrations. Although both morphine and meperidine patient groups were similar in opioid potency of milk, the gastrointestinal absorption, metabolism, and excretion patterns of the 2 drugs are dramatically different. Meperidine, being far more lipid soluble than morphine, is much more rapidly and fully absorbed from the neonatal gastrointestinal tract. In the neonate, meperidine, undergoes first-pass hepatic N-demethylation to form normeperidine, an active metabolite that persists with a prolonged half-life of 63 hours.[62] In contrast, morphine also undergoes hepatic first-pass metabolism, but forms an inactive glucuronide

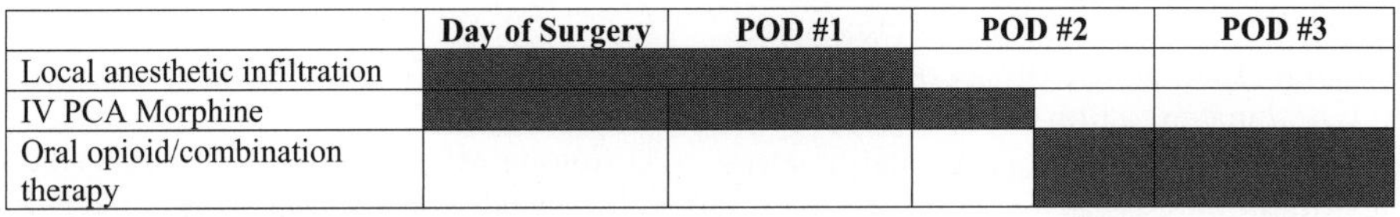

	Day of Surgery	POD #1	POD #2	POD #3
Local anesthetic infiltration	▓	▓		
IV PCA Morphine	▓	▓	▓	
Oral opioid/combination therapy			▓	▓

Figure 32.1: Multimodal therapy: pain management following general anesthesia. Modified with permission from: The Requisites in Anesthesiology: Postcesarean Analgesia, Ferne Braveman, M.D., 2006.

	Day of Surgery	POD #1	POD #2	POD #3
Clonidine (25–50 μg) + Morphine (0.2 mg intrathetcal)	▓	▓		
Ketorolac (15 mg every 6 hours IV RTC)		▓	▓	
Oral opiod/combination therapy			▓	▓

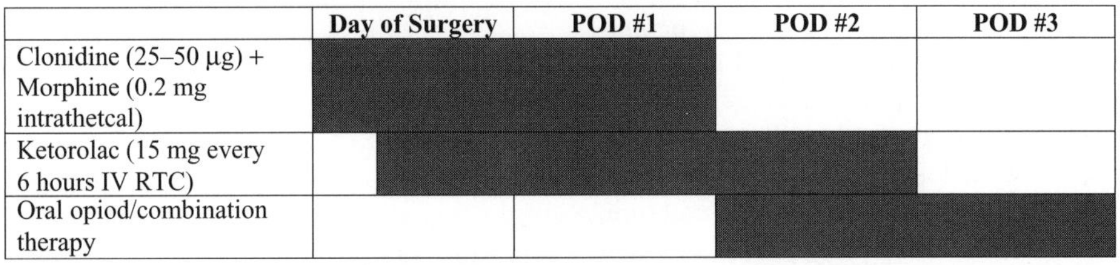

Figure 32.2. Multimodal therapy: pain management following spinal anesthesia. Abbreviation: RTC = around the clock. Modified with permission from: The Requisites in Anesthesiology: Postcesarean Analgesia, Ferne Braveman, M.D., 2006.

	Day of Surgery	POD #1	POD #2	POD #3
DepoDur	▓	▓	▓	
Ketorolac (15 mg IV every 6 hours PRN)		▓	▓	
Oral opioid/combination therapy			▓	▓

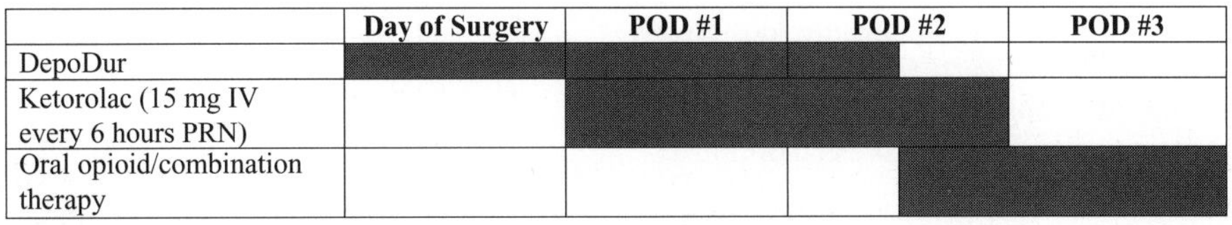

Figure 32.3. Multimodal therapy: pain management following DepoDur. Abbreviation: PRN = as needed. Modified with permission from: The Requisites in Anesthesiology: Postcesarean Analgesia, Ferne Braveman, M.D., 2006.

	Day of Surgery	POD #1	POD #2	POD #3
Morphine (0.2 mg Intrathecal)	▓	▓		
PCEA		▓	▓	
Ketorolac (15 mg IV every 6 hours PRN)	▓	▓	▓	
Oral opioid/combination therapy			▓	▓

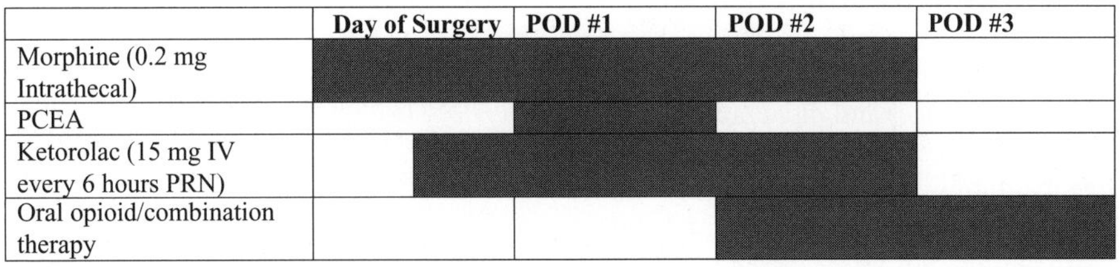

Figure 32.4. Multimodal therapy: CSE-PCEA. Abbreviation: PRN = as needed. Modified with permission from: The Requisites in Anesthesiology: Postcesarean Analgesia, Ferne Braveman, M.D., 2006.

	Day of Surgery	POD #1	POD #2	POD #3
PCEA	▓	▓		
Ketorolac (15 mg every 6 hours PRN			▓	▓
Oral opioid/combination therapy			▓	▓

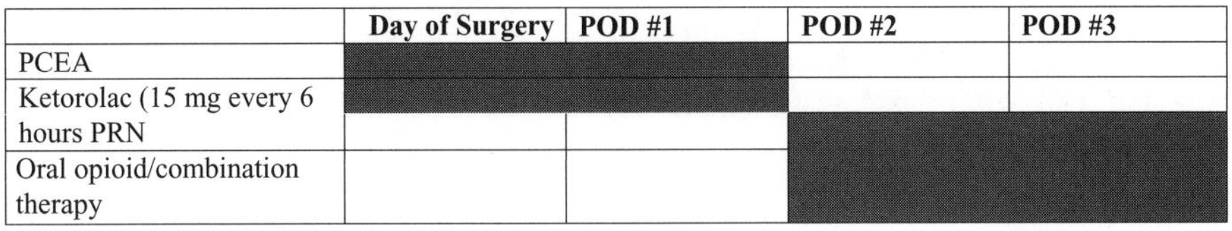

Figure 32.5. Multimodal therapy: PCEA. Abbreviation: PRN = as needed. Modified with permission from: The Requisites in Anesthesiology: Postcesarean Analgesia, Ferne Braveman, M.D., 2006.

metabolite. As a result, neonates are more capable of detoxifying morphine, by glucuronidation, than of detoxifying meperidine, which ultimately depends on renal excretion.

Because PCA with meperidine results in accumulation (in breast milk) of normeperidine and associated neonatal neurobehavioral depression, PCA with morphine may be a better choice for postcesarean analgesia in the parturient who nurses. Especially with a low-birth-weight infant (<2500 g) who is already prone to seizures, neonatal ingestion and accumulation of normeperidine would only exacerbate that risk. Finally, it is important to remember that, among nursing parturients who receive PCA with morphine after cesarean delivery, neonatal neurobehavior is no different from that observed in normal infants with no drug exposure after vaginal delivery.[61]

NSAIDs are used routinely as part of the multimodal postoperative analgesic regimen. Ibuprofen does not enter breast milk in significant quantities. Ketorolac is excreted in breast milk but in insignificant amounts. Acetaminophen is also excreted in small amounts into breast milk. The American Academy of Pediatrics considers all to be compatible with breastfeeding.[64]

SUMMARY OF MATERNAL AND NEONATAL CONSIDERATIONS

The first and omnipresent consideration in managing obstetric pain is that the recipient of care is the parturient-neonate *pair*. Thus, one must assess the optimal choice of therapy by analyzing the risks, benefits, and potential complications of each option as they apply to both the mother and infant.

To provide analgesia after cesarean delivery, one must first determine if the mother will be breastfeeding. If the parturient is nursing, and IV PCA is used, morphine is the best alternative of PCA opioid choices to minimize neonatal morbidity while maintaining maternal analgesia and satisfaction. Most oral therapies are compatible with breastfeeding, and patients should be encouraged to ensure their comfort to allow them to bond with their infant. For parturients that will be bottle feeding, analgesia may be provided by the use of many different opioids, which have subtle differences in terms of advantages and disadvantages.

The ultimate goal of postcesarean section analgesia is to optimize pain relief while maintaining the quality of maternal-neonatal interaction. Breast or bottle feeding, holding and cuddling, and other activities should not be denied because of inadequate analgesia. Neither should the mother be expected to tolerate severe dose-dependent side effects often observed with parenteral administration. The excellent quality of pain relief, low dose requirement, and lack of excessive sedation associated with spinal opioid analgesia are characteristics ideally suited for optimal maternal and neonatal recuperation after cesarean delivery. Pain relief may be provided by several multimodal/multiroute forms of therapy that differ in terms of cost and complexity. The ultimate choice is influenced by analgesic effectiveness, side effect profile, and impact on mother/infant bonding. Common dosing regimens are presented in Figures 32.1–32.5.

REFERENCES

1. Nikolajsen L, Sorensen HC, Jensent TS, et al. Chronic pain following cesarean section. *Acta Anesth Scand.* 2004;48:111–116.
2. Gadsden J, Hart S, Santos AC. Post-cesarean delivery analgesia. *Anesth Analg.* 2005;101(suppl 5):S62–S69.
3. Chen B, Kwan W, Lee C, et al. A national survey of obstetrical postanesthesia care in teaching hospitals (Abstract). *Anesth Anal.* 1993;76:543.
4. Cousins MJ, Mather LE. Intrathecal and epidural administration of opioids. *Anesthesiology,* 1984;61:276–310.
5. Yaksh TL. Spinal opiate analgesia: characteristics and principles of action. *Pain.* 1981;11:293–346.
6. Wong CA, Scavone BM, Peaceman AM, et al. The risk of cesarean delivery with neuraxial analgesia given early versus late in labor. *N Engl J Med.* 2005;352(7):655–665.
7. American College of Obstetricians and Gynecologists Committee on Obstetric Practice. ACOG Committee Opinion. No. 339: analgesia and cesarean delivery rates. *Obstet Gynecol.* 2006;107:1487–1488.
8. Rawal N, Sjostrand U, Christoffersson E, et al. Comparison of intramuscular and epidural morphine for postoperative analgesia in the grossly obese. Influence on postoperative ambulation and pulmonary function. *Anesth Analg.* 1984;63:583–588.
9. Fuller JG, Morland GH, Douglas J, et al. Epidural morphine for postoperative pain after caesarean section: a report of 4880 patients. *Can J Anesth.* 1990;37:636–640.
10. Leicht CH, Kurkan WJ, Fians DH, et al. Postoperative analgesia with epidural morphine: single bolus vs. Daymate elastomeric toninuous infusion technique. *Anesthesiology.* 1990;73:A930.
11. Palmer CM, Nogami WM, Van Maren G, et al. Postcesarean epidural morphine: a dose-response study. *Anesth Analg.* 2000;90(4):887–891.
12. Hartrick CT, Manvelian G. Sustained release epidural morphine (Depodur): a review. *Today's Therapeutic Trends.* 2004;22(3):167–180.
13. Gambling D, Hughes T, Martin G, et al. A comparison of Depodur, a novel, single-dose extended-release epidural morphine, with standard epidural morphine for pain relief after lower abdominal surgery. *Anesth Analg.* 2005;100(4):1065, 1074.
14. Carvalho B, Riley E, Cohen SE, et al. Single-dose, sustained-release epidural morphine in the management of postoperative pain after elective cesarean delivery: results of a multicenter randomized controlled study. *Anesth Analg.* 2005;100:1150–1158.
15. Kotelko DM, Dailey PA, Shnider SM, et al. Epidural morphine analgesia after cesarean delivery. *Obstet Gynecol.* 1984;63:409.
16. Hess PE, Snowman CE, Hahn CJ, et al. Chloroprocaine may not affect epidural morphine for postcesarean delivery analgesia. *J Clin Anesth.* 2006;18:29–33.
17. Meagher L, Glassenberg R, Vaisrup N, et al. The effects of 2% lidocaine with epinephrine versus 0.5% bupivacaine plain on the duration of epidural morphine. *Proc Soc Obstet Anesth Perinatol.* 1987;19:43.
18. Naulty JS, Data S, Ostheimer GW, et al. Epidural fentanyl for postcesarean delivery pain management. *Anesthesiology.* 1985;63:694–698.
19. Sevarino FB, McFarlane C, Sinatra RS. Epidural fentanyl does not influence intravenous PCA requirements in the post-caesarean patient. *Can J Anaesth.* 1991;38:450–451.
20. Robertson K, Douglas MJ, McMorland GH. Epidural fentanyl, with and without epinephrine for post-cesarean section analgesia. *Can Anaesth Soc J.* 1985;32:502–505.
21. Birnbach DJ, Johnson MD, Arcario T, et al. Effect of diluent volume on analgesia produced by epidural fentanyl. *Anesth Analg.* 1989;68:808–810.
22. Youngstrom P, Hoyt M, Herman M, et al. Dose-response study of continuous infusion epidural fentanyl-epinephrine for postcesarean analgesia. *Anesthesiology.* 1990;73:A980.
23. Ellis JD, Millar WL, Reiner LS. A randomized double-blind comparison of epidural versus intravenous fentanyl infusion for analgesia after cesarean section. *Anesthesiology.* 1990;72:981–986.

24. Naulty JS, Ross R. Epidural fentanyl and morphine for post-cesarean delivery analgesia. *Proc Soc Obstet Anesth Perinatol.* 1988;20:178.

25. Palmer CM. Post cesarean analgesia. *Tech Reg Anesth Pain Manag.* 2003;7(4):213–221.

26. Crone LAL, Conly JM, Clark KM, et al. Recurrent herpes simplex virus labialis and the use of epidural morphine on obstetric patients. *Anesth Analg.* 1988;67:318–323.

27. Kotelko DM, Rottman RL, Wright WC, et al. Transdermal scopolamine decreases nausea and vomiting following cesarean section in patients receiving epidural morphine. *Anesthesiology.* 1989;71:675–678.

28. Gieraerts R, Navalgund A, Vaes I, et al. Increased incidence of itching and herpes simplex in patients given epidural morphine after cesarean section. *Anesth Analg.* 1987;66:1321–1324.

29. Davies PW, Vallejo MC, Shannon KT, et al. Oral herpes simplex reactivation after intrathecal morphine: a prospective randomized trial in an obstetric population. *Anesth Analg.* 2005;100:1472–1476.

30. Rosen MA, Dailey PA, Hughes SC, et al. Epidural sufentanil for postoperative analgesia after cesarean section. *Anesthesiology.* 1988;68:448–452.

31. Grass JA, Sakima NT, Schmidt R, et al. A randomized, double-blind, dose-response comparison of epidural fentanyl versus sufentanil analgesia after cesarean section. *Anesth Analg.* 1997;85(2):365–371.

32. Chestnut DH, Choi WW, Isbell TJ. Epidural hydromorphone for post-cesarean analgesia. *Obstet Gynecol.* 1989;68:65–69.

33. Ngan Kee WD, Lam KK, Chen PP, et al. Epidural meperidine after cesarean section: a dose-response study. *Anesthesiology.* 1996;85:289–294.

34. Beeby D, MacIntosh K, Bailey M, et al. Postoperative analgesia for caesarean section using epidural methadone. *Anaesthesia.* 1984;39(1):61–63.

35. Haynes SR, Davidson I, Allsop J. Comparison of epidural methadone with epidural diamorphine for analgesia following caesarean section. *Acta Anaesthesiol Scand.* 1993;37:375–380.

36. Roulson CJ, Bennett J, Shaw M. Effect of extradural diamorphine on analgesia after caesarean section under subarachnoid block. *Br J Anaesth.* 1993;71(6):810–813.

37. Capogna G, Celleno D, Zangrillo A, et al. Addition of clonidine to epidural morphine enhances postoperative analgesia after cesarean delivery. *Reg Anesth.* 1995;20(1):57–61.

38. Sakura S, Sumi M, Morimoto N, et al. The addition of epinephrine increases intensity of sensory block during epidural anesthesia with lidocaine. *Reg Anesth Pain Med.* 1999;24(6):541–546.

39. Abboud TK, Dror A, Mosaad P, et al. Mini dose intrathecal morphine for the relief of post-cesarean section pain: safety, efficacy, and ventilatory responses to carbon dioxide. *Anesth Analg.* 1988;67:137–141.

40. Chadwick HS, Ready LB. Intrathecal and epidural morphine sulfate for Postcesarean analgesia – a clinical comparison. *Anesthesiology.* 1988;68:925–929.

41. Abouleish E, Rawal N, Fallon K, et al. Combined intrathecal morphine and bupivacaine for cesarean section. *Proc Soc Obstet Anesth Perinatol.* 1987;19:16.

42. Dahl JB, Jeppesen IS, Jorgensen H, et al. Intraoperative and postoperative analgesic efficacy and adverse effects of intrathecal opioids in patients undergoing cesarean section with spinal anesthesia: a qualitative and quantitative systematic review of randomized controlled trials. *Anesthesiology.* 1999;91:1919–1927.

43. Dahlgren, Hultstrand C, Jakobsson J, et al. Intrathecal sufentanil, fentanyl, or placebo added to bupivacaine for cesarean section. *Anesth Analg.* 1997;85:1288–1293.

44. Palmer CM, Voulgaropoulos D, Alves D. Subarachnoid fentanyl augments lidocaine spinal anesthesia for cesarean delivery. *Reg Anesth.* 1995;20(5):389–394.

45. Yu S-C, Ngan Kee WD, Kwan ASK. Addition of meperidine to bupivacaine for spinal anaesthesia for caesarean section. *Br J Anaesth* 2002;88(3):379–383.

46. Celleno D. Spinal sufentanil. *Anaesthesia.* 1998;53(suppl 2):49–50.

47. Dahlgren G, Hultstrand C, Jakobsson J, et al. Intrathecal sufentanil, fentanyl or placebo added to bupivacaine for cesarean section. Anesth Analg. 1997;85:1288–1293.

48. Celleno D, Capogna G. Spinal buprenorphine for postoperative analgesia after caesarean sections. *Acta Anaesthesiol Scand.* 1989;33:236–238.

49. Palmer CM. Continuous intrathecal sufentanil for postoperative analgesia. *Anesth Analg.* 2001;92(1):244–245.

50. Hays RL, Palmer CM. Respiratory depression after intrathecal sufentanil during labor. *Anesthesiology.* 1994;81(2):511–512.

51. Ferouz F, Norris MC, Leighton BI. Risk of respiratory arrest after intrathecal sufentanil. *Anesth Analg.* 1997;85:1088–1090.

52. Paech MJ, Pavy TJ, Orlikowski CE. Postcesarean analgesia with spinal morphine, clonidine, or their combination. *Anesth Analg.* 2004;98(5):1460–1466.

53. Abouleish E, Rawal N, Tobon-Randall B, et al. A clinical and laboratory study to compare the addition of 0.2 mg of morphine, 0.2 mg of epinephrine, or their combination to hyperbaric bupivacaine for spinal anesthesia in cesarean section. *Anesth Analg.* 1993;77:457–462.

54. Sinatra RS, Lodge K, Sibert K, et al. A comparison of morphine, meperidine and oxymorphone as utilized in patient-controlled analgesia following cesarean delivery. *Anesthesiology.* 1989;70:585–590.

55. Szeto HH, Inturrisi CE, Houde R, et al. Accumulation of normeperidine, an active metabolite of meperidine, in patients with renal failure or cancer. *Ann Intern Med.* 1977;86:738–741.

56. Sinatra R, Chung KS, Silverman DG, et al. An evaluation of morphine and oxymorphone administered via patient-controlled analgesia (PCA) or PCA plus basal infusion in postcesarean delivery patients. *Anesthesiology.* 1989;71:502–507.

57. Davis KM, Esposito MA, Meyer BA. Oral analgesia compared with intravenous patient-controlled analgesia for pain after cesarean delivery: A randomized controlled trial. *Am J Obstet Gynecol.* 2006;194:967–971.

58. Harrison DM, Sinatra R, Morgese L, et al. Epidural narcotic and patient-controlled analgesia for post-cesarean section pain relief. *Anesthesiology.* 1988;68:454–457.

59. Weintraub SJ, Naulty JS. Acute abstinence syndrome after epidural injection of butorphanol. *Anesth Analg.* 1985;64:452–453.

60. Zohar E, Shapiro A, Eidinov A, et al. Postcesarean analgesia: the efficacy of bupivacaine wound instillation with and without supplemental diclofenac. *J Clin Anesth.* 2006;18:415–421.

61. Wittels B, Scott DT, Sinatra RS. Exogenous opioids in human breast milk and acute neonatal neurobehavior: a preliminary study. *Anesthesiology.* 1990;73:864–869.

62. Edwards JE, Rudy AC, Wermeling DP, et al. Hydromorphone transfer into breast milk after intranasal administration. *Pharmacotherapy.* 2003;23(2):153–158.

63. Kuhnert BR, Kuhnert PM, Philipson EH, et al. Disposition of meperidine and normeperidine following multiple doses during labor. II. Fetus and neonate. *Am J Obstet Gynecol.* 1985;151:410–415.

64. Committee on Drugs, American Academy of Pediatrics. The transfer of drugs and other chemicals into breast milk. *Pediatrics.* 2001;108(3):776–789.

33

Acute Pain Management in Sickle Cell Disease Patients

Jaya L. Varadarajan and Steven J. Weisman

Sickle cell anemia is a genetically inherited group of disorders characterized by large amounts of hemoglobin S in the red blood cells. The sickling hemoglobinopathies include patients with hemoglobin (Hgb) SS, SC, S-β thalassemia, SD, and SO. Affected individuals belong to a variety of ethnic groups that originated in equatorial Africa and Asia and have extended into the Mediterranean basin. In the United States, these disorders are most prevalent among African Americans and Hispanics. Approximately 1 in 400–600 African Americans and 1 in 1500–2000 Hispanic Americans has a sickling hemoglobinopathy. These disorders can also, however, be seen in other individuals, who could have derived from a mixed line owing to the multinational and multiracial nature of our population.

Although sickle cell disease is associated with infection, organ failure, and other comorbid conditions that affect the life expectancy of these patients, it is the painful crises that dominate the patients' lives, affecting their productivity and quality of life. The magnitude of the severity and frequency of painful episodes in these disorders warrants an in-depth discussion of its pain management. Indeed, painful episodes in sickle cell anemia account for the highest proportion of outpatient visits to the emergency room or for inpatient hospitalizations in this population. The pain in this disorder is unpredictable and shows components of both acute and chronic pain syndromes.

This chapter is a review of the pathophysiology of pain in sickle cell anemia, with discussions of the various acute and chronic pain syndromes. Aspects of pain assessment and management, including cognitive-behavioral, medical, and analgesic techniques that are specifically relevant to sickle cell anemia, are also discussed.

PATHOPHYSIOLOGY

Patients with clinically relevant sickling syndromes must inherit two abnormal genes that code for β-globin chain production. Heterozygotes for hemoglobin S, C, or β-thalassemia do not have significant signs or symptoms that can result in pain syndromes. Any combination of two abnormal genes that results in a pre-

dominance of abnormal hemoglobin can result in a patient who has clinical symptoms that can escalate into a painful episode. As these episodes are often recurrent and unpredictable, and can occur in various anatomic locations, the perception of pain in this population is frequently embedded in a very complex psychological milieu.

Clinically, the individual will describe pain in the bones or joints but may also perceive the soft tissues as being affected. The pain can also be visceral in origin, related to events in the spleen, liver, gall bladder, or intestines. Painful episodes or "crises" may involve multiple sites waxing and waning in the context of one major event. Local swelling, redness, and tenderness can certainly accompany the complaints, with patients not infrequently guarding an affected anatomic site. It is possible that as more experience is gained with nuclear medicine scans or with magnetic resonance imaging, these diagnostic tools may help determine the location and extent of infarction. Such knowledge would help target the site of involvement and aid in pain management.

Painful crises, as well as most of the clinical sequelae seen in sickle cell anemia, occur because of vaso-occlusion in the microcirculation. Although the precise mechanism causing vaso-occlusion is a topic of debate among clinical investigators, the irreversibly sickled red blood cell has been universally implicated in the process.[1] The normal human red blood cell, which measures about 8 μm across, must traverse capillaries as small as 5 μm in diameter. The conditions that permit the remarkable deformability and plasticity of the red blood cell are often not present when there are significant amounts of sickling hemoglobin. Hemoglobin S forms rather rigid linear polymers when exposed to low oxygen tension and low pH. In addition, sickle hemoglobin-containing cells with high mean corpuscular hemoglobin concentration (MCHC) are dense cells, more predisposed to polymer formation.[2] These irreversibly polymerized, nondeformable cells are either trapped by precapillary vessel sphincters or may become more adherent to small vessel walls.[3–5] Ultimately the small vessels are occluded, followed by extension of the vascular infarct area into collateral blood vessels, which leads to necrosis and direct nociception of this painful stimulus.[1,6–8] This pathophysiologic process can be precipitated by infection, cold, dehydration, oxygen deprivation, menstruation, and psychological stress. It has been hypothesized that white blood cells also contribute to the pathology of sickle cell disease.[9–11] Pain is more likely to start at night because of nocturnal desaturation or relative dehydration. Physiologic factors that can contribute to the red cell maintaining its deformability include the presence of non-S hemoglobins such as hemoglobin F or A.[12,13] Bone pain is the consequence of the release of inflammatory mediators that result in raised intramedullary pressures and stimulation of nociceptors.[14–16] The mechanism is hypothesized to be a centrally mediated reflex that shunts blood away from the medullary cavity.[17.]

Pain is the hallmark of sickle cell disease and the painful episodes or crises can vary remarkably in severity and duration.[18] In fact, the pain of a vaso-occlusive episode can be perceived to even surpass that of a surgical procedure. The pain can last as little as several hours to as long as several weeks. Most episodes last 3–5 days, with pain occurring all day. However, there are no clear-cut objectives or measurable parameters to define the nature or extent of the vasoocclusive episode. Various hematologic parameters, such as the numbers of dense or sickled cells, have been studied but these and other methods are either not universally available or have not been reproducibly predictive. For example, in the face of seemingly similar hematologic findings, about 30% of patients will experience rare or no pain episodes at all, another 50% will have several painful episodes each year, and about 20% will report frequent and/or excruciating pain crises.[19] There is also great variability in frequency of painful crises. Although some have mildly painful episodes that respond readily to supportive treatment, others have severe crises that require hospitalization for days, and still others have chronic persistent pain with acute exacerbations. The episodes can also vary in the same individual at various times.

As alluded to earlier, pain can occur in virtually any anatomic site. There is, however, some relationship between age and sites of pain. In children under 3–5 years of age, painful swelling of the hands and feet (hand-foot syndrome or dactylitis) is not only common but may also be the first manifestation of the disease itself.[20,21] Prior to more widespread screening for sickle cell disease, many episodes of dactylitis either went unrecognized or misdiagnosed.[22–24] As more experience has been gained with nuclear medicine scans and magnetic resonance imaging, these tools have helped in determining the location and extent of infarction.[25–28] As children enter the school-age and adolescent years, the pain is more commonly localized to the long bones and then, with age, progresses more frequently to the abdomen.[29] Patients will also have neurological complications from their illness.[30–32] The classification of sickle cell pain syndromes is outlined in Table 33.1.

ASSESSMENT OF PAIN

Walco and Dampier[34] evaluated the pain associated with sickle cell vasoocclusive crisis in 17 hospitalized adolescents. They found that the pain associated with crises were quite severe, averaging 7–8 on a 10-point scale during the first 3 days and then dropping off dramatically. Objective signs, however, are often absent especially in the first 1–2 days, making assessment a challenge. This pattern indicates the need for careful and

Table 33.1: Classification of Painful Episodes in Sickle Cell Disease

Pain secondary to the disease itself
  Acute pain syndromes
    Recurrent acute painful episodes (crises)
    Acute chest syndrome
    Hepatic crisis
    Priapism
    Calculus cholecystitis
    Hand-foot syndrome
    Splenic sequestration
  Chronic pain syndromes
    With objective signs
      Avascular necrosis
      Arthropathies
      Leg ulcers
      Chronic osteomyelitis
    Without objective signs
      Intractable chronic pain
  Neuropathic pain
Pain secondary to therapy
  Withdrawal
  Loose prosthesis
  Postoperative pain
Pain as a result of comorbid conditions
  Trauma
  Arthritis
  Peptic ulcer disease
Other conditions

Adapted from Ballas.[33]

frequent assessment throughout the vaso-occlusive crisis, as well as at other times in the patient's life. Therefore, any program that is directly managing sickle cell pain must have, at its core, an adequate assessment regimen.

Issues of pain assessment for children with sickle cell anemia are not unlike those for children with other chronic and acute pain problems. There are, however, some unique aspects of sickle cell anemia that require alternative assessment strategies.

General Considerations in Pain Assessment

The most reliable indicator of pain is the self-report of the person experiencing the pain. Over the age of 7 or 8 years, children can usually use a visual analog or numeric pain rating scale, similar to that used by adults. Such scales can be a line without intervals, a line with intervals where the anchors are *no pain* and *the most pain imaginable* or a 0–10 numeric scale. Most children over 7 years of age can use such scales to rate the intensity of their pain. For children between the ages of 3 and 7 years, pictorial self-report scales have been developed. These include the use of color scales (not recommended), cartoon faces, pain thermometers, and photographs of children in various levels of discomfort and poker chips that represent pieces of hurt.[35,36]

On all of these scales, the child is asked to rate the amount of discomfort he or she is experiencing. Most of these instruments have reliability and construct validity.[37] Although there may be some differences in the subtlety of measurement that each offers, for the most part they do indicate if a patient is in discomfort or not. Which scale is chosen is less important than the fact that routine pain assessment is included as part of the care plan and that caregivers are uniform in their choice of a scale.[38]

For those children who are younger than 3 years or who are unable to verbally communicate their level of discomfort to caregivers, other strategies are required. One such strategy involves the use of behavioral scales that allow us to look at various behaviors infants and young children might demonstrate that are associated with pain. In infants, these include certain facial characteristics or cry patterns that have been identified as associated with pain.[38,39] In older children, various patterns of bodily movements, whimpering, body positions, and so on are often also associated with pain. Scales have been developed, coalescing these variables together to offer us a score that is believed to reflect discomfort.[40]

In addition to behavioral scales, physiologic measures are also available to us. These tend to be the least specific, because many factors can cause a child's blood pressure, heart rate, or respiratory rate to increase. For some children, however, a combination of behavioral and physiologic variables is needed to determine the degree of discomfort they are experiencing.

Sickle Cell–Specific Assessment Issues

Several factors about sickle cell anemia mandate some modifications in our pain assessment strategies. One unique aspect has to do with the fact that we are dealing with pain that exacerbates intermittently, often unpredictably, at home or in the hospital and that it may be superimposed on a certain level of baseline pain. Therefore some mechanism of ongoing pain assessment is often necessary for these children. Shapiro et al[18] and Dampier et al[41,42] have reported on the use of home diaries to provide an ongoing assessment of pain associated with sickle cell disease and identify clues to the early phases of a vasoocclusive episode. Such techniques require not only ongoing monitoring by health care providers but also engaged parents and compliant patients and, as a result, are often hard to implement.

Another unique aspect of sickle cell pain is that there is often discordance between the race of the health care provider and that of the patient. Sickle cell patients are usually African American or Hispanic, whereas health care providers in this country are predominately Caucasian or Asian, although the distribution is somewhat specific to the region. There is an established literature in the health care delivery field that demonstrates that the racial or ethnic background of the provider can have a strong impact on the patient's symptom reporting.[43] We do believe that the gulf between the different ethnic, racial, and socioeconomic groups in this country has an influence on both symptom reporting by patients and the appreciation of those symptoms by health care providers. These differences mandate the need for health care professionals to work at understanding a population that is so different from themselves and provide care in a culturally sensitive fashion. An example of incorporation of cultural/racial sensitivity is reflected in the development of African American and Hispanic oucher scales.[44] Pain in sickle cell patients is unlike postoperative pain or other acute pain problems, which tend to be localized to a specific site. The pain of sickle cell anemia can be widespread. Pains in the chest, extremities, back, and abdomen are all common, and a typical episode may involve any one or all of these areas. The intensity of the pain can vary at each site, however. An adequate assessment must take into account the location of the pain and it's varying intensities and not strictly its overall intensity.[45] Therefore, the use of pain assessment instruments that require the child to report a specific location of discomfort, in addition to the intensity is also important. The Varni-Thompson Pediatric Pain Questionnaire and the Children's Comprehensive Pain Questionnaire both contain body-contour maps that even young children have been able to use to pinpoint the location of their discomfort.[46–49]

MEDICAL MANAGEMENT OF SICKLE CELL PAIN

The management of sickle cell pain is complex and must take into account the disease as a whole.[50] The pain cannot be treated in isolation and the provider cannot make management decisions based solely on the pain behavior.[51–53] A thorough understanding of the issues pertaining to treatment of a progressive disease on a chronic basis is necessary.[54,55]

General Principles

It is universally accepted that aggressive hydration should be a part of any pain management care plan for the patient with sickle cell anemia.[19,56] Increases in intravascular volume should limit vascular sludging in capillary beds, thus reducing pain. Much of the notion regarding copious delivery of fluids during painful episodes is based on in vitro observations of intracellular hemoglobin polymerization and the well-known fact that because of renal damage, sickle cell patients have difficulty concentrating their urine.[57] It is unclear if there are any differences in the effectiveness of hydration by the various routes that fluids are administered. For the euvolemic or mildly hypovolemic patient, oral hydration as an initial step is appropriate.[58,59]

Oxygen has been a part of the algorithm for management of these patients. Without clearly identified hypoxemia, it can be disputed if supplemental oxygen plays a role in the management of a pain crisis. Prospective, randomized, controlled clinical trials have demonstrated that 50% oxygen is associated with significant reductions in the number of reversible sickled red blood cells, compared to patients on room air.[60–62] This reduction does not, however, affect the duration of painful crises, hospital admission rates, or analgesic needs. Oxygen is readily available and inexpensive, making it commonly used in practice. However, in the event that a pulmonary sequestration or clear-cut hypoxemia is present, oxygen is certainly indicated.

Scheduled blood transfusion to patients with sickle cell anemia is avoided as much as possible, because of the numerous side effects of transfusion of any blood product. Simple transfusions to increase hemoglobin levels above 10 g/dL or hematocrit above 30% may actually increase the risk of sickling. Exchange transfusions are employed to decrease hgb S levels to <30%. Regular transfusions may then be provided to maintain a hematocrit no greater than 30%. This has been shown to suppress new Hgb S red cell formation and prevent vasoocclusive episodes.[63,64] In patients who have suffered a stroke, regular transfusion will effectively prevent recurrences and the onset of painful episodes. Such therapy does, however, carry the well-known risk of viral transmission and iron accumulation. In addition, alloimmunization commonly occurs, because of the ethnic variance between the donor pool and the sickle cell recipient population.[65] Finally, repeated chronic transfusion will result in iron overload and ultimately hemochromatosis with death from organ damage.[66] Patients with debilitating, recurrent pain syndromes may benefit from periods of regular transfusion support, if these risks are outweighed by the benefits of pain-free periods. Vichinsky et al and the Preoperative Transfusion in Sickle Cell Study Group compared the perioperative complication rate in sickle cell patients assigned to either an aggressive group (patients transfused to decrease Hgb S to <30% with preop Hgb of 11 gm%) or a conservative group (transfusion to increase Hgb to 10 gm%).[67] Although acute chest syndrome occurred equally in both groups, there was a 2-fold increase in transfusion related complications in the aggressive transfusion group. These included development of a new alloautoantibody, hemolysis, allergic or anaphylactic reactions, fevers, fluid overload, and other minor reactions. This group concluded that a conservative transfusion regimen was as effective as an aggressive regimen in preventing perioperative complications in sickle cell patients.

Over the years, investigators have searched for compounds that inhibit sickling in the red blood cells of affected patients.[68,69] Unfortunately, until recently, almost all such antisickling agents have carried unacceptable toxicity, which preclude their use to prevent painful episodes. It is, however, well known that certain patients who have increased levels of non-S hemoglobin have much less severe sickle cell symptoms. This is particularly true with respect to hemoglobin F. Chemotherapeutic agents such as hydroxyurea (HU) and 5-azacytidine have been used successfully in patients with sickle cell anemia to increase the percentage of hemoglobin F in their blood.[70-77] Although hydroxyurea is licensed in the United States for administration to sickle cell patients who have more than 3 crises a year in steady state, it remains unlicensed in most countries, where it is regarded as an experimental drug. This is not because the clinical efficacy is doubted but because the long-term adverse effects are unknown. Potential long-term toxic effects for HU include teratogenicity, carcinogenesis, and, for young children, impaired cognitive development.[78-80] Omega-3 fatty acids, docosahexaenoic acid, and eicosapentaenoic acid are now being studied in sickle cell patients.[9,81,82] They are believed to confer resistance to hemolysis. This improves hemoglobin levels and reduces blood coagulability, with the end effect being a reduction in vasoocclusive episodes, ischemic organ damage and disease complications. Unlike HU these agents are not cytotoxic, occur naturally, would be more available and affordable especially in developing countries, and be more acceptable to patients and providers. Experiments are also underway to induce production of normal hemoglobin in the erythorcytes of sickle cell patients using various viral transfection models.[83] These do hold promise for the future direction of care in these patients.

Antibiotics are commonly recommended, as there is a high risk of bacterial infections in these patients. Specific painful syndromes, such as cholecystitis or avascular necrosis of the femoral heads, are managed with standard medical-surgical guidelines, including aggressive analgesic therapy. Pain management for specific infections such as pneumonia or osteomyelitis should include treatment of the primary underlying pathologic condition in addition to provision of adequate analgesia.

Table 33.2: Behavioral and Physical Methods for Pain Management

Education and preparation

Psychological

Self-control

Parental involvement

Hypnotherapy and biofeedback

TENS (transcutaneous electrical nerve stimulation)

Physical therapy

NONPHARMACOLOGIC APPROACHES TO PAIN MANAGEMENT

Therapies that reduce sickling, such as hydration, supplemental oxygen, and transfusions, and pain control with analgesics are clearly the mainstay of sickle cell pain management. However, there are several nonpharmacologic techniques that are also beneficial (Table 33.2).

Education and Psychological Techniques

An appreciation of the causes, treatment, and eventual outcome of children with sickle cell disease is helpful to children and their families in understanding what they must face. For children with the potential for lifelong, unpredictable crises, like those associated with sickle cell disease, education about the illness itself replaces the traditional preparation available to children who are about to undergo, or be involved in, a predictable acutely painful situation such as surgery. Several studies suggest that many families of children with sickle cell disease do not, in fact, understand some of its basic principles.[84] Therefore, a more developmentally and psychologically appropriate teaching regimen would appear necessary for most children and their families. Such education would relieve anxiety, which is often associated with increased pain. It could also help make parents more effective advocates in getting their children adequate and appropriate treatment. In addition to education, emotional support is often necessary for children and adults with sickle cell anemia. They have a chronic illness that is fraught with unpredictable episodes of pain that affects their growth, development, and employment opportunities. Such a situation often causes depression or anxiety, which in turn, exacerbates the pain they experience. Support groups, individual psychotherapy, and psychotropic medications should be considered as a part of their comprehensive care. The early teaching of coping skills would be a definite benefit.

Cognitive-Behavioral Techniques

It has been shown that in many situations, increasing the patient's sense of control is helpful in decreasing his or her pain. For children with sickle cell disease in particular, a pattern of learned helplessness often emerges where they feel it is not possible for them to influence the treatment or its outcome.[85] Therefore, activities that increase the child's sense of control are often helpful. One such technique tied to medical therapy is the use of patient-controlled analgesia, described in detail in another section. Another way in which patient control can be increased is through the use of behavioral contracts. Such contracts can be tailored to each patient and can lay out clearly what is expected from the child, such as practicing relaxation exercises and reporting discomfort fairly, and what can be expected from the caregivers, such as rapid response to the child's complaints of discomfort and reminders about practicing relaxation. A pain behavior contract is a treatment modality that is underused and that, particularly for adolescents, may be beneficial.[86] In addition, the use of pain diaries has been helpful in focusing families on improving pain management.[7]

HYPNOTHERAPY AND BIOFEEDBACK

Hypnoanalgesia and biofeedback have well-established efficacy in children with recurrent pain problems such as headaches. There is also evidence for their use in sickle cell disease. Zeltzer[87] described the use of hypnoanalgesia for crisis pain in 2 patients. In addition, Erikson[88] described a controlled, randomized trial of this technique. In this report, 99% of children and adolescents who used this technique reported some pain relief, whereas 56% reported almost complete pain relief, at least some of the time while using these techniques. Cozzi, Tryon, and Sedlacek found that biofeedback decreased the pain patients reported with sickle cell crises and the number of days that analgesics were taken.[89] It did not, however, influence emergency room visits or hospitalizations. These reports indicate that these techniques may be an important part of an overall approach to sickle cell disease management. Because they are noninvasive and essentially free from side effects, their use should be encouraged and further refined.[90–94]

TENS and Physical Therapy

Transcutaneous electrical nerve stimulation (TENS) units have been used for sickle cell pain. Unfortunately, the pain associated with vasoocclusive episodes is often widespread, and TENS units tend to be more effective when used on more localized musculoskeletal pain problems. In one double-blind crossover study on the use of TENS for sickle cell patients, methodological problems precluded an adequate appreciation of its beneficial effect.[58,95] The authors suggested that no substantial benefit from a TENS unit could be demonstrated on pain ratings, but three-fourths of the patients did believe that it was helpful. Physical therapy techniques (eg, exercise, splinting, local application of heat, and so on) also clearly have a role in the treatment of vasoocclusive episodes.

Medical Report Passport System

It has been reported that emergency department personnel often disbelieve the pain reported by children and adults with sickle cell disease.[56,96–98] As a result, these patients are not given adequate analgesia in the emergency department, which leads them to become increasingly melodramatic in displaying their pain to get an effective response. This increased melodrama further convinces the medical staff that these patients are not really experiencing pain but are, in fact, merely drug seeking. This cycle has the potential for creating increased learned helplessness as well as frustration and anger on the part of the patients.[99] Ballas[100–103] has reported on the use of a small plasticized information card that patients with sickle cell disease can carry, with their name, diagnosis, previous complications, and usual pain treatment, both inpatient and outpatient. Such a technique may be helpful in streamlining care and decrease the frustration and tension that this disease produces in both patients and health care providers.[104]

PHARMACOLOGIC APPROACHES

General

Therapy with analgesics can and should be individualized for each patient, but there are certain guiding principles of therapy.[105,106] A stepwise escalating analgesic ladder, much like the one proposed by the World Health Organization for cancer pain, should be used to determine the sequence of analgesic administration for sickle cell patients.[107,108] Nonopioid, peripherally acting agents such as acetaminophen or a nonsteroidal anti-inflammatory drug (NSAID) usually suffice for mild pain. When pain persists or intensifies, addition of an oral opioid analgesic, such as oxycodone or hydrocodone, is usually adequate. The severe pain crises are more challenging to manage. In these instances, potent opioids, administered intravenously or peridurally, can be combined with acetaminophen or an NSAID to provide the level of analgesia needed to control the painful episode. Adjuvants may be added as necessary (Table 33.3).

Nonopioid Analgesics

These include acetaminophen, NSAIDs, topicals, tramadol, and corticosteroids. NSAIDs and acetaminophen may be the drugs of choice, in general, for mild to moderate pain of any etiology.[109] It is unclear how applicable these analgesics are to sickle cell crisis pain, which is often more pronounced in nature. However, these drugs are still invariably the first line of therapy, particularly at home, for the patient with sickle cell anemia, in the initial stages of a crisis.[110,111] Some of the dose-limiting concerns with toxicity are outlined in the accompanying table.

Acetaminophen has analgesic and antipyretic effects but no anti-inflammatory properties. It does have a ceiling effect, a dose above which there is no additive analgesic effect. The maximal daily dose should not exceed 4 g in adults and about 90 mg/kg in children. Higher doses can be toxic to the liver. It is available in combination forms with opioids such as hydrocodone and oxycodone.[112]

NSAIDs include nonselective cyclooxygenase (COX) inhibitors and selective (celecoxib) or partially selective (meloxicam) COX-2 inhibitors. They have an anti-inflammatory component, in addition to their analgesic and antipyretic potential. They also have a ceiling effect above which no further analgesia is obtained and the risk of side effects is increased. If used chronically in patients with sickle cell anemia, the risks of analgesic nephropathy, gastropathy, and hemostatic defects become a concern. COX-2 inhibitors cause significantly fewer gastrointestinal and hemostatic adverse effects, but their effect on renal function is about the same as that of the nonselective NSAIDs.[113] The COX2 inhibitors (coxibs) are useful in these patients in the initial and ending stages of a crisis or even as maintenance therapy. Finally, parenteral nonsteroidals have now become available.[114–118] Ketorolac (Toradol) is approved by the Food and Drug Adminstration for intramuscular and intravenous use in children over 2 years of age and adults for pain management. Although multidose treatment is recommended for only up to 72 hours, it is suggested that one use the lowest effective dose for the shortest duration. Even in adults, treatment with NSAIDs is not recommended for longer than 5 days. Parenteral NSAIDs are definitely an option for inpatient treatment. The concomitant administration of ketorolac with opioids is reported to exert

Table 33.3: Analgesic Management of Sickle Cell Disease Pain

Analgesics for Mild Pain

Drug	Equianalgesic Dose (mg)	Pediatric Dose (mg/kg/dose)	Comments
Acetaminophen	650	10	Minimal anti-inflammatory properties
Aspirin	650	10	Gastritis, antiplatelet effects
Choline magnesium trisalicylate	650	10	Gastritis, usually no antiplatelet effects
Codeine	30–60	0.5–1	Weak opioid, dose-limiting nausea and vomiting; CYP450 metabolism
Ibuprofen/naproxen	400	5–10	Gastritis, antiplatelet effect, hepatic or renal dysfunction

Analgesics for Moderate to Severe Pain

Drug	Dose	Equianalgesic Oral Dose	Pediatric Dose	
Ketorolac	30 mg	30 mg	0.25–0.5 mg/kg IV every 6 hours	Can be given orally 20–30 mg PO every 4–6 hours
Tramadol	50–100 mg		1.0 mg/kg/dose	Every 6 hours

Opioid Analgesics for Moderate to Severe Pain

Drug	Equianalgesic Parenteral Dose	Equianalgesic Oral Dose	Pediatric Doses	Pediatric infusion or Oral Doses
Fentanyl	100 μg	10–15 μg/kg	1–2 μg/kg IV every 1 hour	2–4 μg/kg/hr IV
Hydromorphone	2 mg	10 mg	0.02 mg/kg IV every 3 hours	0.1 mg/kg PO q3h
Meperidine	75 mg	300 mg	0.8–1.0 mg/kg IV every 2 hours 0.8–1.3 mg/kg SC every 3 hours	3–4 mg/kg PO q3h
Methadone	10 mg	20 mg	0.1 mg/kg IV every 12 hours	0.1–0.2 mg/kg PO every 12 hours
Morphine	10 mg	30–60 mg	0.08–0.1 mg/kg IV every 2 hours	0.02–0.05 mg/kg/h IV 0.2–0.4 mg/kg PO every 3 hours
Oxycodone		5 mg (available in various combinations with NSAIDs)	0.1–0.2 mg/kg PO every 4 hours	

The reader should also refer to American Pain Society Guidelines for opioid management of sickle cell pain (http://www.ampainsoc.org/pub/sc. htm) and analgesic guidelines for managing acute sickle cell crisis published in British Journal of Haematology (http://pt.wkhealth.com/pt/re/ bjha/fulltext 00002328-200510010-00019.htm). Abbreviations: IV = intravenously; SC = subcutaneously; PO = per os.

an additive analgesic effect and have opioid-sparing properties. In one study, intramuscularly administered ketorolac provided pain relief comparable to meperidine during sickle cell vasooc-clusive crises. This drug certainly has applicability in children and adolescents in whom there is a concern regarding the use of opioids.[119–121]

Tramadol is a synthetic, centrally acting analgesic, not chemically related to opioids that exerts some of its effects through the μ-receptor.[122] It also stimulates the release of serotonin and inhibits reuptake of both serotonin and norepinephrine, thus displaying the functional properties of an opioid and an antidepressant. It is available in oral form alone in the United States, but a parenteral form is being used in Europe and other countries. A long-acting oral form is also available worldwide. It can be used to manage mild and moderately severe sickle cell pain, but it can lower the seizure threshold that can cause problems in some patients.[114,118] There are concerns about its abuse potential, but tramadol is currently a nonscheduled drug.

OPIOIDS

Many of the opioid agonists, partial agonists, and mixed agonist-antagonists can be used effectively to treat moderate or severe pain in sickle cell disease. They can be administered orally, sub-cutaneously, intramuscularly, intravenously, transdermally and by a patient-controlled pump.[123] Codeine and hydrocodone are opioids that are most commonly employed in the outpatient setting for moderately painful episodes. These two agents carry a fairly high incidence of nausea, vomiting, constipation, and sedation and thus exhibit a relative ceiling effect, which limits their use for severe pain. There are several fixed-ratio preparations with either of these two opioids combined with acetaminophen. Codeine may not be an ideal opioid choice, because it requires sufficient presence of the CYP2D6 isozyme of the P450 cytochrome hepatic enzyme system to undergo conversion to morphine, its active analgesic moiety.[124–126] Oral oxy-codone either alone or in combination with acetaminophen or ibuprofen is an attractive oral opioid. Its potency and formulations permit small volume or tablet dosing.

Meperidine, morphine, and hydromorphone are the major parenteral opioid agonists used. Meperidine may still be the most widely employed potent opioid in patients with sickle cell anemia, especially in adult care.[127] There are, however, several reasons why this drug is an extremely poor choice in these patients. Meperidine, which is often administered on an 4–6 hourly basis, actually has a half-life of about 3 hours, very similar to that of morphine. More importantly, however, is the fact that this drug is metabolized to normeperidine, which has a half-life of 18 hours and is a central nervous system stimulant without analgesic activity.[128–132] When this metabolite accumulates, it can cause nervousness, tremors, myoclonus, and seizures. The effects of meperidine and normeperidine on seizure induction are more pronounced in the presence of renal disease.[133,134] Meperidine kinetics may also be different in sickle cell patients. In fact, blood levels measured using otherwise standard doses seem to be subtherapeutic in sickle cell patients. These observations may account for the poor pain control with meperidine when it is employed in acute sickle cell crisis pain. Finally, there is no direct evidence that meperidine poses a smaller addiction potential than other potent opioids such as morphine. These issues have led to a shift in choice of opioids to morphine and hydromorphone.[135] Fentanyl is anther opioid that is also available in parenteral, transdermal, and transmucosal formulations. It may be very useful in patients with intractable pruritis from the other opioids.

The mixed agonist-antagonist opioid compounds are attractive alternatives for pain management. These agents, such as butorphanol or buprenorphine, may cause less respiratory depression and may result in slower onset of tolerance and physical dependence.[136–141] However, these advantages become apparent only at the very highest analgesic doses, which approach the "ceiling" analgesia characteristic of these agents. There is only limited experience with these agents in sickle cell anemia, and their future role in managing these patients remains to be determined.

Opioid antagonists are often used to counteract some of the troubling side effects of opioid agonists. There have been recent reports that small doses of antagonists in combination with agonists enhance the analgesic effect and prevent or delay tolerance to opioid agonists.[144,145] In addition, troubling pruritis can be treated with low-dose agonist-antagonist or pure antagonist therapy.[144,145] We prefer intravenous nalmefene (0.25–0.5 μg/kg every 8 hours) or naloxone (0.5–2 μg/kg/h) by continuous infusion.

One can successfully manage even severe painful sickle cell episodes by becoming familiar with a limited number of opioid analgesics.[146–152] There are, however, important limitations that should be considered in sickle cell patients.[153,154] Opioids have no ceiling effect (with the exception of codeine or the partial/mixed agonists-antagonists). They are also histaminergic, which can trigger bronchospasm, allergic reactions, or intractable pruritis.[155] However, it is important to remember that most sickle cell patients in crisis will require larger doses than the average population because of the high pain intensity of a crisis, accelerated renal clearance and hepatic metabolism in some, and possible pharmacologic tolerance.[151,156–158]

Opioid therapy hence should be aggressive in sickle cell patients. The usual routes of administration are applicable in the patient with sickle cell anemia.[159] It is essential to remember that children find intramuscular or subcutaneous administration of

analgesics rather unpleasant, and these routes of administration should be avoided if at all possible.[19] Furthermore, because aggressive hydration is invariably a part of the management of a painful crisis, intravenous access is usually present in all inpatients, and should be preferentially employed for analgesic administration.[160]

In the outpatient setting, knowledge of equianalgesic oral and parenteral doses of the opioids is essential so that they can be administered effectively.[161] A well-informed physician can manage vaso-occlusive episodes in a cooperative and compliant patient successfully, sometimes even avoiding the need for repeated hospitalization.[162–164] Both Powers and Friedman have reported on the relative effectiveness of orally administered potent opioids in treating sickle cell pain episodes.[165] In addition, as experience with and availability of long-acting narcotic preparations such as MS-contin and oxycontin has increased, it has become clear these drugs also play a critical role in pain management in this population. Methadone is another long-acting opioid that can be used for maintenance therapy. With its long half-life and slow onset to peak effect, it can substitute for other long-acting preparations in combination with short-acting opioids in selected patients. It can cause QTc prolongation in some patients.[166,167]

When opioids are employed in the hospital, an effective regimen should be developed for each individual patient.[168] One should not make assumptions or generalizations. Nonindividualized care can lead to oversedation of an opioid-naïve patient or under treatment of a patient tolerant to them. In the face of a history of nonresponsiveness to a particular drug, one should try a different one.[169–172] In the older child, adolescent, and adults, patient-controlled analgesia (PCA) may be the method of choice for drug delivery.[173–175] If this is not used, intravenous therapy that avoids swings with analgesic peaks and troughs should be the next option. The use of continuous infusions of opioids, such as morphine or hydromorphone, has many advantages over more traditional intermittent bolus therapy. Pharmacologically, the peaks and troughs that correlate both with analgesic and toxic effects are avoided. This technique or PCA also allow for rapid titration to analgesia. In addition, these dosing methods bypass the required dependency on nursing staff that traditional bolus administration carries. Experience with continuous infusion narcotics has broadened, making it the recommended route of delivery for patients with severe vasoocclusive pain. Guidelines for pharmacological management are presented in Table 33.3.

Patient-Controlled Analgesia in Sickle Cell Disease

Studies have demonstrated that PCA can provide safe and effective postoperative pain relief for children as young as 5 years of age.[176,177] Its usefulness in sickle cell disease, seems obvious. PCA allows patients to administer their own analgesics without being dependant on the health care providers, thus decreasing the potential for conflict and mistrust. It gives them an increased sense of control over their care, which may ameliorate some of the learned helplessness that often accompanies this disease. In comparison to intermittent bolus administration, it allows for the almost instantaneous treatment of discomfort, thus decreasing the amount of time the patient is uncomfortable and potentially decreasing the amount of analgesics that are required to eliminate pain.[178–184]

Available literature strongly indicates that significantly higher doses of opioids may be necessary for relief of vasoocclusive crisis pain as compared to the doses necessary for relief of postoperative pain. In Shapiro's work, an average continuous infusion was 0.04 mg/kg/h with an average bolus dose of 0.05 mg/kg. The average maximal opioid dose (sum of the continuous infusion and bolus dose) on the worst day was 0.1 mg/kg/h, which was approximately twice the typical dose one would use either with a PCA or with a continuous infusion for routine postoperative pain. Shapiro suggests that a continuous infusion should be relied on less for these patients for fear of respiratory depression and reports of increased acute chest syndrome that correlates with opioid use.[185,186] It has been the experience of others, however, that without the use of a continuous infusion, the patients are constantly pushing the button for inadequate pain relief and trying to catch up. These issues clearly require further study. For the present, it seems reasonable to start out with a continuous basal infusion of 0.02 mg/kg/h with a bolus dose of approximately 0.02–0.03 mg/kg. An average lockout period would be 6–8 minutes with an hourly maximum dose of close to 0.1–0.2 mg/kg. The doses would obviously need to be titrated to effect and increased rapidly, if necessary. In summary, patient-controlled analgesia seems to be a helpful modality for use in children and adolescents in sickle cell crisis. Controversies regarding how to most effectively use this modality require further clarification.

Regional Techniques in Pain Management

The use of regional anesthetic techniques has not been formally studied in children with sickle cell disease, but they offer significant theoretic advantages for a select group of these patients. The use of sympathetic blockade to increase blood flow to localized affected areas during a crisis and use of epidural or other regional anesthetic techniques for pain relief appear advantageous. There has been only a few reports of the use of these techniques in sickle cell disease, including a pregnant woman in crisis and several children with chest or abdominal pain.[187–190] There is, however, a broader clinical experience with these techniques than the published literature would indicate. Yaster et al[190] reported on 9 children with 11 vasoocclusive crises, who were treated with epidural analgesia as part of their pain management. Following initial treatment with opioids, NSAIDs, and other adjunctive medications with pain scores of 8–10 on a 10-point scale, these patients received epidurals that resulted in immediate relief of pain with improvement in pain scores to 0–2. Incidentally the SpO_2 increased in 7 of these patients from the mid-1980s to >95%. Clearly these techniques do offer great promise to patients with localized pain in a sickle cell crisis, such as in the lower extremities, abdomen, or chest.[191] They are also useful in those who have problems tolerating systemic opioids in higher doses. However, one has to be cognizant of the fact that when epidural blocks set up, the redistribution of blood flow may lead to transient hypotension that could produce low flow states predisposing to infarction.

Adjuvants

These include antihistamines, antidepressants, benzodiazepines, anticonvulsants, α agonists, and corticosteroids.[192,193] Some of these potentiate the analgesic effects of opioids, treat side effects, and may have their own mild analgesic effect.

Steroids have a limited role. Although they reduce opioid requirement and the duration of analgesic treatment, they also lead to an increase in the rate of rebound attacks. This, with the fear of the long-term complications of steroid therapy has discouraged the use of this treatment strategy.[194,195]

Chronic pain is often accompanied by mood disorders and psychiatric comorbidities that are not uncommon in sickle cell patients.[196,197] A long history of recurrent pain and inadequate treatment can generate feelings of anxiety or depression that can escalate during a painful crisis. These patients can also exhibit aberrant drug-related behaviors that might actually represent an expression of fear or anger or an unsuccessful attempt at coping with a chronic illness. They may use opioids or alcohol in an attempt to lessen anxiety, panic, depression, or insomnia. It is beneficial for sickle cell patients with recurrent pain problems to get involved in a multidisciplinary chronic pain program, thus allowing them the opportunity to get familiar with a physician and psychologist that follows them on a long-term basis. For some, psychiatric consultation may be warranted. In the presence of comorbid conditions, treatment with a tricyclic antidepressant, selective serotonin reuptake inhibitor, or other mood stabilizers may be of benefit.

Gabapentin and other anticonvulsants may be of benefit if there is a suspicion of neuropathic pain in the extremities caused by repeated vasoocclusive episodes.

CHRONIC SICKLE CELL PAIN

Patients with chronic sickle cell pain and those with recurrent acute episodes are best managed with a combination of long-acting opioids and a short-acting opioid for breakthrough pain. We believe that this approach with the active involvement of a team of providers helps decrease the frequency of admissions to the hospital. Emotional distress and behavioral dysfunction are associated with chronic sickle cell pain syndrome, which is often the most difficult to treat. A patient with a chronic pain syndrome maintained on long-acting opioids may develop an acute painful episode over and above the chronic pain. The opioids then need to be escalated to very clinically effective levels to get pain relief and, even then, may not be fully efficacious. The pathophysiology of this chronic pain syndrome is unclear but may be related to central sensitization, a situation where repeated and frequent painful stimuli lower the pain threshold to a point where innocuous stimuli can cause severe pain. Chronic use of high-dose opioids can also result in the phenomenon of hyperalgesia, which is only made worse by the progressive escalation of opioids during an acute episode.[198] These patients are extremely difficult and challenging. It has now been proposed that ketamine is a good choice in treating pain associated with hyperalgesia.[199,200]

BARRIERS TO ADEQUATE TREATMENT

Pediatric pain management has, in the past, been less than adequate in most clinical situations. The reasons for this are complex but essentially revolve around various myths and misconceptions about childrens' perception of pain and inadequate knowledge on the part of health care providers about how to use the available techniques in an effective manner.[201] In addition to these preexisting problems, sickle cell disease brings with it several other unique complexities. The ethnocultural discordance between health care providers and sickle cell patients has created a difficult situation. As a result of ill-founded preconceived notions of drug-seeking behavior in African American

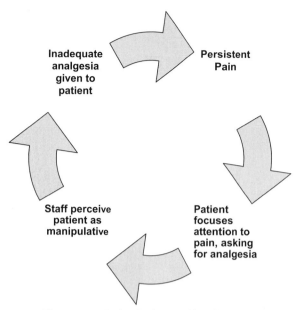

Figure 33.1: Cycle of pain in sickle cell anemia.

Table 33.4: Causes for Inadequate Analgesia

Insufficient knowledge

Medical staff values about the disease

Inadequate pain assessment tools

Fears of addiction/drug abuse

adolescents, many health care providers may be reluctant to administer appropriate doses of opioid analgesics to these patients. However, because of their persistent and often under-treated pain, these patients often develop what is perceived by medical staff as manipulative or clock-watching behavior or pseudoaddiction. Both of these behavior patterns reinforce for the medical staff their previously held notions, and the cycle continues (Figure 33.1).

There are no available data on addiction in patients with sickle cell disease. However, it has been found that physicians and nurses both tend to overestimate the prevalence of addiction in this population.[202–205] The available information in other illnesses that have a chronic pain component, such as cancer, indicates that addiction is a minor problem. Sickle cell patients, however, come with a lifelong history of often inadequate care, a sense of inability to influence the quality of their care, and a life punctuated by unpredictable painful crises, therefore representing a unique problem. Payne,[56] at the University of Cincinnati Comprehensive Sickle Cell Center, has identified approximately 9% of his patients in whom opioid use is problematic. These are either patients who have had a history of drug abuse, have been known to tamper with drug-delivery pumps, or have been involved in illegal drug activity, such as selling prescription drugs or street drugs. Other authors, such as Vichinsky et al[19] and Brozovic et al,[206] report a smaller incidence of this problem. Despite the fact that a relatively small percentage of sickle cell patients have had a history of problems with opioids, there is the perception that there is widespread drug abuse in this population. This perception has negatively influenced aggressive pain management in sickle cell disease (Table 33.4).[207,208]

There are few articles in the literature that report on randomized clinical trials for pain management in sickle cell disease comparing the efficacy of different drug regimens or of different routes of administration in these patients. The American Pain Society (APS) published an evidence-based guideline for pain management in sickle cell disease, *Guideline for the Management of Acute and Chronic Pain in Sickle Cell Disease.*[209] The APS guideline does address sickle cell patients' requests for specific medications and doses. It also recognizes that sickle cell patients and parents are typically very knowledgeable about the medications and dosages that have worked for them in the past, so requests for specific medications at specific dosages alone should not be considered an indicator of drug-seeking behavior. The guideline also addresses tolerance and recommends increasing dosages and shortening intervals between doses as appropriate adjustments to overcome tolerance.

HOW WE MANAGE SICKLE CELL PATIENTS IN OUR PRACTICE

The physician's responsibility is to treat all patients in pain with compassion and avoid causing harm. Patients with sickle cell disease, especially older ones, may have experienced numerous pain crises with inconsistent and often inadequate treatment. Patients that are followed by our pain management service are encouraged to call in during the beginning stages of a crisis and supportive therapy is initiated at home with attempts to keep them out of the hospital. This might include medication management in the form of NSAIDs and opioids. When this is unsuccessful, as in more severe or advanced stages of a crisis, the patients present to the emergency room. Management invariably entails intravenous opioids and NSAIDs, either with or without continuation of the patient's home regimen. The choice of analgesic, dose, and route of administration is often influenced by prior experience with a given patient. Periodic assessment continues with rating of pain as the crisis progresses. We have a readily available database that is on the desktop of our institution's multiple personal computers. As a backup, there is a binder in the emergency department with pertinent disease and analgesic parameters for all of our program's known sickle cell patients. This allows interventions and modifications of the treatment plan to take place rapidly and efficiently. We begin PCA in the ED and thereby avoid the delay in pump procurement and setup on the inpatient units. Patients in true crises remain on parenteral analgesics via PCA until the crisis abates and are then transitioned over to oral pain medications. We commonly discharge patients, after vasoocclusive crisis, on long-acting opioids with breakthrough immediate-release medications based on their in-hospital use. Patients are encouraged to follow up with the chronic pain and sickle cell programs on a regular basis.

REFERENCES

1. Nagel RL, Fabry ME, Billett HH, Kaul DK. Sickle cell painful crisis: a multifactorial event. *Prog Clin Biol Res.* 1987;361–380.
2. Noguchi CT, Torchia DA, Schechter AN. Intracellular polymerization of sickle hemoglobin: effects of cell heterogeneity. *J Clin Invest.* 1983;72:846–852.

3. Baez S, Kaul DK, Nagel RL. Microvascular determinants of blood flow behavior and HbSS erythrocyte plugging in microcirculation. *Blood Cells*. 1982;8:127–137.

4. Hebbel RP. Extracorpuscular factors in the pathogenesis of sickle cell disease. *Am J Pediatr Hematol Oncol*. 1982;4:316–319.

5. Kaul DK, Fabry ME, Windisch P, Baez S, Nagel RL. Erythrocytes in sickle cell anemia are heterogeneous in their rheological and hemodynamic characteristics. *J Clin Invest*. 1983;72:22–31.

6. Chiang EY, Frenette PS. Sickle cell vaso-occlusion. *Hematol Oncol Clin North Am*. 2005;19:771–884.

7. Dampier C, Ely E, Eggleston B, Brodecki D, O'Neal P. Physical and cognitive-behavioral activities used in the home management of sickle pain: a daily diary study in children and adolescents. *Pediatr Blood Cancer*. 2004;43:674–678.

8. Elion JE, Brun M, Odievre MH, Lapoumeroulie CL, Krishnamoorthy R. Vaso-occlusion in sickle cell anemia: role of interactions between blood cells and endothelium. *Hematol J*. 2004;5(suppl 3):195–198.

9. Okpala I. Leukocyte adhesion and the pathophysiology of sickle cell disease. *Curr Opin Hematol*. 2006;13:40–44.

10. Okpala I. The intriguing contribution of white blood cells to sickle cell disease – a red cell disorder. *Blood Rev*. 2004;18:65–73.

11. Schnog JB, Mac Gillavry MR, van Zanten AP, et al. Protein C and S and inflammation in sickle cell disease. *Am J Hematol*. 2004;76:26–32.

12. Dover GJ, Charache S. The effect of increased fetal hemoglobin production on the frequency of vaso-occlusive crisis in sickle cell disease. *Prog Clin Biol Res*. 1987;240:277–285.

13. Vichinsky EP, Lubin BH. Sickle cell anemia and related hemoglobinopathies. *Pediatr Clin North Am*. 1980;27:429–447.

14. Almeida A, Roberts I. Bone involvement in sickle cell disease. *Br J Haematol*. 2005;129:482–490.

15. Ejindu VC, Hine AL, Mashayekhi M, Shorvon PJ, Misra RR. Musculoskeletal manifestations of sickle cell disease. *Radiographics*. 2007;27:1005–1021.

16. Onuba O. Bone disorders in sickle-cell disease. *Int Orthop*. 1993;17:397–399.

17. Kim SK, Miller JH. Natural history and distribution of bone and bone marrow infarction in sickle hemoglobinopathies. *J Nucl Med*. 2002;43:896–900.

18. Shapiro B, Dinges DF, Orne EC. Recording of crisis pain in sickle cell disease. *Adv Pain Res Ther*. 1990;313–321.

19. Vichinsky EP, Johnson R, Lubin BH. Multidisciplinary approach to pain management in sickle cell disease. *Am J Pediatr Hematol Oncol*. 1982;4:328–333.

20. Rao KR, Patel AR, Shah PC, Vohra RM. Sickle cell dactylitis. *Arch Intern Med*. 1980;140:439.

21. Worrall VT, Butera V. Sickle-cell dactylitis. *J Bone Joint Surg Am*. 1976;58:1161–1163.

22. Stevens MC, Padwick M, Serjeant GR. Observations on the natural history of dactylitis in homozygous sickle cell disease. *Clin Pediatr (Phila)*. 1981;20:311–317.

23. Watson RJ, Burko H, Megas H, Robinson M. The handfoot syndrome in sickle-cell disease in young children. *Pediatrics*. 1963;31:975–982.

24. Foucan L, Ekouevi D, Etienne-Julan M, Salmi LR, Diara JP. Early onset dactylitis associated with the occurrence of severe events in children with sickle cell anaemia. The Paediatric Cohort of Guadeloupe (1984–99). *Paediatr Perinat Epidemiol*. 2006;20:59–66.

25. Lutzker LG, Alavi A. Bone and marrow imaging in sickle cell disease: diagnosis of infarction. *Semin Nucl Med*. 1976;6:83–93.

26. Mankad VN, Williams JP, Harpen MD, et al. Magnetic resonance imaging of bone marrow in sickle cell disease: clinical, hematologic, and pathologic correlations. *Blood*. 1990;75:274–283.

27. Rao VM, Fishman M, Mitchell DG, et al. Painful sickle cell crisis: bone marrow patterns observed with MR imaging. *Radiology*. 1986;161:211–215.

28. Aloui N, Nessib N, Jalel C, et al. Febrile osseous pain in children with sickle cell disease: MRI findings. *J Radiol*. 2005;86:1693–1697.

29. Keeley K, Buchanan GR. Acute infarction of long bones in children with sickle cell anemia. *J Pediatr*. 1982;101:170–175.

30. Ohene-Frempong K, Weiner SJ, Sleeper LA, et al. Cerebrovascular accidents in sickle cell disease: rates and risk factors. *Blood*. 1998;91:288–294.

31. Quinn CT, Shull EP, Ahmad N, Lee NJ, Rogers ZR, Buchanan GR. Prognostic significance of early vaso-occlusive complications in children with sickle cell anemia. *Blood*. 2007;109:40–45.

32. Sarnaik SA, Ballas SK. Molecular characteristics of pediatric patients with sickle cell anemia and stroke. *Am J Hematol*. 2001;67:179–182.

33. Ballas SK. Current issues in sickle cell pain and its management. *Hematol Am Soc Hematol Educ Progr*. 2007;2007:97–105.

34. Walco GA, Dampier CD. Pain in children and adolescents with sickle cell disease: a descriptive study. *J Pediatr Psychol*. 1990;15:643–658.

35. Beyer JE, Aradine CR. Content validity of an instrument to measure young children's perceptions of the intensity of their pain. *J Pediatr Nurs*. 1986;1:386–395.

36. Szyfelbein SK, Osgood PF, Carr DB. The assessment of pain and plasma beta-endorphin immunoactivity in burned children. *Pain*. 1985;22:173–182.

37. Finley GA, McGrath PJ. Measurement of pain in infants and children. Seattle, WA: IASP Press; 1998.

38. Manworren RC, Hynan LS. Clinical validation of FLACC: preverbal patient pain scale. *Pediatr Nurs*. 2003;29:140–146.

39. Grunau RV, Craig KD. Pain expression in neonates: facial action and cry. *Pain*. 1987;28:395–410.

40. Katz ER, Kellerman J, Siegel SE. Behavioral distress in children with cancer undergoing medical procedures: developmental considerations. *J Consult Clin Psychol*. 1980;48:356–365.

41. Dampier C, Ely E, Brodecki D, O'Neal P. Home management of pain in sickle cell disease: a daily diary study in children and adolescents. *J Pediatr Hematol Oncol*. 2002;24:643–647.

42. Dampier C, Ely B, Brodecki D, O'Neal P. Characteristics of pain managed at home in children and adolescents with sickle cell disease by using diary self-reports. *J Pain*. 2002;3:461–470.

43. Thomas VJ, Hambleton I, Serjeant G. Psychological distress and coping in sickle cell disease: comparison of British and Jamaican attitudes. *Ethn Health*. 2001;6:129–136.

44. Luffy R, Grove SK. Examining the validity, reliability, and preference of three pediatric pain measurement tools in African-American children. *Pediatr Nurs*. 2003;29:54–59.

45. Johnson CS. The acute chest syndrome. *Hematol Oncol Clin North Am*. 2005;19:857,79, vi–vii.

46. McGrath PA. Pain in the pediatric patient: practical aspects of assessment. *Pediatr Ann*. 1995;24:126, 33, 137–138.

47. McGrath PA. Psychological aspects of pain perception. *Arch Oral Biol*. 1994;39(suppl):55S–62S.

48. McGrath PA. Evaluating a child's pain. *J Pain Symptom Manage*. 1989;4:198–214.

49. Varni JW, Thompson KL, Hanson V. The Varni/Thompson Pediatric Pain Questionnaire. I. Chronic musculoskeletal pain in juvenile rheumatoid arthritis. *Pain*. 1987;28:27–38.

50. Powars DR, Chan LS, Hiti A, Ramicone E, Johnson C. Outcome of sickle cell anemia: a 4-decade observational study of 1056 patients. *Medicine (Baltimore)*. 2005;84:363–376.

51. McGrath PA. The multidimensional assessment and management of recurrent pain syndromes in children. *Behav Res Ther*. 1987;25:251–262.

52. McGrath PA, Speechley KN, Seifert CE, et al. A survey of children's acute, recurrent, and chronic pain: validation of the pain experience interview. *Pain*. 2000;87:59–73.

53. McGrath PJ, Johnson GG. Pain management in children. *Can J Anaesth*. 1988;35:107–110.

54. Miller ST, Sleeper LA, Pegelow CH, et al. Prediction of adverse outcomes in children with sickle cell disease. *N Engl J Med*. 2000;342:83–89.

55. Raphael RI. Pathophysiology and treatment of sickle cell disease. *Clin Adv Hematol Oncol*. 2005;3:492–505.

56. Payne R. Pain management in sickle cell disease: rationale and techniques. *Ann N Y Acad Sci*. 1989;565:189–206.

57. Buckalew V Jr, Someren A. Renal manifestations of sickle cell disease. *Arch Intern Med*. 1974;133:660–669.

58. Alcorn R, Bowser B, Henley EJ, Holloway V. Fluidotherapy and exercise in the management of sickle cell anemia: a clinical report. *Phys Ther*. 1984;64:1520–1522.

59. Okomo U, Meremikwu MM. Fluid replacement therapy for acute episodes of pain in people with sickle cell disease. *Cochrane Database Syst Rev*. 2007;2:CD005406.

60. Embury SH, Garcia JF, Mohandas N, Pennathur-Das R, Clark MR. Effects of oxygen inhalation on endogenous erythropoietin kinetics, erythropoiesis, and properties of blood cells in sickle-cell anemia. *N Engl J Med*. 1984;311:291–295.

61. Schulman LL. Oxygen therapy in sickle-cell anemia. *N Engl J Med*. 1984;311:1319–1320.

62. Zipursky A, Robieux IC, Brown EJ, et al. Oxygen therapy in sickle cell disease. *Am J Pediatr Hematol Oncol*. 1992;14:222–228.

63. Miller ST, Wright E, Abboud M, et al. Impact of chronic transfusion on incidence of pain and acute chest syndrome during the Stroke Prevention Trial (STOP) in sickle-cell anemia. *J Pediatr*. 2001;139:785–789.

64. Thurston GB, Henderson NM, Jeng M. Effects of erythrocytapheresis transfusion on the viscoelasticity of sickle cell blood. *Clin Hemorheol Microcirc*. 2004;30:83–97.

65. Vichinsky EP, Earles A, Johnson RA, Hoag MS, Williams A, Lubin B. Alloimmunization in sickle cell anemia and transfusion of racially unmatched blood. *N Engl J Med*. 1990;322:1617–1621.

66. Fung EB, Harmatz P, Milet M, et al. Morbidity and mortality in chronically transfused subjects with thalassemia and sickle cell disease: a report from the multi-center study of iron overload. *Am J Hematol*. 2007;82:255–265.

67. Vichinsky EP, Neumayr LD, Earles AN, et al. Causes and outcomes of the acute chest syndrome in sickle cell disease: National Acute Chest Syndrome Study Group. *N Engl J Med*. 2000;342:1855–1865.

68. Benjamin LJ, Berkowitz LR, Orringer E, et al. A collaborative, double-blind randomized study of cetiedil citrate in sickle cell crisis. *Blood*. 1986;67:1442–1447.

69. Temple JD, Harrington WJ, Ahn YS, Rosenfeld E. Treatment of sickle cell disease with danazol. *J Fla Med Assoc*. 1986;73:847–848.

70. Goldberg MA, Brugnara C, Dover GJ, Schapira L, Charache S, Bunn HF. Treatment of sickle cell anemia with hydroxyurea and erythropoietin. *N Engl J Med*. 1990;323:366–372.

71. Goldberg MA, Brugnara C, Dover GJ, Schapira L, Lacroix L, Bunn HF. Hydroxyurea and erythropoietin therapy in sickle cell anemia. *Semin Oncol*. 1992;19:74–81.

72. Ballas SK, Dover GJ, Charache S. Effect of hydroxyurea on the rheological properties of sickle erythrocytes in vivo. *Am J Hematol*. 1989;32:104–111.

73. Charache S, Dover GJ, Moore RD, et al. Hydroxyurea: effects on hemoglobin F production in patients with sickle cell anemia. *Blood*. 1992;79:2555–2565.

74. Charache S, Terrin ML, Moore RD, et al. Effect of hydroxyurea on the frequency of painful crises in sickle cell anemia: Investigators of the Multicenter Study of Hydroxyurea in Sickle Cell Anemia. *N Engl J Med*. 1995;332:1317–1322.

75. Dover GJ, Charache S. Stimulation of fetal hemoglobin production by hydroxyurea in sickle cell anemia. *Prog Clin Biol Res*. 1989;316B:295–306.

76. Dover GJ, Charache S. Chemotherapy and hemoglobin F synthesis in sickle cell disease. *Ann N Y Acad Sci*. 1989;565:222–227.

77. Dover GJ, Charache S, Boyer SH, Vogelsang G, Moyer M. 5-Azacytidine increases HbF production and reduces anemia in sickle cell disease: dose-response analysis of subcutaneous and oral dosage regimens. *Blood*. 1985;66:527–532.

78. Moore RD, Charache S, Terrin ML, Barton FB, Ballas SK. Cost-effectiveness of hydroxyurea in sickle cell anemia: Investigators of the Multicenter Study of Hydroxyurea in Sickle Cell Anemia. *Am J Hematol*. 2000;64:26–31.

79. Steinberg MH, Lu ZH, Barton FB, Terrin ML, Charache S, Dover GJ. Fetal hemoglobin in sickle cell anemia: determinants of response to hydroxyurea. Multicenter Study of Hydroxyurea. *Blood*. 1997;89:1078–1088.

80. Vichinsky EP, Lubin BH. A cautionary note regarding hydroxyurea in sickle cell disease. *Blood*. 1994;83:1124–1128.

81. Ren H, Obike I, Okpala I, Ghebremeskel K, Ugochukwu C, Crawford M. Steady-state haemoglobin level in sickle cell anaemia increases with an increase in erythrocyte membrane n-3 fatty acids. *Prostaglandins Leukot Essent Fatty Acids*. 2005;72:415–421.

82. Ren H, Okpala I, Ghebremeskel K, Ugochukwu CC, Ibegbulam O, Crawford M. Blood mononuclear cells and platelets have abnormal fatty acid composition in homozygous sickle cell disease. *Ann Hematol*. 2005;84:578–583.

83. Oh IH, Fabry ME, Humphries RK, et al. Expression of an anti-sickling beta-globin in human erythroblasts derived from retrovirally transduced primitive normal and sickle cell disease hematopoietic cells. *Exp Hematol*. 2004;32:461–469.

84. Mitchell MJ, Lemanek K, Palermo TM, Crosby LE, Nichols A, Powers SW. Parent perspectives on pain management, coping, and family functioning in pediatric sickle cell disease. *Clin Pediatr (Phila)*. 2007;46:311–319.

85. Shapiro BS. The management of pain in sickle cell disease. *Pediatr Clin North Am*. 1989;36:1029–1045.

86. Burghardt-Fitzgerald DC. Pain-behavior contracts: effective management of the adolescent in sickle-cell crisis. *J Pediatr Nurs*. 1989;4:320–324.

87. Zeltzer L, Dash J, Holland JP. Hypnotically induced pain control in sickle cell anemia. *Pediatrics*. 1979;64:533–536.

88. Erickson CJ. Applications of cyberphysiologic techniques in pain management. *Pediatr Ann*. 1991;20:145, 146, 148–150, 152–156.

89. Cozzi L, Tryon WW, Sedlacek K. The effectiveness of biofeedback-assisted relaxation in modifying sickle cell crises. *Biofeedback Self Regul*. 1987;12:51–61.

90. Bodhise PB, Dejoie M, Brandon Z, Simpkins S, Ballas SK. Non-pharmacologic management of sickle cell pain. *Hematology*. 2004;9:235–237.

91. Dinges DF, Whitehouse WG, Orne EC, et al. Self-hypnosis training as an adjunctive treatment in the management of pain associated with sickle cell disease. *Int J Clin Exp Hypn*. 1997;45:417–432.

92. Holbrook CT, Phillips G. Natural history of sickle cell disease and the effects on biopsychosocial development. *J Health Soc Policy*. 1994;5:7–18.

93. Jay S, Elliott CH, Fitzgibbons I, Woody P, Siegel S. A comparative study of cognitive behavior therapy versus general anesthesia for painful medical procedures in children. *Pain*. 1995;62:3–9.

94. Yoon SL, Black S. Comprehensive, integrative management of pain for patients with sickle-cell disease. *J Altern Complement Med.* 2006;12:995–1001.

95. Wang WC, George SL, Wilimas JA. Transcutaneous electrical nerve stimulation treatment of sickle cell pain crises. *Acta Haematol.* 1988;80:99–102.

96. Brookoff D, Polomano R. Treating sickle cell pain like cancer pain. *Ann Intern Med.* 1992;116:364–368.

97. Clare N. Management of sickle cell disease: management would improve if doctors listened more to patients. *BMJ.* 1998;316:935.

98. Shapiro BS, Benjamin LJ, Payne R, Heidrich G. Sickle cell-related pain: perceptions of medical practitioners. *J Pain Symptom Manage.* 1997;14:168–174.

99. Day SW. Development and evaluation of a sickle cell assessment instrument. *Pediatr Nurs.* 2004;30:451–458.

100. Ballas SK. Management of sickle pain. *Curr Opin Hematol.* 1997;4:104–111.

101. Ballas SK. Sickle cell disease: clinical management. *Clin Haematol* 1998;11:185–214.

102. Ballas SK. Ethical issues in the management of sickle cell pain. *Am J Hematol.* 2001;68:127–132.

103. Ballas SK. Pain management of sickle cell disease. *Hematol Oncol Clin North Am.* 2005;19:785, 802, v.

104. Mehta SR, Afenyi-Annan A, Byrns PJ, Lottenberg R. Opportunities to improve outcomes in sickle cell disease. *Am Fam Physician.* 2006;74:303–310.

105. Nagel RL. The challenge of painful crisis in sickle cell disease. *JAMA.* 2001;286:2152–2153.

106. Jacob E, Miaskowski C, Savedra M, Beyer JE, Treadwell M, Styles L. Management of vaso-occlusive pain in children with sickle cell disease. *J Pediatr Hematol Oncol.* 2003;25:307–311.

107. Moussavou A, Vierin Y, Eloundou-Orima C, Mboussou M, Keita M. Sickle cell disease pain management following the World Health Organization's protocol. *Arch Pediatr.* 2004;11:1041–1045.

108. Dunlop RJ, Bennett KC. Pain management for sickle cell disease. *Cochrane Database Syst Rev.* 2006;2:CD003350.

109. Agble YM. Management of sickle cell disease: non-addictive analgesics can be as effective as morphine and pethidine. *BMJ.* 1998;316:935.

110. Beyer JE, Simmons LE. Home treatment of pain for children and adolescents with sickle cell disease. *Pain Manag Nurs.* 2004;5:126–135.

111. Shapiro BS, Dinges DF, Orne EC, et al. Home management of sickle cell-related pain in children and adolescents: natural history and impact on school attendance. *Pain.* 1995;61:139–144.

112. Pollack CV Jr, Sanders DY, Severance HW Jr. Emergency department analgesia without narcotics for adults with acute sickle cell pain crisis: case reports and review of crisis management. *J Emerg Med.* 1991;9:445–452.

113. Simckes AM, Chen SS, Osorio AV, Garola RE, Woods GM. Ketorolac-induced irreversible renal failure in sickle cell disease: a case report. *Pediatr Nephrol.* 1999;13:63–67.

114. Erhan E, Inal MT, Aydinok Y, Balkan C, Yegul I. Tramadol infusion for the pain management in sickle cell disease: a case report. *Paediatr Anaesth.* 2007;17:84–86.

115. Gillis JC, Brogden RN. Ketorolac. A reappraisal of its pharmacodynamic and pharmacokinetic properties and therapeutic use in pain management. *Drugs.* 1997;53:139–188.

116. Goodman E. Use of ketorolac in sickle-cell disease and vaso-occlusive crisis. *Lancet.* 1991;338:641–642.

117. Hardwick W Jr, Givens TG, Monroe KW, King WD, Lawley D. Effect of ketorolac in pediatric sickle cell vaso-occlusive pain crisis. *Pediatr Emerg Care.* 1999;15:179–182.

118. de Franceschi L, Finco G, Vassanelli A, Zaia B, Ischia S, Corrocher R. A pilot study on the efficacy of ketorolac plus tramadol infusion combined with erythrocytapheresis in the management of acute severe vaso-occlusive crises and sickle cell pain. *Haematologica.* 2004;89:1389–1391.

119. Eke FU, Obamyonyi A, Eke NN, Oyewo EA. An open comparative study of dispersible piroxicam versus soluble acetylsalicylic acid for the treatment of osteoarticular painful attack during sickle cell crisis. *Trop Med Int Health.* 2000;5:81–84.

120. Beiter JL, Jr, Simon HK, Chambliss CR, Adamkiewicz T, Sullivan K. Intravenous ketorolac in the emergency department management of sickle cell pain and predictors of its effectiveness. *Arch Pediatr Adolesc Med.* 2001;155:496–500.

121. Perlin E, Finke H, Castro O, et al. Enhancement of pain control with ketorolac tromethamine in patients with sickle cell vaso-occlusive crisis. *Am J Hematol.* 1994;46:43–47.

122. Dayer P, Collart L, Desmeules J. The pharmacology of tramadol. *Drugs.* 1994;47:3–7.

123. Martin WR. Pharmacology of opioids. *Pharmacol Rev.* 1983;35:283–323.

124. Somogyi AA, Barratt DT, Coller JK. Pharmacogenetics of opioids. *Clin Pharmacol Ther.* 2007;81:429–444.

125. Lotsch J, Skarke C, Liefhold J, Geisslinger G. Genetic predictors of the clinical response to opioid analgesics: clinical utility and future perspectives. *Clin Pharmacokinet.* 2004;43:983–1013.

126. Brousseau DC, McCarver DG, Drendel AL, Divakaran K, Panepinto JA. The effect of CYP2D6 polymorphisms on the response to pain treatment for pediatric sickle cell pain crisis. *J Pediatr.* 2007;150:623–626.

127. Richardson P, Steingart R. Meperidine and ketorolac in the treatment of painful sickle cell crisis. *Ann Emerg Med.* 1993;22:1639–1640.

128. Kaiko RF, Foley KM, Grabinski PY, et al. Central nervous system excitatory effects of meperidine in cancer patients. *Ann Neurol.* 1983;13:180–185.

129. Meperidine usage in patients with sickle cell crisis. *Ann Emerg Med.* 1986;15:1506–1508.

130. Abbuhl S, Jacobson S, Murphy JG, Gibson G. Serum concentrations of meperidine in patients with sickle cell crisis. *Ann Emerg Med.* 1986;15:433–438.

131. Hagmeyer KO, Mauro LS, Mauro VF. Meperidine-related seizures associated with patient-controlled analgesia pumps. *Ann Pharmacother.* 1993;27:29–32.

132. Nadvi SZ, Sarnaik S, Ravindranath Y. Low frequency of meperidine-associated seizures in sickle cell disease. *Clin Pediatr (Phila).* 1999;38:459–462.

133. Szeto HH, Inturrisi CE, Houde R, Saal S, Cheigh J, Reidenberg MM. Accumulation of normeperidine, an active metabolite of meperidine, in patients with renal failure of cancer. *Ann Intern Med.* 1977;86:738–741.

134. Tang R, Shimomura S, Rotblatt M. Meperidine induced seizures in sickle cell patients. *Hosp Form.* 1980;76:764–772.

135. Perlman KM, Myers-Phariss S, Rhodes JC. A shift from demerol (meperidine) to dilaudid (hydromorphone) improves pain control and decreases admissions for patients in sickle cell crisis. *J Emerg Nurs.* 2004;30:439–446.

136. Gonzalez ER, Ornato JP, Ware D, Bull D, Evens RP. Comparison of intramuscular analgesic activity of butorphanol and morphine in patients with sickle cell disease. *Ann Emerg Med.* 1988;17:788–791.

137. Lunzer MM, Yekkirala A, Hebbel RP, Portoghese PS. Naloxone acts as a potent analgesic in transgenic mouse models of sickle cell anemia. *Proc Natl Acad Sci USA.* 2007;104:6061–6065.

138. Martin WR. Opioid antagonists. *Pharmacol Rev.* 1967;19:463–521.

139. Martin WR. Pharmacologic factors in relapse and the possible use of the narcotic antagonists in treatment. *IMJ Ill Med J.* 1966;130:489–494.

140. Romagnoli A, Keats AS. Ceiling respiratory depression by dezocine. *Clin Pharmacol Ther.* 1984;35:367–373.

141. Romagnoli A, Keats AS. Ceiling effect for respiratory depression by nalbuphine. *Clin Pharmacol Ther.* 1980;27:478–485.

142. Ballas SK. Sickle cell anaemia: progress in pathogenesis and treatment. *Drugs.* 2002;62:1143–1172.

143. Woods GM, Parson PM, Strickland DK. Efficacy of nalbuphine as a parenteral analgesic for the treatment of painful episodes in children with sickle cell disease. *J Assoc Acad Minor Phys.* 1990;1:90–92.

144. Connelly NR, Rahimi A, Parker RK. Nalmefene or naloxone for preventing intrathecal opioid mediated side effects in cesarean delivery patients. *Int J Obstet Anesth.* 1997;6:231–234.

145. Kendrick WD, Woods AM, Daly MY, Birch RFH, DiFazio C. Naloxone versus nalbuphine infusion for prophylaxis of epidural morphine-induced pruritus. *Anesth Analg.* 1996;82:641–647.

146. Dickerhoff R, von Ruecker A. Pain crises in patients with sickle cell diseases: pathogenesis, clinical aspects, therapy. *Klin Padiatr.* 1995;207:321–325.

147. Forbes K, Hanks GW, Justins DM, Cherry DA. Sickle cell pain crisis. *Lancet.* 1996;347:262.

148. Kotila TR. Management of acute painful crises in sickle cell disease. *Clin Lab Haematol.* 2005;27:221–223.

149. Meltzer BA. Sickle cell pain crisis. *Lancet.* 1996;347:262.

150. Simini B. Sickle cell pain crisis. *Lancet.* 1996;347:261–262.

151. Stinson J, Naser B. Pain management in children with sickle cell disease. *Paediatr Drugs.* 2003;5:229–241.

152. Ward SJ. Sickle cell pain crisis. *Lancet.* 1996;347:261.

153. Cole TB, Sprinkle RH, Smith SJ, Buchanan GR. Intravenous narcotic therapy for children with severe sickle cell pain crisis. *Am J Dis Child.* 1986;140:1255–1259.

154. Conti C, Tso E, Browne B. Oral morphine protocol for sickle cell crisis pain. *Md Med J.* 1996;45:33–35.

155. Wagner MC, Eckman JR, Wick TM. Histamine increases sickle erythrocyte adherence to endothelium. *Br J Haematol.* 2006;132:512–522.

156. Dunlop RJ, Bennett KC. Pain management for sickle cell disease. *Cochrane Database Syst Rev.* 2006;2:CD003350.

157. Kotila TR. Management of acute painful crises in sickle cell disease. *Clin Lab Haematol* 2005;27:221–223.

158. Shapiro BS, Cohen DE, Howe CJ. Patient-controlled analgesia for sickle-cell-related pain. *J Pain Symptom Manage.* 1993;8:22–28.

159. Ballas SK, Viscusi ER, Epstein KR. Management of acute chest wall sickle cell pain with nebulized morphine. *Am J Hematol.* 2004;76:190–191.

160. Robieux IC, Kellner JD, Coppes MJ, et al. Analgesia in children with sickle cell crisis: comparison of intermittent opioids vs. continuous intravenous infusion of morphine and placebo-controlled study of oxygen inhalation. *Pediatr Hematol Oncol.* 1992;9:317–326.

161. Jacobson SJ, Kopecky EA, Joshi P, Babul N. Randomised trial of oral morphine for painful episodes of sickle-cell disease in children. *Lancet.* 1997;350:1358–1361.

162. Dumaplin CA. Avoiding admission for afebrile pediatric sickle cell pain: pain management methods. *J Pediatr Health Care.* 2006;20:115, 122; quiz 123–125.

163. Eaton ML, Haye JS, Armstrong FD, Pegelow CH, Thomas M. Hospitalizations for painful episodes: association with school absenteeism and academic performance in children and adolescents with sickle cell anemia. *Issues Compr Pediatr Nurs.* 1995;18:1–9.

164. Epstein K, Yuen E, Riggio JM, Ballas SK, Moleski SM. Utilization of the office, hospital and emergency department for adult sickle cell patients: a five-year study. *J Natl Med Assoc.* 2006;98:1109–1113.

165. Powers RD. Management protocol for sickle-cell disease patients with acute pain: impact on emergency department and narcotic use. *Am J Emerg Med.* 1986;4:267–268.

166. Krantz MJ, Lewkowiez L, Hays H, Woodroffe MA, Robertson AD, Mehler PS. Torsade de pointes associated with very-high-dose methadone. *Ann Intern Med.* 2002;137:501–504.

167. Kornick CA, Kilborn MJ, Santiago-Palma J, et al. QTc interval prolongation associated with intravenous methadone. *Pain* 2003;105:499–506.

168. Jacob E, Miaskowski C, Savedra M, Beyer JE, Treadwell M, Styles L. Quantification of analgesic use in children with sickle cell disease. *Clin J Pain.* 2007;23:8–14.

169. Ives TJ, Guerra MF. Constant morphine infusion for severe sickle cell crisis pain. *Drug Intell Clin Pharm.* 1987;21:625–627.

170. Harrison JF, Liesner R, Davies SC. Pethidine in sickle cell crisis. *BMJ.* 1992;305:182.

171. Nagar S, Remmel RP, Hebbel RP, Zimmerman CL. Metabolism of opioids is altered in liver microsomes of sickle cell transgenic mice. *Drug Metab Dispos.* 2004;32:98–104.

172. D'Sa S, Parker N. Fast track admission for children with sickle cell crises. Opiates other than pethidine are better. *BMJ.* 1998;316:934–935.

173. Berde CB, Lehn BM, Yee JD, Sethna NF, Russo D. Patient-controlled analgesia in children and adolescents: a randomized, prospective comparison with intramuscular administration of morphine for postoperative analgesia. *J Pediatr.* 1991;118:460–466.

174. Brozovic M, Davies SC, Yardumian A, Bellingham A, Marsh G, Stephens AD. Pain relief in sickle cell crisis. *Lancet.* 1986;2:624–625.

175. McPherson E, Perlin E, Finke H, Castro O, Pittman J. Patient-controlled analgesia in patients with sickle cell vaso-occlusive crisis. *Am J Med Sci.* 1990;299:10–12.

176. McDonald AJ, Cooper MG. Patient-controlled analgesia: an appropriate method of pain control in children. *Paediatr Drugs.* 2001;3:273–284.

177. Rusy LM, Olsen DJ, Farber NE. Successful use of patient-controlled analgesia in pediatric patients 2 and 3 years old: two case reports. *Am J Anesthesiol.* 1997;14:212–214.

178. Dix HM. New advances in the treatment of sickle cell disease: focus on perioperative significance. ∗∗∗*AANA J.* 2001;69:281–286.

179. Gonzalez ER, Bahal N, Hansen LA, et al. Intermittent injection vs patient-controlled analgesia for sickle cell crisis pain: comparison in patients in the emergency department. *Arch Intern Med.* 1991;151:1373–1378.

180. Holbrook CT. Patient-controlled analgesia pain management for children with sickle cell disease. *J Assoc Acad Minor Phys.* 1990;1:93–96.

181. Melzer-Lange MD, Walsh-Kelly CM, Lea G, Hillery CA, Scott JP. Patient-controlled analgesia for sickle cell pain crisis in a pediatric emergency department. *Pediatr Emerg Care.* 2004;20:2–4.

182. Schechter NL, Berrien FB, Katz SM. PCA for adolescents in sickle-cell crisis. *Am J Nurs.* 1988;88:719, 721–722.

183. Schechter NL, Berrien FB, Katz SM. The use of patient-controlled analgesia in adolescents with sickle cell pain crisis: a preliminary report. *J Pain Symptom Manage.* 1988;3:109–113.

184. Shapiro BS, Cohen DE, Howe CJ. Patient-controlled analgesia for sickle-cell-related pain. *J Pain Symptom Manage.* 1993;8:22–28.

185. Buchanan ID, Woodward M, Reed GW. Opioid selection during sickle cell pain crisis and its impact on the development of acute chest syndrome. *Pediatr Blood Cancer.* 2005;45:716–724.

186. Kopecky EA, Jacobson S, Joshi P, Koren G. Systemic exposure to morphine and the risk of acute chest syndrome in sickle cell disease. *Clin Pharmacol Ther.* 2004;75:140–146.

187. Finer P, Blair J, Rowe P. Epidural analgesia in the management of labor pain and sickle cell crisis – a case report. *Anesthesiology.* 1988;68:799–800.

188. McHardy P, McDonnell C, Lorenzo AJ, Salle JL, Campbell FA. Management of priapism in a child with sickle cell anemia; successful outcome using epidural analgesia. *Can J Anaesth.* 2007;54:642–645.

189. Labat F, Dubousset AM, Baujard C, Wasier AP, Benhamou D, Cucchiaro G. Epidural analgesia in a child with sickle cell disease complicated by acute abdominal pain and priapism. *Br J Anaesth.* 2001;87:935–936.

190. Yaster M, Tobin JR, Billett C, Casella JF, Dover G. Epidural analgesia in the management of severe vaso-occlusive sickle cell crisis. *Pediatrics.* 1994;93:310–315.

191. McHardy P, McDonnell C, Lorenzo AJ, Salle JL, Campbell FA. Management of priapism in a child with sickle cell anemia; successful outcome using epidural analgesia. *Can J Anaesth.* 2007;54:642–645.

192. Williams RM, Moskowitz DW. The prevention of pain from sickle cell disease by trandolapril. *J Natl Med Assoc.* 2007;99:276–278.

193. Griffin TC, McIntire D, Buchanan GR. High-dose intravenous methylprednisolone therapy for pain in children and adolescents with sickle cell disease. *N Engl J Med.* 1994;330:733–737.

194. de Abood M, de Castillo Z, Guerrero F, Espino M, Austin KL. Effect of Depo-Provera or Microgynon on the painful crises of sickle cell anemia patients. *Contraception.* 1997;56:313–16.

195. Ahn YS, Fernandez LF, Kim CI, et al. Danazol therapy renders red cells resistant to osmotic lysis. *FASEB J.* 1989;3:157–162.

196. Anie KA. Psychological complications in sickle cell disease. *Br J Haematol.* 2005;129:723–729.

197. Benton TD, Ifeagwu JA, Smith-Whitley K. Anxiety and depression in children and adolescents with sickle cell disease. *Curr Psychiatry Rep.* 2007;9:114–121.

198. Angst MS, Clark JD. Opioid-induced hyperalgesia: a qualitative systematic review. *Anesthesiology.* 2006;104:570–587.

199. Richebe P, Rivat C, Laulin JP, Maurette P, Simonnet G. Ketamine improves the management of exaggerated postoperative pain observed in perioperative fentanyl-treated rats. *Anesthesiology.* 2005;102:421–428.

200. Joly V, Richebe P, Guignard B, et al. Remifentanil-induced postoperative hyperalgesia and its prevention with small-dose ketamine. *Anesthesiology.* 2005;103:147–155.

201. Schechter NL. The undertreatment of pain in children: an overview. *Pediatr Clin North Am.* 1989;36:781–794.

202. Elander J, Marczewska M, Amos R, Thomas A, Tangayi S. Factors affecting hospital staff judgments about sickle cell disease pain. *J Behav Med.* 2006;29:203–214.

203. Labbe E, Herbert D, Haynes J. Physicians' attitude and practices in sickle cell disease pain management. *J Palliat Care.* 2005;21:246–251.

204. Pack-Mabien A, Labbe E, Herbert D, Haynes J, Jr. Nurses' attitudes and practices in sickle cell pain management. *Appl Nurs Res.* 2001;14:187–192.

205. Shapiro BS, Benjamin LJ, Payne R, Heidrich G. Sickle cell-related pain: perceptions of medical practitioners. *J Pain Symptom Manage.* 1997;14:168–174.

206. Brozovic M, Davies SC, Yardumian A, Bellingham A, Marsh G, Stephens AD. Pain relief in sickle cell crisis. *Lancet.* 1986;2:624–625.

207. Silbergleit R, Jancis MO, McNamara RM. Management of sickle cell pain crisis in the emergency department at teaching hospitals. *J Emerg Med.* 1999;17:625–630.

208. Tetrault SM, Scott RB. Five-year retrospective study of hospitalization and treatment of patients with sickle cell anemia. *South Med J.* 1976;69:1314–1316.

209. American Pain Society. *Guideline for the Management of Acute and Chronic Pain in Sickle Cell Disease.* Glenview, IL: American Pain Society; 1999.

34

Acute Pain Management in Patients with Opioid Dependence and Substance Abuse

Sukanya Mitra and Raymond S. Sinatra

In contrast to the "opiophobic" attitudes that existed in America in the 1970s and 1980s,[1] since the late 1990s, there has been a gradual but noticeable shift regarding the use of opioids for the management of severe chronic pain. Both primary care physicians and pain specialists are prescribing opioids to a greater number of patients and in doses appropriate to their needs.[2–6] A number of opioid analgesics and delivery systems have been introduced that have increased patient satisfaction, physician acceptance, and overall use. Nevertheless, along with improvements in pain relief and quality of life, an increasing number of patients are affected by issues related to opioid tolerance and physical dependence. There are only a few published reviews that address the treatment of acute pain in patients with substance use disorders (SUD),[2–4] and fewer focused specifically on perioperative pain management in opioid-dependent patients.[5–7]

Acute pain management of opioid-dependent patients poses a special challenge to primary caregivers, anesthesiologists, and pain specialists alike. This problem emanates from the often-conflicting needs to balance patient rights to adequate analgesia and concerns of safety, diversion and abuse, thus raising important ethical issues.[5–8]

This chapter outlines the settings in which an anesthesiologist or pain specialist may come across patients with chronically high intake of opioids and other psychoactive substances and provides the rationale, principles, and guidelines for acute pain management in this specialized subset of patients, focusing essentially but not exclusively on the perioperative period.

INCREASING RELEVANCE OF THE TOPIC

There are four good reasons why an anesthesiologist or pain specialist is more likely than ever to encounter patients with a high chronic baseline intake of opioids. These are (1) increasing number of chronic pain patients who are on long-term prescription opioids; (2) a high number of substance-abusing patients, including those with opioid dependence and polysubstance abuse; (3) an increasing number of patients stabilized on methadone and, more recently, the partial agonist, buprenorphine, as maintenance therapy for their prior opioid addiction; and (4) a significant minority of those patients with a combination of (1) and (2) (ie, chronic pain patients on prescription opioids, but also with excessive or nonprescription opioid abuse). Any of these patients from the above four categories can need surgical procedures that may or may not be related to their primary condition. Additionally, some of these patients (eg, substance abusers) may develop acutely painful conditions as complications of their primary conditions (eg, accidents and injuries, acute pancreatitis), which then requires acute pain management. Each of these four scenarios is described briefly below.

More Patients on Prescription Opioids

In recent years, the percentage of patients prescribed opioid analgesics for chronic pain has increased dramatically. An Australian study found that 83% of patients with chronic pain, including back pain, other forms of benign pain, and cancer pain, were prescribed opioid analgesics by their general practitioners at the time of referral to a multidisciplinary pain center.[9] Moreover, 47% of these patients were treated with strong opioids such as morphine, oxycodone, and methadone. In another study, long-term opioid use and dose escalation were noted in one-third of patients suffering from chronic noncancer pain.[10]

Overall, 20%–90% of patients with various chronic pain conditions attending pain intervention settings have been reported to receive opioids for chronic pain management.[11] This is reflected in the fact that the annual sales of opioid analgesics on the outpatient basis in the United States increased by nearly 130% between 1999 and 2003, more than double of the sales for the previous decade.[12] Factors responsible for the increased acceptance and prescription of opioid analgesics include physician education, concerns of analgesic undermedication and inadequate pain control, the favorable side-effect profiles of newer semisynthetic and sustained-release opioids, and morbidity associated with nonsteroidal anti-inflammatory drugs (NSAIDs) and selective cyclooxygenase 2 (COX-2) inhibitors despite their potential usefulness in the acute pain setting.[2,3,9,13]

Many Patients with Opioid and Other Substance Abuse

Drug addiction refers to a complex phenomenon with behavioral, cognitive, and physiological components, where the use of a particular drug assumes central importance in the user's life, even in the face of obvious physical or psychological harm.[14] Essentially, the life of the addicted patient centers on the repeated use of opioid and nonopioid substances to experience pleasure or to avoid displeasure (ie, avoiding withdrawal; see below).

According to the 2004 National Survey on Drug Use and Health (NSDUH), 4.4 million persons aged 12 or older were estimated to have used opiate analgesics nonmedically in the past month.[15] The incidence of emergency department (ED) visits related to the use of these medications has been increasing since the 1990s and has more than doubled between 1994 and 2001.[16] In 2001, there were an estimated 90,232 ED visits related to opioid analgesic abuse, a 117% increase since 1994. In 2004, opiate analgesics were implicated in an estimated 158,281 ED visits attributed to drug misuse/abuse.[17]

The repeat NSDUH report of 2005 estimated that 19.7 million Americans aged 12 or older were current (past month) users of illicit drugs, constituting 8% of this population.[18] Marijuana was the most commonly used illicit drug (14.6 million past month users), followed by pain relievers, including opioid analgesics (4.7 million); cocaine (2.4 million); tranquilizers (1.8 million); stimulants, including methamphetamine (1.1 million); and hallucinogens, including club drugs such as MDMA (ecstasy) (1.1 million). Past-month heroin use was reported by 136,000 persons. Although the use of several of these substances remained more or less stable since 2002 survey results, it was of some concern to note that past-month nonmedical use of prescription drugs among young adults actually increased significantly from 5.4% in 2002 to 6.3% in 2005. Further, this increase was primarily because of an increase in pain reliever use, from 4.1% in 2002 to 4.7% in 2005.

Moving on from current use to abuse and dependence, in 2005, an estimated 22.2 million persons (9.1% of the population aged 12 years or older) were classified with substance abuse or dependence in the past year based on the *Diagnostic and Statistical Manual of Mental Disorders* (4th edition, DSM-IV)[19] criteria. The specific illicit drugs that had the highest level of past-year dependence or abuse in 2005 were marijuana (4.1 million), cocaine, and pain relievers (1.5 million each). Most of the prescription pain relievers contained opioids.[18]

Of the various illicit opioids, heroin is the most commonly abused drug. According to a national survey, approximately 1 adult among 3 who tries heroin becomes addicted to this drug.[14] Heroin is readily available on the illicit market but has varying levels of purity. Each 100-mg bag of powder in early 1990 had only 4 mg (0–8 mg range) of heroin, and the rest was inert or sometimes toxic adulterants such as quinine. In the mid-to-late 1990s, street heroin reached 45–80% purity. In some large cities, 90% pure heroin was made available. Thus, heroin, which initially required IV injection, could be smoked or administered intranasally (snorted). As a result, only 37% of new heroin abusers inject the drug.[20] Recent data show that, among students surveyed as part of the 2006 Monitoring the Future Study, 1.4%

of tenth-, eleventh-, and twelfth-graders reported lifetime use of heroin, and, worryingly enough, heroin availability was rated as "fairly easy" to "very easy" by 13%, 17%, and 27% of these three grades, respectively.[21]

Prescribed opioids that provide a desirable "high" (ie, a rapid onset to peak effect and pleasurable feelings of sedation or euphoria) are also commonly abused. These include rapid-acting semisynthetics such as oxycodone, hydrocodone, oxymorphone, and hydromorphone and nonmorphine-like synthetics, including methadone and fentanyl.[14,22] Reports of oxycodone and hydrocodone abuse increased 68% and 31%, respectively, from 1999 to 2000.[20] The sustained-release oxycodone preparation oxycontin, has also gained notoriety for being diverted and abused. Oxycontin was developed as a sustained-release opioid for moderate to severe pain, which avoided peaks and troughs in analgesic plasma concentrations. In most patients, oxycontin provides safe and effective pain relief; however, with tampering (ie, crushing and powdering the preparation), it may be injected or used intranasally to provide a rapid and powerful opioid effect. Methadone (dolophine) is also diverted and abused. It remains unclear if newer second-generation sustained-release morphine (Avinza) and oxymorphone (Opana) preparations are more tamper resistant and less likely to be abused.

The latest phase of nonmedical use of opioid substances happened with fentanyl, with a surge in ED visits between late 2005 and mid-2006. The Community Epidemiologic Work Group (CEWG), monitoring drug use indicators in 20 selected areas of the United States over a number of years, has identified fentanyl and fentanyl-laced heroin as "an emerging drug of abuse" among the key findings in its June 2006 meeting.[23] Such fentanyl-laced heroin has several street names, such as "lethal injection," "drop dead," "fat Albert," and "the bomb," and was confirmed to be responsible for overdose-related deaths in several areas prominently, including Chicago/Cook County, Detroit/Wayne County, New Jersey, Philadelphia, and St. Louis, among others. In its latest report, the CEWG has agreed to keep a close watch on the evolving situation.[23]

More Patients on Opioid Agonist Maintenance Therapy

Treatment of opioid addiction with opioid agonists such as methadone and, more recently, buprenorphine is now well established. Historically, a significant breakthrough in the treatment of opioid addiction occurred with the introduction of methadone in the mid-1960s. Methadone maintenance proved safe and effective and improved the patients' daily functioning. Within a few years of its introduction, however, new federal laws and regulations, such as the Methadone Regulations Act of 1972 and the Narcotic Addict Treatment Act of 1974, essentially restricted methadone maintenance treatment (MMT) to the context of the opioid treatment program (OTP) setting. In essence, the OTP operated as strictly licensed and regulated methadone clinics, with a closed distribution system for methadone that required special licensing by both federal and state authorities. This system severely restricted the access of opioid dependent patients to an OTP.

Efforts to return opioid dependence treatment to the mainstream medical care resulted in the Drug Addiction Treatment Act of 2000 (DATA 2000)[24] that enabled qualifying physicians to obtain a "waiver" from the special registration requirements in the Narcotic Addict Treatment Act of 1974 to treat opioid dependence with opioid agonist drugs. Importantly, under the DATA 2000, such waived physicians can now prescribe and/or dispense these medications in treatment settings other than licensed OTPs, including in office-based settings. This significant change broadened the scope and ease of opioid-dependence treatment in less restricted settings.

On October 8, 2002, two new sublingual formulations of the opioid partial agonist buprenorphine (Subutex, Reckitt Benckiser) and buprenorphine/naloxone combination (Suboxone, Reckitt Benckiser) received Food and Drug Administration (FDA) approval for the treatment of opioid addiction, including in the setting of office-based practices. Physicians who obtain DATA 2000 waivers can treat opioid addiction with Subutex or Suboxone in any appropriate clinical settings in which they are credentialed to practice medicine. Other than destigmatizing opioid addiction treatment, these changes have greatly expanded the available treatment options as well as the availability and accessibility of opioid agonist treatment to the patients in their own locality.

Until recently, the approved upper limit of patients for buprenorphine maintenance therapy under DATA 2000 was only 30 patients per practice. As late as December 2006, the U.S. Congress passed legislation allowing such DATA 2000 waived physicians with 1 year of clinical experience to request an additional exemption within DATA 2000 allowing the limit of 30 patients per practice to be raised to 100 patients per physician.

The upshot of all these developments, from the point of view of the anesthesiologist or pain specialist, is that an appreciably higher number of patients receiving high-dose maintenance buprenoephine will become available in the community and, hence, potentially for acute pain management because of various reasons.

Patients on Prescription Opioids Who also Abuse Opioids

Although it is difficult to ascertain the prevalence of opioid abuse or addiction in chronic pain patients, a study performed by Fishbain and coworkers[25] found that between 3% and 19% of the chronic pain patients suffer an addictive disorder, which is comparable to the lifetime prevalence rate of addictive disorders in general population. It has been suggested that prevalence of addiction may be higher in chronic pain patients because of their background emotional and psychological instability and conditioning behavior resulting from increasing pain intensity and relief resulting from opioid use.[25,26] Of 125 chronic pain patients, a study found 12% to be diagnosable with a substance abuse or dependence disorder using formal *Diagnostic and Statistical Manual of Mental Disorders* (3rd edition, revised, DSM-III-R) criteria.[27] Other studies, using diverse patient populations, but all with chronic pain, and using different definitions and detection methods for substance abuse and addiction, have reported a very wide range of 3%–41%.[2,11,28] In addition, a combination of illicit drug use and abuse of controlled substance was found in 34% of chronic pain patients.[29] A recent prospective study of 500 consecutive patients with chronic pain attending an interventional pain management practice and considered to be stable on prescription opioids detected a rate of 9% for opioid abuse and 16% for illicit drug use.[11] Thus, a significant minority of chronic pain patients on prescription of opioids as controlled substance are also known to have additional problems of opioid or other substance abuse.

ISSUES SPECIFIC TO ACUTE PAIN MANAGEMENT IN THESE PATIENTS

Given the increasing relevance of the topic for pain specialists as outlined above, the question arises as to why these people (on chronic high-dose opioids for medical or nonmedical reasons) should be treated any differently from others regarding acute pain management. The higher demand for analgesic measures in these patients is often blatantly labeled as "drug-seeking behavior," with an obvious or covert pejorative connotation.

Scimeca et al[30] noted the following common problems in pain management in hospitalized patients on MMT (problems that could conceivably be applicable in patients on buprenorphine maintenance treatment and for others consuming high-dose opioids as well):

1. Methadone doses were lowered in the hospital, with resultant opioid withdrawal.
2. Physicians believed that the maintenance methadone dose would itself provide adequate analgesic cover.
3. Clinicians feared that additional analgesics would cause respiratory depression.
4. Clinicians believed that methadone might interfere with surgical or other procedures and hence often ordered methadone withdrawal before such procedures.
5. Patients' methadone dose, if increased to provide analgesia during hospital stay, was often left unaltered after discharge.
6. Some patients complained that opioid antagonists were used inappropriately, thus precipitating acute opioid withdrawal.
7. The stigma of getting branded as a "methadone patient," made some patients conceal their status during emergency or hospital admission, at times resulting in unwanted consequences such as precipitation of acute withdrawal because of injection of pentazocine or other agonist/antagonist drugs.

Four common misconceptions have been noted by Alfred et al,[31] all of which result in undertreatment of acute pain in patients on MMT or other opioid agonist therapy (OAT):

1. The maintenance opioid agonist provides adequate analgesia.

   Actually, pharmacokinetic and dynamic factors at cellular and subcellular levels result in phenomena such as tolerance and opioid-induced hyperalgesia, which not only make the patients immune to the initial analgesic effects of these drugs, but also may actually render them in a hyperalgesic state. Also, patients on OAT are known to have a lower pain threshold and higher pain sensitivity than other patients.[32]
2. Use of opioids for analgesia may result in addiction relapse.

   Actually, there is no evidence to support this common notion in the setting of acute pain management in patients on OAT.[33,34] On the contrary, patients on MMT stated that the experience of chronic severe pain played an important role in their continuing drug use.[35]
3. The additive effects of opioid analgesics and OAT may cause respiratory and CNS depression.

   Again, this concern is not supported by evidence.[31] For example, patients with worsening cancer-related pain who require opioid dose escalations typically do not exhibit respiratory and CNS-depressant effects.[36,37]

4. Demanding more drugs because of reported pain might reflect manipulative or drug-seeking behavior.

This is a difficult and tricky issue, not the least because pain is essentially a subjective phenomenon. Although it is always possible for opioid-addicted or OAT-maintained patients to report pain to obtain additional opioids, the motivation behind such behavior may not be always to obtain a hedonistic reward but simply to obtain relief from, or avoid the recurrence of, intolerable pain. Such phenomena have been variously termed as opioid pseudoaddiction,[38] therapeutic dependence,[39] or pseudo-opioid resistance.[40]

Thus, before coming to the clinical aspects of patient management in these groups of patients, it is useful to gain some understanding of the basic aspects of substance use disorder which can then lead to appropriate patient assessment and, finally, management.

BASIC ASPECTS OF SUBSTANCE USE DISORDER

Criteria and Definitions

Diagnostic and Statistical Manual of Mental Disorders (4th edition, text revision; DSM-IV-TR)[19] defines substance dependence as a maladaptive pattern of substance use, leading to clinically significant impairment or distress, as manifested by at least three of the following 7 criteria, occurring at any time in the same 12-month period: tolerance; withdrawal; taking the substance in larger amounts or over a longer period than was intended; a persistent desire or unsuccessful efforts to cut down or control substance use; long time spent in activities related to the substance; giving up important social, occupational, or recreational activities because of substance use; and, finally, continued use of the substance despite knowledge of having a persistent or recurrent physical or psychological problem that is likely to have been caused or exacerbated by the substance. Further, a diagnostic specifier, "With physiological dependence," is used in case there is evidence of tolerance or withdrawal.

For better understanding, some other helpful definitions can be found in Table 34.1.[19,31,41,42] It may be noted that the terms and their distinctive boundaries are not always very clear, especially terms such as *addiction, dependence, abuse, substance abuse*, and so on. This is partly because these terms have evolved over time in varying historical and sociocultural contexts. They also reflect conflicts regarding appropriate terminology for the complex medical and psychosocial issues that underlie chronic and compulsive substance-using behavior. For example, the strict medical or biological viewpoint that characterizes SUD essentially as a "disease" or "disorder" conflicts with the strictly sociocultural viewpoint that tends to "demedicalize" such behavior and explain it from a social and cultural context.[7] For the purpose of this review, the terms *addiction, SUD*, and *psychological dependence* will often be used interchangeably.

Physical Dependence

The term *physical dependence* describes alterations in physiological response that result from opioid binding and receptor mediated activity in the autonomic nervous system.[22,26] Abrupt discontinuation of oral or parenterally administered opioids leads

to opioid withdrawal syndrome. This syndrome is characterized by heightened sympathetic and parasympathetic responses mediated via the myenteric plexus, brainstem vagal and hypothalamic nuclei. It is clinically characterized by hypertension, tachycardia, diaphoresis, abdominal cramping, and diarrhea, as well as physiologic and behavioral responses such as shaking ("wet dog shakes"), yawning, and leg jerking ("kicking the habit"). When opioid-dependent patients abruptly discontinue their habit they use the term *cold turkey* to describe the appearance of their cold, pale, goose-bumped skin. These symptoms, although very unpleasant and extremely distressing, are rarely life-threatening. They can, however, often confuse clinical diagnosis and care.

Opioid Tolerance

Opioid tolerance is a predictable pharmacological adaptation. Continued opioid exposure results in a rightward shift in the dose-response curve and patients require increasing amounts of drug to maintain the baseline pharmacologic effects. The phenomenon of tolerance develops to analgesic, euphoric, sedative, respiratory depressant, and nauseating effects of opioids but not to their effects on pupil size (miosis) and bowel motility (constipation).[14,22]

The degree or gradation of opioid tolerance is generally related to duration of exposure, daily dose requirement, and receptor association/disassociation kinetics. Depending on their intrinsic efficacy opioid agonists binding to the same receptor may show asymmetric cross-tolerance. For example, patients treated with sufentanil, an agonist having high intrinsic efficacy and requiring low receptor occupancy for a given analgesic effect, develop tolerance more slowly than to opioids having low intrinsic efficacy such as morphine.[43] Although there are no clear gradation guidelines, individuals requiring the equivalent of 1 mg or more intravenous (IV), or 3 mg or more of oral morphine per hour for a period greater than 1 month, may be considered to have high-grade opioid tolerance.[7]

Tolerance is observed in patients legitimately prescribed opioids for pain management as well as in those abusing this class of drug. In general, the higher the daily dose requirement the greater the degree of tolerance development.[22,43] This is of importance for many patients and caregivers who perceive an increasing opioid dose requirement as reflecting harmful addiction rather than a normal adaptation to this class of analgesics.[3,14] The molecular and cellular basis of opioid tolerance is presented in Figures 34.1(a) and 34.1(b).

PATIENT ASSESSMENT ISSUES

The importance of patient assessment and early recognition cannot be overemphasized, because, failing this essential first step, the principles that follow become irrelevant.[2–7] The assessment strategy aims at correct identification of the opioid-abusing patient from dependent individuals suffering from chronic pain conditions. The true abuser should be detected, whereas legitimate users are not to be falsely labeled as addicts. In other words, both false positive as well as false negative rates should be low.[44] This is, however, easier said than done, because drug-seeking behavior, superficially suggestive of addiction, may actually arise in patients who cannot obtain tolerable relief with prescribed doses of opioid and seek alternate sources or increased doses of pain medication ("pseudoaddiction").[38] Alternatively, patients who achieve effective pain control may take extraordinary steps

Table 34.1: Substance Use Disorder: Related Definitions[19,31,41,42]

Addiction	Commonly used term meaning the aberrant use of a specific psychoactive substance in a manner characterized by loss of control, compulsive use, preoccupation, and continued use despite harm; pejorative term, replaced in the DSM-IV-TR[19] in a nonpejorative way by the term *substance use disorder* (SUD) with psychological and physical dependence
Dependence	Psychological dependence: need for a specific psychoactive substance either for its positive effects or to avoid negative psychological or physical effects associated with its withdrawal.
	Physical dependence: A physiological state of adaptation to a specific psychoactive substance characterized by the emergence of a withdrawal syndrome during abstinence, which may be relieved in total, or in part, by readministration of the substance.
	One category of psychoactive substance use disorder
Chemical dependence	A generic term relating to psychological and/or physical dependence on one or more psychoactive substances, classes of psychoactive substances are abused (alcohol; sedatives, hypnotics, and anxiolytics; cannabis; opioids; cocaine; amphetamines and other sympathomimetics; hallucinogens; caffeine; nicotine; phencyclidine)
Substance use disorders	Term of DSM-IV-TR[19] comprising two main groups:
	Substance dependence disorder and substance abuse disorder
	Substance-induced disorders (eg, intoxication, withdrawal, delirium, psychotic disorders)
Tolerance	Normal neurobiological event; a state in which an increased dosage of a psychoactive substance is needed to produce the original effect. Cross-tolerance: induced by repeated administration of one psychoactive substance that is manifested toward another substance to which the individual has not been recently exposed
Withdrawal syndrome	The onset of a predictable constellation of signs and symptoms following the abrupt discontinuation of or a rapid decrease in dosage of a psychoactive substance
Polydrug dependence	Concomitant use of two or more psychoactive substances in quantities and frequencies that cause individually significant physiological, psychological, and/or sociological distress or impairment (polysubstance abuser)
Recovery	A process of overcoming both physical and psychological dependence on a psychoactive substance with a commitment to sobriety
Abstinence	In recovery, nonuse of any psychoactive substance
Maintenance	Prevention of craving behavior and withdrawal symptoms of opioids by permanently acting opioid (eg, methadone, buprenorphine)
Substance abuse	Use of a psychoactive substance in a manner outside of sociocultural conventions; according to this, any use of illicit and licit drugs in a manner not dictated by convention (eg, according to physicians' order) is abuse.
Pseudoaddiction	Behavioral changes in patients that seem similar to those in patients with opioid dependence or addiction, but are secondary to inadequate pain control.
Drug-seeking behaviors	Directed or concerted efforts on the part of the patient to obtain opioid medication or to ensure an adequate medication supply; may be an appropriate response to inadequately treated pain.
Opioid-induced hyperalgesia	A neuroplastic change in pain perception resulting in an increase in pain sensitivity to painful stimuli, thereby decreasing the analgesic effects of opioids.

to maintain an adequate supply of medication. Although indicative of addictive drug seeking, such behavior may in actuality reflect the efforts of an extremely anxious patient to maintain tolerable pain relief and prevent undermedication.[38–40] Table 34.2 outlines the underlying principles that help the clinician differentiate between patients suffering chronic pain and the opioid abusers.

Patients with addiction to alcohol, marijuana, or nicotine show a higher incidence of dependence on other substances than the general population. This phenomenon has been termed *cross addiction* or *polydrug abuse*.[14] Opioid-dependent patients with superimposed cocaine dependence may present additional problems for acute caregivers, including hemodynamic instability and extreme emotional lability. Some opioid-dependent patients are also codependent on benzodiazepines and other anxiolytics. By simply focusing on opioid dependency issues and not accounting for or administering adequate doses of benzodiazepines, these individuals may develop severe withdrawal reactions, including anxiety, agitation, and confusion.

Applying DSM-IV criteria for drug abuse to patients taking prescribed opiates for a chronic pain problem can be difficult.[45] Thus, special assessment criteria need to be developed and applied. Although a few opiate abuse checklists and questionnaires for these patients are available[46,47] (see Table 34.3 for one such checklist), a major problem with these is that some of the criteria used for assessment necessitate prolonged physician contact with the patient and hence may be difficult to apply in acute pain settings.

The anesthesiologist and pain specialist also need to be aware of the rapidly changing profile of opioid-based analgesia. It may be worthwhile to recognize both the names of newly developed opioids and method of action of novel delivery systems, including oral sustained-release, transmucosal, intranasal, and transdermal preparations.

Finally, it is worth emphasizing that acute pain setting is not the optimal time to attempt a detoxification or rehabilitation management for any patient abusing opioids or other substances.[6,7,44] Although obviously important, such issues

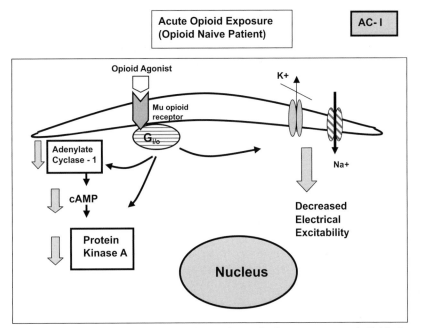

Figure 34.1(a): Molecular and cellular basis of opioid tolerance. In naïve individuals, opioid binding at μ-receptors activate coupled G-proteins (Gi/o), which in turn inhibit the neuronal cyclic adenosice monophosphate (cAMP) pathway, including suppression of adenylate cyclase and reduced production of cAMP and protein kinase-A (PKA). G-protein activation also leads to an inhibition in potassium (K^+) flux, decreased electrical excitability of nociceptive neurons, and pain modulation.

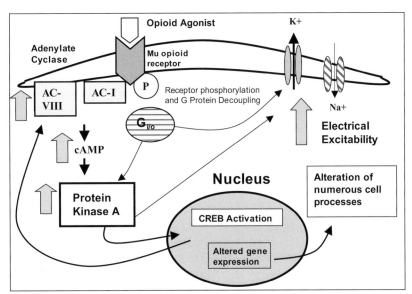

Figure 34.1(b): Continued opioid exposure leads to a variety of intraneuronal changes, including μ-receptor phosphorylation and G-protein decoupling. Activation of a key nuclear regulator, cAMP response element-binding protein (CREB), results in a compensatory upregulation of the cAMP pathway. This involves upregulation of two forms of adenylylate cyclase (AC-I, AC-VIII) and increased production of cAMP and PKA-A. Enhanced PKA-A activity alters gene expression as well as numerous cell processes and is also responsible for increased K^+ flux and increased electrical activity in nociceptive cells. Upregulation of the cAMP pathway would oppose the inhibitory effects of acute opioid exposure and represents physiologic tolerance. On removal of opioids, the upregulated cAMP pathway becomes fully functional and contributes to features of withdrawal. Modified from Nestler and Aghajanian.[22]

Table 34.2: Difference between Chronic Pain and Opioid-Addicted Patients

Chronic Pain Patient	Opioid Addicted Patient
Appropriate use of opioid	Out-of-control with opioids
	Compulsive drug use
	Craving drug when not in pain
	Obtains drugs from nonmedical sources or through illegal activities
	Escalates opioid use without medical instructions
	Supplements prescribed drugs with other opioids
Opioid use primarily concerned with pain relief	Opioid use primarily concerned with pleasure ("kick") or avoiding unpleasantness of withdrawal
No stereotyped demand for specific drug or route of administration so long as pain remains under control	Demands specific opioid drug
	Prefers specific routes of administration
Demand for opioids ceases with effective pain control	Demand for opioids continues despite effective pain control
Opioids improve quality of life	Opioids impair quality of life
Aware of side effects	Unconcerned
Follows treatment plan	Does not follow plan
Has medication saved from prior prescriptions; can regulate use according to supply	Out of medication, "loses" prescriptions, has a "story"

Table 34.3: Opiate Abuse Checklist

The patient displays an overwhelming focus on opiate issues during pain clinic visits that occupy a significant portion of the pain clinic visit and impedes progress with other issues regarding the patient's pain. The behavior must persist beyond the third clinic treatment session.

The patient has a pattern of early refills (3 or more) or escalating drug use in the absence of an acute change in his or her medical condition.

The patient generates multiple telephone calls or visits to the administrative office to require more opiates, early refills, or problems associated with the opiate prescription; a patient may qualify with fewer visits if he or she creates a disturbance with the office staff.

There is a pattern of prescription problems for a variety of reasons that may include lost medications, spilled medications, or stolen medications.

The patient has supplemental sources of opiates obtained from multiple providers, emergency rooms, or illegal sources.

Adapted from Chabal et al.[46]

should be dealt with later when the patient is stable and pain has declined in intensity.

PATIENT MANAGEMENT

Broad Goals and Strategies

The broad goals of acute pain management in opioid-dependent patients are outlined in Table 34.4.[2] The first and foremost of these, as mentioned above (patient assessment), is the correct identification of the population at risk, keeping in mind that this may not always be straightforward, given the stigma, anxiety, and fears associated with drug addiction or even its maintenance treatment with high-dose opioids. Other groups of patients on high-dose opioids also need to specifically identified. The second goal is to avoid the occurrence or precipitation of acute withdrawal and its complications. The third goal is the alleviation or symptomatic management of anxiety and other psychologically distressing symptoms. The next obvious and central goal is the provision of effective, round-the-clock, and comprehensive pain treatment in the acute phase. This is described in detail in the following sections. Finally, after the acute management phase is over, patients need to be brought forward to an acceptable and suitable maintenance therapy (ie, to enter [or reenter] the chronic phase of treatment), which is beyond the scope of this chapter.

There are more specific strategies to provide effective analgesia in this group of patients.[48] An important strategy is to avoid the use of opioid agonist-antagonist drugs (such as pentazocine, nalbuphine, butorphanol, and dezocine) or partial agonists (buprenorphine) in known or suspected patients on chronic high-dose opioid agonists, because the former drugs can precipitate an acute withdrawal.

Other strategies pertain to (1) using multimodal analgesia, including nonopioid medications (such as NSAIDs, acetaminophen, selective COX-2 inhibitors, ketamine, clonidine, etc); (2) while using opioids, maintaining a structured control of access to opioids, judicious use of other routes and techniques (such as local anesthetic techniques, intravenous patient-controlled analgesia, regional anesthesia, opioid rotation, more frequent but regular dosing intervals when necessary rather than as needed [PRN] dosing); (3) maintaining an effective dialog with the patient on various aspects of therapy (eg, gaining confidence, alleviation of anxiety, assuring the patient of adequate pain relief in the acute phase, but also focusing on the end point of treatment on the effectiveness of pain relief itself, encouraging the patient in recovery to enhance his or her recovery program, etc); and, finally, (4) ensuring that the underlying pain-producing disorder as well as any comorbid physical or psychiatric issues are addressed.

Table 34.4: Broad Goals of Acute Pain Management in Opioid-Dependent Patients

Identification of the populations at risk: patients on long-term opioid therapy for various chronic pain situations (musculoskeletal, neuropathic, sickle cell disease, HIV-related disease, and palliative care), drug abusers, recovering addicts in opioid maintenance programs

Prevention of withdrawal symptoms and complications

Symptomatic treatment of psychological affective disorders such as anxiety

Effective analgesic treatment in acute phase

Rehabilitation to an acceptable and suitable maintenance opioid therapy

Reprinted with permission from Mehta and Langford.[2]

Multimodal analgesia with acetaminophen, NSAIDs, and adjuvant drugs remains the cornerstone of acute pain management in these patients just as in those without dependency issues but with one key distinction: the underlying opioid requirement must be continued to be met. Just as assuming that these baseline opioids would do the job of pain control is fallacious, the assumption that nonopioid drugs will obviate the need for baseline opioid requirement is incorrect. NSAIDs and selective COX-2 inhibitors have the advantage of not having central depressant or mind-altering properties; they, however, do have a ceiling effect and should be used cautiously or sparingly in patients with renal, hepatic, or gastric diseases (not uncommon in our index group of patients).

Ketamine, an antagonist of the NMDA receptor that has been implicated in pain mechanisms, in a low dose, has been shown to be effective as an adjunctive treatment in opioid-dependent patients.[49,50]

Clonidine, an agonist of the α_2 adrenergic receptors, has been found to be effective in having a "quietening" effect on heavy users of opioids in the postoperative period when given in a relatively higher dose of 2–4 μg/kg IV (or subcutaneously [SC] if venous access unavailable).[51]

Local anesthetic techniques can provide adequate pain relief in opioid-dependent patients and should be used whenever feasible.[52,53] However, the usual precautions should be kept in mind, and patients may not agree to this procedure.[54,55]

Other than these agents, nonpharmacological measures such as heat/cold application, massage, and manipulation may help.[2] Cognitive-behavioral and other psychotherapeutic interventions may help in addressing comorbid psychological issues.

Opioid Medications

After meeting the baseline opioid requirement, and if nonopioid measures are not adequate (and at times, if the pain if judged to be too severe to be controlled by these measures, even from the beginning), additional opioids should be given. These should be prescribed on a regular rather than PRN basis only, often in frequent intervals so as to provide effective round-the-clock analgesia. Either an additional dose of the same baseline opioid or another potent opioid titrated to the patient's need on

Table 34.5: Advantages and Disadvantages of Patient-Controlled Analgesia

Advantages

Intuitive and easy to use

Accepted standard practice in the acute pain setting

Promotes maintenance of a stable blood opioid concentration, providing uniform pain relief at a lower total dose, thereby avoiding (a) sedation at high peak levels and (b) pain, anxiety, and drug craving at trough levels

Patients appreciate being "in control" and maybe reduced likelihood of confrontational behavior

Disadvantages

Potentially difficult to optimize dose size and lockout time because of wide between-patient variability

Patients might use PCA dose for psychological effects rather than for analgesic purpose

PCA device needs to be tamper-proof, as the patients are aware of the opioid source

Frequent need of opioid might be perceived as drug craving by health care professionals

Associated with serious caregiver and technology related errors in dosing

Use of basal infusion may increase risk of overdose in opioid naive patients

a short-term basis may be given in the acute phase of treatment. Equianalgesic dose charts of alternate opioids (including route equivalence) can be useful but should be used only as an approximate guide because of interindividual differences as a result of issues of tolerance and hyperalgesia. The final arbitrator in this matter has to be the patient's pain response and the safety issues.

The principle of opioid rotation, derived from palliative care settings and based on the phenomenon of incomplete cross-tolerance between various opioids, may also be used in the acute care setting. However, more research is needed for optimal opioid switching.[2] Methadone has been found to be an effective rotation agent after morphine[56,57] and hydromorphone after morphine.[58] Buprenorphine, however, being an partial agonist, carries a potential risk of precipitating withdrawal if administered to patients dependent on large doses of morphine or methadone.[59]

Regarding route of administration, parenteral administration is often favored over the oral route in the acute care setting. Patient-controlled analgesia (PCA) has its advantages and disadvantages (Table 34.5)[2] but has a significant role if risks of abuse are judged not to be serious and if the PCA is set up and monitored by experienced staff.[60] Swenson et al[61] have described a technique based on pharmacokinetic models that can be used to provide safe but effective fentanyl analgesia by PCA. Using specially designed software, first the threshold for the onset of fentanyl-induced respiratory depression is defined in response to a fentanyl challenge. The target analgesic concentration of fentanyl is calculated from this data and the rest of the algorithm, including the PCA settings and lockout interval, are derived from this.

Of the oral preparations, oral transmucosal fentanyl (Actiq) and, more recently, rapidly disintegrating oral fentanyl (Fentora) have been used to control breakthrough pain in patients on chronic high-dose opioid therapy.[62,63]

Patients on Opioid Agonist Maintenance Therapy

As mentioned, the number of such patients (especially those on buprenorphine maintenance treatment, BMT) are on the increase and likely to increase further with recent legislative changes in the scope and capacity of such treatment. As such, this is an issue of ever-increasing clinical importance. The issue of pain management in patients on OAT (MMT or BMT) has been addressed in several recent reviews and experience-based articles,[30,31,64,65] although the research database does not seem impressive at the moment. The anesthesiologist and pain specialist may devote time to allay patient apprehensions that they may lose control and possibly relapse or that their pain will be inadequately controlled. Patients may be reassured that, despite a prior history of opioid dependency, effective pain control is an achievable goal and that the risk of relapse can be minimized.[7,25,26] The patient, OAT physician or prescribing agency, and rehabilitation counselor may meet prior to surgery and develop a management plan. Together they may formulate and agree to follow a realistic protocol that would minimize but not eliminate pain perception while avoiding excessive opioid doses that might lead to recurrence of addictive disorder.

A practical approach might include the use of a medication agreement or contract, setting appropriate goals for pain intensity scores, as well as daily dose of analgesic and method of analgesic administration.[64] Patients' monitoring may include drug screens and pill counts and careful documentation of postoperative course.

Table 34.6[31,64,65] shows the acute pain management guidelines for these patients in the general acute and perioperative settings. A detailed section deals with BMT patients because of the expected increase in their number because of factors mentioned above. The basic general principles all apply as mentioned before (broad goals and strategies). It is essential, in addition, to inform and liaise with the addiction treatment agency responsible for the patient's OAT.

In case of MMT patients, additional analgesics – both nonopioid and short-acting opioids for temporary use – may be given over and above the baseline methadone. There is a potential risk of improper use of methadone in the perioperative setting that might result in either an overdose or, conversely, an acute withdrawal.[64] Most of the patients on MMT take a liquid fixed-concentration preparation such as 5 mg/mL. Although most physicians describe the dose in milligrams, many patients communicate in terms of milliliters. A miscommunication in this regard can potentially result in a single-dose overdose. Further, unlike morphine or other short-acting opioids used in the postoperative setting, methadone has a very long elimination half-life, even though its duration of action as an analgesic is much shorter.[64] Therefore, life-threatening complications may not result from any one single dose, but rather the accumulation of previous doses. The clinical implication is that, in acute postoperative pain management, serious caution should be exercised to titrate the methadone dose according to its analgesic effect while monitoring for signs of sedation, which may be the result of methadone accumulation in the body. A final cau-

tion pertains to drug-drug interactions such as those between methadone and sedative-hypnotic drugs (synergistic effects on the depressant effects of methadone), discontinuation of a potent inhibitor of cytochrome P450 system (CYP450) that is the main metabolizer of methadone (eg, erythromycin) and hence rapid metabolism of methadone precipitating a state of relative opioid withdrawal, or the discontinuation of a potent CYP450 inducer (eg, rifampin or carbamazepine), resulting in slow methadone metabolism with its adverse consequences. To further complicate matters, a minority of these patients may be diverting some or all of their prescribed methadone for sale or trade. In addition, some of the relatively active or unstable patients often also abuse other drugs, notably benzodiazepines, which could have important implications for acute pain management. The keys to dealing with such situations are (1) establishing a good rapport with the patient to the extent possible in an acute pain setting, (2) obtaining as complete a history as possible (both about legally prescribed and illegal consumption of other drugs), and (3) liaising with the MMT agency or physician. Finally, it must be remembered that patients on IV methadone, those receiving very high dose oral methadone (>200 mg/d), and those on additional medications such as haloperidol, amiodarone, and disopyramide are at a higher risk of developing a prolonged QTc interval and hence torsades de pointes.[66] These patients particularly need a high electrocardiographic and clinical vigilance. The FDA has reviewed reports of death and life-threatening adverse events such as respiratory depression and cardiac arrhythmias in patients receiving methadone. These adverse events are the possible result of unintentional methadone overdoses, drug interactions, and methadone's cardiac toxicities (QT prolongation and Torsades de Pointes). Physicians prescribing methadone should be familiar with methadone's toxicities and unique pharmacologic properties. Methadone's elimination half-life (8–59 hours) is longer than its duration of analgesic action (4–8 hours). Methadone doses for pain should be carefully selected and slowly titrated to analgesic effect even in patients who are opioid-tolerant. Physicians should closely monitor patients when converting them from other opioids and changing the methadone dose, and thoroughly instruct patients how to take methadone. Health care professionals should tell patients to take no more methadone than has been prescribed without first talking to their physician.

Clinical experience treating acute pain in patients on BMT is limited and research data are even sparser.[31,65] In these patients, there are essentially two approaches: (1) continue with buprenorphine itself (same or 25% increased dose, preferably in 3–4 divided doses rather than the BMT schedule of once daily dosage, and with or without additional analgesics) or (2) temporarily discontinue BMT, replace with methadone or slow-release morphine as the baseline opioid, use additionally titrated analgesics during the acute phase, and then bring the patient back on the previous BMT once the acute treatment phase has subsided or before discharge from the hospital. Buprenorphine should be reinstituted after about 8 hours after the last methadone or morphine dose to avoid precipitation of acute withdrawal by the buprenorphine itself (it being a mixed agonist-antagonist). In all cases, because of highly variable rates of buprenorphine dissociation from the μ-opioid receptor, naloxone should be available and the level of consciousness and respiratory rate should be frequently monitored. The specific guidelines as given in Table 34.6 are essentially based on expert

Table 34.6: Recommendations for Acute Pain Management in Patients on Opioid Agonist Therapy with Methadone or Buprenorphine Maintenance Therapy

Addiction treatment issues

    Reassure patient that addiction history will not prevent adequate pain management

    Continue with usual dose (or equivalent) of OAT

    Methadone or buprenorphine maintenance doses must be verified by the patient's methadone maintenance clinic or prescribing physician

    Liaise with Hospital-based Alcohol and Drugs Service (HADS) during the period of patient's hospital stay

    Notify the addiction treatment program or prescribing physician regarding the patient's admission and discharge from the hospital and confirm the time and amount of last maintenance opioid dose.

    Inform the addiction treatment maintenance program or prescribing physician of any medications such as opioids and benzodiazepine dose given to the patient during hospitalization because they may show up on routine urine drug screening

Pain management issues

    Relieve patient anxiety by discussing the pain management in a nonjudgmental manner

    Maximize the use of non-opioid treatments to aggressively treat the painful condition

    Opioid cross-tolerance and patient's increased pain sensitivity will often necessitate higher opioid analgesic doses administered at shorter intervals

    Write continuous scheduled dosing orders rather than "as needed" orders

    Avoid using mixed agonist-antagonist opioids

    Closely observe patients for (a) adequate analgesia and (b) adverse effects of sedation or respiratory depression, especially for patients on multiple high-dose opioids. For these patients, have naloxone available at the bedside. Coprescription of sedative-hypnotics is generally inadvisable given the potential for CNS and respiratory depression.

If the patient is receiving MMT and requires surgery

    Continue methadone as before on the day of surgery

    Advise patients to bring their own methadone to hospital

    Establish liaison with MMT physician, agency, or pharmacy

    Preoperative anesthesia consult, investigations especially ECG

    In case of day surgery

        Resume regular dose of methadone after surgery

        Additional analgesic for pain control

    In-patient surgery

        While NPO, alternative analgesic by regional analgesia or patient-controlled analgesia with alternative opioids, including IV methadone after dose adjustment

        Watch for drug interaction

        Resume methadone PO ASAP when patient can tolerate oral fluid well; if greater than 5 days off methadone, resumption of dosing should be with advice from MMT prescriber

If the patient is receiving BMT and requires surgery

Elective admissions

    Minor operations: continue BMT at current dose ± 25% increase

    Major operations

    Continue BMT at current dose + 25% increase, maximize nonopioid analgesia and admit to a high dependency unit (HDU) for titration of high dose i.v. opioids such as fentanyl or morphine.

    OR

    Cease buprenorphine 72 hours preoperatively and commence a full opioid agonist (methadone or sustained-release morphine) 24 hours later (or earlier if opioid withdrawal is noted). Additional doses of a full agonist can then be titrated as required to withdrawal symptoms preoperatively, and analgesic requirements postoperatively. The following starting doses may be used as a guide: BMT buprenorphine dose < 4 mg → commence methadone 20 mg/d or morphine 60 mg/d; buprenorphine dose > 4 mg → commence methadone 40 mg/d or morphine 80 mg/d.

Acute or emergency admissions

    Liaise with HADS

    Maximize nonopioid analgesic treatments

    If pain control not adequate, admit to HDU for titration of high dose IV opioids and close observation to monitor for opioid toxicity as partial agonist effects decline. It may be prudent to use a shorter acting opioid such as fentanyl in this context.

    If the duration of convalescence is expected to be short, buprenorphine may be continued at the usual dose during this period. Otherwise, conversion to a full opioid agonist may be prudent.

Discharge from hospital

    The patient should be stabilized on their preoperative buprenorphine dose ± simple analgesics at the time of discharge.

    They may be transferred to their standard buprenorphine regimen when postoperative analgesic requirements are minimal. Buprenorphine should be administered either 8 hours after the last opioid dose, or when early signs of opioid withdrawal are noted

Adapted from Alfred et al,[31] Peng et al,[64] and Roberts and Meyer-Witting.[65]

opinion, clinical experience, and extrapolation from pharmacological principles rather than rigorous scientific data that are urgently needed.

PERIOPERATIVE MANAGEMENT

Preoperative Period

Perioperative management of opioid-dependent patients begins with preoperative administration of their daily maintenance or baseline opioid dose prior to induction of general, spinal, or regional anesthesia. Patients may be instructed to take their usual dose of oral opioid on the morning of surgery. Because most sustained-release opioids provide 12 hours or more of analgesic effect, baseline requirements will generally be maintained during preoperative and intraoperative periods. Thereafter baseline requirements may be provided orally, particularly following ambulatory surgery, or parenterally for those recovering in hospital from more invasive procedures.[4,67] Unless contraindicated, patients may also be instructed to take their morning dose of COX-2 inhibitor to reduce inflammatory responses to surgery and to augment opioid-mediated analgesia.[13]

Patients who are instructed not to take, or those who forget to take, baseline opioids may be treated with an equivalent loading dose of morphine or hydromorphone, administered preoperatively as an oral elixir (if time permits), or intravenously, either at anesthetic induction or during the operative procedure. Patients may also be instructed to maintain their transdermal fentanyl patch into the operating room. If the preparation was removed, an intravenous fentanyl infusion may be initiated to maintain baseline plasma concentrations. A new patch may then be applied intraoperatively; however, it may take 6–12 hours to reestablish baseline analgesic effects.[68,69] During that time interval, the fentanyl infusion may be gradually decreased in rate and eventually discontinued.

Baseline intravenous opioid infusions may also be maintained preoperatively and then converted to IV PCA following recovery from anesthesia. Epidural and intrathecal opioid infusions delivered by internally implanted devices are generally maintained throughout the perioperative period and are used to maintain baseline pain control. The only exception to this rule applies to patients receiving intrathecal infusions of the nonopioid relaxant lioresal (Baclofen). It may be prudent to discontinue or reduce the intrathecal infusion rate of lioresal during the immediate perioperative period as central effects and peripheral skeletal muscle-relaxing effects of this agent may enhance neuromuscular blockade and increase the incidence of hypotension and excessive sedation.[70]

Intraoperative Period

If the surgical or anesthetic technique permits, it is preferable to continue with oral opioids such as oral transmucosal fentanyl (Actiq), rapidly disintegrating oral fentanyl (Fentora), or "swish and swallow" doses of methadone, during the intraoperative and immediate postoperative period.[71] Patients recovering from ambulatory surgery may initially be treated with intravenous boluses of fentanyl or sufentanil. Following stabilization in the postanesthesia care unit (PACU), they may be restarted on oral opioids in doses higher than baseline requirements depending on the invasiveness of the procedure.[71]

Differences in oral to intravenous dose equivalence must be appreciated to estimate perioperative baseline and supplemental opioid dose requirements. Because parenteral administration bypasses gastrointestinal absorption variables and first-pass hepatic clearance and metabolism, most IV or intramuscular (IM) doses of opioids can be adjusted downward from doses taken orally.[72,73] This is particularly the case with IV morphine and hydromorphone, which have 3 and 2–4 times, respectively, greater bioavailability and systemic potency than equivalent oral doses.[73–75] In contrast, oxycodone and sustained-release oxycontin have high oral bioavailability that approaches 83% of an IV dose, therefore baseline oral dose can be approximated by nearly similar doses of IV morphine (1–1.5 mg oral oxycodone = 1 mg IV morphine).[76,77] Patients treated with transdermal fentanyl (Duragesic) or receiving IV PCA morphine/hydromorphone at home or hospice are more straightforward as their baseline requirement may be supplied with an equivalent IV dose of opioid.[73]

Because there may be significant interpatient variability in opioid dose requirements, intraoperative vital signs, particularly heart rate, respiratory rate, and degree of pupil dilation, need to be closely monitored. The optimal intraoperative dose should avoid both under- and overmedication, both associated with negative perioperative outcomes.[5–7,71] One technique that may help gauge the adequacy of intraoperative opioid dosing is to reverse neuromuscular blockade and allow patients to breathe spontaneously at later stages of the general anesthetic. Patients with respiratory rates greater than 20 breaths per minute and exhibiting slight to markedly dilated pupils generally require additional opioid dosing. Intravenous boluses of morphine, fentanyl, or hydromorphone are titrated as needed to maintain a rate of 12–14 breaths per minute and a slightly miotic pupil.[7]

Postoperative Period

To provide effective postsurgical analgesia, a continuous parenteral opioid infusion or IV PCA provide useful options.[78,79] IV PCA may be started in the PACU as soon as patient becomes oriented and capable of utilizing the device. Initiation in the PACU minimizes the risk of undermedication and breakthrough pain that may occur during patient transport to the surgical care unit. To compensate for opioid tolerance and receptor downregulation, higher than normal doses of morphine or hydromorphone might be considered. A basal infusion equivalent either to the patient's hourly oral dose requirement or 1 to 2 PCA boluses per hour may be added to maintain baseline opioid requirements. Basal infusions may not be required in patients receiving baseline analgesia via transdermal fentanyl patch.

Oral methadone has been advocated for use in patients who experience ineffective post surgical analgesia despite administration of relatively high doses of morphine or synthetic derivatives of morphine.[56] The improved analgesic efficacy may be related to (1) methadone's ability to activate a different spectra of μ-receptor subtypes to which morphine tolerance has not developed; (2) methadone's activity at α-adrenergic receptors may provide useful analgesic effects that are not influenced by high-grade opioid tolerance; and, finally, (3) d-methadone has been shown to block morphine tolerance and opioid-induced hyperalgesia by virtue of its NMDA-receptor antagonistic and α-adrenergic agonistic properties.[80,81] For these reasons, some have even advocated methadone as the IV PCA opioid of choice in opioid-dependent patients.[82,83]

Nonopioid analgesic adjuvants may also be employed to reduce opioid dose requirements and provide multimodal analgesia in the postoperative period, although relatively few evaluations have been performed in opioid-dependent patients. Nonopioid analgesics, including NSAIDs and selective COX-2 inhibitors,[13,84] low-dose ketamine, and clonidine by various routes, have all been studied (see General Patient Management). A recent review on the topic has encouraged the use of multimodal pain management therapy in the perioperative management of chronic pain patients with opioid dependency by using a round-the-clock regimen of NSAIDs, COX-2 inhibitors, acetaminophen, and regional blockade.[75]

Finally, it may be worthwhile to consider the contribution of fear and anxiety to the overall pain syndrome. This is especially true for opioid-tolerant patients and polydrug abusers. Anxiety and fear need to be discussed and treated with appropriate medication as required. Anxiolytic agents, benzodiazepines, and tricyclic antidepressants may be administered to treat symptoms as they arise. Liaison with appropriate agencies (addiction medicine, psychiatry) may become necessary.

Neuraxial Analgesia for Postoperative Pain

Neuraxial administration of opioids offers a more efficient method of providing postsurgical analgesia than parenteral or oral opioids.[85–88] Intrathecal and epidural doses of morphine are roughly 100 times and 10 times more potent than for the same dose of morphine given parenterally.[86] Thus, significantly greater levels of analgesia can be delivered to those patients recovering from more extensive procedures where postsurgical parenteral opioid doses would be expected to be very high. Despite this, there have been few evaluations of neuraxial analgesia in opioid-dependent patients.[89] In contrast to local anesthetic blockade, neuraxial opioid analgesia is influenced by downregulation of spinal opiate receptors and epidural and intrathecal dose requirements are increased proportionally.[86–88]

With intrathecal administration, opioid dose is generally a small fraction of the patient's baseline oral requirement. Despite the fact that patients experience effective pain relief, plasma concentrations and supraspinal receptor binding may decline to the point that acute withdrawal is precipitated, unless supplementary opioids are given.[86] For this reason it is important to maintain baseline opioid requirements either orally or by intravenous PCA in patients who remain nil per os (NPO). Monitoring for complications in particular excessive sedation and respiratory depression is mandatory when administering opioid drugs in higher than normal concentrations and via different routes of administration.

Increasing the concentration of epidurally administered opioids may compensate for spinal receptor downregulation. For patients treated with epidural infusions, an opioid loading dose greater than that used in naïve patients, followed by a more concentrated infusion may improve pain control in highly tolerant patients. Patient-controlled epidural boluses (PCEA) may be added to complement the basal epidural infusion. Local anesthetics such as bupivacaine (0.1%), levobupivacaine (0.1%), or ropivacaine (0.2%) may be added to the epidural infusate to provide selective neural blockade and augment opioid-mediated analgesia.[86] Rescue doses of parenteral and possibly oral opioids might be administered to gain supraspinal analgesic effects

and to prevent withdrawal symptoms. In patients ordered to take nothing by mouth, epidural analgesia is employed for postsurgical pain while baseline requirements are maintained with IV PCA, IV boluses of opioids, or "sip and swallow" doses of methadone. In addition to increasing the epidural opioid infusion concentration, some advocate switching to an opioid that has high intrinsic potency such as sufentanil.[89]

Regional Analgesia for Postoperative Pain

Expert opinion suggests that, whenever possible, opioid-tolerant patients should be offered regional analgesia particularly on procedures performed on the extremities.[7,71] Techniques that may be considered include tissue infiltration and nerve and plexus blockade. Advantages of a regional analgesic approach include reduction in parenteral/oral opioid requirements and improvement in distal perfusion as a result of sympathetic blockade. Regional blockade may offer a useful alternative for most peripheral vascular and reimplantation surgeries and for other procedures requiring graft revision or replacement. For upper extremity procedures, brachial plexus blockade can be performed using interscalene and supraclavicular approaches. Similarly, for lower extremities, sciatic block, lumbar plexus block, continuous femoral block, and ankle block may be performed. Neural blockade may be initiated with bupivacaine or levbupivacaine in standard doses. A continuous infusion of bupivacaine or levobupivacaine may be continued postoperatively. With appropriate protocols and safety guidelines, patients may be discharged home with indwelling brachial plexus catheters and local anesthetic infused for up to 48 hours via disposable pumps. Other interventions include injection of local anesthetics and opioids into knee and other articular joints and injections of local anesthetics into disk spaces or iliac crest for spinal surgery. The goal is to minimize pain perception and reduce, although not completely eliminate, the use of oral or parenteral opioids.[6,71]

Dose Tapering

Following ambulatory surgery, baseline requirements for oral opioids generally need to be supplemented with additional doses, generally 20%–50% increase above baseline, to accommodate pain associated with surgical injury.[71] Oral opioids may then be downtitrated daily over 3–7 days to presurgical amounts, as the intensity of acute pain diminishes.

Although opioid analgesics should never be withheld from dependent patients, some caregivers cautiously underestimate theoretical IV dose equivalencies in patients requiring extremely high baseline doses of oral or transdermal opioids, especially in patients recovering from surgical procedures performed to reduce baseline chronic pain.[6,7,71] For example, only 50% of an intravenous equivalent may need to be given to patients requiring oxycodone doses greater than 200 mg/d, morphine doses greater than 300 mg/d, or transdermal fentanyl doses greater than 150 μg/h. Opioid dosing may be increased as needed if patients do not experience adequate pain control. When pain is markedly reduced following successful spine surgery, neurolysis, or cordotomy, baseline opioid dosing should be gradually tapered rather than abruptly stopped to avoid withdrawal.[6,7,90] Postoperative baseline or maintenance dose may be reduced 25%–50% and administered as divided doses. Dose tapering may proceed by 25%–50% every third day, until the daily dose

Table 34.7: Guidelines for Perioperative Pain Management in Opioid Tolerant Patients

Preoperative

    Evaluation: should include early recognition and high index of suspicion

    Identification: identify factors such as total opioid dose requirement, previous surgery/trauma resulting in undermedication, inadequate analgesia, or relapse episodes

    Consultation: meet with addiction specialists and pain specialists with regard to perioperative planning

    Reassurance: discuss patient concerns related to pain control, anxiety, and risk of relapse

    Medication: calculate opioid dose requirement and mode(s) of administration, provide anxiolytics or other medications: as clinically indicated

Intraoperative

    Maintain baseline opioids (oral, transdermal, intravenous). Have patient take morning dose of sustained duration opioids the day of surgery

    Increase intraoperative and postoperative opioid dose to compensate for tolerance

    Provide peripheral neural or plexus blockade, consider neuraxial analgesic techniques when clinically indicated

    Utilize nonopioids as analgesic adjuncts

Postoperative

    Plan preoperatively for postoperative analgesia; formulate primary strategy as well as suitable alternatives.

    Maintain baseline opioids

    Employ multimodal analgesic techniques

    Patient-controlled analgesia: as primary therapy or as supplementation for epidural or regional techniques

    Continue neuraxial opioids: intrathecal or epidural analgesia

    Continue continuous neural blockade

Postdischarge

    If surgery provides complete pain relief, opioids should be slowly tapered, rather than abruptly discontinued

    Develop a pain management plan prior to hospital discharge; provide adequate doses of opioid and nonopioid analgesics

    Arrange for a timely outpatient pain clinic follow-up or a visit with the patient's addictionologist

Reprinted with permission from Mitra and Sinatra.[7]

has decreased to 10–15 mg of morphine equivalent, after which time it may be stopped.[96] Alternatively, patients can be switched to an equianalgesic dose of methadone, which can then be slowly tapered. Transdermal fentanyl patches are easily maintained and replaced. In patients recovering from back procedures, surgical improvement in analgesia may allow fentanyl dose tapering of 25% within 24–48 hours. Further tapering may continue every 48 to 72 hours as tolerated by the patient. Application of clonidine transdermal patch 0.1–0.2 mg/h may help minimize some of the autonomic aspects of opioid withdrawal if symptoms should become distressing.

Following hospital discharge, opioid-dependent patients should be scheduled for immediate follow-up visit with a pain specialist, who can optimize pain management during rehabilitation and facilitate opioid dose tapering. Some patients may require the expertise of an addictionologist and possibly enrolment into a buprenorphine detoxification program.

Mitra and Sinatra[7] suggested detailed guidelines for perioperative pain management in opioid-tolerant patients. A general guideline for the perioperative period is shown in Table 34.7.

CONCLUSION

In conclusion, it is important to emphasize that opioid-dependent and substance-abusing patients have unique needs in the acute pain setting. Starting with the initial important goals of identifying and assessing such patients, the anesthesiologist and

the pain specialist are responsible for maintaining baseline opioid requirements and for providing effective multimodal analgesia. Withdrawal phenomena because of the abrupt discontinuation of other substances need also be identified and prevented or treated. Comprehensive, round-the-clock pain control remains the prime concern in the acute phase of management, relegating the issue of addiction treatment to a later phase once the patient is clinically more stable and pain free. Liaison with the patient's addiction treatment system is important for this purpose. The liaison issue becomes vitally important in the case of acute pain management for those on methadone or buprenorphine maintenance therapy. The latter scenario (acute pain management in those on BMT) is especially likely to become more commonplace in future. Guidelines for management, as suggested in the accompanying tables, are often based on clinical experience, expertise of people working in this area, and anecdotes rather than rigorous scientific data. Future studies with appropriate methodology are warranted in this respect.

Finally, it must be said that the cornerstone of management of these patients is achieving the balance between the administration of appropriate analgesia, on one hand, and close clinical monitoring for patient safety, on the other.

REPRESENTATIVE CASE MANAGEMENT

The following case reports offer insight and management guidelines for common issues observed in opioid-dependent patients, recognizing that alternative methods of treatment may be provided.

Case 1

Mrs RM, a 77-year-old, with a history of non-insulin-dependent diabetes mellitus, degenerative joint disease, and obesity, was scheduled for elective bilateral total knee arthroplasty. She has been taking oxycontin 20 mg twice a day for 2 years, which was recently increased to 40 mg twice a day. Her anesthesiologist used a combined spinal-epidural (CSE) technique. Intraoperatively she received 0.75% bupivacaine (15 mg) with 0.25 mg of preservative-free morphine (which reflect the standard spinal anesthetic/analgesic dose at our institution) and following completion of the procedure the epidural catheter was tested with 3 mL of 2% lidocaine. Approximately 45 minutes following her arrival in PACU, she began to complain of severe pain (VAS pain intensity of 9). At this point, an epidural bolus of 8 mL of 0.25% bupivacaine resulted in improved pain relief. An epidural infusion with hydromorphone (10 μg/mL) with 0.03% bupivacaine was started at a rate of 10 mL/h. However, within 60 minutes she again complained of severe pain. The pain specialist was notified and suspected that the inadequate level of analgesia noted by the patient was related to high-grade opioid tolerance. An epidural loading dose of hydromorphone (3 mg, usual loading dose is 1 mg), plus 8 mL bupivacaine (0.25%), reestablished effective pain control. A more concentrated epidural infusion containing hydromorphone (30 μg/mL) plus bupivacaine (0.1%) at 12 mL/h plus patient-controlled boluses of 3 mL every 10 minutes as needed maintained analgesia. In addition to neuraxial analgesia, IV morphine (5 mg every 2–3 h PRN) was prescribed to insure adequate central analgesic and sedating effects. Intravenous morphine was discontinued the evening following surgery and oxycontin (20 mg) was initiated. Multimodal analgesic supplementation included administration of a COX-2 inhibitor rofecoxib (50 mg every day), and application of a clonidine patch (0.1 mg every hour). The following morning, her dose of oxycontin was increased to 40 mg twice a day, the epidural infusion was discontinued 48 hours following surgery, and she was advanced to oral analgesics, oxycontin (80 mg twice a day) plus oxycodone (10–20 mg every 4 hours PRN) and rofecoxib (50 mg). The patient remained comfortable on this dose during her additional 2-day stay in the hospital. Following discharge her daily dose of oxycontin was gradually decreased to 20 mg twice a day over a period of 2–3 weeks and the dose of rofecoxib was decreased to 12.5 mg every day.

The major error in this case was to have not recognized that, despite her age, Mrs RM was highly opioid tolerant, therefore doses of opioids employed for neuraxial analgesia should have been increased substantially and supplemented with judicious doses of IV or oral opioids as required.

Case 2

Mr RS is a 48-year-old with chronic low back pain of several years' duration who presents for spinal fusion surgery with iliac crest bone graft. He has required treatment with opioid analgesics for several years and is currently prescribed transdermal fentanyl patch (Duragesic, Janssen; 100 μg/h) and oxycodone (5 mg) with acetaminophen. He was told by his orthopedic surgeon to discontinue transdermal fentanyl the night prior to surgery, as it might interfere with the general anesthetic. During the 3-hour operative procedure performed with an isoflurane-based anesthetic, Mr RS received 400-μg of fentanyl and 10 mg of morphine sulfate. On transfer to the PACU, he was noted to be tachycardic, hypertensive, and screaming in pain. The patient was given 20 mg of morphine in divided doses over a period of 5 minutes yet continued to experience severe pain (pain intensity score of 11 on a 0–10 VAS scale). He was then given an additional 250 μg of fentanyl yet continued to be hyperdynamic and agitated and complaining of severe pain. The pain management team took over care of the patient and titrated 8 mg of IV hydromorphone over a period of 10 minutes. At this time his pain score was reduced to 5 on a 0–10 VAS. The patient was started on IV PCA hydromorphone with a bolus dose of 0.6 mg every 6 minutes and a basal infusion of 0.6 mg/h. Two transdermal fentanyl patches (100 μg/h plus 50 μg/h; total 150 μg/h) were applied to reestablish baseline opioid requirements. In addition the patient was treated with rofecoxib (50 mg every day) and clonidine transdermal patch (0.1 mg/h). (Because rofecoxib has been withdrawn celecoxib [400 mg] offers a suitable alternative.) Approximately 12 hours after the fentanyl patch was applied, the patient was noticeably more comfortable, with a VAS score of 3, and somewhat sedated, therefore the PCA basal infusion was discontinued. The patient remained on PCA hydromorphone for 48 hours; thereafter he was converted to oral opioids. We calculated that he used 26 mg of hydromorphone each day, and converted him to oral hydromorphone 6 mg every 4 hours PRN for pain while continuing transdermal fentanyl (150 μg/h). Over the next 48 hours, his dose of oral hydromorphone was reduced to 2 mg every 4 hours and the transdermal fentanyl patch was reduced to 100 μg/h. Clonidine patch and oral rofecoxib were continued. Mr RS was discharged to home on this dose of opioid and scheduled for a follow-up visit in the pain clinic.

The important point in this case is that patients treated with transdermal fentanyl are opioid tolerant. The patch should be maintained during the perioperative period and supplemented with higher than normal doses of IV or oral opioids for breakthrough pain.

Case 3

Mr JK is a 34-year-old heroin addict (for 5 years) who was otherwise healthy prior to his motor vehicle accident and femur fracture 5 weeks ago. Following open repair of the fracture, he has been off heroin and has been treated with fentanyl transdermal delivery system (Duragesic patch; 100 μg/h) for pain control. He was scheduled for replacement of hardware at the fracture site. The transdermal fentanyl patch was removed the morning of surgery. Intraoperatively, he received epidural anesthesia with 2% epidural lidocaine with fentanyl (100 μg). For postoperative pain control, he received an epidural infusion of bupivacaine 0.1% with fentanyl (5 μg/mL) at the rate of 10 mL/h plus epidural PCA. Mr JK's postoperative pain relief was fair to good, but he used the maximum epidural PCA dose and required two rescue boluses of bupivacaine (0.25%). The next day, during the morning rounds, he was noted to be in moderate discomfort (VAS score of 5 of 10); however, he was also diaphoretic, tachycardic, and complaining of abdominal cramping and diarrhea. Infectious disease was called and a stool sample was obtained to rule out *Clostridium difficile* infection. The orthopedic surgeons suspected infection and possible sepsis and requested that the epidural be removed. The pain management team recognized that the patient was exhibiting classic signs of opioid withdrawal. He was immediately treated with IV hydromorphone (6 mg) and a clonidine patch (0.1 mg/h) was applied. In addition his preoperative dose of transdermal fentanyl was restarted. The patient's symptoms subsided and he made a smooth transition from epidural analgesia to transdermal fentanyl plus oral hydromorphone as needed for breakthrough pain.

The major message associated with this case is that, although neuraxial analgesia may provide effective pain relief, the dose of opioid administered may be too low to maintain baseline plasma concentrations and prevent systemic opioid withdrawal.

Case 4

Mr RM is a 35-year-old male presenting for a right total hip arthroplasty. He was involved in a motor vehicle accident 1 month prior with fracture and dislocation of his right hip. The patient's past medical history is notable for substance abuse of opioids, marijuana, benzodiazepines, and tobacco. It was unclear as to when he last used benzodiazepines. He is otherwise healthy with no known cardiac, respiratory, gastrointestinal, or infectious issues. The patient has been on maintenance methadone, taking 110 mg every morning. He took his methadone on the morning of the operation.

In the operating room, before the induction of general anesthesia, the patient had a lumbar L3-L4 epidural catheter placed. He was given 1 mg of hydromorphone epidurally along with local anesthetic intraoperatively before starting a continuous standard epidural infusion of 10 μg/mL of hydromorphone and 0.031% of bupivacaine at a rate of 12 mL/h.

In the recovery room, the patient was in severe 10/10 pain, complained of muscle spasms, and was diaphoretic. The patient was given a bolus through the epidural pump of 20 mL of the standard epidural infusion with an increase in the rate of the epidural infusion to 18 mL/h. The concentration of the hydromorphone in the epidural infusion was increased to 30 μg/mL and the infusion was run at a rate of 12 mL/h. His pain score decreased to 5/10.

On arrival to the surgical floor approximately 1 hour later, the patient again complained of 10/10 pain that was unbearable and associated with uncontrollable muscle spasms and rigors. The catheter was bolused with bupivacaine (0.25%) and 2 mg of hydromorphone, which provided some relief; however, the patient remained very anxious. Intravenous lorazepam (2 mg) was given in incremental doses. He eventually calmed down, and reported feeling much better at a pain scale of 4/10. The epidural infusion with repeated scheduled doses of lorazepam (2 mg every 4 to 6 hours) eventually provided adequate relief.

This case illustrates how clinicians may focus on, and adequately compensate for, opioid tolerance while restricting or omitting other centrally acting agents that the patient may be dependent on. Placement of the epidural catheter and administration of high doses of hydromorphone was a good option for this patient; he, however, was troubled by excessive anxiety and agitation that worsened his perception of pain. Once his benzodiazepine dependence was uncovered, a nearly continuous administration of lorazepam significantly reduced his pain intensity and agitation. Given the magnitude of his anxiety component, scheduled doses of benzodiazepines should have been administered intraoperatively and in the early postsurgical period.

Case 5

The pain service was asked to consult for a 34-year-old patient suffering severe postoperative discomfort that could not be adequately controlled by the PACU nursing team and orthopedic surgical staff. The patient had a long history of substance abuse, including illicit use of heroin, oxycodone, and cocaine. He enrolled in an opioid detoxification program approximately 3 months prior to the present admission and has been treated with sublingual buprenorphine (8 mg) plus naloxone (Suboxone) daily. The last dose was taken the morning of surgery. He presented to the same-day surgical center with a diagnosis of a left knee meniscal tear with severe pain and underwent an arthroscopic repair with general anesthesia. Despite receiving 400 μg of fentanyl intraoperatively, he complained of severe discomfort (VAS of 10 of 10) that was unresponsive to PACU doses of morphine (15 mg), fentanyl (100 μg), and hydromorphone (3 mg). The pain service recognized that the patient was on BMT (Suboxone), and suspected that ongoing receptor antagonism may have reduced the effectiveness of the opioid-mediated analgesia. To overcome receptor blockade and rapidly gain pain control the patient was treated with sufentanil, a potent opioid with high receptor affinity. After receiving 50 μg in divided doses, he reported a reduction in pain intensity (VAS 8 of 10). The patient refused a femoral nerve block; however, he did agree to a single intra-articular injection of bupivacaine (0.25%, 8 mL) performed by the surgical team. He also received ketorolac (30 mg) to reduce the inflammatory aspects of his acute pain. The patient was admitted to the surgical care unit for overnight pain control. He was provided IV PCA hydromorphone (3-mg loading dose followed by 0.4-mg incremental bolus doses with an 8-minute lockout) and given single dose of celecoxib (400 mg) later in the evening. The following morning, he was converted to oral analgesics (oxycodone [10–15 mg] plus celecoxib [200 mg twice a day]). Methadone (10 mg twice a day) was substituted for suboxone. He was discharged uneventfully and maintained on this prescription for the next 72 hours, whereupon suboxone therapy was reinitiated by his psychiatrist. The patient and his caregivers were instructed that prior to future surgery, methadone should be employed as a temporary substitute for buprenophine/naloxone compounds and, if applicable, regional anesthesia/analgesia techniques should be strongly considered.

REFERENCES

1. Morgan JP. American opiophobia: customary underutilization of opioid analgesics. *Adv Alcohol Subst Abuse.* 1985;5:163–168.
2. Mehta V, Langford RM. Acute pain management for opioid dependent patients. *Anaesthesia.* 2006;61:269–276.
3. Streitzer J. Pain management in the opioid-dependent patient. *Curr Psychiatry Rep.* 2001;3:489–496.
4. May JA, White HC, Leonard-White A, Warltier DC, Pagel PS. The patient recovering from alcohol or drug addiction: special issues for the anesthesiologist. *Anesth Analg.* 2001;92:1601–1608.
5. Jage J, Bey T. Postoperative analgesia in patients with substance use disorders: part I. *Acute Pain.* 2000;3:140–155.
6. Hord AH. Postoperative analgesia in the opioid-dependent patient. In: Sinatra RS, Hord AH, Ginsberg B, Preble LM, eds. *Acute Pain: Mechanisms and Management.* St Louis, MO: Mosby; 1992;390–398.

7. Mitra S, Sinatra RS. Perioperative management of acute pain in the opioid-dependent patient. *Anesthesiology.* 2004;101:212–227.

8. Cohen MJ, Jasser S, Herron PD, Margolis CG. Ethical perspectives: opioid treatment of chronic pain in the context of addiction. *Clin J Pain.* 2002;18(suppl 4):S99–S107.

9. Nissen LM, Tett SE, Cranoud T, Williams B, Smith MT. Opioid analgesic prescribing: use of an audit of analgesic prescribing by general practitioners and the multidisciplinary pain centre at Royal Brisbane Hospital. *Br J Clin Pharmacol.* 2001;52:693–698.

10. Bell JR. Australian trends in opioid prescribing for chronic non-cancer pain, 1986–1996. *Med J Aust.* 1997;167:26–29.

11. Manchikanti L, Cash KA, Damron KS, Manchukonda R, Pampati V, McManus CD. Controlled substance abuse and illicit drug use in chronic pain patients: an evaluation of multiple variables. *Pain Physician.* 2006;9:215–226.

12. IMS H. IMS National sales perspective. 2004 (as cited in reference 61).

13. Stephens J, Laskin B, Pashos C, Pena B, Wong J. The burden of acute postoperative pain and the potential role of the COX-2-specific inhibitors. *Rheumatology.* 2003;42(suppl 3):iii40–iii52.

14. O'Brien CP. Drug addiction and drug abuse. In: Hardman JG, Limbird LE, eds. *Goodman and Gilman's The Pharmacological Basis of Therapeutics,* 10th ed. New York, NY: McGraw-Hill; 2001;621–642.

15. Substance Abuse and Mental Health Services Administration. *Overview of Findings from the 2003 National Survey on Drug Use and Health.* Rockville, MD: Office of Applied Statistics, NSDUH Series h-24, DHHS Publication No. SMA 04-3963; 2004.

16. Crane E. Narcotic analgesics. The Drug Abuse Warning Network (DAWN) report, January 2003. Available at: http://oas.samhsa.gov/2k3/pain/DAWNpain.pdf. Accessed February 15, 2007.

17. US Department of Health and Human Services. Office of Applied Statistics, Substance Abuse and Mental Health Services Administration (SAMHSA). Drug Abuse Warning Network (DAWN). *The DAWN Report: Opiate-related drug misuse deaths in six states: 2003.* Rockville, MD: SAMHSA, 2006: Issue 19.

18. Substance Abuse and Mental Health Services Administration. *Results from the 2005 National Survey on Drug Use and Health: National Findings.* Rockville, MD: Office of Applied Studies, NSDUH Series H-30, DHHS Publication No. SMA 06-4194; 2006.

19. American Psychiatric Association. *Diagnostic and Statistical Manual of Mental Disorders.* 4th ed. Text revision (DSM-IV-TR). Washington, DC: American Psychiatric Association; 2000.

20. US Department of Health and Human Services. Office of Applied Statistics, Substance Abuse and Mental Health Services Administration (SAMHSA). Drug Abuse Warning Network (DAWN). *The DAWN report: year-end 2000 emergency department data.* Rockville, MD: Office of Applied Studies, DAWN Series D-18, DHHS Publication No. SMA 01-3532; 2001.

21. Office of National Drug Control Policy (ONDCP). Drug facts: heroin. Available at: http://www.whitehousedrugpolicy.gov/drugfact/heroin/index.html. Accessed February 15, 2007.

22. Gustin HB, Akil H. Opioid analgesics. In: Hardman JG, Limbird LE, eds. *Goodman and Gilman's The Pharmacological Basis of Therapeutics.* 10th ed. New York, NY: McGraw-Hill, 2001;569–619.

23. US Department of Health and Human Services. National Institutes of Health. Community Epidemiology Work Group. *Epidemiologic trends in drug abuse: advance report June 2006.* Bethesda, MD: National Institute on Drug Abuse NIH Publication No. 06-5878A; 2006.

24. Clark HW. Office-based practice and opioid use disorders. *N Engl J Med.* 2003;349:928–930.

25. Fishbain DA, Rosomoff HL, Rosomoff RS. Drug abuse, dependence, and addiction in chronic pain patients. *Clin J Pain.* 1992;8:77–85.

26. Savage SR. Addiction in the treatment of pain: significance, recognition and treatment. *J Pain Symptom Manage.* 1993;8:265–278.

27. Kouyanou K, Pither CE, Wessely S. Medication misuse, abuse and dependence in chronic pain patients. *J Psychosom Res.* 1997;43:497–504.

28. Hurwitz W. The challenge of prescription drug misuse: a review and commentary. *Pain Med.* 2005;6:152–161.

29. Manchikanti L, Beyer C, Damron K, Pampati V. A comparative evaluation of illicit drug use in patients with or without controlled substance abuse in interventional pain management. *Pain Physician.* 2003;6:281–285.

30. Scimeca MM, Savage SR, Portenoy R, Lowinson J. Treatment of pain in methadone-maintained patients. *Mount Sinai J Med.* 2000;67:412–422.

31. Alfred DP, Compton P, Samet JH. Acute pain management for patients receiving maintenance methadone or buprenorphine therapy. *Ann Intern Med.* 2006;144:127–134.

32. Compton P, Charuvastra VC, Kintaudi K, Ling W. Pain responses in methadone-maintained opioid abusers. *J Pain Symptom Manage.* 2000;20:237–245.

33. Kantor TG, Cantor R, Tom E. A study of hospitalized surgical patients on methadone maintenance. *Drug Alcohol Depend.* 1980;6:163–173.

34. Manfredi PL, Gonzales GR, Cheville AI, Kornick C, Payne R. Methadone analgesia in cancer pain patients on chronic methadone maintenance therapy. *J Pain Symptom Manage.* 2001;21:169–174.

35. Karasz A, Zallman I, Berg K, et al. The experience of chronic severe pain in patients undergoing methadone maintenance treatment. *J Pain Symptom Manage.* 2004;28:517–525.

36. Jasinski DR. Tolerance and dependence to opiates. *Acta Anaesthesiol Scand.* 1997;41:184–186.

37. Bruera E, Macmillan K, Hanson J, MacDonald RN. The cognitive effects of the administration of narcotic analgesics in patients with cancer pain. *Pain.* 1989;39:13–16.

38. Weissman DE, Haddox JD. Opioid pseudoaddiction – an iatrogenic syndrome. *Pain.* 1989;36:363–366.

39. Portenoy RK, Foley KM. Chronic use of opioid analgesics in non-malignant pain: report of 38 cases. *Pain.* 1986;25:171–186.

40. Evers GC. Pseudo-opioid-resistant pain. *Support Care Cancer.* 1997;5:457–460.

41. Steindler EM. ASAM addiction terminology. In: Graham AW, Schultz TK, eds. *Principles of Addiction Medicine.* 2nd ed. Chevy Chase, MD: American Society of Addiction Medicine; 1998;1301–1304.

42. Savage SR, Joranson DE, Covington EC, Schnoll SE, Heit HA, Gilson AM. Definitions related to the medical use of opioids: evolution towards universal agreement. *J Pain Symptom Manage.* 2003;26:655–667.

43. de Leon-Casasola OA, Lema MJ. Epidural sufentanil for acute pain control in a patient with extreme opioid dependency. *Anesthesiology.* 1992;76:853–856.

44. Robinson RC, Gatchel RJ, Polatin P, Deschner M, Noe C, Gajraj N. Screening for problematic prescription opioid use. *Clin J Pain.* 2001;17:220–228.

45. Savage SR. Assessment for addiction in pain-treatment settings. *Clin J Pain.* 2002;18(suppl 4):28–38.

46. Chabal C, Erjavec MK, Jacobson L, Mariano A, Chaney E. Prescription opiate abuse in chronic pain patients: clinical criteria, incidence, and predictors. *Clin J Pain.* 1997;13:150–155.

47. Compton P, Darakjian J, Miotto K. Screening for addiction in patients with chronic pain and "problematic" substance use: evaluation of a pilot assessment tool. *J Pain Symptom Manage.* 1998;16:355–363.

48. Prater CD, Zylstra RG, Miller KE. Successful pain management for the recovering addicted patient. *Primary Care Companion J Clin Psychiatry.* 2002;4:125–131.

49. Clark JL, Kalan GE. Effective treatment of severe cancer pain of the head using low-dose ketamine in an opioid-tolerant patient. *J Pain Symptom Manage.* 1995;10:310–314.

50. Haller G, Waeber JL, Infante NK, Clergue F. Ketamine combined with morphine for the management of pain in an opioid addict. *Anesthesiology.* 2002;96:1265–1266.

51. Mackenzie JW. Acute pain management for opioid dependent patients. *Anaesthesia.* 2006;61:907–908.

52. Liu S, Carpenter RL, Neal JM. Epidural anesthesia and analgesia: their role in postoperative outcome. *Anesthesiology.* 1995;82:474–506.

53. Schug SA, Fry RA. Continuous regional analgesia in comparison with intravenous opioid administration for routine postoperative pain control. *Anaesthesia.* 1994;49:528–532.

54. Wood PR, Soni N. Anaesthesia and substance abuse. *Anaesthesia.* 1989;44:672–680.

55. Scheutz F. Drug addicts and local analgesia – effectivity and general side effects. *Scand J Dental Res.* 1982;90:299–305.

56. Sartain JB, Mitchell SJ. Successful use of oral methadone after failure of intravenous morphine and ketamine. *Anaesth Intensive Care.* 2002;30:487–489.

57. Lawlor PG, Turner KS, Hanson J, Bruera ED. Dose ratio between morphine and methadone in patients with cancer pain – a retrospective study. *Cancer.* 1998;82:1167–1173.

58. Lawlor PG, Turner KS, Hanson J, Bruera ED. Dose ratio between morphine and hydromorphone in patients with cancer pain – a retrospective study. *Pain.* 1997;72:79–85.

59. Walsh SL, Eissenberg T. The clinical pharmacology of buprenorphine: extrapolating from the laboratory to the clinic. *Drug Alcohol Depend.* 2003;70:S13–S27.

60. Savage SR. Principles of pain treatment in the addicted patient. In: Graham AW, Schultz TK, eds. *Principles of Addiction Medicine.* 2nd ed. Chevy Chase, MD: American Society of Addiction Medicine, Inc.; 1998;919–944.

61. Swenson JD, Davis JJ, Johnson KB. Postoperative care of the chronic opioid-consuming patient. *Anesthesiology Clin N Am.* 2005;23:37–48.

62. Fine PG, Marcus M, De Boer AJ, Van Der Oord B. An open label study of oral transmucosal fentanyl citrate (OTFC) for the treatment of breakthrough cancer pain. *Pain.* 1991;45:149–153.

63. Shaiova L, Wallenstein D. Outpatient management of sickle cell pain with chronic opioid pharmacotherapy. *J Nat Med Assoc.* 2004;96:984–986.

64. Peng PWH, Tumber PS, Gourlay D. Perioperative pain management of patients on methadone therapy. *Can J Anesth.* 2005;52:513–523.

65. Roberts DM, Meyer-Witting M. High-dose buprenorphine: perioperative precautions and management strategies. *Anaesth Intensive Care.* 2005;33:17–25.

66. Krantz MJ, Lewcowicz L, Hays H, Woodroffe MA, Robertson AD, Mehler PS. Torsades de pointes associated with very-high-dose methadone. *Ann Intern Med.* 2002;137:501–504.

67. Rapp SE, Ready LB, Nessly ML. Acute pain management in patients with prior opioid consumption: a case-controlled retrospective review. *Pain.* 1995;61:195–201.

68. Sevarino FB, Ning T. Transdermal fentanyl for acute pain management. In: Sinatra RS, Hord AH, Ginsberg B, Preble LM, eds. *Acute Pain: Mechanisms and Management.* St Louis, MO: Mosby; 1992; 364–369.

69. Caplan RA, Ready B, Oden RV, et al. Transdermal fentanyl for postoperative pain management. *JAMA.* 1989;261:1036–1039.

70. Gomar C, Carrero EJ. Delayed arousal after general anesthesia associated with baclofen. *Anesthesiology.* 1994;81:1306–1307.

71. Saberski L. Postoperative pain management for the patient with chronic pain. In: Sinatra RS, Hord AH, Ginsberg B, Preble LM, eds. *Acute Pain: Mechanisms and Management.* St Louis, MO: Mosby; 1992;422–431.

72. Pereira J, Lawlor P, Vigano A, Dorgan M, Bruera E. Equianalgesic dose ratios for opioids: a critical review and proposals for long-term dosing. *J Pain Symptom Manage.* 2001;22:672–687.

73. Foley RM. Opioid analgesics in clinical pain management. In: Herz A, Akil H, Simon EJ, eds. *Handbook of Experimental Pharmacology: Opioids II.* Vol. 104. New York, NY: Springer Verlag: 1993;697–743.

74. Quigley C. Hydromorphone for acute and chronic pain. *Cochrane Database Syst Rev.* 2002;1:CD003447.

75. Brill S, Ginosar Y, Davidson EM. Perioperative management of chronic pain patients with opioid dependency. *Curr Opin Anaesthesiol.* 2006;19:325–331.

76. Poyhia R, Vainio A, Kaiko E. A review of oxycodone's clinical pharmacokinetics and pharmacodynamics. *J Pain Symptom Manage.* 1993;8:63–67.

77. Ginsberg B, Sinatra RS, Adler LJ, et al. Conversion to oral controlled-release oxycodone from intravenous opioid analgesic in the postoperative setting. *Pain Med.* 2003;4(1):31–38.

78. Macintyre PE. Safety and efficacy of patient-controlled analgesia. *Br J Anaesth.* 2001;87:36–46.

79. Parker RK, Holtman B, White PF. Patient-controlled analgesia – does a concurrent opioid infusion improve pain management after surgery? *JAMA.* 1992;266:1947–1952.

80. Pasternak GW. Incomplete cross-tolerance and multiple mu opioid peptide receptors. *Trends Pharmacol Sci.* 2001;22:67–70.

81. Davis AM, Inturrisi CE. D-methadone blocks morphine tolerance and N-methyl-D-aspartate-induced hyperalgesia. *J Pharmacol Exp Ther.* 1999;289:1048–1053.

82. Boyle RK. Intra- and postoperative anaesthetic management of an opioid addict undergoing caesarean section. *Anaesth Intensive Care.* 1991;19:276–279.

83. Fitzgibbon DR, Ready JB. Intravenous high dose methadone administered by patient controlled analgesia and continuous infusion for the treatment of pain refractory to high dose morphine. *Pain.* 1997;73:259–261.

84. Katz WA. Cyclooxygenase-2-selective inhibitors in the management of acute and perioperative pain. *Cleve Clin J Med.* 2002;69(suppl 1):SI65–S175.

85. Harrison DH, Sinatra RS, Chung J, et al. Epidural narcotic and patient-controlled analgesia for post-cesarean section pain relief. *Anesthesiology.* 1988;68:454–457.

86. Cousins MJ, Bridenbaugh PO, eds. *Epidural Neural Blockade in Clinical Anesthesia and Management.* 3rd ed. Philadelphia, PA: Lippincott-Raven; 1998.

87. Wang JK, Nauss LA, Thomas JE. Pain relief by intrathecally applied morphine in man. *Anesthesiology.* 1979;50:149–151.

88. Bromage PR. *Epidural Analgesia.* Philadelphia, PA: W.B. Saunders; 1978.

89. de Leon-Casasola OA, Lema MJ. Epidural bupivacaine/sufentanil therapy for postoperative pain control in patients tolerant to opioid and unresponsive to epidural bupivacaine/morphine. *Anesthesiology.* 1994;80:303–309.

90. Inturrisi CE. Clinical pharmacology of opioids for pain. *Clin J Pain.* 2002;18 (suppl. 4):S3–S13.

Specialist Managed Pain

35

Pain Management Following Colectomy:
A Surgeon's Perspective

Theodore J. Saclarides

Colectomy, whether performed for benign or malignant disease processes, is a potentially morbid operation accompanied by a significant hospital stay, prolonged period of recovery, and extended time off from work. There has been considerable interest recently in determining ways to lessen complications and hasten recovery. Several centers have established clinical pathways and fast-track protocols that attempt to streamline the care of these patients from the minute they walk into the admissions department to the time the discharge order is written. Integral to the optimum management of patients undergoing colon resection is efficient pain control. In fact, pain specialists, whether they are anesthesiologists, nurse anesthetists, or nurse clinicians, have become important team members in these pathway committees.

Successful relief of pain following major abdominal surgery invariably involves the use of parenteral and oral opioids; however, it is well known that narcotics contribute to the formation of an ileus, persistence of which may impair the recovery of patients with respect to restoration of normal bowel function. Consequently, clinicians have sought for ways to minimize the use of systemic narcotics, hasten recovery, and shorten hospital stay without compromising patient comfort or overall satisfaction with respect to their hospitalization. These efforts include neuraxial administration of opioids, using nonnarcotic analgesics, employing minimally invasive surgical techniques, and challenging traditional surgical practices with respect to nasogastric decompression, diet advancement, physical activity, and reliance on old criteria for discharge such as the passage of stool.

POSTOPERATIVE BOWEL DYSFUNCTION

Opioid analgesics are associated with a number of undesirable side effects, including postoperative bowel dysfunction (POBD) and development of ileus. There is no standardized definition for ileus, but Livingston and Passar have defined it as the "functional inhibition of propulsive bowel activity, irrespective of pathogenic mechanism."[1] The Postoperative Ileus Management Council has defined postoperative ileus (POI) as "transient cessation of coor-

dinated bowel motility after surgical intervention, which prevents effective transit of intestinal contents or tolerance of oral intake."[2] Ileus is an expected complication following abdominal surgery and it may normally last for 3 to 4 days. The presence of a complication such as an intra-abdominal infection or anastomotic leak, however, may prolong an ileus. Ileus may follow other types of surgery, and can occur after urologic, gynecologic, orthopedic, and cardiothoracic procedures. It is a very common reason for prolonged hospital stay.

According to 1999–2000 data from the Health Care Financing Administration, in the United States, the overall incidence of postoperative ileus after common abdominal operations was 8.5%. The incidence varies according to specific type of operation performed, being highest for surgery on the small bowel and colon, reaching almost 20%.[2] The actual incidence may actually be higher because adequate documentation in the medical records may be lacking when a retrospective study of this nature is conducted. As stated previously, some reduction in gastrointestinal motility is to be expected during the first few days after an operation. Factors responsible for postoperative bowel dysfunction are outlined in Table 35.1.

The various segments of the gastrointestinal tract recover their normal peristaltic activity at different times. The small bowel is the first to recover its normal motility and it does so usually within the first 24 hours postoperatively. In fact, small bowel peristalsis is visibly apparent during surgery in many cases, and jejunostomy tube feedings may be safely started immediately following completion of the operation. The stomach will recover next, usually within 48 hours. The colon is the last to recover and does so between 48 and 120 hours.[1,3]

Clinically, a patient with a postoperative ileus will complain of abdominal distention, cramping, nausea and vomiting, and delayed passage of flatus and stool. As a consequence of this, resumption of oral intake of nutrients may be delayed and parenteral nutrition may be required. Complications related to a central venous catheter could then occur. Other sequelae of an ileus include delayed ambulation, hypoalbuminemia, poor wound healing, reduced immune function, and nosocomial infections, including pneumonia. The end results are delayed

Table 35.1: Factors Responsible for Postoperative Bowel Dysfunction

Surgical manipulation

    Neurogenic: sympathetic hyperactivity

    Inflammatory: cellular and humoral factors, including endogenous opioid peptides

    Hormonal: corticotrophin releasing factor

Pharmacologic pain management

    Exogenous opioids: used for pain prevention, but also act in the myenteric plexus to directly inhibit GI motility

---

Kehlet H, Holte K. *Am J Surg.* 2001;182 (5A suppl):3S–10S.

Holte K, Kehlet H. *Drugs.* 2002;62:2603–2615.[5]

discharge, increased hospital costs, and reduced overall patient satisfaction (Table 35.2).

The neural regulation of the gastrointestinal tract is governed by both intrinsic (enteric) and extrinsic systems. The former establish the basic motility patterns, that is, the frequency with which migratory peristaltic contractions occur within each segment of the gut. Extrinsic control occurs through the sympathetic and parasympathetic nervous systems, whose function reflect what is occurring at any given moment for a particular patient.[4] Stimulation of the sympathetic nervous system (surgical incisional pain, release of catecholamines as part of the normal response to stress) will have an inhibitory effect on gut function; enhanced parasympathetic activity will have the opposite effect. Alterations in either the intrinsic or extrinsic pathways may contribute to the development of postoperative ileus as may other factors such as infection, inflammation, the extent of surgical manipulation, and opioids. The inflammatory response produced by surgical manipulation and trauma results in activation of macrophages and mast cells that release various inflammatory mediators such as prostaglandins and nitric oxide, a potent inhibitor of gut function. Vasoactive intestinal polypeptide (VIP) and substance P are also released, both of which may contribute to ileus.[5–7]

Table 35.2: Clinical Impact of Postoperative Ileus

Increased postoperative visceral pain

Increased nausea and vomiting

    Increased risk of aspiration

Need for Nasogastric intubation

Prolonged time to oral intake and regular diet

    Delayed wound healing

    Increased risk of malnutrition and catabolism

Prolonged time to mobilization

    Increased pulmonary complications

    Increased risk of DVT

Prolonged hospitalization

    Impaired rehabilitation

    Increased health care costs

From: Kurz A, Sessler DI. *Drugs.* 2003;63:649–671.

Table 35.3: Surgical Techniques: Laparoscopy

Duration of ileus is shortened after less invasive surgery

Reduction in tissue injury leads to less inflammation and sympathetic response

More rapid progression to a solid diet

More rapid hospital discharge

Several studies have shown favorable results

These results may reflect earlier feeding and less reliance on opioid analgesia

---

Holte and Kehlet. *Drugs.* 2002;62(18):2603–2615.[5]

Baig MK, Wexner SD. *Dis Colon Rectum.* 2004;47:516–526.[18]

Endogenous opioids (endorphins, enkephalins, dynorphins) are released as part of the stress response that normally occurs after surgery. Exogenous systemic opioids are potent analgesics and are commonly prescribed following surgery. Both types of opioids activate the same receptor site within the bowel, the μ-receptor, and affect motility, secretion, and transport of fluids and electrolytes. They also profoundly inhibit peristaltic activity, delay gastric emptying, and intestinal transit. The total dose of exogenous opioid administered correlates significantly with the return of bowel function as measured by the return of bowel sounds, time to passage of first flatus, and time to first bowel movement. As expected, return of bowel function correlates with hospital length of stay.[8–10]

MINIMALLY INVASIVE SURGERY

Altering the surgical approach to incorporate minimally invasive technology will have beneficial effects on postoperative pain intensity, analgesic requirements, recovery of bowel function and length of hospital stay. Laparoscopic surgery has been studied extensively and has been compared to open surgery in a randomized fashion. In a meta-analysis of 12 randomized clinical trials published before 2002, 2512 patients were studied. Although laparoscopic surgery took an average of 32.9% longer to complete, there were fewer complications with this approach, specifically with respect to wound complications. The average time to passage of first flatus was reduced by 34% and to tolerance of solid food by 24%. Narcotic usage was reduced by 37%. At 6 hours, pain at rest decreased by 35% and during coughing by 35%. At 3 days, pain at rest was decreased by 63% and during coughing by 40%. Hospital stay was decreased by almost 21%. There were no significant differences in perioperative mortality or oncologic result.[11] Benefits associated with minimally invasive surgery are outlined in Table 35.3.

OPIOID EFFECTS ON BOWEL FUNCTION

When one considers the possible interventions physicians can introduce to shorten the duration of postoperative ileus, hasten return of gastrointestinal function, and shorten hospital stay, the use of opioids is probably one of the easiest and most important modifiable factors. Opioids decrease gastric motility and increase pyloric tone, potentially leading to anorexia, nausea, and vomiting (Table 35.4). They also decrease pancreatic and biliary secretions, reduce small bowel propulsion, and increase

Table 35.4: GI Effects of Opioids[a]

Pharmacologic Impact	Clinical Effect
Decreased gastric motility	Increased GI reflux
Inhibition of small intestinal propulsion	Delayed absorption of medications
Inhibition of large intestinal propulsion	Straining, incomplete evacuation, bloating, abdominal distension
Increased amplitude of nonpropulsive segmental contractions	Spasm, abdominal cramps, and pain
Constriction of sphincter of Oddi	Biliary colic, epigastric discomfort
Increased anal sphincter tone, impaired reflex relaxation, rectal distension	Impaired ability to evacuate bowel
Diminished gastric, biliary, pancreatic and intestinal secretions. Increased absorption of water	Hard, dry stool

[a] If left untreated, opioid-induced bowel dysfunction can lead to pseudo-obstruction of the bowel, fecal impaction, poor absorption of oral drugs, and severe impairment of quality of life. (From: Pappagallo M. *Am J Surg.* 2001;182(suppl):11S–18S; Vanegas G, et al. *Cancer Nurs.* 1998;21:289–297; Kurz A, Sessler DI. *Drugs* 2003;63: 649–671.)

fluid absorption. Within the colon, opioids bind to, and activate, mu receptors in the myeteric plexus. Following activation, these receptors mediate decreased propulsion, increased nonpropulsive contractions, and increased fluid absorption leading to hard and dry stools, bloating, distention, and constipation.

Virtually all anesthetics/analgesics may depress gastrointestinal motility, however the sympathetic blockade and opioid sparing effects associated with epidural local anesthetics may provide clinical benefits Epidural local anesthetics were first administered in the 1920s for the treatment of paralytic ileus. Several studies have demonstrated an improvement in outcome following surgery with respect to pulmonary function, blunting the surgical stress response, and better pain control. Reduced postoperative ileus is a significant benefit of epidural anesthetics/analgesics when compared to general anesthesia and systemic opiates. In fact, bowel function may return 2 to 3 days earlier. This should be taken into consideration when planning clinical pathways and fast-tract protocols for shortening hospital stay.

BENEFITS OF EPIDURAL ANALGESIA

There are several mechanisms by which epidural anesthesia may promote recovery of gastrointestinal motility. These include blockade of noxious afferent fibers, blockade of thoracolumbar sympathetic nerves, release of parasympathetic inhibition, reduced need for postoperative opioids, and increased gastrointestinal blood flow (Table 35.5). It is probably the reduction in postoperative systemic opioids that has the most profound effect.[12–16] Several randomized controlled trials comparing epidural anesthetics/analgesics versus systemic opioids have shown a benefit in favor of the former.[17] Namely, there has been

Table 35.5: Epidural Anesthesia/Analgesia

Blocks sympathetic nervous system efferent tone responsible for inhibiting bowel motility

Minimizes exposure to opioid analgesics

Reduces effort dependent pain, encourages ambulation

Inclusion of local anesthetics is important (Several studies have shown reduction in GI paralysis with epidural local anesthetics alone or combined with opioids as compared with opioids alone[1,3]

Sympathetic blockade with epidural local anesthetics is associated with a higher incidence of hypotension. (Patient must be well hydrated)

Location of catheter important: thoracic application more effective than lumbar or low-thoracic

Steinbrook RA. *Anesth Analg.*1998;86:837–844.

Jorgensen H, et al. *The Cochrane Library.* Issue 3. 2004.

Liu SS. *Anesthesiology.* 1995;83:757–765.

a demonstrable reduction in time to passage of first flatus, first stool, or both. Epidural infusions containing local anesthetics provide greater facilitation of bowel function but are more likely to precipitate hypotension in hypovolemic patients. Liu and coworkers[15] reported that in patients recovering from colonic surgery, infusions containing local anesthetic or dilute local anesthetic plus opioid were associated with more rapid return of bowel function and met criteria for discharge sooner than either epidural solutions containing opioids alone or intravenous patient-controlled analgesia (IV PCA) (Table 35.6). Additional benefits from epidural anesthesia include improved perioperative pulmonary function, blunted surgical stress response, reductions in perioperative cardiac morbidity, and a lower incidence of pulmonary infections and embolism. Complications from epidural catheters include transient paresthesias and the rare case of epidural hematomas. Generally, epidural anesthesia is safe for patients undergoing bowel surgery. Studies have shown that epidurally administered local anesthetics maintain intestinal blood flow and mucosal pH and have a potentially beneficial effect on anastomotic healing rates.[17]

NSAIDS AND COX-2 INHIBITORS

Other pharmacologic methods of reducing systemic opioid use include the administration of nonsteroidal anti-inflammatory drugs (NSAIDs), cyclooxygenase 2 (COX-2) inhibitors (coxibs), and peripheral μ-receptor opioid antagonists. NSAIDs allow one to reduce the dose of systemic opioids by as much as 20%–30%. Blunting the inflammatory response with the use of NSAIDs may lead to a reduction in the influx of macrophages and mast cells into the area of surgical trauma and a reduction in nitric oxide, prostaglandins, and proinflammatory cytokines, all of which potentiate postoperative ileus. Inclusion of NSAIDs into a postoperative pain management protocol has become common, specifically with ketorolac trimethamine. This drug does not reduce colonic contractions, an effect noted with morphine. Postoperative analgesia with ketorolac may cause a faster resolution of ileus compared to analgesia with morphine and ketorolac.[3,18–20] NSAIDs and coxibs provided additive postoperative analgesia and significant opioid-sparing effects following

Table 35.6: Recovery of GI Function and Time until Hospital Discharge[a]

	Epidural Morphine plus Bupivacaine (MB)	Epidural Morphine (M)	Epidural Bupivacaine (B)	IV PCA Morphine (PCA)
Time until first flatus (h)	43 ± 4^{b}	71 ± 4	40 ± 2^{b}	81 ± 3
Time until meeting discharge critera (h)	67 ± 8^{b}	102 ± 13	62 ± 5^{b}	96 ± 7
Time until actual hospital discharge (h)	96 ± 12	130 ± 14	101 ± 11	122 ± 9

Note: values represent mean $\pm$ SE.

Abbreviation: PCA = patient-controlled analgesia.

[a] Liu SS et al: *Anesthesiology.* 1995;83;757–765.

[b] Different from group M and group PCA ($P < .005$).

abdominal surgery. Grass and coworkers[21] found that the addition of ketorolac (15 mg every 6 hours) reduced pain intensity scores and epidural PCA fentanyl requirements in patients recovering from bowel surgery. Patients assigned to the ketorolac group also benefited from faster time to oral diet and bowel movement. Many surgeons are concerned about platelet inhibition and increased risk of perioperative bleeding, with ketorolac and other nonselective NSAIDS. Coxibs have minimal impact on platelet function and have been advocated for postoperative analgesia. Perioperative doses of rofecoxib (50 mg every day) for 5 days reduced IV PCA morphine requirements by 30% while reducing pain intensity scores in patients recovering from abdominal surgery.[22] Rofecoxib treated patients also benefited from significant reductions in sedation scores and more rapid return of bowel function. As rofecoxib has been withdrawn by the manufacturer, celecoxib in doses of 200 mg twice a day offers a suitable alternative

PERIPHERAL OPIOID ANTAGONISTS

The effects of opioids on gut function are mediated primarily through the μ-receptors within the bowel. If one could block the peripheral effects of opioids on the bowel while maintaining their central nervous system effects on analgesia, gut function could be protected while maintaining pain relief. The drugs naloxone and naltrexone reduce opioid-induced bowel dysfunction but reverse analgesia. An ideal preventative measure or treatment of postoperative ileus would be a peripheral opioid μ-receptor antagonist that reverses gut side effects without compromising pain control.

Naloxone does not achieve this. Although naloxone is a competitive μ-receptor antagonist, it readily crosses the blood-brain barrier when given intravenously, reverses analgesia, and may induce opioid withdrawal. Its beneficial effects include reversal of opioid-induced central nervous system depression and respiratory depression, and it may decrease opioid-induced constipation. There are no data to support its use in the prevention or treatment of ileus.

Emerging therapy for POBD and POI include two peripherally selective μ-receptor antagonists, methylnaltrexone and alvimopam (Figure 35.1). Methylnaltrexone is a selective peripheral opioid receptor antagonist that has recently been approved for treatment of opioid induced bowel dysfunction (OBD). Addition of CH_3 (methyl) group to naltrexone, a naloxone-derived, tertiary antagonist, prevents the drug from penetrating the blood-brain barrier. Consequently, it reverses opioid-induced motility problems without reversing analgesia or inducing withdrawal. It is available as an injectable and is currently being evaluated in chronic and postoperative settings.

The effectiveness of this compound provides support for concept that OBD and possibly POI areprimarily brought about by opioid receptors in the GI tract. Intravenous doses of 0.15–0.3 mg/kg have been shown to rapidly initiate a bowel movement (Figure 35.2). While not approved for use in surgical settings, the IV formulation has been advocated for reversal of POI.

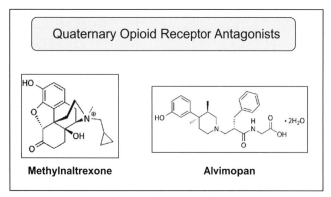

Figure 35.1: Emerging therapy for opioid induced bowel dysfunction: methynaltrexone and alvimopam.

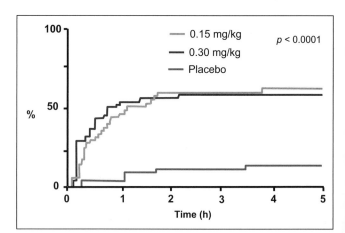

Figure 35.2: Methylnaltrexone in patients with opioid-induced constipation. Time to laxation was significantly more rapid for patients treated with methylnaltrexone when compared to placebo group within the first 5 hours. From: Yuan CS, Israel RJ. *Expert Opin Investig Drugs.* 2006;15(5):541–552.

Alvimopan is a peripherally acting μ-opioid receptor antagonist.[23] Its large molecular weight and polarity do not allow it to cross the blood-brain barrier and thus does not block central opioid receptors.[24] It has a higher potency at the μ-receptor than does morphine or methylnaltrexone and a longer duration of action than methylnaltrexone. Its side effects are currently under investigation and include abdominal pain, flatulence, and diarrhea.[24]

Alvimopan acts by reversing only the peripheral side effects of opioids without interfering with their central effects. Morphine, codeine, hydrocodone, oxycodone, and fentanyl relieve pain by crossing the blood-brain barrier and activating receptors of the central nervous system. This can also produce sedation, respiratory depression, and dependence. Concurrently, peripheral opioid receptors are activated such as those in the gastrointestinal tract potentially leading to alterations in bowel motility. Phases I, II, and III studies with alvimopan have been conducted, the phase III studies have also incorporated a fast-track protocol for all study subjects whereby all potentially innovative means to shorten hospital stay have been utilized. Such methods have included avoidance of nasogastric decompression, initiation of early feedings, and early ambulation. These methods, when employed in a clinical pathway approach, have been shown in a randomized controlled trial to shorten hospital stay when compared to traditional postoperative care. Patient satisfaction, pain control, and patient readmission rate because of complications or failure to progress satisfactorily have not been compromised.[25–27]

Alvimopan was studied in a double-blinded, randomized, placebo-controlled phase III trial involving 34 North American academic, public, and private medical centers to evaluate its effect on postoperative ileus. Enrollment included 510 patients in 3 different study arms: alvimopan (6 mg), alvimopan (12 mg), and placebo.[27] All patients were over the age of 17 years who underwent segmental small or large bowel resection or radical total hysterectomy. All were scheduled to receive intravenous patient-controlled analgesia with opiates and all were scheduled to have the nasogastric tube removed at the completion of surgery. Study medications were given orally at least 2 hours before surgery and then twice a day until hospital discharge or up to 7 days. The primary efficacy end point was time to recovery of gastrointestinal function, as defined by the later of the times that the patient first tolerated solid food and that the patient first passes flatus or stool. An additional end point was the time to when the hospital discharge order was written. The time to recovery of gastrointestinal function was significantly accelerated by alvimopan at both doses compared to placebo; however, a more pronounced effect was noted with the 12-mg dose. The hospital discharge order was written approximately 20 hours earlier for patients receiving the 12-mg dose and 13 hours for those receiving the 6-mg dose. Interestingly, there were fewer instances of nasogastric tube insertion after surgery in patients treated with alvimopan compared to placebo. There were no differences in average daily opiate consumption between the treatment groups and daily and maximum postoperative pain scores were comparable.[26] This is an important point to take note of: pain control and, hence, patient satisfaction was not jeopardized. The incidence of adverse events was similar among the 3 treatment groups, although the incidence of nausea and vomiting was slightly lower in the alvimopan treatment groups compared to placebo. In a second phase III study, similar results

Table 35.7: Summary of Current Therapies for POBD

At present there is no adequate treatment or prevention for POI

Nonpharmacologic therapies have demonstrated no real value in the treatment of POI in clinical trials

Techniques such as laparoscopy are complicated and may not be suitable for all patients

Emerging management and treatment strategies include epidural and regional anesthesia/analgesia, use of COX-2 inhibitors (celecoxib), use of less invasive surgery, introduction of prokinetic opioid antagonists

were noted.[25,27] When the results from the phase III studies are pooled, the alvimopan-treated groups had a lower incidence of nasogastric tube insertion, a lower incidence of postoperative ileus and early postoperative bowel obstruction, a reduction in hospital stay, and a trend toward a lower readmission rate.

As stated, most patients undergoing colectomy require opioids for pain relief. It is not the intention of any of the maneuvers mentioned to totally eliminate the need for opioids, rather the goal of optimum patient management is to minimize the effects of systemic opioids on gut function. At the same time, a primary objective is to relieve patients of pain, eliminate unnecessary suffering, and ensure their satisfaction with their hospital stay. This is achieved by using analgesic techniques and adjuncts which lower the dose of opioid required to alleviate pain. Such therapy includes use of NSAIDs such as ketorolac or a Cox-2 inhibitor such as celecoxib, local anesthetic wound infiltration, oral or IV acetaminophen and epidural blockade. When postoperative gut function returns earlier, hospital stay is shortened. This could have significant implications on the cost of health care. In the United States, the annual burden of postoperative ileus on health care is \$750 million to \$1 billion per year.[3] This is attributable to prolonged need for intravenous fluid administration, nasogastric decompression, extra hospital days, additional nursing care, and laboratory and radiologic tests. If one considers the number of laparotomies performed annually, if the hospital stay could be reduced by even 1 or 2 days for each patient, the cost savings could be enormous. Current strategies for minimizing POBD are outlined in Table 35.7.

CONCLUSION

Surgical concerns regarding postoperative pain management are often complicated by potential adverse effects of analgesics, such as impaired hemostasis with NSAIDs and POBD with opioids, as well as surgical related factors such as hypovolemia and anticoagulation that may contraindicate placement of neuraxial catheters. Nevertheless, the treating physician has a number of ways to reduce pain intensity, shorten hospital stay and hasten gut recovery following colectomy. One can consider altering the technique to include minimally invasive technology, but perhaps the most significant way is to employ a multidisciplinary approach to pain control. Epidural anesthetic agents, NSAIDs/COX-2 inhibitors, and peripheral opioid-receptor antagonists all show promise in reducing the incidence and duration of postoperative ileus.

REFERENCES

1. Livingston EH, Passar EP Jr. Postoperative Ileus. *Dig Dis Sci.* 1990;35:121–132.

2. Delaney CP, Wolff BG, Viscusi ER, et al. Alvimopan, for postoperative ileus following bowel resection. *Ann Surg.* 2007;245(3):355–363.

3. Luckey A, Livingston E, Tache Y. Mechanisms and treatment of postoperative ileus. *Arch Surg.* 2003;138:206–214.

4. Goyal RK, Hirano I. The entire nervous system. *N Engl J Med.* 1996;334:1106–1115.

5. Holte K, Kehlet H. Postoperative ileus: progress towards effective management. *Drugs.* 2002;62:2603–2615.

6. Behm BW, Stollman NH. Postoperative Ileus: etiologies and interventions. *Clin Gastroenterol Hepatol.* 2003;1:71–80.

7. Bauer AJ, Schwartz NT, Moore BA, Turler A, Kalff JC. Ileus in critical illness: mechanisms and management. *Curr Opin Crit Care.* 2002;8:152–157.

8. Prasad M, Matthews JB. Deflating postoperative ileus. *Gastroenterology.* 1999:117;489–492.

9. Bauer AJ, Boeckxstaens GE. Mechanisms of postoperative ileus. *Neurogastroenterol Motil.* 2004;16(suppl 2):54–60.

10. Cali RL, Meade PG, Swanson MS. Freeman C. Effect of morphine and incision length in bowel function after colectomy. *Dis Colon Rectum.* 2000;43:163–168.

11. Abraham NS, Young JM, Solomon MJ. Meta-analysis of short-term outcomes After laparoscopic resection for colorectal cancer. *Br J Surg.* 2004;91:1111–1124.

12. Ogilvy AJ, Smith G. The gastrointestinal tracts after anesthesia. *Eur J Anaesthesiol.* 1995;10(suppl):35–42.

13. Moraca RJ, Sheldon DG, Thirlby RC. The role of epidural anesthesia and analgesia in surgical practice. *Ann Surg.* 2003;238:663–673.

14. Steinbrook RA. Epidural anesthesia and gastrointestinal motility. *Anesth Analg.* 1998;86:837–844.

15. Liu S, Carpenter RL, Neal JM. Epidural anesthesia and analgesia: their role in postoperative outcome. *Anesthesiology.* 1995;82:1474–1506.

16. Ryan P, Schweitzer SA, Woods RJ. Effect of epidural and general anaesthesia compared with general anaesthesia alone in large bowel anastomoses: a prospective study. *Eur J Surg.* 1992;158:45–49.

17. Holte K, Kehlet H. Postoperative ileus: a preventable event. *Br J Surg.* 2000;87:1480–1493.

18. Baig MK, Wexner SD. Postoperative ileus: a review. *Dis Colon Rectum.* 2004;47:516–526.

19. Soybel DI, Zinner MJ. Ileus and the macrophage. *Ann Surg.* 2003;237:316–318.

20. Ferraz AA, Cowles VE, Condon RE, et al. Nonopioid analgesics shorten the duration of postoperative ileus. *Am Surg.* 1995;61:1079–1083.

21. Grass JA, Sakima NT, Valley M, et al. Assessment of ketorolac as an adjuvant to fentanyl patient-controlled epidural analgesia after radical retropubic prostatectomy. *Anesthesiology* 1993;78:642–648.

22. Sinatra RS, Boice J, Loeys TL, et al: Evaluation of perioperative rofecoxib treatment on pain control and clinical outcome in patients recovering from gynecologic abdominal surgery: a randomized, double-blind, placebo controlled clinical study. *Reg Anesth Pain Med.* 2005;31;134–142.

23. Azodo IA, Ehrenpreis ED. Alvimopan (Adolor/GlaxoSmithKline). *Curr Opin Investig Drugs.* 2002;3:1496–1501.

24. Schmidt WK. Alvimopan (ADL 8-2698) is a novel peripheral opioid antagonist. *Am J Surg.* 2001;182(suppl 5A):27S–38S.

25. Taguchi A, Sharma A, Saleem RM, et al. Selective postoperative inhibition of gastrointestinal opioid receptors. *N Engl J Med.* 2001;345:935–940.

26. Wolff BG, Michelassi F, Gerkin TM, et al. Alvimopan Postoperative Ileus Study Group. Alvimopan, a novel, peripherally acting mu opioid antagonist: results of a multi-center, randomized, double-blind, placebo-controlled phase III trial of major abdominal surgery and postoperative ileus. *Ann Surg.* 2004;240:728–735.

27. Delaney CP, Weese JL, Hyman NH, et al. Alvimopan Postoperative Study Group. Phase III trial of alvimopan, a novel, peripherally acting, mu opioid antagonist, for postoperative ileus after major abdominal surgery. *Dis Colon Rectum.* 2005;48:1114–1125.

36

Acute Pain Management in the
Emergency Department

Knox H. Todd and James R. Miner

Emergency physicians provide care for an extraordinary broad range of illnesses and injuries, the majority of which involve some degree of pain. Table 36.1 lists major categories of discharge diagnoses among those presenting to a multicenter emergency department (ED) network with a principal complaint of pain. Emergency physicians also frequently cause pain in the course of performing emergent therapeutic and diagnostic procedures. This chapter considers the prevalence of pain in the emergency department, barriers to its adequate treatment, as well as a variety of treatment modalities. Space limits prohibit a discussion of the wide variety of specific painful conditions that present to the ED. These can be found in other chapters of the text.

PREVALENCE AND ASSESSMENT OF PAIN IN THE EMERGENCY DEPARTMENT

Pain is the presenting complaint for up to 78% of visits to U.S. EDs.[1-3] Although making an accurate diagnosis and choosing the appropriate therapy to treat underlying conditions are principal goals for emergency physicians, those who present to the ED with pain seek recognition of their pain and rapid, effective interventions to control pain. In the United States, the ED serves as a safety net for our fragmented health care system, and pain is but one of many conditions for which emergency physicians not only treat acute clinical presentations but also care for those with chronic or recurrent painful conditions who are unable to access other parts of the health care system.

Pain is inherently subjective and inevitably complex. Patients experience pain and suffering as individuals; clinicians assess it only indirectly. The emergency provider's task is to use a commonly understood vocabulary and classification system in assessing pain so that our findings can be communicated consistently. Only by quantifying the pain experience in meaningful ways can we move beyond practices that are influenced by myth and opinion toward a scientific approach to our many questions regarding the pain experience. This challenge is at the root of our difficulties in treating pain, and not only in the ED setting;

thus issues surrounding pain assessment should have primacy in our attempts to understand the pain experience.

EDs employ a number of practical unidimensional pain assessment tools. Viewing pain as the "fifth vital sign" as encouraged by revised standards of the Joint Commission for Accreditation of Health Care Organizations has fostered the widespread use of such tools. For those without cognitive impairment, pain intensity can be assessed with either an 11-point numerical rating scale (NRS) or a graphical rating scale (GRS). The NRS is sensitive to the short-term changes in pain intensity associated with emergency care.[4,5] GRS or picture scales are particularly useful for populations with limited literacy, including children.[6,7] In one study of patients who have advanced cancer and pain, 81% were able to complete a picture scale, whereas only 75% could complete the VAS.[8] In another study, the authors noted that male patients were uncomfortable with scales depicting severe pain using tears.[9] Picture scales with such depictions might be avoided, because they may be biased in the direction of less severe pain in male patients.

The visual analog scale (VAS) is used by some EDs; however, this instrument is more commonly employed in research settings. There is no advantage in using a VAS over an NRS in the ED settings; both are reliable and valid measures of pain intensity.[10] In fact, certain patient populations find the NRS easier to complete, therefore it is preferred over the VAS for routine use.[4,11]

No matter the specific pain scale used, assessments should be repeated after therapeutic interventions and at the time of ED discharge. One multicenter study suggests that relatively few ED patients are reassessed after an initial pain score, finding that fewer than one-third of ED patients presenting with moderate to severe pain had repeat pain assessments while in the ED.[12]

THE PROBLEM OF EMERGENCY DEPARTMENT OLIGOANALGESIA

Notwithstanding the clinician's duty to provide compassionate care, pain that is not acknowledged and managed appropriately causes anxiety, depression, sleep disturbances, increased

Table 36.1: Major Categories of Diagnoses for 819 Patients Discharged from the ED after Presenting with Moderate to Severe Pain

Diagnosis	N (%)
Wound, abrasion, or contusion	91 (11)
Sprain or strain	90 (11)
Back or neck pain	85 (10)
Abdominal pain	71 (9)
Fracture or dislocation	48 (6)
Headache	47 (6)
Chest pain (noncardiac)	40 (5)
Upper respiratory infection	30 (4)
Abscess or cellulitis	25 (3)
Toothache	19 (2)
Urinary tract infection	16 (2)
Renal colic	14 (2)
Other diagnoses	243 (30)
Total	819 (100)

From: Todd KH, Ducharme J, Choiniere M, et al. Pain in the emergency department: results of the Pain and Emergency Medicine Initiative (PEMI) Multicenter Study. *The Journal of Pain* 2007;8(6):460–466.[12]

Table 36.2: Factors Contributing to ED Oligoanalgesia

Lack of educational emphasis on pain management

Inadequate ED quality improvement systems

Lack of ED pain research, particularly among geriatric and pediatric populations

Emergency providers' concerns regarding opioid addiction and abuse

Fear of opioid adverse effects

Racial and ethnic bias

oxygen demands with the potential for end organ ischemia, and decreased movement with an increased risk of venous thrombosis.[13,14] Failure to recognize and treat pain may also result in dissatisfaction with medical care, hostility toward the physician, unscheduled returns to the ED, delayed complete return to full function, and, potentially, an increased risk of litigation.[15]

Although adequate analgesia in the ED is an important goal of treatment, the underuse of analgesics, termed *oligoanalgesia* by Wilson and Pendleton in 1989, occurs in a large proportion of ED patients.[16–20] A variety of factors are felt to give provenance to pain undertreatment (Table 36.2).[21]

The very young or old often receive less intensive treatment for pain in the ED,[22–24] and studies have documented oligoanalgesia among those of minority ethnicity.[25,26] It has been suggested that patients' expectations for pain treatment and perceptions of pain intensity do not differ by ethnic groups when patients are matched for socioeconomic factors.[27–29] Differences have been noted, however, in the manner in which patients of different cultural backgrounds express their pain.[29] Differences in the interactions of physicians and patients of different ethnic groups have been described and subtle differences within these interactions may affect the physician's pain assessment.[30,31] When affect, actual patient-MD interaction, and cultural expressions of ethnicity are removed from a case presentation, such as through written clinical vignettes, patients with similar pain tend to be similarly treated by physicians.[32] Cultural discordance between the patient and the physician may hinder the ability of patients to confer an understanding of their pain to the physician.

Of course, any treatment of pain is dependent on the physician's accurate assessment of the patient's pain. In fact, the only predictor of treatment that Bartfield and colleagues found for ED patients with back pain was the physician's assessment, regardless of the patients' ethnicity, age, or insurance status.[33] Disparities in the treatment of pain likely result from variations in assessment rather than variations in treatment among patients assessed as having a similar degree of pain.

Although emergency physicians may be reluctant to accept patient report as the most reliable indicator of pain, and disparities between patient's and physician's pain intensity ratings may lead to inadequately treated pain, even patients themselves may be reluctant to report the presence of pain and its intensity. This may be because of low expectations of obtaining pain relief, fear of analgesic side effects, and perhaps the notion that pain is to be expected as part of an underlying disease or from medical treatments. Some patients exhibit an inappropriate fear of addiction when prescribed opioids, or fear the stigma associated with opioid use, even in the short term.

Although federal regulators and state medical boards do not perceive emergency medicine as a specialty prone to inappropriate prescribing resulting in investigations and possible sanctions, emergency physicians express fears of such scrutiny or sanctions related to prescribing or administering opioids. In treating pain in patients receiving chronic opioid therapy, confusion over the concepts of physical dependence, tolerance, addiction, and pseudoaddiction may also constitute barriers to appropriate treatment. The use of standard definitions and widespread dissemination of these terms may be helpful in caring for patients managed with chronic opioids who present to the ED.

ED personnel commonly identify patients who they feel are attempting to obtain opioids for illegitimate purposes. Although drug addiction occurs in all patient populations, it is likely that the ED sees a higher proportion of such patients than a typical office-based practice. Unfortunately, the true prevalence of addiction and aberrant drug-seeking behaviors in the ED is unknown and difficult to measure. When the prevalence of such problems is overestimated, oligoanalgesia is the predictable result.

PAIN TREATMENT AND PROCEDURAL SEDATION IN THE ED

Effective pain management involves both pharmacologic and nonpharmacologic modalities. Simply asking about pain and validating the pain reports affects patients' satisfaction with ED pain management. In one study, patient satisfaction with pain management was predicted more strongly by the perception that ED staff asked about pain than by the actual administration of an analgesic.[34] Other nonpharmacologic modalities, such as reassuring the patient that pain will be addressed, immobilizing and elevating injured extremities, and providing quiet, darkened rooms for patients with migraine headaches are important aspects of quality pain management. Pharmacologic therapies should begin as soon as is practical after presentation to the ED. Analgesic protocols allowing early pain treatment can decrease the time to effective treatment and improve patient outcomes.[35–37]

Analgesics may be administered by a variety of routes; however, the vast majority of medications are administered by the oral or parenteral routes. Oral therapies are most commonly employed, as they are convenient and inexpensive for patients who can tolerate oral intake. When pain is severe, analgesics must be given immediately and titrated to effect, generally by parenteral routes. The intravenous (IV), rather than intramuscular (IM), route is indicated in this context. Intramuscular injections are painful, do not allow for rapid titration, and result in a slower onset of drug action; moreover, absorption is unpredictable. Unless intravenous access is elusive, there is little to recommend the intramuscular route. In general, it is inappropriate to delay analgesic use until a diagnosis has been made. In the case of acute abdominal pain, for which surgical dogma historically discouraged adequate analgesia, a large series of studies report no deleterious effect of intravenous opioid therapy on our ability to make appropriate diagnoses.[38–44]

SPECIFIC TREATMENT MODALITIES

A wide variety of analgesics are used in emergency medicine practice. In a recent -site survey of ED analgesic practice, a total of 735 doses of 24 different analgesics were administered to 506 patients receiving analgesics while in the ED. Analgesics administered to this cohort of ED patients are listed by prevalence in Table 36.3.[12] The majority of analgesics administered were opioids (59%); morphine being the most commonly used analgesic (20%), followed by ibuprofen (17%).

NONOPIOIDS

Commonly used ED analgesics include opioids, acectaminophen, and nonsteroidal anti-inflammatory drugs (NSAIDs). When opioids are required for pain treatment, nonopioids should be included to potentiate the opioid analgesic effect and decrease the severity of side effects. Unfortunately, nonopioid agents exhibit an analgesic ceiling effect and cannot be titrated to effect. This limits their usefulness in the setting of severe or fluctuating pain; however, they should be used as an adjunct to opioid therapies unless otherwise contraindicated.

Acetaminophen is indicated for mild to moderate pain and is often combined with opioid agents. Acetaminophen, unlike NSAIDs, has no antiplatelet activity or anti-inflammatory effect. Although a great deal of attention has been paid to acetaminophen hepatotoxicity, especially in the setting of chronic malnutrition, alcoholism, or liver disease, such effects are uncommon, particularly when contrasted to the underappreciated high prevalence of NSAID-related adverse effects.

NSAIDs, including salicylates, act to inhibit prostaglandin synthesis by interfering with cyclooxygenase (COX) enzymes. They cause platelet dysfunction and can precipitate renal failure in patients with renal insufficiency or volume depletion, a par-

Table 36.3: ED Analgesics Administered to 506 Patients Presenting with Moderate to Severe Pain

Analgesics Administered in the ED (735 doses given to 506 patients)	N (%)
Morphine	148 (20.1)
Ibuprofen	127 (17.3)
Hydrocodone/acetaminophen	93 (12.7)
Oxycodone/acetaminophen	83 (11.3)
Ketorolac	60 (8.2)
Acetaminophen	53 (7.2)
Hydromorphone	36 (4.9)
Antacid	26 (3.5)
Meperidine	24 (3.3)
Fentanyl	23 (3.1)
Metoclopramide	13 (1.8)
Codeine/acetaminophen	12 (1.6)
Oxycodone	10 (1.4)
Naproxen	9 (1.2)
Other	18 (2.4)
Total	735 (100)

From: Todd KH, Ducharme J, Choiniere M, et al. Pain in the emergency department: results of the Pain and Emergency Medicine Initiative (PEMI) Multicenter Study. *The Journal of Pain* 2007;8(6):460–466.[12]

ticular concern in the elderly or those presenting to the ED with hemodynamic instability. Ketorolac, the only parenteral available in the United States, is commonly used in the ED and is felt to be particularly useful in the setting of renal colic. One recent study of renal colic in the ED found that a combination or ketorolac and morphine resulted in superior analgesia and reduced adverse effects when compared to the use of either agent alone.[45]

OPIOIDS

Opioid combination analgesics are commonly used for moderate to severe pain. Although the opioid component in these agents does not exhibit ceiling analgesic effects, the nonopioid component dose must be limited; thus one cannot titrate these analgesics. The convenience of combination therapy must be balanced against this limitation. Hydrocodone and oxycodone combination agents are associated with less nausea and vomiting and are preferable to codeine combinations agents. Also, a significant proportions of the population are poor metabolizers of codeine, which must be metabolized to morphine to manifest analgesic effects, further limiting its effectiveness.

The tramadol/acetaminophen combination agent is indicated for acute pain; however, experience with this agent in the ED setting is limited. In one recent trial of acute ankle sprains presenting to the ED, the tramadol/acetaminophen combination agent had comparable clinical utility to that of hydrocodone with acetaminophen.[46] Tramadol's mechanism of action is unclear: it binds only weakly to opioid receptors, but a metabolite is a more potent opioid and, in addition, it inhibits the reuptake of both norephinephrine and serotonin with analgesic effects like the tricyclic antidepressants.

Opioids are the mainstay of ED therapy for moderate to severe pain and morphine is the standard of comparison for all agents of this class. If contraindicated because of allergy or other sensitivity, hydromorphone or fentanyl may be substituted. These opioids can be rapidly titrated intravenously to control severe pain, allowing early institution of an oral regimen. Fentanyl has the advantage being relatively short acting and is preferred in the setting of multiple trauma, head injury, and potential hemodynamic instability. Intravenous morphine is the standard of treatment for severe pain in the ED. Morphine (0.1 mg/kg bolus) has been found to be safe but not usually adequate to effect pain relief.[47] Repeat boluses of 0.05 mg/kg every 5 minutes until pain relief represents a safe incremental strategy.

Meperidine is a problematic opioid for a number of reasons. Many EDs have eliminated meperidine completely because of its metabolism to normeperidine, a toxic metabolite causing central excitation and seizures. In addition, meperidine is contraindicated in patients taking monoamine oxidase inhibitors as this combination may precipitate a serotonergic crisis.[48] Historically, subtherapeutic doses of intramuscularly administered meperidine have been used to treat a wide variety of acute pain complaints by generations of physicians. The availability of other opioid agents of equal efficacy with fewer contraindications and less adverse effects argues against its routine use.

Agonist-antagonist opioids, such as nalbuphine and butorphanol, have mixed effects on opioid receptor subtypes, exhibiting ceiling effects on both analgesia and respiratory depression. Because clinically important respiratory depression is distinctly rare in the setting of acute pain treatment, it is difficult to justify their routine use. One possible exception is for patients with advanced pulmonary disease. A particular drawback is that one cannot titrate these drugs to maximal effect because of analgesic ceiling effects. Additionally, these drugs are contraindicated and will induce withdrawal symptoms in patients who are physically dependent on opioids, either because of opioid therapy for chronic pain, methadone maintenance therapy, or active opioid addiction.

PATIENT-CONTROLLED ANALGESIA

The use of patient-controlled analgesia (PCA) has been described in emergency medicine for both adults and children.[49,50] Although no specific advantage has been found over the titration of opioids, PCAs are at least as effective in relieving pain. In the setting of high demands on nursing resources, PCAs could serve to ensure that patients' pain treatment needs are addressed in a timely fashion. In addition, patients admitted from the ED to inpatient hospital beds often experience a "pain window" between the last dose of an analgesic in the ED and the first dose administered on the hospital ward. Wider use of ED PCA might obviate this common problem.

ALTERNATIVE DELIVERY ROUTES

Multiple alternative delivery routes for the administration of pain medications have been described. The use of nebulized fentanyl has been described and holds promise as a route of opioid delivery that can be initiated before an IV has been placed.[51–53] Nebulized pain medications, especially for children who have severe pain but has not had an IV placed, could be of use in the ED.

PROCEDURAL SEDATION AND ANALGESIA

Patients often present to the ED in need of painful or complex procedures that require patient cooperation and must be done emergently. Procedural sedation and analgesia (PSA) practices and policies have evolved rapidly in the ED and this is a growing area of emergency medicine research. Unlike most patients who are undergoing sedation in other settings, patients in the ED have unpredictable nil per os (NPO) status, often have concurrent severe systemic disease, and usually are in severe pain before the procedure begins. In addition, unpredictable concurrent events, as well as time and space constraints in the ED, can serve to complicate these procedures.

The indications for ED PSA range from pain control for short painful procedures to the need for patient compliance with complex emergency procedure. Goals for level of sedation during ED PSA range from minimal through moderate to deep sedation, depending on the demands of specific procedures. Although it is acknowledged that deep sedation can inadvertently result in patient's achieving a level of sedation consistent with anesthesia, this is not typically the goal of ED PSA. Minimal sedation, a drug-induced state during which patients respond appropriately to verbal commands (according to their developmental age), is generally performed for procedures that require patient compliance but are not typically intensely painful when performed with local anesthesia. Minimal sedation is typically used for lumbar puncture, evidentiary exams, simple fracture reductions (in combination with local anesthesia), and the incision and drainage of small abscesses.

During minimal sedation, cardiovascular and ventilatory functions are generally well maintained, although patients should be monitored for inadvertent oversedation to deeper levels, using oxygen saturation monitors and close nursing supervision. Agents typically used for minimal sedation include fentanyl, midazolam, combinations of the two, and low-dose ketamine.

Moderate sedation is performed on patients who would benefit from either a deeper level of sedation to augment the procedure or amnesia of the event itself. Moderate sedation is a drug-induced depression of consciousness during which patients respond to verbal commands (appropriately to their developmental age), either alone or with light tactile stimulation. Patients usually have an intact airway and maintain ventilatory function without support. As with minimal sedation, inadvertent oversedation to deeper levels can occur with moderate sedation. Appropriate assessments, including oxygen saturation, cardiac monitoring, and blood pressure measurements, should be done throughout the sedation, and direct observation of the patient's airway should be maintained throughout the procedure. Agents used for moderate sedation in the ED include propofol, etomidate, ketamine, and the combination of fentanyl and midazolam.

Deep sedation is performed on patients who would benefit from a deeper level of sedation, often to complete a procedure already begun. Generally, amnesia of the procedure is similar between moderate and deep sedation, and it is not necessary to sedate patients to a deep level only to obtain amnesia.[54] Deep sedation is achieved in the ED with the same agents as moderate sedation; the difference is in the intended level of sedation. Monitoring requirements for deep sedation are similar to those for moderate sedation.

End tidal carbon dioxide has also been described in ED PSA, but its utility over direct assessment of airway status has not been established.[55] Deeply sedated patients can develop respiratory depression but generally maintain a patent airway and adequate ventilation. Patients sedated to this level can progress to a level of sedation consistent with anesthesia,[56–58] and there is some evidence that this occurs more frequently in patients targeted for deep sedation than in those undergoing moderate sedation.[59] For this reason, it is usually safer to use moderate sedation than deep sedation in the ED unless the procedure requires progressively deeper levels of sedation to complete successfully, such as the reduction of hip dislocations.

Patients who progress to an unintended level of sedation consistent with general anesthesia are not arousable, even to pain. The ability to independently maintain ventilatory function is usually impaired, and patients often require assistance in maintaining a patent airway. Because patients can quickly progress to this level using agents commonly employed for moderate and deep sedation, physicians performing ED PSA must be prepared to provide ventilatory support until the patient has regained consciousness. To decrease the likelihood of aspiration, patients who are undergoing moderate or deep sedation in the ED should be kept NPO. It is difficult to find a consensus on the amount of time a patient should be kept NPO prior to PSA.[60,61] Many departments use 3–6 hours as a minimum.[62]

ED PSA is necessarily used for patients who are medically stable (American Society of Anesthesiologists physical classes 1 and 2) and must be avoided in patients who are ASA 3 or 4. PSA for critically ill children has been described using ketamine[63] and in adults using propofol or etomidate.[64] The degree of respiratory depression noted in these patients was similar to patients with physical status scores of 1 or 2, but an increased rate of hypotension was seen in physical status 3 and 4 patients who received propofol. It may be that ketamine and etomidate are better suited for the emergent sedation of critically ill patients, but there is not yet sufficient data to make a definite recommendation. Both ketamine and propofol can have profound hemodynamic and respiratory effects in the more physiologically compromised patients.

Sedated patients are generally monitored by pulse oximetry, which is a sensitive measure of oxygenation. If a patient receives supplemental oxygen prior to starting PSA, this monitor may not be as sensitive to changes in the patient's ventilatory status.[55,65,66] Preoxygenation is generally recommended for ED PSA; however, there is no evidence that it decreases the incidence of transient hypoxia that has been noted as a complication of PSA. End tidal carbon dioxide has been recommended as an additional modality for the monitoring of sedated patients.[62,67] Monitoring expired carbon dioxide during PSA allows for a graphically display of the patients ventilatory status that can be a detector of respiratory depression before it becomes clinically apparent otherwise.[55] In the event of hypoventilation, the end tidal CO_2 value increases as the respiratory rate decreases. In the event of increasing airway obstruction, the baseline end tidal CO_2 value decreases along with a blunting of the waveform as a result of increased mixing of the nasal expiratory sample with ambient air because of the turbulence from the obstruction.

Ketamine use has been described in adults[68] but is more commonly used for children undergoing ED PSA.[69] Ketamine is a dissociative anesthetic that provides 15–20 minutes of sedation when given intramuscularly, with a return to baseline mental status in 30–60 minutes. It can be given in doses of 1 to 4 mg/kg IM and should be combined with atropine (0.01 mg/kg) to prevent hypersalivation. The addition of 0.1 mg/kg of midazolam to ketamine has been described to prevent emergence phenomena but is of unclear utility.[70] The 1-mg/kg dose achieves light sedation sufficient for such procedures as lumbar puncture, dressing changes, and simple laceration repair. Doses from 2 to 4 mg/kg result in increasingly deeper levels of moderate to deep sedation. Patients sedated with ketamine usually maintain a patent airway and ventilate normally. Patients receiving ketamine should be monitored for respiratory depression and rare occurrences of laryngospasm.[69,71] Emergence phenomena, unpleasant perceptual experiences as patients regain consciousness, have been described in both adults and children.[70,72,73] Intravenous ketamine is also used for ED PSA at doses of 1 mg/kg IV with an onset of 1–2 minutes, followed by moderate sedation lasting 8 to 12 minutes. Side-effect profiles of IV ketamine are similar to those of IM use.

The combination of fentanyl and midazolam has been used for minimal, moderate, and deep sedation in the ED.[55,59,72,74,75] This combination results in longer periods of sedation than other agents and carries a higher rate of dose-related respiratory depression. Although adequate for minimal sedation, this combination is less useful for moderate to deep sedation and its use for these levels of sedation is not recommended. Dosing for minimal sedation has been described as 0.1 mg/kg IV midazolam followed by 0.05 mg/kg IV fentanyl, with repeated fentanyl boluses every 3 minutes until the patient is adequately sedated. The sedation typically lasts 30–60 minutes with a return to baseline mental status by 45 to 120 minutes. This method of PSA requires close respiratory monitoring. Pentobarbital is another agent resulting in similar durations of sedation but without analgesic properties. It is used for minimal to moderate sedation of children for radiologic procedures.[76,77] The medicine is administered at 2.5 mg/kg IV, followed by 1.25 mg/kg IV every 5 minutes until adequate sedation is achieved. Pulse oximetry is required. The rate of respiratory depression is lower than that for other protocols but the sedation level is inadequate for most painful procedures.[78]

Methohexital has been used for moderate and deep PSA.[79–81] It is a very short-acting agent with dense amnestic properties. It is administered at 1 mg/kg IV with 0.5 mg/kg repeat boluses every 2 minutes as needed. It has an onset of 30 seconds, with sedation lasting 2–4 minutes and returning to baseline within 10 to 15 minutes. It has been associated with respiratory depression and a quick progression to deeper levels of sedation than intended, it can cause oversedation even when carefully titrated, therefore close respiratory monitoring is required. When compared directly to propofol, methohexital is similarly effective and safe with single bolus use; however, it is less safe than propofol when multiple doses are required.[79] It should be used principally for very brief procedures expected to last less than 2–4 minutes, such as the reduction of simple fractures and dislocations.

Propofol is well described for ED PSA.[55–59,64,79,82–86] It is administered as a 1-mg/kg bolus with repeat boluses of 0.5 mg/kg

The majority of emergency department (ED) patients require treatment for painful medical conditions or injuries. The American College of Emergency Physicians recognizes the importance of effectively managing ED patients who are experiencing pain and supports the following principles.

1. ED patients should receive expeditious pain management, avoiding delays such as those related to diagnostic testing or consultation.

2. Hospitals should develop unique strategies that will optimize ED patient pain management using both narcotic and nonnarcotic medications.

3. ED policies and procedures should support the safe utilization and prescription writing of pain medications in the ED.

4. Effective physician and patient educational strategies should be developed regarding pain management, including the use of pain therapy adjuncts and how to minimize pain after disposition from the ED.

5. Ongoing research in the area of ED patient pain management should be conducted.

Approved by the ACEP Board of Directors March 2004.

From: Anonymous. Pain management in the emergency department. Annals of Emergency Medicine. 44(2):198, 2004.

Figure 36.1: American College of Emergency Physicians policy on pain management.

every 3 minutes until the patient is adequately sedated. The sedation persists 2–5 minutes after a single bolus, and longer for patients receiving multiple boluses, with a return to baseline within 10–15 minutes. This medication has been associated with rates of clinically apparent respiratory depression from 4.0% to 7.7% in ED PSA, and, again, close respiratory monitoring is required. Propofol causes hypotension in critically ill patients and should be used with caution in hemodynamically unstable patients.[64]

Finally, etomidate is useful for ED PSA.[64,87–92] It is given as a single bolus of 0.1 to 0.3 mg/kg, with an onset of sedation in 30–60 seconds and sedation lasting 7–10 minutes. It is not associated with hypotension, thus is more commonly used when this is an issue; however, its use is associated with myoclonic jerking in up to 25% of patients. This adverse effect can complicate the procedure for which the patient has been sedated, making it a suboptimal sedative for healthy patients.[64] Etomidate, in single boluses of 0.3 mg/kg, has been shown to cause transient adrenal suppression, but no significant changes in cortisol levels occur, and the significance of this finding remains unclear.[93]

EVOLVING ED PAIN MANAGEMENT PRACTICES

Pain management practices in the emergency department continue to evolve. The American College of Emergency Physicians, emergency medicine's principal specialty organization, established its first general policy statement regarding analgesic practices in 2004.[94] Prior to this, data from the National Hospital Ambulatory Medical Care Survey showed that, from 1997 through 2001, there was an impressive 18% increase in analgesic use in US EDs (from 47.2 to 56.2 mentions per 100 visits), with

marked increases in both nonsteroidal anti-inflammatory agents and opioid analgesics (Figure 36.1).[95]

At the local level, adoptions of pain management guidelines and quality improvement processes have demonstrated dramatic improvements in practices. In one 3-site study, rates of ED analgesic treatment increased from 54% to 84% over 1 year as a result of individual and group feedback.[96] In a recent study from one Swiss ED, educational programs and guideline implementation led to marked increases in pain intensity documentation, analgesic administration, reduction in pain intensity scores, and improved patient satisfaction over a 4-month period.[97]

We do not know the reasons for the rapid evolution of ED pain management practice. Policy and regulatory initiatives, institutional quality improvement programs, pharmaceutical marketing campaigns, educational efforts, and new knowledge from basic and clinical research are all likely to be influential factors. No matter the cause, emergency medicine pain research is increasing at a rapid pace, and ED pain management practices will continue to evolve.

REFERENCES

1. Cordell WH, Keene KK, Giles BK, et al. The high prevalence of pain in emergency medical care. *Am J Emerg Med.* 2002;20:165–169.
2. Johnston CC, Gagnon AJ, Fullerton L, et al. One-week survey of pain intensity on admission to and discharge from the emergency department: a pilot study. *J Emerg Med.* 1998;16:377–382.
3. Tanabe P. Buschmann M. A prospective study of ED pain management practices and the patient's perspective. *J Emerg Nurs.* 1999;25:171–177.
4. Paice J, Cohen F. Validity of a verbally administered numeric rating scale to measure cancer pain intensity. *Cancer Nurs.* 1997;20:88–93.
5. Farrar JT, Cleary J, Rauck R, et al. Oral transmucosal fentanyl citrate: randomized, double-blinded, placebo-controlled trial for treatment of breakthrough pain in cancer patients. *J Natl Cancer Inst.* 1998;90:611.
6. Breyer JE, Knott CB. Construct validity estimation for the African-American and Hispanic versions of the Oucher Scale. *J Pediatr Nurs.* 1998;13:20–31.
7. Bellamy N, Campbell J, Syrotuik J. Comparative study of self-rating pain scale in osteoarthritis patients. *Curr Med Res Opin.* 1999;15:113–119.
8. Shannon MM, Ryan MA, D'Agostino N, et al. Assessment of pain in advanced cancer patients. *J Pain Symptom Manage.* 1995;10:274–278.
9. Ramer L, Richardson JL, Zichi Cohen M, et al. Multimeasure pain assessment in an ethnically diverse group of patients with cancer. *J Trans Nurs.* 1999;10:94–101.
10. Todd KH. Pain assessment instruments for use in the emergency department. *Emerg Med Clin North Am.* 2005;23(2):285–295.
11. Stahmer SA, Shofer FS, Marino A, Shepherd S, Abbuhl S. Do quantitative changes in pain intensity correlate with pain relief and satisfaction. *Acad Emerg Med.* 1998;5:851–857.
12. Todd KH, Ducharme J, Choiniere M, et al. Pain in the emergency department: results of the Pain and Emergency Medicine Initiative (PEMI) multicenter study. *J Pain.* 2007;8(6):460–466.
13. Gureje O, Von Korff M, Simon GE, et al. Persistent pain and well-being: a World Health Organization study in primary care. *JAMA.* 1998;280:147–151.
14. Anderson FA Jr, Spencer FA. Risk factors for venous thromboembolism. *Circulation.* 2003;107(23 suppl 1):I9–I16.

15. Furrow BR. Pain management and provider liability: no more excuses. *J Law Med Ethics.* 2001;29:28–51.

16. Wilson JE, Pendleton JM. Oligoanalgesia in the emergency department. *Am J Emerg Med.* 1989;7:620–623.

17. Stalnikowicz R, Mahamid R, Kaspi S, et al. Undertreatment of acute pain in the emergency department: a challenge. *Int J Qual Health Care.* 2005;17(2):173–176.

18. Pines JM, Perron AD. Oligoanalgesia in ED patients with isolated extremity injury without documented fracture. *Am J Emerg Med.* 2005;23(4):580.

19. Neighbor ML, Honner M, Kohn MD. Factors affecting emergency department opioid administration to severely injured patients. *Acad Emerg Med.* 2004;11(12):1290–1296.

20. Fosnocht DE, Swanson ER, Barton ED. Changing attitudes about pain and pain control in emergency medicine. *Emerg Med Clin North Am.* 2005;23(2):297–306.

21. Rupp T, Delaney KA. Inadequate analgesia in emergency medicine. *Ann Emerg Med.* 2004;43(4):494–503.

22. Jones JS, Johnson K, McNinch M. Age as a risk factor for inadequate emergency department analgesia. *Am J Emerg Med.* 1996;14(2):157–160.

23. Friedland LR, Kulick RM. Emergency department analgesic use in pediatric trauma victims with fractures. *Ann Emerg Med.* 1994;23(2):203–207.

24. Selbst SM. Managing pain in the pediatric emergency department. *Pediatr Emerg Care.* 1989;5(1):56–63.

25. Todd KH, Samaroo N, Hoffman JR. Ethnicity as a risk factor for inadequate emergency department analgesia. *JAMA.* 1993;269(12):1537–1539.

26. Todd, KH, Deaton C, D'Adamo AP, et al. Ethnicity and analgesic practice. *Ann Emerg Med.* 2000;35(1):11–16.

27. Miner J, Biros MH, Trainor A, et al. Patient and physician perceptions as risk factors for oligoanalgesia: a prospective observational study of the relief of pain in the emergency department. *Acad Emerg Med.* 2006;13(2):140–146.

28. Pfefferbaum B, Adams J, Aceves J. The influence of culture on pain in Anglo and Hispanic children with cancer. *J Am Acad Child Adolesc Psychiatry.* 1990;29(4):642–647.

29. Greenwald, HP. Interethnic differences in pain perception. *Pain.* 1991;44(2):157–163.

30. Tait RC, Chibnall JT. Physician judgments of chronic pain patients. *Soc Sci Med.* 1997;45(8):1199–1205.

31. Cooper-Patrick L, Gallo JJ, Gonzales JJ, et al. Race, gender, and partnership in the patient-physician relationship. *JAMA.* 1999;282(6):583–589.

32. Tamayo-Sarver JH, Dawson NV, Hinze SW, et al. The effect of race/ethnicity and desirable social characteristics on physicians' decisions to prescribe opioid analgesics. *Acad Emerg Med.* 2003;10(11):1239–1248.

33. Bartfield JM, Salluzzo RF, Raccio-Robak N, et al. Physician and patient factors influencing the treatment of low back pain. *Pain.* 1997;73(2):209–211.

34. Todd KH, Sloan EP, Chen C, et al. Survey of pain etiology, management, and satisfaction in two urban emergency departments. *Can J Emerg Med.* 2002;4(4):252–256.

35. Zohar Z, Eitan A, Halperin P, et al. Pain relief in major trauma patients: an Israeli perspective. *J Trauma.* 2001;51(4):767–772.

36. Kelly AM. A process approach to improving pain management in the emergency department: development and evaluation. *J Accid Emerg Med.* 2000;17(3):185–187.

37. Fry C, Aholt D. Local anesthesia prior to the insertion of peripherally inserted central catheters. *J Infus Nurs.* 2001;24(6):404–408.

38. Attard AR, Corlett MJ, Kidner NJ, et al. Safety of early pain relief for acute abdominal pain. *BMJ.* 1992;305:1020–1021.

39. Pace S, Burke TF. Intravenous morphine for early pain relief in patients with acute abdominal pain. *Acad Emerg Med.* 1996;3:1086–1092.

40. Vermeulen B, Morablia A, Unger PF, et al. Acute appendicitis: influence of early pain relief on the accuracy of clinical and US findings in the decision to operate: a randomized trial. *Radiology.* 1999;210:639–643.

41. Mahadevan M, Graff L. Prospective randomized study of analgesic use for ED patients with right lower quadrant abdominal pain. *Am J Emerg Med.* 2000;18:753–756.

42. Kim MK, Strait RT, Sato TT, et al. A randomized clinical trial of analgesia in children with acute abdominal pain. *Acad Emerg Med.* 2002;9:281–287.

43. Thomas SH, Silen W, Cheema F, et al. Effects of morphine analgesia on diagnostic accuracy in emergency department patients with abdominal pain: a prospective randomized trial. *J Am Coll Surg.* 2003;196:18–31.

44. Gallagher EJ, Esses D, Lee C, Lahn M, Bijur PE. Randomized clinical trial of morphine in acute abdominal pain. *Ann Emerg Med.* 2006;48:150–160.

45. Safdar B, Degutis LC, Landry K, Vedere SR, Moscovitz, HC, D'Onofrio G. Intravenous morphine plus ketorolac is superior to either drug alone for treatment of acute renal colic. *Ann Emerg Med.* 2006;48:173–181.

46. Hewitt DJ, Todd KH, Xiang J, Jordan DM, Rosenthan NR for the CAPSS-216 Study Investigators. Tramadol/acetaminophen or hydrocodone/acetaminophen for the treatment of ankle sprain: a randomized, placebo-controlled trial. *Ann Emerg Med.* 2007;49(4):468–480.

47. Bijur PE, Kenny MK, Gallagher EJ. Intravenous morphine at 0.1 mg/kg is not effective for controlling severe acute pain in the majority of patients. *Ann Emerg Med.* 2005;46(4):362–367.

48. Hershey LA. Meperidine and central neurotoxicity. *Ann Intern Med.* 1983;98(4):548–549.

49. Melzer-Lange MD, Walk-Kelly MD, Lea CM, et al. Patient-controlled analgesia for sickle cell pain crisis in a pediatric emergency department. *Pediatr Emerg Care.* 2004;20(1):2–4.

50. Evans E, Turley N, Robinson N, et al. Randomised controlled trial of patient controlled analgesia compared with nurse delivered analgesia in an emergency department. *Emerg Med J.* 2005;22(1):25–29.

51. Fulda GJ, Giberson F, Fagraeus L. A prospective randomized trial of nebulized morphine compared with patient-controlled analgesia morphine in the management of acute thoracic pain. *J Trauma.* 2005;59(2):383–388.

52. Ballas SK, Viscusi ER, Epstein KR. Management of acute chest wall sickle cell pain with nebulized morphine. *Am J Hematol.* 2004;76(2):190–191.

53. Bartfield JM, Flint RD, McErlean M, et al. Nebulized fentanyl for relief of abdominal pain. *Acad Emerg Med.* 2003;10(3):215–218.

54. Miner JR, Bachman A, Kosman L, et al. Assessment of the onset and persistence of amnesia during procedural sedation with propofol. *Acad Emerg Med.* 2005;12(6):491–496.

55. Miner JR, Heegaard W, Plummer D. End-tidal carbon dioxide monitoring during procedural sedation. *Acad Emerg Med.* 2002;9(4):275–280.

56. Bassett KE, Anderson J, Pribble CG, et al. Propofol for procedural sedation in children in the emergency department. *Ann Emerg Med.* 2003;42(6):773–782.

57. Frazee BW, Park RS, Lowery D, et al. Propofol for deep procedural sedation in the ED. *Am J Emerg Med.* 2005;23(2):190–195.

58. Miner JR, Biros MH, Seigel T, et al. The utility of the bispectral index in procedural sedation with propofol in the emergency department. *Acad Emerg Med.* 2005;12(3):190–196.

59. Miner JR, Biros MH, Heegaard W, et al. Bispectral electroencephalographic analysis of patients undergoing procedural sedation in the emergency department. *Acad Emerg Med.* 2003;10(6): 638–643.

60. Green SM. Fasting is a consideration – not a necessity – for emergency department procedural sedation and analgesia. *Ann Emerg Med.* 2003;42(5):647–650.

61. Agrawal D, Manzi SF, Bupta R, et al. Preprocedural fasting state and adverse events in children undergoing procedural sedation and analgesia in a pediatric emergency department. *Ann Emerg Med.* 2003;42(5):636–646.

62. American College of Emergency Physicians. Procedural sedation in the emergency department. *Ann Emerg Med.* 2005;46(1):103–104.

63. Green SM, Denmark TK, Cline J, et al. Ketamine sedation for pediatric critical care procedures. *Pediatr Emerg Care.* 2001;17(4):244–248.

64. Miner JR, Martel ML, Meyer M, et al. Procedural sedation of critically ill patients in the emergency department. *Acad Emerg Med.* 2005;12(2):124–128.

65. Hart LS, Berns SD, Houck CS, et al. The value of end-tidal CO2 monitoring when comparing three methods of conscious sedation for children undergoing painful procedures in the emergency department. *Pediatr Emerg Care.* 1997;13(3):189–193.

66. Bennett J, Peterson T, Burleson V. Capnography and ventilatory assessment during ambulatory dentoalveolar surgery. *J Oral Maxillofac Surg.* 1997;55(9):921–925; discussion 925–926.

67. Levine DA, Platt SL. Novel monitoring techniques for use with procedural sedation. *Curr Opin Pediatr.* 2005;17(3):351–354.

68. Chudnofsky CR, Weber JE, Colone PD, et al. A combination of midazolam and ketamine for procedural sedation and analgesia in adult emergency department patients. *Acad Emerg Med.* 2000;7(3):228–235.

69. Green SM, Krauss B. Clinical practice guideline for emergency department ketamine dissociative sedation in children. *Ann Emerg Med.* 2004;44(5):460–471.

70. Wathen JE, Roback MG, Mackenzie T, et al. Does midazolam alter the clinical effects of intravenous ketamine sedation in children? A double-blind, randomized, controlled, emergency department trial. *Ann Emerg Med.* 2000;36(6):579–588.

71. Green SM, Nakamura R, Johnson NE. Ketamine sedation for pediatric procedures: Part 1, A prospective series. *Ann Emerg Med.* 1990;19(9):1024–1032.

72. Kennedy RM, Porter FL, Miller JP, et al. Comparison of fentanyl/midazolam with ketamine/midazolam for pediatric orthopedic emergencies. *Pediatrics.* 1998;102(4 Pt 1):956–963.

73. Green SM, Sherwin TS. Incidence and severity of recovery agitation after ketamine sedation in young adults. *Am J Emerg Med.* 2005;23(2):142–144.

74. Pena BM, Krauss B. Adverse events of procedural sedation and analgesia in a pediatric emergency department. *Ann Emerg Med.* 1999;34(4 Pt 1):483–491.

75. Dionne RA, Moore PA, Gonty A, et al. Comparing efficacy and safety of four intravenous sedation regimens in dental outpatients. *J Am Dent Assoc.* 2001;132(6):740–751.

76. Malviya S, Tait AR, Reynolds PI, et al. Pentobarbital vs chloral hydrate for sedation of children undergoing MRI: efficacy and recovery characteristics. *Paediatr Anaesth.* 2004;14(7):589–595.

77. Kienstra AJ, Ward MA, Sasan F, et al. Etomidate versus pentobarbital for sedation of children for head and neck CT imaging. *Pediatr Emerg Care.* 2004;20(8):499–506.

78. Karian VE, Burrows PE, Zurakowski D, et al. Sedation for pediatric radiological procedures: analysis of potential causes of sedation failure and paradoxical reactions. *Pediatr Radiol.* 1999;29(11):869–873.

79. Miner JR, Biros M, Krieg S, et al. Randomized clinical trial of propofol versus methohexital for procedural sedation during fracture and dislocation reduction in the emergency department. *Acad Emerg Med.* 2003;10(9):931–937.

80. Zink BJ, Darfler K, Salluzzo RF, et al. The efficacy and safety of methohexital in the emergency department. *Ann Emerg Med.* 1991;20(12):1293–1298.

81. Bono JV, Rella JG, Zink BJ, et al. Methohexital for orthopaedic procedures in the emergency department. *Orthop Rev.* 1993; 22(7):833–838.

82. Pershad J, Godambe SA. Propofol for procedural sedation in the pediatric emergency department. *J Emerg Med* 2004;27(1):11–14.

83. Burton JH, Miner JR, Shipley ER, et al. Propofol for emergency department procedural sedation and analgesia: a tale of three centers. *Acad Emerg Med.* 2006;13(1):24–30.

84. Symington L, Thakore S. A review of the use of propofol for procedural sedation in the emergency department. *Emerg Med J.* 2006; 23(2):89–93.

85. Guenther E, Pribble CG, Junkins EP Jr, et al. Propofol sedation by emergency physicians for elective pediatric outpatient procedures. *Ann Emerg Med.* 2003;42(6):783–791.

86. Havel CJ Jr, Strait RT, Hennes H. A clinical trial of propofol vs midazolam for procedural sedation in a pediatric emergency department. *Acad Emerg Med.* 1999;6(10):989–997.

87. Falk J, Zed PJ. Etomidate for procedural sedation in the emergency department. *Ann Pharmacother* 2004;38(7–8):1272–1277.

88. Hunt GS, Spencer MT, Hays DP. Etomidate and midazolam for procedural sedation: prospective, randomized trial. *Am J Emerg Med.* 2005;23(3):299–303.

89. Burton JH, Bock AJ, Strout TD, et al. Etomidate and midazolam for reduction of anterior shoulder dislocation: a randomized, controlled trial. *Ann Emerg Med.* 2002;40(5):496–504.

90. Vinson DR, Bradbury DR. Etomidate for procedural sedation in emergency medicine. *Ann Emerg Med.* 2002;39(6):592–598.

91. Keim SM, Erstad BL, Sakles JC, et al. Etomidate for procedural sedation in the emergency department. *Pharmacotherapy.* 2002;22(5):586–592.

92. Ruth WJ, Burton JH, Bock AJ. Intravenous etomidate for procedural sedation in emergency department patients. *Acad Emerg Med.* 2001;8(1):13–18.

93. Schenarts CL, Burton JH, Riker RR. Adrenocortical dysfunction following etomidate induction in emergency department patients. *Acad Emerg Med.* 2001;8(1):1–7.

94. Anonymous. Pain management in the emergency department. *Ann Emerg Med.* 2004;44(2):198. [Editorial]

95. McCaig LF, Burt CW. National Hospital Ambulatory Medical Care Survey: 2001 emergency department summary. Advance data from vital and health statistics. No. 335. Hyattsville, MD: *National Center for Health Statistics*; 2003.

96. Sucov A, Nathanson A, McCormick J, Proano L, Reinert SE. Peer review and feedback can modify pain treatment patterns for emergency department patients with fractures. *Am J Med Qual.* 2005;20(3):138–143.

97. Decosterd I, Hugli O, Tamchès E, Blanc C, Mouhsine E, Givel J, Yersin B, Buclin T. Oligoanalgesia in the emergency department: short-term beneficial effects of an education program on acute pain. *Ann Emerg Med.* 2007.

37

The Nurse's Perspective on Acute Pain
Management

Chris Pasero, Nancy Eksterowicz, and Margo McCaffery

Advances in pain research and technology since the late 1980s have resulted in an exciting expansion in nursing roles in the field of pain management. Although nurses have always cared for patients with pain, the specialty of pain management nursing is relatively new.[1] Among the first to define the nurse's role were nurses designated to coordinate newly established acute pain services in the late 1980s and early 1990s.[2] Pain management is now identified as a nursing specialty[3] that offers nursing certification in the field and a wide variety of opportunities for nurses who want to focus their careers on the care of people with pain, including in the areas of clinical practice, research, and education.

One of the purposes of this chapter is to illustrate the growth and progress nurses have made in the field of acute pain management over the past several years. The chapter focuses on the various nursing roles that have emerged with the identification of pain as a specialty, including an in-depth discussion of the role of the acute pain service clinical coordinator and the education, credentials, and attributes necessary to adequately fulfill the role. The extensive responsibilities of the bedside nurse are also presented. Current pain management issues and challenges that nurses confront in their practices are described and solutions offered.

GROWTH AND PROGRESS

In the late 1980s, anesthesiologists began to extend their services and expertise beyond the operating room to the postoperative setting. Their recognition of the key role bedside nurses would play in assessment and management of acute pain therapies, such as intravenous patient-controlled analgesia (IV PCA) and epidural analgesia, brought about the need for a nurse specialist who could link the two disciplines.[2] Guided largely by anesthesiologists, hospitals across the country began to establish formal acute pain services and designate nurses to coordinate them. Support for this approach was found in publications, most notably the first clinical practice guideline on acute pain management in the United States, which described the importance of a multidisciplinary approach to the management of acute pain.[4] The pub-lication of the first Agency for Health Care Policy and Research (AHCPR) guideline was a defining moment for those who managed acute pain because it emphasized the need to adopt an evidence-based approach to pain management and rely on individuals with unique expertise in the field to insure therapies are delivered safely and effectively.

The American Nurses Association (ANA) and specialty professional nursing organizations, such as the American Society of PeriAnesthesia Nurses and the Oncology Nursing Society, have long supported the nurse's role in pain management with the publication of standards, position papers, and guidelines for nursing care of patients with pain.[5–7] However, in 1990, 7 nurses who at the time were serving as pain service coordinators in various parts of the country recognized the need for a professional nursing organization that could focus entirely on the optimal care of patients with pain and formed the American Society for Pain Management Nursing (ASPMN).[1] This group recognized that increasing numbers of nurses were being employed to fulfill positions in pain management, especially acute pain management, without any formal preparation. The ASPMN is dedicated to the provision of pain education for professionals, development of standards, and the promotion of advocacy and research in pain management nursing. The ASPMN membership today consists of nearly 2000 registered nurses (RNs), most specializing in pain management. Recognizing the frontline nurse's responsibility for implementation of effective pain care, the organization recently opened its membership to all licensed nurses. In 2005 RNs across the country sat for the first pain management nursing certification exam, which validated the specialty and achieved a goal of the organization since its inception.

THE ACUTE PAIN SERVICE CLINICAL COORDINATOR

As acute pain services began to spring up across the country in the early 1990s, the number of nurses assuming the position of clinical coordinator grew rapidly. Nursing departments in community hospitals designated full-time coordinator positions. The department of anesthesiology often directly hired

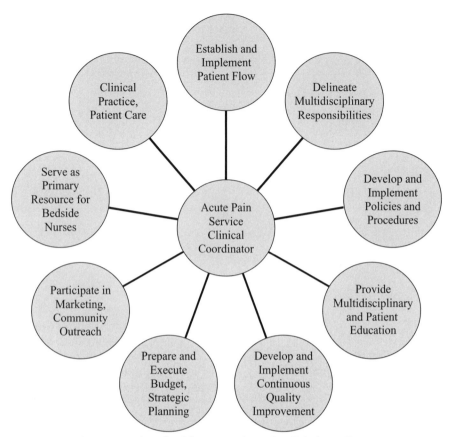

Figure 37.1: The role of the acute pain service clinical coordinator.

nurses to fill the role in academic settings and in some community hospital-based private practices.

Today, the acute pain service clinical coordinator is a key figure in health care institutions and has a vast range of responsibilities, including most obviously the smooth implementation of acute pain therapies (see Figure 37.1). The clinical coordinator serves as the liaison between the pain service and bedside nurses as well as all of the other specialties and departments involved in the delivery of safe and effective pain treatment.

Characteristics of the Clinical Coordinator

Most community hospitals require the acute pain service clinical coordinator to be an RN who holds a bachelor's degree; often a master's degree is preferred. A master's or doctorate degree-prepared nurse is strongly recommended for the position in a large academic setting.[2] Achievement of pain management nursing certification is desirable for all candidates.

The clinical coordinator must have considerable prior experience caring for patients with pain, especially those with postoperative pain, in-depth knowledge of the anatomy and physiology of pain and pharmacology and principles of pain management, and expert assessment skills. The ideal candidate is one who has nursing management background with previous exposure to and understanding of hospital administration and policies as well as budget preparation. An appreciation of the roles of both management and day-to-day bedside nursing is essential for practical strategic planning. The ability to quickly and appropriately adapt to a wide range of scenarios is essential.

Because the clinical coordinator must interface with almost every department in the hospital and gain the trust and support of the many disciplines involved in pain treatment, the candidate must have excellent interpersonal skills. In addition to informal and in-the-moment instruction, formal education of both staff and patients is one of the coordinator's primary responsibilities; therefore, teaching ability is a prerequisite.

The safety and effectiveness of acute pain service therapies depend on the coordinator's ability to insure that nurses in the clinical units individualize therapies to meet each patient's unique needs. This requires the coordinator to have confidence in bedside nurses and the ability to foster a relationship of trust with them. Knowledge and appreciation of the challenges as well as the priorities of bedside nursing are vital to the clinical coordinator's job.

Advanced Practice Registered Nurses

There is a trend toward clinical nurse specialists, certified registered nurse anesthetists (CRNAs), and nurse practitioners electing to specialize in pain management. In most cases, these nurses have a master's or doctorate degree and have achieved advanced practice certification. Advance practice registered nurses (APRNs) may be hired by the anesthesia department or by the institution or university to work with the anesthesia or nursing department to provide acute pain service therapies or coordinate a formal acute pain service.

Depending on state regulations, the APRN may have a collaborative practice agreement with a physician or anesthesia group and be considered a licensed independent practitioner within the institution. These APRNs often are directly reimbursed for their services. Depending upon the State in which they practice, clinical nurse specialists may or may not bill directly for their services; however, they promote the hospital's mission and are recognized as clinical leaders within the institution.

The APRN brings the advantage of complex practice skills such as catheter placement and prescribing authority to the service, which is beneficial, particularly in institutions where there is no formal anesthesia-driven acute pain service. Most have extensive clinical experience and an understanding of the challenges of bedside nursing. Bedside nurses tend to see the APRN as a valuable ally in the effort to better manage pain.

Organizational Structure

There are several options for selecting the department under which the hospital-funded clinical coordinator position can be placed; most of these depend on the coordinator's assigned responsibilities. The clinical coordinator must interface with a wide range of disciplines and departments through established channels of communication, representing anesthesiologists who have limited relationships with departments outside of the operating room. A good example of such interaction is with the department of nursing education. The clinical coordinator will spend a great deal of time educating and supporting the bedside nursing staff. It is, therefore, logical in many community hospitals to place the position under the authority of nursing services or directly under the department of nursing education. In academic settings, the acute pain service clinical coordinator is generally under the department of anesthesia in the organizational structure.

The acute pain service clinical coordinator is a change agent, advising others about matters of significant consequence and influence. It is important that this person be seen as a clinical leader and should, therefore, answer to at least the director level of management in the organizational structure. This will allow the coordinator to confidently interact with a variety of disciplines and earn respect through participation in multidisciplinary educational programs and development of institutional policies and procedures. Clinical nurse specialists are often hired for the coordinator position through the patient care or nursing services department and report to a hospital director. In academic settings the clinical coordinator answers directly to the acute pain service medical staff director.

Responsibilities of the Clinical Coordinator

The responsibilities of the acute pain service clinical coordinator are many and range from administrative duties to the provision of direct patient care. Following is a discussion that illustrates the clinical coordinator's multifarious role.

Establish Patient Flow

The first order of business for the clinical coordinator is to collaborate with the acute pain service medical staff director and establish an efficient mechanism for the delivery of therapies. An excellent place to start is to consider how patients will flow through the service so that every step before, during, and after treatment and the key personnel involved at each step can be identified (see Figure 37.2). How licensed independent practitioners will refer patients to the service must be determined. For example, surgeons in some community hospitals have an agreement with the anesthesia-based pain service to automatically manage their patients' postoperative pain following certain surgical procedures, such as thoracotomy and total joint replacement. Others may require a formal request for consultation.

patient entry to health care system → automatic or formal referral to acute pain service (*licensed independent practitioner*) → pain service consultation (*anesthesiologist, fellow, resident, nurse practitioner, clinical coordinator*) → development of pain treatment plan → patient education (*preadmission and admission personnel*) → acquisition of necessary supplies and equipment (*pharmacy, sterile processing personnel*) → titration to comfort and initiation of therapy (*PACU, ED, ICU, clinical unit personnel*) → ongoing management (*clinical unit personnel*) → transition to alternate analgesia in preparation for discharge → discontinue acute pain service therapy, discharge from acute pain service → evaluate overall response and satisfaction (*QI*)

Figure 37.2: Patient flow through the service.

Centralization of patient enrollment in the acute pain service will help insure smooth patient flow. Therapies can be initiated in a central location. For example, catheters can be placed in the holding area before surgery and IV PCA can be started routinely in the postanesthesia care unit (PACU) to assure seamless transition from one care area to another and optimal pain management. This process is facilitated when the clinical coordinator trains the preadmission nurses to provide patient education. The operating room (OR) or holding room staff is generally responsible for assisting anesthesiologists and CRNAs with catheter placement. The PACU nurses requisition analgesic infusion devices and drugs and insure therapies are initiated. Identification of a central location, such as the bioengineering or material distribution department, for cleaning, storing, dispensing, and tracking analgesic infusion devices is also recommended.

Standardization of therapies as much as possible is a common characteristic of well-organized pain services. Nursing staff express a greater degree of confidence in their ability to manage pain therapies when they know what to expect. The pharmacy department will be able to more efficiently provide analgesic and anesthetic solutions and other medications when the acute pain service has designated standard formulations and side-effect medication regimens for the majority of the therapies it will offer. The use of standardized documentation and computerized or preprinted order forms helps to insure clarity of the treatment plan and better compliance with documentation requirements. Most important, such consistency may help to prevent confusion and error in the clinical setting.

Delineate Responsibilities

The clinical coordinator will need to partner with department managers and directors as well as frontline staff members to define personnel responsibilities in delivering analgesic therapies. For example, direct communication with the pharmacy is crucial; often the coordinator asks a pharmacist or doctor of pharmacy (PharmD) to serve as a liaison to the acute pain service and as a member of the pain care committee.[8]

Some of the many roles that must be described are those of the acute pain service medical staff director, anesthesiologists, CRNAs, licensed independent practitioners (eg, primary physicians, nurse practitioners, and physician assistants), clinical pharmacists, and bedside nursing staff (see Table 37.1). In academic settings, the involvement of residents, fellows, and

Table 37.1: Key Disciplines and Responsibilities for Acute Pain Services

Discipline	Key Responsibilities

Clinical Coordinator	1. Clinical practice
	  ▪ Conducts consultations and rounds
	  ▪ Assists with catheter placement and initiation of therapies
	  ▪ Assesses pain
	  ▪ Titrates and manages/evaluates therapies on an ongoing basis
	  ▪ Discontinues therapies
	  ▪ Manages side effects and complications
	  ▪ Operates and troubleshoots analgesic infusion devices
	  ▪ Documents therapies
	  ▪ Provides follow up with referring service as indicated
	  ▪ Serves as primary pain resource to all departments and disciplines
	  ▪ Coordinates pain resource nurse program
	2. With medical staff director, makes decisions regarding implementation of the pain service
	3. Develops and implements policies and procedures, standards, and guidelines
	4. Provides multidisciplinary, patient, and community education
	  ▪ Pain resource nurse program
	  ▪ Nursing pain management competencies
	  ▪ Medical staff/resident education
	  ▪ Fellowships and preceptorships
	5. Implements continuous quality improvement plan
	6. Participates in research activities
	7. Serves as pain committee chair or co-chair; represents pain service at departmental and committee meetings as indicated
	8. Prepares and executes budget; strategic planning
	9. Participates in marketing and community outreach activities

Pain Service Medical Staff Director	1. Clinical practice
	  ▪ Conducts consultations and rounds
	  ▪ Serves as primary pain medicine resource for residents/medical staff
	  ▪ Supervises and assists residents with patient management, procedures (e.g., catheter placement), and documentation
	2. With clinical coordinator, makes decisions regarding implementation of pain service
	3. Serves as primary contact for clinical coordinator regarding pain service issues
	4. Provides input for development of policies and procedures, standards, and guidelines
	5. Provides multidisciplinary pain education
	  ▪ Reviews (daily) components of the core curriculum for regional analgesia and pain management for residents
	  ▪ Participates in nursing education as indicated
	6. Communicates or delegates responsibility for communicating patient status to referring service
	7. Serves as pain committee chair or co-chair
	8. Participates in continuous quality improvement activities as indicated
	9. Oversees research activities
	10. Represents pain service at departmental and committee meetings as indicated
	11. Provides input into budget preparation and execution; strategic planning

Anesthesiologists/ CRNAs/Fellows/ Residents	1. Clinical practice
	  ▪ Conducts consultations and rounds
	  ▪ Places catheters
	  ▪ Prescribes therapies
	  ▪ Evaluates patient response to therapies
	  ▪ Manages side effects and complications
	  ▪ Discontinues therapies
	  ▪ Documents therapies
	  ▪ Provides follow up with referring service
	  ▪ Serves as a primary pain medicine resource
	  ▪ Serves as primary medicine contact for clinical coordinator and nursing staff regarding patient-specific issues
	2. Provides multidisciplinary education
	3. Provides input for development of policies and procedures, standards, and guidelines
	4. Serves on pain committee as indicated
	5. Participates in continuous quality improvement activities as indicated
	6. Participates in research activities

Discipline	Key Responsibilities

Pharmacist/Doctor of Pharmacy (PharmD)	1. Clinical practice
	   ■ Conducts consultations and rounds
	   ■ Serves as primary pharmacology resource for medical and nursing staff
	2. Insures access to necessary analgesics and other requisite medications
	3. Provides multidisciplinary education
	4. Serves on pain committee
	5. Participates in development of policies and procedures, standards, and guidelines
	6. Participates in continuous quality improvement as indicated
	7. Participates in research activities

Bedside Clinical Nurse	1. Clinical practice: primary pain manager, pain resource nurse
	   ■ Assesses pain
	   ■ Assists with catheter placement
	   ■ Titrates, initiates, and maintains therapies
	   ■ Changes analgesic doses
	   ■ Administers bolus doses
	   ■ Monitors patients and therapies
	   ■ Manages side effects and complications
	   ■ Operates and troubleshoots analgesic infusion devices
	   ■ Discontinues therapies
	   ■ Documents therapies
	2. Provides patient education
	3. Serves on pain committee
	4. Provides input for development of policies and procedures, standards, and guidelines
	5. Participates in continuous quality improvement activities
	6. Participates in research activities

medical students must be clarified. Other critical individuals are support personnel from the departments of material management, biomedical engineering, and accounting as well as those who will provide secretarial (clerical) assistance for the acute pain service. The importance of acquiring input from every department that will be involved in the delivery of therapies cannot be overemphasized as this will help to insure accurate work assignment and their ultimate cooperation and support of the service.

Establish Policies and Procedures

The acute pain service clinical coordinator, with guidance from the medical staff director and others as appropriate, is responsible for establishing policies and procedures, standards, and guidelines for pain treatment. This involves researching the literature and networking with others in the field to determine current standard of care and insure an evidence-based approach is applied to the care of patients with pain. It often requires interfacing with the state board of nursing on scope of nursing practice issues. Policies and procedures should address the Joint Commission (JC) pain treatment and safety standards in hospitals that are surveyed by the JC. Coordinators who are inexperienced in writing policies and procedures and the JC survey process can seek assistance from those who are responsible for addressing these issues in the institution.

Because many of the acute pain management policies and procedures influence and direct activity in other departments, the clinical coordinator should schedule time to meet with department directors to help insure accuracy and ultimate adherence. Among others, acute pain policies and procedures should address (1) patient flow through the service; (2) patient-selection criteria for the various therapies; (3) prescribing guidelines; (4) pain assessment; (5) therapy initiation, maintenance, and discontinuation processes; (6) patient monitoring; (7) side-effect and complication management; (8) medication, equipment, and supply acquisition; (9) infection control; (10) multidisciplinary education; and (11) patient education.

Clinical Practice

Responses to an informal survey of 51 nurses who specialize in pain management and subscribe to a pain management nursing electronic-mail list service revealed that the majority of respondents (82%) spend most of their time in the clinical setting providing direct care to patients receiving analgesic therapies.[9] This care is administered in diverse ways, including initial interviews and consultations, counseling patients and families, rounds both with and without medical and anesthesia staff, assisting bedside nurses in the clinical unit, and troubleshooting analgesic infusion device problems.

Ideally, patient rounds include the acute pain service clinical coordinator, acute pain service anesthesiologist or medical staff director, and additional team members, such as a clinical pharmacist, at least once daily. The team should invite the bedside nurse to provide input on the patient's status prior to or during rounds. At the time evaluations occur, titration decisions are made and orders are written. In the community setting, the coordinator is responsible for follow-up and evaluating changes in therapies, reporting back to the anesthesiologist and assuring that any additional changes in therapies are implemented.

In an academic setting, the clinical coordinator works closely with the attending anesthesiologist and resident assigned to the acute pain service. As an integral member of the team, the coordinator orients each resident to the daily responsibilities and technical skills. Although the attending anesthesiologist

Box 37.1: Nursing Education Content

1. Adverse effects of unrelieved pain
2. Anatomy and physiology of pain
3. Pain assessment and goal setting
4. Pharmacology of pain
5. Selected pain therapies and delivery systems
6. Population-specific considerations, e.g., labor, neonatal, pediatrics, geriatrics
7. Side effect and complication management
8. Transition to alternative analgesia and discontinuation of therapy
9. Appropriate nondrug interventions
10. Documentation
11. Policy and procedure review
12. Clinical skill requirements
    - Pain assessment
    - Titration to comfort prior to therapy
    - Initiation and maintenance of therapy
    - Evaluation of patient response, decision making, and dose adjustment
    - Discontinuation of therapies; removal of various infusion catheters
    - Analgesic infusion device operation

supervises the resident during preoperative catheter insertions, the coordinator covers the incoming pages, assists with patient positioning, and facilitates setting up equipment as needed. The coordinator and resident conduct a second set of patient rounds to evaluate therapy changes. The follow-up rounds also provide the resident with the additional information needed to give an accurate account of the pain treatment plan to pass off to the covering resident.

A significant amount of the clinical coordinator's time is spent serving as a resource to beside nurses as they manage the acute pain service patients' pain. This involves assisting with pain assessment and decision-making with regard to the need for changes in the patient's pain treatment plan, validating psychomotor skills such as analgesic infusion device operation and removal of the various infusion catheters, and managing side effects and complications. The coordinator documents therapies and insures that others document appropriately. Thorough documentation is essential because it ensures continuity of the pain management plan, captures reimbursement, and provides information for quality improvement.

Multidisciplinary Education

A major responsibility of the clinical coordinator is to educate all of the disciplines involved in the delivery of acute pain therapy. Bedside clinical nurses initiate, monitor, maintain, and discontinue acute pain therapies. Their knowledge and skill at completing these activities will determine the safety and effectiveness of the acute pain service. The clinical coordinator is the primary pain nursing resource for the bedside nurses

and responsible for providing the initial and ongoing education required to fulfill their role as primary pain managers. In addition to formal lectures, the coordinator conducts much of the instruction in the clinical unit, often at the bedside, validating the nursing staff's decision-making and skills. It is imperative that the clinical coordinator work with the institution's nursing education department to determine how nurses will achieve their educational requirements (see Box 37.1).

The pain service medical staff director helps identify important pain content and clinical skill requirements for the nursing staff; medical staff directors and anesthesiologists or CRNAs often provide lectures for the nursing staff. In the academic setting, the acute pain service medical staff director oversees the residents' educational process, and the clinical coordinator assists in providing them with both formal and informal education (see Box 37.2).

Box 37.2: Resident Education Content

1. Adverse effects of unrelieved pain; benefits of specific analgesic therapies
2. Anatomy and physiology of pain
3. Patient selection criteria and indications for various therapies
4. Prescribing guidelines
    - Analgesics, anesthetics
    - Adjuvant medications
    - Side-effect management
    - Patient population considerations
5. Initiation of therapies
    - Discuss plan with acute pain service attending and clinical coordinator
    - Discuss plan with referring service as indicated
    - Obtain consent
    - Catheter placement procedures
6. Evaluation of patient response to therapies
    - Pain: evaluate at rest and activity
    - Achievement of functional goals
    - Side effects
    - Analgesic use during past 24 hours
    - Concurrent medication use
    - Problem-oriented physical exam
    - Patient satisfaction
7. Complication management
8. Appropriate nondrug interventions
9. Discharge preparation
    - Transition to alternative analgesia
    - Discontinuation of therapy
    - Transfer care to referring service
10. Communication with nurses, patients, families, referring service
11. Documentation
12. Analgesic infusion device operation

Patient Education

One of the primary reasons for the management of acute postoperative pain is to optimize postoperative patient outcomes, and the patient's active participation in the achievement of recovery goals is critical to this process. This is enhanced when patients understand what they can expect from the health care team and what the team expects of them during the postoperative period. The clinical coordinator must develop and implement a means by which patients receiving acute pain treatment are educated about these important points.

Although not always possible, every effort should be made to conduct education prior to initiation of therapy. Educationally appropriate reading material can be provided to the patient and family to review at home after the surgical planning visit. References and resources for additional details are usually included in these materials. Some acute pain services provide videos or DVDs that can be either shown in the surgeon's office or given to the patient to be viewed at home.

A central location, such as the preadmission testing area, for the majority of in-person patient education is convenient; however, patient education can be reinforced anywhere, including in the preoperative holding area and in the clinical units. Enlisting nursing staff to routinely include defined pain management content in their teaching sessions will help to insure patient education is provided and will ease the clinical coordinator's workload. Important content includes a review of the adverse effects of pain, an explanation of the pain treatment plan, establishment of realistic comfort-function goals,[10] and, if indicated, a demonstration and return demonstration of PCA equipment.

Continuous Quality Improvement

The development and implementation of a continuous quality improvement (CQI) plan that focuses on process and performance will help to insure safe and effective acute pain management is delivered. The clinical coordinator must work with the QI and risk management departments to address among other indicators: (1) pain assessment; (2) analgesic effectiveness (pain reduction and control, goal achievement and outcomes, patient satisfaction); (3) treatment and reduction of side effects; (4) prevention of infection, complications, and safety hazards; (5) multidisciplinary performance; and (6) compliance with JC pain treatment and safety standards.

Data collection can consume a significant amount of time. It is, therefore, advised that the acute pain service clinical coordinator work with the clinical unit managers to incorporate monitoring of pain management indicators into their unit-specific CQI plans. Key to the ongoing and systematic monitoring of these indicators, is the analysis of findings and implementation of action plans aimed at improving care when problems or potential problems are identified.

Other General Responsibilities

The effective acute pain service clinical coordinator becomes the voice for patients with pain in the institution by serving as the nursing representative at pertinent committee meetings and whenever a decision must be made that will affect or be affected by pain management. The coordinator often chairs or cochairs (with the acute pain service medical staff director) the pain committee, which focuses on building institutional commitment to improvements in pain management. They serve on or prepare and present reports to various other committees such as infection control, pharmacy and therapeutics, professional development, and strategic planning. Input from the acute pain service clinical coordinator and medical staff director on the development of clinical practice guidelines is essential.

Other general responsibilities include budget preparation, insuring appropriate evaluation and acquisition of analgesic infusion devices and other pain service equipment and supplies, and working with the marketing department on a variety of activities, including development of patient information material and community outreach programs.

DIVERSITY OF THE NURSE'S ROLE

Changes in health care have brought about interesting diversity in the role of nurses who specialize in pain management. With the advent of managed care in the mid-1990s and subsequent budget cuts across the country, many community hospitals discontinued their formal acute pain services and several clinical coordinators lost their jobs. Others were retained but were assigned additional responsibility for patient care in other areas of the hospital, such as in the PACU or intensive care unit (ICU). Several were assigned responsibility for global institutional pain management issues, such as JC compliance and process improvement rather than as the coordinator of an acute pain service. With the widespread acquisition and merging of hospitals, many clinical coordinators now distribute their time among some or all of the hospitals in the health care system. As a result, the nurse's role in pain management is diverse, and creative strategies for improving pain management and insuring the safe and effective administration of pain therapies have been developed. Following are some examples.

Pain Resource Nurse Programs

Nurses who care for patients in the clinical units have been described as primary pain managers by virtue of their assessment abilities and 24-hour presence.[11] They have a tremendous impact on the delivery of acute pain management therapies. Their involvement spans the continuum of care and encompasses multiple responsibilities (see Table 37.1).

One of the most creative approaches to prepare and support bedside nurses in their role as primary pain managers and to generally improve the management of pain in institutions is the pain resource nurse (PRN) program.[8] The implementation of a PRN program involves the designation of at least one nurse, preferably an RN, per shift on every clinical unit in the hospital to serve as a resource to the other members of the nursing staff regarding pain management issues. PRNs complete an extensive educational program, which is specifically designed to teach them about pain management as well as how to serve as a support person and role model for their peers. This is followed by validation of skill requirements in the clinical setting. The City of Hope National Medical Center in Duarte, California, has presented annual PRN educational programs since the early 1990s and prepared nearly 2000 nurses to assume the PRN role or return to their institutions to establish their own PRN programs.[12]

Common pitfalls of PRN programs are that PRNs often feel as though they do not have enough time to perform educational activities and that they are stretched to address their own patients' pain, much less the pain problems of their coworkers' patients.[8] Sustained success of a program depends on administrative commitment to it, which involves periodically providing additional staffing so that the PRNs have adequate time to educate and assist other nurses in their clinical unit with pain management issues. Programs spearheaded by an identified full-time nurse coordinator are much more likely to succeed.[8] Quite often this coordinator is based in a clinical unit such as the PACU or ICU. If available, the acute pain service clinical coordinator or APRN who specializes in pain often provides the educational support and serves as the point person for the PRNs. The ultimate goal of all PRN programs should be to target every nurse on the clinical unit, rather than a select few, to become proficient in the management of pain.[2,8]

Role Model Programs and Preceptorships

One of the best ways to teach others is through role modeling.[8] A variety of role modeling programs have been offered nationwide over the years whereby dyads of physicians and nurses or other colleagues attend a conference to learn how to improve pain management processes in their institutions. The University of Wisconsin at Madison sees the nurse as the primary change agent in a health care facility and offers the Practice Change Program to prepare nurses for this role.

A few hospitals with particularly well-organized pain services offer preceptorships for nurses who want to observe the service in action. These programs tend to last 2 to 4 days and provide didactic as well as clinical exposure. Attendees are given support materials such as policy and procedure templates to use when they return to their institutions. Those who attend preceptorships consistently cite the firsthand observation of patient flow through a well-managed pain service as invaluable.[13]

Nurse-Based Pain Programs

Nurse-based pain programs have sprung up around the country in response to the need for improved pain management in institutions that do not offer an anesthesia-based acute pain service. Most often a master's-prepared nurse or APRN hired by the health care facility and based in a clinical unit, such as the PACU or ICU, or directly under nursing administration leads the service and works with medicine and surgery colleagues to establish a mechanism for referral to the service. Medical direction may be provided by a variety of specialties, most often the anesthesia or surgery department.

Any licensed independent practitioner may request a formal consultation with the nurse-based pain service; some have established automatic referral for certain surgical procedures and medical conditions. In most institutions the nursing staff may ask for an informal consultation with the nurse-based pain service, which usually leads to treatment recommendations and problem resolution or a formal referral.

Some nurse-based pain services have a staff of nurses available 24 hours a day, who round regularly on referred patients, and all rely on the bedside nurses to provide the majority of care. Similar to the clinical coordinator, the nurses who manage and work for the nurse-based PCA service serve as the bedside nurse's primary pain management resource and provide education and skill development for them. The pharmacy department usually works closely with the service to provide standardized analgesic solutions and side-effect medications as well as patient consultations. Physicians who utilize the nurse-based service often cite

the consistent provision of patient education, ongoing evaluation of their patients' responses to pain treatment, and reliable management of complex pain issues as major benefits of the service.

NURSING ISSUES

As a result of an increased commitment to the management of pain, a number of issues that directly affect nurses have come to the forefront. Most of these are universal among all nurses; however, some have arisen from the needs of specific patient populations. Following is a brief discussion of some of these issues; recommendations and solutions are offered.

Pain Assessment in Nonverbal Patients

The introduction of the JC pain treatment standards in 2000 resulted in recognition of the need for better pain assessment in health care facilities nationwide, even in those that were not JC accredited (see Chapter X). The use of the 0-to-10 numeric pain rating scale quickly became the standard tool for obtaining the patient's report of pain intensity and was incorporated into routine nursing care nationwide. However, it soon became clear to nurses in certain clinical areas that the 0-to-10 scale was inappropriate for many of their patients because of an inability to report pain, such as unconscious, ventilated patients in the ICU.[14] ICU nurses and those who care for infants, toddlers, and cognitively impaired patients expressed frustration with the unrealistic expectation that a pain rating be recorded for every patient under their care. There was also concern that pain assessment seemed to have become reduced to recording a number in the medical record.[14]

In response to this issue, the ASPMN appointed a task force to develop guidelines on the assessment of pain in the nonverbal patient (anyone who could not use a customary self-report pain assessment tool).[15] This included infants, toddlers, the cognitively impaired, and unconscious, ventilated patients. The guideline describes the use of a hierarchy of pain measures, which involves assessment of

- Self-report in patients who can provide it or documentation why the clinician cannot use self-report; single most reliable indicator of pain
- Presence of underlying pathology or procedure that is thought to be painful
- Behavioral indicators of pain, such as grimacing and restlessness, or use of behavioral tools such as the Critical-Care Pain Observation Tool (CPOT)[16] and the Pain Assessment Checklist for Seniors with Limited Ability to Communicate (PACSLAC)[17]
- Surrogate (parent, significant other, or caregiver) report of possible pain behaviors
- Analgesic trial whereby analgesia is administered and any changes in identified behaviors help to confirm the presence of pain

The hierarchy provides nurses with a multidimensional method for assessing pain in patients who are unable to provide a report using a customary self-report tool and establishes a basis for formulating a pain treatment plan. Further, this approach led to the approval in institutions nationwide of the acronym APP (assume pain present) for documentation for patients in whom pathology, behaviors, or other indicators suggest pain.[14]

Patient Monitoring

The emphasis on providing better pain management has led to an increase in the use of opioid analgesics and concerns over an apparent subsequent increase in opioid-induced respiratory depression.[18,19] This, in turn, has led to recommendations for increased patient monitoring, particularly during parenteral and intraspinal opioid therapy.[19] Because nurses provide the bulk of patient monitoring and are responsible for insuring patient safety during opioid therapy, any new recommendations will directly impact their practice.

The observation that increased sedation precedes opioid-induced respiratory depression suggests that more frequent nurse assessment of sedation level during opioid therapy is of the utmost importance.[11] Responses to an informal survey of 63 nurses (representing 66 hospitals) who specialize in pain management and subscribe to a pain management nursing electronic mail list service revealed that 99% of those responding were using some type of sedation scale during IV and intraspinal opioid therapy, the most common being the Pasero Opioid-induced Sedation Scale (POSS) (see Box 37.3).[20] However, only 9% incorporated recommendations for nursing actions at the various levels of sedation.

Box 37.3: Pasero Opioid-Induced Sedation Scale (POSS) with Interventions

S = Sleep, easy to arouse
Acceptable; no action necessary; may administer opioid dose

1 = Awake and alert
Acceptable; no action necessary; may administer opioid dose

2 = Slightly drowsy, easily aroused
Acceptable; no action necessary; may administer opioid dose

3 = Frequently drowsy, arousable, drifts off to sleep during conversation
Unacceptable; decrease opioid dose by 25 to 50%; suggest administration of a nonsedating, opioid-sparing nonopioid, such as acetaminophen or a nonsteroidal antiinflammatory drug; monitor respiratory status and sedation level closely until sedation level is less than 3 and respiratory status is satisfactory.

4 = Somnolent, minimal or no response to physical stimulation
Unacceptable; stop opioid administration; consider administering naloxone; notify pain service, licensed independent practitioner, house officer, or first-response team for orders; monitor respiratory status and sedation level closely until sedation level is less than 3 and respiratory status is satisfactory. When opioid is resumed, decrease the initial dose by 50%.

Used with permission. Copyright, C. Pasero, 1994. *Acute Pain Management Service: Policy and Procedure Guideline Manual.* Los Angeles (CA): Academy Medical Systems.

This survey indicates that nurses understand there is a link between increased sedation and impending opioid-induced respiratory depression and recognize the importance of sedation assessment. Nurses also verify that sedation assessment is simple, convenient, and cost-effective. However, the increase in the incidence of clinically significant opioid-induced respiratory depression also indicates that nurses are not held accountable for sedation assessment and acting when dangerous increased sedation is detected.

It is imperative that all opioid prescriptions be accompanied by clear monitoring guidelines for nursing staff that include sedation assessment at least every 2 hours during at least the first 24 hours of opioid therapy and the expectation that nurses will immediately decrease the opioid dose as soon as a dangerous level of increased sedation is detected (see sedation level 3 in Box 37.3).[11,21] Further, nurses should be expected to observe respiratory status (depth, regularity, rate, and noise during respiration) at this same frequency. Sleeping patients with unacceptable respiratory depth, regularity, or rate and those with noisy respirations (eg, snoring) must be aroused for further assessment. The use of a simple scale, such as the POSS, that focuses solely on opioid-induced sedation and does not include agitation indicators is recommended for assessment of opioid-induced sedation.[21]

Analgesia by Catheter Techniques

Analgesia delivered by catheter techniques, such as intraspinal analgesia and perineural infusions, is common for the management of acute pain. However, there has been some confusion and inconsistency nationwide with regard to the extent to which nurses can monitor and manage these therapies.[22] Nurses often report that they are able to provide complete care for patients receiving analgesia by catheter techniques in one clinical care area but not in another. For example, RNs within the same institution may be allowed to increase the rate of an epidural analgesic infusion in a neonate but are prohibited from doing so in a labor patient.

In response to this issue, the ASPMN developed a position statement reinforcing that it has long been within the scope of nursing practice for an RN to administer analgesia and stating their belief that this scope includes analgesia by catheter techniques such as intraspinal, perineural, and interpleural administration.[22] Personal perception or bias unsupported by scientific evidence is not adequate justification for refusing to care for patients receiving analgesia by catheter techniques. The organization emphasizes that bedside RNs are critical to ensuring safe and effective analgesia by these methods and provides monitoring and management recommendations for the licensed independent practitioner, health care facility, and the RN.

Range Order Administration

Range orders are defined as a medication order in which the dosage or time period or both are specified according to a range.[23] As-needed range orders have been considered an essential method for the management of acute pain for decades.[23,24] In response to JC and other accrediting organizations' concerns about the safety of this practice and the nurse's associated role, the ASPMN and the American Pain Society (APS) issued a consensus statement that reinforced their belief that competent

RNs can safely interpret and implement properly written analgesic range orders.[24] The development of prescribing guidelines and a protocol that outlines patient monitoring and facilitates the nurse's decision making with regard to appropriate dose selection is recommended.[25] Insuring RN competency through didactic and psychomotor skill validation is essential.

Alternative Agent-Controlled Analgesia

There is general acceptance that effective use of PCA requires patients to understand the relationships among pain, self-administration of a dose of pain medication, and pain relief and be cognitively and physically able to use the PCA device (see Chapter X).[11,26] There are many patients who would benefit from PCA but are denied the therapy because they do not meet these criteria. A solution to this dilemma is the authorization of a competent alternate agent, such as a parent or significant other, who is capable of assuming responsibility for using the PCA device to administer analgesic doses to a loved one.[26] The agent is taught how to recognize pain and whether it is safe to administer a dose.

With nurse-activated dosing, the patient's primary nurse serves as the alternate agent and utilizes the PCA device to deliver analgesic doses. This is an ideal therapy in the ICU where patients are too ill to manage their own pain using PCA. A continuous infusion (basal rate) can be administered and the nurse can press the demand button to administer supplemental doses for breakthrough pain and to prepare the patient for painful procedures. This method saves nursing time and assures that the correct opioid dose is administered.[26]

These alternative uses of analgesic infusion devices have been safely administered for several years in both children and adults.[8,26] In 2007, the ASPMN published clinical recommendations in a position statement supporting the nurse's role in the use of these effective pain management methods.[27]

REFERENCES

1. Pasero C, Reed B. The formation and early history of the American Society for Pain Management Nursing. *ASPMN Pathways.* 2003;12(12):2, 8. Available at: http://www.aspmn.org/Organization/history.htm. Accessed January 12, 2007.

2. Pasero C, Preble LM. Role of the clinical nurse coordinator. In: Sinatra RS, Hord AH, Ginsberg B, Preble LM, eds. *Acute Pain. Mechanisms & Management.* St Louis, MO: Mosby;1992;552–559.

3. St Marie B, ed. *Core Curriculum for Pain Management Nursing.* St Louis, MO: Saunders; 2002.

4. Agency for Healthcare Policy and Research (AHCPR). *Acute Pain Management: Operations or Medical Procedures and Trauma. Clinical Practice Guideline.* Rockville, MD: U.S. Public Health Service, AHCPR Publication 92-0032.

5. American Nurses Association (ANA). Position statement on the role of the registered nurse (RN) in the management of analgesia by catheter techniques (epidural, intrathecal, intrapleural, or peripheral nerve catheters). Washington, DC: ANA. Available at: http://www.nursingworld.org/readroom/position/joint/jtcathet.htm. Accessed January 12, 2007.

6. Krenzischek D, Wilson L. Introduction to the ASPAN pain and comfort clinical practice guideline. *J Perianesth Nurs.* 2003; 18(4):228–231.

7. Oncology Nursing Society (ONS). ONS Publications. Retrieved January 10, 2007 from http://www.ons.org/publications/.

8. Pasero C, Gordon DB, McCaffery M, Ferrell BR. Building institutional commitment to improving pain management. In: McCaffery M, Pasero C, eds. 2nd ed. *Pain: Clinical Manual,* St Louis, MO: Mosby; 1999;711–744.

9. Pasero C. Electronic-mail communication with the American Pain Society Nursing Special Interest Group email list service subscribers, February 26 through April 1, 2007.

10. Pasero C, McCaffery M. Comfort-function goals. *Am J Nurs.* 2004;104(9):77–78, 81.

11. Pasero C, Portenoy RK, McCaffery M. Opioid analgesics. In: McCaffery M, Pasero C, eds. *Pain: Clinical Manual.* 2nd ed. St Louis, MO: Mosby; 1999;161–299.

12. Pasero C. Electronic-mail communication with Betty Ferrell, PhD, RN, Research Scientist, City of Hope National Medical Center, Duarte, CA on March 24, 2007.

13. Pasero C. Personal communication with Joan Beard, MS, RN, Director of Pain and Palliative Care, Mercy Medical Center, Des Moines, IA, September 13, 2006.

14. Pasero C, McCaffery M. No self report means no pain intensity. *Am J Nurs.* 2005;105(10):50–53.

15. Herr K, Coyne P, McCaffery M, et al. Pain assessment in the nonverbal patient: position statement with clinical recommendations. *Pain Manag Nurs.* 2006;7(2):44–52.

16. Gelinas C, Fillion L, Puntillo KA, Viens C, Fortier M. Validation of critical-care pain observation tool. *Am J Crit Care.* 2006;15:420–427.

17. Fuchs-Lacelle S, Hadjistavropoulos T. Development and preliminary validation of the pain assessment checklist for seniors with limited ability to communicate (PACSLAC). *Pain Manag Nurs.* 2004;5(1):37–49.

18. Vila H, Smith RA, Augustyniak MJ, et al. The efficacy and safety of pain mnagement before and after implementation of hospital-wide pain management standards: is patient safety compromised by treatment based solely on numerical pain ratings. *Anesth Analg.* 2005;101:474–480.

19. Weinger MB. Dangers of postoperative opioids. *APSF Newslett.* 2006–2007;21(4):63–68.

20. Pasero C. Electronic mail communication with the American Pain Society Nursing Special Interest Group email list service subscribers, March 1 through April 10, 2006.

21. Pasero C, McCaffery M. Monitoring opioid-induced sedation. *Am J Nurs.* 2002;102(2):67–68.

22. Pasero C, Eksterowicz N, Primeau M, Cowley C. Registered nurse management and monitoring of analgesia by catheter techniques. *Pain Manag. Nurs.* 2007;8(2):49–55.

23. Manworren RCB. A call to action to protect range orders. *Am J Nurs.* 2007;106(7):30–33.

24. Gordon DB, Dahl J, Phillips P, Frandsen J, Cowley C, Foster RL, Fine PG, Miaskowski C, Fishman S, Finley RS. The use of "as needed" range orders for opioid analgesics in the management of acute pain: a consensus statement of the ASPMN and the APS. *Pain Manag Nurs.* 2004;5(2):53–58.

25. Pasero C, Manworren RCB, McCaffery M. IV opioid range orders. *Am J Nurs.* 2007;107(2):52–59.

26. Pasero C, McCaffery M. Authorized and unauthorized use of PCA pumps. *Am J Nurs.* 2005;105(7):30–33.

27. Wuhrman E, Cooney M, Dunwoody C, Eksterowicz N, Merkel S, Oakes L. Authorized and unauthorized ("PCA by proxy") dosing of analgesic infusion pumps: position statement with clinical practice recommendations. *Pain Manag Nurs.* 2007;8(1):4–11.

38

Role of the Pharmacist in Acute Pain Management

Leslie N. Schechter

Today's pharmacist responsibilities have expanded beyond the traditional roles of compounding, filling, dispensing prescriptions with accuracy and appropriateness, and pharmaceutical supply management. Pharmacists have been identified as part of a collaborative team that provides appropriate medication therapy management. This team approach benefits patients that receive medications for the treatment of acute pain. Pharmacists also ensure proper preparation of sterile products, adhering to the United States Pharmacopeia (USP) 797 recommendations.[1] In addition, pharmacists provide drug information and critical evaluations of new drug products or devices to the Pharmacy and therapeutics (P&T) Committee. Additional roles for the pharmacist include quality assurance data collection, development of proper medication labeling, medication error reporting, and the development of policies and procedures for appropriate opioid control systems.

MEDICATION THERAPY MANAGEMENT

Pharmacists are well situated in the medication use process to influence patient outcomes from drug therapy.[2] They are usually the last health care provider whom a patient comes in contact with before using a new medication. In addition, community-based pharmacists are easily accessible to patients. Therefore, pharmacists are in a unique position to optimize patient outcomes by identifying, resolving, and preventing medication therapy problems.

Medication therapy problems include improper drug selection, subtherapeutic dosage, overdosage, adverse drug reaction, drug interaction, failure to receive the drug, and drug use without an indication.[3] Drug-related morbidity is costly and prevalent. In 2000, an estimated $177.4 billion was spent in the United States to manage direct costs associated with drug-related morbidity in the ambulatory setting.[4] Pharmacists are in a unique position to help identify, resolve, and prevent drug-related morbidity, thereby optimizing patient outcomes in pain management.

Federal and state regulations have catalyzed the expanding responsibilities of pharmacists in patient care. Pharmacists' legal responsibilities have been expanding since 1990, when most states implemented a federal standard contained in the Omnibus Budget Reconciliation Act of 1990.[5] The Act mandated that pharmacists perform prospective drug use reviews as a condition of participation in the federally funded, but state-administered, Medicaid program. The Act required pharmacists to screen for drug duplication, drug-disease contraindications, drug-drug interactions, incorrect dosage or duration of drug treatment, allergic reactions, and clinical abuse/misuse.[5] Once a problem is identified, the pharmacist contacts the prescriber, initiating a collaborative relationship that will lead to a resolution of the problem.

Patient counseling is an expected service provided by pharmacists to ensure that patients have the information needed to use their medications properly.[6] More recently, with the passage of the Medicare Modernization Act of 2003 and the Medicare Prescription Medication Benefit (Part D), the federal government has begun to develop a plan that incorporates pharmacists, in collaboration with physicians, as being responsible for medication therapy management (MTM).[6] This team approach benefits patients that receive medications for the treatment of acute pain.

MTM has been defined by the pharmacy profession as "a distinct service or group of services that optimize therapeutic outcomes for individual patients that are independent of, but can occur in conjunction with, the provision of drug product."[7] With implementation of MTM, patient outcomes should include appropriate medication use, enhanced patient understanding of their medication regimens, increased patient compliance with prescribed medications, reduced risks for adverse events associated with medication administration, and reduced medical costs.[7] Some states are authorizing collaborative drug therapy management so that pharmacists can order and interpret laboratory tests, modify drug dosage, and initiate new drug therapy under a plan approved by the patient's physician.[8] To date, these types of collaborations are found mostly within hospitals and other institutions but are beginning to extend into community pharmacies and other independent practices.

Another unique role for the pharmacist is with medication reconciliation. Medication reconciliation is defined by the Joint Commission on Accreditation of Healthcare Organizations (JCAHO) as the "the process of comparing the medications that the patient/client/resident is currently taking with the medications that the organization is planning to provide."[9] The intent of medication reconciliation is to provide continuity of care for patients with regard to medication use as they transition in the health care system and to avoid errors in transcription, omission, duplication of therapy, drug-drug and drug-disease interactions. Cornish and colleagues reported that over 50% of patients admitted to a general internal medicine hospital floor had at least one unintended discrepancy between the physician's admission medication orders and a comprehensive medication history obtained through an interview.[10] This has tremendous implications for chronic pain patients treated with complicated regimens, including high-dose opioids, who will be having surgery and experiencing acute on chronic pain. Data from the USP MEDMARX program from September 2004 to July 2005, indicated that more than 2000 medication errors were attributed to failures of medication reconciliation; 22% occurred during hospital admission, 66% during transition/transfer to another level of care, and 12% at hospital discharge.[11]

The Joint Commission National Patient Safety Goal 8 requires that through a collaborative effort, the organization, the patient and/or family, the patient's primary physician, and outpatient pharmacy develop a complete list of medications that the patient is currently taking on admission to the organization.[9] The list must include over-the-counter and alternative therapies as well as prescription medications. The medications must then be compared to the medications ordered at admission and any differences or potential problems, such as omissions, dose changes, duplication of therapy, or drug interactions, must be reconciled. On discharge or transfer to another health care provider, the list is to be given to the patient and to the next care provider. This JCAHO requirement is not intended just for inpatients. Medication reconciliation should occur any time the patient enters a health care organization where medications will be administered. The standard does not specify who must perform the reconciliation or specify any particular documentation. However, a formal and systematic approach to reconciling a patient's medications across the continuum of care with multidisciplinary input from key organizational departments/services is imperative.[11] Pharmacists are critical to establishing an effective medication reconciliation program. They can ensure that medications used for the treatment of pain are continued or converted to an appropriate alternative when transitioning from one organization to another. If a pharmacist notes that a patient is on a long-acting opioid at home and is admitted for surgery, ensuring that the opioid dose is considered in the postoperative pain regimen is crucial. The pharmacist can assist the surgeon with appropriate conversions to intravenous opioids during the immediate postoperative period and then again when the patient is tolerating oral medications.

Pharmacists play an important role in improving the management of acute pain by ensuring that analgesic drug therapies are reconciled, prescribed, dispensed, and administered properly. The need to assess and treat pain appropriately has evolved into the fifth vital sign; that is, pain assessment is documented at a minimum of every eight hours when other vital signs are taken. JCAHO requires organizations to recognize patients' rights to appropriate assessment and management of pain.[12] Healthcare providers must assess the existence, nature, and intensity of pain in all patients and record the results in a way that facilitates regular reassessment and follow-up. In addition, JCAHO requires policies and procedures that support appropriate ordering of pain medications. Patient needs must also be addressed by providing education for patients and families about effective pain management, both in the hospital setting and on discharge. Opportunities for pharmacists to improve pain management may begin with efficient dispensing but must also include becoming a team member in managing the overall care for the patient with pain. Empirical evidence supports this type of collaboration as an effective means to improve therapeutic outcomes, reduce health care costs, and relieve patient suffering.[8]

PAIN MANAGEMENT EDUCATION FOR PHARMACISTS

The topic of pain management is not adequately presented and developed in the curricula of many United States schools of pharmacy. Although pain management is included in some format, it is usually covered in a fragmented way, usually as part of presentations on diseases with pain as a prominent feature, such as cancer.[13] Some schools have specific courses in pain management, but these are usually elective courses, taken by a small percentage of the student body. In addition, instruction about the diagnosis of pain, patient assessment, and physical examination is minimal.[13] Therefore, clinical training of pharmacists in the field of pain management, as with other professionals, needs to be further developed and refined for pharmacists to be effective members of a pain service.

JCAHO pain management standards require education about pain management for all relevant clinical staff, including physicians, nurses, and pharmacists. Educational and competency based programs will ensure that pharmacists become competent in pain management. A program should be available to evaluate the pharmacist's communication skills in effectively talking to patients regarding pain management. In addition, pharmacists must have a basic knowledge of various analgesic medications and their place in pain management. It is imperative that pharmacists understand the differences between addiction, pseudoaddiction, dependence, and tolerance and are able to address patient concerns regarding these topics. This will help to alleviate misconceptions regarding the use of opioids for the management of pain. Pharmacists must also be familiar with the equianalgesic dosing tables and competent in providing guidance to other health care professionals converting patients from one opioid analgesic to another. Although there are clinical pharmacy pain specialists, all pharmacists should be minimally competent in providing effective pain management for their patients.

MANAGEMENT OF SCHEDULE II NARCOTICS

Controlled substances are placed in one of five schedules. Schedule I is for those abusable drugs that are deemed to have no medical utility (eg, heroin). Schedules II through V are for drugs with abuse potential that currently have acceptable medical uses. The lower the schedule number (eg, Schedule II), the higher the risk of abuse. The federal Controlled Substances Act requires all registrants, including pharmacists, to keep complete, accurate, and detailed records of the acquisition and disposition of all controlled substances.[14] These records are to be maintained in a readily retrievable manner so that the inspectors of the Drug Enforcement Administration (DEA) can easily review them. When dispensing controlled substances, pharmacists have a legal responsibility to verify that all prescriptions for controlled substances have been written by a prescriber in the usual course of that prescriber's legitimate medical practice.[14] Violations of the Controlled Substances Act and DEA regulations can subject pharmacists to a variety of sanctions, ranging from an administrative letter of admonition to licensure suspension to criminal prosecution.[14]

The collaborative effort between physicians and pharmacists could have a significant affect on the treatment of patients who are prescribed controlled substances such as opioids for acute pain management. Pharmacists are acutely aware of their "gatekeeper" or "drug police" positions at the end of the drug distribution chain and of their responsibility not to provide drug diverters or addicts with easy access to controlled substances.[8] However, pharmacists are equally mindful of their responsibilities for the appropriate medication therapy management of their patients. Pharmacists strive to fill valid prescriptions and to refuse purported prescriptions, but discerning between the two is not an easy task and some error may occur.

Traditionally, physicians and pharmacists have had a confrontational relationship regarding scheduled narcotics because of stringent regulatory controls over these substances and pharmacists' sometimes unjustified fear of disciplinary action.[8] Even today, some pharmacies will not stock particular medications that have high "street" value. Other pharmacists question the overuse of opioids by the physicians who prescribe them. Just as physicians continue their reluctance to prescribe adequate medications for pain, pharmacists are similarly reluctant to dispense high doses of opioid medications.

Accountability for narcotics within a hospital system must be a coordinated effort among pharmacists, nurses, and physicians. Pharmacists are responsible for ordering and maintaining an adequate central stock of controlled substances within the hospital. When controlled substances are distributed to the patient care areas, nursing personnel are then accountable for conducting controlled substance inventory review and reconciliation every shift, ensuring proper documentation for patient administration and narcotic wastage. When controlled substances are distributed directly to anesthesiology personnel, they are then accountable for the controlled substances. The pharmacy department is ultimately responsible for reviewing nursing and anesthesiology records for accuracy and potential diversion issues.

Replacing this relationship of confrontation with a collaborative agreement would place the responsibility for patient outcomes in the hands of both physician and pharmacist.[8] Together they would determine the appropriate pain management therapy for each patient, based on objective clinical practice guidelines. This will not only assure that patients get the most appropriate medication therapy management but also provide an avenue through which physicians and pharmacists can manage the risk of regulatory scrutiny.[8]

DRUG FORMULARY MANAGEMENT AND POLICY DEVELOPMENT

Drug Formularies

Drug formularies are in place at the hospital, community, and national levels.[15] At the hospital level, the formulary is a list of available drugs meeting the medication needs of the patients serviced at the hospital. This formulary will provide a list of drugs that are considered by the P&T Committee to be the most useful in patient care and provides guidelines for drug use.[16] When formularies were first created in hospitals, they were lengthy lists of all the drugs available for use in a hospital. Modern formularies not only include this list but also reflect organizational policies and procedures for rationale drug use and cost considerations.[17] Hospital formularies may be open with unrestricted prescribing, closed with prescribing strictly controlled and therapeutic substitution as a standard of practice, or mixed.[17] Many hospitals limit therapeutic classes of drugs to specific agents. The decision for selecting one or two drugs in a therapeutic class is usually based on clinical efficacy, safety, and cost factors.[15]

At the community level, general practitioners and pharmacists have implemented formulary programs as a mechanism to ensure the use of cost-effective therapy.[15] In addition, in the community, insurance companies have developed formularies, usually with tier levels. A level one medication will have the lowest copay. The insurance copays increase as the tier level increases. At the national level in many European countries, the formulary is defined by the health authority as the list of drugs that are reimbursable by the national health program.[15] Drugs not included on the list must be paid for by the patient. In addition, certain drugs may be restricted to patients with certain documented pathologies where the additional benefit justifies the additional cost.

In the hospital setting, opportunities for pharmacists to improve MTM in managing pain begin with the availability and dispensing of pain medications. Efficacy and safety are among the primary concerns of the Food and Drug Administration (FDA) before a new drug or device is approved. When a new drug is commercially available, it is the responsibility of the P&T Committee to evaluate the new drug entity based not only on safety and efficacy but also on cost and outcome considerations.[17] The pharmacist's role in evaluating new drugs and drug delivery technologies for formulary addition may involve searching the published literature for clinical trial reports, obtaining additional information from the manufacturer, critically reviewing the data, and preparing drug monographs and reports to the P&T Committee. Pharmacists should be members of the P&T Committee and Institution Review Board (IRB). As a member of the IRB, pharmacists will have the opportunity to become familiar with new drugs before their approval by the FDA.

When reviewing a medication for hospital formulary addition, the P&T Committee should not only review its safety and efficacy based on the results of randomized, controlled trials but also review the pharmacoeconomics (ie, the scientific discipline that compares the value of one pharmaceutical drug or drug therapy to another), pharmacoepidemiology (ie, the use and effects of drugs in large numbers of patients), and outcomes from using the drug. Outcomes should include side effects and therapeutic failure as well as desired therapeutic endpoints. The

Table 38.1: Functions and Scope of the P&T Committee[16,18]

Developing, maintaining, and approving a formulary of medications accepted for use in the organization.

Establishing programs and procedures that help ensure effective, safe, and cost-effective drug therapy; if a medication is only indicated for epidural administration, it should be restricted to those practitioners competent in spinal drug administration, primarily anesthesiologists

Establishing or planning educational programs on medication use for all professional staff

Initiating or directing medication use evaluations to optimize medication use

Participating in quality improvement activities to minimize medication errors

drug under consideration is compared to other drugs in the same class or for the same indication. Comparable efficacy and adverse event profiles must be critically evaluated, as well as reviewing the cost. The cost of the medication should be assessed using a pharmacoeconomic analysis, taking into account not only the price of the drug but also the impact of therapy on other institutional factors such as laboratory testing, staff time management, impact on length of hospital stay, and patient satisfaction and quality of life. For example, the use of a new drug may reduce the adverse effects, nursing staff time, patient recovery time, and the duration of hospitalization compared with other drugs, resulting in cost savings that more than offset the higher cost of the new drug. Pharmacists also have knowledge of special drug acquisition costs and pricing programs. These incentives should be a consideration in the pharmacoeconomic analyses. The functions and scope of the P&T Committee are listed on Table 38.1.[16,18]

Therapeutic Substitution Programs

Developing therapeutic substitution programs and educating prescribers on the use of these policies and protocols can yield substantial cost savings.[19] When two or more drugs have been proven to be therapeutically equivalent, many hospitals and some insurance formularies apply a policy of automatic drug exchange or interchange. In addition, a therapeutic interchange program can be implemented to convert patients receiving intravenous therapy to oral therapy as soon as the patient is able to tolerate oral intake. The decision to have a therapeutic interchange is determined by both the medical and pharmacy staff and approved by the Medical Executive Committee. Generally, hospital pharmacists automatically implement the drug interchange so that the transition to the selected product occurs quickly. This may impact acute pain management if an institution has a therapeutic interchange program for opioids, nonsteroidal anti-inflammatory drugs (NSAIDs), or local anesthetics. Physicians and pharmacists must work together closely to ensure that a therapeutic interchange program will not adversely impact patients that may require a specific drug within a certain drug class. There can be exceptions to therapeutic interchange if a patient does not tolerate the therapeutically equivalent interchange drug.

Medication Guidelines

Development of medication guidelines offers health care providers valuable information on the indications, dosing, monitoring, and equivalencies within therapeutic categories. The development and implementation of pain management guidelines offers prescribers a reference of evidence-based treatment for pain. The guidelines should include important phone numbers for consultations, available formulary medications, including the doses and important prescribing information in all therapeutic classes used to treat pain, medications used to treat side effects, and equivalency tables for converting patients from one opioid to another. These guidelines are approved by the P&T Committee and an educational program is designed to train prescribers on its appropriate use.

INFUSION DEVICE SELECTION CONSIDERATIONS

Although the P&T Committee is responsible for the maintenance of medication policies, the New Products Committee is responsible for evaluating and introducing new devices into the hospital setting. This is generally a multidisciplinary committee consisting of representatives from various departments within the hospital. Medical, nursing, pharmacy, biomedical, and hospital administration staff may all be represented. Any new device is presented to the committee and evaluated similarly to a new medication. Efficient use of technology to ensure that medications are readily available for the patient is imperative. The use of patient-controlled analgesia (PCA), epidural, and local anesthetic delivery devices along with medication storage units should be evaluated. Device selection should be based on safety, accuracy, reliability, ease of use, cost, and compatibility with selected drugs.[20] Appropriate staff education must be provided after a decision is made to purchase or lease new devices.

Many devices are available with differing mechanisms for drug delivery, including syringe pumps, peristaltic devices, and elastomeric reservoir pumps. Syringe pumps are used to deliver the contents of the syringe over a given period of time or on patient activation.[20] The contents of the syringe may be delivered over several hours or several days. This is the most common type pump for PCA use in the treatment of acute postoperative pain. There are commercially available morphine (1 mg/mL) and meperidine (10 mg/mL) prefilled syringes in standard concentrations for use in these types of PCA pumps. When other opioids such as hydromorphone and fentanyl, or when variant concentrations of morphine are used, the pharmacist is responsible for preparing these syringes.

Peristaltic devices deliver drug from a flexible reservoir via administration tubing that is mechanically squeezed to allow the delivery of the drug.[20] These pumps are traditionally used for the administration of IV fluids but have been modified for the administration of epidural infusions. Peristaltic devices can accommodate larger volume infusion solutions because they use a flexible reservoir bag.[21] The capacity of these bags range from 50 mL to 1000 mL. Flow rate capabilities range from 0.1 to 999 mL/hr.

Elastomeric reservoir pumps are usually disposable devices that consist of an inflatable balloon reservoir surrounded by a protective shell with a medication entry port and permanently attached tubing. After the balloon is filled with medication and

Table 38.2: Considerations for Selecting Infusion Devices

Patient population using the device

The maximum reservoir volume

The range of administration rates

Ability to lock a reservoir if the medication contained in the device is a controlled substance

Design of occlusion and end-of-infusion alarms

Cost of disposables

Cost of the pump (renting, leasing, buying)

the tubing is primed, pressure created by the inflated balloon forces the medication through the tubing and into the patient.[22] The flow rate is controlled either by using calibrated lengths of small-bore tubing or with a flow-restricting device located near the end of the tubing.[22] Elastomeric devices are available in different flow rates (50 to 250 mL/hr) and volume capacities (50 to 500 mL). Several devices are available for instillation of local anesthetic into surgical incisions.

When evaluating or selecting any infusion device, many variable issues should be considered. As described previously, safety, accuracy, reliability, and ease of use are imperative. Other important considerations are included in Table 38.2.

Many institutions are evaluating "smart" pumps, infusion devices with drug libraries and decision support.[23] Smart pump technology enables health care providers to set limits in the pumps to help eliminate over- and underadministration of medications. Pharmacists should help to determine the minimum and maximum rates and drug concentrations to be programmed into smart pumps. Pharmacists are a valuable resource for determining stability and proper container size for various pumps. Education programs must be designed to ensure that new technologies are not utilized unless proper education and training of staff is provided. Pharmacists who become knowledgeable about these technologies should be involved in the development of educational programs and policies and procedures (see also Chapter 19, *Patient-Controlled Analgesia Devices and Analgesic Infusion Pumps*).

ROUTE OF ADMINISTRATION CONSIDERATIONS FOR THE TREATMENT OF PAIN

Traditionally, the treatment for acute pain has been intermittent oral, intramuscular (IM), or intravenous (IV) injections. PCA and the use of epidural injections of opioids are improvements in pain management modalities, yet all have limitations. Intermittent analgesia is frequently associated with "analgesic gaps," that is, time periods when the patient's pain level is higher than desired.[24] In addition, IM injections may be painful and provide variable absorption of the medication. Oral medications may be valuable as transition agents but may not be usable in the postoperative setting if a patient cannot take anything by mouth. Because of these limitations, nursing administered intermittent administration of pain medications is usually not recommended.

Intravenous PCA offers convenience by eliminating the need for intermittent dosing by nursing personnel and gives patients some autonomy in the treatment of their pain.[25] Patients deter-

mine when they are ready for a dose, press the PCA administration button to receive the dose, eliminating the waiting time for a nurse to assess the patient, and then obtain and administer the opioid. Different PCA pumps have different configurations. Usually there is a syringe or cartridge containing the analgesic, locked into the PCA pump, that is then programmed to allow administration of a small bolus dose at specified time intervals, with or without an accompanying continuous IV infusion.[26]

When the technique of epidural and intrathecal administration was developed, it was standard of practice to administer these agents as a single bolus or multiple as-needed bolus injections.[21] However, this technique is usually not recommended because it may result in periods of inadequate pain control and has been associated with a higher frequency of side effects resulting from temporary peak levels of drug.[27] Current methods now allow for initial bolus doses followed by a continuous infusion with or without patient-controlled epidural analgesia (PCEA).[28] Like PCA, PCEA allows for infusion of a fixed dose of analgesic with incremental patient demand doses during periods of inadequate pain relief. This method allows for individualization of treatment, increased patient satisfaction, and convenience.[20,28]

Regional anesthetic techniques are also available and widely used for the management of acute postoperative pain. These techniques involve either intermittent or continuous infusions of local anesthetics through an epidural-like catheter directly into nerve sheaths or incision sites.[27,29–31] There is evidence that this method of pain control may be effective in inhibition of the sensitization phenomena associated with postinjury hyperalgesia.[27]

A mechanism must be designed to identify patients receiving local anesthetics epidurally or into incisional wounds. Traditionally, anesthesiologists insert and manage epidural infusions while surgeons insert peripheral catheter devices that infuse local anesthetic directly into the surgical wound site. If local anesthetics are used in both peripheral and epidural sites, caution is warranted because of the potential risk for toxicity with dual administration sites. Pharmacists should be aware of all local anesthetics administered to patients and report any duplication of therapy to both prescribing physicians. Nurses, physicians, and pharmacists should be aware of all pain modalities for any given patient. Methods must be in place to document and identify patients that have received intraspinal analgesics, patients with a continuous infusion through an epidural catheter, and patients with surgical incision site infusions of local anesthetic.

INTRASPINAL SOLUTION PREPARATION, STABILITY, AND STERILITY

Pharmacists must be familiar with the preparation, dosing, and administration techniques for all routes of pain medication administration. Any drug injected or infused into the epidural or intrathecal space must be free of neurotoxic preservatives.[28,32] Injectable drugs that contain preservatives such as methylparaben, benzyl alcohol, methylhydroxybenzoate, propylhydroxybenzoate, phenol, and formaldehyde must be avoided.

Although infection of the epidural or intrathecal space is rare, it can have a high morbidity or be fatal. Preparation of all intraspinal solutions should be performed with strict adherence to sterile aseptic technique. On January 1, 2004, chapter 797 of the USP became the nation's first enforceable standard for the compounding of sterile preparations.[1] This standard was developed in response to a growing demand to hold pharmacies accountable for preparations that are compounded outside of a controlled environment.[33] The chapter provides procedures and requirements for compounding sterile preparations. Sterile compounding requires a clean facility, specific training and testing of personnel in principles and practices of aseptic manipulations, air quality evaluation, and knowledge of sterilization and solution stability principles and practices.[1] The FDA considers chapter 797 an enforceable standard and JCAHO is using it as a standard when surveying hospitals.[33] Therefore, whenever possible, the preparation of any solution being administered in the epidural or intrathecal space should be prepared within the pharmacy, in accordance to USP 797 guidelines. Most pharmacies prepare sterile products in a clean room, within a laminar flow hood.

The stability of morphine, fentanyl, sufentanil, and hydromorphone alone or in combination with bupivacaine, ropivacaine, clonidine, or epinephrine in a variety of syringes and reservoirs has been studied.[34–38] All solutions studied were stable for up to 30 days. However, the risk of microbial contamination in preservative-free solutions is still considered problematic.[21] Guidelines and recommendations from the Centers for Disease Control and Prevention (CDC) and the American Society of Health-System Pharmacists recommend that preservative-free infusion solutions be completely used or discarded within 24 hours of preparation when not refrigerated.[28,39–40] These guidelines also recommend that preservative-free mixed solutions should be stored under refrigeration for no more than seven days.[39–40] After the solution is dispensed for patient use, a 24-hour expiration date must be applied to the label.[39–40]

DRUG SELECTION, DOSAGE, AND ADVERSE EFFECTS

Nonopioid Analgesics

Nonopioids such as aspirin, acetaminophen, and NSAIDs are traditionally used for the treatment of mild to moderate pain and may be combined with opioid analgesics for the treatment of moderate to severe pain. Pharmacists should evaluate postop order sets and ensure that at least one nonopioid analgesic is available to the patient for pain management. In addition, pharmacists should evaluate the number of medications ordered that contain acetaminophen. Opioid combination formulations may contain 500 mg of acetaminophen per tablet. If a patient is receiving two tablets every four hours, this will exceed the recommended maximum daily dosage of acetaminophen (4 grams). Patients may have acetaminophen ordered for elevated temperature. Additional acetaminophen doses may unintentionally be administered, exposing the patient to potential hepatotoxicity. For these reasons, it may be appropriate to prescribe opioids and acetaminophen as separate entities.

Although all NSAIDs have similar mechanisms of action and adverse effect profiles, they do differ in potency, time to onset of action, duration of action, and interpatient tolerance variations.[41] Pharmacists and physicians need to evaluate the efficacy, therapeutic end points, and side-effect profiles of various NSAIDs to determine which NSAIDs will be on the hospital formulary for the treatment of acute pain. Consideration for the inclusion of ketorolac on the formulary, the only injectable NSAID approved in the United States, will be impor-

Table 38.3: Equianalgesic Opioid Conversions Based on Injection Site[a]

Drug	Oral (mg)	Parenteral (mg)	Epidural (mg)	Intrathecal (mg)
Morphine	30	10	1	0.1
Hydromorphone	7.5	1.5	0.15	
Fentanyl		0.1	0.001	

[a] Adapted from Krames ES.[42] These equivalencies are not supported by large-scale, double blinded studies, and are meant as a reference for identifying appropriate conversions.

tant for patients unable to take oral medications. Pharmacists must ensure that ketorolac is ordered appropriately based on the patient's age, renal function, and history of gastrointestinal bleeding. In addition, ketorolac therapy is limited to five days.[26]

Opioids

Opioids are the cornerstone of treatment for moderate to severe acute pain. The choice and dosage for an opioid depends on the patient's pain severity, whether the patient is opioid naïve or tolerant, the route of administration, pharmacokinetics, patient preference, adverse effects, and cost.[26] The pharmacokinetics of the various opioids are important in designing the dosage and frequency of opioids. Pharmacists must assess postoperative pain order sets to ensure the proper dosing and dosing intervals are utilized.

Routes of administration for opioids include oral, sublingual, nasal, intramuscular, intravenous, transdermal, rectal, inhalation, and intraspinal. Depending on the route of administration, the dose of opioid will vary. Pharmacists must be familiar with dosing for all routes of administration. When an opioid is administered epidurally, there will be a maximum infusion rate secondary to the physical characteristics of the epidural space. Administration rates may vary from 4 to 18 mL/hr, and rates above 20 mL/hr are generally not indicated.[21] Administration via the intrathecal route is rarely indicated for acute pain and has even lower infusion rates. Understanding the difference in dosing depending on the route of administration is imperative. Individual hospitals should develop ranges for all medications that may be administered epidurally or intrathecally. Table 38.3 provides a guideline for equianalgesic opioid conversion for intravenous, epidural, and intrathecal routes.[42]

Pharmacists should also be involved in helping physicians select the most appropriate opioid for the treatment of acute pain. Historically, meperidine was commonly used for the treatment of acute pain. It remains one of the most frequently prescribed opioids for procedural sedation; however, its use should be limited for extended treatment of acute pain because of its neurotoxicity, short duration of action, and lower potency relative to morphine. Normeperidine, the major metabolite of meperidine, accumulates with repeated dosing and seizures have been observed even in patients with normal renal function.[43] The American Pain Society now recommends avoiding meperidine for the treatment of acute pain whenever possible.[44] Pharmacists can educate and recommend alternative opioids when meperidine has been included in postoperative order sets. When there is no alternative for meperidine, its use should be limited to 48 hours and no more than 600 mg may be administered per day.[44]

Propoxyphene is generally prescribed for mild to moderate pain. However, because of the risk for toxicity associated with the metabolite norpropoxyphene that may occur in patients with diminished renal function, repeated doses, and in the elderly, its use should be avoided.[45,46] Propoxyphene has no clinical advantage over nonopioid analgesics and has a higher incidence of adverse effects.[47] Again, pharmacists can educate and recommend alternatives to propoxyphene for the treatment of acute pain.

Codeine is generally considered an opioid for mild to moderate pain, with a higher incidence of significant adverse effects such as nausea and constipation compared to other opioids at equianalgesic doses.[44] In addition, codeine must be converted to morphine via the cytochrome P450 2D6 pathway to provide analgesia. A substantial percentage of Caucasians are poor metabolizers due to deficiencies in this isoenzyme.[48] These patients will not be able to convert the codeine to morphine and will therefore receive no analgesic benefit. If codeine is part of a postop order set, pharmacists should ensure that other opioids are ordered for those patients that do not obtain relief from codeine.

Methadone is a unique opioid option. Methadone is a mu-receptor agonist and an N-methyl-D-aspartate (NMDA) receptor antagonist. NMDA receptors can decrease mu-receptor's response to opioids. This added activity may be useful during opioid rotation or when treating known drug abusers for acute pain. Methadone's duration of analgesic action following a single dose is four to six hours.[49] However, because of its high volume of distribution, there can be a substantial increase in duration of action following chronic dosing.[49] Methadone has a long, unpredictable half-life and, with tissue accumulation, serious, life-threatening toxicity can occur. There is limited knowledge on titrating doses and equivalencies. Many equianalgesic tables use equivalencies based on single-dose studies. In reality, studies have indicated that methadone's potency increases in patients on higher doses of opioid.[50] Equianalgesic tables many times fail to consider these unique properties and dose conversion based on the listed ratio may result in a drastic overdose. It is recommended that conversion ratios be based on the total daily dose of morphine (or its equivalent) and adjustments in conversion ratios adjusted as opioid doses increase.[50] Pharmacists and physicians must be cautious when converting patients to methadone and appropriate monitoring is imperative.

Pharmacists play an important role in identifying drug allergies. Many patients state that they have an allergy to a particular opioid, yet genuine allergies to opioids are rare. In many cases, the patient reports an allergy because they experienced a side effect from the opioid. The diagnosis of an opioid allergy is further complicated because many opioids can cause histamine release, manifesting as a drug allergy. Therefore, it is important for the pharmacist to illicit the reaction a patient had with the implicated opioid and determine its significance. Identifying which opioid a patient has tolerated in the past often helps with prescribing opioids for the treatment of new acute pain syndrome.

Pharmacists also play a role in identifying potential adverse effects from opioids and ensuring orders have been placed and processed to help treat opioid-related side effects. Differences in side effects may be related to the opioid ordered, the surgical procedure, the type of anesthesia, and individual patient characteristics. The most frequently reported side effects from opioids are respiratory depression, sedation, nausea, vomiting, constipation, urinary retention, and itching.[48] Other adverse effects include confusion, hallucinations, nightmares, and dizziness. These adverse effects can have a negative impact on recuperation, participation in rehabilitation, and potentially prolong hospital stay. Factors such as age, extent of disease or surgery, concurrent administration of other drugs, prior opioid use, and route of administration can also increase the risk of opioid-related adverse effects.[46]

Respiratory depression is the most serious adverse effect of opioids. When it occurs, it is often in an opioid-naïve patient. The patient generally experiences sedation and mental clouding prior to developing the respiratory depression.[45,48] Patients at increased risk for respiratory depression include obese patients and patients with a history of sleep apnea or airway disease. These patients require additional monitoring that may include pulse oximetry, capnography, and more frequent assessment of sedation levels. This monitoring should be incorporated into all postop order sets. Treatment for respiratory depression may include an opioid antagonist such as naloxone. The pharmacist should ensure that the proper dose of naloxone is administered for the reversal of respiratory depression. The dose used for the treatment of opioid overdose (0.4 to 2 mg IV) is not appropriate for reversing opioid side effects. These doses will also reverse the analgesic effects of the opioid. Initiating administration with small doses of a diluted solution of naloxone (diluting 0.4 mg to a concentration of 0.04 mg/mL) and administering 20 mcg (0.5 mL) to 40 mcg (1 mL) every minute until the respiratory rate increases above 10 per minute is a more appropriate method to reverse respiratory depression. If naloxone doses need to be continued, a naloxone infusion may be started. Doses of 0.25 mcg/kg/hr have been effective in reducing opioid-related side effects while maintaining adequate analgesia.[51–52] This dose offers a starting point for reversal of side effects. The infusion rate may be increased if the patient's status warrants.

Opioid-induced gastrointestinal side effects such as nausea/vomiting and constipation are the most common and, from the patient's perspective, the most troubling postop adverse effect.[53] Switching opioids or route of administration may be beneficial, but most importantly, prevention and treatment should be part of an opioid order set. Transdermal scopolamine, metoclopramide, droperidol, phenothiazines, and serotonin type 3 receptor antagonists have all been used for treatment of nausea and vomiting. Regimens to treat opioid-induced constipation should include stimulant laxatives. Stool softeners and bulk laxatives offer minimal effects. Although not indicated for the management of opioid-induced constipation from short term use of opioids, two peripheral opioid antagonists, methylnaltrexone and alvimopan, have recently been approved by the FDA. In April 2008, methylnaltrexone was approved to help restore bowel function in patients with late-stage, advanced illness who are receiving opioids on a continuous basis for pain management.[54] In May 2008, alvimopan was approved to accelerate the restoration of normal bowel function in patients 18 years and older who have undergone partial large or small bowel resection surgery.[55] In addition, as part of alvimopan's approval under the FDA's new Risk Evaluation and Mitigation Strategy (REMS) rules, it may be given only in hospitalised patients at specially certified facilities.[56] More studies are needed before either agent may be used for the treatment of constipation from the short-term administration of opioids in the post-op setting.

Administering opioids for acute pain management is a balancing act. Patients should be provided with the best pain

Table 38.4: Frequency of Reported PCA Error Events from MAUDE Database[62]

Reported Error	Frequency	Possible Causes of Error
Device related	79.1%	Battery, display board, software failures
		Failure to deliver drug on demand
		Faulty alarm system
		Lack of free-flow
		Error code
		Defective patient on-demand device
Indeterminate events	12.5%	Excessive delivery of drug
		Underdelivery of drug
Possible operating errors	6.5%	Pump programming error (dose, concentration, rate)
		Failure to clamp-unclamp tubing
		Improperly loading syringe or cartridge
		Not responding to safety alarms
		Battery improperly inserted
		Pharmacy medication error
Possible adverse drug reaction	1.2%	Nausea/vomiting
		Sedation
		Respiratory depression
		Pruritus
		Urinary retention
Possible patient-related error	0.6%	Misunderstanding instructions for PCA use

Table 38.5: Frequency and Types of PCA Errors Reported to MEDMARX and USP MER Programs

Type of Error	Percentage Frequency (%)
Improper dose/quantity	38.9
Unauthorized drug	18.4
Omission error	17.6
Prescribing error	9.2
Wrong administration technique	4.8
Extra dose	4.7
Wrong drug preparation	4.2
Wrong time	3.3
Wrong patient	2.5
Wrong dosage form	1.6
Wrong route	0.6
Deteriorated/expired product	0.3

management available, with minimal side effects. Treatment for potential side effects from pain medications should be included in order sets.

ROLE OF THE PHARMACIST IN REDUCING PAIN MEDICATION ERRORS

Medication error prevention is the responsibility of all healthcare providers. However, pharmacists must understand the unique role they have in preventing, detecting, and reporting errors that occur during the medication use process. This should include a systems approach to design an optimum drug delivery system and education of patients and other healthcare providers to ensure a better understanding and compliance with prescription and over-the-counter medications.[57]

When evaluating medication error rates, it is difficult to analyze the literature because different end points are used in various studies. However, the Institute for Safe Medication Practices (ISMP) identified morphine as one of six medications on the very first List of High-Alert Medications published in 1989. In the most current publication of the ISMP's List of High-Alert Medications,[59] opiates remain as a class of drugs that bear a heightened risk of causing significant patient harm when they are used in error. One major error that is reported frequently is inadvertent substitution of hydromorphone for morphine.[60] Many times the error is related to the misconception that hydro-

morphone is the generic name for morphine. A misunderstanding of equivalencies may lead to administration of high hydromorphone doses (1.5 mg of hydromorphone intravenously is approximately equal to 10 mg of morphine).[49] This inadvertent substitution has resulted in patient death.[61] Several steps may be taken within an institution to help prevent this error. When possible, use tall man lettering to emphasize the *Hydro* portion of *Hydromorphone* on pharmacy labels, auxiliary labels, medication administration records, and drug listings on computer screens or automated dispensing cabinets.[61] When computer physician (or prescriber) order entry (CPOE) is available, an information screen can be designed describing the equivalency of hydromorphone to morphine.

In conjunction with opiate medication errors, device errors can also be dangerous and potentially fatal. The Manufacturer and User Facility Device Experience (MAUDE) maintains a database of reports of adverse outcomes for medication devices that is publicly available.[62] PCA-related adverse events were analyzed from the MAUDE database from January 1, 2002, to December 31, 2003. Table 38.4 describes the frequency of reported PCA error events and the possible causes. Adverse events included respiratory depression/arrest (9%), excessive sedation (3%), death (19%), and naloxone administration (58%).[62] PCA errors are also reported to the USP-ISMP Medication Errors Reporting (MER) Program and MEDMARX, a national, Internet-accessible database that hospitals and health care systems use to track and trend adverse drug reactions and medication errors. Five thousand one hundred and ten PCA errors were reported and analyzed from September 1, 1998, through August 31, 2003.[63] Table 38.5 lists the frequency and types of PCA errors reported to MEDMARX and USP MER programs.

ISMP had identified how PCA errors occur (Table 38.6). To help prevent PCA errors, ISMP recommends performing a failure mode and effects analysis (FMEA). FMEA is a procedure for analysis of potential failure modes within a system for the classification by severity or determination of the failure's effect on the system.[65] When using FMEA, consider whether the PCA pump can be programmed easily to deliver desired concentrations, if the pump operation intuitive for the clinician and patient, and if the information displayed appears in logical sequence.[64] Mechanisms to help prevent PCA errors are included on Table 38.7.[66]

Table 38.6: How PCA Errors Occur[64]

Error	Special Considerations
PCA by proxy	Family members and health professionals may not realize the implications of activating the PCA button
	This may result in oversedation, respiratory depression, and death
Improper patient selection	Elderly patients should be evaluated carefully prior to initiating PCA
	Patient must be cognitive and psychologically competent to manage their own pain.
Inadequate monitoring	Ensure guidelines are established for routine monitoring, especially for the first 24 hours and at night.
	Consider pulse oximetry or capnography monitoring
Inadequate patient education	Ensure patient is educated prior to surgery
	Ensure patient is able to identify and utilize the PCA button
Drug product mix-ups	Separate Hydromorphone from morphine
	Separate syringes with standard concentrations of opioid from special concentrations
Practice-related problems and inadequate staff training	Misprogramming of PCA pump
	Incorrect transcription of prescriptions
	Calculation errors
Device design flaws	Default opioid concentrations
	Use of mL versus mg
	Pumps that do not require users to review all settings prior to initiation
	Activation button may look like the nurse call bell
	Patient does not know if they received a dose when they push the button
Prescription errors	Opioid conversion errors
	Prescribed inappropriate opioid
	Dosing errors

Table 38.7: Mechanisms to Help Prevent PCA Medication Errors

Require health care provides to undergo competency testing for prescribing and programming PCA pumps

Establish one standard concentration for each opioid used in PCA

Design standard order sets that include:

    Standard concentrations of opioids

    Patient monitoring

        Frequent monitoring of respiratory rate and sedation level

        If patient is at risk for respiratory depression (eg, history of sleep apnea), provide more intense monitoring

    Treatment for side effects or adverse events

Avoid ordering doses in mL; dose opioids in mcg or mg

Establish patient selection criteria

Ensure patient education prior to surgery and patient competence to utilize PCA postoperatively

Maintain standard PCA syringes in one narcotic storage area. Separate morphine from Hydromorphone

Custom PCA concentrations should be stocked away from the standard concentrations

Require two health care providers to double check right patient, order, drug concentration, and pump settings

Table 38.8: Strategies for Preventing Epidural and Intrathecal Infusion Errors

Pump considerations

    Consider using distinctly different pumps for epidural infusions

    Use "smart pumps" that incorporate drug protocol and maximum dosing limits

    Add a large visible label marked "epidural pump" on the pump infusing the epidural solution

    Avoid the use of dual chamber pumps for both IV and epidural infusions

    Consider placing IV pump and epidural pumps on opposite sides of the patient bed

    If possible, discontinue the IV fluid and insert a heparin lock

Epidural tubing

    Consider infusion tube distinction by either using colored tubing or labeling the tubing with brightly colored "for epidural use only" stickers. Stickers should be placed at distal connecting sites

    Epidural tubing should have no injection ports

Limit the volume of the epidural solution (prepare 100- to 200-mL bags)

Epidural medication errors have frequently been reported in the literature and to ISMP.[28,67,68] In fact, ISMP added epidural and intrathecal medications to the 2007 LT High-Alert Drug List after practitioners were surveyed and requested the addition.[69] Drugs including potassium chloride, theophylline, and antibiotics intended for intravenous administration have been accidentally administered into the epidural or intrathecal space.[28,67,68] Several reports have described infusion rate issues when epidural pumps are identical to IV infusion pumps.[68] Nurses mistakenly set the rate of the epidural pump to the rate that is supposed to be on the IV infusion pump. To help prevent epidural or intrathecal medication errors, Table 38.8 describes strategies for prevention.

Pharmacists should identify opportunities to promote proved strategies to minimize medication errors. Working with physicians and nurses to promote efficient drug ordering, distribution, and administration will help to prevent medication errors.

DEVELOPMENT OF STANDARD ORDER SETS

Pharmacists and the P&T committee are often involved in the development and review of physician order sets, whether for traditional paper charts or CPOE. Order sets should be carefully evaluated for appropriate selection of medications, accuracy of

Table 38.9: Important Elements for Epidural Analgesia Orders Sets[21]

Patient name, birth date, medical record number, room number

Drug(s), concentration(s)

Instructions for administration

   Bolus doses

      Drug with dose to be bolused

      Interval between bolus injections

   Infusions

      Loading dose

      Infusion rate

Treatment for breakthrough pain

Maintenance of intravenous site for administration of fluids and for access for emergency administration of reversal medications if necessary

Order to prevent other services from prescribing CNS depressants

Monitoring instructions for opioid and/or local anesthetic administration.

Specific observations that should be immediately communicated to the anesthesiologist (respiratory rate less than 6, systolic blood pressure less than 90 mm Hg)

Instructions and treatment options for side effects

Contact information if problems occur

Date, time, and physician signature

Table 38.10: Equianalgesic PCA Opioids Used at Thomas Jefferson University Hospital

Opioid	Concentration
Morphine	1 mg/mL
Fentanyl	0.01 mg/mL (10 mcg/mL)
Hydromorphone	0.2 mg/mL
Meperidine (avoid using)	10 mg/mL

Epidural Infusions

The final volume and concentrations for epidural solutions must be considered when standardizing epidural infusions. Decisions regarding standard epidural preparations must take into consideration safety, cost, time for preparation, narcotic accountability, and the reservoir capacity in the infusion device. When possible, using whole rather than partial ampules or vials and using available package sizes of the drugs used in preparation of epidural infusions help to minimize waste.[21] This process is also beneficial in helping to keep narcotic inventories accurate and minimizing the need to document of waste.

When establishing standard epidural solutions, physician preference and stability considerations should be assessed. With adjustments in rate, the majority of patients may be prescribed a standard solution. In patients with a history of opioid use or in patients not receiving adequate analgesia from a standard epidural, a specialized solution may need to be prepared. The anesthesiologist should communicate with the pharmacist regarding the deviation from standard protocol. Table 38.9 provides important elements for epidural analgesia order sets.[21]

PCA Orders

Standardization of PCA orders is imperative to help prevent medication errors. Most institutions will use a standard incremental PCA dose of 1 mg of morphine sulfate every six to eight minutes.[26] Examples of equianalgesic opioid concentrations for PCA syringes that were developed at Thomas Jefferson University Hospital are listed in Table 38.10. An optional nursing bolus or loading dose equal to twice the incremental dose may be administered for breakthrough pain. Another feature of PCA pumps is the "lockout" or maximum dose that may be administered over a specified period of time. The lockout period may be a design feature within the device or may be programmed. A continuous or basal infusion may also be programmed into the PCA pump for patients with higher opioid requirements, particularly the opioid-tolerant patient. A basal or continuous infusion is not recommended for opioid-naive patients because of an increased incidence of respiratory depression. When designing an order entry form or computer program, all of the above criteria must be included. In addition, appropriate patient monitoring and treatment options for side effects such as respiratory depression, itching, and gastrointestinal disturbances must part of the order set. Table 38.11 lists important elements for PCA order sets.[21] If a patient has higher opioid requirements and a higher concentration of opioid is required in the PCA syringe, a nonstandard PCA syringe will be compounded. This syringe will need to be stored in a different location from the standard concentration

dosing, and appropriate patient monitoring based on medications ordered. For pain management, different classes of pain medications should be available to treat pain. Acetaminophen or an NSAID may be used for mild pain. An oral combination product with hydrocodone or oxycodone may be used for moderate pain and injectable opioids may be used for severe pain. If epidural analgesia is employed, the anesthesiologists monitoring the effectiveness of this modality should also be responsible for ordering breakthrough pain medications. Pain assessment and reassessment of the adequacy of the pain medication should be evaluated on a regular basis. Adjustments should be made to drug regimens when adequate pain relief is not obtained.

In addition to the appropriate pain medications, order sets should also include medications to treat the potential adverse effects attributed to these medications. There are several classes of drugs that may be chosen to treat nausea and vomiting, constipation, respiratory depression, and pruritus caused by opioid administration. The age of the patient, patient history, and the adverse effects of these drugs should be taken into consideration. Naloxone orders should include the appropriate dose for reversing respiratory depression while maintaining analgesia, as described previously.

One of the recommendations from the ISMP to help prevent medication errors is to standardize concentrations of injectable medications.[66] Based on this recommendation, PCA syringes, opioid infusions, and epidural solutions should be prepared using standard concentrations. Pharmacists should be familiar with the standardized dosing ranges and carefully evaluate orders that deviate from the established ranges.

Table 38.11: Important Elements for PCA Order Sets[21]

Patient name, birth date, medical record number, room number

Drug(s), concentration(s)

Pump settings

    Incremental dose (PCA dose)

    Lockout interval (time between PCA doses)

    Total hourly limit

    Basal infusion (for opioid tolerant patients)

    Nursing bolus doses for breakthrough pain

Initial loading dose instructions

Maintenance of intravenous site either as heparin lock or for administration of fluids (access for emergency administration of reversal medications if necessary)

Order to prevent other services from prescribing CNS depressants

Monitoring instructions

Specific observations that should be immediately communicated to the anesthesiologist (respiratory rate less than 6, systolic blood pressure less than 90 mm Hg)

Instructions and treatment options for side effects

Contact information if problems occur

Date, time, and physician signature

---

syringes to avoid its inadvertent use in another patient, resulting in a potentially major medication error.

SUMMARY

The pharmacist is a valuable resource in the provision of appropriate pain management strategies. Pharmacists' responsibilities are expanding beyond the roles of compounding, filling, and dispensing prescriptions with accuracy and appropriateness, and pharmaceutical supply management. As a member of a medication management team, the pharmacist can assist in the appropriate treatment for patients with acute pain. Pharmacists can ensure proper preparation of sterile products, adhering to the USP 797 recommendations. Pharmacists can facilitate the identification of medication errors and adapt corrective measures to prevent future misadventures. Having the guidance of an experienced pharmacist as a member of a medication management team can ensure patients receive the most appropriate pain management.

REFERENCES

1. Pharmaceutical compounding-sterile preparations. In: United States Pharmacopeia, and National Formulary, (USP 31-NF 26), Suppl 2. Rockville MD: United States Pharmacopeial Convention; 2008;3700–3734.

2. Hepler CD, Grainger-Rousseau TJ. Pharmaceutical care versus traditional drug treatment: is there a difference? Drugs. 1995;49:1–10.

3. Strand LM, Cipolle RJ, Morley PC. Drug-related problems: their structure and function. DICP Ann Pharmacother. 1990;24:1093–1097.

4. Planas LG, Kimberlin CL, Segal R, et al. A pharmacist model of perceived responsibility for drug therapy outcomes. Soc Science Med. 2005;60:2393–2403.

5. Huang SW. The Omnibus Reconciliation Act of 1990: redefining pharmacists' legal responsibilities. Am J Law Med. 1998;24(4):417–442.

6. McGivney SM, Meyer SM, Duncan-Hewitt W, et al. Medication therapy management: its relationship to patient counseling, disease management, and pharmaceutical care. J Am Pharm Assoc. 2007;47(5):620–628.

7. American Pharmacists Association, National Association of Chain Drug Stores Foundation. Medication therapy management in community pharmacy practice: core elements of an MTM service. Version 1.0. J Am Pharm Assoc. 2005;45:573–579.

8. Brushwood DB. From confrontation to collaboration: collegial accountability and the expanding role of pharmacists in the management of chronic pain. J Law Med Ethics. 2002;29:69–93.

9. F. The Joint Commission. FAQs for the 2008 National Patient Safety goals (updated March 2008). Available at: http://www.jointcommission.org/NR/rdonlyres/F770FD7F-C0F2-4454-B4F8-C8D38D4559BB/0/2008_FAQs_NPSG_08.pdf. Accessed September 08, 2008.

10. Cornish PL, Knowles SR, Marchesano R, et al. Unintended medication discrepancies at the time of hospital admission. Arch Intern Med. 2005;165:424–429.

11. Santell JP. Reconciliation failures lead to medication errors. Jt Comm J Qual Patient Saf. 2006;32(4):225–229.

12. The Joint Commission. History tracking report: 2009 to 2008 requirements. Chapter: provision of care, treatment, and services. Available at: http://www.jointcommission.org/NR/rdonlyres/5DA65D95-B0E4-42E6-ACAF-F867A9A8CDDB/0/OBS_PC_09_to_08.pdf. Accessed September 08, 2008.

13. Singh RM, Wyant SL. Pain management content in curricula of US schools of pharmacy. J Am Pharm Assoc. 2003;43(1):34–40.

14. Branding FH. The impact of controlled substance federal regulations on the practice of pharmacy. J Pharm Prac. 1995;8:130–137.

15. Scroccaro G. Formulary management. Pharmacotherapy. 2000;20(10pt2):317S–321S.

16. American Society of Hospital Pharmacists. ASHP guidelines on formulary system management. Am J Hosp Pharm. 1992;49:648–652.

17. Schechter LN. Advances in postoperative pain management: the pharmacy perspective. Am J Health-Syst Pharm. 2004;61:S15–S21.

18. American Society of Hospital Pharmacists. ASHP statement on the pharmacy and therapeutics committee. Am J Hosp Pharm. 1992;49:2008–2009.

19. Schachtner JM, Guharoy R, Medicis JJ, et al. Prevalence and cost savings of therapeutic interchange among U.S. hospitals. Am J Health-Syst Pharm 2002;59:529–533.

20. Kwan JW. Use of infusion devices for epidural or intrathecal administration of spinal opioids. Am J Hosp Pharm. 1990;47:S18–S23.

21. Carfagno ML, Schechter LN. Regional anesthesia and acute pain management: a pharmacist's perspective. Techn Reg Anesth Pain Manag. 2002;6(2):77–86.

22. Schleis TG, Tice AD. Selecting infusion devices for use in ambulatory care. Am J of Health-Syst Pharm. 1996 53(8):868–877.

23. Rothschild JM, Keohane CA, Cook EF, et al. A controlled trial of smart infusion pumps to improve medication safety in critically ill patients. Crit Care Med 2005;33:533–540.

24. Carr DB, Reines HD, Schaffer J, et al. The impact of technology on the analgesic gap and quality of acute pain management. *Reg Anesth Pain Med* 2005;30:286–291.

25. Viscusi ER. Emerging treatment modalities: balancing efficacy and safety. *Am J Health-Syst Pharm.* 2007;64(suppl 4);S6–S11.

26. Strassels SA, McNicol E, Suleman R. Postoperative pain management: a practical review, part 1. *Am J Health-Syst Pharm.* 2005;62:1904–1916.

27. Holder KA, Dougherty TB, Porche VH, et al. Postoperative pain management. *Int Anesthesiol Clin.* 1998;36:71–86.

28. Littrell RA. Epidural analgesia. *Am J Hosp Pharm.* 1991;48:2460–2474.

29. Peng PWH, Chan VWS. Local and regional block in postoperative pain control. *Surg Clin North Am.* 1999;79:345–370.

30. Paut O, Sallabery M, Scheiber-Deturmeny E, et al. Continuous fascia iliaca compartment block in children: a prospective evaluation of plasma bupivacaine concentrations, pain scores, and side effects. *Anesth Analg.* 2001;92:1159–1163.

31. Zohar E, Fredman B, Phillipov A, et al. The analgesic efficacy of patient-controlled bupivacaine wound instillation after abdominal hysterectomy with bilateral salpingo-oophorectomy. *Anesth Analg.* 2001;93:482–487.

32. Shafer Al, Donnelly AJ. Management of postoperative pain by continuous epidural infusion of analgesics. *Clin Pharm.* 1991;10:745–764.

33. Candy TA, Schneider PJ, Pedersen CA. Impact of Unites States Pharmacopeia chapter 797: results of a national survey. *Am J Health-Syst Pharm.* 2006;63:1336–1343.

34. Tu YH, Stiles ML, Allen LV. Stability of fentanyl citrate and bupivacaine hydrochloride in portable pump reservoirs. *Am J Hosp Pharm.* 1990;47:2037–2040.

35. Oster Svedberg K, McKenzie J, Larrivee-Elkins C. Compatibility of ropivacaine with morphine, sufentanil, fentanyl, or clonidine. *J Clin Pharm Ther.* 2002;27(1):39–45.

36. Christen C. Johnson CE. Walters JR. Stability of bupivacaine hydrochloride and hydromorphone hydrochloride during simulated epidural coadministration. *A J Health-Syst Pharm.* 1996;53(2):170–173.

37. Johnson CE. Christen C. Perez MM. Ma M. Compatibility of bupivacaine hydrochloride and morphine sulfate. *Am J Health-Syst Pharm.* 1997;54(1):61–64.

38. Priston MJ, Hughes JM, Santillo M, Christie IW. Stability of an epidural analgesic admixture containing epinephrine, fentanyl, and bupivacaine. *Anaesthesia.* 2004;59:979–983.

39. Centers for Disease Control. Guideline for prevention of intravascular device-related infections. *Am J Infect Control.* 1996;24:262–293.

40. Anonymous. ASHP guidelines on quality assurance for pharmacy-prepared sterile products. American Society of Health System Pharmacists. *Am J Health-Syst Pharm.* 2000;57(12):1150–1169.

41. Moote C. Efficacy of nonsteroidal anti-inflammatory drugs in the management of postoperative pain. *Drugs.* 1992;44(suppl 5):14–30.

42. Krames ES. Practical issues when using neuraxial infusion. *Oncology.* 1999;13(suppl 2):37–44.

43. Latta KS, Ginsberg B, Barkin RL. Meperidine: a critical review. *Am J Ther.* 2002;9:53–68.

44. Ashburn MA, Lipman AG, Carr D, et al. *Principles of Analgesic Use in the Treatment of Acute Pain and Chronic Pain.* 5th ed. Glenview, IL: American Pain Society; 2003.

45. Inturrisi CE. Clinical pharmacology of opioids for pain. *Clin J Pain.* 2002;18 (suppl 4):S3–S13.

46. Strassels SA, McNicol E, Suleman R. Postoperative pain management: a practical review, part 2. *Am J Health-Syst Pharm.* 2005;62:2019–2025.

47. Carr DB, Jacox AK, Chapman CR, et al. Clinical practice guideline number 1: acute pain management: operative or medical procedures and trauma. Rockville, MD: Agency for Health Care Policy and Research, AHCPR publication no. 92-0032; 1992.

48. Gutstein HB, Akil H. Opioid analgesics. In: Brunton LL, Lazo JS, Parker KL, eds. *Goodman and Gilman's the Pharmacological Basis of Therapeutics.* 11th ed. New York, NY: McGraw-Hill; 2007;569–619.

49. Anderson R, Saiers JH, Abram S, et al. Accuracy in equianalgesic dosing: conversion dilemmas. *J Pain Sympt Manage.* 2001;21:397–406.

50. Ripamonti C, Grof L, Brunelli C, et al. Switching from morphine to oral methadone in treating cancer pain: what is the equianalgesic dose ratio? *J Clin Oncol.* 1998;16:3216–3221.

51. Gan TJ, Ginsberg b, Glass PS, et al. Opioid-sparing effects of a low-dose infusion of naloxone in patient-administered morphine sulfate. *Anesthesiology.* 1997;87(5):1075–1081.

52. Maxwell LG, Kaufmann SC, Bitzer S, et al. The effects of a small-dose naloxone infusion on opioid-induced side effects and analgesia in children and adolescents treated with intravenous patient-controlled analgesia: a double-blind, prospective, randomized, controlled study. *Anesth Analg.* 2005:100(4):953–958.

53. Macario A, Weinger M, Carney S, et al. Which clinical anesthesia outcomes are important to avoid? The perspective of patients. *Anesth Analg.* 1999;89:652–658.

54. U.S. Food and Drug Administration. FDA approves Entereg to help restore bowel function following surgery. Available at: http://www.fda.gov/bbs/topics/NEWS/2008/NEW01838.html. Accessed September 12, 2008.

55. U.S. Food and Drug Administration. FDA approves Relistor for opioid-induced constipation. Available at: http://www.fda.gov/bbs/topics/NEWS/2008/NEW01826.html. Accessed September 12, 2008.

56. Lavine G. New drug to restore bowel function approved under new FDA rules. *Am J Health-Syst Pharm.* 2008;65:1204.

57. Mangino PD. Role of the pharmacist in reducing medication errors. *J Surg Oncol.* 2004;88:189–194.

58. Davis NM, Cohen MR. Today's poisons: how to keep them from killing the patients. *Nursing.* 1989;89:49–51.

59. Institute for Safe Medication Practices. ISMP's List of High-Alert Medications. Available at: http://www.ismp.org/Tools/highalertmedications.pdf. Accessed September 12, 2008.

60. Institute for Safe Medication Practices. High alert medication feature: reducing patient harm from opiates. Available at: http://www.ismp.org/Newsletters/acutecare/articles/20070222.asp. Accessed September 12, 2008.

61. Institute for Safe Medication Practices. An omnipresent risk for morphine-hydromorphone mix-ups. Available at: http://www.ismp.org/Newsletters/acutecare/articles/20040701.asp. Accessed September 12, 2008.

62. U.S. Food and Drug Administration. Manufacturer and User Facility Device Experience Database – (MAUDE). Available at: http://www.fda.gov/cdrh/maude.html#files. Accessed September 12, 2008.

63. U.S. Pharmacopeia Quality Review. Patient-controlled analgesia pumps. Available at: http://www.usp.org/pdf/EN/patientsafety/qr812004-09001.pdf. Accessed September 12, 2008.

64. Institute for Safe Medication Practices. Safety issues with patient-controlled analgesia: part I – how errors occur. Available at:

http://www.ismp.org/Newsletters/acutecare/articles/20030710. asp. Accessed September 12, 2008.

65. Anonymous. Failure mode and effects analysis: a hands-on guide for healthcare facilities. *Health Devices*. 2004;33(7):233–243.

66. Institute for Safe Medication Practices. Part II – How to prevent errors – safety issues with patient-controlled analgesia. Available at: http://www.ismp.org/Newsletters/acutecare/articles/20030724.asp. Accessed September 12, 2008.

67. Institute for Safe Medication Practices. IV potassium given epidurally: getting to the "route" of the problem. Available at:

http://www.ismp.org/Newsletters/acutecare/articles/20060406. asp. Accessed September 12, 2008.

68. Institute for Safe Medication Practices. Epidural-IV route mix-ups: reducing the risk of deadly errors. Available at: http://www.ismp.org/Newsletters/acutecare/articles/2008070360406.asp. Accessed September 12, 2008.

69. Institute for Safe Medication Practices. ISMP 2007 Survey on high-alert medications: differences between nursing and pharmacy perspectives still prevalent. Available at: http://www.ismp.org/Newsletters/acutecare/articles/20070517.asp. Accessed September 12, 2008.

Pain Management and Patient Outcomes

39

Economics and Costs: A Primer for Acute Pain Management Specialists

Amr E. Abouleish and
Govindaraj Ranganathan

Healing is an Art.
Medicine is a Science.
Healthcare is a Business.
 – *Author unknown*

As much as each one of us would like to concentrate only on our patients and their families, the reality is that health care is a business. In addition, your treatment decisions will affect not only your revenue and costs but often the costs of other parties, including your patients, the hospital, and third-party payers. Because these other parties have an economic interest in your medical decisions, if you are not involved in and do not understand the economic issues, then others will make policies and rules that will significantly affect how you practice and what treatment options are available to your patients.

Economics is defined as the science that deals with the production, distribution, and consumption of goods and services. The underlying fact is that resources are limited. Therefore, the economic problems faced by all of us are (1) the goods and services produced, (2) how they will be distributed, and (3) who will consume or use them.

These economic questions are not limited to health care and acute pain management; they also exist for us as a society and for each of us personally. The goal of this chapter is not to present brand new concepts but to explain concepts and principles that each of us use in everyday life and show how these same concepts also exist in our professional life. In addition, the chapter should also provide the right terminology to explain and understand the economic issues in acute pain and health care.

BUSINESS PLANS VERSUS ECONOMIC STUDIES

Before proceeding, the differences in the concepts of business plans and economic studies must be discussed. Simply, business plans are used to convince a person or group of persons that spending money today will result in a return of that money and more in the future, that is, the "return on investment" (ROI) is

worth the risk. Because the plan is about the future, there must be assumptions made in the plan. Assumptions are based on either "current market conditions" (based on surveys or current contracts) or economic studies. The most common studies are cost minimization, cost-benefit, or cost-effective studies. The studies are focused on a specific issue and are not the same as business plans. Further, other assumptions may be considered the best estimate (or "guess"). Therefore, to understand and develop business plans, one must understand the issues of revenue, costs, and economic studies.

PERSPECTIVES

Figures don't lie, liars figure.

There is much truth to this colloquial saying. The basic understanding of perspectives when dealing with economic analysis – business plans, economic studies – is a requirement to avoid drawing the wrong conclusions. Without this understanding, you are at the mercy of the person who is doing the analysis.

Perspective is defined as the following: in any economic analysis, the revenue and costs included depend on what is determined as relevant.

This concept of perspective – personally, professional, hospital, patient, society – will be seen throughout this chapter and is the underlying principle you must understand!

REVENUE

Because a business plan is based on both costs (present and ongoing) and revenue (future), we will cover both of these topics. From the professional perspective, the increase in revenue should be directly proportional to an increase in services as long as those services are billable. The major determinants of the revenue expected are the estimated payer mix, either current or predicted, and the estimated number of procedures. For example, if you predict that you will do 10 epidural catheter placements with initial consult and one follow-up, and the payer mix will be

Table 39.1: Estimated Revenue

	CPT	Fee Weighted Average	Medicare 25%	Medicaid 25%	Commercial 50%
Consult	99253	$112.78	$108.67	$72.83	$134.80
Epidural catheter placement	62319	$238.25	$89.96	$150.02	$356.50
Follow-up	01996	$92.82	$54.63	$46.65	$135.00
Total per epidural		$443.84	$253.26	$269.50	$626.30
Total for 10 epidurals		$4438.40			

Note: Medicare and Medicaid fees are for 2007 Texas; commercial rates are estimates.

25% Medicare, 25% Medicaid, and 50% commercial, then the evaluation would be as in Table 39.1.

However, taking the hospital perspective, the additional acute pain procedure does not change the hospital revenue, that is, the "per diem" payment (commercial payers) or "DRG" payment (governmental payers). Therefore, why should the hospital incur the additional costs and risks of the additional services?

The adequate management of acute pain is important for hospitals for three major economic reasons. First, the Joint Commission on Accreditation Health Care Organizations (JCAHO) has made pain management important in 2000 with the publication of Pain Management Standards for hospitals.[1] Because of these JCAHO standards, hospitals must now incorporate acute pain management in policy and procedures throughout the facility. Therefore, hospitals must commit financial resources toward pain management. Although no direct increase in revenue may occur from an increase in acute pain management services, there is still a nonfinancial benefit to the services. Further, by having

acute pain specialists at the facility, the hospital can rely on them to help with education of staff on pain management.

The second reason is that improved acute postoperative pain management can result in increased patient mobility.[2] Increased mobility has been shown to reduce postoperative complications, (eg, pneumonia, ileus) and length of stay.[3] Further, with adequate pain management, including with the use of regional blocks and indwelling catheters, surgical procedures that have traditionally required inpatient postoperative care can be performed as ambulatory surgery.[4,5] Although there is no change in hospital revenue (assuming the revenue is relatively fixed by procedure), as discussed below, the ambulatory patient reduces the cost and hence the net profit per procedure increase.[6]

Finally, the third reason is that improved acute pain management can be used for marketing of the hospital as well as the all-important "word-of-mouth." What can be a better marketing tool than "painless" surgery. In fact, a surgeon, who may

---

Perspective

Everyday Example

A school decides that a half-day school day (with the other half for staff education) costs the school district nothing and results in no loss of revenue. In fact, there is an added-value of staff education and satisfaction without any costs! The administrators make this conclusion because they focus only on the school's perspective. A half-day results in the same costs as a full day. The revenue from taxes and the government is the same, because it is considered a day of school. So having a half-day does not cost the district anything and, at the same time, allows them to have staff education time (added value to the school employees). However, if the perspective of parents is considered, the conclusions would be different. Working parents must make child care arrangements or even take the day off work, all resulting in costing the parents money and even lost salary.

Hospital Example

A hospital administrator determines that 24-hour epidural services for obstetric patients is a good business decision. The administrator determines that even though there is a small cost (cost of medications and epidural kit), the increase in revenue from increase in market share will easily outweigh the cost. However, if the physician (anesthesiologist) perspective is included in the hospital administrator's evaluation, the costs of providing the service must include the costs of 24-hour on-call services even when no cases are done. From a laboring parturient's perspective, there is no real increase in cost (covered by the patient's third-party payer). Hence, solely from the patient's perspective, the 24-hour labor epidural service is all benefit without cost.

Cost Centers

Everyday Example

Hospital economics are similar to those of a restaurant that offers all-you-can-eat buffet meals. For the restaurant, once the customer has paid his/her entrance fee, the goal is to serve the patient at a cost less than the entrance fee. If the restaurant is successful, then the restaurant makes a profit. Hence, the restaurant manager must view the buffet as a "cost center" rather than a "revenue-center." Fortunately for the restaurant, if the manager calculates the costs correctly, then he/she can set the entrance fee higher than the costs. Without an understanding of costs, the restaurant manager is only guessing (and praying) that he/she set the entrance fee correctly.

be reluctant to have pain management procedures to be done on his or her patients may become the best proponent of the procedures if the benefits of this "word-of-mouth" increases the number of referrals to his or her practice.

COSTS

Unlike revenue, the costs of services is often much more difficult to determine. The final cost analysis is very much dependent on which costs are included and which are excluded (perspective). Without an understanding of costs, you cannot evaluate any business plan properly nor can you be effective in cost analysis projects initiated by your hospital or other entities (eg, government or third-party payers).

As noted above, for many hospitals, the revenue from a patients' procedure or hospitalization is fixed. That is, once the patient arrives at the hospital, one cannot change the revenue expected. Hence, the management challenge is to reduce and control costs to improve the net profit from the stay.

For health care providers, one must know what the costs of a service are to be able to determine what fee is needed to earn a profit. Without understanding costs, the provider is only guessing that the service is profitable or the negotiated fee is a good contract. Unfortunately, with government payers, negotiations are not possible, and one must either reduce costs below the government fee or lose money on every patient.

Costs Definitions[7–9]

Simply viewing costs as the cost of buying a product is incorrect and simplistic. Further, whoever determines what costs are included or excluded will have great influence on the findings of the analysis. Therefore, an understanding of how costs are defined and categorized will allow one to have the tools to be able to participate in any cost analysis efforts effectively.

Costs Are Not Charges

Because hospital costs have not been easy to determine, many analysis have relied on charges and the estimate of costs by the cost to charge ratio. Unfortunately, by using charges, improper findings can occur. Charges may or may not be related to revenue, but they are *not* related to actual costs, because a consistent cost to charge ratio does not exist between hospital services.[7] In a study evaluating the cost of inpatient surgeries, Marcario et al used a cost information system to determine costs of hospital services and the charges associated with each. The overall ratio of cost to charge was 0.42, but this ratio was not consistent. For those departments with a high ratio, charge analysis using the overall ratio would underestimate the costs of these services. For instance, if the departmental ratio was 0.8, then the costs were 80% of the charges. But when the overall ratio is used, the cost of the department would be calculated as 42% of charges and hence underestimating the actual costs. Similarly, a department with a low ratio would be incorrectly viewed as having higher costs. For anesthesia services, the ratio was 0.29 and hence in the past with charge-based analysis, the anesthesia services' costs were overestimated. Fortunately, many hospitals have begun to use cost-accounting systems to track estimated costs rather than simply relying on charge data.

Explicit, Implicit, and Total Cost

Costs can be simply defined is what someone is willing to sacrifice for a good or services. *Explicit costs* are the monetary payment for the goods or services. In contrast, *implicit costs* occurs when no monetary transaction occurs. The *total cost* is the sum of explicit and implicit costs. Explicit costs are easy to determine; simply what someone is willing paying for the good or service. If you are the provider of the good or service, you set the price (or cost to the buyer) based on the market demand and supply. With the introduction of Ebay and other internet selling Web sites, determining value of a good has been simplified! However, implicit costs are not as easily identifiable and are often overlooked.

In addition to implicit and explicit cost categorization, costs can be grouped in two other ways: direct, indirect, and intangible and then fixed and variable. Each grouping is important for evaluating the economics of a project or service.

Total Costs = Explicit + Implicit Costs

Everyday Example: The Cost of Landscaping Your Yard

If you do it yourself, often you only include the explicit costs, that is, the amount you pay at the nursery for supplies (bushes, flowers, dirt, etc). Often, you forget to include your implicit costs (eg, cost of your own labor and the cost of acute back pain).

Acute Pain Management Example: The Cost of IV PCA

Often, the cost of IV PCA is quoted to be a small number (eg, $8 per patient). This cost is limited and includes only one of the explicit costs (ie, the acquisition cost of the morphine PCA cartridge). (Some additional explicit costs are the cost of the actual pump and the tubing.) Implicit costs are often overlooked, for example, labor costs, including nursing (2 nurses are required to check the PCA settings, evaluation of the pain control), pharmacy, biomedical engineering, and transportation.

Direct, Indirect, and Intangible Costs

Acute Pain Management Example

   Direct costs: Labor costs of patient care (physician, nurse practioner, physician assistant, resident, nurse's aide), medications, hospital room (bed days), catheters and kits, IV equipment

   Indirect costs: Laundry, security, hospital president, billing office, loss of workdays (patient and family), loss of livelihood

   Intangible costs: Pain and suffering, stress on family from inadequate pain relief, stress on nursing staff

---

Direct, Indirect, and Intangible Costs

Direct costs are the costs related to directly with the service or goods produced. For health care, these are costs directly involved with patient care. *Indirect costs* are not related directly to patient care but support patient care. Finally, *intangible costs* are costs that are difficult to quantify but are important depending on the perspective of the cost analysis.

When evaluating the net profit (as defined as revenue minus costs), if only direct costs are included, there may be a profit, but when indirect costs are included, there may be a loss. Unfortunately, often a decision is made to close a unit or clinic because of overall loss. This decision may be a poor economic one, if direct costs show a profit. The reason is that the clinic to be closed helps pay some of the allocated indirect administrative costs. Without the clinic, all the other services must now cover this cost. By closing the clinic, one may actually lead to the other clinics going from net profit to net loss because of the increase in indirect costs that are allocated!

As one can see, which costs are included can change the final answer. Further, which intangible costs and how to quantify them becomes extremely important to the analysis. Again, the only way to be assured the costs that you feel are important are included is to be involved in the planning. When asked by an administrator to be involved with committees that examine patient care or budgets, you should respond with a resounding yes.

Fixed and Variable Costs

A *fixed cost* does not change with a change in the quantity of the goods or services provided. In contrast, a *variable cost* does change directly with a change in quantity. For health care, a variable cost increases with each service provided. The most commonly identifiable variable costs are medications. However, fixed costs do not increase with a change in the number of patients. An example is the cost of an anesthesia machine.

Labor costs over the short run are fixed. That is to staff a unit or a pain management service for the next month, the staffing costs are fixed. However, over the long run, staffing can be adjusted. So if there is a projected increase in staff next year, one can vary the staffing given enough time. The use of locums tenens or agency staffing allows for some flexibility but for most positions the above is true.

One of the greatest mistakes that cost analysis studies do is to assume that fixed costs are variable costs. In anesthesia care, we see this mistake when newer agents or equipment wish to tout that their increase costs are offset by saving minutes or even an hour of a stay in a unit, for example, the operating room (OR) or postanesthesia care unit. Just because the hospital charges or allocates costs by time (cost per minutes of stay), this does not mean the actual costs are variable by the minute. If a hospital determines that an OR is to be staffed, then the staffing for that OR is fixed. It does not matter if 1 patient is scheduled for 1 hour or 2 hours, the staffing costs are the same for that day.

Total, Average, and Marginal Costs

The *total cost* of a service has been defined above as the sum of explicit and implicit costs. Another way is to define it as the sum of fixed and variable costs. In this situation, the term *average total costs* is used to signify that the fixed costs is spread out among all the services produced. For example, if in the morning, the fixed costs for an OR staffing is deteremined. If one patient is done, then the fixed costs associated per patient is the fixed costs

---

Fixed or Variable Costs?

It is not often that scientific journals allow sarcasm to illustrate a point, but the editors of *Anesthesiology* made a great decision when they chose to publish the following letter to the editor:

Cost Savings in the Operating Room
by Jay B. Brodsky, MD

To the Editor: Because of the growing costs of medical care, we have been asked to modify our practices to be more fiscally responsible. In our area, the operating room, we have undergone periodic operations improvement (OI) efforts to reduce unnecessary expenses. Nurses have been replaced with technicians, and physicians have been asked to work "more efficiently."

We have found a simple way to significantly reduce expensive operating room time without jeopardizing patient care. Rather than moving patients on the count of three ("1-2-3" move) as had been our practice, we now count only to two ("1-2" move). Because for every case, each patient is moved to and then from the operating room table we now save 2 s per patient. We have 30 operating rooms, each with an average of 3 operations per day, so our projected savings are 180 s or 3 min per day. Approximately 600 min can be saved over the course of a year by this simple maneuver. Our operating room time costs $20/min. Thus, we can save $12,000 per annum by counting only to two. More importantly, the additional 10 h of operating room time is sufficient for another three to five cases to be performed.

With the acceptance and success of the "move-on-two" maneuver, we have initiated a pilot study of a "move-on-one" maneuver. Initial reports suggest that this can be just as safely and successfully done and will lead to a doubling of efficiency (i.e., saving time and money) over the next fiscal year.

Anesthesiology 1998;88:834

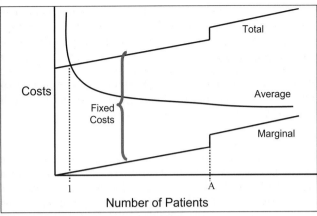

Figure 39.1: Total, average, fixed, and marginal costs.

divided by 1. However, if 3 patients are done, then the fixed costs is divided by 3 and hence the fixed cost per patient is reduced. The *marginal cost* is the change in total costs that results in providing 1 more service. Generally, this is simply the variable costs associated with the additional service. Continuing with the above example, the marginal cost of taking care of 1 more patient once the OR is staffed is simply the variable costs. Hence, the average total cost per patient is the average fixed costs + variable costs (Figure 39.1).

For a given range, this average total costs will continue to decrease as the number of patients increases (a spread of the fixed costs among more patients). At some point, the number of patients will result in a need for increasing staffing (could be a second OR or afternoon shift), and hence the fixed costs will go up. This situation is also true for clinics (hiring more staff and leasing additional space) and for acute pain services (hiring more staff). The most difficult decision is when to hire the additional staff. Does one hire the additional staff to meet expected growth? In this way, one keeps the good level of service that has been seen in the past, but, on the other hand, one takes the risk that the volume will not grow to cover the costs. Or does one wait until the demand is too much for current staff and then hire the additional staff. In this way, one does not take a risk of increased staffing but does risk losing business because of inability to meet the demands in timely manner. In Figure 39.1, this point is "Point A" in the x axis.

The average costs per patient continues to decrease because the fixed costs are spread among more patients. At point A, there is a need to hire more staff and/or more space.

Opportunity Costs

The final category of costs is *opportunity costs*. The definition is simply stated, "If you spend it here, you can't spend it there." Because resources are limited, the decision spend resources on a service or good over another service or good is an example of opportunity costs.

Total, Average, Marginal Costs

Everyday Example

An athletic club is a great example of fixed and marginal costs. When the owners build and equip an athletic club, most of the costs are fixed. The costs of the exercise machines, free weights, the aerobics room, the locker room, and the utilities are fixed. They do not change if one person comes and works out or if 100 do. The staffing costs over the short run are fixed as well. So what is the cost of having 1 more member? That is the marginal cost associated with one more member, which include administrative costs (member data entry, billing), small utilities costs, and maybe some maintenance costs. Hence, each new member will result in profit when examining the marginal costs and the new revenue. If the owner looks at the total costs, initially, each new member will be assigned a net loss because of the fixed costs. But it would be incorrect to say that the owner should then not sign up new members. In fact, in the business plan, the owner has a break-even point where the fixed costs is spread among enough members that the monthly dues result in no loss when total costs are included.

In another example of spreading the costs over a large period is the example of home decorating, specifically, window treatments. We are confident that in many households, the argument for accepting the high cost of window treatments is that the cost is not really for 1 year but for the lifetime of the house (decades and decades). The cost per year is not much. (The same argument is made about furniture and kitchen appliances.)

Anesthesiology Example

When looking at professional charges for anesthesia care, base units per case can be viewed as the fixed "cost" and time units as the "variable costs." The average units billed per hour care is very dependent on surgical duration. For a short case, the base units per case is only spread out over a short period, whereas for long cases, the base units is spread out over many hours. For example, a 1-hour 7-base unit case has an average ASA units per hour of 11 units (7 base + 4 time units divided by 1 hour). However, the same 7-base unit case that takes 4 hours has an average ASA units per hour of less than 6 units (7 base + 16 time units divided by 4 hours).[11]

Opportunity Costs

Everyday Example

Everyday, we make many decisions where we are limited with a resource and decide to spend it on one activity or good over another. These include decisions that require spending or saving money. But we also make these decisions in our time management because time is a limited resource; for example, should I spend time writing a chapter or play golf or play with the kids?

In health care, opportunity costs may be explicit costs (ie, spending dollars on staffing or equipment instead of another service or equipment). Although staffing costs are considered fixed over the short run, what the staff spends time doing can also illustrate opportunity costs. For example, if a patient has adequate pain management from a regional block, then the floor nurse will spend less time managing the patient's pain (eg, assessing pain, answering questions of the family, contacting physician, administering medications, and even witnessing medications-being wasted) and have more time doing other activities (eg, patient education, quality improvement projects, finishing nursing documentation during the shift rather than after the shift is over). Although the improved pain management may not show up as cost savings on the hospital accounts, the opportunity costs of having to spend time on pain management may end up leading to increased costs in long run (eg, with staff dissatisfaction, having to recruit and train new staff).

PERSPECTIVES AND SYSTEM THINKING

As one can see, the costs included in any analysis and possible benefits depend on what perspective is used. Specifically, in examining acute pain management, a larger perspective than simply the service provided should be examined. The improvement in acute pain management improves many aspects of the health care provided and outcomes. Although direct cause and effect is often difficult to establish, even the JCAHO recognizes the connection. When taking a larger perspective, then one begins to use *system thinking*. Although it is easier to view everything from one's own perspective, we all work in a system. For example, if better acute pain management is provided, there may be less chance of developing a chronic pain condition and the associated costs (direct health care costs and indirect in loss of work and livelihood). In the discussions of economic studies, the concepts of system-thinking and perspective will determine what kind of study is performed, and many times, the outcome of the study.

ECONOMIC STUDIES

Three types of economic studies or cost analyses can be done. They are categorized as cost minimization, cost-benefit, and cost-effective. Cost minimization is the easiest to do and understand, but requires that the end point or benefits of treatment are identical between the therapies evaluated. If the end points are not the same, then a cost-benefit or cost-effective study must be performed.

Cost Minimization

The underlying assumption of a cost minimization study is that the end points of care are the same. Hence, the question is which intervention will allow one to get there for the least amount of money. The major advantage is that these studies are easy to understand and do. The major disadvantages are that the equal end points assumption may be disputed and that the costs included or excluded may also be questioned. Often, the only costs included in the study are explicit costs (ie, the costs that the accounting system can identify as money spent). The most common example in the hospital is the evaluation of which medication should be on the formulary. If there are two types of medications that provide the same effect, then the hospital often focuses only on the acquisition costs. The costs of administrating the medications are often ignored (even when one is once a day and another 3 times a day). In addition, for many medications, the end points are not necessarily identical. A worse situation is when this type of analysis is done to two different types of services focused on the same problem. In acute pain management, an administrator may want to do a cost minimization study comparing IV PCA with continuous femoral nerve catheter infusion for acute pain management after total knee replacement surgery. Clearly, these two "services" do not lead to identical end points (as defined as pain management, mobility, physical therapy). But still the analysis may be done. Adding insult to injury, the analysis may only look at acquisition costs rather than total costs!

Cost-Benefit and Cost-Effective

If the end points are not the same, then a cost-benefit or a cost-effective study should be performed. They are relatively the same except that in the benefit studies, the outcomes are assigned a monetary value, whereas in the effectiveness studies, the outcomes are converted to arbitrary units. The advantage is that these types of studies can be used to compare different benefits and the respective costs. The disadvantage is the valuation of costs, benefits, and outcomes are often very subjective.

Cost Minimization versus Cost-Benefit/Cost-Effective Studies

Everyday Example

What kind of car do you drive to work? How do you decide which car to drive? If you believe that any working car will suffice because the end point (ie, arriving to work on time) is identical, then you should use a cost minimization analysis to choose the car. This way you will choose the least expensive car that you can find. If you choose to spend more money on the car, then you have done a cost-benefit or cost-effective analysis without even realizing it. Further, in determining which of the extra features to get with the new car, you also weighed in the opportunity costs.

It is very important to note that these studies are done only if the more expensive service or therapy is more effective or has more benefits. In other words, if the better service or therapy costs less, then why do an analysis? Only when it costs more does one need to determine if it is worth the money spent.

Some of the end points used in cost-effective studies include quality adjusted life-years (QALYs), life-years gained, and days off work. Because QALY is used in looking at long-term outcomes, one needs to be familiar with the term. QALY is used to report on the quality of everyday life (as based on medical conditions) and not simply survivability. In studies that use QALY, a numeric value for a year of life is given with the value of a year of life ranging from 1 (perfect health) to 0 (equivalent to death). The basis of this valuation is the patient. That is, the patient is asked to value what a year living with the medical condition is compared to living a year in perfect health. In most cases, this measurement is used looking at chronic pain conditions (eg, chronic back pain). Most valuations are done using a health survey. In a study comparing surgery to rehabilitation, patients who chose surgery for chronic back pain valued their current state at 0.35 QALY (ie, each year with the pain = 0.35 year of perfect health) and those that chose nonsurgical therapy valued their state at 0.41 QALY.[11] In evaluating costs of therapy, improvements in QALY is used as a denominator to compare \$spent/ΔQALY. For acute pain, this benefit study would be used in the examination of preventing chronic pain syndromes.[12]

In contrast, a cost-benefit study gives monetary values to benefits. In acute pain perspective, how should the valuation of "no pain" be done? Because of the use of survey, the amount patients will pay will be dependent on previous experience of pain, cultural, anxiety, and other factors.[13]

CONCLUSION

As pain management specialist, you can no longer ignore the pressure of cost control that the hospital must respond to to succeed. In fact, changing perspective to a more system thinking approach will allow you to argue that not only is pain management an added-value for the hospital, but the hospital should spend more resources toward pain control! Further, if you are not involved in the process of evaluating and determining where resources will be spent, some one else, including someone who is not a physician, may end up making decisions that affect how you will practice.

REFERENCES

1. Phillips DM. JCAHO pain management standards are unveiled. *JAMA*. 2000;284:428–429.
2. Pham DC, Gautheron E, Guilley J, et al. The value of adding sciatic block to continuous femoral block for analgesia after total knee replacement. *Reg Anesth Pain Med*. 2005;30:128–133.
3. Beaussier M, Weickmans H, Parc Y, et al. Postoperative analgesia and recovery course after major colorectal surgery in elderly patients: a randomized comparison between intrathecal morphine and intravenous PCA morphine. *Reg Anesth Pain Med*. 2006;31:531–538.
4. Williams BA, Kentor ML, Vogt MT, et al. Economics of nerve block pain management after anterior cruciate ligament reconstruction: potential hospital cost savings via associated postanesthesia care unit bypass and same-day discharge. *Anesthesiology*. 2004;100:697–706.
5. Ilfeld BM, Mariano ER, Williams BA, Woodard JN, Macario A. Hospitalization costs of total knee arthroplasty with a continuous femoral nerve block provided only in the hospital versus on an ambulatory basis: a retrospective, case-control, cost-minimization analysis. *Reg Anesth Pain Med*. 2007;32:46–54.
6. Williams BA. For outpatients, does regional anesthesia truly shorten the hospital stay, and how should we define postanesthesia care unit bypass eligibility. *Anesthesiology*. 2004;101:3–6.
7. Macario A, Vitez TS, Dunn B, McDonald T. Where are the costs in perioperative care? Analysis of hospital costs and charges for inpatient surgical care. *Anesthesiology*. 1995;83:1138–1144.
8. Watcha MF, White PF. Economics of anesthetic practice. *Anesthesiology*. 1997:86:1170–1196.
9. Sperry RJ. Principles of economic analysis. *Anesthesiology*. 1997:86:1197–1205.
10. Abouleish AE, Prough DS, Whitten CW, Zornow MH. The effects of surgical case duration and type of surgery on hourly clinical productivity of anesthesiologists. *Anesth Analg*. 2003;97:833–838.
11. Rivero-Arias O, Campbell H, Gray A, Fairbank J, Frost H, Wilson-MacDonald J. Surgical stabilisation of the spine compared with a programme of intensive rehabilitation for the management of patients with chronic low back pain: cost utility analysis based on a randomised controlled trial. *BMJ*. 2005;330:1239–1245.
12. Perkins FM, Kehlet H. Chronic pain as an outcome of surgery: a review of predictive factors. *Anesthesiology*. 2000;93:1123–1133.
13. Macario A, Fleisher LA. Is there a value in obtaining a patient's willingess to pay for a particular anesthetic intervention. *Anesthesiology*. 2006;104:906–909.

40

Evidence-Based Medicine

Tee Yong Tan and Stephan A. Schug

THE GROWING EMPHASIS ON EVIDENCE IN ACUTE PAIN MANAGEMENT

The pharmacology of and techniques in managing acute postoperative pain have improved dramatically since the late 1990s. But despite these advances, acute postoperative pain is still poorly managed, with 29.7% of postoperative patients having moderate-severe pain and 10.9% of postoperative patients having severe pain.[1] In parallel, since the late 1990s, there has been an increased awareness of the suffering associated with acute postoperative pain and the importance of perceiving pain relief as a basic human right. This concept has received widespread endorsement from various international bodies such as the International Association for the Study of Pain (IASP) and the World Health Organization (WHO).[2]

The Australian and New Zealand College of Anaesthetists (ANZCA), in the year 2001, published its statement on patients' rights to pain management.[3] The statement explicitly points out the patients' right of access to appropriate and effective pain management strategies, thus making the link between treatment strategies and supporting data. To further highlight the importance of evidence in the practice of acute postoperative pain management, The Australian and New Zealand College of Anaesthetists and Faculty of Pain Medicine produced the second edition of the book *Acute Pain Management: Scientific Evidence.*[4] This document helps to guide clinicians in their practice of evidence-based medicine (EBM) in the arena of acute postoperative pain management; it will be discussed in more detail later in the chapter.

Thus the understanding of the various principles, methodology, and limitations of EBM is critical to the successful translation of the scientific developments in the area of acute pain medicine into routine clinical care.

WHAT IS EVIDENCE-BASED MEDICINE?

Evidence-based medicine is best understood as a framework for decision-making processes; it involves consideration of the results of research, other forms of scientific evidence, pathophysiologic reasoning, clinician's experience, and patients' preferences when making health care decisions.[5,6] Clinical practice guidelines can be defined as "systematically developed statements to assist in clinicians' and patients' decisions about appropriate healthcare for specific clinical circumstances."[7] Thereby, evidence-based medicine provides both clinicians and patients with a structured process to guide them in making decision to achieve the outcome they desire.[5]

DISTINGUISHING FEATURES OF EBM

In the analysis of evidence, EBM emphasizes the importance of ensuring that any recommendation provided is comprehensive, critical, and explicit.[8]

- Comprehensiveness ensures that all available evidence is examined rather than that of a particular point of view, tradition, or belief.
- Critical appraisal looks into the quality of each of the evidence, its strengths and weaknesses, and its validity in the context of the clinical question.
- Last, explicitness ensures that the process of EBM is transparent and open to scrutiny by both peers and the public.

In the application of EBM, there are two major principles that guide decision-making. First, it is important to realize that pure evidence on its own is often inadequate in the multitude of differing clinical scenarios, and, second, there is always a hierarchy of evidence and no two statements of evidence are equal.[9]

Contrary to common beliefs and fears, EBM does not attempt to convert clinical practice into "cookbook" medicine.[8] Clinicians have to be acutely aware that evidence alone cannot be the sole guide to our clinical practice. There is a need to synthesize the available evidence with a multitude of other factors that will influence the clinicians' decision-making process. Such factors include the strength of the evidence, the potential benefit and associated risk from the intervention, differing values among fellow clinicians, and the patient's expectation and belief systems.[9]

An example would be the heightened concerns among surgeons with regard to the stimulating effects of epidural analgesia on bowel activity perioperatively and its potential risk of anastomotic leakage although there may not be evidence to support these claims.[10] Such beliefs would directly influence the anesthetist's practice with regard to the use of epidural analgesia for bowel surgery.

In supporting decisions, EBM involves in addition to best current evidence the needs of the population and their value system. The needs of a population are influenced by disease patterns in this particular population and the resources available.[11] In situations where resources are scarce, the implication is that any resource spent has an opportunity cost attached to it. Thus, improving acute pain management could diminish resources made available to other aspect of medicine.

Furthermore, the value system of the population, represented frequently by the politicians of the country, will support decisions that best suit the interest of the population – which may not be evidence based but value based.[11] An example would be the availability of opioids in many third-world countries. Although there is wide ranging evidence supporting the use of opioid in acute postoperative pain and cancer pain management, opioids for medical use are still not readily available in a large number of countries. In an attempt to correct this, the WHO, in collaboration with the IASP and the International Narcotics Control Boards, is working on approaches to make decisions on the national availability of opioids more rational and less driven by "opiophobia."[2]

In the formulation of evidence-based guidelines, it is important to understand that there is frequently a lack of available evidence to provide a substantial recommendation.[7] Available evidence may range from poor-quality evidence with limited internal or external validity to well-performed randomized controlled trials. Moreover, grading the quality of the evidence is critical, as is clearly stating or reporting the quality of evidence available. This practice allows clinicians to have a better idea of the presence or absence and level of evidence relevant to their practice. A hierarchy of available evidence will allow clinicians to formulate a clear course of action for the patient.[9]

EVIDENCE-BASED AND EXPERT-BASED OPINION

Evidence-based medicine has the potential of answering questions in situations where our clinical impression can actually cause more harm than good. Thus evidence-based medicine can provide clinicians with the necessary data to help overrule theoretically logical or belief-based, but potentially harmful, decisions.[5] An example would involve the practice of adding a background infusion to intravenous patient-controlled analgesia (PCA) in an attempt to improve pain control and sleep in patients after a major surgical procedure. An examination of this practice using evidence-based techniques reveals that it does not improve pain relief or sleep or reduce the number of PCA demands (RCT based, ie, level II evidence), but increases the risk of respiratory depression (case series based, ie, level IV).[4]

In addition, evidence-based medicine aids medical professional bodies in becoming more transparent in their practices by establishing standards and guidelines. Such changes have proved to be timely in the current global trend of increasing professional accountability.[5]

However, expert opinion will always remain an essential component in all evidence-based guidelines. Such expert input includes the subjective assessment of strength and generalizability of evidence and, when evidence is not available, providing recommendations based on opinion. Often such expert opinions are also needed to fill gaps that result either from areas of medical practice not yet scrutinized by randomized controlled trials or from areas where such evidence will never be obtainable (eg, for ethical concerns or because of the size of RCTs required to identify statistically rare benefits or adverse effects of a therapeutic intervention). The EBM document of ANZCA quoted above has therefore introduced a class of statements described as "Clinical practice points: Recommended best practice based on clinical experience and expert opinion."[4] A typical example of such a statement would be: "Self-reporting of pain should be used whenever appropriate as pain is by definition a subjective experience."

Expert opinion on the other hand is subject to a series of problems on its own. These include the bias, which arises from personal experience, and bias, selective use of evidence and external influence (eg, medicolegal concerns, patient's pressure and business interest).[8]

DEVELOPING EVIDENCE-BASED PRACTICE GUIDELINES

Systematic reviews and meta-analyses have become a widely used technique to aid clinicians in summarizing and expanding their existing medical knowledge. Systematic review is defined as a formal process of identifying, appraising, and evaluating primary studies and other relevant research to draw conclusions to a specific issue.[12] A systematic review becomes a meta-analysis when statistical technique is applied to synthesize the data collected from the numerous trials to generate a pooled estimate of the treatment effect or other end points.[13,14]

In systematic reviews and meta-analyses, as more than one trial is being examined for a particular intervention, the summation of the result should provide the best available evidence.[14] To allow clinicians to practice with confidence, it is important for the clinician to know the processes by which recommendations are generated. These involve 4 main steps, namely[5]:

- asking the right question
- searching the literature (both published and unpublished) for source of data
- appraising and evaluating the data collected
- answering the question posed using the collected data

SYNTHESIZING MEDICAL EVIDENCE

Evidence-based medicine is facilitated by converting information obtained from thousands of individual studies into user-friendly risk estimates.[5] One useful tool that clinicians can readily understand and apply for weighing the benefits and risks of various treatments is the concept of number needed to treat/harm (NNT/NNH), respectively.

The NNT is the number of people who need to be treated for 1 to achieve a specified level of benefit in comparison to placebo treatment. This number can be easily calculated from either raw data or from statistical estimates and applied to various end points.[15] Furthermore, such numbers allow easy comparison between various analgesic agents with a common outcome (at least 50% pain relief compared with placebo). NNT can then be used as a yardstick whereby an alternative therapy can be measure.

But it is also important for users to remember that NNT is always relative to the comparator and applies only to a specified clinical outcome.[16] Further concerns regarding the pooling of data from various different pain models in an attempt to base NNT calculations on the largest possible numbers are discussed later in this chapter.

Another limitation in the usage of NNT is that it can be applied only to data that are dichotomous. This means that the question must be answerable with either a yes or no. In the realm of pain relief, gradual analgesic effects cannot be considered and setting a cutoff at 50% pain relief compared to placebo may at times make this a difficult target to achieve. Thus, if an analgesic is capable of producing 30% pain relief in a patient, which might be a clinically relevant effect, then it will be deemed to be ineffective without due consideration of the clinical circumstances.[16]

QUALITY AND VALIDITY ISSUES

Although each step used in performance of the meta-analysis appears relatively straightforward, users have to be aware of the possible pitfalls in its application. Some of the problems a clinician could face are as follows[14,17]:

- Regression during analysis is often nonlinear, but estimates of effect size can be meaningful only when regressions are linear.
- The effect studied may often have a multivariate relationship rather than a univariate relationship to the intervention. For example, analyzing the effect of an analgesic on postoperative nausea and vomiting is difficult, as it is only one of multiple causes of postoperative nausea and vomiting.
- The clinical relevance of the studies analyzed can be limited by the exclusion criteria that were prespecified in the study design.
- Bad- or poor-quality studies are included in a meta-analysis.
- Data summarized are not homogenous.
- Grouping of different causal factors leads to meaningless estimates of effects.
- Theory-directed approaches in meta-analysis may obscure any discrepancies that existed in the data. Although clarifying the discrepancies is more important than estimating effect sizes, what typically clinicians are more interested in the latter.

To help clinician in deciding the quality of the meta-analysis that is performed, it is possible for the clinician to utilize the 18 items checklist and flow diagram that is suggested by the QUOROM (*quality of reporting of meta-analysis*) statement (available at: http://www.consort-statement.org/QUOROM.pdf).[18,19]

This practice will help clinicians better identify good-quality meta-analyses from those that are poorly done.

Similarly, the CONSORT (*consolidated standards of reporting trials*) statement has provided clinicians with a framework to analyze randomized controlled trials to differentiate the quality of work and thus to see that only valid results are used in clinical practice (available at http://www.consort-statement.org/Downloads/Checklist.doc or http://www.consort-statement.org/Downloads/checklist.pdf).[18,20]

CHALLENGES TO THE PRACTITIONER OF EVIDENCE-BASED MEDICINE

There are two important issues to ensure the successful implementation of evidence-based medicine. First, there is a need to ensure that the available evidences in the area of practice have been adequately reviewed, with evidence-based practice guidelines and recommendations laid out for clinicians. Second, strategies have to be in place for the successful translation of guidelines and recommendations into practice. This would include a paradigm shift in clinical practice and the willingness of clinicians to adopt the recommendations.[9] Knowledge of current best evidence together with willingness to discard outdated practice ideas is needed to ensure that clinicians are armed with the latest state-of-the-art medical care capabilities.[21]

Evidence-based guidelines or recommendations can provide a specific direction to guideline clinical practice. But for changes to be effective, they have to be preceded by learning. This is then followed by incorporating this new information using experience and wisdom.[22]

In a systematic review, it was found that evidence-based guidelines can work and are capable of improving patients' care but often do not achieve this goal.[23] The review further attempts to delineate the common features of guidelines, which achieved successful implementation.

- guidelines covered an area with large variation in clinical practice
- evidence base is fairly secure
- indication for use of the guidelines is common among the clinicians
- clinician is aware of the knowledge gaps in area covered by guidelines
- benefit of implementation is huge

Thus, even with the availability of evidence-based guidelines, it can be seen only as a road map for clinical care. What is more important to a clinician is the intellectual wisdom to apply this road map to patient care. Thus the outcome cannot be based only on its clinical benefit or its biomedical good but also on its ability to translate the practices for the personal good of the patient, in the light of the patient's circumstances and his or her choices. As such, a clinician can no longer be a just mere executor of these evidence-based guidelines; he or she must also be armed with the wisdom to be able to exercise the moral responsibilities endowed on them for the "good" of the practice.[22]

On a much broader view, evidence-based medicine that stimulates much discussion among practicing clinicians regarding how to best gather and assimilate data and translate it into guidelines, and how to implement this evidence for the well-being of the patients, has within the medical community become a positive force in moving health care toward a better future.[24]

LIMITATIONS OF EVIDENCE-BASED MEDICINE

With the exponential growth in the amount of clinical researches and systematic reviews, it is hopeful that the number of "gray zones" in clinical practice would be reduced. Also notable is the fact that there are obvious limitations in the practice of evidence-based medicine that make practicing it imperfect in many ways.

First, there is a lack of evidence in many areas of clinical practice and only a small proportion of medical practice has been tested in well-designed trials.[7] Furthermore, there are areas where study is not feasible. The recommendation that the appropriate treatment of acute neuropathic pain might prevent chronic pain is currently based on expert opinion.[4] Performing a randomized controlled trial in this area will require patients with acute neuropathic pain to be treated with placebo and such a trial may be deemed unethical.

Another area of limitation involves mainly publication bias. It is common that compared to negative trials, trials with positive or statistically significant results get published in medical journals. In addition, certain data are used in multiple articles, resulting in duplication of data. Also, there is an obvious bias against articles that are not published in English language, as these trials tend to be missed in searches.[12]

In addition, there is a lack of a unified definition in many of the trials, which results in many difficulties in trying to compare "apples to apples." The use of sedation as a marker of impending respiratory depression in patients on patient-controlled analgesia (PCA) produced an incidence of between 0% and 25.7%. This relatively wide range demonstrated the importance of a standardized definition to make data collection in clinical trials meaningful.[25] For the outcome of any systematic reviews or meta-analysis can only be as accurate or reliable as the original studies.[12]

Furthermore, the recommendations provided by the author depends largely on the author's interpretation of the results at hand. In two different systematic reviews published in the same year (2003) by two different authors on the same topic (the effects of nonsteroidal anti-inflammatory drugs [NSAIDs] and the risk of operative site bleeding after tonsillectomy), the conclusions were drastically different. One author concluded that the use of NSAIDs increases the risk of reoperation for hemostasis and thus the drug should not be used.[26] By contrast, the other author felt that the evidence of increased bleeding remains ambiguous and, compared to opioids, NSAIDs seem to be equianalgesic with decreased risk of postoperative nausea and vomiting. On the balance of things, the second author concluded that NSAIDs can be used cautiously in tonsillectomy.[27] This difference in recommendation on the level of a meta-analysis (level I) could well create confusion among practicing clinicians.

To add to the confusion, different guidelines use different scales to assign different weightings to the various evidences. Thus similar practices may have different levels of recommendations depending on the source of the guideline.[7] Two different recommendations are outlined below.

The following levels of evidence are adapted from the National Health and Medical Research Council (NHMRC) of Australia for interventional studies[4,28]:

Level of Evidence	Study Design
I	Evidence obtained from a systematic review of all relevant randomized controlled trials.
II	Evidence obtained from at least one properly designed randomized controlled trial.
III – 1	Evidence obtained from well-designed pseudorandomized controlled trials (alternate allocation or some other method).
III – 2	Evidence obtained from comparative studies (including systematic reviews of such studies) with concurrent controls and allocation not randomized (cohort studies), case control studies, or interrupted time series with a control group.
III – 3	Evidence obtained from comparative studies with historical control, two or more arm studies, or interrupted time series without parallel control group.
IV	Evidence obtained from case series, either posttest or pretest and posttest.
Consensus	In the absence of scientific evidence and where the executive committee, steering committee, and review groups are in agreement, the term *consensus* has been applied.

In comparison, the Scottish Intercollegiate Guidelines use a set of evidence recommendations originating from the US Agency for Health Care Policy and Research, which differs from those above. Their guideline is set out in the following table.[29]

Level of Evidence	Study Design
I a	Evidence obtained from meta-analysis of randomized controlled trials.
I b	Evidence obtained from at least one randomized controlled trial.
II a	Evidence obtained from at least one well-designed controlled study without randomization.
II b	Evidence obtained from at least one other type of well-designed quasi-experimental study.
III	Evidence obtained from well-designed nonexperimental descriptive studies, such as comparative studies, correlation studies. and case studies.
IV	Evidence obtained from expert committee reports or opinions and/or clinical experiences of respected authorities.

Comparing the above 2 tables, it is not difficult to understand how confusion can result when 2 different forms of classification are being utilized.

EVIDENCE-BASED MEDICINE IN ACUTE PAIN MANAGEMENT

The most widely internationally endorsed EBM document on acute pain management is *Acute Pain Management: Scientific Evidence*, which was published in an initial version by the National Health and Medical Research Council of Australia (NHMRC) in 1999. This document has been updated by the Australian and New Zealand College of Anaesthetists and its Faculty of Pain Medicine and was then published in 2005 in the form of a paperback book[4] and a PDF file on a Web site (http://www.anzca.edu.au/publications/acutepain.htm).

It has been endorsed not only by the NHMRC but also by the Australian Pain Society, the Royal College of Anaesthetists, and the International Association for the Study of Pain and is recommended by the American Academy of Pain Medicine. It has also been the topic of editorials in a number of journals, including the British Journal of Anaesthesia.[30–32]

It presents the highest ranked, highest quality evidence on all aspects of acute pain management. The aim of the document is to combine the best available evidence in this area with current clinical and expert practice and to present the substantial amount of evidence currently available for the management of acute pain in a concise and easily readable form. It covers all aspects of acute pain, far beyond postoperative pain, and includes evidence-based statements on pain associated with nonsurgical conditions such as spinal cord injury, burns, cancer, acute zoster, neurological diseases, hematological disorders (eg, sickle cell disease), and HIV/AIDS, as well as abdominal (eg, renal and biliary colic), cardiac, musculoskeletal, and orofacial pain and headache.

The main information is summarized in key messages based on highest levels of evidence available. The progress in the area can be shown by the fact that the 1999 document had 34 levels I, II, and III key statements, whereas the edition in 2005 has 108 level I recommendations alone. A consumer document has been developed from this document and is available from the same Web site as well as a version updated to December 2007.

The revision of the document was organized and coordinated by a working party, which also prepared the final version of the document. A panel of contributors was selected to draft sections of the document and a large multidisciplinary consultative committee (including medical, nursing, and allied health and complementary medicine clinicians in addition to consumers) was appointed to review the early drafts of the document and contribute more broadly as required to ensure general applicability and inclusiveness.

Although such guidelines can influence clinical decision-making in a positive way, they generalize the evidence and present no data on specific procedures. However, there is now good evidence that different surgical procedures may result in different types of pain, different intensities of pain, and different locations of pain. These procedural differences lead to different risk-benefit ratios for different analgesic techniques in the different settings. Examples of such differences are the different efficacy of, for example, paracetamol in different pain models.[33] By pooling studies from disparate procedures the confidence intervals for numbers needed to treat from different agents overlap, providing little evidence for their real benefit in a specific procedure.[34] Thereby NNT league tables ignore specific effects of analgesics in different pain models and lead to extrapolations of efficacy that are inappropriate for a specific procedure.[35] Therefore, generalized evidence-based guidelines for postoperative pain treatment may often be insufficient because available evidence does not suggest that different pain models are truly comparable and the efficacy of different agents may vary between procedures.

In response to these issues, another avenue to summarize evidence on acute pain management has been taken by the members of the PROSPECT group.[36] This approach recognizes that different surgical procedures may result in different types of pain, different intensities of pain, and different locations of pain. It is quite obvious that such differences lead to different risk/benefit ratios for different analgesic techniques in the various postoperative settings. This recognition has led to the concept of developing procedure-specific guidelines for postoperative pain management. The PROSPECT approach has followed this guidance and aims to provide health care professionals with procedure-specific information that is up to date and evidence based.[37] The recommendations are presented on a Web site (www.postoppain.org) and provide recommendations for best practice accessible to everybody on this Web site with a user-friendly interface. The development of the PROSPECT recommendations is based on a systematic literature review of procedure-specific data which are then supplemented by evidence from studies of other procedures believed to have a similar pain profile as the procedure under review and by information from clinical practice as far as relevant. The overall information is assessed at a consensus meeting of the PROSPECT Working Group and procedure-specific recommendations for the management of pain after specific procedures are developed.

The methodology underlying the PROSPECT recommendations is published in the peer-reviewed literature.[38] In brief summary, the development of PROSPECT recommendations is based on a systematic literature review. This literature review includes studies that have a definable group of patients undergoing the procedure under review; are randomized trials of an analgesic, anesthetic, or surgical technique aimed at influencing postoperative pain; are appropriately randomized and blinded and where pain scores are reported on a linear pain scale. Such selected procedure-specific data are analyzed qualitatively and pooled where possible for quantitative meta-analysis. Specific outcomes analyzed are VAS scores, supplementary analgesic requirements, the time to first analgesic request, and incidence or severity of postoperative nausea and vomiting. The procedure-specific data thus assembled are supplemented by evidence from studies of other procedures believed to have a similar pain profile as the procedure under review.[39] In addition, information from clinical practice, for example, with regard to aspects of practicality and risk benefit, are also taken into consideration when assessing the data. The overall information condensed in this way is assessed at a consensus meeting of the PROSPECT working group and procedure-specific recommendations for the management of the specific postoperative pain are developed.

These recommendations are then formulated in a way that facilitates clinical decision-making and are provided in a Web-based interface with quick and easy access to the relevant information. This Web site presents the evidence in a tree structure. The evidence and the recommendation for each procedure are contained in folders representing each step in the perioperative care pathway; operative techniques, anesthetic techniques, and analgesic strategies are reviewed. Information is then summarized in an overall set of recommendations for each procedure, which shows a pathway for the continuity of the pre-, intra-, and postoperative pain management. For each step, procedure-specific evidence, transferable evidence from other procedures and clinical practice recommendations are listed, as well as the concluding PROSPECT recommendations. The user is also able to see the original references for each of these recommendations. The user can access the qualitative analysis, the quantitative meta-analysis in a classical graph if available and the details of the underlying references, including their abstracts. The final recommendations for a procedure are presented in the form of a flow diagram.

Currently online are the following surgical procedures: laparoscopic cholecystectomy,[40] primary total hip arthroplasty,[41] abdominal hysterectomy, colonic resection, herniorraphy, thoracotomy, total knee arthroplasty, and mastectomy. Overall, this approach offers a robust foundation for the development of clinical decision support by the use of the Cochrane Collaboration methodology and the inclusion of transferable evidence and clinical practice.

CONCLUSION

As medical science develops, the future promises an expansion of research information. Practicing clinicians will find it more and more difficult to incorporate all new findings into their everyday clinical decision-making because of a lack of time and resources.[42]

Systematic reviews have in recent years aided clinicians in keeping abreast of medical literature by summarizing the huge body of information available and addressing the differences that arise from the various studies.[43] Armed with this new knowledge, clinicians now have the tools to discharge outdated practices and assimilate new guidelines and recommendations into their daily practice.

REFERENCES

1. Dolin SJ, Cashman JN, Bland JM. Effectiveness of postoperative pain management: I. Evidence from published data. Br J Anaesth. 2002;89(3):409–423.
2. Brennan F, Cousins MJ. Pain relief as a human right. IASP Pain Clinical Updates 2004;XII(5).
3. Australian and New Zealand College of Anaesthetists Professional Document. Statement on Patients' Rights to Pain Management. PS45 (2001). www.anzca.edu.au/publications/profdocs/profstandards/index.htm.
4. Australian and New Zealand College of Anaesthetists, Faculty of Pain Medicine. Acute Pain Management: Scientific Evidence. Melbourne: Australian and New Zealand College of Anaesthetists; 2005.
5. Donald A. Evidence-based medicine: Key concepts. MedGenMed. 2002;4(2). Available at: http://www.medscape.com/viewarticle/430709.
6. Cook DJ, Levy MM. Evidence-based medicine: a tool for enhancing critical care practice. Crit Care Clin. 1998;14(3):353–358.
7. Swinglehurst D. Evidence-based guidelines: the theory and the practice. Evidence-Based Healthcare Public Health. 2005;9:308–314.
8. Woolf SH. Evidence-based medicine and practice guidelines – an overview. Cancer Control. 2000;7(4):362–367.
9. Guyatt G, Rennie D. User's Guides to the Medical Literature: A Manual for Evidence-Based Clinical Practice. Washington, DC: AMA Press; 2002.
10. Holte K, Kehlet H. Epidural analgesia and risk of anastomotic leakage. Reg Anesth Pain Med. 2001;26:111–117.
11. Muir Gray JA. Evidence-based and value-based healthcare. Evidence-Based Healthcare Public Health. 2005;9:317–318. [Editorial]
12. Columb MO, Lalkhen A-G. Systematic reviews and meta-analyses. Curr Anaesth Crit Care. 2005;6:391–394.
13. Barker FG, Carter BS. Synthesizing medical evidence: systematic reviews and meta-analyses. Neurosurg Focus. 2005;19(4). Available at http://www.medscape.com/viewarticle/515632
14. Herbert RD, Bø K. Analysis of quality of interventions in systematic reviews. BMJ. 2005;331:507–509.
15. Oulos J, Kam PCA. "Number needed to treat": a tool for summarizing treatment effect, and its application in anaesthesia and pain management. Curr Anaesth Crit Care. 2005;16:173–179.
16. Holdcroft A, Jaggar S. Core Topics in Pain. Cambridge, UK; Cambridge University Press; 2005.
17. Eysenck HJ. Meta-analysis and its problems. BMJ. 1994;309:789–792.
18. Needleman I. Editorial: Is this good research? Look for CONSORT and QUORUM. Evid Based Dent. 2000;2:61–62.
19. Moher D, Cook D J, Eastwood S, Olkin I, Rennie D, Stroup D. Improving the quality of reports of meta-analyses of randomized controlled trials: the QUOROM statement. Lancet. 1999;354:1896–1900.
20. Moher D, Schulz KF, Altman DG for the CONSORT group. The CONSORT statement: revised recommendations for improving the quality of reports of parallel-group randomized trials. Lancet. 2001;357:1191–1194.
21. Linklater D R, Pemberton L, Taylor S, Zeger W. Painful dilemmas: an evidence-based look at challenging clinical scenarios. Emerg Med Clin N Am. 2005;23:367–392.
22. Giordano J. Techniques, technology and tekne: the ethical use of guidelines in the practice of interventional pain management. Pain Physician. 2007;10:1–5.
23. Bazian Ltd. Do evidence-based guidelines improve the quality of care? Evidence-Based Healthcare Public Health. 2005;9:270–275.
24. Cronje RJ, Freeman JR, Williamson OD, Gutsch CJ. Evidence-based medicine: recognising and managing clinical uncertainty. Lab Med. 2004;35(12):724–731.
25. Tan TY, Schug SA. Safety aspects of postoperative pain management. Rev Analg. 2006;9:45–53.
26. Marret E, Flahault A, Samama C M, Bonnet F. Effects of postoperative, nonsteroidal, anti-inflammatory drugs on bleeding risk after tonsillectomy. Anesthesiology. 2003;V98:1497–1502.
27. Møiniche S, Rømsing J, Dahl JB, Tramèr MR. Nonsteroidal anti-inflammatory drugs and the risk of operative site bleeding after tonsillectomy: a quantitative systematic review. Anesth Analg. 2003;96:68–77.
28. Australian Acute Musculoskeletal Pain Guidelines Group. Evidence-based management of acute musculoskeletal pain: a guide for clinicians. Bowen Hills, Queensland: Australian Academic Press; 2004.
29. Scottish Intercollegiate Guidelines Network. Control of Pain in Patients with Cancer: A National Clinical Guideline. Edinburgh, UK: SIGN Publication; 2000.
30. Macintyre PE, Walker S, Power I, Schug SA. Acute pain management: scientific evidence revisited. Br J Anaesth. 2006;96(1):1–4.

31. Macintyre PE, Schug SA, Scott DA. Acute pain management: the evidence grows. An Australian document now has an important role in acute pain management worldwide. *Med J Aust.* 2006;184(3):101–102.

32. Schug SA, Macintyre P, Power I, Scott D, Visser E, Walker S. The scientific evidence in acute pain management. *Acute Pain.* 2005;7(4):161–165.

33. Barden J, Edwards JE, McQuay HJ, Moore AR. Pain and analgesic response after third molar extraction and other postsurgical pain. *Pain.* 2004;107(1–2):86–90.

34. McQuay HJ, Moore RA. *An Evidence-Based Resource for Pain Relief.* Oxford, UK: Oxford University Press; 1998.

35. Gray A, Kehlet H, Bonnet F, Rawal N. Predicting postoperative analgesia outcomes: NNT league tables or procedure-specific evidence? *Br J Anaesth.* 2005;94(6):710–714.

36. Schug SA, Kehlet H, Bonnet F, et al. Procedure specific pain management after surgery – "PROSPECT." *Acute Pain.* 2007;9(2):55–57.

37. Kehlet H, Wilkinson RC, Fischer HB, Camu F. PROSPECT: evidence-based, procedure-specific postoperative pain management. *Best Pract Res Clin Anaesthesiol.* 2007;21(1):149–159.

38. Neugebauer EA, Wilkinson RC, Kehlet H, Schug SA. PROSPECT: a practical method for formulating evidence-based expert recommendations for the management of postoperative pain. *Surg Endosc.* 2007;21(7):1047–1053.

39. Neugebauer E, Wilkinson R, Kehlet H, on behalf of the PROSPECT Working Group. Transferable evidence in support of reaching a consensus. *Z ärztl Fortbild Qual Gesundh.* 2007;101:103–107.

40. Kehlet H, Gray A, Bonnet F, et al. A procedure-specific systematic review and consensus recommendations for postoperative analgesia following laparoscopic cholecystectomy. *Surg Endosc.* 2005;19(10):1396–1415.

41. Fischer HB, Simanski CJ. A procedure-specific systematic review and consensus recommendations for analgesia after total hip replacement. *Anaesthesia.* 2005;60(12):1189–1202.

42. Mulrow CD, Cook DJ, Davidoff F. Systematic reviews: critical links in the great chain of evidence. *Ann Intern Med.* 1997;126(5):389–391. [Editorial]

43. Cook DJ, Mulrow CD, Haynes RB. Systematic reviews: synthesis of best evidence for clinical decisions. *Ann Intern Med.* 1997;126(5):376–380.

41

Effect of Epidural Analgesia on
Postoperative Outcomes

Marie N. Hanna, Spencer S. Liu,
and Christopher L. Wu

Epidural analgesia is a widely accepted analgesic technique for the treatment of postoperative pain. Compared to parenteral opioids, epidural analgesia in general will provide superior analgesia and may confer certain physiologic benefits, including attenuation of perioperative pathophysiologies, which may ultimately contribute to a decrease in perioperative morbidity or even mortality. High-risk surgical patients, such as those who are elderly, have decreased physiologic reserve or, undergoing certain procedures, may especially benefit from postoperative epidural analgesia. However, postoperative epidural management must be optimized to achieve any improvement in postoperative outcomes.

Despite the potential benefits of postoperative epidural analgesia, the superiority of epidural analgesia compared to parenteral opioids is somewhat uncertain, which may be related to conflicting results of relatively small randomized controlled trials (RCTs) and other methodological issues. However, we limit our focus to larger RCTs, meta-analyses of RCTs, and large databases in an attempt to elucidate the benefits of postoperative epidural analgesia on conventional outcomes (eg, mortality, major morbidity) and patient-reported outcomes (eg, satisfaction, quality of recovery, and analgesia).

MORTALITY

The overall advances in anesthesia care have significantly decreased the incidence of mortality since the late 1960s, as reflected in the Institute of Medicine report on medical errors (ie, "anesthesiology has successfully reduced anesthesia mortality rates from two deaths per 10,000 anesthetics administered, to one death per 200,000–300,000 anesthetics administered").[1] Although the incidence of postoperative death is fortunately relatively infrequent, the low incidence is problematic in determining whether an intervention such as perioperative epidural anesthesia and analgesia might be associated with a decrease in perioperative mortality. For instance, data from Medicare surgical patients indicated a 30-day mortality rate of approximately 2.5%.[2] An RCT designed to detect a 50% reduction in incidence

from 2% to 1% would require approximately 4600 patients, which is 3 to 4 times more subjects than the largest available RCT on this topic. In addition, there are other limitations of an RCT in examining the effect of epidural analgesia on mortality.[3] Thus, use of meta-analyses and database analysis may facilitate assessment of the effect of epidural analgesia on postoperative mortality.

The largest meta-analysis of RCTs (Collaborative Overview of Randomised Trials of Regional Anaesthesia, CORTRA) comparing neuraxial anesthesia, including epidural anesthesia and analgesia) to general anesthesia included 141 RCTs with 9559 patients undergoing a variety of surgical procedures.[4] The results of this meta-analysis suggested that perioperative neuraxial anesthesia and analgesia (versus general anesthesia) was associated with a reduction in mortality (1.9% vs 2.8%; odds ratio [OR] = 0.7 with 95% confidence intervals [CI] = 0.54 to 0.90) that was attributed to a reduction of major morbidity in various multiple organ systems. A subset of approximately 5000 patients (66 RCTs) utilized epidural anesthesia and analgesia. Other smaller subsequent meta-analyses, however, have shown no benefit for the use of epidural analgesia in decreasing mortality. A meta-analysis examined 11 RCTs (1173 subjects) that used postoperative epidural analgesia for 24 hours or more after surgery demonstrated no difference in the incidence of mortality between those who received epidural analgesia or systemic opioids (3.1% vs 4.4%, $P = .30$).[5] Other meta-analyses have also noted no difference in death although the authors of many of these meta-analyses acknowledged that it would be difficult to assess a relatively rare outcome such as mortality because of the small numbers of patients studied. A meta-analysis (13 RCTs, 1224 subjects) examining patients undergoing open abdominal aortic surgery compared patients randomized to epidural analgesia or systemic opioid but found similar mortality rates (3.5% vs 4.3%).[6] Another meta-analysis (15 RCTs, 1178 subjects) for patients undergoing coronary artery bypass grafting did not note a reduction in mortality with use of epidural anesthesia (0.7% vs 0.3%).[7] Other meta-analyses on RCTs examining epidural analgesia versus systemic opioids for postoperative analgesia after abdominal surgery (711 subjects)[8] and hip/knee replacement

Table 41.1: Summary of Meta-Analyses and Large Randomized Controlled Trials: Mortality

Author	No. of RCTs	No. of Patients	Type of surgery	Mortality in NA Group (%)	Mortality in GA Group (%)	Odds Ratio (95% CI)	P Value
Rodgers et al (2000)[4]	141	9559	MIX	1.9%	2.8%	0.70 (0.54–0.90)	$P = .0006$
Beattie et al (2001)[5]	11	1173	MIX	3.1%	4.4%	0.74 (0.40–1.37)	$P = .3$
Nishimori et al (2006)[6]	13	1224	ABD	3.5%	4.3%	0.86 (0.48–1.55)	$P = .6$
Liu et al (2004)[7]	15	1178	CABG	0.7%	0.3%	1.56 (0.35–6.91)	$P = .56$
Park et al (2001)[10]	1	1021	ABD	4%	3.4%	n/c	$P = .74$
Rigg et al (2002)[11]	1	915	ABD	5.1%	4.3%	n/c	$P = .67$

Abbreviations: ABD = abdominal (including aortic) surgery; CABG = coronary artery bypass surgery; CI = confidence interval; GA = general anesthesia; MIX = mixed surgical procedures; NA = neuraxial analgesia; n/c: not calculated.

surgery (555 subjects)[9] indicated that there was insufficient evidence for a benefit of postoperative epidural analgesia in decreasing perioperative mortality (Table 41.1).

There have been at least two large multicenter RCTs comparing epidural analgesia to systemic opioids since the publication of the CORTRA meta-analysis with both of these RCTs showing no difference in mortality between the two forms of analgesia. The Veterans Affairs Cooperative Studies Program (VACS) randomized approximately 1000 patients undergoing aortic, gastric, biliary, or colon surgery to combined general/epidural anesthesia followed by epidural morphine or general anesthesia followed by systemic opioids.[10] Overall mortality rates were similar between groups (4% for epidural opioid versus 3.4% for systemic opioids). Another relatively large RCT, the Multicentre Australian Study of Epidural Anesthesia (MASTER), enrolled 915 high-risk patients who underwent abdominal surgical procedures and were randomized to combined general/epidural anesthesia followed by 72 hours of postoperative epidural analgesia with local anesthetic/opioids or general anesthesia followed by systemic opioids.[11] The overall mortality rates were similar between the groups (5.1% for epidural versus 4.3% for systemic opioids); however, there was poor protocol compliance, as only 225 of 447 patients fully adhered to the epidural analgesia protocol. Although both RCTs did not demonstrate a difference in mortality between epidural analgesia and systemic opioids, the studies were not adequately sized to assess a relatively mortality.

In an attempt to circumvent the issue of inadequate sample size, a group of investigators used a 5% random sample of the Medicare claims database to examine patients undergoing a variety of surgical procedures and stratified them according to the presence (n = 12 780 subjects) or absence (n = 55 943) of postoperative epidural analgesia (Table 41.2).[2] Regression analysis revealed that the presence of postoperative epidural analgesia was associated with a significantly lower risk for both 7-day (0.5% vs 0.8%, OR = 0.52 with 95% CI = 0.38 to 0.73) and 30-day (2.1% vs 2.5%, OR = 0.74; 95% = CI 0.63 to 0.89) mortality. However, the benefit of epidural analgesia in possibly decreasing mortality was limited to patients undergoing higher-risk (eg, thoracotomy) rather than lower-risk (eg, joint replacement) surgery. The lack of benefit for epidural analgesia for lower-risk surgery is reflected in a separate Medicare claims analysis in patients undergoing total hip replacement where there was no significant difference in mortality between those who did or did not receive epidural analgesia (0.2% vs 0.4%; OR = 0.6; 95% CI = 0.2 to 1.5).[12]

Thus, the definitive evidence for reduction of perioperative mortality with postoperative epidural analgesia compared to systemic opioids is lacking. Although, the largest sets of data (CORTRA meta-analysis and Medicare claims dataset) suggest a benefit for epidural anesthesia and analgesia in decreasing postoperative mortality, there are limitations to each type of analyses.[3] Procedure specific meta-analyses and individual RCTs have noted no benefit for epidural analgesia in reducing postoperative mortality; however, these studies lack sufficient sample size to assess relatively rare outcomes such as death.

MAJOR MORBIDITY

The perioperative pathophysiologies (eg, neuroendocrine stress response) that result from surgery will affect all organ systems. Use of epidural analgesia may confer many analgesic and physiologic benefits that may theoretically translate into improved patient outcomes postoperatively. Furthermore, because the incidences of complications and major morbidities (eg, cardiovascular, pulmonary, gastrointestinal, coagulation) are generally higher than that seen for mortality in the perioperative period, any benefits for epidural analgesia may be more apparent for these higher frequency events. Many meta-analyses have been conducted examining the efficacy of postoperative epidural analgesia on various patient outcomes.

CARDIOVASCULAR MORBIDITY

Approximately 100 million adults worldwide undergo noncardiac surgery annually, and nearly half of the patients are estimated to have cardiac risk factors.[13] It has been estimated that 5% of these patients will develop some type of perioperative cardiac complication or morbidity.[14] Although the reported incidences of perioperative cardiovascular morbidity varies depending on surgical and patient factors, high-risk patients (eg, elderly, pre-existing comorbidities) or procedures (eg, emergency or cardiac surgery) carry the highest risk of developing cardiovascular morbidity postoperatively. For instance, the incidence of myocardial infarction is higher for emergency surgery in the elderly (approximately 19% vs 0.2% for myocardial infarction)[2,15] and those undergoing major vascular surgery (5%–10% incidence).[7,16]

Postoperative pain control is important in attenuating the perioperative pathophysiology (eg, activation of the sympathetic nervous system, surgical stress response, and coagulation

Table 41.2: Summary of Databases (Medicare) Analyses: Mortality

Author	Procedure	Mortality in GA (%)	Mortality in NA (%)	Odds Ratio (95% CI)	P Value
Wu et al (2004)[2]	Mixed	7 days: 0.8%	7 days: 0.5%	0.52 (0.38–0.73)	$P = .0001$
		30 days: 2.5%	30 days: 2.1%	0.74 (0.63–0.89)	$P = .0005$
Wu et al (2003)[12]	Hip replacement	7 days: 0.39%	7 days: 0.2%	0.6 (0.24–1.48)	$P = 0.27$
		30 days: 0.9%	30 days: 0.6%	0.63 (0.35–1.11)	$P = 0.11$

Abbreviations: CI = confidence interval; GA = general anesthesia; MIX = mixed surgical procedures; NA = neuraxial analgesia.

cascade) that can contribute to cardiovascular morbidity by increasing myocardial oxygen demand (via increases in heart rate, blood pressure, and contractility) or decreasing myocardial oxygen supply (via enhanced perioperative hypercoagulability, coronary thrombosis, or vasospasm).[17,18] Animal data suggest that use of thoracic epidural anesthesia and analgesia with local anesthetics may confer physiologic benefits by reducing sympathetic activation and providing a favorable balance of myocardial oxygen.[19] Clinical data also suggest a physiologic benefit of thoracic epidural analgesia with local anesthetics in patients with multivessel ischemic heart disease.[17,20] It is important to note that lumbar epidural anesthesia may not provide the same physiologic benefits as thoracic epidural anesthesia as there is a compensatory increase in sympathetic activity above the level of blockade for lumbar epidural analgesia,[21] which may be associated with an increased incidence of left ventricular wall dysfunction (compared to thoracic epidural anesthesia).[17] Nevertheless, use of lumbar epidural analgesia may still be preferable to systemic opioids as a small study noted a marked reduction in cardiovascular events (0% vs 19%) in patients with hip fractures randomized to preoperative lumbar epidural analgesia versus systemic analgesia.[15]

There are at least 5 meta-analyses that have examined the efficacy of postoperative epidural analgesia on cardiovascular morbidity either as a primary or secondary outcome (Table 41.3).[5–9] Three meta-analyses that specifically examined the efficacy of postoperative epidural analgesia on cardiovascular morbidity indicated a benefit for thoracic epidural analgesia in decreasing cardiovascular morbidity. The first meta-analysis (9 RCTs, 632 patients) evaluated subjects undergoing a variety of surgical procedures but where epidural analgesia was extended for at least 24 hours postoperatively.[5] The use of thoracic epidural (OR = 0.43; 95% CI = 0.19 to 0.97) but not lumbar epidural (OR = 0.77; 95% CI = 0.31 to 1.92) analgesia provided a significant reduction in the rate of myocardial infarction (3.6% vs 8.5%, rate difference = −5.3% with 95% CI of −9.9% to −0.7%). Another similar but more procedure specific meta-analysis in patients undergoing open abdominal aortic surgery (13 RCTs, 1224 patients) also suggested a significant reduction in risk of cardiovascular complications (relative risk [RR] = 0.74; 95% CI = 0.56 to 0.97) and myocardial infarction (RR = 0.52; 95% CI 0.29 to 0.93) with epidural analgesia compared to that for systemic analgesia.[6] The third procedure specific meta-analysis (15 RCTs, 1178) examined patients undergoing coronary artery bypass surgery[7] and found a significant reduction in the incidence of dysrhythmias with thoracic epidural analgesia (17.8% vs 30%, OR = 0.52; 95% CI = 0.29 to 0.93) compared to systemic opioids. Finally, two other procedure-specific meta-analyses examining effects of

epidural analgesia on abdominal and hip and knee replacement surgery found no benefit for epidural analgesia in decreasing cardiovascular morbidity; however, the authors concluded that there was insufficient evidence in these meta-analyses to analyze cardiovascular complications.[8,9]

The two previously described RCTs (VACS and MASTER trials) did not consistently demonstrate a benefit of epidural analgesia in decreasing postoperative cardiovascular complications. Although the VACS trial overall did not note a significant reduction in cardiovascular complications with use of epidural morphine, the abdominal aortic surgery subgroup had a significantly lower incidence of cardiovascular complications (9.8% vs 17.9%, $P = .03$) primarily due to reduction in myocardial infarction (2.7% vs 7.9%, $P = .05$).[10] The MASTER trial observed no benefit for epidural analgesia in decreasing cardiovascular morbidity (2.6% vs 2.4%) and there were no significant differences in cardiovascular complications in a subgroup analysis of patients undergoing abdominal aortic surgery (4.5% vs 4.7%).[22] Several analyses of the Medicare claims data did not demonstrate a differences in cardiovascular complications between patients with and without postoperative epidural analgesia for a variety of surgical procedures; however, the accuracy of these databases in capturing major morbidity is uncertain as the overall cardiovascular complication rates were quite low (0.8%–4%).[2,12]

Thus, there is consistent evidence that thoracic epidural analgesia may reduce the risk of cardiovascular complications, such as myocardial infarction, in high-risk patients, including those undergoing major vascular surgery. The benefit for thoracic epidural analgesia reflects experimental data demonstrating physiologic benefits of this technique and may also reflect the higher underlying rate of cardiovascular complications for high-risk surgical population (4%–18%). However, there is minimal evidence that epidural analgesia reduces cardiovascular complications in the general (more healthy) surgical population.

PULMONARY MORBIDITY

Postoperative pulmonary complications (PPC) remain a significant problem and may occur at a higher frequency than cardiac morbidity in patients undergoing elective abdominal procedures.[23,24] Like that seen in other systems, the pathophysiology of postoperative pulmonary dysfunction is multifactorial and may include disruption of normal respiratory muscle activity, reflex inhibition of phrenic nerve activity and subsequent decrease in diaphragmatic function, and uncontrolled postoperative pain leading to deceased lung volumes.[24] Use of epidural analgesia, particularly if placed in the thoracic region and

Table 41.3: Summary of Meta-Analyses and Large Randomized Controlled Trials: Cardiovascular

Author	No. of RCT	No. of Patient	Type of Surgery	Rate of CV Events: Epidural	Rate of CV Events: Control	Outcomes Assessment	Odds Ratio (95% CI)	P Value
Beattie et al (2001)[5]	9	632	MIX	T: 7/196	T: 17/201	Overall complications	T: 0.43 (0.19–0.97)	T: $P = .04$
				L: 8/328	L; 12/351		L: 0.77 (0.31–1.92)	L: $P = .06$
Nishimori et al (2006)[6]	13	1224	ABD	ABD: 65/611	ABD: 85/611	Overall complications,	ABD: 0.74 (0.56–0.97)	ABD: $P = .03$
			AAA	AAA: 16/851	AAA: 32/851	MI	AAA: 0.52 (0.29–0.93)	AAA: $P = .03$
Liu et al (2004)[7]	15	1178	CABG	17.8%	30%	Dysrythmias	0.52 (0.29–0.93)	$P = 0.03$
Park et al (2001)[10]	1	1021	ABD	ABD: 26/330 (7.9%)	ABD: 23/317 (7.3%)	Overall complications,	n/c	ABD: $P = .88$
			AAA	AAA: 18/184 (9.8%)	AAA: 34/190 (17.9%)	MI	n/c	AAA: $P = .03$
Peyton et al (2003)[22]	1	915	ABD	ABD: 2.6%	ABD: 2.4%	Overall complications	ABD: 1.09 (0.81–1.48)	ABD: $P = .56$
			AAA	AAA: 4.5%	AAA: 4.7%		AAA: 0.92 (0.50–1.70)	AAA: $P = .79$

Abbreviations: AAA = abdominal aortic aneurysm procedure; ABD = abdominal (non-aortic) procedure; CABG = coronary artery bypass graft; CI = confidence interval; L = lumbar epidural analgesia; MI = myocardial infarction; MIX = mixed surgical procedures; n/c = not calculated; T = thoracic epidural analgesia.

incorporating a local anesthetic-based solution, will confer superior analgesia (vs systemic opioids) and other physiologic benefits, which ultimately may result in improved voluntary pulmonary function.[25] Although the physiologic effects of epidural analgesia on respiratory muscle function are complex,[24] some data indicate that thoracic epidural analgesia with bupivacaine (0.25%) does not impair ventilatory mechanics, inspiratory respiratory muscle strength, or airway flow, even in patients with severe chronic obstructive pulmonary disease.[26,27]

There are at least 4 meta-analyses that examine the effects of epidural analgesia on PPC (Table 41.4). Although the COR-TRA meta-analysis did not specifically examine postoperative epidural analgesia, a large percentage of subjects did receive epidural anesthesia and analgesia, and use of neuraxial block for a variety of surgical procedures was associated with significantly decreased risk of pneumonia (3.1% vs 6%, OR = 0.61; 95% CI = 0.48 to 0.76) with thoracic epidural analgesia demonstrating strong efficacy (OR = 0.48; 95% CI = 0.35 to 0.67) compared to spinals or lumbar epidurals (OR = 0.76; 95% CI = 0.55 to 1.04).[4] One of the first meta-analyses (18 RCTs, 1016 patients) examined the effect of analgesia on PPC noted a reduced risk of overall pulmonary complications (RR = 0.58; 95% CI = 0.42 to 0.80) and infections (RR = 0.35; 95% CI = 0.21 to 0.65) with epidural regimens compared to systemic or epidural opioids.[28] Other procedure-specific meta-analyses also indicated that use of thoracic epidural analgesia (vs systemic opioids) is associated with a significantly decreased risk of respiratory failure (RR = 0.63; 95% CI = 0.51 to 0.79) for open abdominal aortic surgery[6] and PPC (17.2% vs 30.3%, OR = 0.41; 95% CI = 0.27 to 0.60) for coronary artery bypass surgery.[7] Meta-analyses examining use of epidural analgesia in abdominal surgery and total hip-knee replacement surgery concluded there were insufficient subjects to perform analysis on PPCs.[8,9]

For RCTs, the VACS study noted a nonsignificant reduction in respiratory failure for all patients (9.9% for epidural vs 14% systemic analgesics); however, subgroup analysis of patients undergoing abdominal aortic surgery revealed a significant reduction in respiratory failure with use of epidural analgesia (14% vs 28%, $P < .01$).[10] Similarly, the MASTER study noted a lower incidence of respiratory failure for patients randomized to receive epidural analgesia (23% vs 30%, $P = .02$).[11] Analyses of the Medicare claims data revealed no benefit for postoperative epidural analgesia in decreasing the risk of pneumonia or respiratory failure in patients undergoing a variety of surgical procedures although again the authors noted significant limitations of the Medicare database in assessing complications such as PPC.[2,12] Thus, there is consistent evidence from meta-analyses and large RCTs that use of thoracic epidural analgesia with local anesthetics (compared to systemic opioids) is associated with a significantly reduced risk of PPC, particularly in high-risk surgical patients such as those undergoing open abdominal aortic surgery or coronary artery bypass. These benefits are not apparent with use of epidural opioids compared to systemic opioids.

GASTROINTESTINAL MORBIDITY

Postoperative ileus is a common complication, particularly after abdominal surgery, and may result in an increase in resource use and length of stay.[29] Like that seen with other systems, the pathophysiology of postoperative ileus and decreased gastrointestinal (GI) motility is multifactorial. Possible etiologies include neurogenic (spinal, supraspinal adrenergic pathways), inflammatory (ie, local inflammatory responses instigate neurogenic inhibitory pathways), and pharmacologic mechanisms.[30] Use of epidural analgesia with local anesthetics may attenuate several of the mechanisms of postoperative ileus. By decreasing both the degree of postoperative pain (compared to systemic opioids) and amount of systemic opioids used,[25] epidural analgesia may facilitate return of GI function postoperatively. In addition, sympathetic block from epidural local anesthetics may attenuate postoperative reflex inhibition of GI motility, and the

Table 41.4: Summary of Meta-Analyses and Large Randomized Controlled Trials: Pulmonary

Author	No. of RCT	No. of Patients	Type of Surgery	Rate of Pulmonary Events: Epidural	Rate of Pulmonary Events: Control	Outcomes Assessment	Odds Ratio (95% CI)	P Value
Rodgers et al 2000[4]	141	9559	MIX	3.1%	6%	Pneumonia	T: 0.61(0.48–0.76)	n/c
							L: 0.48 (0.35–0.67)	
							I: 0.76 (0.55–1.04)	
Ballantyne et al 1998[28]	18	1016	MIX	n/c	n/c	Overall complications, pneumonia	RR: 0.58 (0.42–0.80)	n/c
							RR: 0.35 (0.21–0.65)	
Nishimori et al 2006[6]	13	1224	ABD	19.8%	30,6%	Respiratory failure, pneumonia	RR: 0.63 (0.51–0.79)	ABD: P = .00004
			AAA	4.8%	7.8%		RR: 0.64 (0.38–1.05)	AAA: P = .08
Liu et al 2004[7]	15	1178	CABG	17.2%	30.3%	Overall complications	0.41 (0.27–0.60)	P < .00001
Park et al 2001[10]	1	1021	ABD	25/330 (7.6%)	18/317 (5.7%)	Overall complications	n/c	ABD: P = .35
			AAA	26/184 (14.1%)	55/190 (28.9%)			AAA: P = .0006
Rigg et al 2002[11]	1	915	ABD	23%	30%	Respiratory failure	n/c	P = .02

Abbreviations: AAA = abdominal aortic aneurysm procedure; ABD = abdominal (nonaortic) procedure; CABG = coronary artery bypass graft; CI = confidence interval; I = intrathecal opioids; L = lumbar epidural analgesia; MI = myocardial infarction; MIX = mixed surgical procedures; n/c = not calculated; RR = relative risk; T = thoracic epidural analgesia.

suppression of the surgical stress response and systemic absorption of epidural local anesthetics may reduce the inflammatory response to attenuate postoperative ileus.[29,30]

Experimental data consistently indicate that epidural analgesia with local anesthetics shortens time of intestinal paralysis without impairing anastomotic healing or increasing risk of anastomotic leakage.[31] There have been numerous RCTs examining the efficacy of epidural analgesia on the return of GI function and many of these were included in a Cochrane Library meta-analysis (22 RCTs with 1023 patients) that examined patients undergoing abdominal surgery.[32] Similarly to that seen in experimental studies, this meta-analysis indicates that epidural analgesia with local anesthetics consistently showed reduced time to return of gastrointestinal function compared to systemic opioids (mean of −37 hours) or epidural opioids (mean of −24 hours). Thus, it appears that epidural analgesia with local anesthetics hastens return of postoperative GI function after abdominal surgery by 24 to 37 hours.

COAGULATION-RELATED MORBIDITY

It is widely recognized that a general state of hypercoagulability occurs following surgical procedures that may increase the risk of coagulation-related complications such as deep venous thrombosis (DVT) or pulmonary embolism (PE). Following surgery, there is a tendency toward thrombosis as the normal process of coagulation becomes unbalanced with increases in levels of tissue factor, tissue plasminogen activator, plasminogen activator inhibitor-1, and von Willebrand factor, all of which contribute to

a hypercoagulable and hypofibrinolytic state postoperatively.[33] Despite the presence of modern practices of thromboprophylaxis, coagulation-related events are still an important cause of perioperative morbidity and mortality.

Intra-operative neuraxial (spinal and epidural) anesthesia with local anesthetic regimens can attenuate perioperative hypercoagulability and may confer physiologic benefits, including increased arterial and venous blood flow, attenuation of perioperative increases in coagulation proteins and platelet activity, and preservation of fibrinolytic activity.[19] In addition, systemic absorption of epidural local anesthetics may confer beneficial rheologic properties, including reduction in platelet aggregation, inhibition of thrombus formation, and reduction in blood viscosity.[34] Thus, use of intraoperative neuraxial anesthesia may prevent some of these coagulation-related complications. However, it is not certain whether these potential benefits can be extended into the postoperative period with use of epidural analgesia as some experimental data suggest that postoperative epidural analgesia using common local analgesic concentrations (≤0.125% bupivacaine) does provides no significant increase in blood flow or decrease in postoperative hypercoagulability.[35] The large numbers of subjects examined in the CORTRA meta-analysis allowed the authors to perform subgroup analyses that revealed that use of neuraxial block was associated with a significant reduction in risk of DVT (2.9% vs 4.7%) and PE (0.6% vs 1.4%) (Table 41.5).[4] However, it may be difficult to apply these data to individual patients as there were a mix of surgical procedures and intraoperative neuraxial anesthesia. Subsequently performed procedure-specific meta-analyses for open aortic surgery, abdominal surgery, and total hip and knee

Table 41.5: Summary of Meta-Analyses and Large Randomized Controlled Trials: Coagulation

Author	No. of RCT	No. of Patients	Type of Surgery	Rate of Coagulation Events: Epidural	Rate of Coagulation Events: Control	Outcomes Assessment	Odds Ratio (95% CI)	P Value
Rodgers et al (2000)[4]	141	9559	MIX	2.9%	4.7%	DVT	0.56 (0.43–0.72)	n/c
				0.6%	1.4%	PE	0.45 (0.29–0.69)	
Christopherson et al (1993)[36]	1	100	LER	4%	22%	Graft failure	n/c	P < .01
Tuman et al (1991)[37]	1	80	LER	2.5%	20%	Graft failure	n/c	P = .013

Abbreviations: CI = confidence interval; DVT = deep venous thrombosis; LER = lower extremities revascularization; MIX = mixed surgical procedure; n/c = not calculated; PE = pulmonary embolism.

replacement were unrevealing as there were insufficient subjects for analysis.[6,8,9] It also must be noted that many of the meta-analyses did not comment on use of thromboprophylaxis, which is important as many of the underlying RCTs were performed prior to the release of currently popular thromboprophylactic agents (ie, only 38 of 141 RCTs were published >1990).[4] Several RCTs have also noted that use of perioperative epidural anesthesia and analgesia may be associated with a lower risk of graft failure in patients undergoing vascular surgical procedures.[36,37] Thus, although *intra*operative neuraxial anesthesia appears to be associated with a reduced risk of coagulation-related events such as DVT, PE, and graft failure, there is minimal evidence that *post*operative epidural analgesia affects risk of DVT and PE. A confounding factor is that very few studies have addressed this question with use of current methods of effective thromboprophylaxis.

OTHER OUTCOMES

Chronic Pain

Chronic pain following surgery can be a significant postoperative complication with the incidence as high as 30%–81% after limb amputation, 22%–67% after thoracotomy, 17%–57% after breast surgery, and 4%–37% after hernia repair.[38,39] The etiology of chronic postoperative pain is most likely multifactorial and may include peripheral and central sensitization. Although the severity of acute postoperative pain is a recognized risk factor for development of chronic postoperative pain[38] and use of epidural analgesia would theoretically confer superior postoperative analgesia that possibly may result in a lower incidence of chronic postsurgical pain, the causality of this relationship is uncertain and the degree of hyperalgesia may be important is determining the extent of chronic postsurgical pain.[40]

Cognitive Decline and Delirium

Postoperative cognitive decline is common, particularly in older patients, with rates of postoperative cognitive decline reported as high as 7%–26% and delirium as high as 10%–60% after certain procedures.[41] Although the etiology of postoperative cognitive decline and delirium is uncertain, it most likely is multifactorial and certain factors, such as the severity of postoperative pain and use of opioids, have been identified as possible risk factors for the development of postoperative delirium in the elderly.[41,42] Despite the theoretical advantages of regional anesthesia and

analgesia, no meta-analyses or systematic reviews show a benefit for this technique in decreasing postoperative cognitive decline and delirium. Also refer to Chapter 31 (*Acute Pain Management for Elderly High-risk and Cognitively Impaired Patients: Rationale for Regional Analgesia*).

Infectious and Immune Complications

Following major surgical procedures, there is an early hyperinflammatory response (eg, release of proinflammatory tumor necrosis factor-α [TNF-α], interleukins, and cytokines) with subsequent cell-mediated immunosuppression.[43] Although use of epidural analgesia with local anesthetics has been shown to reduce lymphocyte suppression, attenuate proinflammatory cytokines, and increase surgical wound oxygen tension,[44,45] no large-scale data exist to demonstrate a translation of these benefits clinically into a decrease rate of infection per se.[46] The CORTRA meta-analysis noted low incidences of wound infections (0.05% vs 0.07%) without differences between those who received neuraxial or general anesthesia.[4] Interestingly, however, there are some experimental studies showing that use of regional anesthesia and analgesia can preserve perioperative immune function that may be of benefit in those undergoing cancer surgery.[47]

PATIENT-REPORTED OUTCOMES

Despite the number of studies examining the effect of postoperative epidural analgesia on patient outcomes, only a few have examined the effect on patient-reported outcomes such as quality of life, postoperative quality of recovery, and patient satisfaction. Patient-reported outcomes are recognized as valid and important end points that are assessed from the patient's perspective. These outcomes, like other common low-morbidity events (ie, medication-related side effects), may become more relevant as the incidence of anesthesiology-related mortality and major morbidity has decreasedsince the late 1960s.[1]

Different analgesic agents and techniques (eg, epidural local anesthetic vs systemic opioids) would be expected to result in different levels of analgesia and incidences of side effects. In general, peripheral and epidural regional analgesic techniques are expected to provide superior analgesia compared to systemic opioids.[48–50] These difference in analgesia may influence patient-reported outcomes as higher levels of postoperative pain may be associated with an overall decrease in mental and psychological function,[51,52] higher levels of postoperative fatigue,[53,54] and disturbances in sleep.[55] Furthermore, the presence of side effects may be an important input into the patient-reported outcomes of health-related quality of life (HQRL), postoperative quality of recovery (QOR), and patient satisfaction. Thus, it is possible that different analgesic agents or techniques may result in different levels of HRQL, QOR, or patient satisfaction in the immediate postoperative period.

Health-Related Quality of Life

Health-related quality of life can be considered as the comprehensive assessment of the medical care received by a patient. This assessment conceptually incorporates the domains of physical functioning, mental health, cognitive functioning, symptoms (eg, pain), role and social functioning, general health perceptions, sleep, and energy. There are many validated HRQL instruments, some of which are generic and others specific. A recent systematic review[56] found 5 RCTs that examined the effect of postoperative analgesia on HRQL but found that only 1 of 5 demonstrated any difference in HRQL between analgesic techniques. The 1 study that showed a difference examined patients undergoing elective colon surgery who were randomized to receive perioperative epidural analgesia vs IV PCA opioids.[57] Those who received epidural analgesia had significantly preserved quality of life (SF-36) at up to 6 weeks after surgery. Despite the presence of this study, no definitive conclusions can be made regarding the effect of the type of analgesic technique, degree of analgesia, and presence of side effects on HRQL.

Postoperative Quality of Recovery

Postoperative QOR specifically assesses postoperative recovery on a daily basis[58] and in some sense may be considered a subset of HRQL in part because of some of the common domains assessed. In fact, changes in postoperative QOR may correlate with long-term changes in HRQL.[59] A recent systematic review[56] found 4 RCTs that examined the effect of postoperative analgesia on QOR; however, none showed any difference in postoperative QOR using different analgesic regimens. There were methodologic issues with these studies and as such, it is not clear whether the type of analgesic technique, degree of analgesia, and presence of side effects may influence postoperative QOR.

Patient Satisfaction

The measurement of patient satisfaction is quite complex and very few studies have examined the effect of postoperative analgesia on satisfaction as a primary outcome. Although there may not be a direct correlation between levels of postoperative pain and satisfaction as there are many inputs into satisfaction, the level of pain may be one of the more important inputs[60] and poor control of postoperative pain (along with the presence of analgesic-related side effects) generally correlates with decreased patient satisfaction.[61,62] A recent systematic review[56] found 95 RCTs assessing satisfaction with different analgesic techniques but only 2 RCTs used a validated instrument to assess patient satisfaction. Approximately half of the RCTs (47 of 95) noted an improvement in satisfaction with one analgesic technique or regimen over another but no definitive conclusions can be made because of the methodologic issues in assessing satisfaction.

ECONOMIC OUTCOMES

Very few studies have incorporated economic assessments in their evaluation of the efficacy of epidural analgesia (versus systemic opioids) on outcomes. Many studies that do incorporate economic assessments, however, generally are not comprehensive in their inputs for costs. Nevertheless, there are some data that can be summarized in the areas of length of stay and a multimodal approach to patient convalescence.

Length of Stay

There are at least 16 RCTs that have examined the effect of postoperative epidural analgesia on length of stay.[56,62] Only a minority used prospectively defined discharge criteria for assessment of length of stay. None of the 5 RCTs that used a multimodal approach to patient convalescence (see Multimodal Approach to Patient Recovery below) showed any difference in length of stay. Thus, the quality of the available data is inconsistent and no definitive conclusion can be made regarding the effect of analgesia on length of stay.

Multimodal Approach to Patient Recovery

Although individual interventions (eg, epidural analgesia, antibiotics, thromboembolism prophylaxis) may be efficacious in reducing some morbidities, a multimodal intervention or approach to patient recovery ("fast track" or accelerated recovery programs) may decrease perioperative morbidity and decrease length of stay.[63] One of the key components of this approach is use of regional anesthetic-analgesic techniques that may provide superior analgesia compared to systemic opioids[48–50] and physiologic benefits that may facilitate convalescence. Other aspects of a multimodal approach to patient recovery include early enteral nutrition, improved perioperative education, and maintenance of oxygen delivery and normothermia.[63] Several RCTs have compared multimodal to conventional care and the vast majority of studies used epidural analgesia with a local anesthetic-based solution as part of the multimodal approach to patient recovery. Although some RCTs demonstrated earlier return of gastrointestinal function and improvement in patient-oriented outcomes with use of a multimodal recovery program, there were no differences between those who received an accelerated with regard to mortality or major pulmonary or cardiovascular morbidity.[54,56]

Thus, use of a multimodal or accelerated recovery program, which typically includes epidural analgesia with a local anesthetic-based solution, may be associated with lower pain scores, increased mobilization, and decreased length of stay when compared to conventional care. There also may be an earlier return of gastrointestinal function, although no difference in other major morbidity or mortality has been found. However, the number and size of available RCTs is relatively small and limited to evaluation in a few surgical procedures and additional studies are needed to provide a definitive answer.

SUMMARY

There are many benefits for the perioperative use of epidural analgesia for the treatment of postoperative pain. Compared to systemic opioids, epidural analgesia provides superior analgesia and certain physiologic benefits. The attenuation of perioperative pathophysiology with perioperative epidural analgesia may result in a decrease in perioperative cardiovascular, pulmonary and gastrointestinal morbidity although any benefit in decreasing coagulation-related morbidity or mortality is uncertain. Although epidural analgesia is associated with lower pain scores, it is unclear whether this benefit may result in any improvement in patient-reported outcomes such as satisfaction, quality of life, and quality of recovery. Further development of instruments assessing patient-reported outcomes in the postoperative period is needed. Finally, the effect of perioperative epidural analgesia on length of stay is uncertain.

REFERENCES

1. Kohn LT, Corrigan JM, Donaldson MS, eds. *To Err Is Human: Building a Safer Health System.* Washington, DC: National Academy Press; 2000.

2. Wu CL, Hurley RW, Anderson GF, Herbert R, Rowlingson AJ, Fleisher LA. Effect of postoperative epidural analgesia on morbidity and mortality following surgery in Medicare patients. *Reg Anesth Pain Med.* 2004;29:525–533.

3. Wu CL, Fleisher LA. Outcomes research in regional anesthesia and analgesia. *Anesth Analg.* 2000;91:1232–242.

4. Rodgers A, Walker N, Schug S, McKee A, et al. Reduction of postoperative mortality and morbidity with epidural or spinal anaesthesia: results from overview of randomised trials. *BMJ.* 2000;321:1493.

5. Beattie WS, Badner NH, Choi P. Epidural analgesia reduces postoperative myocardial infarction: a meta-analysis. *Anesth Analg.* 2001;93:853–858.

6. Nishimori M, Ballantyne JC, Low JHS. Epidural pain relief versus systemic opioid based pain relief for abdominal aortic surgery. *Cochrane Database Syst Rev.* 2006;3:CD005059.

7. Liu SS, Block BM, Wu CL. Effects of perioperative central neuraxial analgesia on outcome after coronary artery bypass surgery: a meta-analysis. *Anesthesiology* 2004;101:153–161.

8. Werawatganon T, Charuluxanun S. Patient controlled intravenous opioid analgesia versus continuous epidural analgesia for pain after intra-abdominal surgery. *Cochrane Database Syst Rev.* 2005:CD004088.

9. Choi PT, Bhandari M, Scott J, Douketis J. Epidural analgesia for pain relief following hip or knee replacement. *Cochrane Database Syst Rev.* 2003:CD003071.

10. Park WY, Thompson JS, Lee KK. Effect of epidural anesthesia and analgesia on perioperative outcome: a randomized, controlled Veterans Affairs cooperative study. *Ann Surg.* 2001;234:560–569.

11. Rigg JR, Jamrozik K, Myles PS, et al. Epidural anaesthesia and analgesia and outcome of major surgery: a randomised trial. *Lancet.* 2002;359:1276–1282.

12. Wu CL, Anderson GF, Herbert R, Lietman SA, Fleisher LA. Effect of postoperative epidural analgesia on morbidity and mortality after total hip replacement surgery in Medicare patients. *Reg Anesth Pain Med.* 2003;28:271–278.

13. Devereaux PJ, Goldman L, Cook DJ, Gilbert K, Leslie K, Guyatt GH. Perioperative cardiac events in patients undergoing noncardiac surgery: a review of the magnitude of the problem, the pathophysiology of the events and methods to estimate and communicate risk. *Can Med Assoc J.* 2005;173:627–634.

14. Mangano DT. Assessment of the patient with cardiac disease: an anesthesiologist's paradigm. *Anesthesiology.* 1999;91:1521–1526.

15. Matot I, Oppenheim-Eden A, Ratrot R, et al. Preoperative cardiac events in elderly patients with hip fracture randomized to epidural or conventional analgesia. *Anesthesiology.* 2003;98:156–163.

16. Mackey WC, Fleisher LA, Haider S, et al. Perioperative myocardial ischemic injury in high-risk vascular surgery patients: incidence and clinical significance in a prospective clinical trial. *J Vasc Surg.* 2006;43:533–538.

17. Meissner A, Rolf N, Van Aken H. Thoracic epidural anesthesia and the patient with heart disease: benefits, risks, and controversies. *Anesth Analg.* 1997;85:517–528.

18. Warltier DC, Pagel PS, Kersten JR. Approaches to the prevention of perioperative myocardial ischemia. *Anesthesiology.* 2000;92:253–259.

19. Liu S, Carpenter RL, Neal JM. Epidural anesthesia and analgesia. Their role in postoperative outcome. *Anesthesiology.* 1995;82:1474–1506.

20. Nygard E, Kofoed KF, Freiberg J, et al. Effects of high thoracic epidural analgesia on myocardial blood flow in patients with ischemic heart disease. *Circulation.* 2005;111:2165–2170.

21. Taniguchi M, Kasaba T, Takasaki M. Epidural anesthesia enhances sympathetic nerve activity in the unanesthetized segments in cats. *Anesth Analg.* 1997;84:391–397.

22. Peyton PJ, Myles PS, Silbert BS, Rigg JA, Jamrozik K, Parsons R. Perioperative epidural analgesia and outcome after major abdominal surgery in high-risk patients. *Anesth Analg.* 2003;96:548–554.

23. Qaseem A, Snow V, Fitterman N, et al. Risk assessment for and strategies to reduce perioperative pulmonary complications for patients undergoing noncardiothoracic surgery: a guideline from the American College of Physicians. *Ann Intern Med.* 2006;144:575–580.

24. Warner DO. Preventing postoperative pulmonary complications: the role of the anesthesiologist. *Anesthesiology.* 2000;92:1467–1472.

25. Wu CL, Cohen SR, Richman JM, et al. Efficacy of postoperative patient-controlled and continuous infusion epidural analgesia versus intravenous patient-controlled analgesia with opioids: a meta-analysis. *Anesthesiology.* 2005;103:1079–1088.

26. Gruber EM, Tschernko EM, Kritzinger M, et al. The effects of thoracic epidural analgesia with bupivacaine 0.25% on ventilatory mechanics in patients with severe chronic obstructive pulmonary disease. *Anesth Analg.* 2001;92:1015–1019.

27. Groeben H, Schafer B, Pavlakovic G, Silvanus MT, Peters J. Lung function under high thoracic segmental epidural anesthesia with ropivacaine or bupivacaine in patients with severe obstructive pulmonary disease undergoing breast surgery. *Anesthesiology.* 2002;96:536–541.

28. Ballantyne JC, Carr DB, de Ferranti S, et al. The comparative effects of postoperative analgesic therapies on pulmonary outcome: cumulative meta-analyses of randomized, controlled trials. *Anesth Analg.* 1998;86:598–612.

29. Mythen MG. Postoperative gastrointestinal tract dysfunction. *Anesth Analg.* 2005;100:196–204.

30. Bauer AJ, Boeckxstaens GE. Mechanisms of postoperative ileus. *Neurogastroenterol Motil.* 2004;16(uppl 2):54–60.

31. Kehlet H, Jensen TS, Woolf CJ. Persistent postsurgical pain: risk factors and prevention. *Lancet.* 2006;367(9522):1618–1625.

32. Jorgensen H, Wetterslev J, Moiniche S, Dahl JB. Epidural local anaesthetics versus opioid-based analgesic regimens on postoperative gastrointestinal paralysis, PONV and pain after abdominal surgery. *Cochrane Database Syst Rev.* 2000:CD001893.

33. Bombeli T, Spahn DR. Updates in perioperative coagulation: physiology and management of thromboembolism and haemorrhage. *Br J Anaesth.* 2004;93:275–287.

34. Moraca RJ, Sheldon DG, Thirlby RC. The role of epidural anesthesia and analgesia in surgical practice. *Ann Surg.* 2003;238:663–673.

35. Bew SA, Bryant AE, Desborough JP, Hall GM. Epidural analgesia and arterial reconstructive surgery to the leg: effects on fibrinolysis and platelet degranulation. *Br J Anaesth.* 2001;86:230–235.

36. Christopherson R, Beattie C, Frank SM, et al. Perioperative morbidity in patients randomized to epidural or general anesthesia for lower extremity vascular surgery. Perioperative Ischemia Randomized Anesthesia Trial Study Group. *Anesthesiology.* 1993;79:422–434.

37. Tuman KJ, McCarthy RJ, March RJ, DeLaria GA, Patel RV, Ivankovich AD. Effects of epidural anesthesia and analgesia on coagulation and outcome after major vascular surgery. *Anesth Analg.* 1991;73:696–704.

38. Perkins FM, Kehlet H. Chronic pain as an outcome of surgery. A review of predictive factors. *Anesthesiology.* 2000;93:1123–1133.

39. Macrae WA. Chronic pain after surgery. *Br J Anaesth.* 2001;87:88–98.

40. Lavand'homme P, De Kock M, Waterloos H. Intraoperative epidural analgesia combined with ketamine provides effective preventive analgesia in patients undergoing major digestive surgery. *Anesthesiology.* 2005;103:813–820.

41. Fong HK, Sands LP, Leung JM. The role of postoperative analgesia in delirium and cognitive decline in elderly patients: a systematic review. *Anesth Analg.* 2006;102:1255–1266.

42. Vaurio LE, Sands LP, Wang Y, Mullen EA, Leung JM. Postoperative delirium: the importance of pain and pain management. *Anesth Analg.* 2006;102:1267–1273.

43. Sido B, Teklote JR, Hartel M, Friess H, Buchler MW. Inflammatory response after abdominal surgery. *Best Pract Res Clin Anaesthesiol.* 2004;18:439–454.

44. Buggy DJ, Doherty WL, Hart EM, Pallett EJ. Postoperative wound oxygen tension with epidural or intravenous analgesia: a prospective, randomized, single-blind clinical trial. *Anesthesiology.* 2002;97:952–958.

45. Beilin B, Shavit Y, Trabekin E, et al. The effects of postoperative pain management on immune response to surgery. *Anesth Analg.* 2003;97:822–827.

46. Yokoyama M, Itano Y, Katayama H, et al. The effects of continuous epidural anesthesia and analgesia on stress response and immune function in patients undergoing radical esophagectomy. *Anesth Analg.* 2005;101:1521–1527.

47. Exadaktylos AK, Buggy DJ, Moriarty DC, Mascha E, Sessler DI. Can anesthetic technique for primary breast cancer surgery affect recurrence or metastasis? *Anesthesiology.* 2006;105:660–664.

48. Block BM, Liu SS, Rowlingson AJ, Cowan AR, Cowan JA Jr, Wu CL. Efficacy of postoperative epidural analgesia: a meta-analysis. *JAMA.* 2003;290:2455–2463.

49. Wu CL, Cohen SR, Richman JM, et al. Efficacy of postoperative patient-controlled and continuous infusion epidural analgesia versus intravenous patient-controlled analgesia with opioids: a meta-analysis. *Anesthesiology.* 2005;103:1079–1088.

50. Richman JM, Liu SS, Courpas G, et al. Does continuous peripheral nerve block provide superior pain control to opioids? A meta-analysis. *Anesth Analg.* 2006;102:248–257.

51. Wu CL, Naqibuddin M, Rowlingson AJ, Lietman SA, Jermyn RM, Fleisher LA. The effect of postoperative analgesia on quality-of-life measurements. *Anesth Analg.* 2003;97:1078–1085.

52. Royse C, Royse A, Soeding P, Blake D, Pang J. Prospective randomized trial of high thoracic epidural analgesia for coronary artery bypass surgery. *Ann Thorac Surg.* 2003;75:93–100.

53. DeCherney AH, Bachmann G, Isaacson K, Gall S. Postoperative fatigue negatively impacts the daily lives of patients recovering from hysterectomy. *Obstet Gynecol.* 2002;99:51–57.

54. Anderson AD, McNaught CE, MacFie J, Tring I, Barker P, Mitchell CJ. Randomized clinical trial of multimodal optimization and standard perioperative surgical care. *Br J Surg.* 2003;90:1497–504.

55. Cronin AJ, Keifer JC, Davies MF, King TS, Bixler EO. Postoperative sleep disturbance: influences of opioids and pain in humans. *Sleep.* 2001;24:39–44.

56. Liu SS, Wu CL. Effect of postoperative analgesia on major postoperative complications: a systematic update of the evidence. *Anesth Analg.* 2007;104:689–702.

57. Carli F, Mayo N, Klubien K, Schricker T, Trudel J, Belliveau P. Epidural analgesia enhances functional exercise capacity and health-related quality of life after colonic surgery: results of a randomized trial. *Anesthesiology.* 2002;97:540–549.

58. Myles PS, Hunt JO, Nightingale CE, et al. Development and pyschometric testing of a quality of life recovery score after general anesthesia and surgery in adults. *Anesth Analg.* 1999;88:83–90.

59. Leslie K, Troedel S, Irwin K, et al. Quality of recovery from anesthesia in neurosurgical patients. *Anesthesiology.* 2003;99:1158–1165.

60. Sauaia A, Min SJ, Leber C, Erbacher K, Abrams F, Fink R. Postoperative pain management in elderly patients: correlation between adherence to treatment guidelines and patient satisfaction. *J Am Geriatr Soc.* 2005;53:274–282.

61. Myles PS, Williams DL, Hendrata M, Anderson H, Weeks AM. Patient satisfaction after anaesthesia and surgery: results of a prospective survey of 10811 patients. *Br J Anaesth.* 2000;84:6–10.

62. Jamison RN, Ross MJ, Hoopman P, et al. Assessment of postoperative pain management: patient satisfaction and perceived helpfulness. *Clin J Pain.* 1997;13:229–236.

63. Kehlet H, Dahl JB. Anaesthesia, surgery, and challenges in postoperative recovery. *Lancet.* 2003;362:1921–1928.

42

Research in Acute Pain Management

Craig T. Hartrick and Garen Manvelian

The current revision of this textbook is a testament to the ongoing evolution of new techniques, agents, and devices specifically for the management of acute pain. Medical practice generally has concurrently evolved to a state where clinical practices are increasingly guided by thoughtful review of the best available evidence. Consequently, the ability to judge the evidence from clinical trials, no longer the exclusive province of editors and academics, is now of primary importance to all clinicians.

Clinical analgesic trials serve two masters. Regulatory agencies require evidence of safety and efficacy. Practitioners require clinically relevant evidence to establish or modify best practices in caring for their patients. The resultant jargon, acronyms, and procedural peculiarities that accompany the merger of these two purposes can present a challenge to clinicians not familiar with research methods as they attempt to judge the quality and practical applicability of this evidence. Similarly, the terminology used to provide the rationale behind the clinical trial process can seem like a language unto itself. The purpose of this chapter is to briefly translate some of the more common terms, explain the rationale behind their use and misuse, and point out frequently encountered pitfalls in trial design. Our intention in this brief introduction to the interpretation of clinical trials is to assist the research naïve clinician to better evaluate the quality of published analgesic studies.

WHAT IS THE PURPOSE OF A CLINICAL TRIAL?

A clinical trial is a prospective research study to evaluate effects of intervention, pharmacologic, or biological product(s) or use of a device in human volunteers. A clinical trial can be initiated by various public or private organizations, government agencies, universities, and/or individual investigators. The clinical trials vary significantly based on goals they are set to pursue. When designed and executed appropriately, the clinical trials generate valid data, which in turn play a very important (if not the most important) role in evidence-based medicine.

There are international and country-specific regulations governing the conduct of clinical trials in human subjects, such as the Declaration of Helsinki and the Guidelines for Good Clinical Practice (GCP) of the International Conference of Harmonization (ICH). Even though basic principles of these regulations, such as " . . . ethical and scientific quality standard for designing, conducting, recording and reporting trials . . . "[1] are applicable to all clinical trials, they are specifically aimed for trials to be submitted to regulatory authorities for marketing approval of new products. These clinical trials are commonly classified as phase 1, 2, 3, or 4, with the understanding that the drug/device product progresses through these phases gradually. Sometimes it is difficult to classify a clinical trial into 1 phase or another, but general study phase objectives are outlined below.

Phase 1 clinical trials are usually performed in healthy male volunteers (not patients) in a specialized clinic providing around-the-clock observation. These trials are designed to determine pharmacologic actions of a drug with specific emphasis on clinical pharmacology related to absorption, distribution, metabolism, and elimination (ADME). Also, phase 1 trials may evaluate drug exposure with respect to certain subpopulations (eg, gender, age, subjects with impaired hepatic or renal function) and food effect. Further, phase 1 clinical trials may evaluate effect of certain concomitant medications on metabolism of a drug or effect of a drug on selected concomitant medications. Another important goal of a phase 1 trial can be to establish tolerability to a drug product at dose levels higher than the projected clinical dose. Phase 2 clinical trials are conducted in patients and usually are controlled and blinded. They are designed to begin the evaluation of the effectiveness of the drug for a particular indication and to determine short-term side effects and risks associated with the drug. Importantly, the goal of these trials is to estimate safe and effective doses and explore relevant study methodologies for future phase 3 studies. After establishing the initial pharmacokinetics and understanding basic safety and efficacy, phase 3 studies commence with selected doses. Phase 3 trials, also usually controlled and blinded, are conducted in patients under "real-life" conditions. They are designed to confirm the efficacy and safety profiles in a specific target population. Phase 4 clinical trials, which typically take place after marketing approval, further refine safety and efficacy in the general population and, in additional sub-populations, address dose recommendations in specific clinical situations, identify less common adverse effects, and evaluate new end points (eg, pharmacoeconomics).

HOW DO WE KNOW THE TRIAL WAS CONDUCTED APPROPRIATELY?

All clinical trials must adhere to high ethical standards. It is seldom that all subjects/patients participating in a clinical trial benefit from it directly because of the fact that the currently accepted standard for clinical trials employs randomization with the consequent chance of being assigned to a placebo treatment arm or to inadequate treatment due to dose evaluation. As a result, every clinical protocol must have built-in criteria for adequate rescue medications or intervention or patient withdrawal on demand from the trial. When there is a conflict between the needs of the particular clinical trial and the needs of the subject/patient, the best interest of the subject should always prevail.

To ensure that procedures employed by the protocol are consistent with sound research methodology, and to evaluate the risk/benefit ratio to subjects, each protocol must be evaluated by an Institution Review Board (IRB). Responsibilities of the IRB do not end with the initial approval. IRB must continue evaluating the clinical trial at intervals appropriate to the degree of risk associated with the trial but not less that once per year. In addition to the protocol review and approval, the IRB must ensure that the informed consent presented to the subject adequately describes the clinical trial at a language level (eighth grade) understandable to the subject or the representative. With rare exception, no subject can be involved in a clinical trial without obtaining effective informed consent of the subject or the subject's legally authorized representative. This consent needs to be obtained under circumstances that provide the prospective subject or representative sufficient opportunity to consider whether to participate while minimizing the possibility of coercion or undue influence. In light of the above, administration of the consent to the subject the morning of surgery for a clinical trial evaluating a pre-, intra- or postoperative investigational product may be viewed as inadequate unless additional efforts are made to ensure ample time is given to the subject to evaluate his/her participation in the trial (eg, presentation and discussion of the protocol by study personnel in advance by phone or during earlier visit or by simply mailing the consent form to the subject).

The pharmaceutical industry has been long criticized as biased by publishing and promoting only positive trial results. In a response to this critique, the Pharmaceutical Research and Manufacturers of America (PhRMA) announced their commitment for timely communication of meaningful results of controlled clinical trials of marketed or investigational products that are approved for marketing, regardless of outcome. This initiative is voluntary and is not guaranteed.[2] Further, in addressing this issue the International Committee of Medical Journal Editors (ICMJE) member journals require authors to register their trial in a registry that meets several criteria. The registry must be accessible to the public at no charge. It must be open to all prospective registrants and managed by a not-for-profit organization. There must be a mechanism to ensure the validity of the registration data and the registry should be electronically searchable. An acceptable registry must include at minimum the

data elements in the following table (Table 42.1). Trial registration with missing fields or fields that contain uninformative terminology is inadequate.[3] One such database meeting these requirements was established by the U.S. National Institutes of Health (NIH), through its National Library of Medicine (NLM). This database (ClinicalTrials.gov)[4] was developed in collaboration with the Food and Drug Administration (FDA) as a result of the FDA Modernization Act, which was passed into law in November 1997. In May 2007, ClinicalTrials.gov contained over 36 000 clinical studies sponsored by the National Institutes of Health, other federal agencies, and private industry. Finally, all participants in the peer review and publication process must disclose all relationships that could be viewed as presenting a potential conflict of interest.[5]

In addition, FDA requires sponsors to collect and file with a new drug application financial disclosure of investigators participating in pivotal registration trials. As a rule, pharmaceutical companies check the debarment list published by FDA for firms or persons debarred from assisting or performing clinical investigation.[5]

DID THE AUTHORS ESTABLISH A TESTABLE, CLINICALLY RELEVANT STUDY QUESTION?

The trial objectives, both primary and secondary, must be clearly stated a priori. The subsequent trial design and its end points must establish the framework as to how these objectives are to be assessed and define the patient population on which the clinical trial is to be conducted. The objectives of the trial must be very specific, such as "to evaluate pharmacokinetic profile of . . . ," "to compare efficacy of medicine X vs. Y," or "to assess dose response of . . . ," and so on. It is important to keep in mind that if many objectives are built into a single clinical trial, the subsequent data analyses may be cumbersome or impossible (not adequate patient representation) and it may impact statistical power of the study. Noncritical, secondary objectives may be presented in the trial for exploratory purposes only, which in turn may help to design subsequent trial(s). When primary objectives fall short, the tendency to seek positive findings through multiple comparisons, subgroup analyses, and other data chasing maneuvers reduces the clinical impact accordingly, even when statistically significant.

The nature of the compound under evaluation (eg, nonsteroidal anti-inflammatory drugs [NSAIDs] vs opioids) will determine the appropriate patient population and choice of the comparator or control. As the following sections will show, the ideal study question should be feasible, novel, ethical, and relevant.[6] Pitfalls related to each of these factors are possible.

HOW WAS THE PRIMARY EFFICACY VARIABLE DEFINED?

After the establishment of the study question, there is perhaps no more important feature of a clinical report than a clearly defined primary efficacy variable. The reader should at once be able to see that the measure selected accurately captures the most salient efficacy information and that this information will answer the study question. Feasibility then relates to the ability of the primary outcome variable to be directly measured. It is paramount

Table 42.1: Minimal Registration Data Set.[a]

	Item	Comment
1.	Unique trial number	The unique trial number will be established be the primary registering entity (the registry)
2.	Trial registration date	The date of registration will be established by the primary registering entity
3.	Secondary IDs	May be assigned by sponsors or other interested parties (there may be none)
4.	Funding source(s)	Name of the organization(s) that provided funding for the study
5.	Primary sponsor	The main entity responsible for performing the research
6.	Secondary sponsor(s)	The secondary entities, if any, responsible for performing the research
7.	Responsible contact person	Public contact person for the trial, for patients interested in participating
8.	Research contact person	Person to contact for scientific inquiries about the trial
9.	Title of the study	Brief title chosen by the research group (can be omitted if the researchers wish)
10.	Official scientific title of the study	This title must include the name of the intervention, the condition being studied, and the outcome (eg, The International Study of Digoxin and Death from Congestive Heart Failure)
11.	Research ethics review	Has the study at the time of registration received appropriate ethics committee approval (yes/no)? (It is assumed that all registered trials will be approved by an ethics board before commencing.)
12.	Condition	The medical condition being studied (eg, asthma, myocardial infarction, depression)
13.	Intervention(s)	A description of the study and comparison/control intervention(s) (for a drug or other product registered for public sale anywhere in the world, this is the generic name; for an unregistered drug, the generic name or company serial number is acceptable). The duration of the intervention(s) must be specified.
14.	Key inclusion and exclusion criteria	Key patient characteristics that determine eligibility for participation in the study.
15.	Study type	Database should provide drop-down lists for selection. This would include choices for randomized versus nonrandomized, type of masking (eg, double-blinded, single-blinded), type of controls (eg, placebo, active), and group assignment, (eg, parallel, crossover, factorial)
16.	Anticipated trial start date	Estimated enrollment date of the first participant
17.	Target sample size	The total number of subjects the investigators plan to enroll before closing the trial to new participants.
18.	Recruitment status	Is this information available (yes/no) (If yes, link to information).
19.	Primary outcome	The primary outcome that the study was designed to evaluate Description should include the time at which the outcome is measured (e.g., blood pressure at 12 months)
20.	Key secondary outcomes	The secondary outcomes specified in the protocol. Description should include time of measurement (e.g., creatinine clearance at 6 months).

[a] The data fields were specified at a meeting convened by the WHO in April 2005; the explanatory comments are largely from the ICMJE.

that the primary efficacy variable be defined in advance of the conduct of the study as it is the key to the design of the entire study. Consequently, the validity of the result is severely compromised when failure to firmly establish the primary efficacy variable turns the study into a fishing expedition.

Making objective assumptions about a subjective pain experience is the Achilles' heel of analgesic clinical trials. Although positron emission tomography, functional magnetic resonance imaging, and other technologies may allow us to quantitatively measure sensory and affective elements of analgesic trials independently,[7] the patients' interpretation of the overall integrated pain experience is best reflected by their response. A number of scales have been validated as a means of assessing pain levels at a given point in time. Other scales assess alternative dimensions of the pain experience such as pain relief or impressions of change and require subjects to remember their previous pain state and then make the appropriate judgments. Self-reports of pain, relief of pain, and global assessments of pain relief remain the best, although imperfect, measures by which analgesics are judged.

Pain Measurement

Pain measurements can be nominal (yes or no), categorical (often arranged as Likert scales with increasing degrees of pain), or continuous measures that may have ratio characteristics. Previously referred to as the gold standard for self-reported pain in analgesic studies, the visual analog scale (VAS) is an example of the latter. Typically the VAS for pain is a 10-cm horizontal line anchored at the left with the number 0 and the comment *no pain* and anchored on the right with the number 10 and the comment *worst pain possible*. The subject is asked to place a single vertical mark on the line at the point that corresponds to their present pain intensity. The resultant score determined by measuring the distance from the left-hand anchor (0) to the point where the vertical line crosses the horizontal. Because subjects are free to choose any point along the line, a continuous range of choices is available and in most circumstances the VAS is considered a *ratio* measure.[8] Continuous ratio variables may be manipulated arithmetically, which is a major advantage.

The numeric rating scale (NRS) has certain similarities to the VAS. Here the subject verbally reports a score on an 11-point scale, from 0 to 10, again where 0 represents *no pain* and 10 represents the *worst pain possible*. Clearly NRS scores should never be intermingled with VAS scores: the VAS is continuous; the NRS uses 11 discrete, ranked, whole number responses. Still, the NRS has often been considered a ratio measure and thus a suitable substitute for VAS.[9] Caution must be advised, however, as this ratiolike relationship does not apply in all circumstances.[10] Unless the NRS has been demonstrated to be a ratio measure in the specific study situation, it would be arguably better treated with nonparametric statistical methods, thus avoiding assumptions regarding the population distribution.

Ordered categorical pain measurement instruments commonly used include assessment of present pain intensity using the 4-point verbal rating scale (VRS: none = 0; mild = 1; moderate = 2; severe = 3), and for evaluating change in pain intensity the 5-point pain relief scale (no relief = 0; a little = 1; moderate = 2; a lot = 3; complete = 4), and a 7-point patient global impression of change scale (PGIC). The assignment of numerical values is arbitrary: arithmetic operations involving these values should be limited. Continuous and categorical pain measurement scales are presented in Chapter 11, *Qualitative and Quantitative Assessment of Pain*.

Significant Pain Reduction

To study pain, some pain must be present. How much pain needs to be present to ensure studies performed are sufficiently sensitive to evaluate analgesics remains a significant issue. A clinically analogous dilemma arises when one considers how much pain should be present before an intervention is offered. The VAS is often used to determine the point at which pain intervention may be required. Just as some trial designs may require moderate pain or a VAS pain score of "4 cm" prior to subject randomization, institutional credentialing bodies may determine that pain scores at or above "4 cm" ethically require intervention. This breakpoint is commonly considered the division between "mild" and "moderate" pain. The pathophysiology underlying this, however, may relate to the nature of the nociceptors themselves or to

psychometric peculiarities wherein subjects are unconsciously relaying additional embedded satisfaction information. Consequently, an exponential rise in response may occur once a certain stimulus threshold is reached. There is no reason to assume that any simple arithmetic relationship holds up, for example, in the transition from "moderate" to "severe" pain, as once the threshold is crossed the rise in reported pain might not be linear with increasing stimulus intensity.[11] This highlights the need to avoid the common mistake of treating values artificially assigned to *ordinal* measures with simple arithmetic manipulations.

Fortunately, when used to make individual patient comparisons of *pain relief*, a remarkably linear response does seem to apply. Bernstein et al[12] reported that when simultaneously using the VAS and the 5-point pain relief scale the difference between *no relief* and *mild relief, mild relief* and *moderate relief,* and *moderate relief* and *a lot of relief* was 2.2, 1.8, and 1.8 cm on the VAS, respectively. This finding has other practical implications in trial design. The minimally clinically meaningful change in pain is commonly defined as 2 cm,[13] which correlates nicely with movement from one pain relief category to another. Additionally, PGIC categories of *much improved* and *very much improved* have been used to determine the minimally significant change in NRS.[14] A 30% reduction in NRS was needed regardless of the initial pain level. Therefore higher baseline pain levels required larger reductions making the NRS, as previously noted, nonlinear.[10]

Still, there is a long history of assigning numerical scores to categorical measures for pain and then manipulating these scores arithmetically as if they were ratio measures.[15] The justification has been that good correlations have been observed between these Likert scales for pain (perhaps even more so for *pain relief* scales) and continuous measures. In analyzing individual patient data from 11 postoperative pain trials, including in excess of 1000 subjects, Collins et al[16] reported the VAS (100-mm scale) for moderate pain was 49±17 mm (mean±SD) and for severe pain was 75±18 mm. Nevertheless, despite seemingly good correlation at these two specific points (*moderate* and *severe*), intermediate points on the Likert scales were not examined. Therefore one should not necessarily assume a linear relationship from 0 to 100 mm. Other possibilities exist, such as a sigmoid-shaped curve with an inflection point at 50 mm. It should therefore be borne in mind that categorical variables with arbitrarily assigned numerical values for pain, although frequently manipulated as if they were continuous variables, are not ratio measures. This becomes of further practical significance when we go on to add, subtract, divide, and otherwise manipulate these arbitrary values; the more the values are remanufactured, the greater the disparities between computed and actual results may become.

Although self-report is by far the preferred method of assessment, observational methods are needed when subjects have cognitive impairment, are under the influence of sedatives or anesthetic agents, or have not yet reached the developmental age required for abstract reasoning needed to understand of the concept of proportions. In contrast to the limited number of observational pain scales for cognitively impaired adults, a number of age-specific observational scales are used in pediatrics. There is also evidence that some scales may be preferred in distinguishing painful from nonpainful (related to anesthetic emergence, separation-anxiety, etc.) postoperative situations.[17] Importantly, regardless of how they are scored, observational pain scores must be treated as ordinal measures.

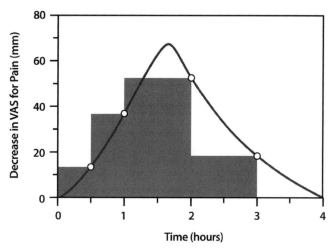

Figure 42.1: In this example, the curve represents the theoretical analgesic effect of a treatment. Intermittent pain measurements taken at 30 minutes, 1 hour, and 2 and 3 hours following administration resulted in decreases in VAS for pain from the baseline measurement (at time = 0) of 16, 36, 52, and 18 mm, respectively. The product of the elapsed time since the last measurement and the change in VAS represent TOTPAR (total pain relief; shaded area), which approximates the area under the curve (AUC).

Summary Measures

Thus far the pain measures discussed have been derived from snapshots in time. Although differences in pain scores following specific interventions are calculated, no understanding of the total amount of suffering, or at any time points between the measurements can be inferred. Attempts to quantify a total "amount" of pain could theoretically be derived by continuously measuring a ratio measure of pain over a period of time and then using calculus to integrate the curve, thus establishing a "total quantity" of pain suffered (area under the curve, AUC) over the entire study. Aside from the fact that near-continuous assessments are impractical, they also would affect the outcome, thus confounding the measurements. However, regularly spaced assessments are used in this fashion as a crude approximation to better capture the overall pain experience. One must be mindful of the fact that the spacing of the assessments can unwittingly skew the results, especially when the measurement intervals are unequal, even when properly weighted. Additional philosophical questions also arise with practical clinical relevance: is a prolonged period with a VAS of 5 worse than a brief period at 10?

One commonly used summary measure is total pain relief (TOTPAR). When reductions in pain intensity (ie, pain relief), as measured ideally using the VAS (or other validated ratio measure), are measured over time, the time-weighted resultant summation value (approximating the AUC) is termed TOTPAR (Figure 42.1). The related measure, summed pain intensity difference (SPID), considers differences in baseline pain intensity. SPID is calculated in an analogous fashion to TOTPAR, but instead of using pain relief scores, SPID uses PID (pain intensity difference scores). PID scores are derived by subtracting each subsequent score from the baseline value. Positive PID scores are also a measure of "pain relief." Various other mathematical manipulations are commonly used, such as %SPID, where SPID is divided by the maximum possible SPID that would be obtained if the subject were pain free throughout the entire observation

period. The justification for this further manipulation is a correction to account for the potentially much larger reduction in pain in subjects starting with higher initial pain scores.

The concept of a percentage of subjects experiencing the maximum analgesic effect (%maxTOTPAR) has been used to compare analgesics and as a means of combining data to perform meta-analyses.[18] It can also be used to calculate number needed to treat (NNT) values. The number of patients you would need to treat to have one patient with at least 50% pain relief is one definition of NNT that on the surface would appear to have clear clinical implications. The addition of 95% confidence interval (95%CI; if repeated, 19 of 20 confidence intervals on average would contain the population mean) places the NNT data in perspective. Yet direct extrapolation of NNT data from a given study to other pain models remains clinically suspect.[19] Agents with differing modes of action might behave differently in various clinical circumstances, making direct comparisons only valid for similar settings. For example, an agent with strong anti-inflammatory properties may work better than a strong opioid in inflammatory pain settings but less well in the absence of inflammation. The commonly accepted use of pooled TOTPAR values derived from categorical measures, instead of continuous measures, might also contribute to the difficulties in generalization.

The odds ratio (OR) represents an alternative method for analgesic efficacy comparisons. The odds of a given event occurring (such as the odds of experiencing at least 50% relief), divided by the odds of an alternative event (the placebo or comparator analgesic producing at least 50% relief) defines the OR. As with the NNT, OR analysis lends itself to the analysis of dichotomous adverse events, such as the presence or absence of nausea. For example, if treatment A resulted in 4 of 10 subjects becoming nauseated (6 subjects not nauseated; odds of nausea 4/6 or 0.67), and treatment B resulted in nausea in 6 of 10 subjects (odds of nausea 6/4 or 1.5), then the OR is 0.44 (0.67 divided by 1.5). An odds ratio of 1 represents even money, equal odds. An odds ratio of less than 1 means the event is less likely in the first group; conversely an odds ratio of greater than 1 means the event is more likely in the first group. Once again the confidence interval provides needed perspective. Not only does the CI reflect a dichotomous (yes or no) judgment regarding the statistical significance, the magnitude of its range provides a sense of precision, potentially affecting the clinical significance. A narrow range, as may be seen in large studies with many subjects, suggests greater credibility. Again, if the 95%CI includes the value 1, then the chance of "even money" (ie, no significant difference between groups) falls within that range of probability. Relative risk (RR), defined as the ratio of probabilities (example above: 4/10 divided by 6/10), is perhaps more intuitive but not always easily determined because we often arbitrarily assign subjects into equal groups, thus distorting true incidence (and probability) information. Odds, rather than probabilities, are the basis for a number of statistical approaches. Moreover, the reciprocal relationship between the odds in favor and the odds against an event are additional mathematical benefits. These mathematical advantages often translate into greater utility in the clinical setting.

In an attempt to evaluate the performance of investigational drugs in clinical trial settings, Silverman et al[20] proposed an integrated assessment of the pain scores and rescue morphine used during the same evaluation period. Each parameter is expressed as a percent difference from the mean rank for that variable in the overall study population. The percentage differences for each parameter are summated on a per-subject basis. The data can be analyzed comparing the treatment groups with standard statistical tests. Although unpublished, we have successfully utilized this method in several clinical trials.

The Initiative on Methods, Measurement, and Pain Assessment in Clinical Trials (IMMPACT) group recommended the adoption of 6 core outcomes in chronic pain analgesic studies (pain, physical functioning, emotional functioning, ratings of improvement and satisfaction with treatment, symptoms and adverse effects, and subject disposition).[21] Health-related quality of life (HRQoL), functional outcomes, time to discharge, ease of care, and pharmacoecomomic measures are increasingly frequent secondary outcomes in acute pain analgesic trials. HRQoL share certain characteristics with global indices wherein they rely on the subjects' memory for pain and other health-related measures. Although memory for pain has long been regarded with skepticism, recent evidence supports its use in the design and implementation of pain assessment instruments.[22]

HOW DOES THE STUDY DESIGN AFFECT INTERPRETATION?

Ethical considerations require that all subjects be afforded access to analgesics in the presence of conditions that are expected to be painful. The analgesic-sparing or *morphine-sparing* design is common. With this approach subjects in each group may be afforded equal opportunity for analgesia in which theoretically may result in equivalent pain scores. In this case, comparisons are made with respect to the amount of additional rescue analgesic required (or spared) to achieve adequate pain control. As a result, various end points can be defined with respect to the lower bound of the CI corresponding to inferiority, equivalence, or superiority. These designs can be used with active comparator agents, yet do not preclude the use of placebo, as a sham/placebo group also has access to rescue analgesia. Interpretation of trial results based on this endpoint from the clinician's standpoint is difficult, because "clinically meaningful" opioid-sparing effect is not defined. Further, regulatory agencies are reluctant to accept this as a primary end point.

Randomized controlled trials (RCT), especially when double blinded and placebo controlled, are considered to provide the highest level of evidence in the establishment of best practice. This gold standard has recently come into question, especially as it relates to the study of invasive analgesic techniques.[23] Double-blind, double-dummy designs generally have two treatment groups. One group receives active treatment A and sham treatment B, whereas the other group receives active treatment B and sham treatment A. Double-blind, double-dummy designs, although cumbersome, offer the advantage of canceling out the "novelty" factor associated with new technology. Additional ethical considerations involving the use of placebo in clinical trial design are discussed elsewhere.[24]

The a priori determination of how missing data (inevitable in longitudinal studies) will be handled is critical to study design. The proper handling of missing data is not only important because of a loss of power (fewer observations), but data missing "not at random" can introduce bias that complicates interpretation of the study results. For example, subjects may withdraw because of factors related to an outcome measure. Whether missing data values will be ignored or imputed, either based on data

points before and after the missing point or by carrying forward the last recorded value, can have significant effects of summated measures. The choice of one approach over another should be dictated by the clinical relevance and will vary depending on the variable being measured.

Although there can be many definitions, commonly the intention-to-treat (ITT) analysis considers all subjects randomized, regardless of whether they follow or complete the protocol. With this definition the pendulum has swung to the extreme. In an attempt to guard against bias introduced when dropout is related to outcome, subjects are included in the treatment group who may not have actually been exposed to the treatment if that is where they were originally assigned. At worst this process can confuse the interpretation of the results and at best it dilutes the results if one assumes that dropouts, because of events unrelated to the outcome, will occur in equal frequencies in all groups. The addition of a Consolidated Standards of Reporting Trials (CONSORT diagram) is of significant benefit in interpreting RCT trials and is required by many journal editors.[25] The progress of subjects through a trial and the reasons for discontinuation are clarified using the CONSORT diagram, thus aiding interpretation and clinical application (Figure 42.2).

Bias control for confounding effects extends beyond randomization and the use of placebo and sham. The observers may affect the subjects' response in ways that might not be readily apparent. For example, both the gender and professional status of the observer can affect subjects' pain score.[26] In an experimental pain setting, subjects tolerated pain longer when they were tested by an observer of the opposite sex and when the observer was considered a professional. Further, higher pain intensities were reported when tested by females. Other subtle cues can bias responses, making specific scripting when questioning subjects ideal.

Finally, crossover trials are sometimes used to control for bias introduced by interindividual differences in subjects. Instead of matching subjects in different groups for comparison, each subject serves as his/her own control by sequentially receiving both treatments. Inherent in the design is the assumption that the order of treatment has no bearing on the results. This assumption can be valid only if there is no carryover effect from the initial treatment that might contaminate the results of the subsequent treatment. Typically a "washout" period is defined in an attempt to reduce carryover effects. The clinical relevance of this interval must be carefully assessed as other motivations in the design of the trial may be at play to shorten this period. The ethical need to limit periods without treatment and to reduce dropout of subjects due to reduced satisfaction when the trial periods are drawn out are practical design considerations. Moreover, although the crossover design lends itself well to the comparison of 2 alternative treatments, analysis and interpretation are somewhat more complicated when 3 or more groups are studied, such as in dose-finding trials or combination therapy trials. As in the examples previously mentioned, assuring that the appropriate nonparametric tests are used for categorical measures that account for period effects, when necessary, is critical to the believability of the results.

ARE THE RESULTS BELIEVABLE?

Unfortunately, published reports where the authors have statistically treated categorical measurements as if it were normally

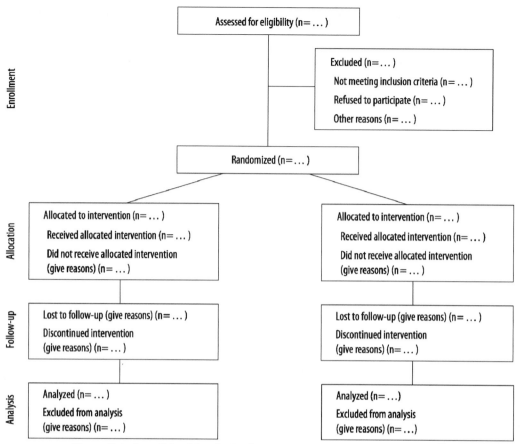

Figure 42.2: Consolidated Standards of Reporting Trials (CONSORT) diagram.[22]

distributed continuous values is not a rare occurrence. Although one expects the peer review process and editorial oversight to identify these errors before publication, vigilance in carefully dissecting clinical reports cannot be overemphasized. Yet believability goes beyond recognition of whether the correct statistical tests are selected for the type of data being analyzed. The results must be viewed within a clinically relevant context. Confidence intervals are aptly named and as previously mentioned help add perspective. But exactly what is the chance that the results presented in a clinical trial are spurious? This assessment requires consideration of several factors.

Most readers are familiar with type I errors, false positives, where a difference between groups is falsely declared. The risk of making this type of error is defined by the P value. A P value of .05 is most common, where the risk of a type I error (α) is 5% (ie, a 1 in 20 risk that the difference between groups is at least as large as that observed if the null hypothesis were true, no difference between groups). Although the statistical significance level is often set at 0.05, it too is arbitrary.[27] Clinically significant differences may well be accepted at other levels depending on the alternative risks. However, one might expect these significance levels to be defined prior to the onset of the trial and not raised later using terms such as *trend* to describe results that fail to meet predefined expectations.

Another approach is to consider the introduction of prior experience to guide the analysis. This could potentially be especially helpful for trials involving invasive techniques, as the approach might allow researchers to limit unnecessary exposure to sham procedures.[28] Bayesian statistical methods use this common sense approach based on prior experience but are infrequently used as researchers and editors often lack familiarity.[29] In this approach a "prior probability" (often based on previous clinical experience) is assigned and then modified after considering the study results to derive a "posterior probability." The probability that a given treatment is at least as good as another, although having no meaning when constrained by frequentist statistical analysis (testing against a null hypothesis), it is quite meaningful in Bayesian analysis.

Type II errors, false negatives, occur when a true difference exists between groups that goes undetected. This relates directly to the sample size because very small studies may not produce statistically significant results unless the difference between groups is very large. The risk of making this type of error (β) is commonly set at 0.20, meaning 2 times of 10 a true difference will be missed. Obviously this may be unacceptable in some circumstances. Clinically, if the risk of making this error is considered grievous, then the value can be appropriately adjusted, at the expense of exposing a greater number of subjects to the study. The *power* of a study is $1 - \beta$, often set at 80%. However, by way of example, if the risk of having a false negative result is set at 0.1, then the power is 0.9 or 90%. These values should be set prospectively and are used, along with assumptions as to the variability of the data (eg, standard deviations in the primary efficacy measure), to determine sample size. Failure to perform a power analysis before the study begins compromises the results, especially when negative findings are reported. Secondary end points, unless the study was powered to evaluate these outcomes should be, as the term *secondary* implies, viewed as lower tier findings. Suppose 20 different outcomes are examined: A P value of .05 would presume that perhaps 1 outcome would demonstrate a significant difference between groups purely by chance. The simplest method, although by no means the only way of dealing with multiple simultaneous comparisons, is the *Bonferroni correction*, where the α value is divided (for the entire set of comparisons) by the number of comparisons. This is arguably the most conservative approach to avoiding spurious conclusions.

The type of data and the nature of the comparisons to be made between groups dictate the appropriate statistical treatments. As mentioned previously, data can be nominal (dichotomous: yes or no), categorical (no relief, mild or a little relief, moderate relief, lots of relief, complete relief), or continuous (where a range of possible values exist: weight, blood pressure, VAS, etc). Further, the types of tests selected depend on whether the data set fits a normal (bell-shaped curve) or other well-defined distribution. Finally, repeated measures over time require special handling.

The most commonly used test for the comparison of two means is the t test. The validity of this approach depends on the equality of the standard deviations of each population. When the standard deviations for the 2 groups are very different and the sample size is small, alternative methods of analysis should be used. When the data consist of pairs of measurements, as in matched case-control studies, or when the same subject is exposed to 2 different treatments, paired t tests may be appropriate. When a well-characterized distribution of outcomes cannot be expected, such as when categorical variables are measured, nonparametric methods based on ranks must be used. In this sense, the Wilcoxon signed rank test is the nonparametric counterpart to the paired t test. Examining differences between multiple groups requires alternative methods such as the 1-way analysis of variance (ANOVA) or the nonparametric Kruskal-Wallis 2-way ANOVA. Correlations are similarly handled with parametric (correlation coefficient) or nonparametric (Spearman's rank correlation) approaches. Time to event measures are commonly assessed using Kaplan-Meier survival curves. Although many alternative methods are used, the distinction between parametric methods and nonparametric methods is of paramount importance. Critically, the aforementioned tests, although demonstrating relationships, do not assure causality. Common sense must always be the final check.

Assessing the relevance and, thus, the importance to everyday clinical practice likewise requires a pragmatic approach. The quality of individual published reports is greatly dependent on an impartial peer review process. Yet how specific reports then affect the larger body of work in an area of study speaks to the study's impact. Regardless of how impact is measured, conceptually a high-impact study is one that affects the clinicians' decision-making process. Redefining clinical pathways based on such evidence often requires synthesis of many, often conflicting, reports. The most commonly applied tool to facilitate this process is termed *meta-analysis*.

Meta-analyses attempting to assimilate quality data from many studies are themselves, however, prone to possible bias. Sampling bias can result from publication bias as well as bias introduced by indexing and search strategies. Selection bias as result of inclusion criteria should be clearly defined, whereas selector bias (when study results are considered as nonstated inclusion criteria) may be more difficult to detect. Bias introduced in the analysis itself may also affect the clinical applicability of the conclusions. Quality score bias is very possible unless the scoring system is strictly defined and the method of resolving disagreements between observers is defined. Length of follow-up is also difficult to control for, leading to time-dependent differences in conclusions drawn.

CONCLUSION

As is often the case, more questions have been raised than answers provided. One may rightly wonder that if a sham procedure produces a beneficial effect by virtue of both expectation and reward,[30] is it ethical to perform clinical trials that eliminate these effects? If so, are the results obtained, depriving the subjects of this added "placebo" benefit, clinically relevant because the clinical treatment of patients by its nature always comes with a certain context that may itself have meaning?[31] One might also question whether RCTs are in fact a gold standard, whether categorical pain assessments may be more clinically relevant that VAS scores, or whether P values actually have any value at all.

The design of clinical trials is beyond the scope of this discussion. Certainly future study designs that address these complex issues will emerge. The use of a "cumulative proportion of responders analysis" as a method to make clinical trial data more clinically relevant has recently been proposed and may represent one such advance.[32] Instead we have attempted to provide the reader with some insight into what to look for when reading the published report of a clinical trial, how to identify weaknesses or strengths that may decrease or bolster enthusiasm for the findings, and how to assess the clinically applicability of the results.

REFERENCES

1. ICH Harmonised Tripartite Guideline: Guideline for Good Clinical Practice, E6(R1). International Conference on Harmonisation. 1996. Available at: http://www.ich.org/LOB/media/MEDIA482. pdf. Accessed September 2, 2008.
2. Pharmaceutical Research and Manufacturers of America. Mission Statement. PhRMA: New Medicines, New Hope. 2008. Available at: http://www.phrma.org/mission_statement/. Accessed September 2, 2008.
3. International Committee of Medical Journal Editors. Obligation to Register Clinical Trials. Uniform Requirements for Manuscripts Submitted to Biomedical Journals: Writing and Editing for Biomedical Publication. 2007. Available at: http://www.icmje.org/ #clin_trials. Accessed September 2, 2008.
4. United States National Institutes of Health. Protocol Registration System. ClinicalTrials.gov. 2008. Available at: http://prsinfo. clinicaltrials.gov/. Accessed September 2, 2008.
5. Food and Drug Administration. Code of Federal Regulations: Title 21 – Food and Drugs; 21CFR1404.800. 2008. Available at: http://frwebgate4.access.gpo.gov/cgi-bin/waisgate.cgi? WAISdocID=37473784732+37+0+0&WAISaction=retrieve. Accessed September 2, 2008.
6. Cummings SR, Browner WS, Hulley SB. Conceiving the research question. In: Hulley SB, Cummings SR, eds. *Designing Clinical Research: An Epidemiologic Approach*. Baltimore, MD: Williams & Wilkins; 1988;12–17.
7. Geha PY, Baliki MN, Chialvo DR, Harden RN, Paice JA, Apkarian AV. Brain activity for spontaneous pain of postherpetic neuralgia

and its modulation by lidocaine patch therapy. *Pain*. 2007;128:88–100.

8. Price, DD, McGrath, PA, Rafii, A, Buckingham, B. The validation of visual analogue scales as ratio scale measures for chronic and experimental pain. *Pain*. 1983;17:45–56.

9. Breivik, EK, Bjornsson, GA, Skovlund, E. A comparison of pain rating scales by sampling from clinical trial data. *Clin J Pain*. 2000;16:22–28.

10. Hartrick CT, Kovan JP, Shapiro S. The numeric rating scale for clinical pain measurement: a ratio measure? *Pain Pract*. 2003;3:310–316.

11. Price, DD, Bush, FM, Long, S, Harkins, SW. A comparison of pain measurement characteristics of mechanical visual analogue and simple numerical rating scales. *Pain*. 1994;56:217–226.

12. Bernstein SL, Chang A, Esses D, Gallagher EJ. Relationship between intensity and relief in patients with acute, severe pain. *Acad Emerg Med*. 2005;12:158–159.

13. Farrar JT, Portenoy RK, Berlin JA, Kinman JL, Strom BL. Defining the clinically important difference in pain outcome measures. *Pain*. 2000;88:287–294.

14. Farrar JT, Young JP Jr, LaMoreaux L, Werth JL, Poole RM. Clinical importance of changes in chronic pain intensity measured on an 11-point numerical pain rating scale. *Pain*. 2002;96:410–411.

15. McQuay HJ, Moore RA. Postoperative analgesia and vomiting, with special reference to day-case surgery: a systematic review. *Health Technol Assessment*. 1998;2:17–21.

16. Collins SL, Moore A, McQuay HJ. The visual analogue pain intensity scale: what is moderate pain in millimeters? *Pain*. 1997;72:95–97.

17. Hartrick CT, Kovan JP. Pain assessment following general anesthesia using the Toddler Preschooler Postoperative Pain Scale: a comparative study. *J Clin Anesth*. 2002;14:411–415.

18. Moore A, Moore O, McQuay H, Gavaghan D. Deriving dichotomous outcome measures from continuous data in randomised controlled trials of analgesics: use of pain intensity and visual analogue scales. *Pain*. 1997;69:311–315.

19. Gray A, Kehlet H, Bonnet F, Rawal N. Predicting postoperative analgesia outcomes: NNT league tables or procedure-specific evidence? *Br J Anaesth*. 2005;94:710–714.

20. Silverman DG, O'Connor TZ, Brull SJ. Integrated assessment of pain scores and rescue morphine use during studies of analgesic efficacy. *Anesth Analg*. 1993;77:168–170.

21. Dworkin RH, Turk DC, Farrar JT, et al. Core outcome measures for chronic pain clinical trials: IMMPACT recommendations. *Pain*. 2005;113:9–19.

22. Jamison RN, Raymond SA, Slawsby EA, McHugo GJ, Baird JC. Pain assessment in patients with low back pain: comparison of weekly recall and momentary electronic data. *J Pain*. 2006;7:192–199.

23. Cahana A. Ethical and epistemological problems when applying evidence-based medicine to pain management. *Pain Pract*. 2005;5:298–302.

24. Koshi EB, Short CA. Placebo theory and its implications for research and clinical practice: a review of the recent literature. *Pain Pract*. 2007;7:4–20.

25. Moher D, Schulz KF, Altman D. The CONSORT Statement: revised recommendations for improving the quality of reporting for parallel-group randomized trials. *JAMA*. 2001;285:1987–1991.

26. Kallai I, Barke A, Voss U. The effects of experimenter characteristics on pain reports in women and men. *Pain*. 2004;112:142–147.

27. Goodman SN. Toward evidence-based medical statistics. 1. The P value fallacy. *Ann Intern Med*. 1999;130: 995–1004.

28. Hartrick CT. Low back pain: best evidence – best tools. *Pain Pract*. 2005;5:151–152.

29. Goodman SN. Toward evidence-based medical statistics. 2. The Bayes factor. *Ann Intern Med*. 1999;130:1005–1013.

30. Amanzio M, Benedetti F. Neuropharmacological dissection of placebo analgesia: expectation-activated opioid systems versus conditioning-activated specific subsystems. *J Neurosci*. 1999;19:484–494.

31. Moerman, Daniel E. The meaning response: thinking about placebos. *Pain Pract*. 2006;6:233–236.

32. Farrar JT, Dworkin RH, Max MB. Use of the cumulative proportion of responders analysis graph to present pain data over a range of cut-off points: making clinical trial data more understandable. *J Pain Symptom Manage*. 2006;31:369–377.

43

Quality Improvement Approaches in Acute Pain Management

Christine Miaskowski

Rapid advances in scientific knowledge and technology mandate that all clinicians actively engage in processes that evaluate the quality of care that they provide to patients and their family caregivers. Nearly a decade ago, the Institute of Medicine released two landmark reports on health care safety and quality, namely *To Err is Human* and *Crossing the Quality Chasm*.[1,2] These reports mobilized the health care system, as well as the public to demand changes in health care delivery when they noted that medical errors cause 44,000 to 98,000 deaths annually in the United States. In addition, differences in what should be done for patients and what actually is done accounts for more than $9 billion per year in lost productivity and nearly $2 billion per year in health care costs.[1,3]

Although these two Institute of Medicine reports helped to articulate a broad agenda for quality improvement in health care, progress in improving the quality of care has been relatively slow.[4] What appears to be slow progress is somewhat understandable because several recent reviews have acknowledged that the creation of reliable and sustained quality improvement approaches in acute care pose numerous challenges for clinicians.[3,5] Quality improvement efforts often require clinicians to change the structures and processes surrounding the delivery of patient care. However, clinicians may not have received education and training in how to develop and implement quality improvement initiatives. The purposes of this chapter include providing an overview of the basics of quality improvement, highlighting the major methodologies that can be used in quality improvement initiatives, and describing guidelines for and approaches to improve the quality of acute pain management.

DEFINITION OF QUALITY

Quality of health care was defined by the Institute of Medicine as care that is safe, timely, efficient, effective, equitable, and patient centered.[2] These terms are defined in Table 43.1. In addition, the Agency for Healthcare Research and Quality defined quality health care as doing the right thing, at the right time, in the

right way, for the right person – and having the best results.[6] These definitions need to guide the development of all quality improvement initiatives.[7,8]

Initial systematic efforts to evaluate quality came from industry's efforts to develop quality control standards for manufactured products. In the early 1980s, Deming recognized that the quality of a product was the primary driver for industrial success and introduced systematic measures to evaluate the quality of a variety of products to Japanese engineers and executives. The strategic application of these quality measures produced considerable growth, particularly in the Japanese automobile industry, and led to subsequent worldwide recognition of the importance of quality in the manufacturing of goods and services.[9,10]

MEASUREMENT OF QUALITY IN HEALTH CARE

Avedis Donabedian is considered to be the father of quality measurement in health care. In a recent review,[11] he described and evaluated the current methods for evaluating the quality of health care. He acknowledged that the measurement of quality in health care rests on a conceptual and operationalized definition of what "quality of health care" means. In addition, he noted that there will never be a single comprehensive criterion by which to measure the quality of patient care.

Donabedian championed the idea that quality measurement involved an evaluation of the structures, processes, and outcomes of care. Structural measures assess the availability and quality of resources, management systems, policies, guidelines, and organizational approaches to the provision of care. Structural measures are critical to sustaining processes of care over time. Process measures use the actual processes of health care delivery as an indicator of the quality of care. Usually, process measures examine what clinicians do or analyze the activities of clinicians to determine whether patient care is practiced according to specific standards or guidelines. Outcome indicators measure the end results of care. They depend not only on the results of patient care but also on genetic, environmental, and behavioral factors.

Table 43.1: Institute of Medicine's Definitions of the Elements of Quality Health Care

Aim	Definition
Safe	Freedom from accidental injury. To improve patient safety, health care organizations and professionals must establish and improve systems to minimize the likelihood of errors that do occur, and prevent or mitigate harm from errors that reach the patient.
Effective	The disciplined use of systematically-acquired knowledge to provide services that are likely to benefit patients and refrain from providing services not likely to benefit patients.
Patient centered	Health care that respects and honors patients' individual wants, needs, and preferences, and that assures that individual patients' values guide all decisions.
Timely	The flow of care, free of undesired waits and delays for both those who receive care and those who give care. The process flows smoothly and waiting times are continually reduced for both patients and those who give care.
Efficient	The continual reduction of waste in health care, especially waste stemming from errors and overuse of ineffective tests, medications, procedures, technologies, and other interventions. Waste includes any resource use that fails to help meet patients' needs including materials, supplies, time, forms, measurements, reports, motion, duplicated efforts, ideas not used and information that is lost.
Equitable	The care of populations and individuals. At a population level, the goal of a health care system is to improve health status for all Americans and to do so in a manner that reduces disparities among particular subgroups. For individuals, the provision of health care services should be based on individual needs and not on personal characteristics unrelated to their health condition. In particular, the quality of care should not differ solely because of such characteristics as sex, race, ethnicity, income, education, disability, sexual orientation, or location of residence.

Adapted from: Committee on Quality Health Care in America, Institute of Medicine. *Crossing the Quality Chasm: A New Health System for the 21st Century.* Washington, DC, National Academy Press; 2001.

In many quality of care studies, outcome indicators are presented based on an evaluation of a group of patients rather than as individual cases.[3,5,11] A list of the strengths and limitations of structure, process, and outcome indicators, as well as examples of each type of indicator relative to acute pain management, are presented in Table 43.2.

QUALITY IMPROVEMENT METHODOLOGIES

A shift has occurred in the evaluation of the quality of care from quality assurance to continuous quality improvement.[12–15] Continuous quality improvement promotes the principle that an opportunity for improvement exists in every process of care and on every occasion. Unlike the old quality assurance initiatives, continuous quality improvement initiatives focus on the development of strategies to improve the quality of patient care and not on the identification of individuals who did not perform to some standard of care. The implementation of continuous quality improvement initiatives requires that a health care organization makes a commitment to constantly improve operations, processes, and activities to meet patient care needs in an efficient, consistent, and cost-effective manner. The continuous quality improvement model emphasizes the view of health care as a process and focuses on the system rather than on the individual when considering how to improve the delivery of patient care.[3,12] The process of continuous quality improvement provides organizations with the ability to collect benchmark data, determine the effectiveness of various processes of care, and evaluate whether systematic changes in processes of care improve the quality of care that patients receive.[16,17]

To achieve the goal of continuous quality improvement in health care, specific methodologies need to be considered and used depending on the goal of the quality improvement initiative. The three most commonly used quality improvement methodologies in health care are plan-do-study-act (PDSA), six sigma, and lean strategies. The choice of a particular methodology depends on the nature of the quality improvement project and on the training of individuals within an organization in a particular methodology. Most of the methodologies use similar techniques. In addition, most of the methodologies include iterative testing of ideas and redesigns of a process of care based on the lessons learned from the quality improvement evaluation.[3] Each of these methodologies is summarized below.

PDSA Cycle

The PDSA cycle is the most common quality improvement methodology used to date. As illustrated in Figure 43.1, it involves a sequence of four repetitive steps (ie, plan, do, study, act) that is carried out repeatedly in a series of small cycles and eventually leads to exponential improvements. The planning part of the PDSA cycle involves the development of the objectives for the quality improvement study and the development of an action plan to carry out the study. In this phase of the PDSA cycle, the most critical step is the determination of which measures will be used to evaluate a specific structure, process, and/or outcome indicator. In the do phase of the cycle, the evaluation study is done and initial analysis of the study findings occur. As part of the study phase of the PDSA cycle, the study findings are reviewed and evaluated in the context of the outcome indicators. In the act phase, the study findings are presented to clinicians. During this phase, the findings are discussed, an action plan is developed with input from all of the relevant clinicians and stakeholders, and the action plan is implemented. Those individuals involved in the quality improvement initiative will determine when the next PDSA cycle will be repeated to evaluate the magnitude of the improvements that occurred as a result of the action plan. More specific details on implementing the PDSA approach within the context of a continuous quality improvement initiative for acute pain management are provided in subsequent sections of this chapter.

Selection of Quality Measures

As mentioned, one of the most difficult tasks within the PDSA cycle is the selection of quality measures based on the quality indicators chosen for a particular project. Quality indicators

Table 43.2: Strengths and Limitations of Structure, Process, and Outcome Quality Indicators and Examples of Acute Pain Management Indicators

Indicator	Strengths	Limitations	Example of an Acute Pain Management Indicator
Structure	Deals with concrete information and accessible information	The relationship between structure, process, and outcome measures are not well established	Patient controlled analgesia pumps are available on all surgical units
Process	Emphasis is placed on whether or not what is known to be "good patient care" was applied Requires that attention be given to specifying the relevant dimensions, values, and standards to be used in the assessment	The estimates of quality may be less stable and less final than those that derive from outcome measures	Pain intensity is documented at frequent intervals
Outcome	Frequently used indicator Validity of the outcome measure is not questioned Outcome measures tend to be concrete measures important to patients	Is it the most relevant measure to evaluate the quality of patient care (eg, survival in the context of palliative care) Many factors other than patient care can influence or confound an outcome measure Some outcomes (e.g., patient satisfaction) are difficult to measure	Acute pain is prevented and controlled to a degree that facilitates function and quality of life

can be classified as structure, process, or outcome indicators that require different types of quality measures. The specific features that define a good quality measure are listed in Table 43.3.[18,19] Although members of the team that will evaluate the quality of acute pain management do not need to test the validity, reliability, and responsiveness of every quality measure, they need to ascertain that the specific measures they choose to use as part of a quality improvement project have all of these features. Specific quality measures for acute pain management are discussed later in this chapter.

Six Sigma

A recent methodology to promote and enhance quality that has caught the attention of the health care field is six sigma. This approach was developed by Motorola and refined over the past

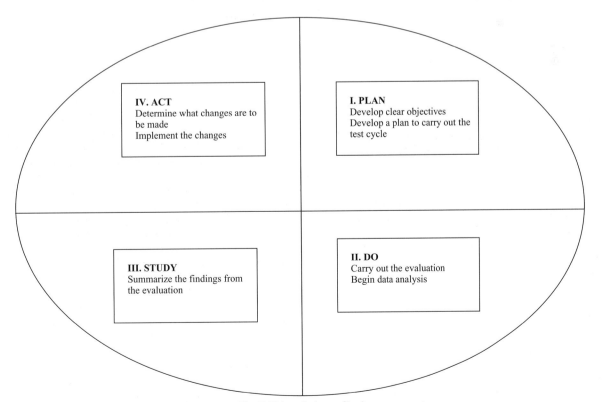

Figure 43.1: The PCSA cycle in quality improvement.

Table 43.3: Features of a Good Quality Measure

Feature	Description
Important	For outcome indicators
	High prevalence outcomes
	Outcomes associated with significant consequences (e.g., morbidity, mortality)
	For structure and process indicators:
	Measure must be linked to clinically important outcomes
	Individuals involved in the quality improvement project need to consider the quality measure important
	Different measures may need to be selected to meet the need of various constituencies (e.g., patients, family members, clinicians, administrators)
Valid	A valid measure refers to the extent to which a measure reflects what it is supposed to measure.
Reliable	A reliable measure refers to the extent to which a measure yields the same result when assessed by a different rater (interrater reliability) or the extent to which repeated measurement provides the same result when the factor being measured has not changed (intrarater reliability).
Responsive	A responsive measure refers to the extent to which a measure is sensitive to change introduced by the quality improvement process.
	Needs to be room for improvement in the measure chosen
	Measure chosen needs to be able to detect the improvement
Interpretable	An interpretable measure is easily understood by the target audience.
Feasible	A feasible measure is useful because it is relatively easy to obtain and be collected with available resources.

10 years by top corporations like General Electric, Sony, and Allied Signal.[3,20–23] Sigma is the Greek letter used to designate a standard variation in a process. The higher the sigma, the fewer are the number of errors or defects. One sigma equals 690 000 defects per million opportunities and two sigma equates with 308 537 defects per million. However, six sigma equals just 3.4 defects per million opportunities or as close to perfection as one can get in the everyday world.[21]

In an excellent review article,[20] Chassin summarized how the use of six sigma, as a quality improvement methodology, could be applied to health care. As shown in Table 43.4, he summarized the level of defects per million that correspond to different sigma levels and gave examples of health care quality studies that documented the incidence of specific problems. In this review, he noted that one health care specialty that reduced serious defects to rates that are close to 3.4 per million is surgical anesthesia. In the 1970s and 1980s, anesthesia-related death rates ranged from 1 in 10 000 to 20 000 or 25 to 50 per million.[24] Through a variety of initiatives, current estimates of anesthesia-related deaths are at about 5 per million cases.[25,26]

Six sigma is a process improvement methodology that uses data and statistical analyses to identify and fix problems. Theoretically, once defects per million opportunities is calculated, sigma values can be looked up in tables in common statistics books. Quality improvement teams can then identify the level of intended magnitude of improvement. Over the past 10 years, the use of the six sigma methodology has delivered a variety of sustainable benefits to companies from many industries. Some of these benefits have included reduced costs, increased revenues, strengthened customer relationships, increased processing speed, and introduction of more efficient production processes.[23]

The six sigma methodology differs from more traditional continuous quality improvement approaches like PDSA in that six sigma is more of a business tool, in which a control phase is built in to focus on sustaining improvements. In contrast, total quality management approaches like PDSA are focused primarily on quality initiatives.[23] Six sigma is achieved through a series of steps that are outlined in Table 43.5 and abbreviated as DMAIC. The first step (define) entails the creation of a project charter. This charter defines the customers' needs, scope of the project, goals of the project, success criteria, team members, and project deadlines. In the second step (measurement), a data collection plan for the process is developed and data are collected from several sources to determine the depth of the defects or errors (ie, defects per million opportunities) in the system. Control charts are created to study the process further. In the third step (analyze), data analysis occurs, deviations from standards are identified, key drivers that lead to the current process performance are identified, and the target for the improved performance is identified. In the fourth step (improve), created solutions and implementation plans are developed. Finally, in the sixth step (control), the process is controlled by implementing policies, guidelines, and error-proofing strategies to make reverting to the old process impossible. Quality controls are developed to monitor the new process and prevent backsliding.[3,23]

Lean Methodology

Lean methodology was developed by Taiichi Ohno, a Toyota Motor Corporation engineer. Lean methodology is driven by the identified needs of the customer and aims to improve processes by removing non-value-added activities. These non-value-added activities, also referred to as waste, do not add to the business margin or to the customer's experience and customers are not willing to pay for them. Seven different types of waste have been identified, including overproduction or underproduction; wasted inventory, reworks, or rejects (ie, mistakes in assembly); wasted motion (eg, poor work area ergonomics); waste associated with waiting (eg, patients waiting to be seen for appointments); waste associated with processing (eg, outdated policies and procedures); and waste from transport or handling (eg, transporting patients when it is not necessary). Lean tools maximize value-added steps in the best possible sequence to deliver continuous flow. Services and products are delivered when the customer needs them and how the customer requests them.[3,27] Although the PDSA methodology has been used for a number of years to improve the quality of patient care, six sigma[21–23,28] and lean methodology[27,29] have only recently been used in health care. To date, neither of these two methodologies has been used to improve the quality of acute pain management.

Table 43.4: Selected Health Care Quality Problems Viewed as Defects per Million Compared with Quality Performance in Selected Industries

Sigma Level	Defects per Million Opportunities	Selected Health Care Examples	Selected Industrial Examples
6	3.4	–	Allied Signal: 3 model factories Publishing: one misspelling in all of the books in a small library
	5.4	Deaths caused by anesthesia during surgery	–
	10–16	–	Two Siebe plants in Italy and the United Kingdom that make temperature controls for refrigerators
5	230	–	Airline fatalities
4	6210	–	Airline baggage handling Restaurant errors
	10 000	1% of hospitalized patients injured by negligence	–
3	66 800	–	Publishing: 7.6 misspelled words per page in a book
	210 000	21% of ambulatory antibiotics for colds	–
2	308 000	–	–
	580 000	58% of patients with depression not detected or treated adequately	–
1	690 000	–	–
	790 000	79% of eligible heart attack survivors fail to receive beta blockers	–

Adapted from: Chassin MR. Is health care ready for Six Sigma quality? *Milbank Q.* 1998;76(4): 565–591, 510.

AN HISTORICAL PERSPECTIVE ON QUALITY IMPROVEMENT INITIATIVES IN ACUTE PAIN MANAGEMENT

In the late 1980s, the first guidelines to be used to evaluate the quality of acute pain management were published by the American Pain Society.[30] Since that time, these guidelines were revised twice.[31,32] The impetus for the development of these quality improvement guidelines was the overwhelming evidence that postoperative pain[33–35] is not well managed and that the under treatment of pain results in deleterious consequences[36,37] and may lead to the development of chronic pain.[38]

In fact, these early studies of the undertreatment of acute pain provided the impetus for the Agency for Health Care Policy and Research to publish a clinical practice guideline on the management of acute postoperative pain.[39] One of the recommendations in this guideline was that after its implementation, the quality of acute pain management should be evaluated.

Another impetus for the development of quality improvement initiatives in acute pain management was the publication of pain standards by the Joint Commission for the Accreditation of Health Care Organizations. These pain standards, published in 2001, represented a landmark initiative by the Joint Commission.[40–42] In addition, they represented a rare and important opportunity for widespread and sustainable improvements in how pain is to be managed in the United States. The requirements contained within the Joint Commission's pain standards are enumerated in Table 43.6.

Based on the need to meet the final pain standard listed in Table 43.6, many health care organizations have developed quality improvement committees that focus on an evaluation of the quality of acute pain management. In addition, many of these pain standards have become structure, process, and outcome indicators for various quality initiatives related to acute pain management. For example, many health care organizations have developed a policy that all clinicians (ie, physicians, nurses, allied health professionals) must receive education about pain management. In addition, most hospitals who are accredited by the Joint Commission have policies and procedures that govern universal screening for pain as well as the initial and ongoing assessment of pain. Ongoing quality improvement programs within health care organizations focus on evaluating whether these types of initiatives improve the quality of acute pain management.

DEVELOPMENT, IMPLEMENTATION, AND MAINTENANCE OF A CONTINUOUS QUALITY IMPROVEMENT PROGRAM FOR ACUTE PAIN MANAGEMENT

As noted, to change the quality of patient care, health care organizations must implement the process of continuous quality improvement. The continuous quality improvement process

Table 43.5: Five Phases of Six Sigma

Phase	Deliverables
Define	Identify process customers and their requirements
	Identify the boundaries of the project using high-level process map
	Complete an approved project-charting document
Measure	Develop an accurate system for measuring the process result
	Develop a detailed drill down on the process flow
	Report the current process performance for the targeted customer requirement
Analyze	Compare the current process performance with customer requirements
	Identify key drivers that lead to the current process performance
	Identify target for the improved performance
Improve	Determine the statistical relationship between the key process drivers and the process outcome
	Propose and pilot potential solutions
	Determine operating ranges for the process drivers
Control	Ensure accurate measurement of the improved key process drivers
	Confirm that improved drivers are delivering the targeted process results in actual practice
	Develop a tracking and rapid reaction plan to detect and correct any process backsliding to ensure that gains are sustained

Adapted from: Elberfeld A, Bennis S, et al. The innovative use of Six Sigma in home care. *Home Healthc Nurse.* 2007;25(1):25–33.

provides organizations with the ability to collect benchmark data on various aspects of acute pain management; determine the effectiveness of various acute pain management practices or processes of care, and evaluate whether systematic changes in the processes and practices surrounding acute pain management improve the quality of care that patients with acute pain receive.

Individuals who work to develop and maintain a continuous quality improvement program in pain management need to remember that continuous quality improvement is a *process.* The emphasis on the term *process* underscores the fact that continuous quality improvement efforts take time and perseverance. Although it is easy to become frustrated with an apparent lack of progress on the part of administrators or clinicians, the quality improvement committee for acute pain management needs to have a long-term vision, clear goals and objectives, and a flexible timeline to complete their quality improvement plan.[16,17]

The steps to develop, implement, and maintain a continuous quality improvement program for acute pain management are outlined in Table 43.7. Following the publication of the pain standards by the Joint Commission for the Accreditation of Health Care Organizations, most health care organizations established quality improvement programs in acute pain management. These quality improvement programs were often mandated by hospital administrators to help facilitate the organization's adherence with the new pain standards.

Table 43.6: Pain Standards from the Joint Commission for the Accreditation of Health Care Organizations

Recognize the right of patients to appropriate assessment and management of their pain

Identify patients with pain in an initial screening assessment

Perform a more comprehensive assessment if pain is identified

Record the results of the assessment in a way that facilitates regular assessment and follow-up

Educate relevant providers in pain assessment and management

Determine and assure staff competency in pain assessment and management

Address pain assessment and management in the orientation of all new staff

Establish policies and procedures that support appropriate prescription or ordering of effective pain medications

Ensure that pain does not interfere with the process of rehabilitation

Educate patients and families about the importance of effective pain management

Address patient needs for symptom management in the discharge planning process

Collect data to monitor the appropriateness and effectiveness of pain management

Development of a Continuous Quality Improvement Program for Acute Pain Management

The development of a continuous quality improvement program for acute pain management requires an enormous commitment from the health care organization, as well as from the members of the quality improvement committee. The initial development of the quality improvement program usually begins with one or more individuals who have already made a commitment to improving pain management within the health care organization. The establishment of a formal quality improvement program in acute pain management allows these individuals an opportunity to develop a more structured approach to achieve specific programmatic goals.

Initial development of the quality improvement program needs to center on enlisting the support of key administrators within the organization. Without this level of administrative support, the initiative will not be successful. Once administrative support is secured, a multidisciplinary committee needs to be constituted to begin to develop the quality improvement program for acute pain management. At a minimum, the committee membership should include physicians, nurses, pharmacists, and administrators. Careful consideration should be given to who serves as chair of the committee. In some cases, it may be advantageous to have cochairs who represent key constituencies within the organization. In addition, in some cases, it may be advantageous to invite the participation of individuals who might be most resistant to change their acute pain management practices. An additional area that warrants consideration, in terms of committee membership, is that all of the key areas in the hospital and all of the key job titles are represented on the committee. Some quality improvement committees have included patients and family caregivers as members to insure that these

Table 43.7: Steps to Develop, Implement, and Maintain a Continuous Quality Improvement Program for Acute Pain Management

Development of a Continuous Quality Improvement Program

  Do background work on acute pain management structures, processes of care, and patient and system outcomes

    Enlist the aid and support of key opinion leaders and stakeholders

    Enlist the aid and support of key administrators within the organization and various departments who play critical roles in acute pain management (eg, chief executive officer, chief nursing officer)

  Constitute a multidisciplinary committee to develop the continuous quality improvement program for acute pain management

    Identify the key stake-holders in acute pain management and establish their support for the program and the continuous quality improvement plan

    Develop a multidisciplinary committee that should include at a minimum – physicians, nurses, pharmacists, and administrators

      Consider carefully who should chair or co-chair the committee

      Consider the mix of job titles needed to do the work of the committee (eg, senior level administrators, middle management, staff) when developing the list of committee members

      Consider the areas of the hospital and specialty areas that need to be represented on the committee (eg, nursing units, radiology, pediatrics, post anesthesia care unit)

    Invite the participation of individuals who might be most resistant to change their acute pain management practices

    Include patient and family member participation when appropriate

  Perform an *initial* analysis of acute pain management practices within the organization

    Identify areas for improvement in acute pain management based on brainstorming sessions with the continuous quality improvement committee

    Collect some initial data and analyze the data to verify the need for improvement in a variety of pain management practices

      Evidence of areas for improvement in acute pain management facilitates the buy-in of key opinion leaders and administration for the establishment of a quality improvement program

  Develop an *initial* continuous quality improvement plan for acute pain management

    Establish the overall goals of the quality improvement program

    Prioritize potential projects and choose the *initial* projects

      High-volume problems

      High-risk problems

      High-cost problems

    Develop a timeline for completion of *initial* projects

    Do an environmental scan to understand the current climate within the organization relative to a specific quality improvement project

      Potential barriers

      Potential opportunities

      Potential resources for the project

    Develop the specific approaches needed to complete the initial quality improvement project(s)

      Create and test the data collection tools and systems

      Create and test the data analysis methods

      Create and test the methods that will be used to report findings and obtain feedback from clinicians on the findings from the quality improvement project

Implementation of a Continuous Quality Improvement Program

  Present findings from initial quality improvement projects to key stakeholders and opinion leaders

    Obtain a buy-in to move forward with a comprehensive quality improvement program for acute pain management

  Develop a comprehensive quality improvement program for acute pain management

    Develop a plan to "institutionalize" acute pain management

    Establish a timeline for completion of major goals and projects

    Determine which acute pain management policies and procedures need to be written, revised, and disseminated

      Pain assessment policies and procedures

      Use of pharmacologic interventions for acute pain management

      Use of nonpharmacologic interventions for acute pain management

      Use of technology for acute pain management

      Safety considerations with acute pain management

(*continued*)

Table 43.7 (*continued*)

    Develop and obtain approval for a budget to implement and maintain the continuous quality improvement program

  Establish accountability for acute pain management within the health care organization

    Determine which staff and which administrators will be responsible for each aspect of the quality improvement program in acute pain management

    Incorporate effective pain management into the mission statement of the health care organization

    Develop competency based assessment tools to evaluate staff performance

    Integrate the principles of effective acute pain management and assign responsibility for pain management into policies, procedures, and job descriptions

  Provide education to all personnel involved in acute pain management

    Provide education on pain assessment

    Provide education on both pharmacologic and nonpharmacologic interventions for acute pain management

    Provide education on the use of new technologies for acute pain management

    Provide education on patient safety issues related to acute pain management

    Provide education on discharge planning considerations related to acute pain management

  Provide education to patients and family caregivers about acute pain management

    Provide education on admission of their right to prompt acute pain treatment

    Explain to patients and family caregivers why acute pain management is an important part of their care

    Teach patients and family caregivers how to report pain using established pain assessment tools

    Provide patients and family caregivers with discharge teaching about acute pain management

  Establish ongoing systems to collect and report data for ongoing quality improvement projects

  Develop approaches to change clinicians' behaviors and to change organizational systems that will lead to improvements in acute pain management

Maintenance of a Continuous Quality Improvement Program

  Determine if the quality improvement indicator is changing based ongoing evaluations

    Use different quality improvement methodologies (e.g., PDSA, six sigma) and tools (eg, medical record reviews, adherence with policies and procedures, competency evaluations of staff, patient interviews) to collect and analyze data

  Modify approaches to change clinicians' behaviors and system issues on a regular basis

  Develop strategies to sustain the enthusiasm and collaboration among the members of the multidisciplinary quality improvement committee

  Maintain ongoing communication with and support from key stake holders, key opinion leaders, and hospital administration

---

perspectives are taken into account as the quality improvement plan develops. Taking the time to obtain the appropriate "mix" of committee members will help to insure that the findings and recommendations from the quality improvement committee are accepted by all of the relevant constituencies.

Once the quality improvement committee is formed, its *initial* efforts need to focus on an analysis of acute pain management practices within the organization. One way to begin this process is to have committee members identify key areas for improvement. These brainstorming efforts can be used to build consensus among committee members on the key acute pain management issues that face the organization. Once a list of the key areas for improvement is identified, some initial data can be collected and analyzed to verify the need to a more detailed and comprehensive quality improvement initiative. This initial investigation provides preliminary data on opportunities for improvement that are specific to acute pain management. In addition, these data can be presented to key opinion leaders and administrators to facilitate their acceptance and buy-in for the quality improvement program.

Once the initial evaluation of acute pain management practices is completed, the quality improvement committee in a sense has "the lay of the land" and can begin the development of the initial continuous quality improvement plan for acute pain management. The first step is to establish the overall goals for the quality improvement program. As part of this step, the committee needs to determine the scope of their quality improvement program. Decisions need to be made about whether the committee will focus only on quality improvement studies or whether they will choose to have a larger scope that includes a variety of activities related to acute pain management (eg, development of policies and procedures for acute pain management, clinician education, patient and family caregiver education, development of competency-based performance evaluations). The choices that the committee makes about the scope of the program will influence the goals and objectives of the quality improvement program for acute pain management.

Once the goals of the quality improvement program are established, the committee needs to determine the specific topics for the initial quality improvement project or projects. As mentioned previously, the choice of topic for a quality improvement study is often based on the identification of high-volume, high-risk, or high-cost problems. Additional considerations for the choice of topic for the initial project might include the interest level of clinicians in a particular topic, the availability of valid and reliable tools to measure the problem, the ease and

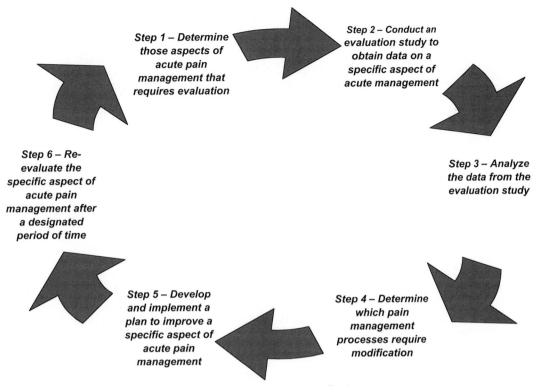

Figure 43.2: The process of continuous quality improvement.

rapidity with which data can be collected, the potential impact that improvement in this area of practice would have on patient care, and the ease with which behavioral strategies to improve this area of practice could be implemented.

Once the initial quality improvement projects are identified, the committee needs to develop and implement the project. This part of the process can be accomplished using the steps outlined in Figure 43.2. One of the critical steps in this part of the process is the development of the data collection tools. The types of tools that are developed often depend on the type of data that are going to be collected. For example, for a chart review, the tool will need to be developed based on the type of data that are available in the medical record. For a patient or staff member interview, the tool may contain more open-ended questions. All of these tools should be piloted tested before the larger quality improvement study is launched. Pilot testing of a tool provides the committee with an opportunity to refine the measure, as well as to refine the instructions that are given to the individuals who will collect the study data.

Following data collection, the results of the study are analyzed and presented to the quality improvement committee. This initial presentation provides the committee with the opportunity to begin to interpret the study findings, as well as to consider additional analyses that may be needed to strengthen the interpretation of the study findings. Once the quality improvement committee is satisfied with the data analysis, they need to determine how the data will be presented to various key stake holders and clinicians. Feedback from clinicians needs to be obtained prior to the development of the quality improvement plan. In many cases, clinicians can identify specific aspects of care that can be modified to improve various aspects of acute pain management.

Once the data are presented and the specific aspects of acute pain management that require modification are determined, the quality improvement committee needs to develop and implement a plan to improve that aspect of acute pain management. The final step in the process of continuous quality improvement is to reevaluate that specific aspect of acute pain management after a designated period of time has elapsed. The quality improvement committee needs to establish the timeline for the reevaluation and how much improvement they expect to achieve following the implementation of their plan to change clinicians' behaviors or systems of care.

Implementation of a Continuous Quality Improvement Program in Acute Pain Management

As outlined in Table 43.7, the implementation of a continuous quality improvement program in acute pain management is a large undertaking that requires a substantial commitment of financial and personnel resources on the part of a health care organization. One of the major goals for this phase of the quality improvement program is the development of a plan and methodologies to institutionalize acute pain management practices. A variety of activities need to be accomplished to achieve this goal. In most health care organizations, quality improvement committees write, revise, and disseminate acute pain management policies and procedures. This activity is part of the scope of the quality improvement program because the members of the quality improvement committee are often the most knowledgeable clinicians within the organization about various aspects of acute pain management. In addition, these individuals have the knowledge to insure that the policies and procedures are in compliance with the mandates or requirements of various accreditation bodies (eg, State Health Department, Joint Commission for the Accreditation of Health Care Organizations).

An important consideration to insure the success of a quality improvement program in acute pain management is the actual resources that are allocated to the program. The quality improvement committee needs to develop a realistic budget that reflects the scope and magnitude of the proposed program. Both financial and personnel resource allocation needs to be consider in terms of the time needed to plan the quality improvement studies, the time needed to collect and analyze the data, the time needed to present the data to various constituencies, and the resources needed to develop and implement the action plan. The quality improvement committee needs to consider which of its functions can be delegated to other groups within the organization (eg, staff development department to disseminate the findings from the quality improvement studies and educate clinicians on new pain management practices).

A critical component of an effective quality improvement program is the establishment of accountability within an organization for acute pain management. The quality improvement committee often takes the lead in the determination of which staff and administrators are responsible for which aspects of acute pain management. In many health care organizations, the mission statement of the organization is revised to incorporate effective pain management as a stated goal of the organization. In addition, many health care organizations are including specific competencies regarding acute pain management (eg, pain assessment, use of pain management technologies) into staff members' job descriptions and performance evaluations. These types of changes within an organization emphasize the importance of pain management within the organization and demonstrate an institutional commitment to acute pain management.

Numerous studies have documented that one of the key factors that contributes to the undertreatment and inappropriate management of pain is lack of clinician,[43–48] patient,[49–51] and family caregiver[52,53] education about pain management. Many quality improvement committees will establish as one of their goals to improve clinician, patient, and family caregiver education about acute pain management. This goal is in concert with the pain standards published by the Joint Commission for the Accreditation of Health Care Organizations. Again, the members of the quality improvement committee have the knowledge and expertise to achieve this goal. However, substantial personnel and financial resources need to be allocated to achieve this goal. Initial educational efforts often need to focus on clinicians. Successful quality improvement programs have incorporated clinician education on pain management into all orientation programs. In addition, the quality improvement committee often facilitates annual updates on pain management within the health care organization.

Maintenance of a Continuous Quality Improvement Program in Acute Pain Management

One of the most challenging aspects of any quality improvement program is the maintenance of momentum and enthusiasm for the program. The major goal of the maintenance phase of the program is to determine if the indicator(s) that were selected for improvement have improved. The reevaluation component of the program, that needs to be done on an *ongoing* basis, is

the most challenging aspect of any quality improvement program. The quality improvement committee needs to be actively engaged in selecting the types of quality improvement methodologies (eg, PDSA, six sigma) that are employed within the health care organization. In addition, they need to be involved in the development of the tools and approaches that will be used to collect data on the various aspects of acute pain management. In many cases, the quality improvement committee can use a variety of tools to collect data. The choices of tools (eg, chart review, clinician interviews, patient interviews) that are used can enrich the breadth of the data that are obtained and provide new directions for quality improvement initiatives.

The committee must engage in processes that maintain members' enthusiasm for the projects and goals of the quality improvement program. In addition, they must think of methodologies to sustain multidisciplinary collaboration and maintain the growth and development of the program. Areas to consider in this regard include turnover of committee chairs, turnover of committee members, periodic retreats to evaluate accomplishments as well as redefine the long-term goals and objectives of the program, and solidification of the ongoing commitment of the institution to the quality improvement program.

QUALITY IMPROVEMENT INDICATORS AND MEASURES IN ACUTE PAIN MANAGEMENT

Initial efforts to improve the quality of acute pain management came through the publication of a specific set of recommendations for monitoring the quality of acute pain management by the Agency for Health Care Policy and Research and the American Pain Society.[30,39] These recommendations included a patient outcome questionnaire that could be used or adapted to evaluate the quality of acute or cancer pain management. Several studies were done with the original or modified versions of the patient outcome questionnaire.[32,54–60] The major finding across all of these studies was that patients reported high levels of satisfaction with pain management despite significantly high levels of pain and long waiting times for pain medications. This paradox suggested that the evaluation of patient satisfaction was not a valid and reliable measure to use to judge the quality of acute pain management.

In 1995, the American Pain Society's Quality of Care Committee revised these quality improvement guidelines based on the published reports and clinical experience.[31] This interdisciplinary committee concluded that efforts to improve the quality of acute pain management must move beyond the assessment of pain and documentation of pain assessments to implementation and evaluation of improvements in pain treatment that are timely, safe, evidenced based, and multimodal. As shown in Table 43.8, the American Pain Society's Quality of Care Committee identified 5 key components that should guide the development of quality improvement programs in acute pain management. In addition, a revision of the patient outcome questionnaire was included in the article. The main revisions to the patient outcome questionnaire were the addition of 6 items on how pain interferes with function from the Brief Pain Inventory[61] and 7 items from the Patient Barriers Questionnaire.[62] In addition, emphasis was placed on the use of continuous quality improvement approaches to improve the quality of acute pain management within health care organizations.

Table 43.8: American Pain Society's Key Components for a Quality Improvement Program in Acute Pain Management

Assure that a report of unrelieved pan raised a "red flag" that attracted clinicians' attention

Make information about analgesics convenient where orders are written

Promise patients responsive analgesic care and urge them to communicate pain

Implement policies and safeguards for the use of modern analgesic technologies

Coordinate and assess implementation of these measures

Adapted from: American Pain Society Quality of Care Committee. Quality improvement guidelines for the treatment of acute pain and cancer pain. *JAMA.* 1995;274(23):1874–1880.

Results of Studies That Evaluated the Quality of Acute Pain Management Using the Indicators and Measures Developed by the American Pain Society

Over the next decade, a number of studies were published that used the revised patient outcome questionnaire to evaluate the quality of acute and cancer pain management.[63–66] In addition, Gordon and colleagues summarized the findings from the majority of the quality improvement studies in acute pain management.[60] The purpose of their extensive review was to determine which indicators were being used for quality improvement, compare findings across these studies, and develop specific recommendations to simplify and standardize future measurement of quality for hospital-based quality improvement initiatives in pain management.

As part of this review,[60] the results of 20 studies performed at 8 large hospitals in the United States were evaluated and compared. In the majority of these studies, convenience samples of patients who had pain were recruited. Patients and records were surveyed either within 3 days of surgery or admission to the hospital or in the 3 days before discharge. The purpose of each of the studies was to gather baseline data, discover targets for improvement, or monitor changes in pain management overtime as part of ongoing hospital-wide quality improvement initiatives.

As listed in Table 43.9, the specific measures used in the patient surveys and medical record audits were derived from structure, process, and outcome indicators recommended for monitoring in the early 1990s.[30,39] Measures included pain intensity, interference with function, patient satisfaction, patient beliefs, documentation of pain assessment, and the range and appropriateness of pain treatments. Analyses of the data across the 20 studies led to consensus on 6 quality indicators for hospital-based pain management programs. The authors of the review concluded that a comprehensive evaluation of the quality of pain management involves both practice patterns and patient outcomes. Although the use of the American Pain Society's patient outcome questionnaire combined with a comprehensive medical record review tool represented more than 100 potentially distinct data points, more and different quality improvement indicators and measures needed to be investigated.[60] For example, acts of omission and the identification of patient safety issues in pain management needed to be investigated in detail.[34]

Table 43.9: Key Indicators and Measures Used in Initial Studies of the Quality of Acute Pain Management

Quality Indicator	Quality Measure
Outcome	Patient comfort (pain intensity)
Outcome	Impact of pain on function
Outcome	Patient and family satisfaction with pain management
Process	Documentation of pain assessments
Structure	Range and appropriateness of options available for acute pain management
Process and Outcome	Effectiveness of pain management options used to prevent and treat pain
Outcome	Prevalence and severity of side effects and complications associated with acute pain management
Structure and process	The quality of pain management across points of transition in the provision of services

Adapted from: Gordon DB, Pellino TA, et al. A 10-year review of quality improvement monitoring in pain management: recommendations for standardized outcome measures. *Pain Manag Nurs.* 2002;3(4):116–130.[60]

American Pain Society Recommendations for Improving the Quality of Acute and Cancer Pain Management

Based on the findings from this review, as well as clinician feedback, in 2005, the American Pain Society Quality of Care Task Force published a revision of their Recommendations for Improving the Quality of Acute and Cancer Pain Management.[67] The differences between the 1995[3] and 2005 recommendations are summarized in Table 43.10. The American Pain Society recommendations specify that all care settings need to formulate structured multilevel systems' approaches to ensure prompt recognition and treatment of pain, involvement of patients and family members in the pain management plan, improved treatment patterns, regular reassessments and adjustments of the pain management plan as needed, and measurement of the processes and outcomes of pain management. The main emphasis in this document is that efforts to improve the quality of pain management must move beyond the assessment and communication about pain to the implementation and evaluation of improvements in pain treatments that are timely, safe, evidenced based, and multimodal.

Based on the work by Gordon and colleagues,[60] the American Pain Society Quality of Care Task Force recommended 6 new quality indicators and several measures that can be used to evaluate the quality of acute pain management. These indicators and measures are summarized in Table 43.11. Additional research is warranted to determine if these indicators and measures are useful tools to evaluate the quality of acute pain management.

Additional Considerations in the Development and Implementation of Quality Improvement Programs for Acute Pain Management

Patient Safety

As noted previously, the major impetus for the publication of pain standards by the Joint Commission for the Accreditation

Table 43.10: Comparison of the 1995 American Pain Society (APS) Quality Improvement (QI) Guidelines and the 2005 APS Recommendations

1995 APS QI Guidelines	*2005 APS Recommendations*
Recognize and treat pain promptly	Recognize and treat pain promptly
Routine assessment of pain intensity	Emphasis on comprehensive pain assessment
Routine documentation of pain intensity	Emphasis on the importance of the prevention of pain
	Emphasis on prompt recognition and treatment of pain
Make information about analgesics readily available in places where clinicians write medication orders	Involve patients and families in the pain management plan
	Emphasis on the need to customize the pain management plan
	Emphasis on the importance of having the patient participate in the pain management plan
Promise patients attentive analgesic care	Improve treatment patterns
Urge patients to report pain to clinicians	Eliminate inappropriate practices
	Emphasis on the need to provide multimodal therapy
Develop explicit policies for analgesic technologies	Reassess and adjust pain management plan as needed
Patient controlled analgesia	Emphasis placed on the need to respond not only to pain intensity scores but to changes in patient's functional status and side effects
Spinal administration of opioids and anesthetics	
Examine the processes and outcomes of pain management with the goal of continuous quality improvement	Monitor processes and outcomes of pain management
	Emphasis on new standardized QI indicators

Adapted from: Gordon DB, Dahl JL, et al. American Pain Society recommendations for improving the quality of acute and cancer pain management. *Arch Int Med.* 2005;165(14):1574–1580.[67]

of Health Care Organizations was the overwhelming evidence on the under treatment of acute[33,35,68] and cancer pain.[69–71] The need exists to continue these efforts to improve the management of acute and cancer pain because studies continue to document the undertreatment of acute and cancer pain in both inpatient and outpatient settings.

However, recent studies completed after the publication of the pain standards by the Joint Commission for Accreditation of Health Care Organizations suggest that careful evaluation of pain management practices is required to insure quality care and patient safety. In one study,[72] following the implementation of a routine numeric pain scoring system in the postanesthesia care unit, an overall increase in the average consumption of opioids was observed (ie, 10.5 ± 10.4 mg versus 6.5 ± 7.3 mg, $P < .001$). This increase in opioid use was not associated with an increased length of stay, an increase in the requirement for naloxone, or an increase in treatment for postoperative nausea and vomiting. The authors concluded that the increase in opioid use as a result of a quality improvement initiative was not associated with additional opioid-induced morbidity in the immediate postoperative period. In contrast, in another study that reported on a quality improvement initiative for acute pain management,[73] the incidence of opioid-induced adverse events increased from 11 to 25 per 100 000 inpatient days at the medical center. Of note, the majority of the adverse drug reactions were preceded by a documented decrease in patient's level of consciousness because of opioid-related sedation. Findings from these studies suggest that quality improvement initiatives related to acute pain management should be evaluated in terms of improvements in

the quality of acute pain management, as well as in terms of potential adverse effects.

Within the context of patient safety, it should be noted that based on the findings from the Institute of Medicine's study on medical errors,[1] Congress passed and the President signed the Patient Safety and Quality Improvement Act in 2005. This act encourages the voluntary reporting of medical errors by providing legal protections to those who report the errors. The idea is to have these errors recorded in databases for subsequent analyses. These analyses should identify patterns in these errors and result in strategies to reduce errors.[74] Of note, the Institute for Healthcare Improvement has noted that 58% of medication-related injuries are because of high-alert medications. The 4 high-alert medications most responsible for injuries are anticoagulants, sedatives, opioids, and insulin (see http://ihi.org/IHI/Programs/Campaign). Therefore, it behooves clinicians and administrators involved in quality improvement programs for acute pain management to include indicators that evaluate various aspects of patient safety associated with analgesic medications, as well as adverse events.

Quality Indicators and Measures in Day Surgery Settings

In an excellent review, Shnaider and Chung[75] summarized the results of published studies on the outcome measures that can be used to assess the quality of ambulatory surgery and anesthesia. In this review, they noted that postoperative pain is one of the most frequent adverse events that occurs following ambulatory surgery. It is associated with a longer postoperative stay and delays patients' return to normal function. In

Table 43.11: Quality Indicators and Measures for Acute Pain Management

Quality Indicator	Measures
Intensity of pain is documented	Is there any documentation of pain in the medical record?
Numeric rating scale (ie, 0 to 10)	
Descriptive rating scale (ie, none, mild, moderate, or severe)	In charts with documentation of pain, was a pain rating scale used?
Pain intensity is documented at frequent intervals	How many pain intensity ratings were documented in a 24-hour period?
Pain is treated by a route other than intramuscular injection	Percentage of patients who received an intramuscular injection of an analgesic in the postoperative period
Pain is treated with regularly administered analgesics	Percentage of patients who received an analgesic on a regular schedule
	Percentage of patients who received meperidine
Pain is treated, when possible, with multimodal approaches	Percentage of patients who received only a single analgesic modality
	Percentage of patients who received combinations of therapeutic approaches (nonopioid, opioid, local anesthetic, regional techniques)
	Percentage of patients who received both pharmacologic and nonpharmacologic approaches
Pain is prevented and controlled to a degree that facilitates function and quality of life	Measurement of worst pain in past 24 hours
	Amount of time the patient was in moderate to severe pain in the past 24 hours
	Level of pain's interference with sleep, walking ability, mood (0 = does not interfere to 10 = completely interferes)
Patients are adequately informed and knowledgeable about pain management	Patient's rating of the adequacy of information received about pain and pain management while in the hospital (1 = poor to 5 = excellent)

Adapted from: Gordon DB, Pellino TA, et al. A 10-year review of quality improvement monitoring in pain management: recommendations for standardized outcome measures. *Pain Manag Nurs.* 2002;3(4):116–130.[60] Gordon DB, Dahl JL, et al. American Pain Society recommendations for improving the quality of acute and cancer pain management. *Arch Int Med.* 2005;165(14):1574–1580.[67]

addition, postoperative pain is one of the most common causes for unanticipated admission and readmission.[76] Quality improvement projects need to be designed and implemented that focus on improving the management of acute pain in the ambulatory surgery setting.

EFFECTIVE APPROACHES TO CHANGE CLINICIANS' BEHAVIORS

The fundamental goal of all quality improvement programs is to improve the quality of patient care. In many cases, to achieve improvements in the quality of patient care, clinicians need to change their behaviors. However, even in the era of evidence-based practice, little is known about the most effective approaches to use to change clinicians' behaviors in general and in relationship to pain management in particular. In one of the most comprehensive reviews published to date, Grimshaw and colleagues[77] attempted to synthesize the evidence from systematic reviews of professional education or quality improvement

interventions that were designed to improve the quality of patient care. Forty-one reviews were identified that covered a wide range of approaches to behavior change. In general, the conclusion was that passive approaches (eg, continuing education programs) were ineffective and did not result in changes in clinicians' behaviors. The most promising interventions were multifaceted and targeted different barriers to behavior change. Systematic investigations are warranted to determine the most appropriate interventions to change clinicians' behaviors in terms of safe and effective pain management.

SUMMARY AND CONCLUSIONS

The need to improve, on an ongoing basis, the quality of patient care is firmly established within the health care system. Caregivers who are involved in acute pain management need to evaluate the quality of acute pain management from multiple perspectives. Patients deserve the most effective and safest pain management that is possible within the context of their medical condition and the setting in which they receive their care.

REFERENCES

1. Kohn LT, Corrigan JM, et al, eds. *To Err Is Human: Building a Safer Health Care System*. Washington, DC: National Academy Press; 2000.

2. Committee on Quality Health Care in America, Institute of Medicine. *Crossing the Quality Chasm: A New Health System for the 21st Century*. Washington, DC: National Academy Press; 2001.

3. Varkey PM, Reller K, et al. Basics of quality improvement in health care. *Mayo Clin Proc*. 2007;82(6):735–739.

4. Berwick DM, Calkins DR, et al. The 100,000 lives campaign: setting a goal and a deadline for improving health care quality. *JAMA*. 2006;295(3):324–327.

5. Curtis JR, Cook DJ, et al. Intensive care unit quality improvement: a "how-to" guide for the interdisciplinary team. *Crit Care Med*. 2006;34(1):211–218.

6. Agency for Healthcare Research and Quality, United States Department of Health and Human Services. Your guide to choosing quality health care: a quick look at quality. Available at: www.ahrq.gov/consumer/qnt/qntqlook.htm. Accessed December 29, 2007.

7. Shine KI. Health care quality and how to achieve it. *Acad Med*. 2002;77(1):91–99.

8. McGlynn EA, Cassel CK, et al. Establishing national goals for quality improvement. *Med Care*. 2003;41(1 suppl): I16–I29.

9. Deming EW. *Out of Crisis*. Cambridge, MA: MIT Center for Advanced Engineering; 2002.

10. James, C. Manufacturing's prescription for improving healthcare quality. *Hosp Top*. 2005;83(1):2–8.

11. Donabedian A. Evaluating the quality of medical care. *Milbank Q*. 2005;83(4):691–729.

12. Berwick DM. Continuous improvement as an ideal in health care. *N Engl J Med*. 1898;320(1):53–56.

13. Berwick DM. A primer on leading the improvement of systems. *Br Med J*. 1996;312(7031):619–622.

14. Berwick DM. Developing and testing changes in delivery of care. *Ann Int Med*. 1998;128(8): 651–656.

15. Berwick DM, James B, et al. Connections between quality measurement and improvement. *Med Care*. 2003;41(1 suppl):I30–I38.

16. Miaskowski C. Monitoring and improving pain management practices: a quality improvement approach. *Crit Care Nurs Clin North Am*. 2001;13(2):311–317.

17. Miaskowski C. New approaches for evaluating the quality of cancer pain management in the outpatient setting. *Pain Manag Nurs*. 2001;2(1):7–12.

18. McGlynn EA. Introduction and overview of the conceptual framework for a national quality measurement and reporting system. *Med Care*. 2003;41(1 suppl):I1–I7.

19. McGlynn EA. Selecting common measures of quality and system performance. *Med Care*. 2003 41(1 suppl):I39–I47.

20. Chassin MR. Is health care ready for Six Sigma quality? *Milbank Q*. 1998;76(4):565–591.

21. Simmons JC. Using Six Sigma to make a difference in health care quality. *Qual Lett Healthc Lead*. 2002;14(4):2–10.

22. Chan AL. Use of Six Sigma to improve pharmacist dispensing errors at an outpatient clinic. *Am J Med Qual*. 2004;19(3):128–131.

23. Elberfeld A, Bennis S, et al. The innovative use of Six Sigma in home care. *Home Healthc Nurse*. 2007;25(1):25–33.

24. Ross AF, Tinker JH, eds. Anesthesia risk. In: *Anesthesia*. New York, NY: Churchill-Livingston; 1994.

25. Lunn JN, Devlin HB. Lessons from the confidential enquiry into perioperative deaths in three NHS regions. *Lancet*. 1987;2(8572):1384–1386.

26. Eichhorn JH. Prevention of intraoperative anesthesia accidents and related severe injury through safety monitoring. *Anesthesiology*. 1989;70(4):572–577.

27. Kim CS, Spahlinger DA, et al. Lean health care: what can hospitals learn from a world-class automaker? *J. Hosp Med*. 2006;1(3):191–199.

28. Hagland M. Six sigma practices: a strategy based on data is perfect fit for healthcare. *Healthc Inform*. 2006;23(1):27–28, 30.

29. de Koning H, Verver JP, et al. Lean six sigma in healthcare. *J Healthc Qual*. 2006;28(2):4–11.

30. American Pain Society Committee on Quality Assurance. Quality assurance standards for relief of acute and cancer pain. In: Bond MR, Charlton JE, Woolf CJ, eds. *Proceedings of the VI World Congress on Pain*. Amsterdam: Elsevier; 1991.

31. American Pain Society Quality of Care Committee. Quality improvement guidelines for the treatment of acute pain and cancer pain. *JAMA*. 1995;274(23):1874–1880.

32. Dahl JL, Gordon D, et al. Institutionalizing pain management: the Post-Operative Pain Management Quality Improvement Project. *J Pain*. 2003;4(7):361–371.

33. Warfield CA, Kahn CA. Acute pain management: programs in U.S. hospitals and experiences and attitudes among U.S. adults. *Anesthesiology*. 1995;83(5):1090–1094.

34. McNeill JA, Sherwood GD, et al. Assessing clinical outcomes: patient satisfaction with pain management. *J Pain Symptom Manage*. 1998;16(1):29–40.

35. Apfelbaum JL, Chen C, et al. Postoperative pain experience: results from a national survey suggest postoperative pain continues to be undermanaged. *Anesth Analg*. 2003;97(2):534–540.

36. Breivik H. Postoperative pain management: why is it difficult to show that it improves outcome? *Eur J Anaesthesiol*. 1998;15(6):748–751.

37. Foss NB, Kristensen MT, et al. Effect of postoperative epidural analgesia on rehabilitation and pain after hip fracture surgery: a randomized, double-blind, placebo-controlled trial. *Anesthesiology*. 2005;102(6):1197–1204.

38. Perkins FM, Kehlet. Chronic pain as an outcome of surgery: a review of predictive factors. *Anesthesiology*. 2000;93(4):1123–1133.

39. Acute Pain Management Guideline Panel. Acute pain management in adults: operative procedures. Quick reference guide for clinicians. *Medsurg Nurs*. 1994;3(2):99–107.

40. Berry PH, Dahl JL The new JCAHO pain standards: implications for pain management nurses. *Pain Manag Nurs*. 2000;1(1):3–12.

41. Phillips DM. JCAHO pain management standards are unveiled. *JAMA*. 2000;284(4):428–429.

42. Berry PH. Getting ready for JCAHO – just meeting the standards or really improving pain management. *Clin J Oncol Nurs*. 2001;5(3):110–112.

43. Jacobsen R, Sjogren P, et al. Physician-related barriers to cancer pain management with opioid analgesics: a systematic review. *J Opioid Manag*. 2007;3(4):207–214.

44. Matthews E, Malcolm C. Nurses' knowledge and attitudes in pain management practice. *Br J Nurs*. 2007;16(3):174–179.

45. Michaels TK, Hubbartt E, et al. Evaluating an educational approach to improve pain assessment in hospitalized patients. *J Nurs Care Qual*. 2007;22(3):260–265.

46. Sun VC, Borneman T, et al. Overcoming barriers to cancer pain management: an institutional change model. *J Pain Symptom Manag*. 2007;34(4):359–369.

47. Xue Y, Schulman-Green D, et al. Pain attitudes and knowledge among RNs, pharmacists, and physicians on an inpatient oncology service. *Clin J Oncol Nurs*. 2007;11(5):687–695.

48. Zanolin ME, Visentin M, et al. A questionnaire to evaluate the knowledge and attitudes of health care providers on pain. *J Pain Symptom Manage.* 2007;33(6):727–736.

49. Bender JL, Hohenadel J, et al. What patients with cancer want to know about pain: a qualitative study. *J Pain Symptom Manage.* 2008;35(2):177–187.

50. Ochroch EA, Troxel AB, et al. The influence of race and socioeconomic factors on patient acceptance of perioperative epidural analgesia. *Anesth Analg.* 2007;105(6):1787–1792.

51. Silver J, Mayer RS. Barriers to pain management in the rehabilitation of the surgical oncology patient. *J Surg Oncol.* 2007;95(5): 427–435.

52. Letizia M, Creech S, et al. Barriers to caregiver administration of pain medication in hospice care. *J Pain Symptom Manage.* 2004;27(2):114–124.

53. Lin CC, Chou PL, et al. Long-term effectiveness of a patient and family pain education program on overcoming barriers to management of cancer pain. *Pain.* 2006;122(3):271–281.

54. Miaskowski C, Nichols R, et al. Assessment of patient satisfaction utilizing the American Pain Society's Quality Assurance Standards on acute and cancer-related pain. *J Pain Symptom Manage.* 1994;9(1):5–11.

55. Ward SE, Gordon. Application of the American Pain Society quality assurance standards. *Pain.* 1994;56(3):299–306.

56. Bookbinder M, Coyle N, et al. Implementing national standards for cancer pain management: program model and evaluation. *J Pain Symptom Manage.* 1996;12(6):334–347; discussion 331–333.

57. Ward SE, Gordon DB. Patient satisfaction and pain severity as outcomes in pain management: a longitudinal view of one setting's experience. *J Pain Symptom Manage.* 1996;11(4):242–251.

58. Bostrom BM, Ramberg T, et al. Survey of post-operative patients' pain management. *J Nurs Manag.* 1997;5(6):341–349.

59. Lin CC. Applying the American Pain Society's QA standards to evaluate the quality of pain management among surgical, oncology, and hospice inpatients in Taiwan. *Pain.* 2000;87(1):43–49.

60. Gordon DB, Pellino TA, et al. A 10-year review of quality improvement monitoring in pain management: recommendations for standardized outcome measures. *Pain Manag Nurs.* 2002;3(4):116–130.

61. Daut RL, Cleeland CS, et al. Development of the Wisconsin Brief Pain Questionnaire to assess pain in cancer and other diseases. *Pain.* 1983;17(2):197–210.

62. Ward, SE, Goldberg N, et al. Patient-related barriers to management of cancer pain. *Pain.* 1993;52(3):319–324.

63. Mann C, Beziat C, et al. Quality assurance program for postoperative pain management: impact of the Consensus Conference of the French Society of Anesthesiology and Intensive Care. *Ann Fr Anesth Reanim.* 2001;20(3):246–254.

64. Idvall E, Hamrin E, et al. Patient and nurse assessment of quality of care in postoperative pain management. *Qual SafHealth Care.* 2002;11(4):327–334.

65. Dihle A, Helseth S, et al. Using the American Pain Society's patient outcome questionnaire to evaluate the quality of postoperative pain management in a sample of Norwegian patients. *J Pain.* 2006;7(4):272–280.

66. Stevenson KM, Dahl JL, et al. Institutionalizing effective pain management practices: practice change programs to improve the quality of pain management in small health care organizations. *J Pain Symptom Manag.* 2006;31(3):248–261.

67. Gordon DB, Dahl JL, et al. American Pain Society recommendations for improving the quality of acute and cancer pain management: American Pain Society Quality of Care Task Force. *Arch Int Med.* 2005;165(14):1574–1580.

68. McNeill JA, Sherwood GD, et al. The hidden error of mismanaged pain: a systems approach. *J Pain Symptom Manag.* 2004;28(1):47–58.

69. Miaskowski C, Dodd M, et al. Randomized clinical trial of the effectiveness of a self-care intervention to improve cancer pain management. *J Clin Oncol.* 2004;22(9):1713–1720.

70. Cleeland CS. The measurement of pain from metastatic bone disease: capturing the patient's experience. *Clin Cancer Res.* 2006;12(20 Pt 2):6236s–6242s.

71. Villars P, Dodd M, et al. Differences in the prevalence and severity of side effects based on type of analgesic prescription in patients with chronic cancer pain. *J Pain Symptom Manag.* 2007;33(1):67–77.

72. Frasco PE, Sprung J, et al. The impact of the joint commission for accreditation of healthcare organizations pain initiative on perioperative opiate consumption and recovery room length of stay. *Anesth Analg.* 2005;100(1):162–168.

73. Vila H Jr, Smith, RA, et al. The efficacy and safety of pain management before and after implementation of hospital-wide pain management standards: is patient safety compromised by treatment based solely on numerical pain ratings? *Anesth Analg.* 2005;101(2):474–480.

74. Kinnaman K. Patient Safety and Quality Improvement Act of 2005. *Orthop Nurs.* 2007;26(1):14–16; quiz 17–18.

75. Shnaider I, Chung F. Outcomes in day surgery. *Curr Opin Anaesthesiol.* 2006;19(6):622–629.

76. Pavlin DJ, Chen, et al. A survey of pain and other symptoms that affect the recovery process after discharge from an ambulatory surgery unit. *J Clin Anesth.* 2004;16(3):200–206.

77. Grimshaw JM, Shirran L, et al. Changing provider behavior: an overview of systematic reviews of interventions. *Medical Care.* 2001;39(8 suppl 2):II2–II45.

44

The Future of Acute Pain Management

Brian Durkin and Peter S. A. Glass

The management of acute pain has come a long way since Roe asked, in his landmark 1963 article, "are postoperative narcotics necessary?"[1] It would be difficult to imagine the past several decades without opioids in our arsenal for the treatment of postoperative pain, but what about the next several decades? Have we really improved in our management of postoperative pain and are too many patients still suffering? This book covers our present management of acute pain, and this chapter covers the future management of acute pain. Before we look into the future, we should reflect on and learn from the past.

ACUTE PAIN MANAGEMENT IN THE PAST

From the mid-1960s and early 1970s, we saw the initiation of patient-controlled analgesia developing from concept to actual commercial delivery systems. Although the idea existed it took time to develop the technology. It thus took 10 years for the concept to reach fruition for daily use in patients and another 10 years for the practice of intravenous patient-controlled analgesia (IV PCA) to enter mainstream use in the United States.

In the mid-1960s, in Houston, Texas, Sechzar[2] instituted a demand system where the patient would push an alert button and the nurse would administer small intravenous doses of morphine. In a 1969 lecture, Scott[3] reported 5 years of success with his device that delivered small intravenous boluses of meperidine to laboring women at the University of Leeds. Forrest,[4] from the Palo Alto Veterans Administration Hospital, developed the "Demand Dropmaster," and Keeri-Szanto[5] from London, Ontario, developed his "Demanalg" device. The first commercially available PCA device, the "Cardiff Palliator," came from Rosen's group[6] in Wales and came to market in 1976 (Figures 44.1 and 44.2).

Prior to the early 1970s, postoperative pain control was not recognized as an integral part of the recovery process. The landmark 1973 article by psychiatrists Marks and Sachar[7] brought to light the gross disregard of patients' pain complaints and set in motion events in the entire field of medicine to focus on relief of pain for various reasons. These reasons ranged from humani-

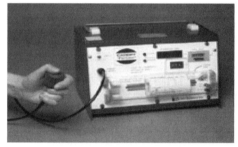

Figure 44.1: Cardiff palliator.

tarian, in the cases of terminal cancer patients, to adequate pain control for discharge home from ambulatory surgery.

The discovery of central nervous system opioid receptors in 1973 by Pert[8] led to the discovery of neuraxial opioid analgesia in humans by Wang[9] in 1979. The safe use of epidural anesthesia and analgesia in obstetrical patients made the conversion to epidural anesthesia and analgesia for postoperative pain rather easy. The 1980s were marked by the beginning of an abundance of literature on postoperative epidural analgesia with, first, intermittent bolus opioids[10] and then combination opioid and local anesthetic infusions.

The 1980s represented an exciting time for anesthesiologists interested in treating acute pain. Technology in the form of

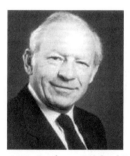

Figure 44.2: Professor Michael Rosen.

microprocessors caught up with demand for intravenous PCA and large medical device companies were able to mass produce safe and viable PCA machines for use around the world. The development of Acute Pain Services[11] led by anesthesiologists working in collaboration with clinical pharmacists and nurses in large teaching centers paved the way for the growth of intravenous PCA, as well as dedicated pain services throughout the various regions in the United States. For the first time, the treatment of acute pain was a dedicated profession while the treatment and disability status of chronic pain patients was argued in the federal government.[12]

The 1990s were a time of massive research and growth of the acute pain specialty. Peripheral nerve blocks joined the mainstream. The federal government produced a mandate for the treatment acute pain.[13] The American Society of Anesthesiologists produced their practice guidelines on acute pain management in 1995,[14] and the decade ended with the Joint Health Commission's[15] impact on making pain "the fifth vital sign." This was a time when multimodal analgesia and preemptive analgesia became buzzwords, and we started using analgesics other than morphine, meperidine, acetaminophen, and local anesthetics for acute pain control. At the same time technology was enhancing the route and mode of delivery of analgesics. The treatment of chronic pain grew as well, and the prescription of opioids for nonmalignant chronic pain became accepted in many parts of the United States.[16] Opiates and PCA became the mainstay of acute pain management. However, we began to realize that this practice might not be optimal. As early as 1988, White[17] pointed out that intravenous PCA causes harm to some patients and may be associated with human programming error. Also, claims began to surface that the JHACO guideline of pain as a vital sign might be causing practitioners to strive toward unsafe levels of analgesia.[18]

We have thus been prompted in this early part of the 21st century of acute pain management to focus largely on improving outcomes by minimizing side effects of opioid analgesia. It is well established that opioid reduction must be at least 30% to provide a reduction in opioid side effects and attain a difference in outcome. This reduction in opiate use has been shown in numerous studies to reduce hospital stay and increase patient satisfaction.

As aggressive pain treatment with opioid analgesics in the chronic pain setting has become more prevalent, so, too, has iatrogenic opioid addiction and dependence.[19,20] This phenomenon has made acute pain management more challenging. Chronic pain patients are presenting for routine surgery and tolerance has made their opioid requirement substantially larger than the usual. We are learning that these patients are better managed with a multimodal plan including regional and neuraxial anesthetics and postoperative nerve and epidural catheters.[21] Adjuvant medications, such as ketamine, gabapentin, acetaminophen, and nonsteroidal anti-inflammatory drugs (NSAIDs),[22] have been very beneficial in this group of patients.

Today, outpatient surgery accounts for the majority of operations done in the United States. In the past, patients stayed in the hospital for many days after surgery that today is done on an ambulatory basis. The growth of minimally invasive surgery is mirrored by the growth in day surgery. The management of postoperative pain has had to adjust, as well. The greater impact of opiate side effects in the ambulatory patient has fostered the practice of multimodal analgesics to minimize their use. The use of peripheral nerve blockade has become increasingly popular in the ambulatory patient and catheter placement for home use has been implemented successfully in some parts of the country.[23]

How is the practice and profession of acute pain management going to change in the next 5 years? This is the question we will try to answer. Paradigms shift every so often. We saw this in the 1960s and 1970s when acute pain management did not get much attention. Often technology must advance further for ideas to be realized. We saw this occur in the 1980s when PCA machines were finally safer and more accessible. Today, we are seeing new technology, in the form of iontophoresis,[24] that may displace the use of intravenous PCA in the future. The 1990s saw another paradigm shift insofar as patients could go home after surgery. Acute pain management adjusted to fulfill this need. The decade thus far is leading to, perhaps, another paradigm shift. Can the management of acute pain today affect patient outcomes weeks, months, or even years later?

WHO WILL MANAGE POSTOPERATIVE PAIN IN THE FUTURE?

Several models exist throughout the world regarding the composition of the acute pain service. In the United States, traditionally, the service has been anesthesiologist led with specialized nursing assistance. Health care payers have lessened or eliminated reimbursement for acute pain management services and procedures in various parts of the United States. Surgeons are managing PCA analgesia more often now while pain services focus on regional and epidural catheter placement and the challenging pain patients. In Europe, a nursing-based service with anesthesiologist consultation is the predominate model and is less expensive to run.[25]

We believe future management of acute pain will involve anesthesiologists, surgeons, and nurses working in collaboration with allied professionals, including physical therapists, pharmacists, social workers, and psychologists. This will differ from our present model of a designated team focusing primarily on the acute postoperative pain needs; rather, this will be a collaborative effort by a multidisciplinary team that designs an overall management plan unique to the patient and will cover management from the time surgery is planned through full recovery and rehabilitation. Thus, this collaboration will be more on a grand scale with both the development of hospital-wide policies created by pain management committees and individual plans generated in advance of any procedure. Pain will need to be addressed prior to even presenting to the hospital. The term *prehabilitation* will take on more meaning as patients are identified prior to admission and worked into better shape physically for a more productive rehabilitation.[26] With our increasing understanding of genetics and genomics and the potential ability to identify patient-specific receptor subtypes, pain pathways, and the development of patient-specific designer drugs, this is likely to include individuals with expertise in these areas becoming involved as members of the pain team. Perioperative pain control will continue to include many of our present techniques and drugs (including many new ideas as described below). Specialists in regional anesthesia will continue as part of this larger pain team to provide nerve blocks and epidurals. The anesthesia team taking care of the patient during the operation will continue to be part of the grand plan to make postoperative pain and side effects minimal. It is important in this model that the anesthesia

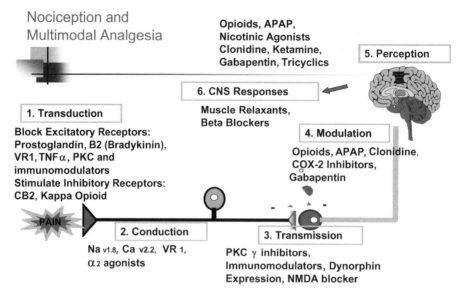

Figure 44.3: Pain pathway.

team actually doing the anesthetic is included in the perioperative plans and tailors the anesthetic appropriately. We as pain specialists must show health care payers tangible results of these efforts and justify our existence as an integral and cost-effective part of the patients perioperative care. Patient satisfaction and good outcomes should be part of this equation.

FUTURE PHARMACEUTICALS

Today, we are on the verge of the next exciting time in acute pain management. The arsenal of weapons used to combat pain is ready for enormous growth. As the discovery of new receptors in the pain pathway continues, so does the development of new pharmaceuticals to block or modify these receptors. Cannabinoids, vanilloids (TRPV1 – transient receptor potential V1) peripheral κ-opioid agonists, melatonin, and acid-sensing ion channels (ASICs) are all terms that may be well known to the acute pain management world in the near future.

The dilemma facing acute pain physicians has been treating pain while minimizing side effects of medications. All medications, whether they are opioids, NSAIDs, or other adjuvants, such as gabapentin, have side effects that may limit their use. We must find a balance between these medications and the side effects they cause to reach the best results for pain relief. Future medications will target the dilemma from multiple angles. New medications will be developed to (1) minimize the side-effect profile of current medications and (2) target more specifically newly discovered pain pathways to either decrease the traditional doses or possibly eliminate the need for medications commonly used today.

REDUCTION OF SIDE EFFECTS

Present development is occurring in the management of opioid-induced side effects. The use of methylnaltrexone and alvimopan for opioid-induced ileus and constipation will likely be in use in the very near future. These μ-opioid antagonists do not cross the blood-brain barrier and act on peripheral opioid receptors to reverse common opioid side effects without affecting the central pain relieving action. Alvimopan has been shown to significantly accelerate gastrointestinal recovery and time to discharge in patients after bowel resection.[27] These new μ-opioid antagonists may make postoperative opioid-induced ileus a term of the past.

The most concerning side effect of opioid analgesia is respiratory depression. Morphine-6-glucuronide (presently in commercial development), an active metabolite of morphine, has been shown to have less ventilatory depression than equipotent analgesic morphine doses.[28] Another exciting development in the prevention of opioid-induced respiratory depression is work on the 5-HT4(a) receptor. This receptor may be prove to be the magic bullet needed to prevent/reverse opioid-induced ventilatory depression. Treatment of rats with 5-HT4(a) receptor agonist has been shown to reverse fentanyl-induced respiratory depression without loss of fentanyl-induced analgesia.[29] However, rats behave very differently from humans, and we wait in anticipation of the same benefit crossing over to humans.

NEW ANALGESICS

The pain pathway has many points where intervention can be made. As shown in Figure 44.3, there are many pieces of the pain puzzle that have been filled, but there are several, particularly in the first 3 steps, that will need to be filled in the future. The pain pathway begins with transduction from the point of insult and is then conducted to the central nervous system. Many opportunities exist for future pharmaceuticals to intervene and block or modulate pain perception at these levels and prevent the CNS from ever knowing there was an injury. This section will focus on some of these new analgesics and their possible use in the future (Figure 44.3).

Sometimes old things become new again. With the growth of minimally invasive surgery, we are seeing procedures performed that several years ago would require a long convalescence and today are being done as an outpatient. Acetaminophen was once the standard medicine for mild to moderate acute pain, and with the intravenous form available, its use is well established in

Europe, for mild to moderate perioperative pain and its release is anticipated soon in the United States. There is a large potential for the perioperative use of intravenous acetaminophen in ambulatory surgery where the use of opioids is best minimized and oral intake is not optimal.[30] Nonsteroidal anti-inflammatories will be used, as well, and likely include intravenous diclofenac, which provides a more rapid onset of action compared to ketorolac. The hysteria regarding the cyclooxygenase 2 (COX-2) inhibitors will likely calm in the near future, and it is likely that intravenous COX-2 inhibitors will make their debut in the United States, eventually, and add to the multimodal analgesic arsenal.

Peripheral κ-opioid receptor agonists represent another potential class of opioids that may show promise in postoperative pain control in the near future. The current members of the class, butorphanol and nalbuphine, are limited in their use by their partial μ-opioid receptor agonist activity. Experimental κ-opioid receptor agonists have been shown to improve chronic visceral pain[31] and may prove to be useful in the pain associated with postoperative abdominal distention that is difficult to treat with μ-opioid receptor agonists and can create or intensify an ileus making the distention worse.

The search for new nonopioid analgesics continues, and two well-known substances may soon contribute to the perioperative management of pain in new ways. Cannabinoids may become a new class of adjuvant analgesics for chronic neuropathic pain or acute inflammatory pain. Much work has been done looking for pain relief with various derivatives of the active ingredient of marijuana, but no firm results have yet been elucidated. Experiments in the 1970s showed the pain-relieving properties of 9-tetrahydrocannabinol (THC) in humans; however, dysphoric side effects limited their use.[32] Further work has shown the synergistic effect of combining THC with opioids to enhance pain relief resistant to opioid alone.[33]

Perhaps the most promising agent to be derived from the cannabinoids is ajulemic acid. It has been shown to be effective in both inflammatory and neuropathic pain treatment, and it lacks psychotropic side effects and withdrawal symptoms after 1 week of use in human volunteers.[34] It works like the NSAIDs on the inflammation pathway but is devoid of their side effects, including gastric irritation and renal artery constriction.

Melatonin may be an interesting addition to the management of acute pain. Melatonin is secreted by the pineal gland in a diurnal manner with increased secretion occurring in the evening.[35] There has been a well-known observation throughout time that humans with pain have less of that pain at night. Melatonin has been shown to release endogenous β-endorphin[36] and is being studied for its anti-inflammatory action. Anesthesia in conjunction with surgery has been shown to decrease the normal circadian release of melatonin, and, perhaps, in the future supplementation may prove to be beneficial in postsurgical patients.

Capsaicin is currently used for treatment of chronic pain and works by opening the transient receptor potential V1 ion channel found on peripheral C fibers. This channel opening allows calcium influx and attenuates C-fiber sensation. Resiniferatoxin is a more potent capsaicin analog and has been shown to decrease pain response in rats.[37] This peripheral response may someday be translated in humans and be beneficial in orthopedic and incisional pain reduction.

The ASIC family is a potential target for new pain medicines. The ASIC family consists of 6 subunits (1 a, 1b, 2 a, 2b, 3, and 4), which are expressed in peripheral neurons with the ASIC 1b and ASIC 3 subunits showing a high degree of selectivity in sensory neurons. Acidic nociception is likely to occur in many inflammatory and ischemic pain conditions such as rheumatoid arthritis and vascular ischemia, as well as in the routine perioperative setting. NSAIDs have been shown to attenuate the large expression of ASIC in sensory neurons induced by inflammation, as well as directly inhibiting sensory neuron ASIC current.[38] The diuretic amiloride has been shown to weakly block ASIC under mild acidic conditions (pH 7.2–6.0) in humans, resulting in attenuated pain perception.[39] Work is currently underway on a more selective and potent ASIC blocker without the limitations of amiloride and could potentially be an effective agent in the treatment of inflammatory and ischemic acute or chronic pain in the future.[40]

With the growing use of low-molecular-weight heparin (LMWH) products, the use of epidural catheters has declined because of the risk of spinal hematoma formation. The risk of deep venous thrombosis (DVT) in many surgical patients is high, and prophylaxis is surely needed. Epidural analgesia has been shown to decrease the incidence in DVT generation by increasing lower extremity blood flow, enhancing postoperative fibrinolysis, and enhancing rehabilitation and patient mobility. However, there is no evidence that the risk reduction of DVT provided by epidural analgesia is better, worse, or no different than that provided by LMWH. The drug manufacturers obviously are in favor of their drugs, so we need to determine ourselves through controlled trials (with the cooperation of surgeons) if LMWH or epidurals are more beneficial in the prevention of deep vein thrombosis, or whether multimodal treatment that includes epidural analgesia and, possibly, LMWH is better. Until this question is answered it would be beneficial to enable the use of epidural anesthesia with its attendant benefits even when LMWH is indicated. An alternative would be to develop long-acting analgesics that do not require indwelling epidural catheters.

There have been several attempts to develop encapsulated extended release local anesthetics. Although none have so far come to fruition newer technologies are likely to make these a reality.[41] An encapsulated form of mepivacaine formulation is in phase II trials currently. Thus it is likely that extended release forms of local anesthetic may in the future be used as a single shot dose in conjunction with encapsulated, long-lasting opioids for procedures where epidural catheters left postoperatively are contraindicated. These extended release local anesthetics would also likely make continuous peripheral nerve catheters obsolete along with their inherent risks of infection and nerve damage.

Genomic research is enlightening our knowledge of disease and medicine, and this is being translated into knowledge of pain and pain medicine. As we learn more about genetics and coding for opioid receptors, we are finding reasons why there is variability in individual pharmacodynamics and pharmacokinetics. This knowledge has resulted in the development of the field of pharmacogenomics, a field with expanding importance in the future.

There will be a time in the future when a quick scan of an individual's DNA will aid dramatically in their postoperative pain control. Perhaps, during preoperative testing, the patient's buccal mucosa will be swabbed and analyzed. The genetic information will be used to tailor treatment not just in pain management but also for all of perioperative medicine. It is known that people respond differently to all kinds of medications, and part of the reasons, likely, will be found in their genetics.

The ability to perceive pain is actually a heritable trait, and there are families in the world with the ability to feel no pain. This may or may not be a beneficial trait to have. The congenital indifference to pain condition is a rare and inheritable condition that was first documented in 1932 after the observation of a circus performer who could pierce his body with knives and feel no pain. Recently, the gene mutation SCN9 A has been identified in multiple families around the globe and implicates the loss of function of the sodium channel Na_v 1.7.[42] Gain of function of this sodium channel has been linked with familial erythermalgia, which is an extremely painful condition of the extremities.[43] Current sodium channel blocking medications include the local anesthetics, but they are limited in their selectivity for the Na_v 1.7 channel and have cardiac and central nervous system limits. In the future, novel pharmaceuticals will target this channel specifically and may actually lead to the "Holy Grail" of pain management leaving all other medications redundant.

FUTURE DELIVERY MECHANISMS

The traditional routes of pain medicine administration are being challenged. Oral, intravenous, and subcutaneous routes will, likely, never be replaced, but the nasal, inhaled, and transcutaneous routes do offer advantages in some situations. As mentioned previously, liposomal-encapsulated medications may offer benefit in the future and offer a longer lasting mode of delivery of opioids, local anesthetics, and anti-inflammatories.

Transcutaneous delivery of medications offers several benefits over the more traditional routes of drug delivery. The need for intravenous access is diminished, and the ability to be free of poles and machinery may enhance the rehabilitation process by increasing patient mobility.

The concept of iontophoresis to deliver medicine transcutaneously can be traced to Veratti, who described the idea in 1747. In the early 1900s, Leduc demonstrated the concept by delivering strychnine iontophoretically to rabbits, thus inducing convulsions.[44] The technique relies on placing drug on the skin in an electrode of the same charge as the drug. An electric current is applied, and the drug is carried with the charge to the deep tissue layers, where it is absorbed by capillaries.

The E-trans system currently using fentanyl at a fixed 40-μg bolus could be modified in the future to deliver other doses or medications. The benefit of the system is its portability and, probably, its safety. Most safety issues with intravenous PCA have been traced to programming error, and with a fixed dose device, that error is exponentially reduced. The new E-trans fentanyl system is the result of more than 15 years of research looking for effective demand delivery of transdermal opioids. The technology uses low-intensity direct current to transport fentanyl from the hydrogel reservoir through the dermis and into the circulation, where it travels to the central nervous system. The device resembles a small roach motel and its adhesiveness to the skin allows for easy portability. It has been shown to be as effective as standard morphine IV PCA dosing.[24] It is likely that many pain medicines will eventually have the option to be delivered by these unconventional routes, and it is not unimaginable that the transcutaneous administration of opioids could replace intravenous PCA in all but the most opioid-tolerant patients (Figure 44.4).

The intranasal route of drug administration also has several unique benefits when compared to the more traditional

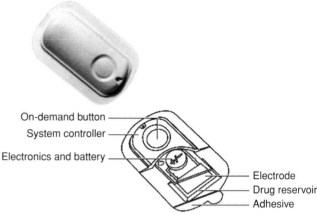

On-demand button
System controller
Electronics and battery
Electrode
Drug reservoir
Adhesive

Figure 44.4: Ionosys fentanyl demand system.

routes. The avoidance of needles and their waste, onset of action almost comparable to intravenous delivery, and the avoidance of the gastrointestinal tract and liver, thus reducing first-pass metabolism, are some of the advantages. The intranasal cavity by design provides an excellent drug delivery route. The mucosal surface area is extensive with the turbinates, providing ample space for drug absorption. The epithelium is highly vascularized and provides for rapid uptake of absorbed drug.[45] However, only small, lipophilic drugs are readily absorbed, whereas large, polar medications are not and are at risk for enzymatic degradation.[45] The development of one particular delivery system uses chitosan, which is derived from the chitin found naturally in crustacean shells. This protein has been used in extended-release tablets and has been found to be safe and bioadhesive and has demonstrated improved absorption across nasal mucosa.

Inhaled fentanyl and intranasal and inhaled morphine are new methods of rapid onset analgesia and could find a place in the acute pain world. Inhalation of opioids has occurred successfully for centuries for both medicinal and recreational reasons. Physical therapy on postoperative day 1 is very common in orthopedics and the need for rapid analgesia in these situations makes inhaled dosing a viable alternative in patients when intravenous PCA is seen as a hindrance to mobility. Often, in these situations, pain is well controlled while patients are in bed but need to be controlled when activity occurs (Figures 44.5 and 44.6).

Intranasal ketamine is another development that will likely show benefit in perioperative pain control. The US military is helping to fund this form of ketamine drug delivery as an easily administered, rapid-acting analgesic with a low side-effect profile in the 10- to 50-mg dosing range. Ketamine is well known to decrease postoperative opioid consumption, in some instances up to 50%, and would be an excellent adjuvant for patients with opioid tolerance or side effects.[46] The perioperative use of ketamine is currently limited in the United States to intravenous or intramuscular dosing as there is no manufacturer of tablets for oral intake. Ketamine may be an underused tool in the perioperative period and with a convenient intranasal application, it could be highly beneficial to pain management in the future.

Liposomal-encapsulated morphine for epidural use has been marketed already and will likely be the first of a host of products that rely on bioerodable delivery systems to extend duration of action of common pain medicines. The ability to provide single-shot dosing of medication to last up to 48 hours may improve

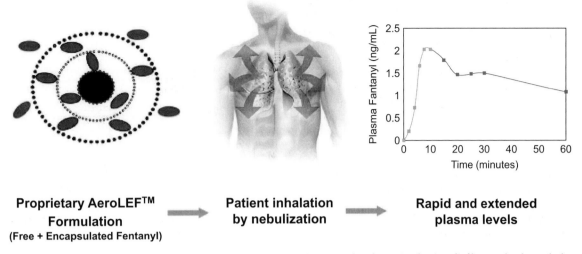

Figure 44.5: Inhaled fentanyl via proprietary AeroLEF system results in rapid and sustained pain relief by uptake through the lungs.

on the current standards and diminish the need for both epidural and peripheral indwelling catheters. The use of medications, such as NSAIDs and other adjuvants, will enable patients to sustain effective pain relief long after discharge and when pain is at its peak. Currently, a proprietary bioerodable system delivering meloxicam is in development with a targeted duration of action of 2 weeks post orthopedic surgery. Although there are several attempts to provide long-lasting (>24 hour) analgesics, the value of such prolonged duration is not fully established. As the pain cycle is relatively short in the acute postoperative setting, the need for drugs lasting longer than 24 hours may actually have disadvantages (eg, more rapid tolerance) and thus we caution that in this setting drugs lasting longer than 24 hours need to demonstrate improvement in pain management.

DOES UNCONTROLLED ACUTE PAIN EFFECT OUTCOMES?

This is a question that will be answered in the next 5 years. We believe that it does, and the consequences of poor pain control will surprise the medical field and society, in general. Much focus has been directed at trying to show that poor acute pain control leads to chronic pain. There are, however, limited data to support what many of us believe is an inherent truth.

There are certain types of operations (amputation, thoracotomy, mastectomy, herniorraphy) that are associated with a high incidence of chronic pain syndromes and seem to be related by their inherent high risk of nerve injury. The ability to diminish the risk of chronic pain postsurgically has been shown in several studies, but they have not been uniformly replicated. Obata et al[47] showed that preincisional injection of epidural local anesthetic, combined with postsurgical epidural analgesia reduced pain at 6 months from 67% to 33%. Uncontrolled acute postthoracotomy pain has been shown to be a significant predictor of postthoracotomy pain syndrome.[48]

Orthopedic extremity surgery has associated with it the dreaded complex regional pain syndrome (CRPS). The incidence is reported to range from 1% to 11% in orthopedic extremity injuries[49] and is probably below 5% of all orthopedic extremity surgeries. Whatever the actual percentage is, there are a very large number of patients who may be at risk for this debilitating

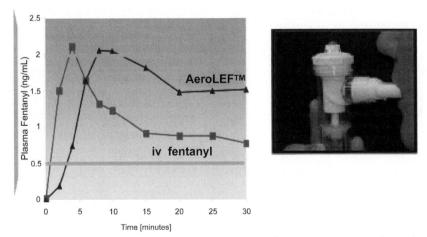

Figure 44.6: AeroLEF inhaled fentanyl has similar rapid onset to intravenous fentanyl, but results in higher fentanyl blood concentration for a longer time period.

disease. Other operations at risk for postoperative chronic pain include spinal fusion and iliac crest harvest.[50] Reuben[51] has shown that a perioperative multimodal analgesic regimen combined with an accelerated rehabilitation program can prevent chronic knee pain after anterior cruciate ligament repair at 6 months postoperatively. The use of celecoxib 1–2 hours preoperatively and then every 12 hours for 14 days was associated with decreased CRPS, anterior knee pain, flexion contracture, and scar tissue requiring rearthroscopy. It was also shown that the celecoxib group returned to a higher activity level and full sports participation after 6 months. This type of study on a well-defined population with a well-defined multimodal analgesic regimen that looks beyond the traditional anesthesiologist definition of the perioperative period (6 months) is what has been lacking over the years and what is needed in the future.

We have seen many studies fail to show significant outcome differences, using various pain control techniques ranging from oral acetaminophen to epidural PCA for surgery ranging from tooth extraction to coronary bypass. To obtain meaningful results it is essential that studies are better controlled and they are extended further into the future to show that we can make a difference in long-term outcomes. These outcomes may be more important than even preventing chronic pain. We believe that effective acute pain control has even more important outcomes (eg, cancer prevention, DVT prevention) associated with it. The challenge will be in proving it.

Good acute pain management means more than lowering pain scores and decreasing nausea. It means getting people back to their lives sooner and in better shape than they were before, therefore the perioperative team must put in a lot more thought and effort for this to occur. Plans for pain management must consider preoperative, intraoperative, and postoperative elements. Pain specialists in the future will consider optimal pain treatment beyond discharge, and all will tailor therapy to optimize quality of life rather than just pain. JHACO had good intentions with their 1999 recommendations regarding pain assessment and treatment; hospitals needed an objective measure and the pain score was born. We believe the future of pain management will need to forget about the pain score and instead look for something that really measures the outcomes that patients desire. What good is a pain score of zero when the patient is just lying in bed for 3 days? Acute pain teams should become "acute rehab teams" or "acute let's get you home and back to work teams."

The ability to prevent cancer recurrence or myocardial infarction months to years after surgery by controlling the neuroendocrine and sympathetic response to surgical insult with regional anesthesia, analgesia, or targeted pharmaceuticals will elevate the acute pain management field to levels never before imagined. Inflammatory response is something that can and should be avoided perioperatively.[52] Liebeskind's well-known mantra "pain can kill" will soon be shown to be true (Figures 44.7 and 44.8).[53]

A recent retrospective analysis of breast cancer surgery patients revealed a siginificant difference in outcome regarding cancer recurrence. The groups were separated by anesthetic technique; one group received general anesthesia and IV PCA morphine postoperatively, whereas the other group received paravertebral blockade combined with general anesthesia. The paravertebral block group had significantly less recurrence and metastasis at both 24- and 36-month follow-up.[54] Whether the difference in outcome can be attributed to the unilateral sympathetic blockade, improved pain control or diminished use of general anesthetic inhalational agents remains to be learned. This study should provide impetus for further research. The surgical manipulation of cancer cells is bound to set some of these cells off into the circulation during the operation and optimizing the patients immune system to fight off these threats is likely beneficial. Sympathetic blockade by local anesthetic delivered via patient-controlled epidural anesthesia has been shown to improve the immune system response[55] and with this improvement it would be expected that both infectious and cancerous complications would be attenuated.

PAIN CAN KILL

Bonica has argued for many years that the term "chronic benign pain" (used in distinction to pain associated with cancer) is seriously misleading (Bonica text, p 20; see also Boas Pain 2: 359, 1976). Chronic pain is never benign, he contends; it can devastate its victims' lives and even lead to suicide. Recently, evidence from laboratory experiments has begun to accumulate suggesting that pain can cause cancer and accelerate its growth. It appears that the dictum "pain does not kill", used by some to justify the inadequate treatment of pain (as documented by Angell), may be dangerously wrong.

Continuing a line of research to which many laboratories have made significant contributions (Ader book), we have recently shown in rats that pain and stress can profoundly inhibit immune function, enhance tumor growth, and increase percent mortality after tumor inoculation (Raz rev). In one paradigm, we used a tumor known to be particularly sensitive to the cytotoxic capability of natural killer (NK) cells (Ben-Eli). We found that even a single exposure to stress (forced swimming) significantly decreases NK cytotoxicity against this tumor in an in vitro assay and significantly increases the number of lung surface metastases10 days after intravenous injection of this tumor in the corresponding in vivo assay. We have also noted that rats made deficient in NK cells by administration of an NK antibody prior to stress fail to show the increase in metastatic growth, suggesting that the NK-suppressive effect of stress is responsible for the increase in tumor development. Using this same model, we are now finding that rats injected with this tumor 3 hours after a standard surgery (laparotomy) show significantly more lung surface metastases 10 days later than do controls subjected only to the anesthetic.

The precise stimulus conditions necessary to produce these effects, whether it is the pain itself or the stress reaction caused by it, need still to be determined, as do the endocrinological and/or neurochemical mediators. What is clear is that pain of adequate intensity and duration can, directly or indirectly, suppress immune mechanisms normally used by the body to defend itself against tumors and can, apparently in consequence, cause a marked increase in tumor growth.

Figure 44.7: *Pain Can Kill* early manuscript, 1990.

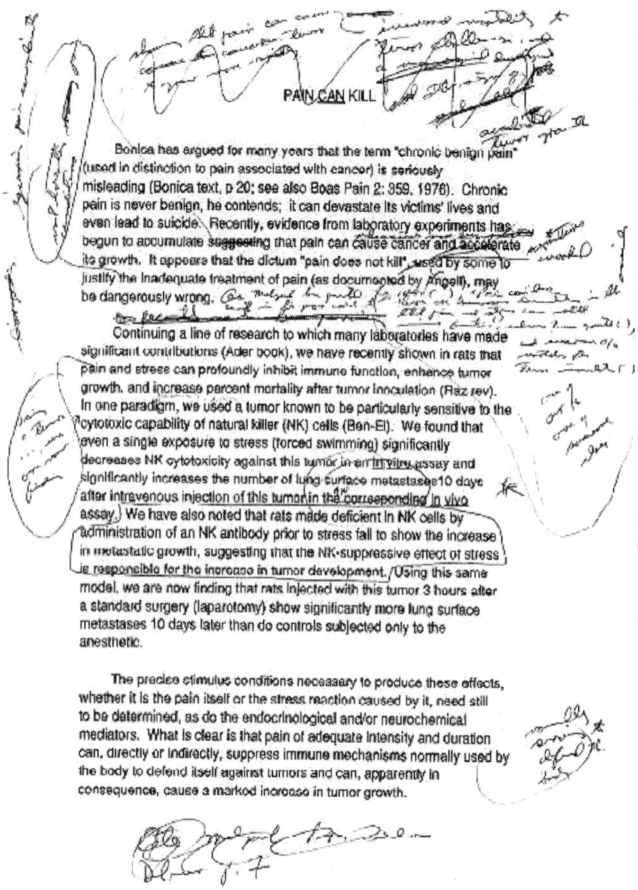

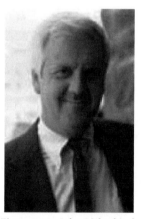

Figure 44.8: John Liebeskind.

The importance of optimal perioperative pain management must be researched further to look for differences in outcomes that go beyond pain scores, morphine consumption, and patient satisfaction. Granted, these outcomes are important in the routine management of acute pain, but there are higher aspirations to achieve in this field. Well-controlled studies must be constructed with large numbers of patients and followed for years in advance to show relevant differences in outcomes such as cancer recurrence, pulmonary embolism, and myocardial infarction. Perhaps the newly formed American Society of Regional Anesthesia AcutePOP (postoperative pain) initiative will be the platform for collection of data to gain the large numbers needed to find outcome differences that are statistically significant.[56]

CONCLUSIONS

Acute pain management has a bright future. There are many new and exciting pharmaceuticals and delivery mechanisms on the horizon that will improve the management of all types of pain. We can look at the past and see that it takes many years for great ideas to be realized in the world of both acute pain management and medicine as a whole. Technology must catch up before ideas like IV PCA, peripheral nerve blocks, and epidural analgesia can reach a wide market. Our knowledge of the pain pathway is growing daily and new medicines and delivery mechanisms are being developed to take further steps toward eliminating pain. Pharmacogenomics will continue to develop to the point where very specific therapies will be initiated and unwanted side effects eliminated or reduced. There may even be a time when our patients' DNA is analyzed and the exact pain receptor targeted for optimal patient pain relief. We can achieve nearly zero pain with regional and epidural analgesia; there will be a time when we can do the same with future pain medicines.

Acute pain management is a relatively new subspecialty to medicine and, to continue its vitality, must prove its worth. The development of databases that can pool data from various locations across the country will enable researchers to gain the numbers necessary to find that effective acute pain management does make a difference in patient outcomes.

We as a specialty are continuously being infringed on by the pharmaceutical and medical device industries in both positive and negative ways. Acute pain physicians must be the leaders for industry. There will be many new advances in technology in the next several years and industry will continue to apply pressure to sell their products. We as a specialty must continue to be the gatekeepers and do what is best for our patients.

Most patients do very well after surgery – or do they? Surgery and anesthesia have become very safe over the years and morbidity and mortality in the perioperative period continue to decline. However, we do not know whether patients are suffering insults that occurred perioperatively because of poor pain management that manifests months or years later. Our views of what exactly constitutes perioperative morbidity and mortality may be limited at the present time. It may be time for a new paradigm shift regarding acute pain management and its effect on outcomes.

We do know that most of our surgical patients do not have the optimal outcomes we have defined above. Patients still hurt months to years after undergoing what they thought would be "routine surgery." Global recovery including pain relief, patient satisfaction, good health, and perhaps even sustained life must be the essential elements we strive for in the management of acute pain. We as a specialty can make a difference in all of our patients, and we must work harder to prove it.

REFERENCES

1. Roe BB. Are postoperative narcotics necessary? *Arch Surg.* 1963;87:912–915.
2. Sechzer PH. Patient-controlled analgesia (PCA): a retrospective. *Anesthesiology.* 1990;72(4):735–736.
3. Scott JS. Obstetric analgesia: a consideration of labor pain and a patient-controlled technique for its relief with meperidine. *Am J Obstet Gynecol.* 1970;106(7):959–978.
4. Forrest WH Jr, Kienitz ME. Self-administration of intravenous analgesics. *Anesthesiology.* 1970;33:363–365.
5. Keeri-Szanto M. Apparatus for demand analgesia. *Can Anaesth Soc J.* 1971;18(5):581–582.
6. Evans JM, et al. Apparatus for patient-controlled administration of intravenous narcotics during labour. *Lancet.* 1976;1(7949):17–18.
7. Marks RM, Sachar EJ. Undertreatment of medical inpatients with narcotic analgesics. *Ann Intern Med.* 1973;78(2):173–181.
8. Pert CB, Snyder SH. Opiate receptor: demonstration in nervous tissue. *Science.* 1973;179(77):1011–1014.
9. Wang JK, Nauss LA, Thomas JE. Pain relief by intrathecally applied morphine in man. *Anesthesiology.* 1979;50(2):149–151.
10. Cousins MJ, Mather LE. Intrathecal and epidural administration of opioids. *Anesthesiology.* 1984;61(3):276–310.
11. Ready LB, et al. Development of an anesthesiology-based postoperative pain management service. *Anesthesiology.* 1988;68(1):100–106.
12. Report of the Commission on the Evaluation of Pain. *Soc Secur Bull.* 1987;50(1):13–44.
13. Carr DB, Jacox A, Chapman CR, et al. Acute pain management: operative or medical procedures and trauma. Clinical Practice Guideline. AHCPR Pub. No. 92-0032. Rockville, MD: Agency for Health Care Policy and Research, Public Health Service, U.S. Department of Health and Human Services; 1992.
14. Practice guidelines for acute pain management in the perioperative setting. A report by the American Society of Anesthesiologists Task Force on Pain Management, Acute Pain Section. *Anesthesiology.* 1995;82(4):1071–1081.
15. Phillips DM. JCAHO pain management standards are unveiled: Joint Commission on Accreditation of Healthcare Organizations. *JAMA.* 2000;284(4):428–429.
16. Turk DC, Okifuji, A. What factors affect physicians' decisions to prescribe opioids for chronic noncancer pain patients? *Clin J Pain.* 1997;13(4):330–336.
17. White PF. Mishaps with patient-controlled analgesia. *Anesthesiology.* 1987;66(1):81–83.
18. Vila H Jr, et al. The efficacy and safety of pain management before and after implementation of hospital-wide pain management standards: is patient safety compromised by treatment based solely on numerical pain ratings? *Anesth Analg.* 2005;101(2):474–480, table of contents.
19. Wasan AD, et al. Iatrogenic addiction in patients treated for acute or subacute pain: a systematic review. *J Opioid Manag.* 2006;2(1):16–22.
20. Gilson AM, Joranson DE. Controlled substances and pain management: changes in knowledge and attitudes of state medical regulators. *J Pain Symptom Manage.* 2001;21(3):227–237.

21. Mitra S, Sinatra RS. Perioperative management of acute pain in the opioid-dependent patient. *Anesthesiology.* 2004;101(1):212–227.

22. Carroll IR, Angst MS, Clark JD. Management of perioperative pain in patients chronically consuming opioids. *Reg Anesth Pain Med.* 2004;29(6):576–591.

23. Swenson JD, et al. Outpatient management of continuous peripheral nerve catheters placed using ultrasound guidance: an experience in 620 patients. *Anesth Analg.* 2006;103(6):1436–1443.

24. Viscusi ER, et al. Patient-controlled transdermal fentanyl hydrochloride vs intravenous morphine pump for postoperative pain: a randomized controlled trial. *JAMA.* 2004;291(11):1333–1341.

25. Rawal N. Organization of acute pain services – a low-cost model. *Acta Anaesthesiol Scand Suppl.* 1997;111:188–190.

26. White PF, et al. The role of the anesthesiologist in fast-track surgery: from multimodal analgesia to perioperative medical care. *Anesth Analg.* 2007;104(6):1380–1396, table of contents.

27. Delaney CP, et al. Alvimopan, for postoperative ileus following bowel resection: a pooled analysis of phase III studies. *Ann Surg.* 2007;245(3):355–363.

28. Romberg R, et al. Pharmacodynamic effect of morphine-6-glucuronide versus morphine on hypoxic and hypercapnic breathing in healthy volunteers. *Anesthesiology.* 2003;99(4):788–798.

29. Manzke T, et al. 5-HT4(a) receptors avert opioid-induced breathing depression without loss of analgesia. *Science.* 2003;301(5630):226–229.

30. White PF. The changing role of non-opioid analgesic techniques in the management of postoperative pain. *Anesth Analg.* 2005;101(5 suppl):S5–S22.

31. Eisenach JC, Carpenter R, Curry R. Analgesia from a peripherally active kappa-opioid receptor agonist in patients with chronic pancreatitis. *Pain.* 2003;101(1–2):89–95.

32. Noyes R Jr, et al. Analgesic effect of delta-9-tetrahydrocannabinol. *J Clin Pharmacol.* 1975;15(2–3):139–143.

33. Cichewicz DL. Synergistic interactions between cannabinoid and opioid analgesics. *Life Sci.* 2004;74(11):1317–1324.

34. Karst M, et al. Analgesic effect of the synthetic cannabinoid CT-3 on chronic neuropathic pain: a randomized controlled trial. *JAMA.* 2003;290(13):1757–1762.

35. Karkela J, et al. The influence of anaesthesia and surgery on the circadian rhythm of melatonin. *Acta Anaesthesiol Scand.* 2002;46(1):30–36.

36. Shavali S, et al. Melatonin exerts its analgesic actions not by binding to opioid receptor subtypes but by increasing the release of beta-endorphin an endogenous opioid. *Brain Res Bull.* 2005;64(6):471–479.

37. Kissin EY, Freitas CF, Kissin I. The effects of intraarticular resiniferatoxin in experimental knee-joint arthritis. *Anesth Analg.* 2005;101(5):1433–1439.

38. Voilley N, et al. Nonsteroid anti-inflammatory drugs inhibit both the activity and the inflammation-induced expression of acid-sensing ion channels in nociceptors. *J Neurosci.* 2001;21(20):8026–8033.

39. Ugawa S, et al. Amiloride-blockable acid-sensing ion channels are leading acid sensors expressed in human nociceptors. *J Clin Invest.* 2002;110(8):1185–1190.

40. Jones NG, et al. Acid-induced pain and its modulation in humans. *J Neurosci.* 2004;24(48):10974–10979.

41. Cereda CM, et al. Liposomal formulations of prilocaine, lidocaine and mepivacaine prolong analgesic duration. *Can J Anaesth.* 2006;53(11):1092–1097.

42. Cox JJ, et al. An SCN9A channelopathy causes congenital inability to experience pain. *Nature.* 2006;444(7121):894–898.

43. Sheets PL, et al. A Nav1.7 channel mutation associated with hereditary erythromelalgia contributes to neuronal hyperexcitability and displays reduced lidocaine sensitivity. *J Physiol.* 2007.

44. Helmstadter A. The history of electrically-assisted transdermal drug delivery ("iontophoresis"). *Pharmazie.* 2001;56(7):583–587.

45. Anez Simon C, et al. Intranasal opioids for acute pain. *Rev Esp Anestesiol Reanim.* 2006;53(10):643–652.

46. Subramaniam K, Subramaniam B, Steinbrook RA. Ketamine as adjuvant analgesic to opioids: a quantitative and qualitative systematic review. *Anesth Analg.* 2004;99(2):482–495, table of contents.

47. Obata H, et al. Epidural block with mepivacaine before surgery reduces long-term post-thoracotomy pain. *Can J Anaesth.* 1999;46(12):1127–1132.

48. Katz J, et al. Acute pain after thoracic surgery predicts long-term post-thoracotomy pain. *Clin J Pain.* 1996;12(1):50–55.

49. Gradl G, et al. Acute CRPS I (morbus sudeck) following distal radial fractures – methods for early diagnosis. *Zentralbl Chir.* 2003;128(12):1020–1026.

50. Joshi A, Kostakis GC. An investigation of post-operative morbidity following iliac crest graft harvesting. *Br Dent J.* 2004;196(3):167–171; discussion 155.

51. Reuben SS, Ekman EF. The effect of initiating a preventive multimodal analgesic regimen on long-term patient outcomes for outpatient anterior cruciate ligament reconstruction surgery. *Anesth Analg.* 2007;105(1):228–232.

52. Carli F. Postoperative metabolic stress: interventional strategies. *Minerva Anestesiol.* 2006;72(6):413–418.

53. Liebeskind JC. Pain can kill. *Pain.* 1991;44(1):3–4.

54. Exadaktylos AK, et al. Can anesthetic technique for primary breast cancer surgery affect recurrence or metastasis? *Anesthesiology* 2006;105(4):660–664.

55. Volk T, et al. Postoperative epidural anesthesia preserves lymphocyte, but not monocyte, immune function after major spine surgery. *Anesth Analg.* 2004;98(4):1086–1092, table of contents.

56. Liu SS, et al. Announcing the Official Formation of ASRA AcutePOP (Acute Postoperative Pain) Initiative. *Reg Anesth Pain Med.* 2007;32(3):265–266.

Index